Prostate Diseases

Prostate Diseases

HERBERT LEPOR, MD

Professor of Urology
Medical College of Wisconsin
Froedtert Memorial Lutheran Hospital
Milwaukee, Wisconsin

RUSSELL K. LAWSON, MD

Chairman, Department of Urology
Medical College of Wisconsin
Froedtert Memorial Lutheran Hospital
Milwaukee, Wisconsin

W.B. SAUNDERS COMPANY

A Division of Harcourt Brace & Company

PHILADELPHIA—LONDON—TORONTO—MONTREAL—SYDNEY—TOKYO

W.B. SAUNDERS COMPANY
A Division of Harcourt Brace & Company
The Curtis Center
Independence Square West
Philadelphia, Pennsylvania 19106

Library of Congress Cataloging-in-Publication Data

Prostate diseases / [edited by] Herbert Lepor, Russell K. Lawson.

p.   cm.

ISBN 0–7216–4545–3

1. Prostate—Diseases.   I. Lepor, Herbert.   II. Lawson, Russell K.
   [DNLM: 1. Prostatic Hypertrophy—diagnosis.   2. Prostatic Hypertrophy—
   therapy.   3. Prostatic Neoplasms—diagnosis.   4. Prostatic Neoplasms—
   therapy.   5. Prostatitis—diagnosis.   6. Prostatitis—therapy.   WJ 752
   P96555]

RC899.P693 1993
DNLM/DLC   92-49620

PROSTATE DISEASES   ISBN 0–7216–4545–3

Printed in the United States of America.

Last digit is the print number: 9   8   7   6   5   4   3   2   1

CONTRIBUTORS

MALCOLM A. BAGSHAW, M.D.
Henry S. Kaplan and Harry Lebeson Professor in Cancer Biology, Emeritus, Department of Radiation Oncology, Stanford University School of Medicine; Staff, Radiation Oncology, Stanford University Hospital, Stanford, California
The Challenge of Radiation Treatment of Carcinoma of the Prostate

MICHAEL J. BARRY, M.D.
Assistant Professor, Department of Medicine, Harvard Medical School; Associate Physician, Massachusetts General Hospital, Boston, Massachusetts
Epidemiology and Natural History of Benign Prostatic Hyperplasia

FRANK P. BEGUN, M.D.
Associate Professor, Department of Urology, Medical College of Wisconsin; Staff, Froedtert Memorial Lutheran Hospital and Milwaukee County Medical Complex; Chief of Urology, Veterans Affairs Medical Center, Milwaukee, Wisconsin
Epidemiology and Natural History of Prostate Cancer

WILLIAM D. BELVILLE, M.D
Associate Professor, Department of Urology, University of Michigan Medical Center, Ann Arbor, Michigan
The Diagnosis of Obstructive Uropathy

BETSY D. BENNETT, M.D., Ph.D.
Professor and Vice-Chair, Department of Pathology, University of South Alabama College of Medicine, Mobile, Alabama
Histopathology and Cytology of Prostatitis

DAVID L. BLUESTEIN, M.D.
Resident in Urology, Mayo Graduate School of Medicine, Rochester, Minnesota
Hormonal Therapy in the Management of Benign Prostatic Hyperplasia

MICHAEL K. BRAWER, M.D.
Associate Professor, Department of Urology, University of Washington School of Medicine; Chief, Section of Urology, Seattle Veterans Administration Medical Center, Seattle, Washington
The Role of Tumor Markers in the Diagnosis and Treatment of Prostate Cancer

REGINALD C. BRUSKEWITZ, M.D.
Professor, Department of Surgery, University of Wisconsin Medical School and University of Wisconsin Hospital and Clinics, Madison, Wisconsin
Benign Prostatic Hyperplasia: Clinical Manifestations and Indications for Intervention

EARL CHENG, M.D.
Resident in Urology, Department of Urology, Northwestern University Medical School, Chicago, Illinois
Endocrinology of the Prostate

DONALD S. COFFEY, Ph.D.
Professor, Departments of Urology, Oncology, and Pharmacology, The Johns Hopkins University School of Medicine, Baltimore, Maryland
The Molecular Biology of the Prostate

CHARLES J. DAVIS, JR., M.D.
Colonel, Medical Corps, U.S. Army, Associate Chairman, Department of Genitourinary Pathology, Armed Forces Institute of Pathology, Washington, D.C.
Histopathology of Prostate Cancer

MICHAEL J. DROLLER, M.D.
Professor and Chairman, Department of Urology, Mount Sinai Medical School, New York, New York
Anatomy of the Prostate

WILLIAM J. ELLIS, M.D.
Assistant Professor, Department of Urology, University of Washington School of Medicine; Assistant Chief, Section of Urology, Veterans Administration Medical Center, Seattle, Washington
The Role of Tumor Markers in the Diagnosis and Treatment of Prostate Cancer

WILLIAM A. GARDNER, JR., M.D.
Professor and Chairman, Department of Pathology, University of South Alabama College of Medicine, Mobile, Alabama
Histopathology and Cytology of Prostatitis

JOHN GRAYHACK, M.D.
Professor, Department of Urology, Northwestern University Medical School; Attending Physician, Northwestern Memorial Hospital, Chicago, Illinois
Endocrinology of the Prostate

NIELS HAUGAARD, Ph.D.
Professor Emeritus, Department of Pharmacology, University of Pennsylvania School of Medicine; Research Scientist, Division of Urology, University of Pennsylvania School of Medicine, Philadelphia, Pennsylvania
Experimental Studies on Bladder Outlet Obstruction

VAHAN S. KASSABIAN, M.D.
Assistant Professor, Department of Urology, Emory University School of Medicine, Atlanta, Georgia
Management of Local Recurrence of Prostate Cancer

ARNON KRONGRAD, M.D.
Assistant Professor, Departments of Urology and Medicine, University of Miami; Chief, Section of Urology, Miami Veterans Administration Medical Center, Miami, Florida
Anatomy of the Prostate

RUSSELL K. LAWSON, M.D.
Professor and Chairman, Department of Urology, Medical College of Wisconsin, Milwaukee, Wisconsin
A Historical View of Prostate Disease; Etiology of Benign Prostatic Hyperplasia

CHUNG LEE, Ph.D.
John T. Grayhack Professor of Urological Research and Professor of Cell, Molecular, and Structural Biology, Northwestern University Medical School, Chicago, Illinois
Endocrinology of the Prostate

HERBERT LEPOR, M.D.
Professor, Departments of Urology, Pharmacology, and Toxicology, Medical College of Wisconsin, Milwaukee, Wisconsin
The Role of Alpha Blockade in the Therapy of Benign Prostatic Hyperplasia; Nerve-Sparing Radical Retropubic Prostatectomy

ROBERT M. LEVIN, Ph.D.
Research Professor, Department of Urology, University of Pennsylvania School of Medicine, Philadelphia, Pennsylvania
Experimental Studies on Bladder Outlet Obstruction

CHRISTOPHER J. LOGOTHETIS, M.D.
Professor, Department of Medicine, University of Texas M.D. Anderson Cancer Center; Staff Internist and Chief, Section of Genitourinary Oncology, Department of Medical Oncology, University of Texas M.D. Anderson Cancer Center, Houston, Texas
Management of Androgen-Independent Prostate Carcinoma

PENELOPE A. LONGHURST, Ph.D.
Research Associate Professor, Departments of Urology and Pharmacology, University of Pennsylvania School of Medicine, Philadelphia, Pennsylvania
Experimental Studies on Bladder Outlet Obstruction

BERNARD LYTTON, M.B., F.R.C.S.
Donald Guthrie Professor of Surgery/Urology, Yale University School of Medicine, New Haven; Attending Urologist, Yale–New Haven Hospital, New Haven; Consulting Urologist, Veterans Affairs Medical Center, West Haven, Connecticut
Open Prostatectomy

EDWARD J. McGUIRE, M.D.
Professor and Chairman, Department of Urology, University of Michigan Medical Center, Ann Arbor, Michigan
The Diagnosis of Obstructive Uropathy

EDWIN M. MEARES, Jr., M.D., F.A.C.S.
Charles M. Whitney Professor and Chairman, Division of Urology, Department of Surgery, Tufts University School of Medicine; Chairman, Department of Urology, and Urologist-in-Chief, New England Medical Center Hospitals, Boston, Massachusetts
Nonbacterial Prostatitis and Prostatodynia

WINSTON K. MEBUST, M.D.
Professor and Chairman, Department of Urology, University of Kansas Medical Center, Kansas City, Kansas
Transurethral Resection of the Prostate and Transurethral Incision of the Prostate

RICHARD G. MIDDLETON, M.D.
Professor, Department of Surgery, and Chairman, Department of Urology, University of Utah School of Medicine; Chief of Urology, University of Utah Medical Center, Salt Lake City, Utah
Treatment of Locally Advanced Prostate Cancer

FREDERICK C. MONSON, M.D.
Research Assistant Professor, Division of Urology, Hospital of the University of Pennsylvania, University of Pennsylvania School of Medicine, Philadelphia, Pennsylvania
Experimental Studies on Bladder Outlet Obstruction

F. K. MOSTOFI, M.D.
Chairman, Department of Genitourinary Pathology, Armed Forces Institute of Pathology, Washington, D.C.; Clinical Professor, Department of Pathology, Georgetown University School of Medicine, Washington, D.C., University of Maryland School of Medicine, Baltimore, Maryland, and F. Edward Hébert School of Medicine of the Uniformed Services University of the Health Sciences, Bethesda, Maryland; Associate Professor, Department of Pathology, The Johns Hopkins University School of Medicine, Baltimore, Maryland
Histopathology of Prostate Cancer

JOSEPH E. OESTERLING, M.D.
Assistant Professor, Department of Urology, Mayo Medical School; Consultant, Department of Urology, Mayo Clinic and Mayo Foundation, Rochester, Minnesota
Hormonal Therapy in the Management of Benign Prostatic Hyperplasia

DAVID F. PAULSON, M.D.
Professor, Department of Surgery, Duke University School of Medicine; Chief, Division of Urology, Department of Surgery, Duke University Medical Center, Durham, North Carolina
Radical Perineal Prostatectomy; Treatment of Localized Carcinoma of the Prostate (Clinical Stages A and B)

PAUL C. PETERS, M.D.
The E.E. and Greer Garson Fogelson Distinguished Chair in Urology and Professor and Chairman, Division of Urology, University of Texas Health Science Center at Dallas, Southwestern Medical School, Dallas; Chief of Service, Parkland Memorial Medical Center and Zale Lipshy University Hospital, Dallas; Attending Physician, Children's Medical Center, Veterans Administration Medical Center, Baylor University Medical Center, and St. Paul Hospital, Dallas, Texas
Staging, Clinical Manifestations, and Indications for Intervention in Prostate Cancer

PRATAP K. REDDY, M.D.
Professor, Department of Urology, University of Minnesota Medical School; Chief, Urology Section, Veterans Affairs Medical Center, Minneapolis, Minnesota
Balloon Dilation/Hyperthermia/Prostatic Stents for Benign Prostatic Hyperplasia

MARTIN I. RESNICK, M.D.
Lester Persky Professor of Urology and Chairman, Department of Urology, Case Western Reserve University School of Medicine, Cleveland, Ohio
Imaging of the Prostate; Screening for Prostate Cancer

PATTI H. RICHARDSON, M.D.
Assistant Professor, Department of Pathology, University of South Alabama College of Medicine, Mobile, Alabama
Histopathology and Cytology of Prostatitis

MORTEN RIEHMANN, M.D.
Research Fellow, University of Wisconsin Medical School, Department of Surgery, Division of Urology, Madison, Wisconsin
Benign Prostatic Hyperplasia: Clinical Manifestations and Indications for Intervention

PETER T. SCARDINO, M.D.
Professor and Chairman, Department of Urology, Baylor College of Medicine, Houston, Texas
Management of Local Recurrence of Prostate Cancer

ANTHONY J. SCHAEFFER, M.D.
Chairman, Department of Urology, Northwestern University Medical School; Staff, Northwestern Memorial Hospital, Chicago, Illinois
Clinical Manifestations and Diagnosis of Prostatitis

FRITZ H. SCHRÖDER, M.D.
Professor and Chairman, Department of Urology, Erasmus University; Staff, Academic Hospital, Rotterdam, The Netherlands
Hormonal Therapy for Prostate Cancer

ISABELL A. SESTERHENN, M.D.
Senior Pathologist, Department of Genitourinary Pathology, Armed Forces Institute of Pathology, Washington, D.C.
Histopathology of Prostate Cancer

ELLEN SHAPIRO, M.D.
Professor, Departments of Urology and Pediatrics, Medical College of Wisconsin, Milwaukee, Wisconsin
Prostatic Morphogenesis, Stromal-Epithelial Interactions, Zonal Anatomy, and Quantitative Morphometry

ERIC M. SMITH, M.D.
Resident in Urology, Case Western Reserve University School of Medicine, Cleveland, Ohio
Imaging of the Prostate

JOHN D. STRANDBERG, D.V.M., Ph.D.
Associate Professor and Director, Division of Comparative Medicine, The Johns Hopkins University School of Medicine, Baltimore, Maryland
Comparative Pathology of Benign Prostatic Hyperplasia

SAMUEL T. THOMPSON, M.D.
Chief Resident in Urology, Case Western Reserve University School of Medicine, Cleveland, Ohio
Screening for Prostate Cancer

ALAN J. WEIN, M.D.
Professor and Chairman, Division of Urology, University of Pennsylvania School of Medicine; Chief of Urology, Hospital of the University of Pennsylvania, Philadelphia, Pennsylvania
Experimental Studies on Bladder Outlet Obstruction; Criteria for Assessing Outcome Following Intervention for Benign Prostatic Hyperplasia

PREFACE

Over the past several years, the diagnosis and treatment of benign and malignant diseases of the prostate have been in a state of constant evolution. The application of existing diagnostic modalities and treatment strategies has been redefined, and entirely new diagnostic and treatment options have been introduced. For example, PSA is now widely used for the screening of prostate cancer, and ultrasensitive PSA assays have been developed to enhance the assessment of disease progression. Technologic advances in ultrasound and magnetic resonance imaging have improved the ability to image the prostate. Medical and minimally invasive therapies for BPH have received a great deal of attention and are currently widely used for the treatment of this very common condition. Although the treatment strategies for managing carcinoma of the prostate have not changed dramatically, the optimal application of existing treatment options continues to be debated. Concepts such as complete androgen ablation, early versus delayed hormonal therapy, hormonal downstaging, and adjuvant radiotherapy have recently been revisited.

The textbook *Prostate Diseases* is intended to serve as a comprehensive and authoritative state-of-the-art reference for the clinician. The introductory chapters review the anatomy, embryology, physiology, endocrinology, and molecular biology of the prostate. The remainder of the textbook focuses on topics and issues related to the diagnosis and management of prostate diseases. The editors made a concerted effort to select pertinent topics and invite internationally recognized authorities to prepare both comprehensive and state-of-the-art manuscripts. The contributors, representing a wide range of expertise, include radiotherapists, medical oncologists, genitourinary pathologists, veterinary pathologists, basic research scientists, and urologists. We are grateful that all of the contributors completed their assignments in a timely manner to assure that the textbook will indeed serve as a state-of-the-art reference. The editors are also grateful for the time, efforts, and creativity that each of the contributors put forth on behalf of this textbook. It was a pleasure to work together with the entire staff at the W.B. Saunders Company. They shared our commitment to excellence, and their guidance and technical expertise were invaluable.

The production of a textbook, from the selection of topics and contributors to publication, represents, at a minimum, a two-year process. During this relatively short period of time, preliminary data and observations presented in the present edition of *Prostate Diseases* have matured, and several new diagnostic and treatment modalities have entered into early stages of investigation. The new advances related to prostate disease reflect the high level of accomplishment, enthusiasm, commitment, and ingenuity of many investigators in this field. We regret that these new topics are not included in the textbook. We will look forward to including these and other developments related to prostate disease in future editions of this textbook.

HERBERT LEPOR, M.D.
RUSSELL K. LAWSON, M.D.

CONTENTS

Section IV
PROSTATITIS

Section I

INTRODUCTION

Chapter 1

A HISTORICAL VIEW OF PROSTATE DISEASE

RUSSELL K. LAWSON

The first description of prostate anatomy dates back to the third century B.C. The discovery and treatment of diseases of the prostate also has a long and interesting history. Herophilus is credited with being the first to provide an anatomic description of the prostate. Born about 300 B.C., he was a physician in the newly founded city of Alexandria. Herophilus carried out dissections of the human body, and he is often called the father of human anatomy. He described the prostate as the prostatae glandulosae and the prostatae cirsoides. He may have confused the ampulla of the vas deferens and the seminal vesicles in man with the bifid prostate seen in some animals. Unfortunately, the writings of this early anatomist were lost in a fire that destroyed the library in Alexandria in A.D. 391. Galen, a physician who lived from A.D. 131 to 200 and practiced in Rome, described several morbid changes in the prostatic urethra that suggest that he was familiar with the pathophysiology of prostatic enlargement. He pointed out that urinary obstruction could be caused by a mass that compresses the urethra. Galen recognized that urinary obstruction could also result from inflammation and abscess in the region of the bladder neck and prostatic urethra. The first accurate anatomic description of the prostate was provided by the Venetian physician Nicolo Massa in 1536. He showed the relationships of the prostate to the bladder neck, seminal vesicles, and ampulla of the vas deferens, and he correctly described the gross anatomy of the gland.

The first scientific description of the pathophysiology of prostatic enlargement is attributed to Jean Riolanus. He pointed out that obstruction causes thickening of the bladder wall and difficulty in emptying the bladder. His description of the effects of prostatic obstruction appeared in *Opera Anatomica* in 1649 (Fig. 1–1).[18] An excellent, detailed description of the pathology of prostatic enlargement with the resulting changes in the bladder and upper urinary tracts is found in the studies of Morgagni.[15] He held the chair of anatomy at the University of Padua in Italy. Two excerpts from his book, *The Seats and Causes of Diseases,* published in 1769, follow:

> From the posterior border of that orifice, from whence the urethra begins, two white, hard, hemispherical, prominences, small in their size, but of equal magnitude, and contiguous to each other, protuberated within the bladder: in cutting which longitudinally, together with the prostate gland, I found them to be continued thereto, and to be made up of the same substance and although one part of the prostate gland was not of that whiteness and hardness yet the remaining substance thereof and especially that which arose up on the sides of the seminal caruncle was perfectly like that of the double prominence, into which it was produced. So that if these prominences were scirrhous, the largest part of the prostate might seem to be no less scirrhous.
>
> But also because it was easy to conceive, that when the patient began to be affected with a tumor and hardness of the prostate, he began also to be attacked with the beginning, as it were, of retention of urine and that then the tumor was, at length, increased to such a great degree, an unusual slowness of circulation, through this gland and around and about this gland, coming suddenly on the canal which passed through it, could not be sufficiently opened for the discharge of urine unless by introducing the catheter which was a solid body.

John Hunter, the famous pathologist, made several important observations in 1786 about prostate growth

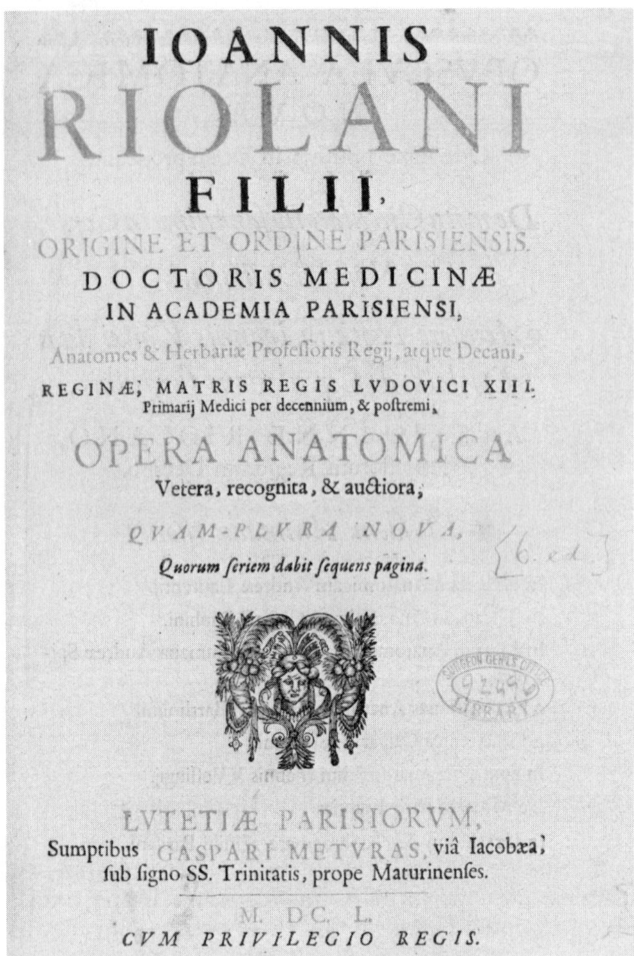

FIGURE 1–1. Title page of paper by Riolanus from *Opera Anatomica.* (Courtesy of the National Library of Medicine.)

that were very much ahead of their time. He described lateral and middle lobe hyperplasia, bladder trabeculation, and upper tract changes that result from lower tract obstruction. His most innovative contribution to our understanding of the developmental biology of the prostate was the discovery that castration of prepubertal rats prevents prostate development and that castration of adult animals causes atrophy of the gland.[11]

The early concepts of Morgagni and Hunter in the 18th century were replaced in the late 19th and early 20th centuries by considerably less scientific speculations on the causes of prostate disease. A small book titled *The Nonsurgical Treatment of Prostatic Disease* by G. W. Overall appeared in 1903.[16] An excerpt follows:

> Men are by nature much more sensuously inclined than women: and when they cultivate libidinous impulses and associate with prostitutes, are liable to indulge their sexual propensities to such an extent as to develop passions that may lead to grave moral vices, like excessive intercourse or masturbation resulting in lesions of the prostate, or some form of nervous disease.
>
> Just as mental disturbances influence sexual conditions, so in like manner do diseases of the prostate gland cause such various forms of mental disorders as inactiv-

ity, depression, and numerous other neurotic aberrations.

I have especially noticed that men between the ages of 40 and 70, suffering from chronic prostatitis lose the keen mental activity they formerly possessed. Their prospective reasoning faculties become sluggish and inactive.

Deaver, in his book *Enlargement of the Prostate: Its Diagnosis and Treatment,* which was published in 1905, states that

> Over-indulgence in sexual intercourse has long been considered a possible factor (in causing an enlarged prostate). From the enlarged and tender prostate of the young masturbator, to the similar organ of the old man who marries a young wife,—it has been common to blame the sexual excitement as the efficient cause; but, as remarked by J. William White it is probably quite as logical, if not more so, to blame the enlarged prostate with exciting unnatural desires.[6]

As a corollary to this belief, Tobin states in a paper published in 1902 that persistence of sexual desire in old men is an indication for castration.[21]

The medical literature from the late 1800s and early 1900s contains an amazing number of possible causes for enlargement of the prostate. Excessive intercourse, continence, masturbation, increased sexual desire, lascivious reading and libidinous thoughts, alcohol, protracted indulgence in withdrawal, wet feet and cold weather, horseback riding, bicycle riding, motorcycle riding, perverted indulgences, and high living are all suggested as possible causes for prostate disease. It must have been difficult for men in that time to discuss their symptoms of prostatic obstruction and prostatitis considering the implication that the problem was brought on by an undesirable lifestyle.

Between 1900 and 1930 a number of papers appeared in the literature that had a more rational basis for the assertions made by their authors. Ciechanowski believed that prostatic enlargement occurred from prostatic duct scarring and obstruction caused by gonorrhea.[4] The obstruction was thought to result in retention of prostatic secretions, which caused enlargement of the gland. It is interesting that one current hypothesis regarding the cause of benign prostatic hyperplasia (BPH) is that microinjury to the prostatic ducts from voiding, ejaculation, or infection may cause stromal proliferation in the periurethral area of the gland. Virchow stated that prostatic enlargement is a neoplasm just like neoplastic growth in other areas of the body.[22] Wade, in 1914, published a paper suggesting that BPH is caused by the action of one or more internal secretions.[24] Much of the research into the cause of BPH over the past 20 years has been to study the role of sex hormones and growth factors in prostate growth.

One of the difficulties in tracing the history of prostate disease is that prior to 1930 there was often confusion regarding the cause of urinary obstruction. BPH, carcinoma of the prostate, bladder stones, infections of the prostate, and urethral strictures were often not distinguished from one another because of the final common pathway of urinary obstruction. From ancient times to the 20th century, bladder stones and infections of the prostate and bladder were much more common than they are today. Consequently, even after the excellent anatomic descriptions by Morgagni and Hunter of the pathophysiology of prostatic obstruction, there continued to be a problem distinguishing bladder stones from prostatic obstruction. During the 19th century, carcinoma of the prostate was thought to be an uncommon problem, and it is quite likely that many of the reports discussing various treatment methods for BPH were in fact incorporating a significant number of patients with carcinoma. It was not until the 20th century that surgeons began to realize that carcinoma of the prostate is a far more common problem than previously recognized. For example, in 1895, White reported on a series of 111 patients treated for BPH with bilateral orchiectomy with good effect on the obstructive voiding symptoms.[27] A number of these men may have had urinary obstruction caused by carcinoma and experienced improved urinary flow because of the effect of androgen withdrawal on the tumor.

Although antedated by Hunter's studies on the effects of castration in rat prostate by more than 100 years, the modern era of research on prostate cancer and BPH began with the pioneering work of Charles Huggins.[9] The discovery that prostate cancer regresses following androgen withdrawal firmly established the role of sex hormones in prostate cancer growth. Huggins also studied the histology of BPH in men with prostate cancer treated by castration.[10] He found atrophy in some parts of the prostate, but the effect was variable. He noted an increased number of acini per microscopic field, smaller acinar lumina, fewer papillary infoldings in acini, and decreased height of the epithelium lining the acini in castrated men. These findings suggested that atrophy of the glandular tissue of BPH takes place with androgen withdrawal. Wendel et al reviewed this topic in 1972 and added data from their own patients who had undergone needle biopsy of the prostate following hormonal treatment for prostate cancer.[26] They found that the BPH present in these glands was of lower grade than that seen in men not treated with hormones or orchiectomy. They concluded that androgens play a role in the maintenance of prostate epithelial cell function in BPH.

In 1944, Moore reviewed a group of 28 patients who were eunuchs or eunuchoid or had pituitary infantilism, and found no evidence of BPH.[14] Observations made on the effects of sex hormones on the prostate by the mid-1940s strongly suggested that benign prostatic hyperplasia is an endocrinologic problem that might be caused by a change in the ratio of androgen to estrogen in the aging male. These studies served as the basis for much of the research work done on the cause of BPH over the last 50 years. There is little doubt that testes must be present for BPH to develop, but the exact role of testosterone, dihydrotestosterone (DHT), and estrogen in the growth of epithelium and stroma has still not been determined.

The important role of the androgens in the growth and maintenance of prostatic epithelial function led to the discovery by Walsh and Wilson that BPH can be produced in the dog by administration of androgen.[25] This work was reported in 1976 and established the dog as the primary animal model for the study of BPH. The dog model has served an important role in the study of the effect of hormones on prostatic growth and maintenance of prostate function. Another landmark discovery was reported by Cunha in 1972.[5] The first of a series of papers appeared that described the strong inductive effect of embryonic urogenital mesenchyma on adjacent epithelial cells to differentiate a prostate epithelial cell phenotype. These studies established the important interaction between the stroma and epithelium in the prostate and served as the beginning for a major area of research in both BPH and prostate cancer.

The early work showing that the glandular compartment of the prostate is androgen dependent led to the study of a number of strategies for treating BPH by androgen deprivation. Castration was used by Rand to treat BPH in two patients in 1895.[17] In the same year, White reported a series of 111 cases of BPH treated by castration.[27] He stated that the treatment was successful in most patients, but he noted an operative mortality of 18 per cent! Androgen deprivation of prostate epithelial cells continues to play an important role in the clinical management of BPH. Previous work has shown that testosterone must undergo conversion to DHT by the enzyme 5α-reductase in order to be an effective stimulator of prostate epithelial function. It is interesting to note that a majority of this enzyme activity occurs in the stroma, showing the important interrelationship between stroma and epithelium. The important role of DHT in maintaining prostatic epithelial cell function has led to the development of a 5α-reductase inhibitor for treating BPH.[13] Finasteride is the drug currently used clinically to cause shrinkage of the prostate and improvement in the symptoms of BPH.

A new and clinically important area of BPH research is the discovery that alpha-adrenergic blockade results in significant improvement in obstructive voiding symptoms and uroflow in men with BPH. Caine et al were the first to report a clinical series of patients treated with the alpha blocker phenoxybenzamine.[2] His work served as the basis for the development of alpha blockers that are more specific for prostatic smooth muscle. The alpha-1 receptor subtype is the predominant adrenergic receptor in BPH and the alpha-1 blocker, terazosin, has proved to be more effective than phenoxybenzamine for treating BPH with fewer side effects.[12] The two pharmacologic strategies for treatment of BPH are totally different in their mode of action, which raises the possibility that a combination of these two drugs may be significantly more effective than either agent alone. The combination drug therapy is currently under investigation.

Prostate cancer often causes symptoms of urinary obstruction that are indistinguishable from those of benign prostatic hyperplasia. Published reports on the incidence of prostate cancer prior to the 20th century indicated that it was an uncommon disorder. When histopathologic examination became routine in the study of prostate disease, the incidence of prostate malignancy was found to be far greater than previously thought. Von Recklinghausen was the first to note that prostate cancer has a predilection for metastasizing to bone.[23] He pointed out that the primary focus of prostate cancer is often small compared with the widespread growth of metastatic deposits in bone. The observations that prostate cancer contains a large amount of acid phosphatase and that men with metastatic prostate cancer often exhibit high serum levels of acid phosphatase were made by Gutman et al in 1936 and Robinson et al in 1939.[8, 19] This early work established the clinical utility of serum acid phosphatase as a marker for metastatic prostate cancer and served as the foundation for later investigations on the use of prostatic acid phosphatase and prostate-specific antigen as markers for the presence of prostate cancer.[1, 20]

Huggins and Hodges, in their seminal paper in *Cancer Research* in 1941, showed that metastatic prostate cancer usually causes an elevation of serum acid phosphatase and alkaline phosphatase levels. They reported that androgen withdrawal by orchiectomy or the administration of large doses of estrogen causes prostate cancer to regress and the phosphatase levels to return to normal in a majority of cases.[9] This was the first report demonstrating that a human tumor regresses by chemical manipulation, and it ushered in the era of cancer chemotherapy. Dr. Huggins was awarded the Nobel Prize in 1966 for this work. Hormonal manipulation has been commonly used in the management of advanced prostate cancer. The pioneering work of Huggins and Hodges has served as the basis for much of the current research into the cause and treatment of prostate cancer. The many new modalities of hormonal manipulation of prostate cancer such as the luteinizing hormone–releasing hormone agonists and androgen receptor blockers have their origin in the fundamental work by these early pioneers in prostate cancer research.

The concept that some cancers of the prostate are "latent" and have little, if any, potential to develop into clinically active disease was introduced by Franks in 1954.[7] This work is generally accepted by the urologic community, but some investigators believe that latent prostate cancer does not exist. There are compelling arguments in support of prostate cancer as a two-stage disease—a long, latent clinically benign stage that may progress in some men to a rapidly growing, metastasizing, clinically malignant stage.[3] The observation that men of different racial backgrounds have a similar incidence of latent prostate cancer at various ages but a substantially different incidence of clinically active disease supports this hypothesis. A number of studies are being conducted to determine if an environmental factor may play a role in the activation of latent prostate cancer. A number of explanations have been offered for this phenomenon, but the proposal that prostate cancer may remain latent and clinically benign is an important conceptual advance that has significant clinical implications.

The studies of the normal prostate and prostate diseases have covered many centuries. Much of the early work was hampered by a lack of histologic verification of the disease processes. The landmark work by Morgagni on the pathophysiology of prostatic obstruction was the beginning of the scientific study of urinary obstruction caused by benign and malignant growth of the prostate. Studies in the rat reported by John Hunter in 1786 established the role of hormones in prostate development and maintenance of prostatic function. The elegant studies on androgen deprivation in men with prostate cancer, reported in 1941 by Huggins and Hodges, not only was the beginning of the modern era of cancer chemotherapy but has served as the basic foundation for research in prostate growth for the past 50 years.

REFERENCES

1. Bruce A, Mahan D, Sullivan LD, et al: The significance of prostatic acid phosphatase in adenocarcinoma of the prostate. J Urol 125:357, 1981.
2. Caine M, Perlberg S, Meretyk S: A placebo-controlled double-blind study of the effect of phenoxybenzamine in benign prostatic obstruction. Br J Urol 50:551, 1978.
3. Carter HB, Piantadosi S, Isaacs JT: Clinical evidence for and indications of the multistep development of prostate cancer. J Urol 143:782, 1990.
4. Ciechanowski S: BPH caused by infection. Med Chir 7:183, 1901.
5. Cunha GR: Tissue interactions between epithelium and mesenchyme of urogenital and integumental origin. Anat Rec 172:529–541, 1972.
6. Deaver JB: Enlargement of the Prostate, Its Diagnosis and Treatment. Philadelphia, P Blakiston's Son & Co, 1905.
7. Franks LM: Latent carcinoma of the prostate. J Pathol Bacteriol 68:603, 1954.
8. Gutman EB, Sproul EE, Gutman AB: Significance of increased phosphatase activity at the site of osteoplastic metastases secondary to carcinoma of the prostate gland. Am J Cancer 28:485–495, 1936.
9. Huggins C, Hodges CV: Studies on prostatic cancer: The effect of castration, of estrogen and of androgen injection on serum phosphatases in metastatic carcinoma of the prostate. Cancer Res 1:293, 1941.
10. Huggins C, Stevens RA: The effect of castration on benign hypertrophy of the prostate in man. J Urol 43:705–714, 1940.
11. Hunter J: Treatise on the venereal disease. London, 1788.
12. Lepor H, Knapp-Maloney G, Wozniak-Petrofsky J: The safety and efficacy of terazosin for the treatment of benign prostatic obstruction. Int J Clin Pharmacol Ther Toxicol 27:392, 1989.
13. McConnell J: Androgen ablation and blockade in the treatment of benign prostatic hyperplasia. Urol Clin North Am 17:661, 1990.
14. Moore RA: Benign hypertrophy and carcinoma of the prostate: Occurrence and experimental production in animals. Surgery 16:152–167, 1944.
15. Morgagni GB: The Seats and Causes of Disease. Translated by B. Alexander. Mt. Kisco, NY, Futura Publishing Co, 1960, pp 426–483. (Facsimile of the London, 1769, edition).
16. Overall GW: A non-surgical treatise on diseases of the prostate gland and adenea. Chicago, Marsh and Grant Co, 1903.
17. Rand HW: A contribution to the surgery of the hypertrophied prostate. Ann Surg 22:1–80, 1895.
18. Riolanus JF: Opera Anatomica. Lutetiae Parisiorum, 1649.
19. Robinson JN, Gutman EB, Gutman AB: Clinical significance of increased serum "acid" phosphatase in patients with bone metastases secondary to prostatic carcinoma. J Urol 42:602–618, 1939.
20. Stamey TA, Yang N, Hay AR, et al: Prostate specific antigen as a marker for adenocarcinoma of the prostate. N Engl J Med 317:909, 1987.
21. Tobin RH: Treatment of senile hypertrophy of the prostate. Br Med J 1:774, 1902.
22. Virchow R: Die krankhoften geshioulste. 3:133, 1862–63.
23. Von Recklinghausen F: Die Fibrose oder deformirende Ostitis die Osteomalacie und die osteoplastische Carcinese in ihren gengenseitigen Beziehungen. *In* Festschrift Rudolf Virchow zu

seinem 71, Geburtstage. Berlin, Georg Reimer Publ, 1891, pp 22–35, 81–85.

24. Wade H: Prostatism (original memoirs). Ann Surg 59:321–359, 1914.

25. Walsh PC, Wilson JD: The induction of prostatic hypertrophy in the dog with androstanediol. J Clin Invest 57:1093, 1976.

26. Wendel EF, Brannen GE, Putong PB, Grayhack JT: The effect of orchiectomy and estrogens on benign prostatic hyperplasia. J Urol 108:116–119, 1972.

27. White JW: The present position of surgery of the hypertrophied prostate. Ann Surg 18:152, 1895.

Chapter 2

PROSTATIC MORPHOGENESIS, STROMAL-EPITHELIAL INTERACTIONS, ZONAL ANATOMY, AND QUANTITATIVE MORPHOMETRY

ELLEN SHAPIRO

Before we discuss these matters in more detail, let me remind you of the normal structure of the gland.

L. M. Franks, M.B., B.S.
ROYAL COLLEGE OF SURGEONS OF ENGLAND
NOVEMBER 24, 1953

MORPHOGENESIS OF THE PROSTATE

The septation of the cloaca by the urorectal septum begins at about 28 days.[57] The rectum and primitive urogenital sinus (UGS) are present by the 44th day of gestation. The primitive UGS proximal to the mesonephric duct develops into the vesicourethral canal. The region distal to the mesonephric duct becomes the definitive UGS. The UGS adjacent to the bladder (pelvic urethra) is narrow and becomes the lower portion of the prostatic and membranous urethra.[23] Embryologically, the cranial half of the pelvic urethra is derived from endodermal UGS.

The prostate is derived from endodermal UGS just below the developing bladder. The ductal network within the prostate originates from solid epithelial outgrowths, or prostatic buds, that grow around müllerian mesoderm, which develops into the utricle, and the mesonephric mesoderm, which develops into the ejaculatory ducts.[26, 28–30, 32]

In the human fetus, the first endodermal buds develop from the lining of the pelvic portion of the UGS at around the 10th week of development. The secretion of testosterone by the embryonic testis stimulates the growth and development of the prostate, resulting in the lengthening, arborization, and canalization of the prostatic ducts.[43, 49, 56, 63, 65] By 13 weeks of gestation, 70 primary ducts are present which exhibit secretory cytodifferentiation.[28, 32]

Posteriorly, a component of mesonephric mesoderm originating from the bladder becomes incorporated into the pelvic urethra (superficial layer of the trigone). Later in development, this mesenchyme becomes smooth muscle that is continuous with the bladder (trigone). The caudal half of the pelvic urethra originates entirely from the UGS.[34, 35]

A detailed anatomic description of the time course of ductal development in the fetal prostate was reported by Lowsley in 1912.[32] He serially sectioned human fetal prostate and noted that by 12 weeks the branching ductal network consisted of five distinct groups. He termed these ductal groups the posterior, lateral (two), anterior, and middle lobes. The ducts of the posterior lobes originate from the floor of the prostatic urethra distal to the openings of the ejaculatory ducts and grow posteriorly. The epithelial buds of the two lateral lobes branch lateral to the verumontanum. The ducts of the middle lobe originate on the posterior urethra proximal to the openings of the ejaculatory ducts. The anterior lobe buds branch anterior to the verumontanum. The anterior lobe is prominent until the 16th week and then involutes by 22 weeks.

Although Lowsley's work in the fetus was meticulous and precise, it cannot be extrapolated to explain the morphology of the adult prostate gland. The distinct boundaries between the five prostate lobes that Lowsley defined cannot be identified after 2.5 months.[26] Nor do the five distinct lobes exist in the prepubertal and normal young adult prostate. Nonetheless, the terms *posterior, lateral, middle,* and *anterior* continue to be used to describe the lobes of the prostate, even though the middle and lateral lobes exist only in the aging male.

Although Lowsley's study emphasized the structural changes in the fetal prostate gland, Zondek and Zondek and others examined the continuous influence of maternal placental and fetal hormones on prostatic growth.[67] The investigators noted periodic acid-Schiff (PAS)–positive staining in the prostate as early as 14 weeks, which correlates with secretion and growth activity in the fetus. The incidence and degree of PAS-positive reactions increase as fetal development progresses. Squamous metaplasia is found in the prostatic tubule epithelium at 22 weeks' gestation and increases as the fetus matures. The squamous metaplasia resolves by acantholysis and exfoliation, resulting in the disappearance of most foci by birth. This process appears to depend upon a delicate balance of estrogen and testosterone. In congenital anomalies such as anencephaly, the fetus is exposed to excessive levels of circulating estrogen in the face of abnormally low testosterone production due to the absence of gonadotropin stimulation. The prostates of fetuses with this anomaly contain extensive squamous metaplasia and cyst formation.

Zondek and Zondek also examined tubular proliferation in the fetus.[67] The fetal prostate is composed of only a few tubules widely separated by stroma. By term, glandular epithelium proliferates and interspersed stromal elements decline.

More recently, Xia et al examined prostate growth, histogenesis, and secretory activity in 107 specimens from normal fetuses ranging in age from 20 weeks gestation to 1 month (postnatal).[66] No sharply delineated "lobules" were recognized, but two zones were apparent. There was the inner (submucosal) zone (IZ), characterized by a concentric mass of fibromuscular connective tissue. This mass contained ducts at various stages of development. A peripheral zone (PZ) contained less concentrically organized fibromuscular connective tissue with secondary ducts, gland buds, and groups of acinar glands. The PZ was further divided into anterior, posterior, and two lateral regions.

These investigators also recognized three stages of development.[66] During the bud stage (20 to 30 weeks), the buds at the ends of the ducts were simple, solid, and cellular and contained no lumen. Columnar cells were seen basally, and spindle-shaped cells were found near the bud center. The bud-tubule stage (31 to 36 weeks) was characterized by small collections of cellular buds and acini in both the PZ and IZ. The histomorphogenesis of the fetal prostate further develops into the acinotubular stage (37 to 42 weeks), in which distinct acinotubular gland clusters arise from tubules with dis-

tinct lumina. Other investigators have noted that progression of ductal formation occurs except in the periurethral zone. There, primitive rounded glands persist.

Xia et al also observed the presence of a glandular pattern in 25 per cent of the fetal prostates, which resembled "budding" atypical hyperplasia with "back-to-back" glands as described in the adult prostate.[66] This pattern was seen as early as 24 weeks but occurred more frequently in the 37- to 42-week gestational age glands. PAS staining intensity was directly related to gestational age, with the region of greatest staining activity in the lateral lobes of the PZ.

Prostate-specific antigen (PSA) was identified in only about 20 per cent of the specimens.[66] When it was identified, it was usually seen in the older fetal or newborn gland. Squamous metaplasia was also noted. It was always seen in association with the utricle and posterior wall of the urethra. Regions of involvement of the ducts with squamous metaplasia were variable. As the fetus progressed in gestational age, the areas of squamous metaplasia became less prominent.

To date, this study is the most comprehensive examination of the embryologic development of the fetal prostate. Our understanding of prostate development has evolved from Lowsley and Venero's concept of five lobes and the organized progression of ductal budding to zonal histogenesis (IZ and PZ).[32] These studies focus primarily on the ductal development of the gland. Popek et al examined not only development of the epithelium but also the qualitative morphologic changes that occur in the mesenchyme or stroma during development.[44] They observed that the primitive mesenchyme is initially very loose, with the epithelium budding into the stroma. As the ductal network progresses, the loose peripheral primitive mesenchyme is replaced by concentrically organized smooth muscle bundles around acini. The stroma maintains its primitive appearance in the periurethral region and does not undergo a change to smooth muscle. Two distinct smooth muscle bands are also noted; one is in association with the anterior fibromuscular stroma and one surrounds the utricle and ejaculatory ducts and is continuous with the smooth muscle of the seminal vesicles. Skeletal muscle is also seen peripherally in association with the prostatic capsule. Muscle-specific actin staining was noted as early as week 16, but mesenchymal expression was more notable by week 22. Prostate-specific acid phosphatase staining was seen in the larger ducts and cannulated acini by 17 weeks. PSA was generally absent in ductal and acinar cellular cytoplasm but was detected in areas of squamous metaplasia by 32 weeks.

STROMAL-EPITHELIAL INTERACTIONS

Although the exact mechanisms for the induction of prostate organogenesis and cytodifferentiation at the cellular and molecular levels are not known, experimental evidence suggests that these phenomena are associated with interactions between testosterone, mesenchyme, and epithelium. The inductive role of the stromal cells in the adult prostate resulting in new nodule formation has been termed "an embryonic reawakening" by McNeal.[37] The investigations by Cunha and Chung have examined the interaction between epithelium and mesenchyme, as well as the androgenic mediation of the events that lead to prostatic growth and development.[5–12]

Fundamental to understanding the stromal and epithelial interactions is the fact that the development of the prostate, as well as the male internal ductal system, is androgen dependent.[15] Chemical or surgical castration of the fetus during critical periods of sexual development inhibits development of the prostate and other male accessory sex glands.[4, 16, 20, 21, 27, 40, 41, 48] During the postnatal period, androgen remains important for prostate growth, as castration at this time inhibits its growth and development.[15, 33, 45] Although the fetal testis elaborates testosterone, dihydrotestosterone, produced by the enzymatic reduction of testosterone by 5α-reductase, is the active intracellular androgen responsible for prostatic morphogenesis. This enzyme has been found in the urogenital sinus and external genitalia of humans.[11, 56, 64] Inhibition of this enzyme in the male rat results in feminization of the external genitalia and urethra and partial inhibition of prostatic development.[24] Although dihydrotestosterone is important for prostatic growth, the developing prostate may be responsive to exceedingly low levels of dihydrotestosterone or other androgens.[24] Also, some aspects of postnatal prostatic growth may be independent of androgens, as castration in the rat during this period does not completely inhibit prostatic development.[15, 33, 45]

A human model to study the sexual differentiation of males who lack dihydrotestosterone can be found in individuals with 5α-reductase deficiency.[25, 60] The 5α-reductase deficiency syndrome is a form of autosomal recessive male pseudohermaphroditism characterized by severe penoscrotal hypospadias, a blind vaginal pouch, and normal testes with normal epididymides, vasa deferentia, and seminal vesicles. The ejaculatory ducts terminate in the blind-ending vagina, and the prostate is small or undetectable. Overall, the phenotypic appearance is female without breast development. Because the defect in virilization during embryogenesis is limited to the urogenital sinus and the anlage of the external genitalia, the selective effects of testosterone and dihydrotestosterone can be understood.

Testicular feminization syndrome (Tfm) is another disorder resulting in complete failure of prostatic development.[22] Androgen receptors are defective or absent in this syndrome. The wolffian ducts undergo degeneration. Although the testes elaborate normal amounts of testosterone, the external genitalia are feminized.

Testicular feminization and 5α-reductase deficiency syndromes provide a clinical basis for understanding the profound effect of dihydrotestosterone on prostate morphogenesis. Although androgens are prerequisite for prostatic development, animal studies have provided strong evidence to underscore the importance of the inductive potential of embryonic stroma on normal adult prostatic epithelial cells. Cunha et al have demonstrated that embryonic UGS mesenchyme of mice can induce adult bladder epithelial cells to replicate in vivo and form prostate-like glandular structures.[13] This induction capability is sensitive to the hormonal status of the host and does not occur in the castrated animal. These studies show that adult epithelial cells can be induced by stroma in a hormonally favorable environment.

Further evidence for the mesenchymal mediation of androgenic effects upon epithelium has been presented in the analysis of tissue recombinant experiments using Tfm mice. These mice have defective androgen receptors and fail to develop prostates.[42] When tissue recombinants constructed of wild-type mesenchyme and Tfm epithelium are exposed to physiologic androgen levels as a result of grafting the recombinants into intact male hosts, normal prostatic morphogenesis proceeds. Prostates do not form when the Tfm mesenchyme is used with either the Tfm or the wild-type epithelium.[8, 12, 31] These results from experiments using recombinants of tissue from normal and androgen-insensitive animals suggest that the stroma responds to androgen stimulation and induces the classic epithelial response to androgen. The importance of dihydrotestosterone in prostatic development is further supported by the presence of dihydrotestosterone receptor–binding sites in wild-type urogenital sinus.[50, 51, 59, 61] Such binding sites are absent in the Tfm urogenital mesenchyme.[12] Also, androgen-induced DNA synthesis is similar in prostates that are completely wild-type or are composed of wild-type mesenchyme and Tfm epithelium.[11, 58] This finding further supports the concept that a variety of aspects of epithelial differentiation are regulated by androgens indirectly through androgen-dependent mediators of stromal origin.[5–7, 18, 19]

ZONAL ANATOMY

The endocrinology and developmental biology of the prostate have been explored over the past decade by McNeal, who has expanded our knowledge of adult prostate morphology.[34–37] He described the zonal anatomy of the prostate based on examination of the gland in different planes of section.

The urethra represents the primary anatomic reference point, dividing the prostate into an anterior fibromuscular and a posterior glandular portion.[36, 37] The urethra angulates sharply (35 degrees). This point of angulation divides the urethra into proximal and distal segments of about equal length (Fig. 2–1). The two principal regions of the glandular prostate are defined as the peripheral zone (approximately 75 per cent of the total glandular volume) and the central zone (approximately 25 per cent of the total volume). The two regions have unique morphometric properties. The central zone and its ductal orifices are closely associated with the ejaculatory ducts and their orifices near the verumontanum in the distal urethral segment, which extends from the prostatic apex to the verumontanum. The peripheral zone ducts enter the urethra separately from those of the central zone and are associated primarily with the distal urethral segment.

The acinar morphology of the central and peripheral zones is also unique.[36, 37] The central zone is composed of ducts that branch into large, irregularly contoured acini, whereas the peripheral zone ducts branch into small, round, regular acini. The epithelial cells in the central zone have granular cytoplasm and enlarged nuclei located at various levels from the basement membrane, whereas the epithelial cells of the peripheral zone have clear cytoplasm and small, dark nuclei located uniformly along the basal aspect of the basement membrane. Finally, the stroma of the central zone is long and compact and closely associated with the acini, whereas that of the peripheral zone is random, with loose interconnections. These morphologic and histologic differences between the peripheral and central zones may be explained by the different embryonic origins. The ejaculatory ducts traverse the center of the central zone, and the epithelium of the central zone is similar to that of the seminal vesicle, suggesting a wolffian duct origin. The peripheral zone is presumed to derive from the urogenital sinus.

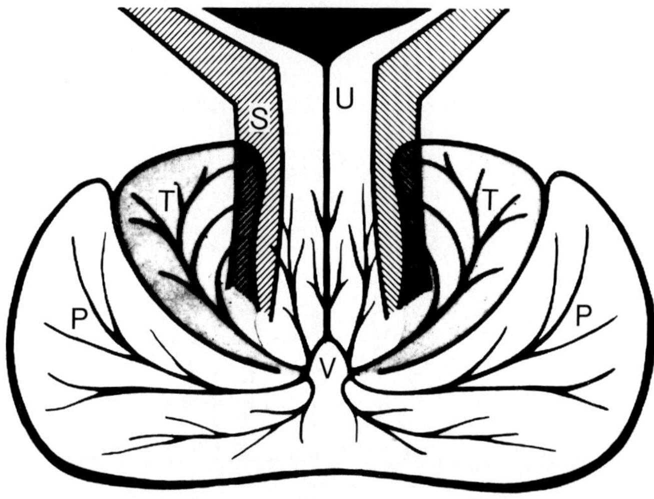

FIGURE 2–2. Oblique coronal plane of prostate subdivided by the preprostatic sphincter (S) into transition zone (T) and periurethral region (U). Main transition zone ducts arise from the urethra at the base of the verumontanum (V) and pass around the distal border of the sphincter as they arborize toward the bladder. P = Peripheral zone of glandular prostate. (From JE McNeal: Origin and evolution of benign prostatic enlargement. Invest Urol 15:340–343, © by Williams & Wilkins, 1978; with permission.)

The anatomic area of the prostate represented by the transitional zone accounts for less than 5 to 10 per cent of the glandular volume and is intimately related to the proximal urethral segment.[36, 37] The cylinder of striated muscle surrounding the proximal urethral segment is termed the *preprostatic sphincter*. Its function is to prevent the retrograde flow of semen by contracting during ejaculation. Just lateral to this sphincter are two small lobes that histologically are similar to the peripheral zone. The stroma in the transitional zone is dense and compact. The transitional zone is adherent to the external aspect of the preprostatic sphincter, and its glands penetrate the sphincter, whereas the peripheral fibers of the sphincter penetrate the transitional zone stroma. The preprostatic sphincter and the transitional zone are less well developed in the prepubertal prostate. Only the proximal extent of the sphincter near the bladder neck is apparent, with a smaller, less well defined transitional zone.

The periurethral gland region of the glandular prostate is less than 1 per cent of the total volume (Fig. 2–2).[36, 37] This region contains tiny ducts arising from the proximal urethral segment that are embedded in the periurethral smooth muscle. The periurethral glands are histologically similar to those of the peripheral and transitional zones, and the transitional zone and periurethral gland region have a common embryonic urogenital sinus origin. These two areas are the exclusive sites of origin of benign prostatic hyperplasia (BPH) (Fig. 2–3). Hyperplastic nodules develop in these areas as early as the fourth decade. Periurethral nodules are stromal and resemble embryonic mesenchyme, whereas transitional zone nodules are glandular.

Nodule genesis is focal and occurs randomly within areas of susceptibility. The initial abnormality in nodule

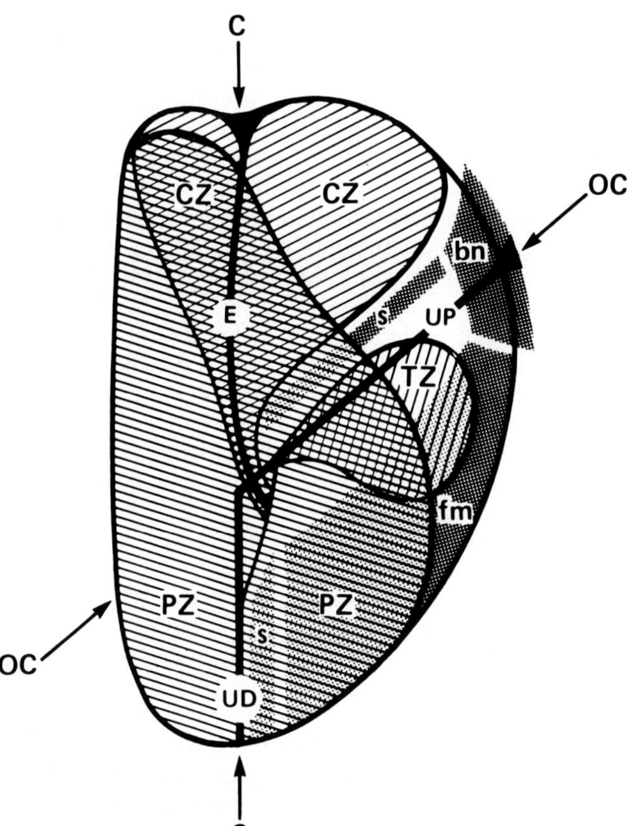

FIGURE 2–1. Sagittal diagram of distal prostatic urethral segment (UD), proximal urethral segment (UP), and ejaculatory ducts (E) showing their relationships to a sagittal section of the anteromedial nonglandular tissues [bladder neck (bn), anterior fibromuscular stroma (fm), preprostatic sphincter (s), distal striated sphincter (s)]. These structures are shown in relation to a three-dimensional representation of the glandular prostate [central zone (CZ), peripheral zone (PZ), transitional zone (TZ)]. Arrows indicate the coronal plane (C) along distal urethral segment, which is the plane of greatest extent of glandular prostate, and the oblique coronal plane (OC) along proximal urethral segment. (From McNeal JE: Normal histology of the prostate. Am J Surg Pathol 12:619, 1988; with permission.)

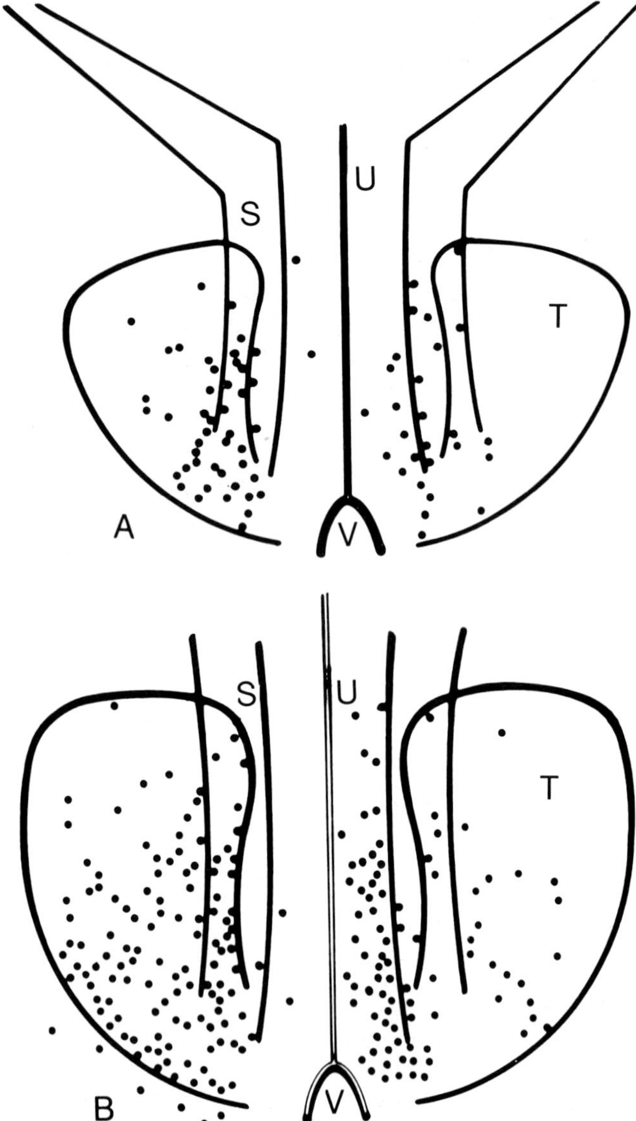

FIGURE 2–3. *A,* Prostate with few nodules superimposed on an oblique coronal diagram of Figure 2–2. Centers of glandular nodules are plotted and lie primarily within the transition zone (T), especially near or within the sphincter (S). Stromal nodules are plotted at right. They are fewer in number and are often periurethral (U) or in the medial sphincter. *B,* Prostate with many nodules and diffusely enlarged transition zone. Glandular nodules (*left*) are generally located within the transition zone. Stromal nodules (*right*) occur primarily in the periurethral region. (From JE McNeal: Origin and evolution of benign prostatic enlargement. Invest Urol 15:340–343, © by Williams & Wilkins, 1978; with permission.)

genesis may be spontaneous reversion of a clone of stromal cells to the embryonic state. Growth potential can then be mediated through coordinated stromal-epithelial interactions. This postulation is supported by the morphologic peculiarities seen in ducts that are tangent to nodule borders. These ducts may show epithelial hyperplasia and budding of new branches on only the duct wall facing the center of the nodule. These eccentric effects suggest that an induction or interaction is occurring on only one side of the duct. The hallmark of embryonic development is the formation of new

architecture. It seems logical that the development of BPH nodules, which is repressed until the fourth or fifth decade of life, may be a "reawakening of embryonic capabilities" in the adult.[37]

QUANTITATIVE MORPHOMETRY

Studies of neonatal and pathologic growth of the prostate have postulated the importance of stromal-epithelial interaction in the control of prostatic growth. A technique has been developed that permits the quantification of the stromal and epithelial components of the prostate gland. Morphometrics is a method that provides a quantitative histologic analysis of fixed tissue sections.[62] Stereologic analysis allows measurements to be taken from a representative number of two-dimensional samples (tissue sections) and used to estimate quantitatively the internal structure of a three-dimensional object (prostate).[2, 62] Stereologic results are expressed as densities that relate a volume, a surface area, or a number of tissue or cellular components to a unit or reference volume. Quantitative morphometry complements qualitative descriptions obtained from light microscopy and yields objective and reproducible values for morphologic structures that allow statistically defined comparisons.

In 1977, Bartsch applied stereologic techniques to light microscopic prostatic tissue sections.[2] He examined hematoxylin and eosin–stained paraffin sections of normal prostate glands from six men (<30 years old) and seven patients undergoing suprapubic prostatectomy for bladder outlet obstruction due to BPH. The tissue was divided into morphologically defined compartments, with inner and the outer dimensions as described by Franks.[17] The normal gland was subdivided into the acinar parenchyma and the interstitial fibromuscular (stromal) tissue. The BPH acinar component of the tissue was further subdivided into the lumina and glandular cells. Stereologic analysis involves superimposing an ocular grid on a microscopic field and counting points of intersection of the grid with the various components of the tissue. This method provides the percentage distribution of each tissue component within the area of interest, and this can be converted into percentage of section volume. An extension of this methodology, termed *biomorphometrics,* has been reported by De-Klerk and Coffey in a study of rat ventral prostate.[14] This technique determines the ratio of various cellular types determined by standard morphometric analysis and the total number of cells in the gland obtained by knowledge of the total DNA content in the gland and DNA per cell nucleus. This eliminates the differential effects of fixation, dehydrating, and embedding of sections on volume and shapes of different tissue components. This type of analysis is useful as an index of hyperplastic growth and can be performed in animal studies in which the whole gland is available for DNA analysis.

Bartsch et al performed elegant stereologic analysis using the point-counting method.[3] They showed that in normal human prostate the volume density of the stroma, glandular cells, and acinar lumina was 0.45, 0.21, and 0.34, respectively. In BPH, these values were 0.6, 0.12, and 0.28, respectively. The ratio of stroma:epithelium in BPH and normal prostates was 5:1 and 2:1, respectively. These studies suggest that BPH results in a primarily stromal composition.

Siegel et al recently used a point-counting stereology method to determine the cellular composition of human prostate.[55] Prostate specimens were obtained from nine men undergoing prostatectomy for BPH. The tissue sections were stained with hematoxylin and eosin. The area densities of prostatic connective tissue, smooth muscle, vascular elements, and epithelium were 47 per cent, 7 per cent, 3 per cent, and 18 per cent, respectively. Twenty-five per cent of the adenoma was edema, leukocytes, nerve, lymphatics, and other poorly defined tissues. The relative proportion of stroma to epithelium was 4.6:1, which is consistent with Bartsch's observation. Although these studies have provided the foundation of our knowledge about normal and pathologic morphogenesis, application of this point-counting technique is cumbersome.

Shapiro et al recently reported the application of computer image analysis that adapts Weibel's multipurpose test grid and line intersect stereologic analysis to quantify the relative amounts of stroma and epithelium in BPH.[52] The grey-density computer image analysis discriminates the epithelial and stromal elements of prostatic tissue sections stained with hematoxylin and eosin. Prostatic adenoma specimens were obtained from 12 subjects undergoing transurethral resection of the prostate (TURP), 12 subjects undergoing open prostatectomy, and 6 subjects undergoing cystoprostatectomy. Prostatic biopsies were performed on 9 additional subjects before they received medical therapy for clinical BPH. Uroflowmetry and symptom scores were determined on all patients prior to surgery or biopsy. A staff pathologist confirmed the histologic diagnosis of BPH in all specimens.

The mean stromal:epithelial ratios in the TURP, open prostatectomy, pharmacotherapy, and cystoprostatectomy groups were 5.1 ± 0.4, 3.2 ± 0.1, 5.7 ± 0.8, and 2.7 ± 0.1, respectively. The grey-density computer image analysis confirmed previous observations that BPH is primarily a stromal process. The baseline clinical data demonstrated that the subjects undergoing TURP, open prostatectomy, and pharmacotherapy had clinical (symptomatic) BPH, whereas the subjects undergoing cystoprostatectomy had no clinical evidence of BPH (asymptomatic BPH). The age and prostate size of the TURP/pharmacotherapy and cystoprostatectomy groups were similar. The mean stromal:epithelial ratios in the TURP/pharmacotherapy and cystoprostatectomy groups were 5.5:1 and 2.7:1, respectively. The morphometry study suggested that the development of clinical BPH is related to the stromal:epithelial ratio of the prostate adenoma. The age and severity of clinical BPH in the subjects undergoing TURP/pharmacotherapy and open prostatectomy were similar. The mean stromal:epithelial ratios in the TURP/pharmacotherapy and open prostatectomy groups were 5.7:1 and 3.2:1, respectively. The

morphometry study suggested that the histologic compositions of large prostates ultimately requiring enucleation prostatectomy and smaller prostates obtained from males with asymptomatic BPH are similar. The large prostates presumably did not cause obstruction at an earlier stage in the hyperplastic process, since the histology did not predispose to obstruction.

Shapiro et al recently developed a technique for quantifying the cellular elements of the prostate.[53] The technique involves double immunoenzymatic staining and color-assisted computer image analysis. The epithelium and smooth muscle were labeled with rabbit antidesmin and a mouse anti–human prostatic acid phosphatase (PSAP), respectively. A rabbit peroxidase-antiperoxidase complex was linked to the rabbit antidesmin by a secondary antibody to rabbit antibody. The peroxidase-antiperoxidase complex was labeled brown using the chromogen DAB. A mouse alkaline phosphatase–antialkaline phosphatase (APAAP) complex was linked to the mouse anti-PSAP by a secondary antibody to mouse antibody. The APAAP complex was labeled using the chromogen fast red. The epithelium, epithelial lumen, smooth muscle, and connective tissue stained red, colorless, dark brown, and light brown, respectively, using the double immunoenzymatic staining technique. The thresholds for the color-assisted computer image analysis were set to discriminate the different staining properties of the prostatic cellular elements. The area densities of the cellular elements of the prostate were originally determined in eight transrectal biopsy specimens obtained from men with clinical BPH prior to initiating pharmacotherapy. The area densities of smooth muscle, connective tissue, epithelium, and epithelial lumen were 22 ± 4 per cent, 54 ± 4 per cent, 16 ± 6 per cent, and 9 ± 1 per cent, respectively. The ratio of stroma:epithelium was 4.8:1. This study demonstrated that a significant component of prostate adenoma is smooth muscle. Shapiro et al recently reported that mouse antiactin is a more sensitive label for prostate smooth muscle than is rabbit antidesmin. Double immunoenzymatic staining was performed on 19 transrectal biopsy specimens obtained from men with clinical BPH using mouse antiactin/rabbit antihuman PSAP and rabbit antidesmin/mouse antihuman PSAP. The area densities of smooth muscle, connective tissue, epithelium, and epithelial lumen in the antiactin/antihuman PSAP–stained tissues were 39 ± 3 per cent, 38 ± 3 per cent, 12 ± 1 per cent, and 11 ± 1 per cent, respectively. The area densities of smooth muscle, connective tissue, epithelium, and epithelial lumen in the antidesmin/antihuman PSAP were 19 ± 2 per cent, 59 ± 2 per cent, 12 ± 1 per cent, and 11 ± 1 per cent, respectively.

Literature examining the morphometry of the prepubertal prostate is scarce.[1, 38] In 1951, Andrews reported on the histology of prepubertal prostates. He noted that from birth until the end of the first month, no significant changes occurred in the gland, but between the first and fourth months, a gradual regression in the epithelium occurred. The only other notable change was in the size of the prostate. Between the fourth month and puberty, the increase in prostate size was attributed to an increase in stroma. The only comprehensive study of prostatic

TABLE 2–1. MORPHOMETRY OF THE PROSTATE

	PER CENT AREA DENSITIES BY AGE GROUP				
GROUP **HISTOLOGIC COMPONENT**	**I** (0–1 yr) n=9	**II** (1–8 yr) n=14	**III** (9–14 yr) n=7	**IV** (15–20 yr) n=9	**V** (21–40 yr) n=3
Smooth muscle	48.9 ± 1.3	41.1 ± 0.6	32.7 ± 2.9	41.4 ± 2.9	48.7 ± 0.3
Connective tissue	30.7 ± 2.0	38.4 ± 1.0	44.4 ± 5.2	31.2 ± 2.7	28.3 ± 2.4
Glandular epithelium	15.9 ± 1.2	14.7 ± 1.1	16.7 ± 1.9	18.6 ± 1.6	15.7 ± 0.3
Glandular lumen	4.6 ± 0.4	5.9 ± 0.4	6.0 ± 1.5	9.0 ± 1.3	7.3 ± 2.2

$*P < .05.$

morphometry in the prepubertal male has recently been reported by Shapiro et al.[54] Quantitative morphometric studies were performed on pediatric prostates obtained from autopsy examinations. Double immunoenzymatic staining using antiactin and anti-PSAP, as described previously, was used to label the tissue components. Color image analysis was performed to discriminate the staining properties of the epithelium, smooth muscle, connective tissue, and lumen. The results are shown in Table 2–1. This study demonstrated age-related changes in the density of smooth muscle that appear to parallel the postnatal testosterone surge (age, 30 to 60 days) and the rise in testosterone at the onset of puberty (Fig. 2–4). The density of prostate smooth muscle was significantly increased in the first year of life. A progressive decrease in smooth muscle was observed throughout childhood and puberty, with a subsequent increase in the density of smooth muscle following puberty. No significant changes were seen in the epithelium or glandular lumen. These studies demonstrate that the pediatric prostate is a dynamic gland, and these changes in relationship to the hormone milieu may be important to our understanding of the development of BPH.

In addition to these dynamic changes in morphometry, the early testosterone surge in the young infant may be a critically important "imprinting" event that may have an impact on the gland's propensity for future abnormal prostatic growth and disease. Hormonal imprinting has been studied in the rat.[46, 47] Naslund et al showed that early hormonal surges are requisite for normal adult prostate growth in the rat and that an alteration in the normal endocrine events that occur shortly after birth can have significant and permanent effects on the androgen sensitivity and growth of the adult prostate.[39] These hormonal surges are thought to affect prostatic growth by altering the properties of the prostatic stem cells. The absolute number of these stem cells is important because it ultimately determines the size of the gland. Therefore, hormonal events occurring before puberty can imprint or program the prostatic size, androgen sensitivity, and function and maintenance of the stem cells.

REFERENCES

1. Andrews GS: The histology of the human foetal and prepubertal prostates. J Anat 85:44–54, 1951.
2. Bartsch G: Stereology, a new quantitative morphological approach to study prostatic function and disease. Eur Urol 3:85–95, 1977.
3. Bartsch G, Muller HR, Boerholzer M, Rohr HP: Light microscopic stereologic analysis of the normal human prostate and benign prostatic hyperplasia. J Urol 122:487–491, 1979.
4. Burns RK: Role of hormones in the differentiation of sex. *In* Young WC (ed): Sex and Internal Secretions. Baltimore, Williams and Wilkins, 1961, pp 76–158.
5. Cunha GR: Epithelio-mesenchymal interactions in primordial gland structures which become responsive to androgenic stimulation. Anat Rec 172:179, 1972.
6. Cunha GR: Support of normal salivary gland morphogenesis by mesenchyme derived from accessory sexual glands of embryonic mice. Anat Rec 173:205, 1972.
7. Cunha GR: Epithelial-stromal interactions in development of the urogenital tract. Int Rev Cytol 47:137, 1976.
8. Cunha GR, Lung B: The possible influences of temporal factors in androgenic responsiveness of urogenital tissue recombinants from wild-type and androgen-insensitive (Tfm) mice. J Exp Zool 205:343, 1978.
9. Cunha GR, Lung B, Reese B: Glandular epithelial induction by

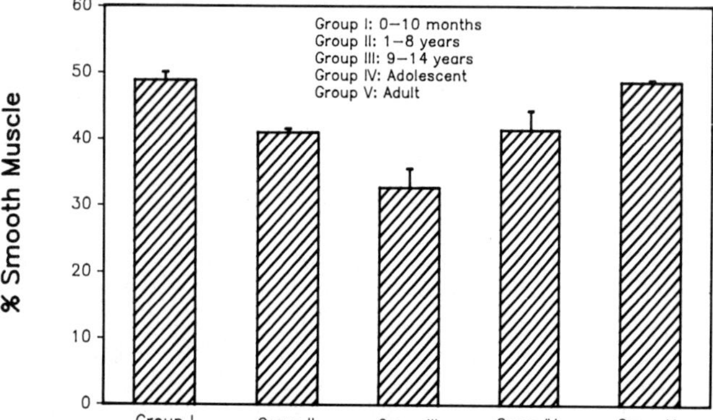

FIGURE 2–4. Bar graph illustrating age-related changes in the area density of smooth muscle in the prostate.

embryonic mesenchyme in adult bladder epithelium of Balb/C mice. Invest Urol 17:302, 1980.

10. Cunha GR, Chung LWK, Shannon JM, et al: Stromal-epithelial interactions in sex differentiation. Biol Reprod 22:19, 1980.

11. Cunha GR, Chung LWK: Stromal-epithelial interactions: Induction of prostatic phenotype in urothelium of testicular feminized (Tfm/y) mice. J Steroid Biochem 14:1317, 1981.

12. Cunha GR, Donjacour AA: Mesenchymal-epithelial interaction in the growth and development of the prostate. *In* Lepor H, Ratliff TL (eds): Urologic Oncology. Boston, Kluwer Academic Publishers, 1989, pp 159–155.

13. Cunha GR, Chung LWK, Shannon JM, Fujji H: Hormonal induced morphogenesis and growth: Role of the mesenchymal-epithelial interactions. Recent Prog Horm Res 39:559–598, 1983.

14. DeKlerk DP, Coffey DS: Quantitative determination of prostatic epithelial and stromal hyperplasia by a new technique: Biomorphometrics. Invest Urol 16:240–245, 1978.

15. Donjacour AA, Cunha GR: The effect of androgen deprivation on branching morphogenesis in the mouse prostate. Dev Biol 128:1–14, 1988.

16. Elger W, Graf KJ, Steinbeck H, et al: Hormonal control of sexual development. Adv Biosci 13:41, 1974.

17. Franks LM: Benign nodular hyperplasia of the prostate: A review. Ann Coll Surg Engl 14:92–106, 1954.

18. Franks LM, Barton AA: The effects of testosterone in the ultrastructure of the mouse prostate in vivo and in organ cultures. Exp Cell Res 19:35, 1960.

19. Franks LM, Riddle PN, Carbonell AW, et al: A comparative study of the ultrastructure and lack of growth capacity of adult human prostate epithelium mechanically separated from its stroma. J Pathol 100:113, 1970.

20. Greene RR: Hormonal factors in sex inversion: The effects of sex hormones on embryonic sexual structures of the rat. Biol Symp 9:105, 1940.

21. Greene RR, Burrill MW, Ivy AC: The effects of estrogens on the antenatal sexual development of the rat. Am J Anat 67:305, 1939.

22. Griffin JE, Wilson JD: Disorders of sexual differentiation. *In* Walsh PC, Gittes RF, Perlmutter AD, Stamey TA (eds): Cambell's Urology, 5th ed. Philadelphia, WB Saunders Company, 1986, pp 1819–1855.

23. Hamilton WJ, Mossman HW: The urogenital system. *In* Human Embryology: Prenatal Development of Form and Function, 4th ed. New York, Macmillan, 1976, p 201.

24. Imperato-McGinley J, Binienda Z, Arthur A, et al: The development of a male pseudohermaphroditic rat using an inhibitor of the enzyme 5α-reductase. Endocrinology 116:807, 1985.

25. Imperato-McGinley J, Guerrero L, Gautier T, et al: Steroid 5α-reductase deficiency in man: An inherited form of pseudohermaphroditism. Science 186:1213, 1974.

26. Johnson FP: The later development of the urethra in the male. J Urol 4:447, 1920.

27. Jost A: Problems of fetal endocrinology: The gonadal and hypophyseal hormones. Recent Prog Horm Res 8:379, 1953.

28. Kellokumpu-Lehtinen P: The histochemical localizations of acid phosphatase in human fetal urethral and prostatic epithelium. Invest Urol 17:435, 1980.

29. Kellokumpu-Lehtinen P: Development of sexual dimorphism in human urogenital sinus complex. Biol Neonate 48:157, 1985.

30. Kellokumpu-Lehtinen P, Santti R, Pelliniemi LJ: Correlation of early cytodifferentiation of the human fetal prostate and Leydig cells. Anat Rec 196:263, 1980.

31. Lasnitzki I, Mizuno T: Prostatic induction and interaction of epithelium and mesenchyme from normal wild-type and androgen-insensitive mice with testicular feminization. J Endocrinol 85:423, 1980.

32. Lowsley OS: The development of the human prostate gland with reference to the development of other structures at the neck of the urinary bladder. Am J Anat 13:299, 1912.

33. Lung B, Cunha GR: Development of seminal vesicles and coagulating glands in neonatal mice. 1. The morphogenetic effects of various hormonal conditions. Anat Rec 199:73, 1981.

34. McNeal JE: The prostate and prostatic urethra: A morphologic synthesis. J Urol 107:1008, 1972.

35. McNeal JE: Developmental and comparative anatomy of the prostate. *In* Grayhack JT, Wilson JD, Scherbenske MJ (eds): Benign Prostatic Hyperplasia. Bethesda, DHEW Publication No. NIH 76-1113, 1976, pp 1–5.

36. McNeal JE: The zonal anatomy of the prostate. Prostate 2:35, 1981.

37. McNeal JE: The prostate gland: Morphology and pathobiology. Monogr Urol 9(3), 1988.

38. Moore RA: The histology of the newborn and prepubertal prostate gland. Anat Rec 66:1–7, 1936.

39. Naslund MJ, Coffey DS: The differential effects of neonatal androgen, estrogen and progesterone on adult rat prostate growth. J Urol 136:1136–1140, 1986.

40. Neumann F, Elger W, Steinbeck H: Antiandrogens and reproductive development. Phil Trans R Soc Lond (Biol) 25:179, 1970.

41. Neumann F, Graf KJ, Elger W: Hormone-induced disturbances in sexual differentiation. Adv Biosci 13:71, 1974.

42. Ohno S: Major Sex Determining Genes. New York, Springer-Verlag, 1979, pp 1–140.

43. Pointis G, Latreille MT, Cedard L: Gonado-pituitary relationships in the fetal mouse at various times during sexual differentiation. J Endocrinol 86:48, 1980.

44. Popek EJ, Tyson RW, Miller GJ, Caldwell SA: Prostate development in prune belly syndrome (PBS) and posterior urethral valves: Etiology of PBS—Lower urinary tract obstruction or primary mesenchymal defect? Pediatr Pathol 11:1–29, 1991.

45. Price D: Normal development of the prostate and seminal vesicles of the rat with a study of experimental postnatal modifications. Am J Anat 60:79, 1936.

46. Rajfer J, Coffey DS: Sex steroid imprinting of the immature prostate: Long-term effects. Invest Urol 16:186–190, 1978.

47. Rajfer J, Coffey DS: Effects of neonatal steroids on male sex tissues. Invest Urol 17:3–7, 1979.

48. Raynaud A, Frilley M: Destruction de cerveau des embryos de souris au treizième jour de la gestation, par irradiation au moyen des rayon X. Comp Rend Soc Biol 141:658, 1947.

49. Resko JA: Androgen secretion by the fetal and neonatal Rhesus monkey. Endrinology 87:680, 1978.

50. Shannon JM, Cunha GR: Autoradiographic localization of androgen binding in the developing mouse prostate. Prostate 4:367, 1983.

51. Shannon JM, Cunha GR, Vanderslice KD: Autoradiographic localization of androgen receptors in the developing urogenital tract and mammary gland. Anat Rec 199:232, 1981.

52. Shapiro E, Hartanto V, Becich MJ, Lepor H: The relative proportion of stromal and epithelial hyperplasia is related to the development of symptomatic BPH. J Urol 147:1293, 1992.

53. Shapiro E, Hartanto V, Lepor H: Quantifying the smooth muscle content of the prostate using double-immunoenzymatic staining and color assisted image analysis. J Urol 147:1167–1170, 1992.

54. Shapiro E, Hartanto V, Perlman E, Lepor H: Morphogenesis of the prostate. Abstract #93. American Academy of Pediatrics Section of Urology, New Orleans, 1991.

55. Siegel YI, Zaidel L, Hanmel I: Morphometric evaluation of benign prostatic hyperplasia. Eur Urol 18:71–73, 1990.

56. Siiteri PK, Wilson JD: Testosterone formation and metabolism during male sexual differentiation in the human embryo. J Clin Endocrinol Metab 38:113, 1974.

57. Stephens FD: Congenital Malformations of the Urinary Tract. New York, Praeger Publishers, 1983.

58. Sugimura Y, Cunha GR, Bigsby RM: Androgenic induction of deoxyribonucleic acid synthesis in prostate-like glands induced in the urothelium of testicular feminized (Tim/y) mice. Prostate 9:217, 1986.

59. Takeda H, Miguno T, Lasnitzki I: Autoradiographic studies of androgen-binding sites in the rat urogenital sinus and postnatal prostate. J Endocrinol 104:87, 1985.

60. Walsh PC, Madden JD, Harrod MJ, et al: Familial incomplete male pseudohermaphroditism, type 2. Decreased dihydrotestosterone formation in pseudovaginal perineoscrotal hypospadias. N Engl J Med 291:944, 1974.

61. Wasner G, Hennermann I, Kratochwil K: Ontogeny of mesenchymal androgen receptors in the embryonic mouse mammary gland. Endocrinology 113:1771, 1983.

62. Weibel ER: Stereological techniques for electron microscopic morphometry. *In* Hagar MA (ed): Principles and Techniques of Electron Microscopy, Vol 3. New York, Van Nostrand Reinhold, 1973.
63. Weniger JP, Zeis A: Sur la secretion precoce de testosterone par le testicule embryonnaire de souris. Comp Rend Acad Sci Paris 275:1431, 1972.
64. Wilson JD, Griffin JE, Leshin M, et al: Role of gonadal hormones in development of the sexual phenotypes. Hum Genet 58:78, 1981.
65. Winter JSD, Faiman C, Reyes F: Sexual endocrinology of fetal and perinatal life. *In* Austin CR, Edward RG (eds): Mechanisms of Sex Differentiation in Animal and Man. New York, Academic Press, 1981, pp 205–254.
66. Xia T, Blackburn WR, Gardner WA: Fetal prostate growth and development. Pediatr Pathol 10:527–537, 1990.
67. Zondek T, Zondek LH: The fetal and neonatal prostate. *In* Goland M (ed): Normal and Abnormal Growth of the Prostate. Springfield, IL, Charles C Thomas, 1975, pp 5–28.

Chapter 3

ANATOMY OF THE PROSTATE

ARNON KRONGRAD and MICHAEL J. DROLLER

The prostate is an accessory reproductive gland found in all orders of male mammals.[43, 60, 71] Although physiologic parallels may abound, anatomic parallels are few. In the dog, as in man, for example, the prostate is intimately associated with the bladder neck, whereas in the opossum many prostatic glands are disseminated along the urethra (Fig. 3–1). In some mammals, such as the rat, the prostate is actually a combination of glandular, paired organs that share the suprasphincteric urethra as their outlet. Even the prostates of the non-human primates, with the possible exception of the gorilla, are grossly different from the human prostate.[47]

Female homologues of the prostate, known as Skene's glands, have been described in several mammalian species, including humans.[79] Although these are similar to the male prostate with respect to general location, glandular structure, and even histochemistry,[84, 97] they are generally far smaller than the male prostate and, from a clinical point of view, of almost no known significance.

In most mammals the prostate is not thought to be of great pathologic significance. In the human, this is not the case. There have been reports of bladder outlet obstruction in women due to hyperplasia of a glandular organ situated at the bladder neck, with the histologic appearance of hyperplastic prostate.[28] Such cases are exceedingly rare. In men, by contrast, the prostate exhibits marked propensity for pathologic behavior. Because to date most therapies for prostatic disease have been surgical, a great deal of attention has been lavished on prostatic anatomy.

Traditionally, prostatic anatomy has been explored by surgical dissection. Recent developments in radiographic techniques have led to the reinvestigation of prostatic anatomy. Although they perhaps add to our diagnostic capabilities, these studies have added little to our com-

prehension of prostatic anatomy.[4, 48] The purpose of this chapter is to review the surgically relevant anatomy of the prostate. The concepts illustrated are based on anatomic dissection.

ANATOMIC ONTOGENY

The prostate is thought to originate primarily from the urogenital sinus,[23, 54] with some evidence of contribution by the wolffian duct.[60, 74] The individual glands begin as mesenchymal outpouchings that extend from the urethra into the surrounding connective tissue stroma (Fig. 3–2). The mesenchyme surrounding the pelvic urogenital organs and the rectum differentiates into the musculature and connective tissue of each of these structures. As the glandular epithelium of the prostate differentiates, the mesenchyme, which invests each acinus, differentiates into the musculature of the glandular acini and their ductules.[21, 63, 64] The prostatic buds coalesce, and the prostate gland grows, incorporating striated muscle fibers from the urethral sphincter primordium into the stroma and capsule.[21, 23, 70, 88]

The adult prostate is a truncated cone, with its base at the urethrovesical junction and its apex at the urogenital diaphragm (Fig. 3–2). The prostate changes little in size until puberty, when it undergoes rapid growth,[63, 83] reaching an age-dependent mean adult weight of more than 40 grams by age 80.[40, 52] By the fifth decade, benign prostatic hyperplasia (BPH) more than compensates for involution of peripheral tissue.[63]

The prostate is pierced by the urethra, which angles forward at the verumontanum, and by the paired ejaculatory ducts, which join the urethra at its point of angulation.[59] By classic description, the parenchyma of the prostate is contained within a fibromuscular capsule

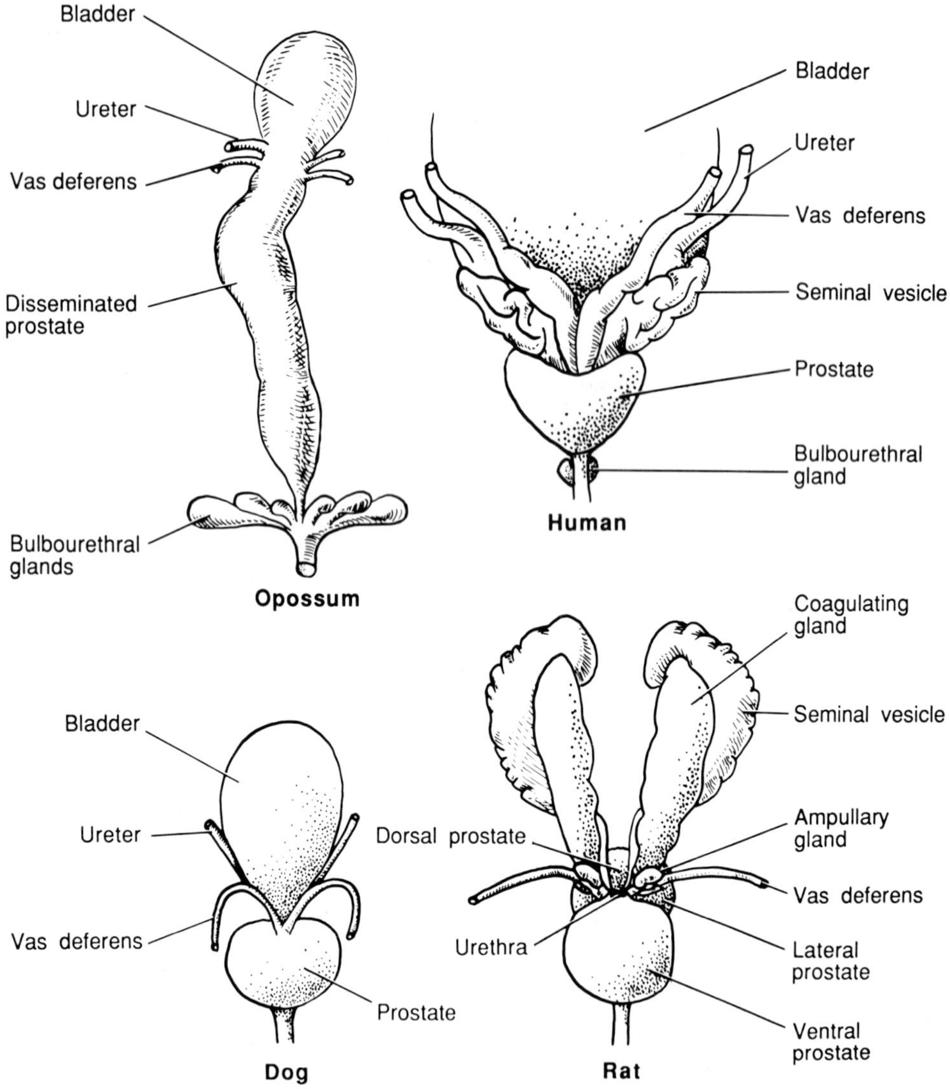

FIGURE 3–1. Comparative prostatic anatomy. Dorsal view of opossum, human, and dog and ventral view of rat accessory reproductive organs. Many anatomic features in this region are constant. Each animal has one bladder and urethra, with paired ureters and vasa deferentia. By contrast, the number, shape, and location of the seminal vesicles, prostate(s), and coagulating and ampullary glands are highly variable.

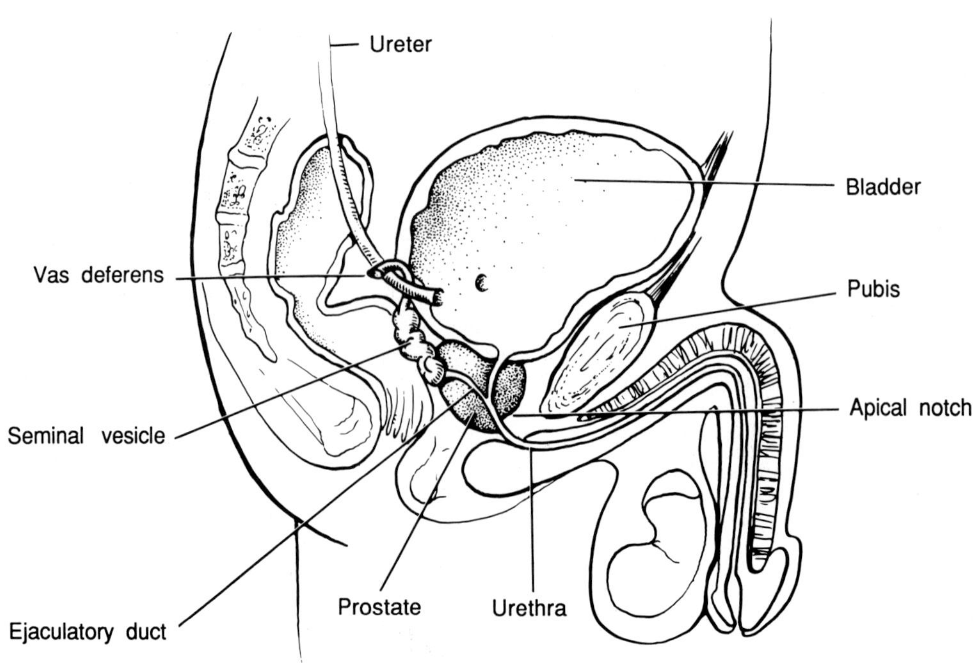

FIGURE 3–2. Adult prostate and surrounding structures. Sagittal view of adult male pelvis. The prostatic base abuts the bladder neck, and its notched apex is situated inferiorly against the urogenital diaphragm (not shown). The urethra pierces the prostate and angles forward at the verumontanum. Posterosuperior to the prostate are the paired, paramedial seminal vesicles. These give rise to ejaculatory ducts that join the urethra at its point of angulation.

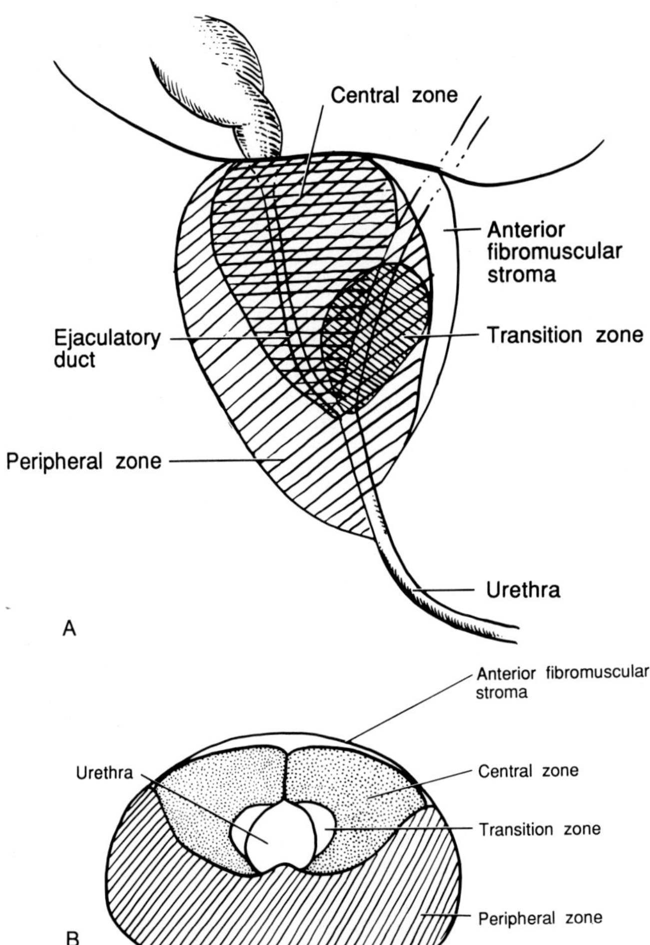

FIGURE 3–3. Prostatic zones. Lateral (*A*) and coronal (*B*) views of prostatic zones. The prostate is composed of four histologically different zones. Anteriorly is a fibromuscular stroma, which has not been linked to a specific pathogenic process. Posteriorly and extending anterolaterally is the peripheral zone, which has been implicated in prostatic neoplasia. Interiorly, immediately adjacent to the urethra, are a pair of transition zones. These comprise the smallest prostatic zone in the presenile prostate but with age give rise to multiple adenomas, which in turn give rise to benign hyperplasia (see Fig. 3–4). Recent evidence suggests that cancer may also originate in these zones. Between the transition and peripheral zones are the central zones, which have not been implicated in a specific pathologic process.

that consists of an outer collagenous layer, two smooth muscle layers (one circular and the other longitudinal), and an inner, dense collagen layer that sends septae into the glandular tissue, uniting with interacinar fibromuscular tracts.[86] A recent reinvestigation suggests that the capsule is really no more than an inseparable outer fibromuscular band that does not cover the apex. Thus, by definition, it is not a capsule.[8] For the surgeon, this is probably no more than a semantic point.

Lowsley proposed a lobar orientation of fetal prostatic parenchyma, but the relevance of this concept to adult anatomy remained unclear for years.[54] Indeed, despite the observations of zone-dependent responses to hormonal stimulation,[5, 45] no discrete anatomic lobes were identified in the adult prostate until 1975, when Tissel and Salander reported three sets of anatomically dis-

tinct, paired lobes in the presenile prostate, which were arranged in an "onion pattern" around the urethra (Fig. 3–3).[52] These anatomic distinctions have since been reproduced by other investigators.[31] Using histologic techniques, McNeal has shown that the urethra receives the so-called preprostatic (i.e., "central") group of ducts proximal to the verumontanum and the ducts of the prostatic (i.e., "peripheral") group distal to the verumontanum.[59]

ANATOMY OF PROSTATIC PATHOLOGY

Although Morgagni referred to benign prostatic adenomas in the early 18th century,[29] it was not until the turn of this century that detailed anatomic observations on the prostatic urethral ducts and glands in the adult were published. In 1902, Albarran and Motz described a "central" group of submucosal glands, situated along the proximal prostatic urethra, that were separated from the peripheral "true" prostatic glands by smooth muscle.[2] Motz and Perearneau then suggested that the "central" glands and their stroma are the anatomic origin of BPH.[66]

Clinically detectable BPH nodules arise from a variety of microscopic adenomas in the periurethral "transition zone" (Fig. 3–4).[58, 63] As the adenomas grow, they encroach on the adjoining smooth muscle, which may result in severe distortion and dysfunction of the muscle (Fig. 3–4).[2, 46, 55, 58, 65, 66] Some have suggested that this dysfunction allows the bladder neck to remain open following surgical resection of the adenoma,[14, 49, 93] so that ejaculation occurs in retrograde fashion.[37, 94] BPH also causes distortion of the ejaculatory ducts, while the prostatic stroma becomes fibrosed and the glandular tissue becomes flattened and atrophic.[65, 66, 70, 78, 86, 88, 89, 96]

A "surgical capsule" develops between the compressed glandular tissue and the hyperplastic nodules, serving as a plane of cleavage that is useful in the surgical removal of the adenoma.[70, 78] This so-called

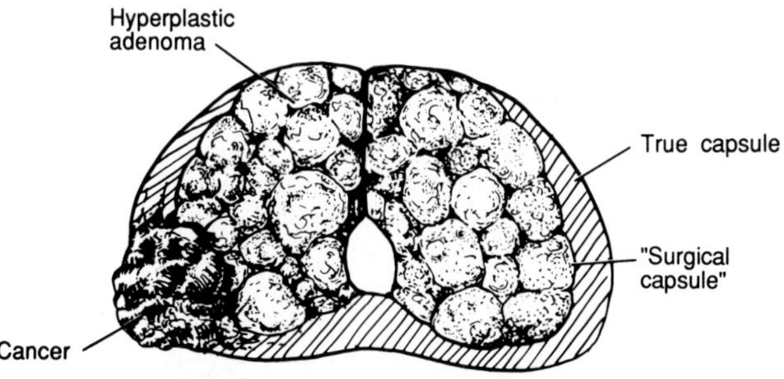

FIGURE 3–4. Pathologic anatomy of the prostate. Coronal view of the senile prostate. With age, the prostate undergoes dramatic anatomic changes. The transition zone adenomas enlarge and obliterate the central zones. Frequently, the anterior fibromuscular stroma and peripheral zones are compressed. A so-called surgical capsule develops around the hyperplastic adenomas, which serves as a convenient plane of cleavage during enucleation of the adenomas. This "capsule" may be continuous in the midline with the anterior true capsule. Prostate cancer has traditionally been regarded as a disease of the peripheral zone, as represented here. Evidence suggests that it may also arise more interiorly.

capsule, which does not exist in the absence of hyperplasia, represents condensed concentrically arranged, fibromuscular interacinar trabeculae. The fascia may be continuous with the anterior fibromuscular prostatic capsule by means of a fibrous septum (Fig. 3–4).[78, 89] It is within this surgical capsule that prostatic calculi most often form.[96] Similar condensations of fibromuscular trabeculae may also form around the larger adenomas, with corresponding atrophy and flattening of the intervening tissue.[70] Smaller adenomas may be found at the surgical capsule, and these may serve as foci for recurrence of benign hyperplasia.[65]

Investigation of the anatomic origin of prostatic carcinoma has emerged more recently, probably in association with the substaging of stage A prostate cancer and the use of transrectal sonographically guided biopsies in staging prostate cancer. Studies of surgical specimens show that prostate carcinoma is a multifocal disease that may originate in the peripheral or transition zones, or even in hyperplastic nodules (Fig. 3–4).[36, 61] Pathologic behavior of these tumors apparently depends somewhat on their points of origin. Primary tumors of the outer (peripheral) zone display less differentiation and a greater propensity for extraprostatic extension than do those of the inner (transition) zone.[36, 51, 62, 77] Unlike the predictable distortion caused by BPH, carcinoma may grow in many directions, spreading by direct extension through the capsule or, in the case of less aggressive tumors, by perineural extension.[51, 87] In late stages, it may involve surrounding organs, typically the periprostatic fat and seminal vesicles, but even the rectum may be involved (Fig. 3–4).

FASCIAL COMPARTMENTS AND ATTACHMENTS OF THE PROSTATE

The pelvic fascia is made up of parietal and visceral layers.[20] The parietal portion is continuous with the psoas and iliac fasciae and is attached to the promontory of the sacrum and the iliopectineal "white line." It passes down over the posterior pelvic walls as the "fascia lunata" to cover the sacral and pudendal plexuses of nerves. The visceral portion, the so-called endopelvic fascia, extends inward from the iliopectineal white line on each side to the posterior surface of the bladder, where it turns onto the base and sides of the bladder to form the lateral or true ligaments of the bladder. This fascia splits into two layers when it reaches the prostate. One layer passes up over the bladder; the other passes downward to envelop the prostate in a loose fibrous sheath. The separate aspects of this sheath are known as the anterior, lateral, and posterior periprostatic fasciae, or aponeuroses. The inner or visceral fascial layer is thus a continuation of the pelvic fascia, and it becomes a membranous diaphragm separating the pelvic cavity from the perineum.[9, 20, 50, 92, 95] This layer passes downward and inward upon the pelvic surface of the levator ani muscles and then extends over the surface of the prostate gland, seminal vesicles, bladder, and rectum.

The prostatic capsule is separated from the peripros-tatic sheath by a venous plexus.[9, 30] This sheath, known as the *loge aponeurotique,* is derived from a coalescence of pelvic fascia and muscular aponeuroses.[2, 9, 92] These mesodermal derivatives anchor the prostate to the bladder sheath superiorly, the urogenital diaphragm inferiorly, the superomedial surface of the levator ani laterally, the rectovesical fascia posteriorly, and the deep dorsal venous plexus and pubis anteriorly.[95] These structures compartmentalize the areas surrounding the prostate and may play a significant role in limiting perineal suppurations and urinary extravasations.[7, 33, 85, 96]

The anterior periprostatic fascia, which is also known as the puboprostatic fascia of Denonvillier or the fascia of Zuckerkandl or Delbet, extends from the anterior surface of the bladder to the posterior surface of the pubis at its lower border and covers the venous plexus of Santorini (Fig. 3–5).[33] This sheath blends laterally with the aponeuroses of the levator ani (the endopelvic fascia) and fuses posteriorly with the prevesical fascia of Charpy. This fascia occupies the space between the anterior puboprostatic ligaments, which extend from the prostate to the posterior surface of the pubis. The deep dorsal vein of the penis extends between the two anterior aponeuroses to reach the venous plexus at the base of the bladder anteriorly. The lowest portion of this sheath is separated from the prostate by the striated muscle fibers of the external sphincter and the posterior urethra in the region of the apex of the prostate.

Anteriorly, the periprostatic sheath is attached to the periosteum of the pubis by the avascular puboprostatic ligaments (see Fig. 3–9). Some have suggested that these ligaments are extensions of the smooth muscle of the bladder and are composed primarily of collagen; they clearly also contain variable amounts of smooth muscle.[3, 57]

Posteriorly, the developing bladder, seminal vesicles, and prostate are separated from the rectum by separate layers of fetal mesenchyme. The pelvic continuation of the peritoneal cavity, consisting of its own mesothelium-lined sac surrounded by a thin layer of subjacent mesenchyme, lies between these two layers of mesenchyme. As the pelvic viscera grow and change in position during embryogenesis, the caudal end of the cul-de-sac of peritoneum is progressively obliterated by approximation and fusion of the two mesothelial surfaces (Fig. 3–5).[11, 85, 92] The mesenchyme originally subjacent to the mesothelial surfaces gradually differentiates into a fibrous membrane known as Denonvillier's fascia. Continued growth and distention of the pelvic organs cause cephalad closure of the peritoneal cul-de-sac. With growth of the seminal vesicles cephalolaterad, the peritoneum extends for only a short distance between the bladder and the seminal vesicles.

In the adult, Denonvillier's fascia is composed of two layers: (1) the rectal fascia immediately external to and mingled with the external longitudinal musculature of the rectum, and (2) a thicker fibroelastic membrane anterior to the connective tissue around the rectum, extending from the pelvic floor to that portion of the peritoneum covering the cephalic surfaces of the pelvic organs. The apex of Denonvillier's fascia, which in sagittal section takes the form of a V, attaches to the

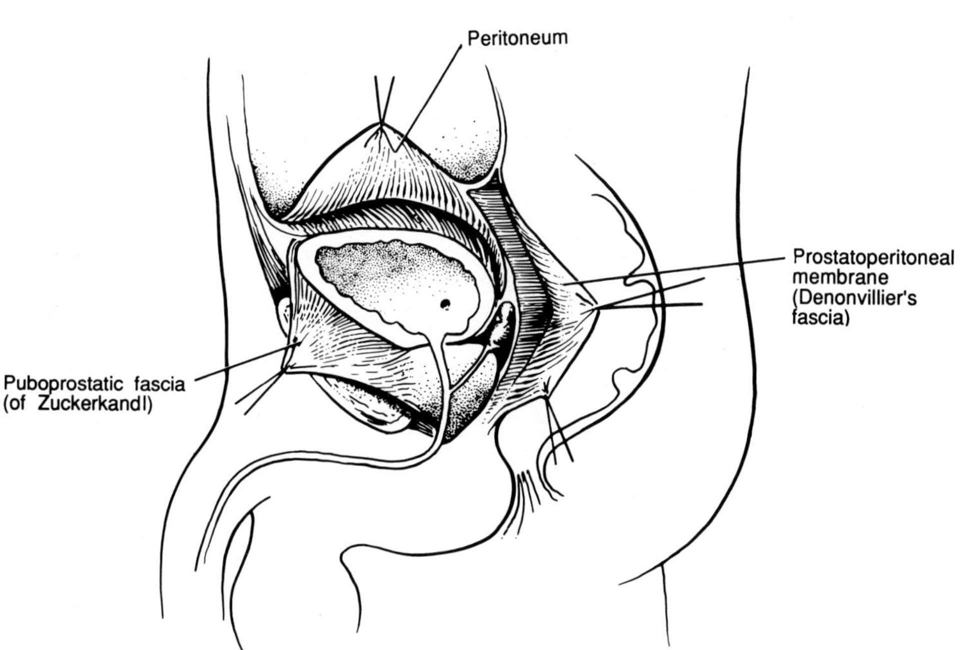

FIGURE 3–5. Periprostatic fasciae. Lateral view of the fascial layers immediately adjacent to the prostate. Anteriorly and covering the venous plexus of Santorini (not shown) is a rather flimsy puboprostatic fascia. This fascia extends from the prostatic apex to the bladder. Posteriorly is the relatively well developed prostatoperitoneal membrane, commonly known as Denonvillier's fascia. This fascia extends from the peritoneum superiorly to the superior aspect of the urogenital diaphragm, covering the posterior surfaces of the prostate and seminal vesicles, where it has a glistening white appearance.

superior layer of the urogenital diaphragm and extends from the prostate to cover the posterior surface of the seminal vesicles (Fig. 3–5). It fuses with the true prostatic capsule at the junction of the ampullae of the vasa deferentia and the ejaculatory ducts to the prostate.

The thickest part of Denonvillier's fascia occurs at the posterior surface of the prostatic capsule, where it has a glistening white appearance. This is a result of its high concentration of elastic fibers. The fascia is much thinner where it extends over the posterior surface of the seminal vesicles and laterally around the sides of the rectal fascia.

The portion of Denonvillier's fascia extending around the external rectal musculature establishes the cleavage plane used in freeing and retracting the rectum backwards in a perineal approach to the prostate.[12] Its intermixing with the external layer of the rectal connective tissue may predispose its dissection to rectal injury. Indeed, if the space between the rectal fascia and the rectal musculature is actually entered inadvertently during dissection, this same fascia can be used advantageously in repair of the rectal tear or resultant fistula.[85]

It has been suggested that Denonvillier's fascia is an important barrier in limiting the spread of cancer regionally or in preventing cancer from spreading posteriorly to the rectum. In addition, the spaces defined by Denonvillier's fascia may direct the flow of pus from a prostatic abscess or the extravasation of urine from a ruptured urethra. Correspondingly, diagnostic tracking by radiographic contrast material may permit identification of the site of rupture when extravasated pus or urine is found in the perineum, pelvis, or retroperitoneum.[7, 33, 85, 96]

The connective tissue that constitutes the true capsule around the sides and front of the prostate is derived from mesenchyme that originally surrounded the neck of the bladder. This tissue is distinct from the mesenchyme of Denonvillier's fascia. The endopelvic fascia,

covering the superior surface of the urogenital diaphragm, fuses with lateral sides of the V-shaped fibrous extension of Denonvillier's fascia as they course laterally and behind the seminal vesicles. Additional fibrous bands extend from the superior border of the seminal vesicles and the posterosuperior surface of the bladder to the pelvic fascia.

MUSCLE GROUPS AROUND THE PROSTATE

Posteriorly, the smooth rectourethralis muscle has its origin in the thickened, anterior, longitudinal band of the rectum, beginning at the level of the verumontanum (Fig. 3–6).[50, 91, 95] These muscles pass over the posterior surface of the prostate and fuse with the raphe of the striated external sphincter. The levator ani muscles, which are distinct from the external sphincter, do not contribute any fibers to the rectourethralis muscle.

Lateral to the prostate are the levator ani muscles, which arise from the posterior surface of the pubis near the symphysis and from the spine of the ischium.[50, 95] Between these points, the levator ani muscles originate from the pelvic fascia along the line of attachment of the obturator fascia. The muscle fibers pass downward and inward toward the midline of the floor of the pelvis. Although some of the muscle fibers fuse with the external vesical sphincter and the deep transverse perineal muscles, the bulk of the levator ani muscles remain separate from the prostate (Fig. 3–6).

Inferiorly, the prostate is bounded by a so-called urogenital diaphragm (Fig. 3–6), which consists of inferior and superior fascial layers that enclose the deep transverse perineal muscle.[9, 92] The concept of a diaphragm has been popular, but the diaphragm is not always easily reproduced anatomically and may be better thought of as a conceptual model for understanding the

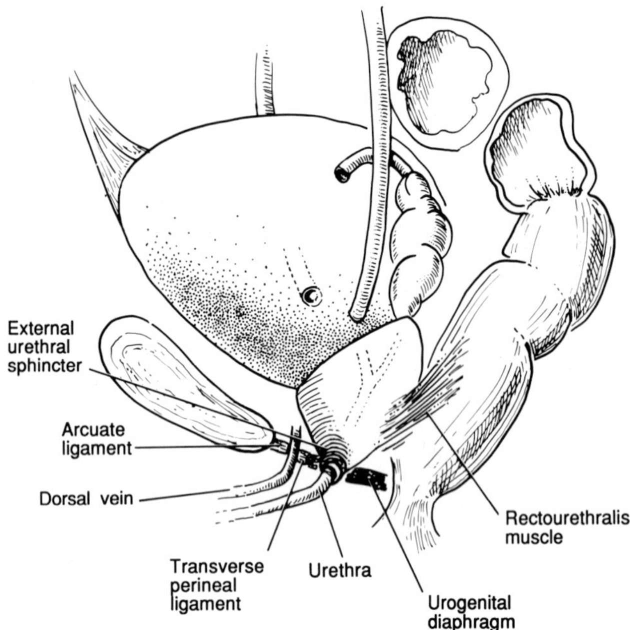

FIGURE 3–6. Periprostatic muscles. Lateral view of the muscles surrounding the prostate. Posteriorly, extending from the anterior longitudinal band of the rectum to the inferoposterior prostate, is the rectourethralis muscle. This muscle is distinct from the levator ani. Inferior to the prostate is the so-called urogenital diaphragm. Although the concept of a diaphragm has been popular, its existence as a distinct entity has been disputed by some anatomists, and it may represent the distal extensions of levator muscles that originate on the lateral pelvic walls. These muscles are separated from the external sphincter by a fibromuscular septum. Within these muscles lie Cowper's glands and the pudendal arteries and nerves (not shown). In the immediate subpubic region the muscular portion of the diaphragm gives way to ligaments stretching horizontally between the two pubic bones under the symphysis. These are pierced by the dorsal vein of the penis.

perineal physiology than as an actual anatomic model.[69] Anteriorly, the urogenital diaphragm is bounded by the transverse perineal ligament, the deep dorsal vein of the penis, and the subpubic arcuate ligament.[92] Inferiorly, this diaphragm borders on the bulbospongiosus and rectourethralis muscles. Connective tissue extensions of the perineal muscles converge inferior to the urogenital diaphragm on the perineal body, which anchors the anorectal region to the pelvic bones.[95] According to this model, the "deep transverse perineal muscle" (urogenital diaphragm), which contains the branches of the pudendal arteries and nerves, is pierced by the membranous urethra from which it is separated by a fibromuscular septum.[68]

Within the fibromuscular septum of the "deep transverse perineal muscle" is a circular, striated urethral sphincter, which may be important in the preservation of urinary continence (Fig. 3–7).[16, 35] It should be noted that the latter muscle is vertically oriented and continuous from the bladder, in association with the urethra and prostate, to its insertion on the perineal membrane.[69] It is distinct from the periurethral striated muscle in both nerve supply and histochemistry[34] and may intermingle with the dorsal vein complex anteriorly, Denonvillier's fascia posteriorly, and even the peripheral zone interiorly.[39, 68]

Muscle configuration in this region may relate to variations in the shape of the apical prostate (see Fig. 3–2).[68] Prostates with substantial hypertrophy anterior to the urethra, with large lateral lobes and no notch, appear to have the external sphincter lying within the transverse urogenital diaphragm, but not in continuity with it. If lateral lobe hypertrophy has not been too great or there has been less hypertrophy of anterior prostatic tissue, the apical notch may appear to be greater, and the external sphincter striated muscle fibers may actually appear to extend more proximally.

The presence of a prominent prostatic notch may allow the urethra to exit more proximal to the prostatic apex. Striated muscle fibers from the external sphincter, extending from the bladder base to the tunica albuginea of the corpus spongiosum, may remain undisturbed in the absence of significant prostatic hyperplasia and may also extend proximal to the prostatic apex in such instances. Transverse transection of the urethra at the apex of the prostate may sacrifice more of the proximal external fibers of the external striated sphincter and potentially compromise urinary continence following radical prostatectomy if more distal exit of the urethra (a smaller notch in lateral lobe or anterior hyperplasia) induces sacrifice of proportionally more external sphincter fibers.[91] Unfortunately, the need to preserve apical anatomy for the sake of continence is superseded by the need for cancer excision. One study suggests that apical

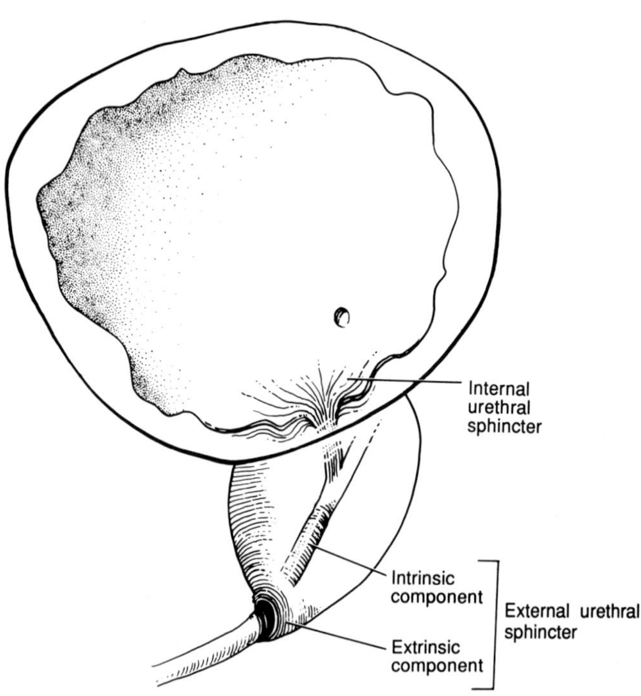

FIGURE 3–7. Urethral sphincters. Anterolateral view of the sphincteric muscles around the prostate. Extending submucosally from the trigone is the smooth internal urethral sphincter. This muscle terminates at the point of urethral angulation and is thought to be relevant in continence and ejaculation. At the prostatic apex and covering the notch is the striated external urethral sphincter. This muscle is distinct from the urogenital diaphragm and extends along the anterior surface of the prostate as far as the bladder. This muscle also has a component that extends interiorly along the urethra.

tumors may be highly represented among tumors with positive surgical margins and, in fact, recommends excision of all tissues from the proximal membranous urethra to the levator muscles, including both neurovascular bundles.[82]

In addition to the so-called intrinsic and extrinsic components of the external sphincter, an internal sphincter extends from the trigone, through the bladder neck, to the region of the verumontanum.[59] This "preprostatic sphincter" may also be relevant in continence, as well as ejaculation, although there is little, if any, direct evidence of this.

VASCULAR STRUCTURES OF THE PROSTATE

The prostate receives most of its blood supply from branches of the prostatovesical arteries (Fig. 3–8). These arteries, which have variable origins from the internal iliac arteries, course along the anteroinferior surface of the bladder and send a variable number of branches to the prostate and the bladder.[13, 17, 22, 27] Additional arteries course along the ejaculatory ducts and supply the urethra adjacent to the verumontanum.[18]

The prostatic arteries actually enter the prostate at the prostatovesical junction,[10, 22, 27, 52] where they may divide to send smaller branches to the rectum. Although the arterial supply to the prostate is localized primarily at the posterolateral bladder neck, arteries to the prostate may course along and penetrate all aspects of the capsule.[18, 22]

Once inside the capsule, the arteries subdivide into longitudinal capsular and urethral branches, with interconnecting intermediate branches.[6, 27] The urethral branches develop only moderately from infancy to adulthood but increase substantially with BPH. Arteriosclerosis, which is thought to cause prostatic infarction, appears to be less common in hyperplastic adenomas.[44, 65]

The periprostatic veins originate in the deep dorsal vein of the penis and course between the periprostatic sheath and the fibromuscular capsule (Fig. 3–9). These receive the venous drainage of the prostatic parenchyma.[18] The deep dorsal vein of the penis penetrates the urogenital diaphragm and trifurcates under the arcuate ligament into a dorsal branch, which proceeds onto the anterior surface of the bladder, and right and left prostatic branches, which constitute the plexus of Santorini.[1, 10, 24–26, 41, 75] These branches communicate in turn with the venous drainage of the perineum, lower extremities, and spine. The dorsal branch most often proceeds directly to the vesicovenous plexus but may also bifurcate, with branches going to the pelvic side walls and the vesicovenous plexus.[67]

Because the periprostatic veins anastomose freely, unintentional lacerations can lead to severe bleeding. It has been shown that in young men all veins are valved at their entrance to the pelvis.[24] The deep dorsal vein of the penis is trebly valved at the arcuate ligament. The other periprostatic veins are also heavily valved. In addition, so-called tourniquet muscles beneath the puboprostatic ligaments presumably compress the venous

plexus of Santorini and prevent blood regurgitation. In older men the findings are inconsistent. Although a number of studies have been unable to document the presence of valves,[1, 10] one study has documented numerous anatomic variations of the veins, particularly in patients with BPH in whom valves were observed radiographically at the base of the deep dorsal vein of the penis as well as in the deep pelvic veins.[25] The exception was in men unable to sustain erections, in whom valves of the deep dorsal vein were frequently absent.

NEUROLOGIC STRUCTURES OF AND IN PROXIMITY TO THE PROSTATE

The nerves to the prostate originate in the perirectal pelvic plexus.[34] These nerves travel posterolaterally out-

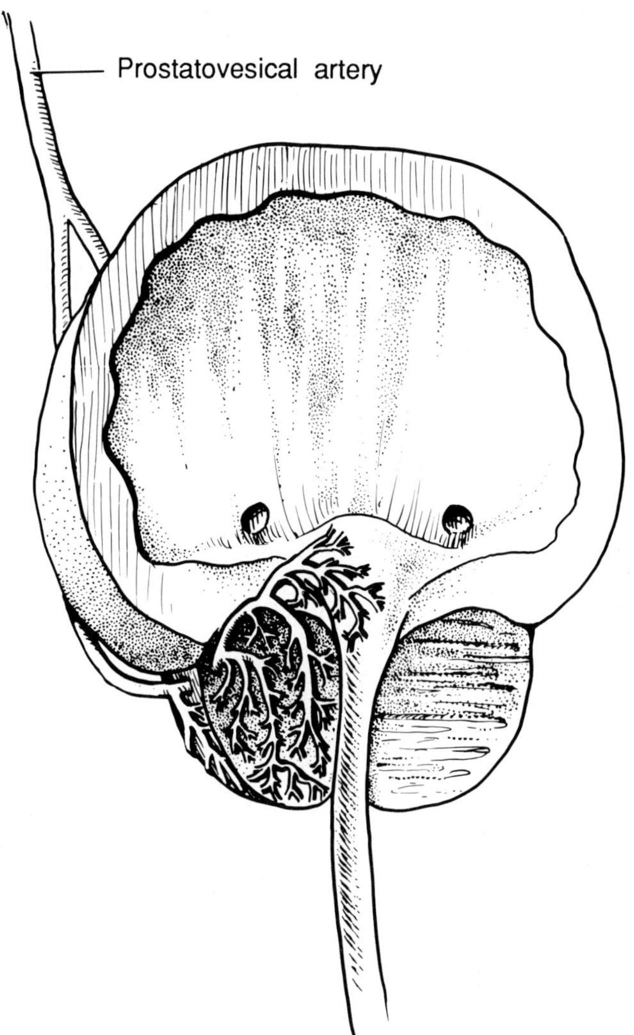

FIGURE 3–8. Arterial supply of the prostate. Coronal view of the arterial supply of the prostate. Vessel size has been exaggerated in order to better demonstrate ramifications. The prostate receives most of its blood from paired arteries originating in the hypogastric arteries. The main branches of these arteries perforate the prostatic capsule posterolaterally at the prostatovesical junction. They then divide further into capsular and urethral branches. Other arteries may perforate the capsule more distally. Additional arteries course along the ejaculatory ducts and supply the urethra adjacent to the verumontanum (not shown).

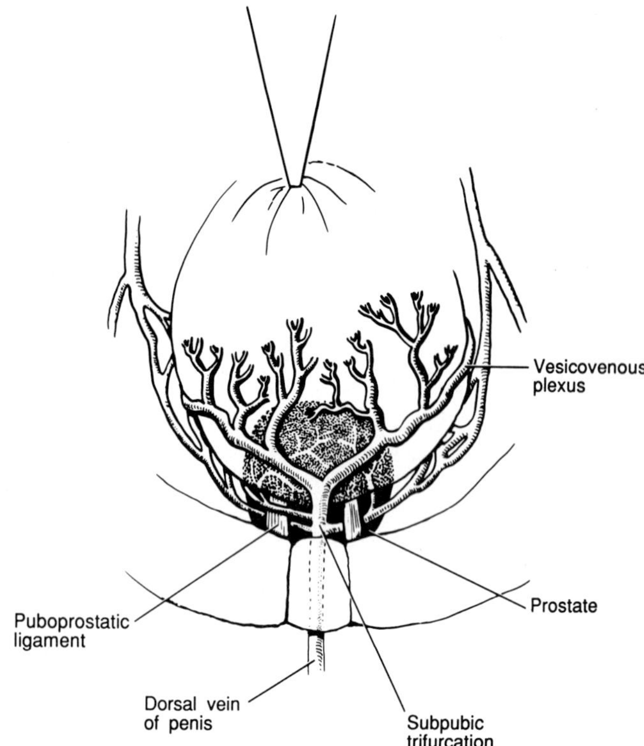

FIGURE 3–9. Venous drainage of the prostate. Anterior view of the periprostatic veins. The deep dorsal vein of the penis penetrates the urogenital diaphragm between the puboprostatic ligaments. It typically branches both before and after crossing the ligaments. These veins receive the venous drainage of the prostate and course between the prostatic capsule and the periprostatic sheath to constitute the venous plexus of Santorini.

side the capsule in the periprostatic sheath, eventually perforating the urogenital diaphragm at the 3 and 9 o'clock positions in relation to the urethra (Fig. 3–10). Along the way they send branches to the prostate, which then ramify within the gland.[42] Perineural spaces may serve as conduits of "least resistance" for transcapsular tumor extension and positive surgical margins, in particular in the case of stage B cancers, and especially at the prostatic apex where the distance from the capsule to the neurovascular bundle is shortest.[87]

Because the prostatic nerves are microscopic, the surgeon must depend on the visual identification of the accompanying vascular branches, which serve as a scaffold upon which the finer nerves course in the pelvis. By ligating and incising the smaller neurovascular branches to the prostate, which course within the periprostatic fascial compartments (see above), the surgeon may separate the prostate from the main neurovascular trunks that innervate the corpora cavernosa and thereby minimize the chances of impotence following radical prostatectomy.[53, 56, 90] Preservation of both neurovascular bundles is especially important to preserving potency in men over 50 years of age.[72]

PROSTATIC LYMPHATICS

It has long been thought that an interacinar lymphatic network in the prostate, which coalesces in a peripros-

tatic subcapsular network, drains prostatic lymph into a series of lymphatic channels and pelvic lymph nodes.[15, 19, 55, 76] In the 1970s, based partly on a theoretical explanation for the prevalence of so-called occult prostate carcinoma, a controversy raged in the urologic literature regarding the existence of prostatic lymphatic channels.[32a] This challenge to traditional dogma proposed that tumor antigen presentation by lymphatics to the immune surveillance system was at the very least faulty, if it indeed existed. Although refuted by some subsequent investigations,[73, 80, 81] this model was anatomically vindicated by an ultrastructural study that demonstrated an absence of lymphatics in subepithelial locations, where small "occult" tumors would arise (Fig. 3–11).[32]

Lymph drainage patterns, as well as lymphaticovenous shunts in the case of severe metastatic prostate carcinoma, have been well characterized. The lymphatic network of the prostate is drained by four primary trunks (Fig. 3–11). The external iliac group arises from the superior and upper part of the posterior surface of the prostate and ascends along the medial border of the seminal vesicles, terminating in one of the nodes of the external iliac chain. The hypogastric pedicle arises from

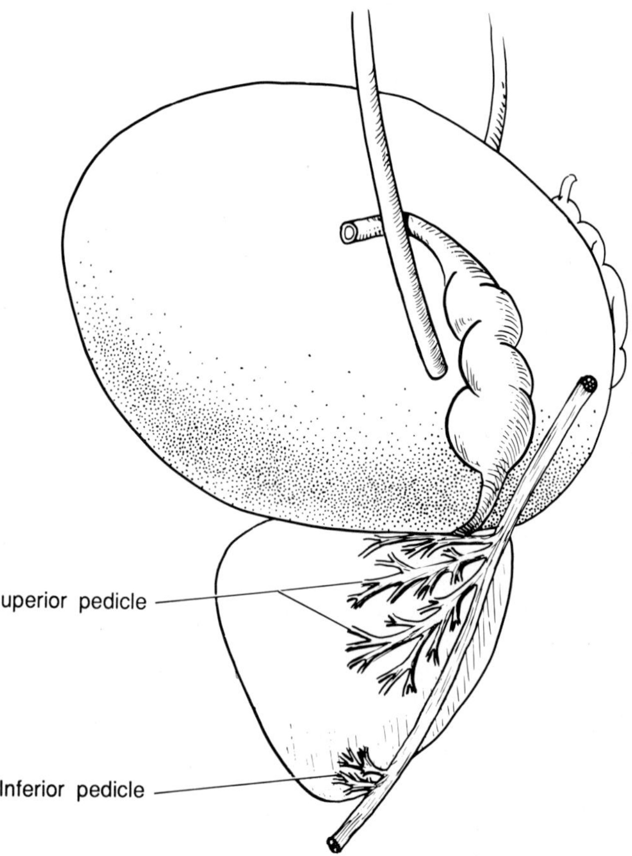

FIGURE 3–10. Prostatic nerves. Posterolateral view of the nerve supply to the prostate. The nerves to the prostate travel posterolaterally outside the prostatic capsule and give off branches to the prostate in association with arterial and venous branches in a so-called neurovascular bundle. It has been suggested that these nerves act as guides for extracapsular tumor extension, particularly at the apex where the nerve branches are short.

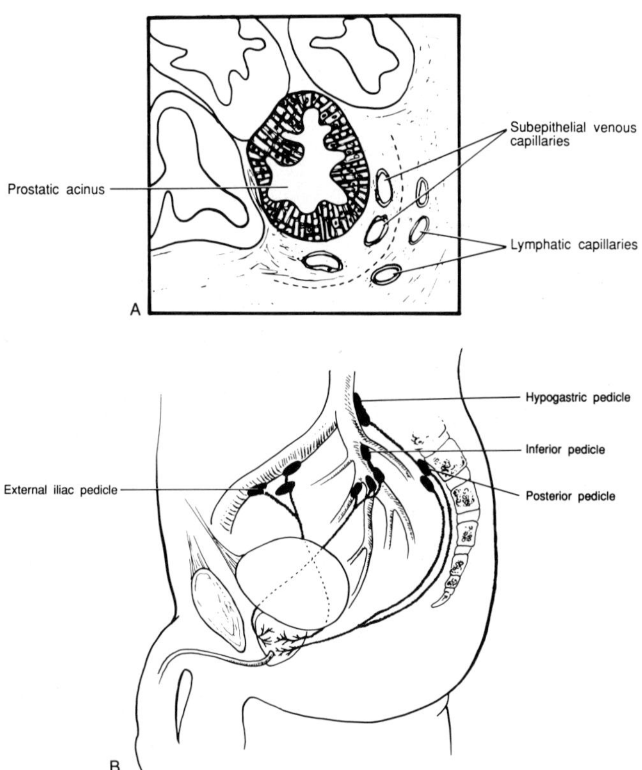

FIGURE 3–11. Prostatic lymphatics. *A,* Histologic subdistribution of prostatic lymphatics. Periacinar spaces exhibit distinct compartmentalization of venous and lymphatic capillaries, with the venous capillaries located closer to the acinus. *B,* Lateral view of lymphatic chains draining the prostate. There are four primary lymphatic chains. The external iliac group arises from the superior and upper part of the posterior surface of the prostate and ascends along the medial border of the seminal vesicles, terminating in one of the nodes of the external iliac chain. The hypogastric pedicle arises from the inferior part of the prostate and ascends onto the posterior surface toward the superior surface of the gland, running along the prostatic artery and terminating in one of the hypogastric nodes. The posterior pedicle arises from the posterior surface of the prostate and courses in the medial aspect of the rectovesical fascia toward the sacrum, terminating in lymph nodes located on the medial side of the second sacral foramen in the region of the sacral promontory. The inferior pedicle is formed by a trunk that descends from the anterior border of the prostate to the floor of the perineum and then follows the internal pudendal artery, terminating in one of the hypogastric nodes near the origin of the internal iliac artery.

the inferior part of the prostate and ascends onto the posterior surface toward the superior surface of the gland, running along the prostatic artery and terminating in one of the hypogastric nodes. The posterior pedicle arises from the posterior surface of the prostate and courses in the medial aspect of the rectovesical fascia toward the sacrum, terminating in lymph nodes located on the medial side of the second sacral foramen in the region of the sacral promontory. The inferior pedicle is formed by a trunk that descends from the anterior border of the prostate to the floor of the perineum and then follows the internal pudendal artery, terminating in one of the hypogastric nodes near the origin of the internal iliac artery.[38]

Two major lymphatic chains drain the prostate: the external group and the internal iliac (hypogastric) group. The external iliac lymphatics consist of three chains: (1) an external (lateral) chain, which runs along the lateral aspect of the external iliac artery; (2) an intermediate (middle) chain, which lies between the external iliac artery and external iliac vein; and (3) an internal (medial) chain, which lies medial to the external iliac vein, superior to the obturator nerve, and dorsal to the external iliac vein. The obturator nodes, which have been described as the "primary echelon" of drainage of the prostate, are anatomically part of the internal group of nodes in the external iliac chain.

The internal iliac or hypogastric lymphatics are located along the distribution of the internal iliac artery and its branches. This group is generally divided into a parietal group of nodes, which drain the musculoskeletal portions of the pelvis, and a visceral group of nodes, which drain the pelvic viscera. Unfortunately, pedal lymphangiography rarely visualizes these nodal clusters. Indeed, the most frequently opacified node of the entire internal iliac group is the lateral sacral node, which is seen in only 50 per cent of normal lymphangiograms.

The three trunks of the external iliac lymphatics communicate extensively with each other at the level of the common iliac artery. Cross communication between left and right common iliac lymphatics, however, occurs in only 50 per cent of cases.[38] The medial lymphatic chain serves as the most important pathway between the pelvic visceral structures and the abdominoaortic region.

The lymphatics of the prostate communicate directly

with those of the bladder, the seminal vesicles, and the rectum. Of the regional lymph nodes, only the external iliac nodes are demonstrated on lymphangiography. Occasionally, hypogastric nodes near the origin of the internal iliac artery may be visualized. Opacification of the sacral promontory node is generally unpredictable.

SUMMARY

Information on the inter-relationship between the vascular, lymphatic, neurologic, fascial, and muscular groups surrounding the prostate guides surgical approach to the prostate. Techniques based on full comprehension of prostatic and periprostatic anatomy maximize the benefit to the patient while minimizing risk. Recent examples of technical innovation based on anatomic principles include the nerve-sparing radical prostatectomy and its subsequent modifications, and an awareness of variability of the prostatic apex and the surrounding sphincteric musculature. Appreciation of anatomic subtleties may be critical to the success or failure of prostatic surgery.

REFERENCES

1. Abeshouse BS, Ruben ME: Prostatic and periprostatic phlebography. J Urol 68:640–646, 1952.
2. Albarran J, Motz B: Contribution a l'etude de l'anatomie macroscopique de la prostate hypertropiee. Ann Mal Org Genitourinaries 20:769–817, 1902.
3. Albers DD, Faulkner KK, Cheatham WN, et al: Surgical anatomy of the pubovesical (puboprostatic) ligaments. J Urol 109:388–392, 1973.
4. Allen KS, Krerssel HY, Arger PH, Pollack HM: Age-related changes of the prostate: Evaluation by MR imaging. AJR 152:77–81, 1989.
5. Andrews GS: The histology of the human foetal and prepubertal prostates. J Anat 85:44–54, 1951.
6. Aumuller G: Zur Gefass-und Muskelarchitektur der menschlichen Prostata. Z Anat Entwickl Gesch 135:88–100, 1971.
7. Aversenq and Dieulafe: Aponevroses et espaces periprostatiques: Suppurations perioprostatiques. Ann Mal Org Genitourinaries 29:1–43, 1911.
8. Ayala AG, Ro JY, Babian R, et al: The prostatic capsule: Does it exist? Its importance in the staging and treatment of prostatic carcinoma. Am J Surg Pathol 13:21–27, 1989.
9. Barnes AR: The pelvic fascia. Anat Rec 22:37–55, 1921.
10. Beneventi FA, Noback GJ: Distribution of the blood vessels of the prostate gland and urinary bladder: Application to retropubic prostatectomy. J Urol 62:663–671, 1949.
11. Benoit G, Boccon-Gibod L, Steg A: Anatomical study of total cystoprostatectomy. Eur Urol 11:228–232, 1985.
12. Boccon-Gibod L, Steg A: Total cystectomy for bladder carcinoma: Denonvillier's fascia as a landmark. Urology 19:386–388, 1982.
13. Bumpus HC, Antonopol W: Distribution of blood to the prostatic urethra. J Urol 32:354–358, 1934.
14. Caine M, Edwards D: The peripheral control of micturition: A cineradiographic study. Br J Urol 30:34–42, 1958.
15. Caminiti: Recherches sur les lymphatiques de la prostate humaine. Ann Mal Org Genitourinaires 2:1441–1460, 1905.
16. Chilton CP: The distal urethral sphincter mechanism and the pelvic floor. In Mundy, AR, Stephenson TD, Wein AJ (eds): Urodynamics: Principles, Practice and Application. Edinburgh, Livingstone, 1984.
17. Clegg EJ: The arterial supply of the human prostate and seminal vesicles. J Anat 89:209–216, 1955.
18. Clegg EJ: The vascular arrangements within the human prostate gland. Br J Urol 28:428–435, 1956.
19. Connolly JG, Thomson A, Jewett MAS, et al: Intraprostatic lymphatics. Invest Urol 5:371–378, 1968.
20. Derry DE: On the real nature of the so-called "pelvic fascia." J Anat Physiol 41:97–106, 1907.
21. Droes JTPM: Observations on the musculature of the urinary bladder and the urethra in the human foetus. Br J Urol 46:179–185, 1974.
22. Duclos JM, Chanzy M, Alexandre JH: Contribution a l'etude de la vasclarisation prostatique. Arch Anat Pathol 20:355–358, 1972.
23. Evatt EJ: A contribution to the development of the prostate in man. J Anat Physiol 43:314–321, 1909.
24. Fenwick EH: The venous system of the bladder and its surroundings. J Anat Physiol 19:320–327, 1885.
25. Fitzpatrick TJ: Venography of the deep dorsal venous and valvular systems. J Urol 111:518–520, 1974.
26. Fitzpatrick RJ, Orr LM: Pelvioprostatic venography: Preliminary report. J Urol 68:647–651, 1952.
27. Flocks RH: The arterial distribution within the prostate gland: Its role in transurethral prostatic resection. J Urol 37:524–548, 1937.
28. Folsom AI, O'Brien HA: The female obstructing prostate. JAMA 121:573–580, 1943.
29. Franks LM: Benign nodular hyperplasia of the prostate: A review. Ann R Coll Surg Eng 14:92–106, 1954.
30. Freyer PJ: A clinical lecture on total extirpation of the prostate for radical cure of enlargement of that organ: With four successful cases. Br Med J 2:125–134, 1901.
31. Fritjofsson A, Kvist U, Ronquist G: Anatomy of the prostate in relation to lobar structure. Scand J Urol Nephrol (Suppl) 107:5–13, 1988.
32. Furusato M, Mostofi FK: Intraprostatic lymphatics in man: Light and ultrastructural observations. Prostate 1:15–23, 1980.
32a. Gittes RF, McCullough DL: Occult carcinoma of the prostate: An oversight of immune surveillance—a working hypothesis. J Urol 112:241, 1974.
33. Goldstein AE, Abeshouse B: Prevesical, perivesical and periprostatic suppurations. Review of literature and report of cases. Surg Gynecol Obstet 49:477–502, 1929.
34. Gosling JA: Autonomic innervation of the prostate. In Hinman F Jr: Benign Prostatic Hypertrophy. New York, Springer-Verlag, 1984.
35. Gosling JA, Dixon JS, Critchley HOD, Thompson SA: A comparative study of the human external sphincter and periurethral levator ani muscles. Br J Urol 53:35–41, 1981.
36. Greene DR, Egawa S, Neerhut G, et al: The distribution of residual cancer in radical prostatectomy specimens in stage A prostate cancer. J Urol 145:324–329, 1991.
37. Hargreave TB, Stephenson TP: Potency and prostatectomy. Br J Urol 49:683–688, 1977.
38. Harrison DA: Normal anatomy. In Clouse DA: Clinical Lymphography. Baltimore, Williams & Wilkins, 1977.
39. Hasui Y, Shinkawa T, Osada Y, Sumiyoshi A: Striated muscle in the biopsy specimen of the prostate. Prostate 14:65–69, 1989.
40. Haugen OA, Harbitz TB: Prostatic weight in elderly men. An analysis in an autopsy series. Acta Pathol Microbiol Scand 80:769–777, 1972.
41. Hayashi T, Taki Y, Hiura M, et al: Simplified technique for management of Santorini plexus and puboprostatic ligaments during radical retropubic prostatectomy. Urology 28:322–323, 1986.
42. Higgins JRA, Gosling JA: Studies on the structure and intrinsic innervation of the normal human prostate. Prostate (Suppl) 2:5–16, 1989.
43. Hirsch EW: A note on the comparative anatomy of the prostate gland. J Urol 25:669–671, 1931.
44. Hubly JW, Thompson GJ: Infarction of the prostate and volumetric changes produced by the lesion. J Urol 43:459–467, 1940.
45. Huggins C, Webster WO: Duality of human prostate in response to estrogen. J Urol 59:258–266, 1948.
46. Hutch JA, Rambo ON: A study of the anatomy of the prostate, prostatic urethra and the urinary sphincter system. J Urol 104:443–452, 1970.

47. Jacobs SC, Beehler BA, Boese G, et al: The prostate of the gorilla. Prostate 5:597–603, 1984.
48. Koslin DB, Kenney PJ, Koehler RE, Van Dyke JA: Magnetic resonance imaging of the internal anatomy of the prostate gland. Invest Radiol 22:947–953, 1987.
49. Krahn HP, Morales PA: The effect of pudendal nerve anesthesia on urinary continence after prostatectomy. J Urol 94:282–285, 1965.
50. Lawson JON: Pelvic anatomy. I. Pelvic floor muscles. Ann R Coll Surg Engl 54:244–252, 1974.
51. Lee F, Siders DB, Torp-Pederson ST, et al: Prostate cancer: Transrectal ultrasound and pathology comparison. A preliminary study of outer gland (peripheral and central zones) and inner gland (transition zone) cancer. Cancer 67:1132–1142, 1991.
52. Leissner KM, Tisell LE: The weight of the dorsal, lateral and medial prostatic lobes in man. Scand J Urol Nephrol 13:223–227, 1979.
53. Libman E, Fichten CS: Prostatectomy and sexual function. Urology 29:467–478, 1987.
54. Lowsley OS: The development of the human prostate gland with reference to the development of other structures at the neck of the urinary bladder. Am J Anat 13:299–349, 1912.
55. Lowsley OS: The gross anatomy of the human prostate gland and contiguous structures. Surg Gynecol Obstet 20:183–192, 1915.
56. Lue TF, Zeineh SJ, Schmidt RA, Tanagho EA: Neuroanatomy of penile erection: Its relevance to iatrogenic impotence. J Urol 131:273–280, 1984.
57. Manley CB: The striated muscle of the prostate. J Urol 95:234–240, 1966.
58. McNeal JE: Origin and evolution of benign prostatic enlargement. Invest Urol 15:340–345, 1978.
59. McNeal JE: The prostate and prostatic urethra: A morphologic synthesis. J Urol 107:1008–1016, 1972.
60. McNeal JE: Relationship of the origin of benign prostatic hypertrophy to prostatic structure of man and other mammals. *In* Hinman F Jr: Benign Prostatic Hypertrophy. New York, Springer-Verlag, 1984.
61. McNeal JE, Redwine EA, Freiha FS, Stamey T: Zonal distribution of prostatic adenocarcinoma. Correlation with histologic pattern and direction of spread. Am J Surg Pathol 12:897–906, 1988.
62. McNeal JE, Villers AA, Redwine EA, et al: Capsular penetration in prostate cancer. Significance for natural history and treatment. Am J Surg Pathol 14:240–247, 1990.
63. Moore RA: The evolution and involution of the prostate gland. Am J Pathol 12:599–624, 1936.
64. Moore RA: The histology of the newborn and prepubertal prostate gland. Anat Rec 66:1–9, 1936.
65. Moore RA: Benign hypertrophy of the prostate: A morphological study. J Urol 50:680–710, 1943.
66. Motz B, Perearneau: Contribution a l'etude de l'evolution de l'hypertrophie de la prostate. Ann Mal Org Genitourinaires 23:1521–1548, 1905.
67. Myers RP: Anatomical variation of the superficial preprostatic veins with respect to radical retropubic prostatectomy. J Urol 145:992–993, 1991.
68. Myers RP, Goellner JR, Cahill DR: Prostate shape, external striated urethral sphincter and radical prostatectomy: The apical dissection. J Urol 138:543–550, 1987.
69. Oelrich TM: The urethral sphincter muscle in the male. Am J Anat 158:229–246, 1980.
70. Page BH: The pathological anatomy of digital enucleation for benign prostatic hyperplasia and its application to endoscopic resection. Br J Urol 52:111–126, 1980.
71. Price D: Comparative aspects of development and structure in the prostate. NCI Monographs #12, 1963, pp 1–27.
72. Quinlan DM, Epstein JI, Carter BS, Walsh PC: Sexual function following radical prostatectomy: Influence of preservation of neurovascular bundles. J Urol 145:998–1002, 1991.
73. Raghavaiah NV, Jordan WP: Prostatic lymphography. J Urol 121:178–181, 1979.
74. Reese JH, McNeal JE, Redwine EA, et al: Differential distribution of pepsinogen II between the zones of the human prostate and the seminal vesicle. J Urol 136:1148–1152, 1986.
75. Reiner WG, Walsh PC: An anatomical approach to the surgical management of the dorsal vein and Santorini's plexus during radical retropubic prostatectomy. J Urol 121:198–200, 1979.
76. Rouviere H: Anatomy of the Human Lymphatic System. Translated by M J Tobias. Ann Arbor, Edwards Brothers, 1938.
77. Scardino PT, Greene D, Taylor S, Wheeler T: DNA ploidy of separate foci prostate cancer. Presented at the 105th meeting of the American Association of Genitourinary Surgeons, Naples, Florida, 1991.
78. Semple JE: Surgical capsule of the benign enlargement of the prostate: Its development and origin. Br Med J 6:1640–1643, 1963.
79. Shehata R: Female prostate and urethral glands in the home rat, *Rattus norvegicus*. Acta Anat 107:286–288, 1980.
80. Shridhar P: The lymphatics of the prostate gland and their role in the spread of prostatic carcinoma. Ann R Col Surg Engl 61:114–122, 1979.
81. Smith MJV: The lymphatics of the prostate. Invest Urol 3:439–444, 1966.
82. Stamey TA, Villers AA, McNeal JE, et al: Positive surgical margins at radical prostatectomy: Importance of the apical dissection. J Urol 143:1166–1173, 1990.
83. Swyer GIM: Post-natal growth changes in the human prostate. J Anat 78:130–145, 1944.
84. Tepper S, Jagirdar J, Heath D, Geller SA: Homology between the female paraurethral (Skene's) glands and the prostate. Arch Pathol Lab Med 108:423–425, 1984.
85. Tobin CE, Benjamin JA: Anatomical and surgical restudy of Denonvillier's fascia. Surg Gynecol Obstet 80:373–388, 1945.
86. Udeh FN: Structure and architecture of the prostatic capsule. Int Urol Nephrol 14:35–43, 1982.
87. Villers A, McNeal JE, Redwine EA, et al: The role of perineural space invasion in the local spread of prostatic adenocarcinoma. J Urol 142:763–768, 1989.
88. Wallace CS: An anatomical criticism of the procedure known as total prostatectomy. Br Med J 6:239–245, 1904.
89. Wallace CS: Total prostatectomy: Deductions to be drawn from the presence of striated muscle fibre in the "capsule" of the parts removed. Br Med J 6:1187, 1904.
90. Walsh PC: Racial prostatectomy with preservation of sexual function: Evolution of a surgical procedure. AUA Update Series V, Lesson 5, 1986.
91. Walsh PC, Quinlan DM, Morton RA, Steiner MS: Radical retropubic prostatectomy. Improved anastomosis and urinary continence. Urol Clin North Am 17:679–684, 1990.
92. Wesson MB: Fasciae of the urogenital triangle. JAMA 81:2024–2030, 1923.
93. Whitaker RH: The fate of the prostatic cavity after retropubic prostatectomy. Br J Urol 43:722–727, 1971.
94. Windle R, Roberts JBM: Ejaculatory function after prostatectomy. Proc R Soc Med 67:46–48, 1974.
95. Wilson PA: Anchoring mechanisms of the ano-rectal region. S Afr Med J 41:1127–1132, 1138–1143, 1967.
96. Young HH, Davis DM: Young's Practice of Urology. Based on the Study of 12,500 Cases. Philadelphia, WB Saunders, 1926.
97. Zaviacic M: The adult human female prostate homologue and the male prostate gland: A comparative enzyme-histochemical study. Acta Histochem 77:19–31, 1985.

Chapter 4

THE MOLECULAR BIOLOGY OF THE PROSTATE

DONALD S. COFFEY

THE MEDICAL IMPORTANCE OF THE PROSTATE AND SEMINAL VESICLES

The immense medical problems caused by the prostate gland are increasing at a most alarming rate,[34] and their full magnitude and impact have only recently been established.[163] Much of the physiology, biochemistry, and molecular biology of the prostate remains to be elucidated, and yet new understanding of basic anatomy[215] has already led to important surgical considerations. The identification of prostate-specific antigen (PSA)[217] and its presence in the sera of prostatic cancer patients[121, 122, 171] has proved to be a most useful marker for clinical monitoring.[36, 116, 121, 196] The contributions of these basic research findings to clinical applications and to approaches to the study of the prostate gland have been reviewed and debated in detail at excellent international meetings and are available in book form.[35, 51]

Aberrations in growth and infections in the human prostate gland produce some of the most common, costly, and devastating diseases that occur in the male. In total, the annual treatment of prostate diseases in the United States requires 4.4 million physician visits and 836,000 hospitalizations, with 39,215 deaths, and costs over $3 billion (Table 4–1). For example, abnormal overgrowth of the human prostate resulting in benign prostatic hyperplasia (BPH) occurs in almost 80 per cent of men by the age of 80, and 25 per cent require surgery at some time in their lives to alleviate urinary obstruction caused by this overgrowth. To correct this obstruction, more than 400,000 surgical procedures are required each year in the United States, making BPH the second most common cause of surgery in the male.

Clinical prostatic cancer develops in one in every 11 white males and one in every 10 black males in the United States during their lifetimes, and it has now become the most commonly diagnosed cancer in men, even exceeding lung cancer. Prostate cancer is often associated with a long protracted course and is the second leading cause of cancer deaths in men in the United States. At present, more than 100,000 new cases are diagnosed and more than 36,000 deaths occur each year, and the mortality rate has been increasing steadily over the last three decades and will continue to do so as our population ages.[34] This is only the tip of the iceberg; an alarming 10 to 30 per cent of all men over 50 years of age harbor silent evidence of a microscopic form of the cancer, assumed to be latent prostate cancer cells that reside asymptomatically within their glands. It is calculated that more than 11 million of these latent forms of cancer currently exist within the male population in the United States, and it appears that the vast majority of cancers may grow very slowly or remain smoldering and silent, therefore never manifesting themselves clinically within the lifetime of the patient.

What causes this tremendous prevalence of latent prostate cancer, and why does most of it remain dormant? What molecular events are required to activate progression to a more malignant form? Why, in comparison, is there so little prostate cancer clinically manifested in Asian men but almost the same amount of latent or dormant forms? Why does the rate of clinical prostate cancer in Japanese men increase dramatically when they migrate to the United States? These questions

This chapter is adapted from Walsh PC, Retik AB, Stamey TA, Vaughan ED Jr (eds.): Campbell's Urology, 6th ed. Philadelphia, WB Saunders Company, 1992, pp 221–266.

TABLE 4–1. IMPACT OF PROSTATE DISEASES IN THE UNITED STATES*

| | ANNUAL RATES | | | COST IN BILLIONS |
PROSTATE DISEASE	Physician Visits	Hospitalizations	Mortality	(DOLLARS)
Benign prostatic hyperplasia	1,709,053	482,349	2,339	$1.82
Prostate cancer	887,341	246,201	36,204	$0.97
Prostatitis	1,850,593	108,024	672	$0.29
Total	4,446,987	836,573	39,215	$3.08

*Calculated by the National Kidney and Urological Diseases Advisory Board, 1990, from data for 1985.
From Coffey DS: The molecular biology, endocrinology, and physiology of the prostate and seminal vesicles. *In* Walsh PC, Retik AB, Stamey TA, Vaughan ED Jr (eds): Campbell's Urology, 6th ed. Philadelphia, WB Saunders, 1992, p 222.

are critical to answer because of the threat that environmental changes may be activating more of these cancers, causing the continuing increase in their incidence. Reviews of epidemiologic factors predisposing to prostate cancer yield scant firm evidence but do point to the tremendous opportunities to resolve these issues.[33]

Surprisingly, all of these abnormalities of prostate growth, including BPH and prostate cancer, are common only to humans and dogs. It is still a mystery why all of the many other species, such as bulls, horses, cats, and rodents, are essentially free of abnormal growth of the prostate, because these animals do share much of our environment. In fact, it is not understood why in humans the prostate gland is the only common site within the sex accessory tissues for these diseases. For example, the seminal vesicles are spared and are almost devoid of any significant incidence of abnormal growth, such as benign or malignant hyperplasia. On first examination, it appears that because of proximity, both the prostate and seminal vesicles might receive essentially the same endogenous blood-borne hormones and might be subjected to the same pathologic insults by carcinogens and pathogens. Some believe that the difference in disease in the two glands may be due to differences in the embryonic origins, the prostate arising from the urogenital sinus and the seminal vesicles from the wolffian ducts. Whether the marked difference between the pathology of the prostate and seminal vesicles resides in intrinsic factors within the gland or in extrinsic environmental or pathologic factors must obviously await further study and understanding.

INFECTIONS AND THE ROLE OF SEX ACCESSORY TISSUES IN THE TRANSMISSION OF ACQUIRED IMMUNODEFICIENCY SYNDROME (AIDS)

Of great current importance is the mechanism of transport of pathogens such as the human immunodeficiency virus (HIV-1) into human semen. The ejaculate is one of the major routes of sexual transmission of these important viruses in the pathogenesis of AIDS, and yet we have little knowledge of exactly how or where the viruses enter the semen, whether in free virus form[27] or carried within cells that appear in the ejaculate.[5–7] If the virus enters the semen distally from the testes or epididymides, vasectomy would stop transmission of AIDS through the ejaculate.[70] The prostate is one of the leading organs in the male for other types of infections and inflammatory processes producing both acute and chronic bacterial prostatitis and the more common nonbacterial prostatitis that is of unknown origin. The influx of lymphocytes and inflammatory cells within the prostate and their presence in semen are still a mystery because these cells can be present in both normal heterosexual males (Table 4–2) and apparently asymptomatic homosexual men who are either HIV serum positive or serum negative.[6] Because these lymphocytes and inflammatory cells in the ejaculate can carry HIV as a major route of sexual transmission of AIDS in heterosexuals and homosexuals, it is obviously of great medical and social importance to understand these mechanisms and the role that the prostate and seminal vesicles play in pathogen transmission.[222]

THE BIOLOGIC IMPORTANCE OF THE SEX ACCESSORY TISSUES

At present, we lack firm insight into the specific biologic functions of the sex accessory tissues such as the prostate, seminal vesicles, and bulbourethral glands (Cowper's glands), other than the simple observation that they provide the bulk of the volume of the ejaculate. The rich secretions of these glands constitute most of the volume and chemical composition of the seminal plasma; fluids from other parts of the male reproductive tract, such as the testes and epididymides make up less than 1 per cent of the total semen volume. These sex accessory tissues produce extremely high concentrations of many important and potent biologic substances in seminal plasma, such as prostaglandin (200 µg/ml), spermine (3 mg/ml), fructose (2 mg/ml), citric acid (4 mg/ml), and extremely high concentrations of zinc (150 µg/ml); proteins (40 mg/ml); and specific enzymes such as immunoglobulins, proteases, esterases and phosphatase.

At present, we have only limited knowledge of the physiologic functions of any of these potent secretory products in the seminal plasma, with the exception of some roles in the clotting and lysing processes occurring with seminal plasma that have unknown physiologic functions. Many investigators even question the necessity for these sex accessory secretions in the fertilization process, because in some mammals it has been observed that spermatozoa removed from the epididymis are capable of fertilizing the ovum; therefore, the sperm are

TABLE 4–2. COMPARISON OF WHITE BLOOD CELLS (WBCs) IN SEMEN OF HETEROSEXUALS AND HOMOSEXUALS (MEDIAN VALUE/ml)

| | HETEROSEXUAL CONTROLS | HOMOSEXUALS | | |
	N = 17	N = 20	N = 12	N = 7
Human immunodeficiency virus (HIV) serum	—	—	+	+
Acquired immunodeficiency syndrome (AIDS) symptomatic	—	—	–	+
Total WBC count	48,751	163,800	431,620	1,067,000
Macrophages	14,828	32,535	65,427	101,000
CD4⁻ lymphocytes	1,182	684	2,450	14,000
CD8⁻ lymphocytes	640	2,012	10,500	50,000

Adapted from Anderson DJ, Wolff H, Pudney J, et al: Presence of HIV in semen. *In* Alexander NJ, Gabelnick HL, Spiler JM (eds): Heterosexual Transmission of AIDS. New York, Alan R. Liss, 1990, pp 167–180. Copyright © 1990. By permission of John Wiley & Sons, Inc.

N = Number of subjects studied.

capable of fertilization without ever having made contact with the secretions of the prostate or seminal vesicles. In addition, the surgical removal of some lobes of the rodent prostate or seminal vesicles (but not both) does not abolish male fertility, and these surgical ablations have been studied on uterine sperm motility.[174] Although the seminal plasma may not contain factors that are absolutely essential for fertilization, the secretions nevertheless may optimize conditions for fertilization by providing a buffer effect or by increasing sperm motility and survival and enhancing transport in both the male and female reproductive tracts. It is suggested that the high concentrations of sugars, such as fructose, and lipids in the seminal plasma provide nutrients or beneficial substrates to the sperm. The seminal plasma, therefore, may extend viability and decrease environmental shock to the sperm. The role of the sex accessory secretions in male infertility has long been suspected, but no single factor has been clearly implicated.[173]

It remains to be resolved what biologic materials, drugs, and biohazards can be transported from the serum into the seminal plasma. Our knowledge of the mechanisms and types of transport of ions, drugs, and natural products in and out of the secretions of the sex accessory tissues is very sparse. In animal studies, it was shown that seven of eight carcinogens tested could be sequestered by transport into prostatic fluid and could reside in the lumen and thus might potentially induce epithelial neoplasias.[193]

The prostate may itself serve with other sex accessory tissues in forming secretions that may protect the lower urinary tract and reproductive system from the insults of pathogens that may invade via the urethra. These sex accessory glands are well positioned to block or intercept the entrance of pathogens by secreting potent biologic substances into the urethra, such as metal ions like zinc or spermine and proteases like lysozymes, as well as secretory immunoglobulins. The mechanical washing of the urethra by these secretions, as well as the establishment of a hostile milieu to invading pathogens, may be one of the primary functions of the sex accessory tissues and may account for their large variability in structure and composition between species. Of all the organs in evolution, the sex accessory organs vary the most; for example, the seminal vesicles are large in the human, European rabbit, rat, and hamster but are absent from the dog, cat, cottontail rabbit, bear, and aquatic mammals. Is this evolutionary selection of a wide range of sex accessory tissue structure and function between species required because of variations in environmental factors or pathogens, or have they been selected for roles in reproductive behavior? In some species, the size and function of the sex accessory tissues are seasonally regulated to coincide with periods of rutting and thus may suggest their primary role in reproductive behavior or fertilization.

The purpose of the aforementioned is to draw attention to some of the critical issues and unsolved problems with respect to the importance of the prostate and seminal vesicles. Many important questions need to be resolved for urology, oncology, and reproductive biology because diseases related to the prostate have a profound medical and social impact. This chapter provides the reader with a basic understanding of the molecular biology and physiology that form the basis of our present progress in understanding the prostate and seminal vesicles. New molecular concepts now appearing in the literature are defined and explained with schematics to introduce both the clinician and the urologic researcher to important background material and to supply a reference source. The prostate gland receives the major portion of attention.

For a more in-depth analysis of other basic concepts, several reference books should be consulted.[13, 15, 50, 139] Two definitive treatises on the seminal vesicles are also available.[13, 220]

ORGANIZATION AND CELL BIOLOGY

Embryonic Development

Aumüller[13] has provided a detailed review of the embryology, histology, and endocrinologic aspects of the development of both the prostate and seminal vesicles. These glands are very different with regard to their embryonic origin and the type of steroid that induces their developmental growth. The wolffian ducts develop into the seminal vesicles, epididymis, vas deferens, ampulla, and ejaculatory duct, and the developmental growth of this group of glands is stimulated by fetal testosterone, not dihydrotestosterone (DHT). The growth of these wolffian-derived sex accessory glands is completed primarily by the 13th week. In contrast, the prostate first appears and starts its development from the urogenital sinus during the third month of fetal growth, and development is directed primarily by DHT, which is produced from the metabolic conversion of fetal testosterone through the action of the enzyme 5α-reductase, which is located within the urogenital sinus. Five epithelial buds form in a paired manner on the posterior side of the urogenital sinus on both sides of the verumontanum, and they then invade the mesenchyme to form the prostate. The top pairs of buds form the inner zone of the prostate and appear to be of mesoderm origin; the lower buds form the outer zone of the prostate and appear to be of endoderm origin. This is of potential importance because the inner zone gives tissue of BPH origin, whereas the outer zone contains the primary origin of cancer. These two zones of the prostate develop as concentric circles around the urethra. The long branched ducts on the outside form the thick outer layer of the true prostate gland. The center portion contains the mucosal and submucosal glands and the ejaculatory ducts as well as the small remnant of the müllerian duct, the utriculum prostaticus, which forms the small prostatic utricle. The prostate is well differentiated by the fourth month.

There have been many debates and divergent views on the development of the zones of the prostate. These have been described in detail by McNeal[147a] and in an in-depth historical review by Aumüller.[13] The full embryology of the prostate in relation to its zones still necessitates modern biologic and molecular techniques for a precise definition.

The prostate forms acini and collecting ducts that branch into the urethra and may be visualized as similar to a small tree, with the growth occurring primarily on the tips as the ducts extend and branch during development. This clear indication that dynamic growth processes occur along a budding and branching system was developed from studies on the mouse prostate.[201]

During the development of the prostate from the urogenital sinus, a close reciprocal interaction occurs between the stromal and epithelial tissue components. Dihydrotestosterone is produced from testosterone by both the epithelium and the mesenchyme; however, the epithelium appears to make much larger amounts of DHT. In contrast, the stromal cells appear to contain larger amounts of androgen receptor. Cunha and colleagues[57] believed that during development the androgen receptor is exclusive to the mesenchyme. It is visualized that a reciprocal action occurs, in that DHT is formed in the epithelial cells and diffuses to the DHT receptor in the stromal nuclei of the mesenchymal cells, which then produce an unknown inductive factor that drives the morphogenesis of the epithelial cells. This is thought to be accomplished in part by the DHT induction of specific soluble growth factors and alterations in the insoluble extracellular matrix components binding the stromal and epithelial cells. Resolving the exact growth factors in these temporal developmental events is an important research frontier. In the development of other organs, it is apparent that growth factors are multifunctional and can be either stimulators or inhibitors of growth, depending upon their dose combinations and sequence of presentation to target cells. For example, the interaction and combination of epidermal growth factor with transforming growth factor-β (TGF-β) and insulin-like growth factor (IGF) as well as gonadotropins have been shown to affect the differentiation of other types of reproductive cells, and it is expected that similar roles will soon be elucidated for prostate cells.[22] Growth factors are discussed later in this chapter, but it is important to note that the müllerian-inhibiting substance (MIS), which is expressed early in gonadal differentiation of the male, causes the regression of the müllerian duct as a prerequisite for virilization in the male.[109] The requirement for MIS in human male development is well established; the human gene has been isolated, the primary amino acid sequence of MIS has been determined, and it now appears that it is closely related to a family of proteins that include TGF-β, which is a very potent inhibitor of growth and function of a wide variety of cell types.

The temporal events involved in the development of the male reproductive tract and the involvement of both steroids and growth hormones are of fundamental importance in developmental biology but also may be of great interest to pathology of the prostate. It has been proposed by McNeal[147] that BPH may be caused by an embryonic reawakening of dormant embryonic growth potential of the adult stroma and that the proliferation of the stromal elements in the periurethral region of the human prostate can stimulate the ingrowth of epithelial cells to produce a benign growth. Animal models have been made by constructing "sandwiches" of chimeric tissue implants composed of embryonic urogenital mesenchyme and adult prostate tissues, and it does appear that in these models the fetal mesenchyme can drive both the differentiation and growth of adult urogenital cells.[43–46, 48, 57, 58, 206]

Postnatal Development and Hormone Imprinting of Growth

At birth, the majority of the acini are lined with squamous epithelium metaplasia and scattered secretory activity and cyst formation.[11, 13] This stimulation is believed to be under the control of residual maternal steroids such as estrogens, and there is a postnatal involution phase that occurs over the first 5 months following birth.

Large transient surges of serum levels of androgen, estrogen, and progesterone normally occur very early in life both in rats and in humans. In the human male neonate, a surge in testosterone is observed that peaks between 2 and 3 months of age; during this period, blood testosterone levels rise to 60 times that of normal prepubertal levels and reach the adult range of about 400 ng/dl.[80, 170] Serum estradiol levels are very high at birth in both humans and rats but fall to very low levels in the first few days after birth; there is a subsequent transient surge prepubertally in the rat but not in the human. Progesterone levels are high at birth in humans and are believed to be from placental progesterone production. A second transient progesterone surge occurs in humans at approximately 2 months of age.[80]

Studies in the rat have shown that neonatal and prepubertal steroids are of critical importance in setting the long-term growth regulation of the prostate; this can occur later in life when the organ is subjected to testosterone stimulation.[29, 47, 117, 157, 161, 162, 177, 178, 202] The ability of neonatal and prepubertal steroids to imprint the prostate has been established as a critical factor in these animal studies but has not been determined for the human prostate.

It is important to note that there are critical differences in the postnatal development of the male reproductive tract between human and rodents, but the correlation of these prepubertal surges in both the rat and human to steroid blood levels might indicate that similar imprinting can be expected in the human. Naslund and Coffey[161, 162] proposed that neonatal imprinting may be an important factor in setting the response of the prostate in later adult life and may have implications for BPH. Higgins and co-authors[94] have shown that differentiation of the rat prostate, as determined by DNA methylation of specific genes in the seminal vesicles and ventral prostate, is determined by similar types of imprinting phenomena, and this may provide the molecular mechanism for these effects.

Structure of the Prostate

Prostate Cell Types

EPITHELIAL CELLS

A summary of the tissue elements and organization of the prostate is listed in Table 4–3. The prostatic epithelium in the human is composed of three major cell types: secretory epithelial cells, basal cells, and neuroendocrine cells. In most glands with cell-renewing populations, there is a steady-state flow of cells from reserve quiescent stem cells to a more rapidly dividing transient proliferating population that finally proceeds to the formation of the fully mature nondividing terminally differentiated secretory cells, which are then programmed to senesce and die off. It is still unclear how this generalized scheme functions in the normal and hyperplastic prostate.[103]

In the prostate, the most common tall (10 to 12 μm) columnar secretory epithelial cells are terminally differentiated and are easily distinguished by their morphologic structure and abundant secretory granules and enzymes that stain abundantly with PSA, acid phosphatase, and other enzymes such as leucine amino peptidase. These tall columnar secretory cells appear like rows of a picket fence resting next to each other, connected by cell adhesion molecules and with their base attached to a basement membrane through integrin

TABLE 4–3. SUMMARY OF THE ANATOMY AND CELL BIOLOGY OF THE PROSTATE GLAND

COMPOUNDS	PROPERTIES
Development	
Seminal vesicles	From wolffian ducts via testosterone stimulation
Prostate	From urogenital sinus via DHT stimulation
Prostate Zones	
Anterior fibromuscular	30% of prostate mass, no glandular elements, smooth muscle
Peripheral	Largest zone, 75% of prostate glandular elements, site of carcinomas
Central	25% of prostate glandular elements, surrounds ejaculatory ducts, may be of wolffian duct origin, seminal vesicle–like
Preprostatic	Smallest, surround upper urethra, complex, sphincter
Transition	5% of prostate glandular elements, site of BPH
Epithelial Cells	
Basal	Small undifferentiated, keratin-rich (type 4, 5, 6) pluripotent cells, less than 10% of epithelial cell number
Transient proliferating	Incorporate thymidine
Columnar secretory	Terminal differentiated, nondividing, rich in acid phosphatase and PSA; 20 μ tall, most abundant cell, keratin types 8, 18, 19
Neuroendocrine	Serotonin-rich, APUD type
Stroma Cells	
Smooth muscle	Actin-rich
Fibroblast	Vimentin-rich and associated with fibronectin
Endothelial	Associated with fibronectin, alkaline phosphatase–positive
Tissue Matrix	
Extracellular	
Basement membrane	Type IV collagen meshwork, laminin-rich, fibronectin
Connective tissue	Type I and Type III fibrillar collagen, elastin
Glycosaminoglycans	Sulfates of dermatan, chondroitin, and heparan; hyaluronic acid
Cytomatrix	Tubulin, actin, and intermediate filaments of keratin
Nuclear matrix	DNA tight-binding proteins, RNA, and residual nuclear proteins

Abbreviations: APUD = amine precursor uptake decarboxylase cell; DHT = dihydrotestosterone; BPH = benign prostatic hyperplasia; PSA = prostate-specific antigen.

From Coffey DS: The molecular biology, endocrinology, and physiology of the prostate and seminal vesicles. *In* Walsh PC, Retik AB, Stamey TA, Vaughan ED Jr (eds): Campbell's Urology, 6th ed. Philadelphia, WB Saunders, 1992, p 227.

receptors. The nucleus is at the base just below a clear zone (2 to 8 μm) of abundant Golgi apparatus, and the upper cellular periphery is rich in secretory granules and enzymes. The apical plasma membrane facing the lumen possesses microvilli, and secretions move out into the open collecting spaces of the acinus. These epithelial cells ring the periphery of the acinus and produce secretions into the acini which drain into the ducts that connect to the urethra.

In androgen ablation, the typical secretory cells decrease by 90 per cent in total numbers, become cuboidal, and shrink by 80 per cent in cell volume and 60 per cent in cell height.[64] Kastendieck[113] suggested more than three types and identified five prostatic epithelial cell types:

Type I, the basal cell
Type II, the immature nonsecretory glandular cell
Type III, the mature secretory glandular cell
Type IV, the nonsecreting predegenerative glandular cell
Type V, the degenerating glandular cell

BASAL AND STEM CELLS

In contrast to secretory epithelial cells, basal cells are much smaller and less abundant in number and are present in less than 10 per cent the number. These small cells are not columnar, are more round with little cytoplasm, and contain large, irregularly shaped nuclei. They are less differentiated and almost devoid of secretory products such as acid phosphatase. These basal cells are always resting on the basement membrane and appear wedged between the bases of adjacent tall columnar epithelial cells. The plasma membrane is rich in ATPase, suggesting that these cells may be involved in active transport. These basal cells are rich in 5-nm tonofilaments and stain brightly with fluorescent antibodies to keratin.[104] It was mistakenly believed that these cells were myoepithelial,[81] but this may not be the case because they are not rich in actin or myosin. It is believed that these undifferentiated basal cells give rise to secretory epithelial cells and as such function as a type of stem cell.[148] Evans and Chandler[79] used pulse chase DNA labeling experiments to challenge the concept of the basal cell as a stem cell for secretory epithelial cells. Basal cell proliferation has been measured in relation to BPH.[65] The importance of understanding the biology of these basal cells is realized because of the growing evidence that many neoplasias, both benign and malignant, really represent stem cell diseases. The stem cell concept of normal and abnormal growth has been reviewed by Isaacs and Coffey.[103]

The proper identification in the prostate of stem cells and the transient proliferating cells has not been realized. Indeed, there may be several types of stem cells as well as several types of secretory cells. Functional and immunologic markers are needed to answer these questions. Lectins as cell markers have been used to identify some types of basal and secretory cells.[192] Merk and associates[149] have presented evidence that canine prostatic epithelial cells have a pluripotentiality of response and can change their keratin pattern, secretory

granules, and phenotype base on treatment with estrogens and/or androgens.

NEUROENDOCRINE CELLS

Significant populations of neuroendocrine cells also reside among the more abundant secretory epithelium in the normal prostate gland. These cells are found in the epithelium of the acini and in ducts of all parts of the gland as well as in the urothelium of the prostatic urethral mucosa.[1, 2, 61] The distribution, morphologic patterns, and secretory products of these cells have been studied in both normal and BPH tissues.[67, 68] There are three types of prostate neuroendocrine cells, with the major type containing both serotonin and thyroid-stimulating hormone (TSH). The two minor cell types contain calcitonin and somatostatin.[1] Neuroendocrine cells are also termed APUD (amine precursor uptake decarboxylase) cells and bring about their regulatory activity by the secretion of hormonal polypeptides or biogenic amines such as serotonin (5-hydroxytryptamine [5-HT]), which is a common marker for these cells. High-pressure liquid chromatography measurements have shown that normal human prostate tissue contains approximately 1400 ng of serotonin/gram of tissue, and this would certainly emphasize the importance of these cells.[61] It is most probable that these neuroendocrine cells are involved in the regulation of prostatic secretory activity and cell growth. Chung and his co-workers[48] have shown that the rat ventral prostatic growth can be uncoupled from secretory function by transplanting the ventral prostate subcutaneously and that the synthesis of prostatin, a secretory protein, can be restored by a β-agonist treatment using L-isoproterenol, thus suggesting β-adrenergic receptors in the regulation of prostatic epithelial cells.[90] It was also demonstrated that norepinephrine has a direct mitogenic effect on cultured prostatic stromal cells, in that norepinephrine and 5-HT were greatly increased in the prostate of castrated animals and the level of the biogenic amine was regulated reversibly by androgens.[48, 90, 207]

Higgins and Gosling[93] have studied the structure and intrinsic innervation of the normal human prostate and have observed acetylcholine esterase in nerves associated with smooth muscle in both the peripheral and central parts of the prostate. In addition, they have shown that the majority of the acini in the peripheral and central regions possess a rich plexus of autonomic nerves and have found vasoactive intestinal polypeptide (VIP)–positive nerve fibers in relation to the epithelial lining acini in the central and peripheral regions of the gland. They concluded that autonomic innervations of peripheral and central regions of the gland are indistinguishable, and they were unable morphologically to find a distinct transitional zone. In contrast, Reese and co-authors[179] found plasminogen activator as a marker for functional zones within the human prostate gland.

Lepor and Kuhar[133] characterized and studied the location of the muscarinic cholinergic receptor in human prostate tissue and localized it to the epithelial cells; this is consistent with the neuropharmacology of muscarinic cholinergic agonist having a marked effect on increasing prostatic secretion. In addition, the α_1-adrenergic receptor has also been studied in the human prostate. This is of great clinical importance because of the use of selected α_1-adrenergic antagonists to alleviate bladder outlet obstruction secondary to BPH.[132, 134, 135]

The Stroma and Tissue Matrix

The epithelial cells rest upon the basement lamina or membrane, which is about 100 nm thick and surrounds the acini. The basement membrane is not a membrane but a complex structure containing collagen types IV and V, glycosaminoglycans, complex polysaccharides, and glycolipids. It forms an interface with the stromal compartment that consists of a structural extracellular matrix, a ground substance, and a variety of stromal cells, including the fibroblasts, capillary and lymphatic endothelial cells, smooth muscle cells, neuroendocrine cells, and axons.[14, 145] The smooth muscle cells are clustered around the acinar structure and the capsule; they are believed to be involved in the mechanical expression of ejaculate fluid under neural stimulation. These smooth muscle cells change their structure in association with BPH in the plasma reticulum, and Golgi apparatus appear to be enlarged as measured by morphometric techniques.[182] It is hypothesized that under hormonal stimulation the smooth muscle is stimulated, producing collagen, which forms part of the extracellular matrix and enhances epithelial growth by a stromal-epithelial type of interaction (see later discussion).

A tissue matrix system is defined as a biologic scaffolding or residual skeleton structure that organizes and locates cells and their polarity and interactions within the organ.[82] The tissue matrix system forms an interacting three-dimensional framework and is one of the most active areas of modern cell biology; it involves the interaction of the matrix components, including the extracellular matrix, cytoskeleton, and nuclear matrix. The epithelial cell rests upon the basement membrane, which is connected by an extracellular matrix to the stromal cells. Structural phase shifts and communication through these matrix elements may play a central role in controlling prostatic development and function of the prostate and in transmitting structural signals from the cell periphery to the DNA, thus playing a central role in regulating chromatin structure and gene expression.[82]

All mammalian cells are composed of a cytomatrix or cytoskeleton network that is formed from a network of microtubules of 20 nm (tubulins), microfilaments of 6 nm (actins), and intermediate filaments of 10 nm (keratin, desmin, vimentin). *Tubulin* is ubiquitous in all cells as a microtubular structure that appears to anchor many cellular structures and is a critical factor in determining the shape of the cell. The microfilaments are composed primarily of *actin,* one of the major proteins in all cells. Actin has the ability to polymerize and depolymerize, and as such it makes one of the important structural chemomechanical systems when it interacts with myosin within the cell. The *cytomatrix,* composed of these filaments, is involved in a central way with transport of

particles and components within the cell and with cell motility.

Several types of intermediate filaments of the cytomatrix are extremely important because they vary in type and composition with differentiation and appear to define the various cell types within the body. For example, one of the intermediate filaments *(desmin)* is a central component of all muscle cells, whereas the intermediate filament *vimentin* is found in all fibroblasts. The intermediate filaments, made of *keratins,* are universal as major components of the cytomatrix of all epithelial cells. In the fibroblast or muscle cells, there is usually just one type of vimentin and desmin. In the epithelial cells, in contrast, the keratins represent more than 20 different molecular types that vary with the state of cellular differentiation and the types of epithelial cells ranging from stratified squamous to simple epithelial cells. Keratins can change in prostatic epithelial cells with disease or hormone action.[3, 28, 73, 104, 149, 176] Of particular interest is the combination of cytoskeletal studies with steroid receptor and secretory function that have been carried out on the human prostate, comparing the keratin patterns in the epithelium of the prepubertal and pubertal prostate with those found in BPH and prostatic adenocarcinoma.[218]

The cytomatrix *(cytoplasmic skeleton),* just described, terminates in the center of the cell by direct attachment to the nuclear matrix (Fig. 4–1). The prostatic epithelial cell, therefore, has direct structural linkage via the matrix systems from the DNA to the plasma membrane. The cytomatrix then makes direct contact to the basement membrane and extracellular matrix and to the ground substance of the stroma. This entire interlocking tissue scaffolding or superstructure—the *tissue matrix*[82]—may have dynamic properties in ordering biologic processes and the transport of secretion from the sex accessory tissues.

Understanding the biologic components of the tissue matrix system within sex accessory tissues is of paramount importance.[82] The epithelial cell is anchored to the basement membrane or basement lamina by an extracellular matrix protein called *laminin.* The laminin proteins are glycoproteins of the extracellular matrix that mediate attachment of cells to the type IV collagen of the basement membrane. Laminin is produced by epithelial cells, but not by fibroblasts, and is a large molecule with molecular domains that interact with the type IV collagen of the basement membrane and the integrin type of receptors within the cell surface glycocalyx of the epithelial cell. Laminin surrounds the basement membrane of prostate acinar epithelial cells, capillaries, smooth muscle and nerve fibers, but not lymphatics, lymphocytes, or fibroblasts, and the laminin distribution is disrupted in higher-grade prostate neoplasias.[191]

A second type of important prostatic glycoprotein that is involved in cell adherence to the extracellular matrix is *fibronectin,* which also binds to the family of cell integrin type receptors. Fibronectin is secreted primarily by prostatic fibroblasts and forms an adhesive material that makes a binding interface of mesenchymal and epithelial cells to various types of collagen and proteo-

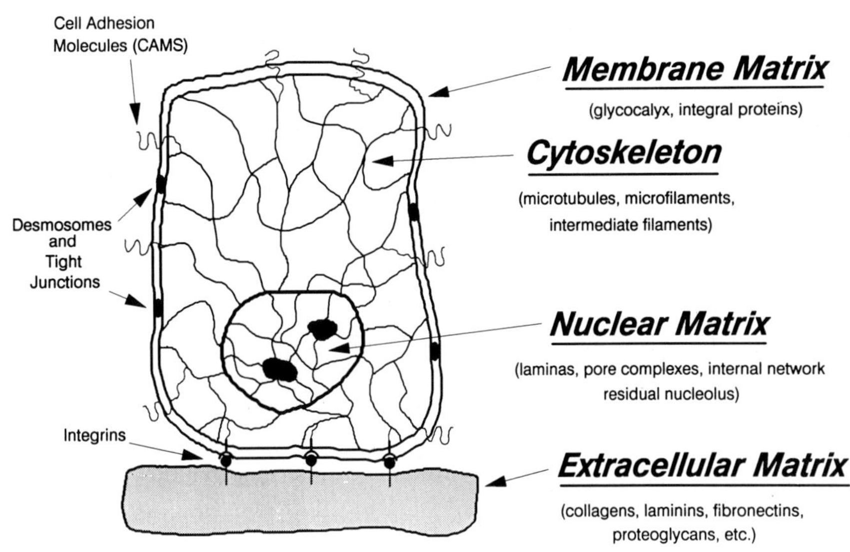

FIGURE 4–1. The tissue matrix system. A superstructure scaffold network connects the extracellular matrix components to the integrin receptors that extend through the plasma membrane and connect directly to the cytomatrix structures. The cytomatrix couples directly to the nuclear matrix, which attaches and organizes the DNA. The cell adhesion molecules (CAMs) and desmosomes connect neighboring cells. (From Getzenberg RH, Pienta KJ, Coffey DS: The tissue matrix: Cell dynamics and hormone action. Endocr Rev 11:399–416, 1990. © The Endocrine Society.)

glycans of the extracellular matrix. There are several types of fibronectin, and it has been proposed that they play a key role in morphogenesis and control of cell growth.

The connective tissue of the prostate is primarily collagen of types I and III, which form the interstitial collagen.[21] Type IV and type V are found primarily in the basement membrane, woven through the stroma and connective tissue of the extracellular matrix in a complex network of glycosaminoglycans (GAGs) and complex polysaccharides. Glycosaminoglycans are large, negatively charged polymers *(polyanions)* that have proved to be critical factors in signaling extracellular matrix events in many different tissues.[92] These latter polysaccharide polymers have long been proposed to play an important role in prostatic growth.[12] DeKlerk[62] isolated and quantitated these important GAGs from the normal and benign human prostates and reported that dermatan sulfate is the predominant (40 per cent) GAG, followed by heparin (20 per cent), chondroitin (16 per cent), and hyaluronic acid (20 per cent). Fetal prostates are devoid of dermatan, and chondroitin sulfate increases with BPH. Chan and Wong[37, 38] studied the histochemical distribution in the guinea pig lateral prostate and identified three types of proteoglycan fibers in different tissue compartments. It will be of interest to determine the role of GAGs in sex accessory tissue function. It has been shown that synthesis of proteoglycans can be regulated in the rat prostate by androgens.[95, 118]

In the near future, one of the most active areas of unraveling the control of sex accessory tissue function will revolve around achieving a clearer understanding of the interactions of these complex tissue matrix components. At present, there have been several important studies[44–46, 57, 58, 62, 208] that all point to the importance of these structural elements. Of particular importance are the studies that have shown the localization of keratins, laminin, fibronectin, and actin within the various cell types of the prostate and other studies[21, 208] on the collagens of the prostate.[145]

REGULATION OF PROSTATIC GROWTH AT THE CELLULAR LEVEL BY HORMONES AND GROWTH FACTORS

It now appears that many levels of cell regulation include hormone action and direct cell-cell communication and growth factors, and these are also at the research forefront of biologic regulation of sex accessory tissue. These types of growth control are usually accomplished by several generalized systems, as depicted in Figure 4–2. They include:

1. *Endocrine factors* or long-range signals arriving at the prostate by serum transport of hormone originating from the secretions of distant organs. This includes serum hormone-like steroids, such as testosterone, estrogens, and serum polypeptide hormones like prolactin, and insulin, as discussed above.

2. *Neuroendocrine signals* originating from neural stimulation such as 5-HT, acetylcholine, and norepinephrine.

3. *Paracrine factors* or soluble tissue growth factors that stimulate or inhibit (chalones) growth and are elaborated over short ranges between neighboring cells within the prostate tissue compartment (e.g., b-fibroblast growth factor, epidermal growth factor).

4. *Autocrine factors*, soluble growth factors that are released by a cell and then feed back on the same cell to regulate growth or function such as autocrine motility factor.

5. *Intracrine factors*, autocrine factors that are not released but work inside the cell.

6. *Extracellular matrix factors*, insoluble tissue matrix systems; these make direct and coupled contact by being attached through integrins and adhesion molecules to the basal membrane and the extracellular matrix components, including the glycosaminoglycans (e.g., heparan sulfate).[82]

7. *Cell-cell interactions* of the epithelial or stromal cells occurring through tight membrane junctions on

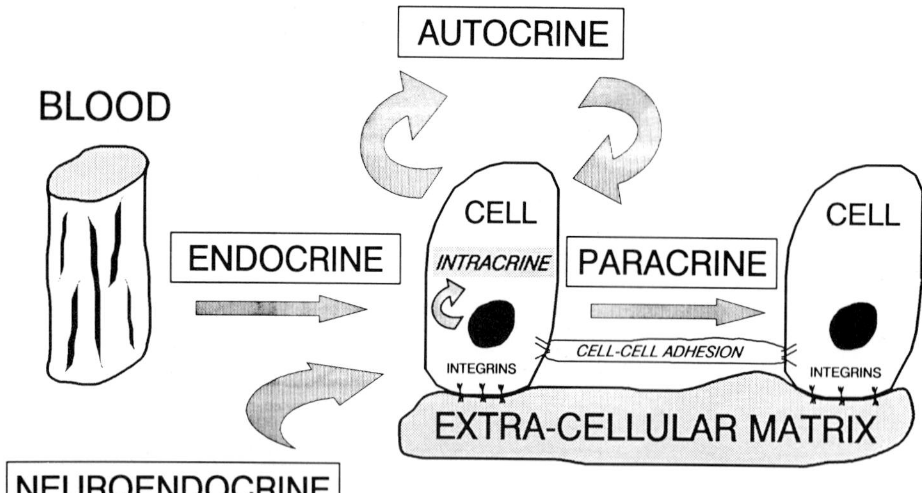

FIGURE 4–2. Types of growth control. Endocrine signals are carried through the circulation from distant organs. Paracrine signals are produced in close proximity by neighboring cells. Autocrine signals feed back on the cells from which they are produced by being secreted or by working internally as intracrine factors. Cell adhesion molecules directly link neighboring cells that are bound through integrin receptors to the extracellular matrix. (From Coffey DS: The molecular biology, endocrinology, and physiology of the prostate and seminal vesicles. *In* Walsh PC, Retik AB, Stamey TA, Vaughan ED Jr [eds]: Campbell's Urology, 6th ed. Philadelphia, WB Saunders, 1992, p 236.)

intramembrane proteins, such as the cell adhesion molecules (CAMs), like *uvomorulin,* that couple neighboring cells.

Of these seven growth control systems, the first studied on the prostate was the endocrine effect of androgenic steroid in the regulation of prostatic growth via changes in serum testosterone levels and steroid receptor interactions. However, rapid progress has recently been made in the understanding of the other systems, particularly the growth factors. At present, structural elements in cellular control involving the tissue matrix are being

developed. These mechanisms, starting with androgen action at the prostate cell level beginning with the arrival of testosterone, are now reviewed.

Androgen Action at the Cellular Level

Testosterone in the serum arrives at the prostate bound to albumin and to the steroid-binding globulins, as depicted in Figure 4–3. Only the free testosterone enters the prostate cell by diffusion, where it is then subjected to a variety of steroid metabolic steps that

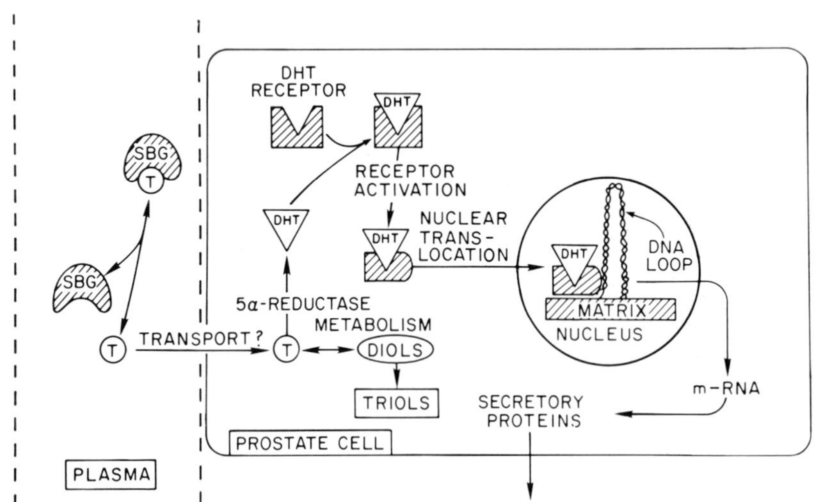

FIGURE 4–3. Schematic diagram depicting the effects of testosterone in inducing growth in an epithelial cell. In the plasma, testosterone is bound to serum-binding globulins (SBGs), such as testosterone-binding globulin and albumin. Unbound testosterone is transported by diffusion into the prostate, where it is enzymatically converted to dihydrotestosterone (DHT) through the action of 5α-reductase and further metabolized to diols (3α or 3β) and irreversibly metabolized into the inactive triols (6α or 7α). Dihydrotestosterone binds to a cytoplasmic receptor (which may actually be nuclear; see text), which is then activated and translocated to the nucleus. There, the DHT receptors interact with the acceptors on the nuclear matrix and with DNA. This nuclear binding of the receptor brings about a stimulation of expression of specific gene messenger RNA synthesis that is translated at the ribosomes in the cytoplasm to form secretory proteins. (From Coffey DS: The molecular biology, endocrinology, and physiology of the prostate and seminal vesicles. *In* Walsh PC, Retik AB, Stamey TA, Vaughan ED Jr [eds]: Campbell's Urology, 6th ed. Philadelphia, WB Saunders, 1992, p 237.)

appear to regulate the activity and, finally, the inactivation of the steroid hormone. The temporal sequence of intracellular events (Figs. 4–3 and 4–4) is as follows:

1. Cellular uptake of testosterone occurs.

2. Testosterone is converted to DHT by metabolism of 5α-reductase.

3. DHT or testosterone is bound to specific androgen receptors in the nucleus.

4. Activation of the steroid receptor occurs in the nucleus by conformational change and phosphorylation, the binding of the receptor to androgen-receptor elements (AREs) that are short specific sequences of DNA, and the binding of the receptor to tissue-specific proteins of the nuclear matrix.

5. Receptor-induced changes in DNA loop topology and chromatin structure take place.

6. The receptor acts as a transcription factor; when bound to the DNA and matrix in proximity to androgen target genes, it increases the RNA polymerase transcription of the DNA into messenger RNA (mRNA).

7. The transcribed message (mRNA) is very large and contains introns, exons, and a poly(A) tail section. The intron portion is removed, and only the exon portion is retained in the final message. The trimming and processing of the mRNA are accomplished on the nuclear matrix as it is transported through the nucleus and out through the nuclear pore complex.

8. The stabilized mRNA is transported into the cytoplasmic compartment to be translated at the ribosome into protein.

9. The proteins are transported to specific cellular sites, and the subsequent post-translational modification occurs.

10. The protein stored in secretory granules is poised for secretion into the lumen on neurologic command during the process of ejaculation.

The epithelial cell is the primary unit in secretion, but specific genes are also activated in the stromal cells. These events are also regulated by testosterone, estrogens, and growth factors in a similar chain of events, as just discussed. Not all cells respond the same to androgens or estrogens. For simplicity, these steps are discussed in relation to the epithelial cells because differences between the cell types are important but have not yet been resolved. Androgens and estrogens, both together and separately, can affect prostate cells through the interaction with receptors, and estrogens may have their primary effect on the stromal cells. These aforementioned events in androgen action within the prostate are now presented in more detail and are described at the molecular level.

5α-Reductase and Androgen Metabolism Within the Prostate

After the free testosterone in the plasma has entered the prostatic cells through diffusion, it is rapidly metabolized to other steroids by a series of prostatic enzymes.[31, 99–102] More than 90 per cent of the testosterone is *irreversibly* converted to the main prostatic androgen, DHT (Fig. 4–5), through the action of nicotinamide-adenine dinucleotide phosphate (NADPH) and the enzyme 5α-reductase (EC 1.3.99.5) located on the endoplasmic reticulum and on the nuclear membrane. The enzyme 5α-reductase reduces the unsaturated bond in testosterone between the 4 and 5 positions to form the 5α-reduced product DHT. The Michaelis constant (K_m) for testosterone is 8.3 nM, and the serum level of testosterone is only in the range of 0.5 to 3.0 nM, indicating that the enzyme cannot be saturated because the testosterone substrate would be less than the K_m value.[31] 5α-Reductase can also convert androstenedione or progesterone to the 5α-reduced form.

Bruchovsky and Dunstan-Adams[31] reported a 10-fold

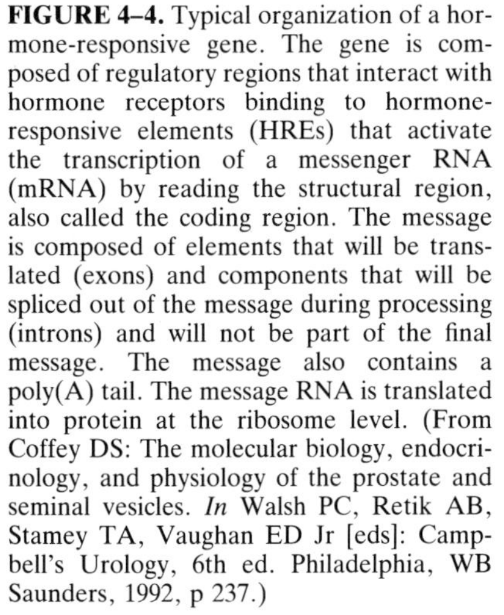

FIGURE 4–4. Typical organization of a hormone-responsive gene. The gene is composed of regulatory regions that interact with hormone receptors binding to hormone-responsive elements (HREs) that activate the transcription of a messenger RNA (mRNA) by reading the structural region, also called the coding region. The message is composed of elements that will be translated (exons) and components that will be spliced out of the message during processing (introns) and will not be part of the final message. The message also contains a poly(A) tail. The message RNA is translated into protein at the ribosome level. (From Coffey DS: The molecular biology, endocrinology, and physiology of the prostate and seminal vesicles. *In* Walsh PC, Retik AB, Stamey TA, Vaughan ED Jr [eds]: Campbell's Urology, 6th ed. Philadelphia, WB Saunders, 1992, p 237.)

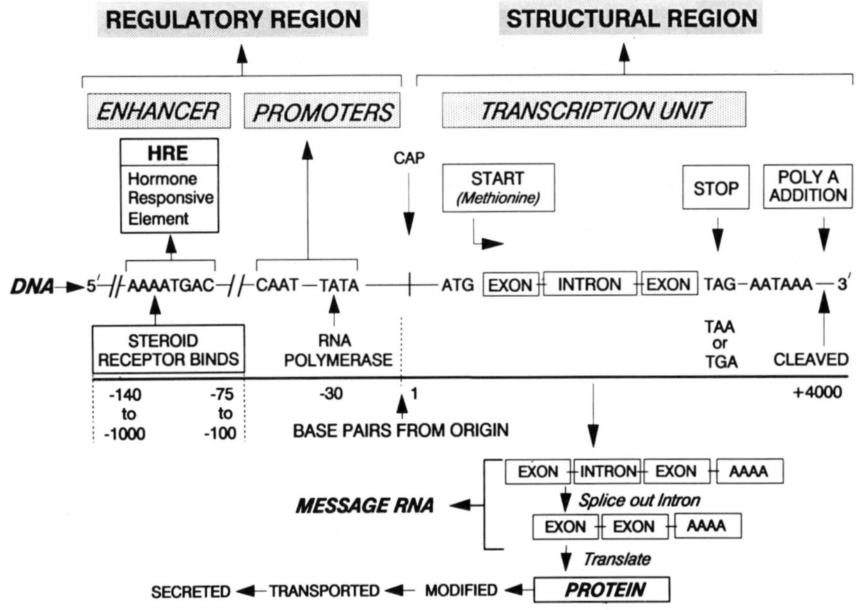

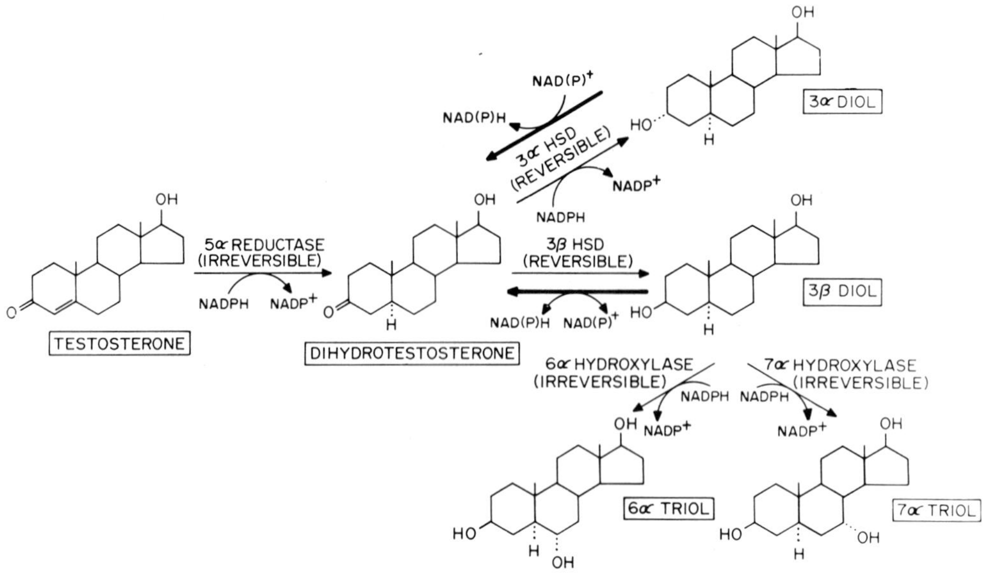

FIGURE 4–5. Metabolic pathways for testosterone within the prostate. Testosterone is irreversibly metabolized by 5α-reductase to the active androgen dihydrotestosterone (DHT), which is then reversibly converted into 3α-diol and 3β-diol. The 3β-diol is irreversibly inactivated to the more soluble 6α-triol and 7α-triol. (From Coffey DS: The molecular biology, endocrinology, and physiology of the prostate and seminal vesicles. *In* Walsh PC, Retik AB, Stamey TA, Vaughan ED Jr [eds]: Campbell's Urology, 6th ed. Philadelphia, WB Saunders, 1992, p 238.)

increase in the maximal velocity, V_{max}, which indicates an activity showing 262 pmol of DHT formed per 30 minutes/mg protein from testosterone when measured in the stroma and less than 10 per cent of that amount with a V_{max} of 19 for the epithelium. The stromal K_m was 76 nM and the epithelial 13. It is not known why these values are different in normal men and those with BPH or cancer, but it is intriguing that there may be alterations occurring in the enzyme or in its regulatory mechanism.

Human and rat 5α-reductase genes have been cloned and expressed.[9] The enzyme is a hydrophobic protein of 259 amino acids with a molecular weight of 29,462. Rat and human 5α-reductase has a 60 per cent homology. The 5α-reductase inhibitor 4-aza-steroids demonstrated marked differences in their ability to inhibit the human and rat steroid 5α-reductase, with it being far more inhibitory on the rat enzyme. The 4-aza-steroids of importance are MK-906 (finazteride, or Proscar), which is 17β-(*N*-t-butyl)carbamyl-4-aza-5α-androst-1-en-3-one, and a related compound called 4MA. These inhibitors work as competitive inhibitors for 5α-reductase. The enzyme is present primarily in the prostate, other sex accessory tissues, liver, and adrenal glands.

5α-Reductase is of great importance because the product DHT is important in the differentiation of the prostate during fetal development, and mutations in 5α-reductase give rise to a rare form of pseudohermaphroditism. In prostate physiology, expression of the 5α-reductase gene is regulated by androgens in both the prostate and liver. It is also believed that the 5α-reductase is involved in male pattern baldness and acne and hirsutism as well as often postulated to be involved in BPH. The 5α-reductase inhibitor MK-906 is being tested for use in the control of BPH.

After DHT is formed from testosterone in the prostate, it is subjected to a series of reversible metabolic reactions to form 3α-diol (5α-androstane-3α, 17β-diol) and 3β-diol (5α-androstane-3β, 17β-diol) (Fig. 4–5). The enzymes that perform this transformation of DHT are 3α- and 3β-hydroxysteroid oxidoreductases (3α-HSOR and 3β-HSOR). These enzymes utilize NADP as a cofactor, but in contrast to 5α-reductase they can also utilize NAD. The equilibrium for the metabolism of DHT favors the formation of DHT, that is, the oxidation of the 3-hydroxy group of 3α- and 3β-diol to the 3-ketone that is present in DHT. Administering 3α-diol to an animal results in a strong androgenic effect through its rapid conversion to the effective DHT. On the other hand, 3β-diol is not very effective as an androgen because it is rapidly and irreversibly converted to the triol form by hydroxylation in the 6α position or the 7α position (Fig. 4–5). The triols are "dead end" products of testosterone metabolism, are very water-soluble, are inactive as androgens, and cannot re-form DHT. Steroids also can form glucuronide or sulfate conjugates and be secreted in a more soluble form. In summary, testosterone is irreversibly metabolized to DHT that is in equilibrium with other reduced steroids primarily through oxidation and reduction at the 3 position. The steroids are inactivated by being irreversibly hydroxylated to the inactive triols.

Estrogens and Estrogen-Androgen Synergism

Estrogens do not block androgen-induced growth of the prostate cell but, on the contrary, may even synergize androgen effects. This has been well documented in the canine prostate, first by Walsh and Wilson[216] and subsequently DeKlerk and co-workers,[63] Tunn and colleagues,[213] and Juniewicz and associates.[110] In the aforementioned studies, the simultaneous administration of estradiol to castrated dogs receiving 5α-androstane metabolites, such as DHT or 3α-diol, produced a twofold to fourfold enhancement in the size of the prostate that was due to an increase in total cell number and was a true glandular hyperplasia. The mechanism of the androgen-estrogen synergism on prostatic growth is not understood; however, it has been shown that estrogens increase the androgen nuclear receptor content in the prostate cell, which might be an important factor in this phenomenon.[211] Estrogen combined with DHT also induces other changes such as increase in steroid metabolism toward DHT formation, collagen formation, and alternation in cell death modification. These changes have been summarized by Coffey and Walsh in relation to BPH.[53]

The synergism of estrogens on androgen-induced growth in the dog prostate is observed only with the 5α-reduced androgens such as DHT or 3α-diol and is not observed when testosterone is administered.[63, 154, 216] In addition, this synergism with androgens and estrogens in the dog does not occur in the rat prostate.[72] Whether this species difference is due to the fact that BPH develops in the dog but not the rat is a matter of conjecture.

Estrogens are capable, either directly or indirectly, of stimulating the stromal elements of the prostate. These studies have been performed in animal models such as the monkey[91] and the guinea pig.[85, 141, 146, 166] Young males receiving androgen blockade with antiandrogens combined with estrogen therapy did not have enlarged prostates, but their stromal elements were markedly enhanced, whereas the epithelial component was involuted.[66] In human BPH nuclei, total assayed estrogens in stromal nuclei (58 fmol/mg of DNA) are six times higher than those found in epithelial nuclei (9 fmol/mg of DNA).[119] It is not known what this large amount of estrogen is bound to in the nucleus.

The distribution of estrogen receptors and binding in the prostate is heterogeneous, but it is clear that stroma is a major target for these estrogens.[71, 120, 152, 187, 188] It is still uncertain whether the very modest amounts of estrogen receptor in the prostate[69, 152] can account for any of the pathologic growths that occur in the prostate. Of great interest will be the localization of estrogen receptors in specific cellular compartments of the prostate, particularly with regard to their role in stem cell growth, cell death, and the secretion of extracellular matrix components such as collagen. It is also still not clear whether the prostate can make any significant amount of estrogens and whether antiestrogens would be an effective treatment for abnormal prostatic growth.[91, 166, 169, 198] It is apparent that estrogens do imprint prostatic growth, and their role in development may be of paramount importance.[161, 162] Estrogens can cause a florid squamous cell metaplasia in prostatic growth that can be offset by androgens.[63, 110] How this is regulated by stem cells is of paramount importance for the role of estrogen in abnormal growth.[63, 148] Estro-

gens may have other actions, including their effect on prostatic secretion and water and electrolyte transport,[100] as well as the potential for affecting urethral musculature and its neurologic control.[186]

Steroid Receptors

In almost all cells in the body, steroids can enter the nucleus, but only a few cells can retain this steroid within their nuclei for any length of time. The cells that retain the steroid have receptors that are specific and can activate specific androgen-sensitive genes within the nucleus to increase the expression of certain protein products that are under steroid control. Earlier, many investigators focused their attention on the cytoplasmic receptor instead of the nuclear compartment, where the androgen action is believed to occur. In fact, the cytoplasmic receptor appears to be an extraction artifact, and most receptors may actually reside within the nucleus. For years it was believed that steroids get into the cell and bind specific cytoplasmic receptors, which by a temperature-sensitive step are activated and then translocated into the nucleus, where they bind to a mysterious nuclear acceptor. The androgen receptor's affinity for the nuclear acceptor site to which it binds in the nucleus, which is probably a compilation of binding to specific sequences on DNA and to the nuclear matrix, is strongly regulated by the presence of the androgen ligand bound to the receptor. When androgens are not present, the receptor decreases its affinity for nuclear binding and can be easily removed; indeed, under castrate conditions, some receptors may leak out into the cytoplasm.[97] Immunohistochemical techniques indicate that the nucleus is the primary place in which the receptor resides.

The prostate and seminal vesicles contain steroid-specific and high-affinity (10^{-9} to 10^{-10} M K_d) saturable (100 to 1000 fmol of receptor/mg DNA equivalents of tissue) androgen receptors. There are 5000 to 20,000 molecules of these receptors per cell. The androgen receptors in the nucleus are believed to bind to specific nuclear acceptors that include chromatin, DNA, and the nuclear matrix. The properties and hormonal regulation of androgen receptors as well as their uses have been reviewed in detail.[20]

The cloning of the human androgen receptor and its expression was a hallmark in the study of the mechanism of hormone action.[39, 137, 138] This has led to the study of the sequence of the gene and its protein product and how this is altered in inherited androgen insensitivity syndromes as well as receptor function.[40, 120a, 137, 138, 140, 210] This powerful new technique is providing the resolution to many questions of andrology.[30, 209]

The gene that codes the androgen receptor is on the X chromosome between the centromere and q13. The coding sequence that will make the protein is divided into eight DNA sections called *exons* (Fig. 4–6). Exons are those parts of the DNA coding sections of the gene that have the final information to be transcribed into message RNA and then subsequently translated into

RECEPTOR	TRANSCRIPTION DOMAIN	DNA BINDING		STEROID BINDING				
	EXON 1	2	3	4	5	6	7	8
ANDROGEN	1607	152	117	288	145	131	158	153
PROGESTERONE	1202	152	117	303	145	131	158	153
ESTROGEN	452	191	117	336	139	134	184	237

FIGURE 4–6. Comparison of base pair numbers in eight exons from various steroid receptors. Steroid receptors are similar and contain eight portions of the genes, called exons, which are translated into amino acid components that make up the receptor. Each exon is composed of a number of nucleotide base pairs. Close homology exists between the various steroid receptors with regard to their size and composition. (From Coffey DS: The molecular biology, endocrinology, and physiology of the prostate and seminal vesicles. *In* Walsh PC, Retik AB, Stamey TA, Vaughan ED Jr [eds]: Campbell's Urology, 6th ed. Philadelphia, WB Saunders, 1992, p 241.)

protein amino acid sequences. They are called exons because this information will exit the nucleus. The exon sections are separated in the gene by intervening *introns,* which are also translated into mRNA but are subsequently deleted from the final message by splicing that occurs in the nucleus. The exon and intron DNA makes a large gene for the androgen receptor that spans a minimum of 54 kilobases (kb).[140] Only the information contained in the eight exons is translated into the receptor. This is very similar to the organization of many other steroid receptors that also contain information from eight exons, such as the progesterone and estrogen receptor (Fig. 4–6). The large androgen receptor gene (54 kb) of DNA is translated into a message of RNA (mRNA) that is only 17 per cent as large as the gene, being only 9.6 kb. This contains an added tail of poly(A) RNA that aids in translation (Fig. 4–7). This mRNA is then translated into a hormone receptor protein with a molecular weight (MW) of approximately 110,000 that contains 917 amino acids. In summary, the gene for making the androgen receptor is very large at 54 kb, but only 17 per cent of these nucleotide bases actually form message. The other 83 per cent of the gene is used for regulatory control and represents sites that are binding to protein to control its translation into RNA. Only a small fraction of the mRNA is translated into

protein, and this portion represents the 2751 base pairs located in the eight exons. Therefore, the final protein is only 5 per cent of the genetic information in the gene, and the other 95 per cent is involved in processing and regulation (Fig. 4–7).

Near the central region of the eight exons is information to code for amino acids in the receptor designed to interact with AREs in DNA located in areas of other genes that are regulated by the presence of the androgen receptor (Fig. 4–4). This DNA-binding domain of the androgen receptor contains 72 amino acids that are rich in cysteine and have a sequence indicating that they form several small loops of protein of 12 to 13 amino acid sequences anchored at their base by complexing with zinc molecules (Fig. 4–8). These small finger loops are referred to as "zinc fingers" and are commonly found in all types of steroid receptors and many other types of transcription-activating factors. These fingers on the receptor that bind directly to the DNA must recognize specific sequences in what is called a *hormone-responsive element* (HRE); this instructs the gene to be androgen-activated (Fig. 4–4). This DNA-binding domain of fingers in the steroid receptor molecule is highly conserved. Therefore, there is a high evolutionary conservation of amino acid sequence homology in this DNA-binding domain between all classes of steroid

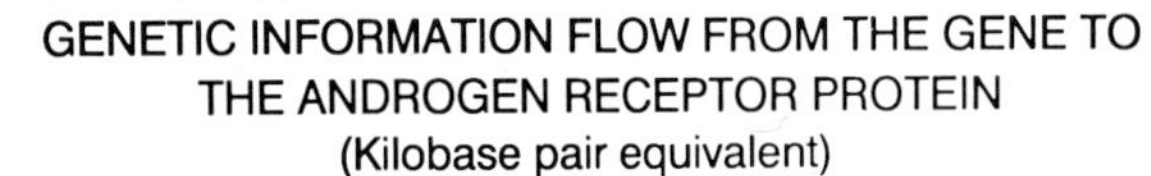

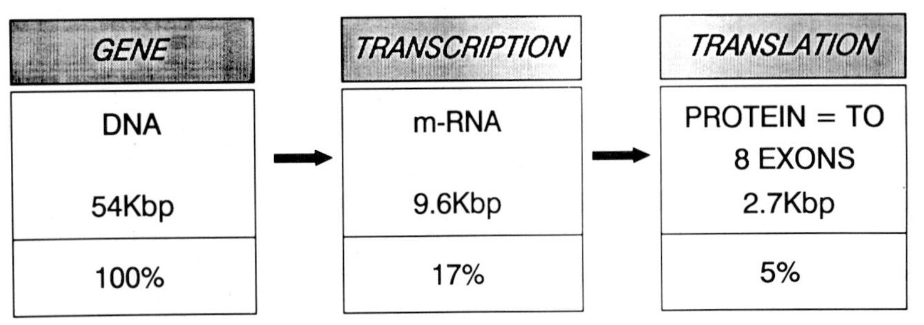

FIGURE 4–7. Ninety-five per cent of genetic information is not translated into protein. Information located in the gene for the androgen receptor is reduced during formation of the final receptor message. The gene contains 54,000 base pairs of nucleotides. This vast amount of information is used for regulation, with only 5 per cent reaching the final message of eight exons that will be translated into the receptor protein. (From Coffey DS: The molecular biology, endocrinology, and physiology of the prostate and seminal vesicles. *In* Walsh PC, Retik AB, Stamey TA, Vaughan ED Jr [eds]: Campbell's Urology, 6th ed. Philadelphia, WB Saunders, 1992, p 241.)

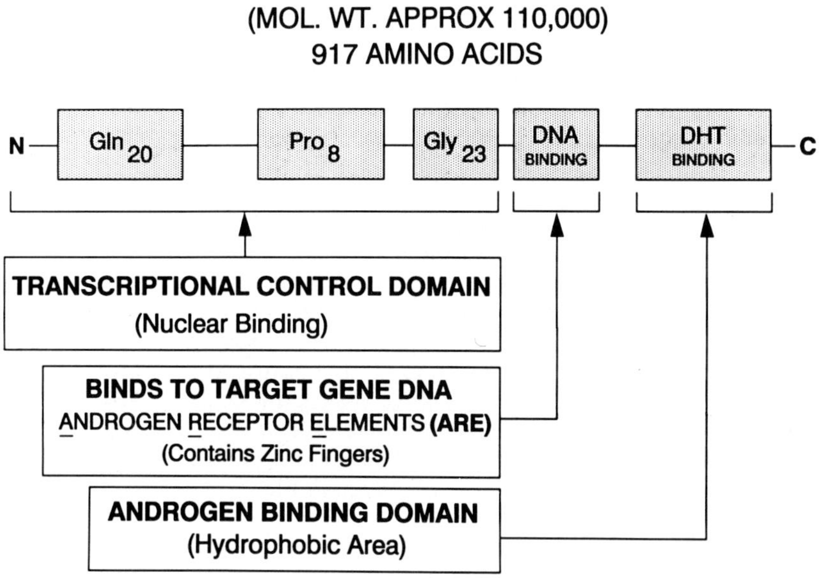

(MOL. WT. APPROX 110,000)
917 AMINO ACIDS

FIGURE 4–8. Structure of the human androgen receptor protein showing the repetitive amino acid components that make up the three domains that regulate transcription, DNA binding, and steroid specificity. (From Coffey DS: The molecular biology, endocrinology, and physiology of the prostate and seminal vesicles. *In* Walsh PC, Retik AB, Stamey TA, Vaughan ED Jr [eds]: Campbell's Urology, 6th ed. Philadelphia, WB Saunders, 1992, p 242.)

receptors. In this region, there is a 79 per cent homology to the progesterone receptor, 76 per cent with the glucocorticoid receptor, and 56 per cent with the estrogen receptor.[40] The closest homology of the androgen receptor is with the progesterone receptor.[39, 40, 137, 138, 140] Mutations of amino acids in this area of the androgen receptor can make the receptor unable to activate androgen-sensitive genes.[87]

The receptor must have steroid specificity and the androgen-binding domain is on the carboxylic acid or C-terminal end of the receptor. It is believed that binding of either DHT or testosterone to this region changes the conformation of the protein and that this permits the receptor to act as a transcription factor by increased binding to target genes, a general process called "*trans*-activation." If certain activations or deletions occur in this C-terminal portion of the molecule, the receptor is able to constitutively activate target genes and *trans*-activate even in the absence of steroids.[140] Marcelli and his colleagues[140] observed that mutations in the androgen receptor at amino acid 587 or 794 are inactive in the assay for androgen binding and for transcriptional activation. However, the removal of amino acids from 708 to the carboxyl end at 917 leads to the synthesis of a receptor protein that does not bind the androgen receptor but is still constitutively active in functional assays as a *trans*-activating factor without needing androgens. This may have profound implications on how prostate cancer may become androgen insensitive and continues to grow in the absence of androgens by producing a steroid receptor that functions without a steroid.

What directs the androgen receptor to activate specific target genes? The target genes are believed to contain an HRE that is a specific sequence of bases that recognize and bind to the zinc fingers of the receptor, and therefore the search is under way to find the DNA sequences of the specific ARE. The identification of an ARE has not yet been fully realized, although in the rat

prostate near the target gene that is under androgen receptor control for forming a secretory protein called *prostatein,* there is an androgen HRE that appears very similar to the glucocorticoid receptor recognition element (GRE) and the progesterone receptor recognition element (PRE); these may be the first identified AREs as described by Tan and associates.[203] These ARE sequences were located both 5′ upstream to the gene and also within the intron.

It is of interest that an androgen receptor is capable not only of activating specific target genes but also of autoactivating its own gene that makes the androgen receptor. Frequently, as the tissue levels of androgen increase, the mRNA levels for the androgen receptor decrease, but mysteriously the androgen receptor still remains high in the tissues. This mechanism of autoregulation of the receptor gene and the receptor stability and turnover in tissue need to be resolved.

The binding of steroids to the receptor is important. The dissociation constant (K_d) for the androgen receptor is 0.2 to 4 nM, and it must be determined whether this affinity for steroid can be modulated by modification of the receptor. Androgen receptors, like all steroid receptors, are known to bind to heat-shock proteins that are ubiquitous and are believed to be involved in sequestering the receptor. In addition, many steroid receptors are regulated by the level of phosphorylation of tyrosine or serine residues on the receptor. It has been shown that the androgen receptor can be phosphorylated in the rat ventral prostate, and it has been reported to occur through a nuclear cyclic adenosine monophosphate (*c*AMP)–independent protein kinase.[86] It has been suggested that the rich acid phosphatases in the prostate may be acting on phosphotyrosyl residues of the androgen receptor, thus playing a role in dephosphorylation and inactivation of androgen receptors.[84]

What produces the tissue specificity in receptor action? Two cell types in different tissues from the same animal can contain the same androgen receptors present in their nuclei, but a cell in one tissue type responds to the receptor by making one type of androgen-induced protein, whereas another cell in a different tissue produces a second type of androgen-induced protein. For example, in the rat, the ventral prostate and the seminal vesicles both have androgen receptors and in the presence of DHT they bind to the same genome (DNA) in their nuclei; however, the prostate makes a different pattern of androgen-controlled gene expression of secretory proteins from the secretory proteins induced by androgen in the seminal vesicles. How two cells with the same DNA respond to the same receptor in a totally different manner remains a mystery. Is it because the receptors are different in these two tissues in some subtle way or that certain DNA sequences have been slightly modified by methylation or changes in topology or chromatin structure? This is one of the major frontiers of endocrine molecular biology.

Part of the tissue and gene specificity in the recognition of receptors and DNA may depend on the organization of the DNA within different nuclei.[82] The steroid receptor complex can interact only with genes that are in regions that are "open" or in the transcriptionally active form, which means that they are susceptible to digestion by incubation with the enzyme DNase I. This indicates that the DNA in this region is in an accessible form to the DNase enzyme. Studies show that these open regions of chromatin with altered conformation extend up to 100,000 base pairs in length, or more than 10-fold the size of a gene that usually ranges from 1000 to 10,000 base pairs. It is not known how such a large range of DNA is altered in conformation, but it may be through binding to structures like the nuclear matrix that can order large-loop domains in the region of 60,000 to 120,000 base pairs.

A typical gene in the open regions of DNA appears to be composed of two major areas: (1) the *structural region*, which is going to be transcribed and becomes part of the message RNA, and (2) a large *regulatory region* of DNA, which contains the control sites for the activation of this gene (Fig. 4–4) and is adjacent to the structural region and upstream toward the 5′ end.

The structural region is called the *coding area* of the gene. Starting on its 5′ end, where it initiates transcription, the nucleotide bases are numbered as + 1 and increase as they move to the right (downstream) into the gene and toward the 3′ end. As one moves away from the gene and to the left of the initiation site and upstream in the 5′ direction, the nucleotide bases are numbered from right to left, starting with −1 and increasing in negative value as one moves to the left of the gene.

The regulatory region includes a *promoter element* that is present in all genes. This promoter element specifies the site to which RNA polymerase II attaches to the DNA and determines the accuracy point for the initiation of transcription. The RNA polymerase copies or transcribes the DNA code into mRNA, a process called *transcription*. This promoter area starts at − 16 nucleotides to −32 upstream from the gene initiation site. This region of −32 to −16 was originally referred to as the Goldberg-Hogness box and has a consensus sequence of TATAAAAG. The RNA polymerase II enzyme binds to this TATA box as one of the initial steps in transcription. Further upstream from the TATA box is a second gene control element, the HRE, which has been identified in many genes regulated by steroid hormones and is the site where the receptor binds to the DNA. In androgen-regulated genes, this area is the ARE; in estrogen, the ERE; and in glucocorticoid, the GRE. This HRE area may contain several discrete sequences, but its overall role is to modulate the frequency of transcription initiation.

In summary, the TATA box tells where RNA polymerase binds and where transcription is to start. The HRE regulates how frequently it is to be transcribed when it is bound to a hormone receptor. Because the HRE element of DNA sequence has been shown to be independent of its position or its orientation, it resembles what has been called the transcription *enhancer element,* which has been found in many other types of genes. The HRE section can vary in its location upstream from the initiation of the gene from − 20 to − 2600 for various types of hormones. With the steroid hormones, it appears to reside about − 140 nucleotides upstream from the initiation site. For example, in the GRE, the site for GRE is approximately − 140 and contains a sequence of nucleotides of AAAATGGAC. This DNA sequence that binds a specific receptor may vary, depending on the type of steroid receptor, and a generalized sequence is presented in Figure 4–4. Deletion mapping experiments have indicated that the receptor-binding domain located in the HRE is indeed required for receptor binding and is necessary for steroid-mediated control of transcription.

Once the DNA is transcribed into mRNA, a series of adenine units is added to the end—the poly(A) tail—and the mRNA is cut and spliced on small nuclear particles (called splicesomes) located on the nuclear matrix. This splicing removes the intron portion of the message. The final mRNA is shipped out of the nucleus, believed to occur on the structural components of the nuclear matrix, and passes through the pore complexes of the nucleus and out to the ribosomes, where the mRNA is then translated into protein product, a step called *translation.* The proteins have specific amino acid sequences that instruct the cell where to ship the protein in relation to secretory granules or to the membrane area. The protein can also be modified after translation by the subsequent addition of carbohydrates, such as sugars, to become glycoproteins or can be phosphorylated by enzymes called kinases; this is called *post-translational modification.* Under appropriate signals, such as neurologic control, secretory proteins can then be excreted into the lumen of the prostate. This process occurs when secretory proteins of the prostate and seminal vesicles are formed into the ejaculate. An example of this process, shown in Figure 4–4, includes the elaboration of PSA and acid phosphatase as well as many other protein products that are regulated in their synthesis by androgens.

The nucleus is where the genetic information of the genes, the androgen receptor interactions, and mRNA processing occur and are integrated. This is within a highly ordered structure of the nucleus that is determined by a residual scaffolding framework, the *nuclear matrix,* which provides three-dimensional organization to both the nucleus and the DNA.

Role of the Nuclear Matrix in Androgen Action

The DNA may be similar in every cell of different tissues in the body, but it appears to be organized in a different three-dimensional array in these various cell types. This spatial organization of DNA appears to be determined by nuclear architecture and structure dictated by the scaffolding element, the *nuclear matrix.* Therefore, more than just a steroid receptor and a DNA sequence with an ARE may be required to determine the high tissue specificity of androgen hormone action; regulation of DNA conformation and three-dimensional structure may be necessary. It is known that there are great regions of at least 100 kb of DNA which are larger than many genes that are in an open conformation and that this varies between cells with the same genome. Strong evidence exists that structural components of the nucleus may organize the DNA into different topologic constraints that permit specific steroid receptor interactions themselves. These structural modifications of topology of DNA may be an integral part of differentiation. The nuclear matrix has been proposed to be an important structural element in this type of DNA organization.[82] The nuclear matrix is an important site that binds hormone receptor complexes and organizes the location of active genes that can be expressed by the action of the steroid receptor. The matrix facilitates the location of target genes, their conformation, and their co-interaction with steroid receptors. For this reason, it is important to describe the properties and structure of the nuclear matrix.

Barrack and Coffey[18, 19] first showed that the nuclear matrix is a major target for androgen and estrogen receptor binding. Because the matrix has been implicated in many important nuclear events, it provides an ideal target for androgen action. The matrix also organizes DNA, and alterations in chromatin structure are known to be affected by hormonal action.

The nuclear matrix has been defined as the dynamic structural subcomponent of the nucleus that directs the functional organization of DNA into loop domains and provides sites for the specific control of nucleic acids.[82, 164] Conceptually, it can be viewed as the nuclear equivalent to the cytomatrix or cytoskeleton. The nuclear matrix contains residual nuclear elements, including the pore-complex-lamina, the residual nucleolus, and an internal ribonucleoprotein particle (RNP) network attached to a dynamic fibrous protein mesh.[23] The nuclear matrix may be isolated by sequential extractions employing nonionic detergent, brief digestion with DNase I, and a hypertonic salt buffer wash. The residual nuclear matrix structures represent only 15 per cent or less of the original total nuclear mass. More than 98 per cent of the DNA, 70 per cent of the RNA, and 90 per cent of the nuclear proteins have been extracted, and the remaining structure is essentially devoid of histones and lipids.

The nuclear matrix has been implicated as an important structural component in a wide variety of important biologic functions (Table 4–4). It serves an important role in DNA organization. There are approximately 50,000 DNA loop domains in a nucleus, each containing about 60 kilobase pairs (kbp) of DNA, and these loops are attached at their bases to the nuclear matrix.[172, 214] This loop organization is maintained during interphase and throughout metaphase.[164] Topoisomerase II, an enzyme that modulates DNA twisting and topology, is associated with the nuclear matrix and the mitotic chromosome scaffold. Hormones are known to activate genes and alter DNA structure. Many studies with a wide variety of systems have demonstrated that active genes are associated with the nuclear matrix, whereas transcriptionally inactive genes are not in close proximity to the matrix. This location of active genes on the matrix provides evidence that the matrix plays an important organizing role in differentiation, placing genes in different configuration.

Androgens can activate DNA synthesis and cell replication in target tissues. The nuclear matrix also serves an important role in DNA replication. The matrix contains fixed sites for DNA synthesis[172] located at the base of the DNA loop. During DNA synthesis, the DNA loop domains are reeled down through the attached replicating complex that is fixed on the matrix. Therefore, the DNA replication fork, DNA polymerase, and newly replicated DNA have been shown to be

TABLE 4–4. REPORTED FUNCTIONS OF THE NUCLEAR MATRIX

Nuclear Morphology: The nuclear matrix contains structural elements of the pore complexes, lamina, internal network, and nucleoli, which give the nucleus its overall three-dimensional organization and shape.

DNA Organization: DNA loop domains are attached to the nuclear matrix at their bases, and this organization is maintained during interphase and metaphase. The nuclear matrix shares proteins with the chromosome scaffold. Topoisomerase II, an enzyme that modulates DNA topology, is associated with the nuclear matrix and chromosome scaffolds. The matrix organizes chromatin structure.

DNA Replication: The nuclear matrix has fixed sites for DNA replication, containing the DNA replication fork. DNA polymerase α, and newly replicated DNA.

RNA Synthesis: The nuclear matrix contains transcriptional complexes, newly synthesized hnRNA, and snRNA. RNA processing intermediates are bound to the nuclear matrix. Actively transcribed genes are associated with the nuclear matrix; inactive genes are not.

Nuclear Regulation: The nuclear matrix has specific sites for steroid hormone receptor binding. The nuclear matrix is a cellular target for transformation proteins, such as the large T antigen, EIA protein, and the *myc* gene product. The nuclear matrix proteins are regulated by phosphorylation.

From Coffey DS: The molecular biology, endocrinology, and physiology of the prostate and seminal vesicles. *In* Walsh PC, Retik AB, Stamey TA, Vaughan ED Jr (eds): Campbell's Urology, 6th ed. Philadelphia, WB Saunders, 1992, p 244.

associated with the nuclear matrix. It is easy to visualize how hormone action and alteration in the nuclear matrix structures can impinge on the androgen regulation of DNA synthesis and growth in a prostate cell.

The nuclear matrix is also associated with mRNA synthesis during transcription. Transcriptional complexes have been identified on the nuclear matrix. O'Malley and colleagues[49] observed that more than 95 per cent of the unprocessed mRNA precursor for ovalbumin was associated with nuclear matrix of the chick oviduct. When the intron portions of the RNA were spliced out, the mature mRNA was released from the nuclear matrix. This led them to suggest that the nuclear matrix is involved in RNA processing. Mariman and van Venrooij[143] have reported that all RNA cleavage products and RNA processing intermediates are firmly bound to nuclear matrix. Once again, alterations in nuclear matrix structures with steroid receptor interactions may alter important steps in transcription and RNA processing. The nuclear matrix contains the attachment sites for the small nuclear ribonucleoprotein particles (snRNPs) that are part of the nuclear splicesome system, which is central to the nuclear processing of RNA to the final mRNA that is transported out to the cytoplasm to be translated.

In conclusion, the nuclear matrix is an important modulator of nuclear regulation and is an ideal target for hormonal regulation. Indeed, the nuclear matrix is a major site of steroid hormone receptor binding.[4, 16, 19, 69, 150, 221] In the prostate, more than 60 per cent of all nuclear androgen receptors are associated with the nuclear matrix.[19] The matrix is also a target for many other types of regulatory interactions, including the nuclear products of oncogenes and viral proteins, which can also induce growth regulation similar to hormone-induced growth. For example, the nuclear matrix is reported to be a cellular target for the retrovirus *mvc* oncogene protein, the adenovirus E1A-transforming protein, and the polyoma large T antigen. All of these transformation proteins that bind to the nucleus are believed to be early molecular events in carcinogenesis or transformation. Therefore, the observation that androgen receptors interact with the matrix has precedence with the matrix as a common target in factors that regulate cell structure and function. For a more detailed review of the matrix in hormone action, see the review of Getzenberg and colleagues[82]; for a review of the role in cancer, see Pienta and co-workers.[175]

Stromal-Epithelial Interactions

The noncellular stroma and connective tissue of the prostate compose what is termed the *ground substance* and *extracellular matrix,* first proposed by Arcadi[12] to play an important role in prostate function and pathology. The extracellular matrix has long been recognized as one of the important inductive components during normal development of many different types of cells.[25, 89, 92] The extracellular matrix is far more than a supporting scaffolding for cells because it has been shown to play a central role in development and the control of cellular function.[92] It now appears that the extracellular matrix is just one of the three major matrix systems that interact and form the overall tissue matrix system of the prostate.[82, 98]

Cell-cell interactions can modify the response of a cell to hormones and growth factors. There has been increasing interest in the role of stromal tissue elements in inducing the growth of the sex accessory tissue because of the early suggestions of Franks[81] in 1970 that epithelial cells require stroma for their growth; in addition, the classic experiments of Cunha and co-authors,[57, 58] Chung and Cunha,[43] and Biller and associates[24] have clearly shown the direct importance of the embryonic mesenchyma in the induction of the differentiation of the normal prostatic epithelial cells (see discussion in earlier section). McNeal[147] proposed that in BPH the stroma may be reactivated in adult life to an embryonic state, thus stimulating abnormal growth; this concept has generated a great deal of interest and effort to understand these tissue components of the prostate. To test whether adult prostate cells could be stimulated by embryonic factors, Chung and others[44, 45] transplanted a fetal urogenital sinus into an adult rat prostate and induced a large hyperplastic overgrowth of adult prostatic tissue that was apparently stimulated by the presence of the factors from the fetal tissue. It is not known whether direct contact with an insoluble embryonic extracellular matrix and/or soluble diffusible growth factor(s) and steroids are responsible for these observations. Figure 4–9 depicts the pathways of coupling stromal-epithelial interactions involving both soluble (growth factors and steroids) and insoluble (extracellular matrix and integrin) interactions.

Cell-matrix interactions can also brake or limit growth. Muntzing[159] proposed that collagen of the prostate might limit prostatic growth. Mariotti and Mawhinney[142] and Thornton and associates[208] have provided evidence that collagen synthesis and degradation can be important events in accompanying limitations on prostatic growth in animals. A clear effect of collagen on normal prostatic growth and function has not been fully established, but several types of collagens are critical components of the extracellular matrix.

The extracellular matrix is becoming a major target for understanding how the phenotype of a cell is regulated. Membrane receptors on the cell surface extend out through the plasma membrane and form a bridge directly connecting the cell skeleton with proteins on the extracellular matrix. These transmembrane receptors are called *integrins* and are made up of two subunits, alpha and beta. These integrins serve externally with contact to the extracellular matrix as receptors for fibronectin and laminin as well as GAGs in the proteoglycans of the extracellular matrix. The integrin receptor domains inside the cell compartment serve as focal points for determining the structure and organization of the cytoskeleton. In addition, other types of transmembrane receptors also extend through the cell to make direct contact with the neighboring cell by recognizing similar receptors and forming hormone-dimer bonds. This permits direct cell-cell interaction; these receptors

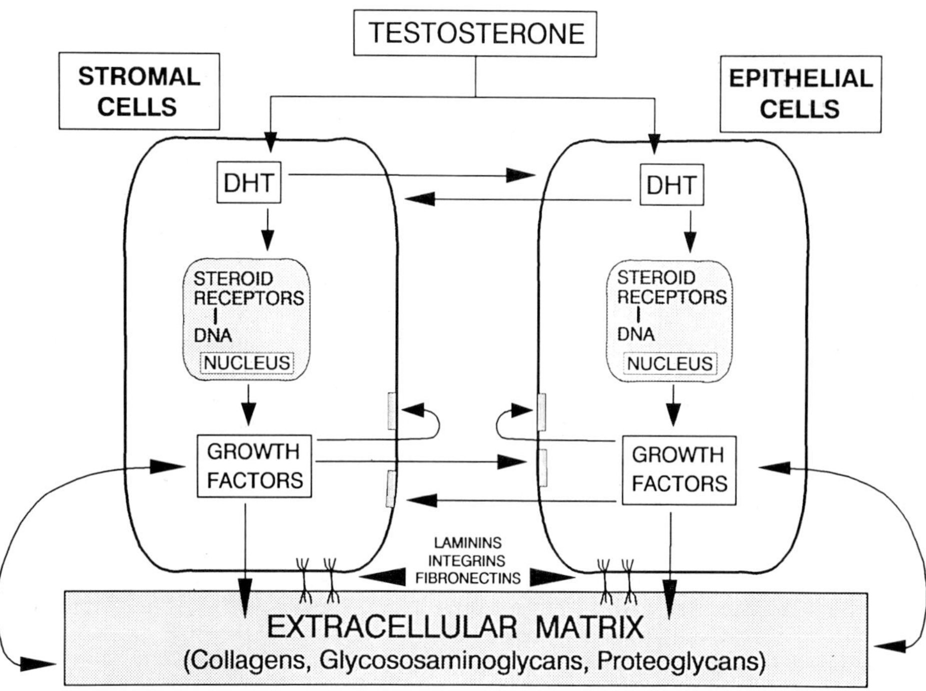

FIGURE 4–9. Types of stromal-epithelial interactions in information transfer and regulation within the prostate. Testosterone and growth factors interact on and between stromal and epithelial cells. The formation of dihydrotestosterone (DHT), the production of growth factors, and extracellular matrix components regulate stromal-epithelial interactions. (From Coffey DS: The molecular biology, endocrinology, and physiology of the prostate and seminal vesicles. *In* Walsh PC, Retik AB, Stamey TA, Vaughan ED Jr [eds]: Campbell's Urology, 6th ed. Philadelphia, WB Saunders, 1992, p 244.)

to neighboring cells, the CAMs, require calcium for their action. One type of CAM of growing importance, uvomorulin, appears to bind many types of epithelial cells together, including the prostate. These interlocking matrix systems interact to form a structural network extending (1) externally, from cell-cell contact and extracellular matrix interactions; (2) internally, to cytoskeleton organization; and (3) centrally, terminating by contact with the nuclear matrix and DNA. The interactions of the tissue matrix regulate many aspects of DNA functions that are involved in growth and differentiation, and the study of this system is at the forefront of molecular endocrinology.[82] These types of tissue matrix interactions are essential to the understanding of stromal-epithelial interactions because they form direct structural linkages and communications between the stroma and epithelial nuclear DNA.

Elements of the stroma and tissue matrix can be isolated as a *biomatrix,* and when this is used as a substratum for epithelial growth in tissue culture, it is apparent that it has the ability to regulate the growth and function of the prostatic epithelial cells.[104] Canine prostatic epithelial cells grow rapidly as primary outgrowth on plastic and do not require stromal elements; however, when these cells are growing on prostatic biomatrix, they reduce their growth and maintain their morphology and secretory ability and more closely approximate what is occurring in vivo.[104] This indicates that the stromal elements can also act as a braking system for growth and therefore limit proliferation and maintain the state of functional differentiation and secretion. Indeed, in normal prostate and in BPH where there is stromal-epithelial interaction, there is usually very little growth and mitotic figures are rare. Removing cells from this normal state (and placing them on plastic)

removes the brake and permits the epithelial cells to grow. The extent of disruption in these braking systems in BPH and cancer is a developing area of tumor biology.

Cancer cells can migrate out of the prostate and are capable of growing elsewhere in the body as metastatic lesions; therefore, they either can use stromal elements from other tissues to support their growth or are free of stromal cell restraints, possibly because of autocrine factors. Chung and his colleagues have shown that the development and establishment of transplanted cancer cells depend upon their transplantation with collagen and either live or dead fibroblasts.[42]

In summary, different components of matrix interactions can have either an inhibitory role in negative regulation of normal prostatic growth and/or a positive role in establishing tumor growth. There have been many hypotheses concerning the mechanism of these epithelial-stromal interactions, but they have yet to be fully resolved.[82, 159, 205]

The discussion to this point has concerned primarily insoluble elements in inducing stromal-epithelial interactions, but soluble hormones, such as steroids and growth factors, are also important. The prostatic stroma does contain steroid receptors and does respond to both androgens and estrogens (see earlier discussion), and the stroma has an androgen-metabolizing ability to form DHT almost equal to that of the epithelium. Steroids can alter the formation of collagen and other extracellular matrix components.

Prostatic Growth Factors and Growth Suppressors

Because the normal adult prostate does not grow rapidly or increase in size, one would not anticipate an abundance of active growth factors in the normal prostate. However, this is a paradox because many adult tissues, not rapidly growing like the prostate, still have high levels of growth factors that can be demonstrated by extracting the tissues and showing that they contain soluble factors that can stimulate in vitro fibroblast growth.

It has been proposed that many of these prostatic growth factors may not be active because they are sequestered by binding to components of the extracellular matrix, such as heparin or heparan sulfates that are part of the GAGs. Indeed, it is known that heparin binding to growth factors is one of the most efficient ways to remove and purify many growth factors such as those in the basic fibroblast growth factor family. If the prostate growth factors are sequestered at the extracellular matrix, it would be important to know what mechanisms are involved in their binding and in their release. Therefore, the simple measuring of total growth factor levels in the prostate is, in itself, not sufficient to define their actual biologic activity in the prostate. In all types of growth, there appears to be a balance between factors that activate growth and factors that suppress growth. These latter inhibitory or braking elements have been labeled "suppressor." In this regard, the extracellular matrix could be termed a "suppressor element" in regard to its ability to sequester growth factors. In addition, extracellular matrix interactions with cells can determine or direct the response of a cell to a mitogen like a growth factor.

Both stromal and epithelial cells themselves can synthesize and respond to growth factors in a reciprocal and interactive manner (Fig. 4–9). Many of these growth factors appear to be under hormonal regulation, particularly in response to androgens, estrogens, and other endocrine factors. Androgens and growth factors can also stimulate the synthesis and degradation of extracellular matrix components that can alter a cell's response to steroids and growth factors. Therefore, the interactions of steroids, growth factors, and the extracellular matrix with the cell are reciprocal and dynamic and can have either positive or negative effects in regulating cell growth.

The combination of steroid hormones and different growth factors and their temporal sequence on different cells of the prostate at various times of development are complex—and it is certainly too early to draw conclusions about mechanisms—but it will be an important area in understanding the biology and pathology of the prostate. In this regard, the effects and mechanism of growth factors on any cell are complicated, and they are generically described with the various pathways in Figure 4–10. Not all steps are realized with each growth factor, but they are usually modifications of the generalized scheme and pathways and involve four phases of regulation: synthesis, secretion, target cell interactions, and effects.

The cell is signaled to produce synthesis of a growth factor by environmental signals that include cell-cell extracellular matrix communications and hormonal levels. The genes for making the growth factors are activated, making mRNAs that can be processed to various forms that are then translated, usually to an inactive or pro-growth factor form. Proteolysis activates the growth factor, which then either can work internally in the cell (intracrine) or can be secreted extracellularly to serve as soluble signals—to its own cell in which it was synthesized (autocrine) or to stimulate a nearby cell (paracrine).

After being secreted, the growth factor can be sequestered by binding to the extracellular matrix; upon release, however, it is capable of binding to specific growth factor receptors that reside on the plasma membrane of the target cell. The degree of occupancy of these membrane growth factor receptors activates a series of second-messenger signals that involve protein kinases, membrane phospholipases, or G protein pathways. The early result of binding to the receptor is the

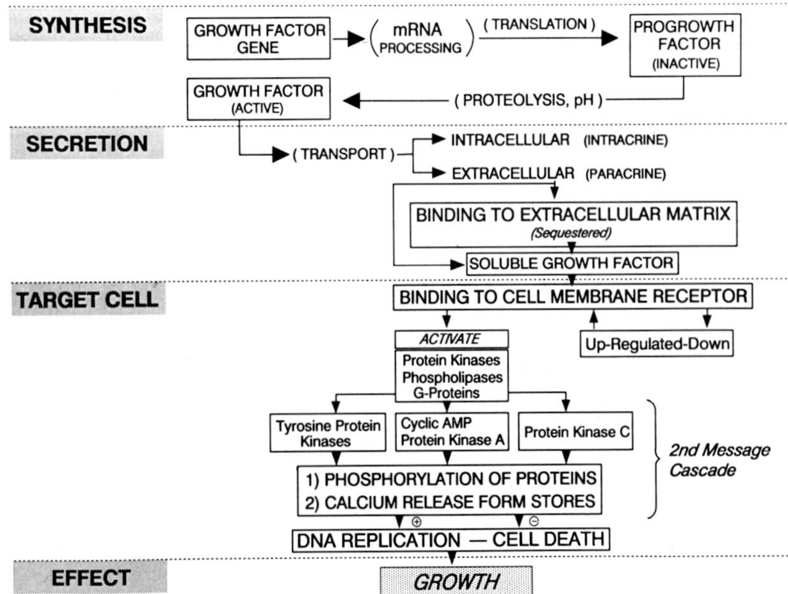

FIGURE 4–10. Mechanisms involved in growth factor action. The synthesis, secretion, and interaction with target cells of growth factors can be quite variable, but in general they follow this schematic. The growth factor requires activation and binding to target cell receptors. This binding activates a series of kinases that release calcium and that phosphorylate specific regulatory proteins. The final effect is to increase DNA replication or cell death to regulate growth (see text). (From Coffey DS: The molecular biology, endocrinology, and physiology of the prostate and seminal vesicles. *In* Walsh PC, Retik AB, Stamey TA, Vaughan ED Jr [eds]: Campbell's Urology, 6th ed. Philadelphia, WB Saunders, 1992, p 246.)

activation of one of these three general types of enzymes that phosphorylate proteins called *kinases*. These kinases are tyrosine kinase, cAMP protein kinase A, and protein kinase C. They either are part of the growth factor receptor itself or are located adjacent to the receptor in the plasma membrane. The growth factor-induced activation of these kinases and second messengers causes a cascade of phosphorylation of specific target regulatory proteins and often the subsequent release of calcium ions from the mitochondria and endoplasmic reticulum. Usually in concert, this cascade brings about the final signal to the nucleus to turn on the expression of specific growth factor-activated genes or to induce DNA synthesis and cell replication. Overall growth is always a net balance between the rate of cell replication and the rate of cell death, and growth factors can either stimulate or suppress growth by affecting this balance.

Fibroblast Growth Factor

The same growth factors often received a wide variety of names, as they were first isolated from different tissues, and this has caused much confusion. For example, basic fibroblast growth factor (bFGF) is the same as, or very similar to, prostatic growth factor, osteoblastic growth factor, a form of tumor angiogenesis factor, endothelial growth factor, uterine growth factor, seminiferous growth factor, and keratinocyte growth factor—to name just a few. Fibroblast growth factors (FGFs) can be isolated from many tissues and come from cells of embryonic mesoderm or neuroectoderm origin. They can also be found in a wide variety of tumors and are produced by many cells in culture. In 1979, a prostatic growth factor shown to be a mitogenic factor present in human prostatic extracts was identified.[106, 107, 126]

There are seven related genes that code for a family of related FGFs; for specific details, consult the review of Goldfarb.[83] In general, there are two major types, both basic and acidic forms, of the growth factor. The acidic form is found primarily in neural tissue, such as the brain and hypothalamus; the basic form (bFGF) may be more important in the prostate. Both of these growth factors bind very tightly to heparin and are sometimes referred to as heparin-binding growth factors. FGF is very mitogenic for mesoderm-derived cells and stimulates capillary growth; it is often therefore called the "tumor angiogenesis factor" and may be involved in neovascularization in any rapidly growing or developing tissue. The acidic and basic FGFs have a 55 per cent amino acid sequence homology. The gene for basic FGF codes for a precursor form of 155 amino acids, and if the protein is kept at neutral pH in the presence of protease inhibitors, 154 amino acid units can be isolated from the prostate[126]; however, the usual form isolated is often 146 amino acids. The ability of the prostate to manufacture its own growth factors, such as bFGF[160] and TGF-β2,[155] and the changes of these levels with pathologic growth, such as BPH and cancer, are obviously of great interest.

Oncogenes are genes that are aberrant in expression or form in cancer cells. One of the oncogenes, *int*-2, is very similar to FGF, but it is larger, containing 239 amino acids. It has now been possible to clone out this gene and to place it into germ cells that upon fertilization produce a mouse that can overexpress the *int*-2 gene. Transgenic mice produce high levels of *int*-2 product, causing epithelial overgrowth as the mice develop. In females, this overproduction produces a mammary gland hyperplasia; in the male, it produces a dramatic prostatic epithelial hyperplasia, but the stromal components do not produce a fibromuscular hyperplasia.[158] The *int*-2 gene is expressed in normal cells of other tissues during embryogenesis, but it is usually not found in adult tissues. Whether the re-expression of *int*-2 or a similar growth factor gene occurs as an embryonic "reawakening" in human BPH needs to be determined.

The membrane receptor that binds bFGF has a molecular weight of approximately 100,000 and extends through the membrane, with the cytoplasmic domain having a tyrosine kinase function that permits the receptor to act as an enzyme phosphorylating tyrosine protein residue.

Thus, FGFs are broad-spectrum mitogens that can stimulate angiogenesis. Because they also induce the expression of plasminogen activator, it has been suggested that they have the properties to support tumor growth and enhance its ability to invade; however, this has not yet been established. It seems a paradox that normal adult prostate tissue that is not growing still contains remarkably high concentrations of these growth factors; this may be because the growth factor is sequestered, inactivated, or incapable of function because of receptor limitations.

Epidermal Growth Factor

Urogastrone, a growth factor that is a polypeptide of 53 amino acids, was first found in the urine and is now known to be similar to mouse epidermal growth factor (EGF) (16,000 MW).

High levels of bFGF are found in all prostates, but the EGF level is usually much lower. This has led to the conclusion that EGF is not the major growth factor in the human prostate[199]; indeed, mRNA for EGF has been difficult to detect in normal or abnormal growth of the human prostate.[155] In contrast, EGF may be prevalent in the rat ventral prostate.[105] It has been reported that EGF-related mitogen with a slightly higher molecular weight than EGF is present in the dorsal prostate of the rat.[167] It has also been reported that the prostatic EGF receptor can be regulated by androgens in the prostate.[212]

There is still much conflict over the role of EGF in the human prostate because prostate cancer cells in culture (LNCaP) do have significant levels of EGF that are 100 times the TGF-α level when measured intracellularly.[54] Morris and Dodd[156] have measured the level of EGF and its receptor EGF-R in the human prostate and have shown the highest levels to be in prostate cancer tissues, thus emphasizing the potential importance of EGF in cancer.

The EGF receptor extends through the plasma membrane and has a molecular weight of 170,000; like bFGF, the receptor is an enzyme tyrosine kinase.

Transforming Growth Factor-α

The TGFs were named because of their ability to promote cell colony formation in suspension cultures, and it therefore was an operational definition. TGF-α is made as a precursor of 160 amino acids and is processed to 50 amino acids (5600 MW). TGF-α is structurally similar to EGF and is believed to bring about most of its effects by interacting with the EGF receptor. TGF-α has been shown to stimulate the growth of human prostate cancers in culture.[219] TGF-α is present in breast cancer and is thought to be an autocrine growth factor stimulated by estrogen treatment. Female transgenic mice that overexpress TGF-α produce both mammary cancers; such male mice produce an epithelial hyperplasia in the prostatic lobe called the *coagulating gland.*[108]

Transforming Growth Factor-β

Transforming growth factor-β is not related to TGF-α, and the similarity in names causes confusion. There are two genes for TGF-β, 1 and 2, and they have a 70 per cent homology. There are three combinations possible between these two genes when a dimer is formed. TGF-β is made as a precursor of 391 amino acids that is inactive in a latent form, and it can be activated by proteolysis, such as plasminogen activator, or by acid to produce a growth factor of 1 monomer each with 112 amino acids (25,000 MW). Although both TGF-β_1 and TGF-β_2 are expressed in prostate tissue, TGF-β_2 has been shown to be significantly increased in expression in BPH in contrast to the normal prostate, whereas TGF-β_1 is not.[155] TGF-β is of paramount interest because it may function as a braking system in negatively regulated epithelial cell growth while being a positive factor in stimulating stromal cell growth. These generalizations may be changed in cancers or BPH tissues where the epithelial cells have changed their response to TGF-β. This may be mediated by changes in the function of the receptors or TGF-β. At present, three of these receptors have been identified and they appear to function through G proteins activating cAMP pathways. The down-regulation of these receptors may release the brake on epithelial growth. This is a complex area because both alternate splicing of the mRNA for TGF-β and the multiple receptor action can produce multiple effects for these important growth factor systems. In addition, TGF-β is also an angiogenesis factor and can regulate neovascularization, which is essential to tumor growth.

Two other growth factors related to the TGF-β family are *müllerian inhibitory substance,* a 140,000 MW protein that causes regression in the müllerian ducts, and *inhibin,* a peptide involved in feedback control of FSH. Inhibin has been reported to be present in the human prostate and seminal plasma and is synthesized in the rat ventral prostate under hormonal control.[185, 190]

Insulin-like Growth Factors I and II (Somatomedin)

Insulin-like substances have also been detected in the prostate.[195] Insulin-like growth factors, termed somatomedin, occur in two closely related forms, type I and type II, and are single-chain polypeptides (75,000 MW) that share sequence homology with human proinsulin. These growth hormones can be found in circulating blood and therefore are endocrine factors, and with their production in target tissue, they therefore are growth factors. These growth factors bind to receptors on the cell membrane that are similar to the insulin receptor consisting of two alpha chains and two beta chains. This receptor has a tyrosine kinase activity. IGF-I is locally produced in connective tissue, such as the chondrocyte, and has an anabolic effect on bone formation through the stimulation of osteoblasts. Many growth factors affect the synthesis of other growth factors, and TGF-β_1 has the ability to strongly stimulate the production of IGF-I in bone and cartilage. Of interest has been the observation that IGF-II and cathepsin-D both have a common type of receptor on breast cancer cells that involves a mannose-6-phosphate receptor, and this may indicate the importance of proteolytic enzymes in functioning also as growth factors. High cathepsin D levels are seen in breast cancer and in the involuting prostate following androgen withdrawal.

Platelet-Derived Growth Factor

Platelet-derived growth factor (PDGF) is expressed in many tissues and is found in the urine. Although it is related primarily to derivation from platelets, it is expressed by the *c-sis* oncogene. PDGF has a strong mitogenic effect on connective tissue cells and makes cells competent to respond to other growth factors. It has been shown to be expressed in prostate tumor models and cells in culture[181, 194] but has not received as much attention as bFGF.

Other Types of Prostate Growth Factors

The growth factors common to the prostate and other tissues are summarized in Table 4–5. In addition, other identified growth factors are claimed to originate in the prostate, but there is no proven growth factor that is unique to the prostate that could be termed a true prostate-specific structure that does not exist in other tissues. It is possible that growth factors may be altered in processing so as to produce increased specificity for an organ, but this is not established. Crabb and colleagues[56] have reported the complete primary structure of a prostatic EGF that they have termed *prostatropin.* Much work will be required to prove that any growth factor is only in the prostate and to eliminate the possible contamination of other known growth fac-

TABLE 4–5. PROPERTIES OF GROWTH FACTORS

ABBREVIATION	TYPE	SIZE	COMMENT
FGF-β	Basic fibroblast growth factor (prostate growth factor, endothelial growth factor, tumor angiogenesis factor, osteoblastic factor)	155 amino acids, 17.6 kDa	Present in normal prostate; elevated in BPH; in tissues of mesoderm origin, stromal elements
	Related to int-2 oncogene	27 kDa	Overexpression produces prostate epithelial hyperplasia but not stromal hyperplasia in transgenic mice
EGF	Epidermal growth factor; urogastrone	67 kDa, single chain	Controversial in normal human prostate but elevated in cancer; prevalent in rat VP
TGF-α	Transforming growth factor–α; 30% similar to EGF, not related to TGF-β	5.6 kDa	Low levels in human prostate, overexpression in transgenic mouse causes epithelial hyperplasia
TGF-β	Transforming growth factor–β; 2 genes (1 + 2), 3 combinations: TGF-$β_1$, TGF-$β_2$, TGF-$β_1$	25 kDa dimer, disulfide	Inhibitor of epithelial growth; stimulates growth of fibroblast; TGF-$β_2$ elevated in BPH; related to MIS, inhibin, and activin
MIS	Müllerian-inhibiting substance	140 kDa, dimer of two identical 70-kDa units	Causes repression of müllerian ducts
IGF	Insulin-like growth factor I–II; somatomedin family	7.5 kDa, single chain	Related to proinsulin
PDGF	Platelet-derived growth factor	30 kDa, dimer	Mitogen for connective tissue cells

Abbreviations: BPH = benign prostatic hyperplasia; VP = ventral prostate; kDa = kilodaltons.

From Coffey DS: The molecular biology, endocrinology, and physiology of the prostate and seminal vesicles. *In* Walsh PC, Retik AB, Stamey TA, Vaughan ED Jr (eds): Campbell's Urology, 6th ed. Philadelphia, WB Saunders, 1992, p 249.

tors. Proteases in the prostate can also clip and modify known growth factors to produce altered forms.

Other growth factors, such as insulin, that originate in distant organs and are transported by the blood are usually termed "endocrine" and not growth factors; however, this is only a matter of classification and does not diminish their importance. For example, prolactin has been shown to have an effect on the increase in DNA synthesis and isolated human BPH tissue.[125] Receptors for many pituitary factors, including prolactin, luteinizing hormone–releasing hormone (LHRH), growth hormone, somatostatin, and thyroid-stimulating hormone, have been sporadically reported in the prostate, but most of the attention has focused on the prolactin and LHRH receptors.[111, 112] It is still unclear how these endocrine and pituitary factors might act as growth hormones in direct interaction on the prostate cells.

Grayhack and his colleagues have long proposed that there is a second factor released by the testes other than testosterone that may be involved in prostatic growth in both the rat and dog, but this factor has not been isolated or characterized.[60]

REGULATION OF PROSTATE GROWTH: BALANCE OF CELL REPLICATION AND CELL DEATH

There is little doubt that most tissues are susceptible to stimulation by growth factors or by inhibition of growth by growth factors and poorly defined tissue chalones, and the actions of these positive and negative growth factors are in a dynamic balance. The net balance between the rate of cell growth and cell death maintains the steady-state size of the prostate; it appears to be under hormonal and growth factor control, and it is age-dependent. Resolving the mechanisms that control this normal growth balance is most crucial to understanding the imbalance that occurs in tumor growth (Fig. 4–11).

For cells to grow, they must first undergo DNA synthesis, and this can be determined on human prostatic tissue by the incorporation of precursors into the DNA, such as thymidine,[151] iododeoxyuridine,[144] or bromodeoxyuridine.[165] Other markers for growth include antibodies against nuclear proteins associated with proliferation, such as KI-67, histones, topoisomerase enzymes, and counting mitotic indices. These techniques have been very helpful in working out the temporal sequence of events that occur in the growth of the prostate under hormonal stimulation in animal models.[52, 64, 75–78, 96, 136, 200] Castration causes a 90 per cent loss in the total number of prostatic epithelial cells and a slower but less complete reduction of approximately 40 per cent in the number of stromal cells. In castrates, following androgen treatment, there is a delay of 1 day before the onset of DNA synthesis, which reaches a maximum rate at 2 to 3 days and then subsides back to normal levels, even in the continued presence of androgen stimulation.[52, 200] It is not known why the rapid synthesis of DNA stops after the gland is restored to its full size. Buttyan and his colleagues[32] have studied the sequence of events occurring following testosterone repletion and preceding the onset of DNA synthesis. They demonstrated that the oncogene c-*fos* showed the earliest transient rise, increasing threefold within 1 hour, followed by an increase in *ras* oncogenes with 2 hours, followed by the transient transcription of both *myc* and

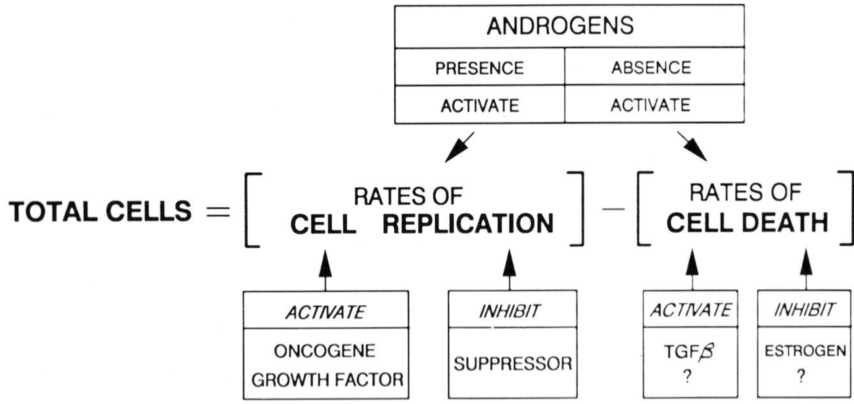

FIGURE 4–11. Cell growth is a balance between replication and cell death. The net size of an organ is the result of the total cell number established by this balance. Androgens, oncogenes, and growth factors induce cell replication and decrease the rate of cell death, and this results in the net increase in organ size. Both benign prostatic hyperplasia and cancer result from a loss of this balance, which exists in normal tissues. (From Coffey DS: The molecular biology, endocrinology, and physiology of the prostate and seminal vesicles. *In* Walsh PC, Retik AB, Stamey TA, Vaughan ED Jr [eds]: Campbell's Urology, 6th ed. Philadelphia, WB Saunders, 1992, p 249.)

myb within 6 to 8 hours. This is typical of many other tissues that are stimulated to grow when similar transient rises in oncogenes precede the onset of DNA synthesis.

There are many normal expressions of oncogenes during growth and development, and it has been proposed that mutated oncogenes, or aberrant forms, may be at the heart of genetic expression in cancer. The *ras* oncogene is the most common oncogene mutated in many human solid tumors, but this has not been shown to have a high incidence in human prostate cancer. Deletion of genetic materials has been shown to release the brake that holds tissues and growth in check. This genetic material has been designated suppressor genes, which means that their absence induces growth; so far, the only suppressor gene implicated in prostatic tissues in culture has been the retinoblastoma gene.[26] This will obviously be an active area of pursuit in the future as allelotyping identifies specific areas of deletion in human prostate cancer.

It was long believed that cell death following androgen withdrawal was simply the choking off of an important biologic factor required to maintain the life of the cell. Studies have shown that this involution is an active rather than a passive process. For example, Grayhack and Lee[88] were the first to report that if protein or RNA synthesis is blocked following castration, the rate of prostate gland involution is markedly reduced.[74, 127, 128, 197] This suggested that specific proteins might be required to be expressed to produce active cell death following androgen deprivation. This process is reminiscent of the system that occurs in bacteria when the synthesis of more than a dozen specific proteins is required to kill the bacteria. It now appears that a similar process of specific protein synthesis is required for prostate involution following androgen withdrawal. This process is termed programmed cell death.

A series of proteins is induced in prostatic involution following castration, and the most actively studied is trpm-2.[153] This has been aided by the characterization and cloning of this gene.[130, 131] The trpm-2 protein was dramatically increased 48 hours following castration and has proved to be one of the most reliable indicators of epithelial cell involution in the prostate. The role of trpm-2 in cell death is still not certain, and it is not known whether trpm-2 is merely a secondary marker

associated with, but not causing, involution. The trpm-2 protein has been shown to be similar to *clusterin*, a sulfated glycoprotein-2 normally found in Sertoli cells and present in human seminal plasma, and it may be important in fertility.[168]

Proteolytic enzymes, such as cathepsin D, are activated during castration-induced involution in the rat prostate.[189, 204] Plasminogen activators are also increased following castration,[180] and three forms are increased following castration in the prostate epithelial cells.[10]

Several groups have studied the appearance of two-dimensional protein patterns that were altered by castration or androgen treatment.[8, 128, 129] The colleagues of Liao[183] showed that specific messages and products are required to be synthesized in the prostate during the process of involution. Saltzman and associates[183] demonstrated that androgen withdrawal causes the production of a 29,000 MW protein and its mRNA during the involution of the rat ventral prostate. Glutathione S-transferase is induced following castration[41]; this is an enzyme located at the cell nucleus that appears to be a DNA-binding protein.

As a cell prepares to undergo programmed cell death, dramatic changes are seen in the nucleus, with a clear zone forming in the perinuclear area.[223] This process, termed *apoptosis,* is a major pathway in prostatic involution.[59, 77, 115, 123, 124, 184]

Isaacs and his colleagues reported that a calcium influx activates a calcium-dependent DNase that causes fragmentation of the DNA molecule; this is an early event in programmed cell death.[77, 123, 124] The timing of these events has been studied,[77] and the role of cell calcium levels has become paramount.[55, 123] Buttyan and associates[32] studied the cascade of induction of a series of oncogenes and heat-shock proteins that follows castration and precedes cell loss.

Kyprianou and Isaacs[124] found an increase in TGF-β receptors during castration that may regulate cell death from a growth factor standpoint. Barrack and Berry[17] studied DNA synthesis in canine prostates induced to massive growth by the combination of androgens and estrogens and found that there is a decrease in the amount of DNA synthesis per unit amount of DNA required to maintain a large gland when 5α-reduced androgens and estrogens are given simultaneously. This led them to suggest that estrogens decrease the rate of cell death in the prostate in the presence of 5α-reduced androgens and that there is not an increase in proliferation. What determines the set-point for the level of cells in the prostate and their rates of growth and death is of paramount importance in understanding BPH and prostate cancer.

REFERENCES

1. Abrahmsson PA, Lilija H: Partial characterization of a thyroid-stimulating hormone-like peptide in neuroendocrine cells of the human prostate gland. Prostate 14:71–81, 1989.
2. Abrahmsson PA, Wadstrom LB, Alumets J, et al: Peptide hormone-serotonin-immunoreactive cells in normal and hyperplastic prostate glands. Pathol Res Pract 181:675–683, 1986.
3. Achstatter TH, Moll R, Moore B, Franke WW: Cytokeratin polypeptide patterns of different epithelial cells from human male urogenital tract: Immunofluorescence and gel electrophoretic studies. J Histochem Cytochem 33:415–426, 1985.
4. Alexander RB, Greene GL, Barrack ER: Estrogen receptors in the nuclear matrix: Direct demonstration using monoclonal antireceptor antibodies. Endocrinology 120:1851, 1987.
5. Anderson DJ, Hill JA: CD4 (T4$^+$) lymphocytes in semen of healthy heterosexual men: Implication for the transmission of AIDS. Fertil Steril 48:703, 1983.
6. Anderson DJ, Wolff H, Pudney J, et al: Presence of HIV in semen. *In* Alexander NJ, Gabelnick HL, Spiler JM (eds): Heterosexual Transmission of AIDS. New York, Alan R. Liss, 1990, pp 167–180.
7. Anderson DJ, Yunis EJ: "Trojan horse" leukocytes in acquired immunodeficiency syndrome (AIDS). N Engl J Med 309:984, 1983.
8. Anderson KM, Baranowski J, Ekonomous SG, Rubenstein M: A qualitative analysis of acetic proteins associated with regressing, growing or dividing rat ventral prostate cells. Prostate 4:151–166, 1983.
9. Andersson S, Russell DW: Structural and biochemical properties of cloned and expressed human and rat steroid 5α-reductases. Proc Natl Acad Sci USA 87:3640–3644, 1990.
10. Andreasen PA, Kristensen P, Lund LR, Dano K: Urokinase-type plasminogen activator is increased in the involuting ventral prostate of castrated rats. Endocrinology 126:2567–2577, 1990.
11. Andrews GS: The histology of the human fetal and prepubertal prostate. J Anat 85:44–54, 1951.
12. Arcadi JA: Role of ground substance in atrophy of normal and malignant prostatic tissue following estrogen administration in orchiectomy. J Clin Endocrinol Metab 14:1113, 1954.
13. Aumüller G: Prostate Gland and Seminal Vesicles. Berlin, Springer-Verlag, 1979.
14. Aumüller G: Morphologic and endocrine aspects of prostatic function. Prostate 4:195, 1983.
15. Aumüller G, Krieg M, Senge T: New Aspects in the Regulation of Prostatic Function. Munich, W. Zuckschwerdt Verlag, 1989.
16. Barrack ER: Steroid hormone receptor localization in the nuclear matrix: Interaction with acceptor sites. J Steroid Biochem 27:115, 1987.
17. Barrack ER, Berry SJ: DNA synthesis in the canine prostate: Effects of androgen and estrogen treatment. Prostate 10:45–56, 1987.
18. Barrack ER, Coffey DS: Specific binding of estrogens and androgens to the nuclear matrix of sex hormone responsive tissue. J Biol Chem 255:7265, 1980.
19. Barrack ER, Coffey DS: Biological properties of the nuclear matrix: Steroid hormone binding. Recent Prog Horm Res 38:133, 1982.
20. Barrack ER, Tindall DJ: A critical evaluation of the use of androgen receptor assays to predict the androgen responsiveness of prostate cancer. *In* Coffey DS, et al (eds): Current Concepts and Approaches to the Study of Prostate Cancer. New York, Alan R. Liss, 1987, pp 155–187.
21. Bartsch G, Brungger A, Schweikert U, et al: The importance of stromal tissue in benign prostatic hyperplasia: Morphological, immunofluorescence and endocrinological investigations. *In* Kimball FA, Buhl AE, Carter DB(eds): New Approaches to the Study of Benign Prostatic Hyperplasia. New York, Alan R. Liss, 1984, p 179.
22. Bendell JL, Dorrington JH: Epidermal growth factor influences growth and differentiation of rat granulosa cells. Endocrinology 127:533–540, 1990.
23. Berezney R, Coffey DS: Nuclear matrix: Isolation and characterization of a framework structure from rat liver nuclei. J Cell Biol 73:616–637, 1977.
24. Biller GH, Runner MN, Chung LWK: Tissue interactions in prostatic growth: Morphological-biochemical characterization of adult mouse prostatic hyperplasia induced by fetal urogenital sinus implants. Prostate 6:241–253, 1985.
25. Bissell MJ, Hall HG, Perry G: How does the extracellular matrix direct gene expression? J Theor Biol 99:31, 1982.
26. Bookstein R, Shew JY, Chen PL, et al: Suppression of tumorigenicity of human prostate carcinoma cells by replacing a mutated RB gene. Science 247:712–715, 1990.
27. Borzy MS, Connell RS, Kiessling AA: Detection of human immunodeficiency virus in cell-free seminal fluid. J AIDS 1:1–6, 1989.
28. Brawer MK, Peehl DM, Stamey T, Bostwick DG: Keratin immunoreactivity in the benign and neoplastic human prostate. Cancer Res 45:3663–3667, 1985.
29. Bronson FH, Whisett MJ, Hamilton TH: Responsiveness of accessory glands of adult mice to testosterone: Priming with neonatal injections. Endocrinology 90:10–16, 1972.
30. Brown TR, Lubahn DB, Wilson EM, et al: Deletion of the steroid-binding domain of the human androgen receptor gene in one family with complete androgen insensitivity syndrome: Evidence for further genetic heterogeneity in this syndrome. Proc Natl Acad Sci USA 85:8151–8155, 1988.
31. Bruchovsky N, Dunstan-Adams E: Regulation of 5α-reductase activity in stroma and epithelium of human prostate. *In* Bruchovsky N, et al (eds): Regulation of Androgen Action. Proceedings of an International Symposium, Berlin, Congressdruck R. Bruckner, 1985, pp 31–34.
32. Buttyan R, Zacker Z, Lochshin R, Wolgemuth D: Cascade induction of c-fos, c-myc and heat-shock 70k transcript during regression of the rat ventral prostate gland. Mol Endocrinol 2:650–657, 1988.
33. Carter BS, Carter HB, Isaacs JT: Epidemiologic evidence regarding predisposing factors to prostate cancer. Prostate 16:187–197, 1990.
34. Carter HB, Coffey DS: The prostate: An increasing medical problem. Prostate 16:39–48, 1990.
35. Catalona WJ, Coffey DS, Karr JP: Clinical Aspects of Prostate Cancer: Assessment of New Diagnostic and Management Procedures. New York, Elsevier, 1989.
36. Chan DW, Bruzek DJ, Oesterling JE, et al: Prostate-specific antigen as a marker of prostatic cancer: A monoclonal and a polyclonal immunoassay compared. Clin Chem 33:1916–1920, 1987.
37. Chan L, Wong YC: Cytochemical characterization of cuprolinic blue stain proteoglycans in the epithelial-stromal interface of the guinea pig lateral prostate. Prostate 14:133–145, 1989.
38. Chan L, Wong YC: Ultrastructural localization of proteoglycans by cationic dyes in the epithelial-stromal interface of the guinea pig lateral prostate. Prostate 14:147–162, 1989.
39. Chang C, Kontis J, Liao S: Molecular cloning of human and rat complementary DNA in coding androgen receptors. Science 240:324–326, 1988.
40. Chang C, Kontis J, Liao S: Structural analysis of the complementary DNA in amino acid sequence of human and rat androgen receptor. Proc Natl Acad Sci USA 85:7211–7215, 1988.
41. Chang GC, Saltzman AG, Sorensen MS, et al: Identification of a glutathione S-transferase Yb_1 mRNA as an androgen-re-

pressed mRNA by cDNA cloning and sequence analysis. J Biol Chem 262:11901–11903, 1987.

42. Chung LWK, Chang SM, Bell C, et al: Co-inoculation of tumorigenic rat prostate mesenchymal cells with non-tumorigenic epithelial cells results in the development of carcinosarcoma in syngeneic and athymic animals. Int J Cancer 43:1179, 1989.

43. Chung LWK, Cunha GR: Stromal-epithelial interactions: II. Regulation of prostatic growth by embryonic urogenital sinus mesenchyme. Prostate 4:503, 1983.

44. Chung LWK, Matsuura J, Rocco AK, et al: A new mouse model for prostatic hyperplasia: Induction of adult prostatic overgrowth of fetal urogenital sinus implants. *In* Kimball FA, Buhl AE, Carter DB (eds): New Approaches to the Study of Benign Prostatic Hyperplasia. New York, Alan R. Liss, 1984.

45. Chung LWK, Matsuura J, Rocco AK, et al: Tissue interactions in prostatic growth: A new mouse model for prostatic hyperplasia. Ann NY Acad Sci 438:394–404, 1984.

46. Chung LWK, Matsuura J, Runner MR: Tissue interactions and prostatic growth: I. Induction of adult mouse prostatic hyperplasia by fetal urogenital sinus implants. Biol Reprod 31:155–163, 1984c.

47. Chung LWK, McFadden DK: Sex steroid imprinting and prostatic growth. Invest Urol 17:337, 1980.

48. Chung LWK, Thompson TC, Chao H, et al: Catecholamines are involved in stromal-epithelial interactions in the rat ventral prostate gland. *In* Rodgers CH, Coffey DS, Cunha G, et al (eds): Benign Prostatic Hyperplasia, Vol. II. Bethesda, National Institutes of Health, Publication No. 87-2881, U.S. Department of Health and Human Services, 1987, pp 27–33.

49. Ciejek EM, Nordstrom JL, Tsai M, O'Malley BW: Ribonucleic acid precursors are associated with the chick oviduct nuclear matrix. Biochemistry 21:4945–4953, 1982.

50. Coffey DS, Bruchovsky N, Gardner WA Jr, et al: Current Concepts and Approaches to the Study of Prostate Cancer. New York, Alan R. Liss, 1987.

51. Coffey DS, Resnick MI, Dorr FA, Karr JP: A Multidisciplinary Analysis of Controversies in the Management of Prostate Cancer. New York, Plenum Press, 1988.

52. Coffey DS, Shimazaki J, Williams-Ashman HG: Polymerization of deoxyribonucleotides in relation to androgen-induced prostatic growth. Arch Biochem Biophys 124:184–198, 1968.

53. Coffey DS, Walsh PC: Clinical and experimental studies in benign prostatic hyperplasia. Urol Clin North Am 17:461–476, 1990.

54. Connolly JM, Rose DP: Production of epidermal growth factor and transforming growth factor-α by the androgen responsive LNCaP human prostate cancer cell lines. Prostate 16:209–218, 1990.

55. Connor J, Sawczuk IS, Benson MC, et al: Calcium channel antagonists delay regression of androgen-dependent tissues and suppress gene activity associated with cell death. Prostate 13:119–130, 1988.

56. Crabb JW, Armes LG, Carr SA, et al: Complete primary structure of prostatropin, a prostate epithelial cell growth factor. Biochemistry 225:4988–4993, 1986.

57. Cunha GR, Chung LWK, Shannon JM, et al: Hormonal induced morphogenesis and growth: Role of the mesenchymal-epithelial interactions. Recent Prog Horm Res 39:559, 1983.

58. Cunha GR, Fujii H, Neubauer BL, et al: Epithelial-mesenchymal interactions in prostatic development: I. Morphological observations of prostatic induction by urogenital sinus mesenchyma in epithelium of the adult rodent urinary bladder. J Cell Biol 96:1662–1670, 1983.

59. Dahl E, Kjaerheim A: The ultrastructure of the accessory sex organs of male rats: II. Post-castration involution of the ventral, lateral and dorsal prostate. Zellforsh Mikrosk Anat 144:167–170, 1973.

60. Dalton DP, Lee C, Huprikar S, Grayhack JT: Non-androgenic role of testes in ventral prostate growth in rats. Prostate 16:225–233, 1990.

61. Davis NS: Determination of serotonin and 5-hydroxyindoleacetic acid in guinea pig and human prostate using HPLC. Prostate 11:353–360, 1987.

62. DeKlerk DP: Glycosoaminoglycans of benign prostatic hyperplasia. Prostate 4:73, 1983.

63. DeKlerk DP, Coffey DS, Ewing LL, et al: Comparison of spontaneously and experimentally induced canine prostatic hyperplasia. J Clin Invest 64:842, 1979.

64. DeKlerk DP, Heston WDW, Coffey DS: Studies on the role of macromolecular synthesis in the growth of the prostate. *In* Grayhack JT, Wilson JD, Scherbenske MJ (eds): Benign Prostatic Hyperplasia. Proceedings of a workshop sponsored by the Kidney Disease and Urology Program of the NIAMDD. Washington, DC, US Government Printing Office, 1976, pp 43–51.

65. Dermer GB: Basal cell proliferation in benign prostatic hyperplasia. Cancer 41:1857–1862, 1978.

66. deVoogt HJ, Rao BR, Geldof AA, et al: Androgen action blockade does not result in reduction in size but changes the histology of the normal human prostate. Prostate 11:305–311, 1987.

67. diSant-Agnese PA, deMesy-Jensen KL: Endocrine-paracrine cells of the prostate and prostatic urethra: An ultrastructural study. Hum Pathol 15:1034–1041, 1984.

68. diSant-Agnese PA, deMesy-Jensen KL, Churukien CJ, Agarwall MM: Human prostatic endocrine-paracrine (APUD) cells: Distribution analysis for the comparison of serotonin and neuron-specific amylase immunoreactivity in silver stains. Arch Pathol Lab Med 109:607–612, 1985.

69. Donnelly BJ, Lakey WH, McBlain WA: Estrogen receptors in human benign prostatic hyperplasia. J Urol 130:183, 1984.

70. Dym M, Orenstein J: Structure of the male reproductive tract in AIDS patients: *In* Alexander NJ, Gabelnick HL, Spieler JM (eds): Heterosexual Transmission of AIDS. New York, Wiley-Liss, 1990, pp 181–196.

71. Eaton CL, Hamilton TC, Kenvyn K, Pierrepoint CG: Studies of androgen and estrogen binding in normal canine prostatic tissue and epithelial stromal cell lines derived from the canine prostate. Prostate 7:377, 1985.

72. Ehrlichman RJ, Isaacs JT, Coffey DS: Differences in the effects of estradiol on dihydrotestosterone induced growth of the castrate dog and rat. Invest Urol 18:466–470, 1981.

73. Ellis DW, Leffer S, Davies J, Meek NG: Multiple immunoperoxidase markers in benign prostatic hyperplasia and adenocarcinoma of the prostate. Am J Clin Pathol, 81:279–284, 1984.

74. Engels G, Lee C, Grayhack JT: Acid ribonuclease in rat prostate during castration-induced involution. Biol Reprod 22:827–831, 1980.

75. English HF, Drago JR, Santen RJ: Cellular response to androgen depletion and repletion in the rat ventral prostate: Autoradiography and morphometric analysis. Prostate 7:41–51, 1985.

76. English HF, Kloszewski ED, Valentine EG, Santen RJ: Proliferative response of the Dunning R3327-H experimental model of prostatic adenocarcinoma to conditions of androgen depletion and repletion. Cancer Res 46:839–844, 1986.

77. English HF, Kyprianou N, Isaacs JT: Relationship between DNA fragmentation and apoptosis in programmed cell death in the rat prostate following castration. Prostate 15:233–250, 1989.

78. English HF, Santen RJ, Isaacs JT: Response of glandular vs. basal rat ventral prostatic epithelial cells to androgen withdrawal and replacement. Prostate 11:229–242, 1987.

79. Evans GS, Chandler JA: Cell proliferation studies in the rat prostate: II. The effects of castration and androgen-induced regeneration upon basal and secretory cell proliferation. Prostate 11:339–351, 1987.

80. Forest MG: Plasma androgens (testosterone and 4-androstenedione) and 17-hydroxyprogesterone in the prenatal, prepubertal and peripubertal periods in the human and the rat: Differences between species. J Steroid Biochem 11:543–548, 1979.

81. Franks LM: Benign nodular hyperplasia of the prostate: A review. Ann R Coll Surg 14:92, 1954.

82. Getzenberg RH, Pienta KJ, Coffey DS: The tissue matrix: Cell dynamics and hormone action. Endocr Rev 11:399–416, 1990.

83. Goldfarb M: The fibroblast growth factor family. Cell Growth Differentiation 1:439–445, 1990.
84. Golsteyn EJ, Graham JS, Goren HJ, LeFebvre YA: Phosphorylation status of the nuclear cytosolic androgen receptors in the rat ventral prostate. Prostate 14:91–101, 1989.
85. Goodwin WE, Cummings RH: Squamous metaplasia of the verumontanum with obstruction due to hypertrophy: Long term effects of estrogen on the prostate in aging male to female transsexuals. J Urol 131:553–554, 1984.
86. Goueli SA, Holtzman JL, Ahmed K: Phosphorylation of the androgen receptor by a nuclear cAMP-independent protein kinase. Biochem Biophys Res Comm 123:778–784, 1984.
87. Govindan MV: Specific region in hormone binding domains is essential for hormone binding and trans-activation by human androgen receptor. Mol Endocrinol 4:417–427, 1990.
88. Grayhack JT, Lee C: Evaluation of prostatic fluid and prostatic pathology. *In* Murphy GP, Sandberg AA, Karr JP (eds): The Prostate: Cell Structure and Function, Part A. New York, Alan R. Liss, 1981, p 231.
89. Grobstein C: The developmental role of the intracellular matrix: A retrospective and prospective. *In* Slavkin HC, Greulich RC (eds): Extracellular Matrix Influence on Gene Expression. New York, Academic Press, 1975, pp 9–16.
90. Guthrie PD, Freeman MR, Liao S, Chung LWK: Regulation of gene expression in rat prostate by androgen and β-adrenergic receptor pathways. Mol Endocrinol 4:1343–1353, 1990.
91. Habenicht UF, el Etreby MF: The periurethral zone of the prostate of the cynomolgus monkey is the most sensitive prostate part for an estrogenic stimulus. Prostate 13:305–316, 1988.
92. Hay ED: The Cell Biology of the Extracellular Matrix. New York, Plenum Press, 1981.
93. Higgins JRA, Gosling JA: Studies of the structure and intrinsic innervation of the normal human prostate. Prostate (Suppl) 2:5–16, 1989.
94. Higgins SJ, Smith SE, Wilson J: Development of secretory protein synthesis in the seminal vesicle and ventral prostate of the male rat. Mol Cell Endocrinol 27:55–65, 1982.
95. Hiler L: The effects of hormones on the proteoglycans of the rat prostate. Thesis. Baltimore, University of Maryland, 1987.
96. Humphries JE, Isaacs JT: Unusual androgen sensitivity of the androgen-independent Dunning R3327-G rat prostatic adenocarcinoma: Androgen effects on tumor cell loss. Cancer Res 41:3148–3156, 1982.
97. Husmann DA, Wilson CM, McPhaul MJ, et al: Anti-peptide antibodies to two distinct regions of the androgen receptor localize the receptor protein to the nuclei of target cells in the rat and human prostate. Endocrinology 126:2359–2368, 1990.
98. Isaacs JT, Barrack ER, Isaacs WB, Coffey DS: The relationship of cellular structure and function: The matrix system. *In* Murphy GP, Sandberg AA, Karr JP (eds): The Prostate Cell: Structure and Function, Part A. New York, Alan R. Liss, 1981.
99. Isaacs JT, Berry SJ: Changes in dihydrotestosterone metabolism in development of benign prostatic hyperplasia in the aging beagle. J Steroid Biochem 18:749–757, 1983.
100. Isaacs JT, Brendler CB, Walsh PC: Changes in the metabolism of dihydrotestosterone in the hyperplastic human prostate. J Clin Endocrinol Metab 56:139–146, 1983.
101. Isaacs JT, Coffey DS: Changes in dihydrotestosterone metabolism associated with the development of canine benign prostatic hyperplasia. Endocrinology 108:445, 1981.
102. Isaacs JT, Coffey DS: Androgen metabolism of the prostate: New concepts related to normal and abnormal growth. *In* Everett JE, Altwein G, Bartsch G, Jacoby GH (eds): Antihormones. Munich, W Zuckschwerdt Verlag, 1981.
103. Isaacs JT, Coffey DS: Etiology and disease processes of benign prostatic hyperplasia. Prostate (Suppl) 2:33–50, 1989.
104. Isaacs WB: Structural and functional components in normal and hyperplastic prostate. Doctoral Thesis. Baltimore, The Johns Hopkins University, 1984.
105. Jacobs S, Storey M, Sasse J, et al: Characterization of growth factors derived from the rat ventral prostate. J Urol (in press).
106. Jacobs SC, Lawson, RK: Mitogenic factors in human prostate extracts. Urology 16:488–491, 1980.
107. Jacobs SC, Pikna D, Lawson RK: Prostatic osteoblastic factor. Invest Urol 17:195, 1979.
108. Jhappan C, Stahle C, Harkins R, et al: TGFα overexpression in transgenic mice induces liver neoplasia and abnormal development of the mammary gland and pancreas. Cell 61:1137–1146, 1990.
109. Jost A: Hormonal factors in development of the fetus. Cold Spring Harb Symp Quant Biol 19:167, 1954.
110. Juniewicz PE, Lemp BM, Barbolt TA, et al: Dose-dependent hormonal induction of benign prostatic hyperplasia (BPH) in castrated dogs. Prostate 14:341–352, 1989.
111. Kadar T, Ben-David M, Pontes EJ, et al: Prolactin and luteinizing hormone-releasing hormone receptors in human benign prostatic hyperplasia and prostate cancer. Prostate 12:299–307, 1988.
112. Kadar T, Redding TW, Ben-David M, Schally AV: Receptors for prolactin, somatostatin and luteinizing hormone-releasing hormone (LH-RH) on experimental prostate cancer after treatment with analogs of LH-RH and somatostatin: Decrease in prolactin binding sites. Proc Natl Acad Sci USA, 85:890–894, 1988b.
113. Kastendieck H: Ultrastrukturpathologie der menschlichen prostatadruse: Cyto- und histomorphogeneses von atrophie, hyperplasie, metaplasie, dysplasie und carcinom. Veroff Pathol H 106. Stuttgart, Fischer, 1977.
114. Katz A, Wise G, Olsson C, et al: A map of molecular events during the early phase of prostate growth (abstr No 380). J Urol 142:380, 1989.
115. Kerr JFR, Searle J: Deletion of cells by apoptosis during castration-induced involution of the rat prostate. Virchows Arch (Cell Pathol) 13:87–102, 1973.
116. Killian CS, Yang N, Emrich JL, et al: Prognostic importance of prostate-specific antigen for monitoring patients with stages B2 to D1 prostate cancer. Cancer Res 45:886–891, 1985.
117. Kincl FA, Folch Pi AF, Herrera Lasso LH: The effect of estradiol benzoate treatment in the newborn male rat. Endocrinology 72:966–968, 1963.
118. Kofoed JA, Tumilasci OR, Curbelo HM, et al: Effect of castration androgens upon prostatic proteoglycans in rats. Prostate 16:102, 1990.
119. Kozak I, Bartsch W, Krieg M, Voigt K: Nuclei of stroma: Site of highest estrogen concentration in human benign prostatic hyperplasia. Prostate 3:433–438, 1982.
120. Krieg M, Klotzl G, Kaufmann J, Voigt KD: Stroma of human benign prostatic hyperplasia: Preferential tissues for androgen metabolism and estrogen binding. Acta Endocrinol (Copenh) 96:422–432, 1981.
120a. Kuiper GGJM, Faber PW, van Rooij HC, et al: Structural organization of the human androgen receptor gene. J Mol Endocrinol 2:R1–R4, 1989.
121. Kuriyama M, Wang MC, Lee CL, et al: Use of human prostate-specific antigen in monitoring prostate cancer. Cancer Res 41:3874–3876, 1981.
122. Kuriyama M, Wang MC, Papsidero LD, et al: Quantitation of prostatic-specific antigen in serum by a sensitive enzyme immunoassay. Cancer Res 40:4658–4662, 1980.
123. Kyprianou N, English HF, Isaacs JT: Activation of calcium-magnesium dependent endonuclease as an early event in castration-induced prostate cell death. Prostate 13:103–117, 1988.
124. Kyprianou N, Isaacs JT: Activation of programmed cell death in the rat ventral prostate after castration. Endocrinology, 122:552–562, 1988.
125. Launoit Y, Kiss R, Jossa V, et al: The influence of dihydrotestosterone, testosterone, estradiol, progesterone or prolactin on the cell kinetics of human hyperplastic prostatic tissue and organ culture. Prostate 13:143–153, 1988.
126. Lawson RK, Storey MT, Jacobs SC, Begun FI: Growth factors in benign prostatic hyperplasia. *In* Ackermann R, Schroeder FH (eds): Prostatic Hyperplasia: Etiology, Surgical and Conservative Management. Berlin, de Gruyter, 1989, pp 73–80.
127. Lee C, Tsai Y, Harrison H, Sensiber J: Proteins of the rat

prostate: I. Preliminary characterization by 2-dimensional electrophoresis. Prostate 7:171–182, 1985.

128. Lee C, Hopkins D, Holland JM: Reduction in prostate concentration of endogenous dihydrotestosterone in rats by hyperprolactinemia. Prostate 6:361–367, 1985.

129. Lee C, Sensibar J: Proteins of the rat prostate: II. Synthesis of new proteins in the ventral lobe during castration-induced regression. J Urol 138:903–908, 1987.

130. Leger JG, Guellec RL, Tenniswood M: Treatment with antiandrogens induces an androgen-repressed gene in the rat ventral prostate. Prostate 13:131–142, 1988.

131. Leger JG, Montpetit ML, Tenniswood M: Characterization and cloning of androgen-repressed mRNAs from rat ventral prostate. Biochem Biophys Res Comm 147:196–203, 1987.

132. Lepor H: Role of long-acting selective α_1 blocker in the treatment of benign prostatic hyperplasia. Urol Clin North Am 17:651–659, 1990.

133. Lepor H, Kuhar MJ: Characterization and localization of the muscarinic cholinergic receptor in human prostate tissue. J Urol 132:397–402, 1984.

134. Lepor H, Shapiro E: Characterization of the alpha$_1$ adrenergic receptor in human benign prostatic hyperplasia. J Urol 132:1226–1229, 1984.

135. Lepor H, Shapiro E, Gup DI, Baumann M: Laboratory assessment of terazosin and alpha$_1$ blockade in prostatic hyperplasia. Urology (Suppl) 32:21, 1988.

136. Lesser B, Bruchovsky N: The effects of testosterone, 5α-dihydrotestosterone and adenosine 3′,5′ monophosphate on cell proliferation and differentiation in rat prostate. Biochim Biophys Acta 308:426–437, 1973.

137. Lubahn DB, Josephs DR, Sar M, et al: The human androgen receptor: Complementary deoxyribonucleic acid cloning sequence analysis and gene expression in prostate. Mol Endocrinol 2:1265–1275, 1988.

138. Lubahn DB, Josephs DR, Sullivan PM, et al: Cloning of the human androgen receptor complementary DNA and localization to the X chromosome. Science 240:327–330, 1988.

139. Mann T, Mann CL: Male Reproductive Function and Semen. New York, Springer-Verlag, 1981.

140. Marcelli M, Tilley WD, Wilson CM, et al: Definition of the human androgen receptor gene structure permits the identification of mutations that cause androgen resistance: Premature termination of the receptor protein at amino acid residue 588 causes complete androgen resistance. Mol Endocrinol 4:1105–1116, 1990.

141. Mariotti J, Mawhinney MG: Hormonal control of accessory sex organ fibromuscular stroma. Prostate 2:397, 1981.

142. Mariotti J, Mawhinney MG: Androgenic regulation of estrogenic action on accessory sex organ smooth muscle. J Urol 129:180–185, 1983.

143. Mariman EC, van Venrooij WJ: The nuclear matrix and RNA processing: Use of human antibodies. *In* Schmuckler EG, Claussen GA (eds): Nuclear Envelope Structure and RNA Maturation. New York, Alan R. Liss, 1985, pp 315–319.

144. Masters JRW, O'Donoghue EPN: Human benign prostatic hyperplasia in organ culture: Studies on iododeoxyuridine uptake. Prostate 4:167–178, 1983.

145. Mawhinney M: The extracellular matrix and cellular proliferation in etiology of benign prostatic hyperplasia. *In* Ackermann R, Schroeder FA (eds): Prostatic Hyperplasia: New Developments in Biosciences, Vol 5. Berlin, deGruyter, 1989, pp 55–62.

146. Mawhinney MG, Neubauer BL: Action of estrogens in the male. Invest Urol 16:409–420, 1979.

147. McNeal JE: Origin and evolution of benign prostatic enlargement. Invest Urol 15:340–345, 1978.

147a. McNeal JE: Anatomy of the prostate: An historical survey of divergent views. Prostate 1:3, 1980.

148. Merk FB, Ofner P, Kwan PWL, et al: Ultrastructural and biochemical expression of divergent differentiation in prostates of castrated dogs treated with estrogens and androgens. Lab Invest 47:437, 1982.

149. Merk FB, Warhol MJ, Kwan P, et al: Multiple phenotypes of prostatic glandular cells in castrated dogs after individual or combined treatment with androgens and estrogens. Lab Invest 54:442–456, 1986.

150. Metzger DA, Korach KS: Cell-free interactions of the estrogen receptor with mouse uterine nuclear matrix: Evidence of saturability, specificity and resistance to KCl extraction. Endocrinology 162:2190, 1990.

151. Meyer JS, Sufrin G, Martin SA: Proliferative activity of benign human prostate, prostatic adenocarcinoma and seminal vesicles evaluated by thymidine labeling. J Urol 128:1353–1356, 1982.

152. Mobbs BJ, Johnson LE, Liu Y: The quantitation of cytosolic and nuclear estrogen and progesterone receptors in benign, untreated and treated malignant human prostatic tissue by radioligand binding and enzyme immunoassays. Prostate 16:235–244, 1990.

153. Montpetit ML, Lawless KR, Tenniswood M: Androgen repressed messages in the rat ventral prostate. Prostate 8:25–36, 1986.

154. Moore RJ, Gazak JM, Quebbeman JF, Wilson JD: Concentration of dihydrotestosterone in 3α-androstanediol in naturally occurring and androgen induced prostatic hyperplasia in the dog. J Clin Invest 64:1003, 1979.

155. Mori H, Maki M, Oishi K, et al: Increased expression of genes for basic fibroblast growth factor: A transforming growth factor type β2 in human benign prostatic hyperplasia. Prostate 16:71–80, 1990.

156. Morris GL, Dodd JG: Epidermal growth factor receptor: mRNA levels in human prostatic tumors and cell lines. J Urol 143:1272–1274, 1990.

157. Morrison RL, Johnson DC: The effects of androgenation in male rats castrated at birth. J Endocrinol 34:117–123, 1966.

158. Muller WJ, Lee FS, Dickson C, et al: The int-2 gene product acts as an epithelial growth factor in transgenic mice. EMBO J 9:907–913, 1990.

159. Muntzing J: Androgen and collagen as growth regulators of the rat ventral prostate. Prostate 1:71, 1980.

160. Mydlo JK, Bulbul MA, Richon VM, et al: Heparin binding growth factors isolated from human prostatic extracts. Prostate 12:343–355, 1988.

161. Naslund MJ, Coffey DS: The differential effects of neonatal androgens, estrogens and progesterones on adult rat prostate growth. J Urol 136:1126–1140, 1986.

162. Naslund MJ, Coffey DS: The hormonal imprinting of the prostate and the regulation of stem cells in prostatic growth. *In* Rodgers CH, Coffey DS, Cunha G, et al: (eds): Benign Prostatic Hyperplasia, Vol. II. Bethesda, US Department of Health and Human Services, National Institutes of Health, Publication No. 87-2881, 1987, pp 73–83.

163. National Kidney and Urological Disease Advisory Board, 1990: Long-Range Plan Window on the 21st Century. Bethesda, US Department of Health and Human Services, National Institutes of Health, Publication No. 90-583, 1990.

164. Nelson WG, Pienta KJ, Barrack ER, Coffey DS: The role of the nuclear matrix in the organization and function of DNA. Annu Rev Biophys Chem 15:457–475, 1986.

165. Nemoto R, Hattori K, Uchida K, et al: S-phase fraction of human prostate adenocarcinoma studied with *in vivo* bromodeoxyuridine labeling. Cancer 66:509–514, 1990.

166. Neubauer B, Bisser T, Jones CD, et al: Antagonism of androgen and estrogen effects in the guinea pig seminal vesicle, epithelium and fibromuscular stroma by keoxifene (LY 156758). Prostate 15:273–286, 1989.

167. Nishi N, Matuo Y, Wada F: Partial purification of the major type of rat prostatic growth factor: Characterization as an epidermal growth factor related mitogen. Prostate 13:209–220, 1988.

168. O'Bryan MK, Baker HWG, Saunders JR, et al: Human seminal clusterin (SP-40, 40). J Clin Invest 85:1477–1486, 1990.

169. Oesterling JE, Juniewicz PE, Walters JR, et al: Aromatase inhibition in the dog: II. Effects of growth, function and pathology of the prostate. J Urol 139:832–839, 1988.

170. Pang S, Levine L, Chow D, et al: Dihydrotestosterone and its relationship to testosterone in infancy and childhood. J Clin Endocrinol Metab 48:821–826, 1979.

171. Papsidero LD, Wang MC, Valenzuela LA, et al: A prostate antigen in sera of prostatic patients. Cancer Res 40:2428–2432, 1980.

172. Pardoll DM, Vogelstein B, Coffey DS: A fixed DNA replication in eukaryotic cells. Cell 19:527–536, 1980.

173. Parsons SJ, Lipshultz LI: The effects of prostatic secretions on male fertility. *In* Fitzpatrick JM, Krane RJ: The Prostate. New York, Churchill Livingstone, 1989, pp 53–59.

174. Peitz B, Olds-Clark EP: Effect of seminal vesicle renal fertility and uterine sperm motility in the house mouse. J Reprod 35:608–617, 1986.

175. Pienta KJ, Partin AW, Coffey DS: Cancer as a disease of DNA organization and dynamic cell structure. Cancer Res 49:2525–2532, 1989.

176. Purnell DM, Heatfield BM, Trump BF: Immunocytochemical evaluation of human prostatic carcinomas for carcinoembryonic antigen, nonspecific crossreacting antigen, beta-chorionic gonadotropins and prostate-specific antigen. Cancer Res 44:285–292, 1984.

177. Rajfer J, Coffey DS: Sex steroid imprinting of the immature prostate: Long term effects. Invest Urol 16:186, 1979.

178. Rajfer J, Coffey DS: Effects of neonatal steroids on sex tissues. Invest Urol 17:3, 1979.

179. Reese JH, McNeil JE, Redwine EA, et al: Tissue type plasminogen activator marker for functional zones, within the human prostate. Prostate 12:47–53, 1988.

180. Rennie PS, Bouffard R, Bruchovsky N, Chang H: Increased activity of plasminogen activators during involution of rat ventral prostate. Biochem J 221:171–178, 1984.

181. Rijnders AWM, van der Korput JA, van Steenbrugge GJ, et al: Expression of cellular oncogenes in human prostatic carcinoma cell lines. Biochem Biophys Res Commun 132:548–554, 1985.

182. Rohr HP, Bartsch G: Human benign prostatic hyperplasia. A stromal disease? Urology 16:625–633, 1980.

183. Saltzman AG, Hiipakka RA, Chang C, Liao S: Androgen repression of the production of a 29-kilodalton protein and mRNA in the rat ventral prostate. J Biol Chem 262:432–437, 1987.

184. Sandford ML, Searle JW, Kerr JFR: Successive waves of apoptosis in the rat prostate after repeated withdrawal of testosterone stimulation. Pathology 16:406–410, 1984.

185. Sathe VA, Sheth AR, Sheth NA: Biosynthesis immunoreactive inhibin-like material (IR-ILM) by rat prostate. Prostate 8:401–408, 1986.

186. Schreiter F, Fuchs P, Stockamp K: Estrogenic sensitivity α-receptors in the urethra musculature. Urol Int 31:13, 1976.

187. Schulze H, Barrack ER: The immunocytochemical localization of estrogen receptors in the normal male and female canine urinary tract and prostate. Endocrinology 121:1773–1783, 1987.

188. Schulze H, Barrack ER: The immunocytochemical localization of estrogen receptors in spontaneous and experimentally induced canine prostatic hyperplasia. Prostate 11:145–162, 1987.

189. Sensibar JA, Liu X, Patai B, et al: Characterization of castration-induced cell death in the rat prostate by immunohistochemical localization of cathepsin D. Prostate 16:263–276, 1990.

190. Sheth AR, Pan SE, Vaze AY, et al: Inhibin in the human prostate. Arch Androl 6:317–321, 1981.

191. Sinha AA, Gleason DF, Wilson MJ, et al: Immunohistochemical localization of laminin in basement membranes of normal, hyperplastic and neoplastic human prostate. Prostate 15:299–313, 1989.

192. Sinowatz F, Gabius HJ, Hellmann KP, et al: Expression of endogenous receptor for neoglycoproteins in Dunning R-3327 rat prostatic carcinoma. Prostate 16:173–184, 1990.

193. Smith ER, Hagopian M: Uptake in secretion of carcinogenic chemicals by the dog and rat prostate. *In* Murphy GP, Sandberg AA, Karr JP (eds): The Prostate Cell: Structure and Function, Part B. New York, Alan R. Liss, 1981, pp 131–163.

194. Smith RG, Syms AJ, Nag A, et al: Mechanisms of the glucocorticoid regulation and growth of the androgen-sensitive prostate-derived R3327 H-G8-A1 tumor cells. J Biol Chem 260:12454–12463, 1985.

195. Stahler MS, Pansky B, Budd GC: Immunocytochemical demonstration of insulin or insulin-like immunoreactivity in the rat prostate gland. Prostate 13:189–198, 1988.

196. Stamey TA, Wang N, Hay AR, et al: Prostate-specific antigen as a serum marker for adenocarcinoma of the prostate. N Engl J Med 317:909–916, 1987.

197. Stanisic T, Sadlowski R, Lee C, Grayhack JT: Partial inhibition of castration-induced ventral prostate regression with actinomycin D and cyclohexamide. Invest Urol 16:15–18, 1978.

198. Stone NN, Fair WR, Fishman J: Estrogen formation in human prostatic tissue from patients with and without benign prostatic hyperplasia. Prostate 9:311, 1986.

199. Storey MT, Jacobs SC, Lawson RK: Epidermal growth factor is not the major growth-promoting agent in extracts of prostatic tissues. J Urol 130:175, 1983.

200. Sufrin G, Coffey DS: A new model for studying the effects of drugs on prostatic growth: I. Antiandrogens in DNA synthesis. Invest Urol 11:45–54, 1973.

201. Sugimura Y, Cunha GR, Donjacour AA, et al: Whole mount autoradiography studies of DNA synthetic activity during postnatal development and androgen-induced regeneration in the mouse prostate. Biol Reprod 34:985, 1986.

202. Swanson HE, Vanderwer FF, Werff ten Bosch JJ van der: Sex differences in growth of rats and their modification by a single injection of testosterone propionate shortly after birth. J Endocrinol 26:197–207, 1963.

203. Tan JA, Marschkek B, French FS: Androgen receptor stimulated transcriptional activation mediated by GRE/PRE-like sequences within the prostate in C3 subunit gene. Abstract, Endocrine Society Meeting, June, 1990.

204. Tanabe E, Lee C, Grayhack JT: Activities of cathepsin D in rat prostate during castration-induced involution. J Urol 127:826–828, 1982.

205. Tenniswood M: Role of epithelial-stromal interactions in the control of gene expression in the prostate: An hypothesis. Prostate 9:375–385, 1986.

206. Thompson TC, Chung LWK: Regulation of overgrowth and expression of prostatic binding protein in rat chimeric prostate gland. Endocrinology 118:2437–2444, 1986.

207. Thompson TC, Zhau H, Chung LWK: Catecholamines are involved in the growth and expansion of prostatic binding protein by the rat ventral prostatic tissue. Prog Clin Biol Res 239:239–248, 1987.

208. Thornton MO, Frederickson R, Matal J, Mawhinney M: Preliminary studies on the relationship between collagen and the growth of the male accessory sex organ epithelial cells. *In* Kimball FA, Buehl AE, Carter DP (eds): New Approaches to the Study of Benign Prostatic Hyperplasia. New York, Alan R. Liss, 1984.

209. Tilley WD, Marcelli M, McPhaul MJ: Recent studies of the androgen receptor: New insights into old questions. Mol Cell Endocrinol 68:C7–C10, 1990.

210. Tilley WD, Marcelli M, Wilson JD, McPhaul MJ: Characterization and expression of cDNA in coding the human androgen receptor. Proc Natl Acad Sci USA 86:327–331, 1989.

211. Trachtenberg J, Hicks LL, Walsh PC: Methods for the determination of androgen receptor concentration in human prostatic tissue. Invest Urol 18:349, 1981.

212. Traish AM, Wotiz HH: Prostatic epidermal growth factor receptors and their regulation by androgens. Endocrinology 121:1461–1467, 1987.

213. Tunn S, Senge TH, Schenck B, Neumann F: Biochemical and histological studies on prostates in castrated dogs after treatment with androstanediol, estradiol and cyproterone acetate. Acta Endocrinol 91:373–384, 1979.

214. Vogelstein B, Pardoll DM, Coffey DS: Supercoiled loops in eukaryotic DNA replication. Cell 22:79–85, 1980.

215. Walsh PC: Techniques for radical retropubic prostatectomy with preservation of sexual function: An anatomical approach. *In* Skinner DJ, Lieskovsky G (eds): Diagnosis and Management of Genitourinary Cancer. Philadelphia, WB Saunders Co, 1988, pp 735–778.

216. Walsh PC, Wilson JD: The induction of prostatic hypertrophy in the dog with androstanediol. J Clin Invest 57:1093, 1976.

217. Wang MC, Valenzuela LA, Murphy GP, Chu TM: Purification of a human prostate specific antigen. Invest Urol 17:159–163, 1979.
218. Wernert TN, Dohm G: Immunohistochemistry of the prostate and diverse prostate carcinomas. *In* Aumuller G, Krieg K, Senge TH (eds): New Aspects in the Regulation of Prostatic Function. Cansteiner Colloquium, Schloss Canstein. Munich, Zuckschwerdt, 1989, pp 69–81.
219. Wilding G, Valvaerius E, Knabbe C, Gelman EP: The role of transforming growth factor α in human prostate cancer cell growth. Prostate 15:1–2, 1989.
220. Williams-Ashman HG: Regulatory features of the seminal vesicle development and function. Curr Topics Cell Regul 22:201–275, 1983.
221. Wilson EM, Colvard DS: Factors that influence interaction of the androgen receptor with nuclei and nuclear matrix. Ann NY Acad Sci 438:85, 1984.
222. Wolff H, Anderson DJ: Male genital tract inflammation is associated with increased numbers of potential human immunodeficiency virus host cells in semen. Andrologia 20:404–405, 1988.
223. Wyllie AH, Kerr JFR, Currie AR: Cell death: The significance of apoptosis. Int Rev Cytol 68:251–306, 1986.

ACKNOWLEDGMENTS: I gratefully acknowledge Ruth Middleton for her expertise in the preparation of the manuscript and Donald Vindivich for his help in the preparation of the illustrations.

Chapter 5

ENDOCRINOLOGY OF THE PROSTATE

EARL CHENG, CHUNG LEE, and JOHN GRAYHACK

The prostate, the major accessory sex gland in the male, has exocrine but no established endocrine secretory function.[65] The adult gland, however, contains endocrine responsive tissue and its growth is hormone-dependent, with the most important of these hormones being androgen. Numerous other hormones such as estrogens, prolactin, and insulin are also known to influence prostatic growth. Despite this, testosterone and other androgens are clearly the most important and essential hormones in cellular proliferation and growth of the prostate, as well as maintenance of the adult prostate in its mature and differentiated state. The importance of androgens in prostate physiology is exemplified by our current management of benign prostatic hyperplasia (BPH) and carcinoma of the prostate, in which much of our therapy is directed toward the elimination of androgen or the altering of its effects on prostatic tissue. This chapter reviews the relevant anatomy, histology, and physiology of the prostate pertinent to our discussion of endocrinology of the prostate. We then discuss in detail our current knowledge of the various hormones known to influence prostatic growth. Last, we briefly summarize our current understanding of the effects of androgen on prostatic growth and differentiation on a cellular level.

RELEVANT ANATOMY, HISTOLOGY, AND PHYSIOLOGY

The topics of anatomy, histology, and physiology of the prostate are discussed at length in another section of this book, but certain aspects of these topics need to be highlighted and emphasized in our discussion of endocrinology of the prostate. Knowledge of these pertinent points allows one to better understand the effect and role that certain hormones have in the regulation of prostatic growth. Because much of our understanding of the physiology and morphology of the prostate has come from information derived from studies using various animal models, we discuss not only the human prostate but also some of the animals used as models in the study of the prostate.

Anatomy

The human prostate is a compound tubuloalveolar gland that lies at the base of the bladder. The normal internal architecture is an area of great interest and has pathophysiologic significance with respect to the origin of various disease processes. Lowsley in the early 1900s studied the fetal prostate and was able to divide the prostate into five discrete lobes.[116, 117] Since then, it has become clear from the work of Franks and McNeal that the adult prostate does not retain this lobar architecture.[57–59] Based on three-dimensional reconstruction of the adult prostate (prior to the development of BPH), McNeal observed that the urethra separates the prostate into the ventral (fibromuscular) and dorsal (glandular) portions. The glandular prostate can be further separated into four distinct regions: peripheral zone, central zone, transitional zone, and periurethral gland region.[125, 126, 128–131] The clinical significance of these zones is that carcinoma is believed to arise primarily in the peripheral zone, whereas BPH initially develops in the transitional zone and periurethral glands. Numerous animal models have been used in the past to study the physiology and hormonal responsiveness of the prostate; the majority of these studies have been conducted in the rat and the dog. Like the human prostate, the adult canine prostate does not have discrete lobes but, unlike the human, the gland is relatively homogeneous throughout, with no histologic evidence of any discrete zones. In the rat and other rodents, the prostate is divided into individual and encapsulated lobes: ventral, dorsal, lateral, and anterior prostate. Each lobe has a separate set of compound ducts with distinctive branching patterns.[169]

Histology

Histologically, the human prostate consists of 30 to 50 branching tubuloalveolar glands with an intervening stroma.[111, 197] The acinar epithelium consists of two cell types: (1) glandular or secretory cell, which is tall, columnar, and luminal in orientation, and (2) a nonsecretory basal cell, which is flattened and cuboidal and abuts a distinct eosinophilic basement membrane. This basement membrane separates the epithelial cells from the stromal cells, and its importance will become more apparent in our discussion later on epithelial-stromal cell interaction. The glandular or secretory epithelium predominates in the human prostate and has numerous secretions, many of which are hormone dependent and have become markers of hormone activity (see section on physiology). Numerous roles of the basal cell have been postulated, including (1) stem cells capable of differentiating into columnar secretory cells,[120, 132, 176] (2) cells capable of transporting material from the stroma to the secretory cells and vice versa,[86] and (3) origin of various disease processes and target of neoplastic agents.[18, 48] The stroma of the prostate consists predominantly of smooth muscle cells, fibroblasts, lymphocytes, and neuromuscular tissue, all embedded within an extracellular matrix.[10] These smooth muscle cells and the fibroblasts are in close approximation to the aforementioned basement membrane, with the smooth muscle cells most likely involved in epithelial–smooth muscle cell interaction.[173]

Physiology

The exact role that the prostate plays in the reproductive process is not entirely clear. The prostate is known to be an exocrine gland whose secretions are somewhat unique and are involved in the process of insemination. The metabolic activity and subsequent products of the prostatic epithelial cell are endocrine responsive and controlled. These secretions are highly complex and heterogeneous.[180] Two-dimensional electrophoresis has demonstrated literally hundreds of distinct moieties, of which only a fraction have been well delineated. Some of these have been better characterized than others and are pertinent to our discussion of endocrinology of the prostate; these include citrate, prostate-specific antigen (PSA), and prostatic acid phosphatase (PAP). Citrate is an important carbohydrate found in prostatic fluid and human seminal plasma. In humans, it may act as a major chelating agent for metal ions. In animals, it has been used as a biologic marker of hormonal stimulation in numerous investigations.[119]

PAP and PSA are two enzymes present in prostatic secretions which have found great clinical use as markers in following disease progression in carcinoma of the prostate. Both are androgen dependent and have also been used as markers of prostate cell differentiation in both in vivo and in vitro experiments. As its name implies, PAP splits organic phosphate with optimal activity at a pH range of 4 to 6. In the dog, the concentration of this enzyme in prostatic secretions seems to reflect biologic androgen stimulation. In man, the mean concentration of PAP decreases progressively with aging.[66] Despite its clinical importance, a unique or essential role for PAP in prostatic growth and function has yet to be identified. PSA, although used in a similar clinical fashion to PAP, is biologically and immunologically distinct.[135] PSA is a kallikrein-like serine protease that is produced exclusively by the secretory epithelial cells lining the acini, either benign or malignant.[112, 190] PSA is responsible for the liquefaction of the seminal coagulum that is formed at the time of ejaculation.[113] Numerous other secretory products of the prostate epithelial cell are currently being investigated with respect to their actions and hormone responsiveness. These include various polyamines, prostate-binding protein, spermine-binding protein, and others. Further description of these is beyond the scope of the present discussion.

HORMONES INFLUENCING PROSTATIC GROWTH

The human prostate undergoes an increase in size and develops histologic evidence of stimulated growth during three periods of life: (1) prior to and at birth, (2) during puberty, and (3) with achievement of advancing age.[171] During these times, the prostate is maintained and functions in a multihormonal environment. How each one of these hormones influences the maintenance and growth of the prostate is not entirely known. We do know, however, that the most important of these hormones is androgen. Androgens are clearly essential because the prostate cannot develop, differentiate, or maintain its size or function in their absence.[72] Although other hormones may have an active role, none of these thus far has been found to be as critical or important as testosterone and other androgens. In this section, we review our current knowledge of androgens and other hormones influencing prostatic growth. This includes a discussion of each hormone's action on the prostate, biochemistry, physiology, and regulation. We also investigate the possible existence of a nonandrogenic testicular factor involved in the stimulation of prostate growth.

The Effect of Androgens on the Prostate

One cannot overemphasize the importance of androgens in our current understanding of the regulation of prostatic growth. Androgens clearly have an active and permissive role in normal and most pathologic types of prostatic growth. This androgen dependence of prostatic development is evident both prenatally and postnatally. Abundant human and animal data support this. Prenatally, the development of the prostate, as well as other male internal accessory structures, is androgen dependent. Ablation of the fetal testis prior to sexual differentiation inhibits the development of the prostate and other male internal sex glands.[93] The fetal testis produces testosterone as its primary androgen, but its conversion to dihydrotestosterone (DHT) by 5α-reductase is necessary for development of the prostate and male external genitalia. Therefore, deficiency of this enzyme, as is present in certain identified families of male pseudohermaphrodites in the Dominican Republic, results in feminization of the external genitalia and a rudimentary or absent prostate.[87–90] 5α-Reductase activity and androgen receptors have been located in the urogenital sinus in both animals and humans.[100, 161, 163, 172, 195, 196]

Postnatally, androgen is also necessary for further development of the prostate. When neonatal rats are castrated, further growth and development of the prostate are inhibited; this can be reversed by the administration of testosterone.[16, 41, 145] Also, if exogenous testosterone is given to immature rats, accelerated prostatic growth occurs such that maximal size is reached precociously. Once this occurs, additional androgen administration does not result in further increased prostatic size, cell number, or DNA content.[16, 146] Further demonstrating the need for androgen in the neonatal and postnatal periods is the fact that when intact and castrate neonatal rats are treated with estradiol, ventral prostatic growth is severely diminished during this time; in addition, response to exogenous androgens administered during adulthood is very limited when compared with control animals.[150]

Much of our knowledge of how androgen regulates prostatic cell proliferation and gene expression has come from the study of the castrate rat ventral prostate. Numerous proteins are contained within the secretions of the rat ventral prostate, with the most prominent of these being prostate-binding protein (PBP). PBP, also known as prostein,[102] α-protein,[32, 33] prostatic secretory protein,[144] or estramustine-binding protein,[55] is the major protein secreted by the rat ventral prostate and has been used along with spermine-binding protein as a marker of androgenic stimulation and action. In the normal intact rat, C1-C3 peptides (subunits) of PBP account for 30 to 50 per cent of the total proteins synthesized by the rat ventral prostate, whereas castration results in a 1000-fold decrease in C1-C3 mRNA, making the postcastration contribution of PBP to the total protein content less than 1 per cent.[29, 76, 137, 138, 142]

With the administration of testosterone to the castrated rat, numerous well-described events occur which result in the restoration of prostate size and function. Following the administration of testosterone, PBP mRNA, as well as evidence of other RNA synthesis, is detectable within 2 hours.[139] Biochemical analysis of prostate homogenates after treatment of castrate rats with testosterone demonstrates that the DNA synthetic rate markedly increases after a lag time of approximately 48 hours, with a peak activity at 72 hours.[22, 34, 36, 163] Similar to the observations made in the immature rat prostate, further stimulation with androgen results in prolonged stimulation of DNA synthesis for 4 to 5 days, with a return to basal levels once prostatic cell number returns to normal precastrate levels. These results indicate that, although androgen is necessary for the development of the prostate, as well as restoration of the prostate following castration, another regulating factor (steroidal or nonsteroidal) may be involved in controlling cellular division as well as the initiation of further cell proliferative processes such as BPH or carcinoma of the prostate. Although the most pronounced proliferative activity of prostatic cells in response to androgen has been observed in prostatic epithelial cells (in vivo), increased replication has also been demonstrated in cells of the connective tissue and vasculature.[46, 52]

Currently, it is not clear how the coupling of androgen and androgen receptors results in the initiation of DNA synthesis, production of proteins, and subsequent cellular proliferation. Also needing clarification is the regulatory process controlling the number of androgen receptors present within the cell. Despite this, it seems reasonable at this time to conclude that androgens are essential for prostatic cell proliferation but that other influential factors exist with regard to the control of cell proliferation.

Many of the above investigations demonstrating the importance of androgen in the development of the prostate used testosterone as the primary androgen. It is now known that testosterone in the prostate most likely functions as a prehormone for DHT, which is the active androgen involved in prostatic growth. In 1968, Bruchovsky and Wilson demonstrated that DHT, not testosterone, is the major intracellular androgen in the prostate.[3, 23, 24] Once converted to DHT in the cytoplasm of target cells, both testosterone and DHT may individually bind to an androgen receptor, resulting in a steroid-receptor complex (Fig. 5–1). The exact location of the androgen receptor is an issue of current controversy. Evidence indicates that under normal physiologic conditions, it most likely is located in the nucleus, whereas in the castrated state, there may be some partial redistribution to the cytosol.[14, 96, 191] Nevertheless, this complex then binds to specific DNA sites in the nucleus, giving rise to the formation of various secretory and regulatory proteins. This androgen receptor is unique among steroid receptors in that it exhibits a two- to three-fold higher binding affinity for DHT than testosterone.[143] With regard to benign prostatic hyperplasia, it was initially thought that DHT levels in BPH tissue were three to four times that of normal tissue, but more recent work by Walsh et al in 1983 and 1984 demonstrated no significant differences in DHT tissue levels between BPH and peripheral prostate tissue.[186, 188] On the other hand, DHT receptor content may be increased in the nucleus and cytoplasm of BPH tissue.[13] Whether or not differential activity of 5α-reductase on androgen plays a role in the development of BPH or carcinoma of the prostate remains to be seen.

In the adult prostate, androgen plays a role in the maintenance of the gland in a mature and differentiated

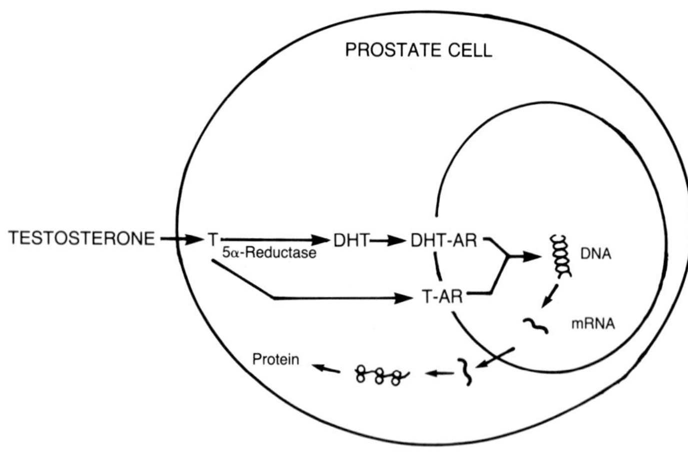

FIGURE 5–1. Androgen action in the prostate: Testosterone (T) diffuses into the prostate cell, where it is converted to dihydrotestosterone (DHT) by 5α-reductase. The androgen receptor (AR) then individually binds T or DHT (with preferential binding of DHT) to form a steroid-receptor complex. This complex then gives rise to the transcription of mRNA, which in turn results in the production of androgen-dependent regulatory and structural proteins.

state. The prostate, prior to the occurrence of BPH, is maintained by homeostatic mechanisms that are androgen dependent. The fact that the adult rat prostate does not enlarge despite the administration of exogenous androgens, but maintains its normal size, suggests a delicate balance of cell death and cell renewal during this time despite high concentration of androgen.[16, 91] In contrast, if the majority of androgen is eliminated, as in castration, striking regression occurs. Castration has long been known to halt prostate growth and cause shrinkage of the prostate.[26, 69, 85, 193] In fact, prior to prostatectomy, castration was used for the treatment of BPH. Interestingly, early trials utilizing castration for relief of bladder neck obstruction secondary to BPH yielded inconsistent therapeutic results. Some patients had immediate marked improvement in their symptoms, whereas others had minimal to no improvement.[47, 83]

Histology demonstrated that castration results in a decrease in the epithelial component in BPH, but not the stromal component.[184, 192] Therefore, those with predominantly stromal BPH would not benefit well from bilateral orchiectomy, suggesting that perhaps growth of stroma is irreversible.[107] The differences that exist between the stromal and epithelial response to hormonal manipulation are extremely important and are discussed below.

The prostate regression that is seen after castration is not simply the result of a single biologic phenomenon that is the direct result of the cessation of the anabolic activities in the prostatic tissue in the absence of testicular androgens. The requirement of an active metabolic process for tissue atrophy in a regressing prostate was first postulated by Bruchovsky and associates in 1975.[2] They observed that the rapid rate of cell loss in a regressing prostate was greater than the expected normal cell turnover rate, which was only 8 per cent in 3 days. Since then, Lee et al have demonstrated that this rapid rate of cell death following castration depends upon the synthesis of specific macromolecules or degradative enzymes that can be partially blocked by the inhibition of RNA and protein synthesis.[106] These and other investigations have led to the concept of "programmed cell death" in the prostate, or apoptosis. More than likely, under normal physiologic conditions, some cells in the

prostate are undergoing programmed cell death, balancing those that are proliferating. Some investigators have postulated that androgen may have a protective effect on the remaining cells and inhibits their active cell death under normal conditions. The removal of androgen would therefore result in active programmed cell death in these formerly "protected" cells.

This rapid response of prostate tissue to castration gained tremendous clinical application when Huggins, in his classic experiments in 1940, introduced the concept of androgen dependence of carcinoma of the prostate.[81, 82] Since that time, despite numerous advances in our knowledge of prostate cancer and endocrinology of the prostate, castration remains a major therapeutic option in the treatment of prostate cancer. The fact that certain cells survive following the removal of androgen from castration suggests that these cells may be independent of the effects of androgen and may be the cells responsible for further disease progression in prostate cancer patients following castration.

Regulation of Androgen

The amount of androgen in the serum available for tissue use is regulated mainly by the hypothalamic pituitary axis. The hypothalamus lies at the base of the brain just above the pituitary gland and has extensive links to other brain areas important in visceral, autonomic, and behavioral function. The median eminence or infundibulum is a highly vascular structure that serves as a communication between the hypothalamus and pituitary through which the pituitary receives humoral messages from the hypothalamus and its rich blood supply. The pituitary gland is divided into two parts: adenohypophysis and neurohypophysis. The adenohypophysis (anterior pituitary) secretes several hormones, including gonadotropins, adrenocorticotropin, prolactin, somatotropin, and thyrotropin. On the other hand, the neurohypophysis (posterior pituitary) has more of a storage role than a secretory role, storing vasopressin and oxytocin, which are secreted from the hypothalamus.[152] The previously mentioned gonadotropins—follicle-stimulating hormone (FSH) and luteinizing hormone (LH)—are involved in the regulation of androgen production. FSH and LH are glycoproteins secreted by the gonadotrophs of the anterior pituitary; the gonadotrophs are also known as "castration cells" because of their marked enlargement following removal of the gonads. Current evidence indicates that the gonadotrophs are capable of secreting either or both of these gonadotropins. Both LH and FSH contain an α and a β chain. The α chain of each is identical, containing 96 amino acids. This α chain is also identical to the ones contained in thyroid-stimulating hormone and human choriogonadotropin. The β chain of each of these hormones is unique and conveys hormonal specificity and biologic activity.[95] FSH and LH both have gonadotropic influences on the testis, the major source of androgen. Although this interaction between FSH, LH, and the testis is very complex, simplistically speaking, FSH promotes spermatogenesis whereas LH stimulates secretion of androgen from testicular Leydig cells.[94]

Secretion and release of LH and FSH from the anterior pituitary with subsequent androgen production from the testis is modulated by two separate mechanisms: (1) trophic influence from the hypothalamus and (2) negative feedback from circulating sex steroids. With regard to the first mechanism, luteinizing hormone–releasing hormone (LHRH) is secreted by the hypothalamus and stimulates the pituitary to then secrete LH and, to a somewhat lesser extent, FSH. LHRH, also known as gonadotropin-releasing hormone (GnRH), is released from the hypothalamus in a pulsatile fashion, thus giving rise to pulsatile and rhythmic secretion of pituitary gonadotropins. The hypothalamus has an overall stimulatory effect on pituitary secretion of LH, FSH, and subsequent androgen production from the testis (Fig. 5–2). The negative feedback of the sex steroids on gonadotropin release comes from the testis and occurs at both the hypothalamic and pituitary level. Castration and elimination of this negative feedback result in a marked rise in FSH and LH. Both testosterone and estradiol are capable of exerting this negative feedback, although probably by separate mechanisms and pathways. Both testosterone and estradiol seem to exert their effect at the level of the hypothalamus, where they slow the hypothalamus pulse generator and subsequent release of LH. Testosterone, in addition, is also able to decrease LH secretion by exerting a negative feedback mechanism directly at the level of the pituitary gland. Despite this, it has been demonstrated in male and female castrated rats that the overall decrease in synthesis and release of gonadotropins is greater with estrogen than that of testosterone.[35] Also, testosterone preferentially inhibits LH relative to FSH, whereas estrogen produces parallel inhibition of both LH and FSH. Inhibin, a protein product of the Sertoli cells in the testis, is also able to inhibit the production of FSH but has minimal, if any, effect on LH secretion[45] (Fig. 5–2).

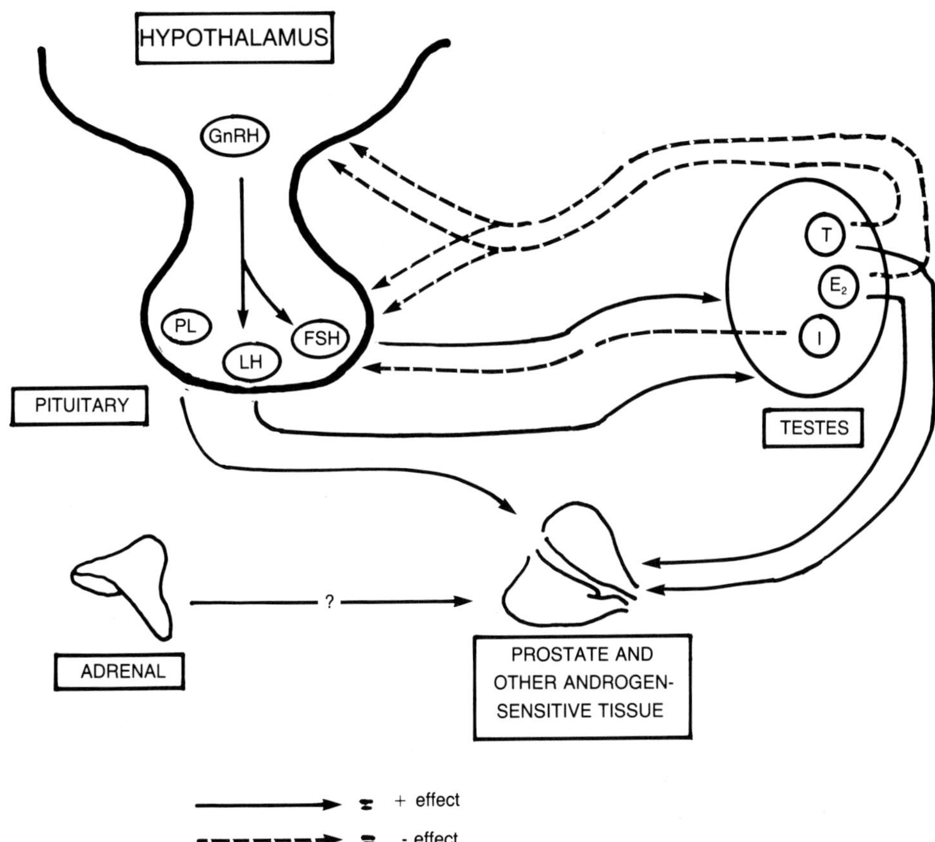

FIGURE 5–2. Endocrine relationship between the hypothalamus, pituitary, prostate, testis, and adrenal (see text for details). GnRH = Gonadotropin-releasing hormone; LH = luteinizing hormone; FSH = follicle-stimulating hormone; PL = prolactin; T = testosterone; E_2 = estradiol; I = inhibin.

The overall regulation of androgen production by the hypothalamus and pituitary gland is somewhat complex. A clear understanding of this system is necessary for the practicing urologist and others involved in the management of prostate diseases because much of our current therapy for BPH and prostate cancer is based upon our current knowledge of androgen regulation. Hormonal and pharmacologic manipulation of the prostate in BPH and prostate cancer is discussed further in other chapters in this text.

Testicular Androgens

Under normal circumstances, testosterone is the major circulating androgen in the male responsible for prostatic growth. Greater than 95 per cent of this is of testicular origin. Testosterone is synthesized from cholesterol by testicular Leydig cells. Five enzymes are needed for the conversion of cholesterol to testosterone. The rate-limiting and crucial step in this process is the conversion of cholesterol to pregnenolone. This step seems to be governed by pituitary LH, which binds to a membrane receptor on Leydig cells and gives rise to cyclic AMP via adenylate cyclase. This in turn activates Leydig cell protein kinase, which stimulates the conversion of cholesterol to pregnenolone.

The testosterone concentration in the spermatic veins (10,000 to 60,000 ng/dl) is approximately 75 times higher than that of peripheral venous serum (300 to 1000 ng/dl). Minimal concentrations of other androgens are also produced by the testis and leave via the spermatic vein. These include androstanediol, androstenedione, and dehydroepiandrosterone (DHEA). In the plasma, testosterone circulates in three forms: 2 per cent is free, 45 to 75 per cent is bound to testosterone-binding globulin (TeBG), and 30 to 55 per cent is bound to albumin. Because the testosterone bound to TeBG dissociates poorly and is unavailable for tissue uptake, the percentage of total testosterone available for tissue use is around 40 to 50 per cent. This represents the fraction of testosterone that is free and albumin bound. This available testosterone then follows one of three major pathways.

1. Testosterone acts as a prohormone for target cells (e.g., prostate), where conversion to DHT occurs in the cytoplasm of these cells via 5α-reductase.

2. Conversion of testosterone to the following weak and inactive androgens: DHEA (a weak adrenal androgen), androsterone (by hepatic 5α reduction), and etiocholanolone (hepatic 5β reduction).

3. Conversion of testosterone to 17β-estradiol by aromatization in peripheral tissues.[94]

As described earlier, testosterone in the prostate is then converted to DHT by 5α-reductase, which gives rise to a cascade of events resulting in the production of various regulatory proteins.

Adrenal Androgens

The adrenal gland is capable of primarily secreting three relatively weak androgens: DHEA, dehydroepi-androsterone sulfate (DHEAS), and androstenedione; and testosterone. All of these adrenal androgens are synthesized from cholesterol and acetate and are C19 steroids. Of these, the principal adrenal androgens are DHEA and androstenedione. Adrenal androgens are not considered a source of potent androgens, either because of their inherent activity or because of their small amount of conversion to stronger androgens. DHEA is itself a weak androgen and may be converted to the more potent androgen testosterone, but less than 1 per cent of plasma testosterone is derived from DHEA. Recent work by Labrie, however, has demonstrated that DHEA and androstenedione may be converted to testosterone by 17β-hydroxy steroid dehydrogenase in prostatic tissue.[99, 175] DHEAS can be converted by prostatic tissue to potent androgen metabolites such as DHT after sulfatase and 5α reductive reactions. This conversion is extremely low, however. Therefore, DHEAS itself is very unlikely to be a potent androgen.

Whether or not adrenal androgens contribute significantly to prostatic growth is still an area of great interest and controversy. Adrenalectomy alone in rats has little effect on prostatic size, DNA, growth, or morphology of sex tissue.[9, 133] Castration without adrenalectomy results in 90 per cent reduction in prostate size without any restoration later. In castrated rats, the addition of adrenalectomy did not result in further reduction in cell number or DNA synthesis. This seems to indicate that adrenal androgens are unable to compensate for the loss of testicular androgen with respect to prostatic growth.[35] On the other hand, in castrated animals, increasing levels of ACTH by exogenous administration results in increased prostatic growth.[9, 177, 181, 187]

Although much of our evidence concerning the role of adrenal androgens on prostate growth comes from animal experiments, it is generally agreed that under normal physiologic conditions in man, adrenal androgens play little role in prostatic growth.[122] In the setting of prostate cancer, clinical evidence regarding a limited role for adrenal androgens in promoting or maintaining growth of the neoplasm has recently been a source of intense controversy and investigation. Several studies in prostate cancer patients involving the suppression or end-organ blockade of adrenal androgens following the elimination or suppression of testicular androgens (total androgen blockade) have recently been reported or are in progress. Early results are conflicting; some show a slightly prolonged survival in patients receiving total androgen blockade, whereas others do not.[38, 156, 158, 159] Additional knowledge regarding the metabolism of adrenal androgens in prostate tissue is needed to clarify further the role of adrenal androgens in prostatic growth and prostate cancer. Further discussion of the role of adrenal androgens in prostate cancer and the results of recent clinical trials are detailed in Chapter 27.

Estrogen

Most of the estrogen in the male is derived from the peripheral conversion of androstenedione and testosterone to estrone and estradiol.[80, 118] This aromatization occurs in peripheral tissue, most likely adipose tissue. Up to 75 to 90 per cent of the estrogen in male serum is derived in this fashion. A small amount of estrogen is also secreted into the blood directly from the testis. The cells responsible for this are probably the Sertoli cells.[50]

Estrogen is known to have two separate effects on prostatic growth, one that is permissive and one that is suppressive. The latter results from the inhibition of LH secretion that estrogen is able to exert on the hypothalamic-pituitary axis through the negative feedback system previously described. The resultant drop in serum testosterone and involution of prostatic epithelium have been demonstrated by numerous investigators.[15, 81, 192] On the other hand, in the dog, estrogen in combination with androgen has been shown to cause increased prostatic growth beyond what would be expected with androgen alone.[92, 182, 183] Thus, estrogen has a permissive and synergistic action with androgen in the growth of the prostate. This was also demonstrated in the rat, in which lateral lobe prostatic growth and citric acid production were increased with the addition of estrogen to androgen.[63] This synergistic effect of estrogen with androgen in the rat is most likely created by estrogen's ability to cause a marked increase in release of prolactin from the anterior pituitary. Prolactin, as discussed later, is known to have a positive effect on prostatic growth. This mechanism was supported by a study by Lee et al, which demonstrated that estrogen did not enhance androgen-stimulated prostatic growth in hypophysectomized rats.[108]

Estrogen also has direct actions on the prostate, including stimulation of fibromuscular tissue[4, 11, 60, 178, 185] and the induction of squamous metaplasia of prostate epithelium.[11, 25, 84, 103, 104, 121, 147, 179] This induced squamous metaplasia is reversible in the adult with estrogen withdrawal, whereas in the neonate it may be irreversible.[8, 124] Estrogen receptors have been identified in both epithelial and stromal cells of humans and various animals. A higher concentration of estrogen receptors in the stromal tissue has been reported and has thus prompted the postulation that this is the primary site of action for estrogen.[12, 30, 61, 98, 114] In the canine prostate, immunocytochemical studies have identified a greater localization of estrogen receptors in the stromal and ductal epithelium in the periurethral region as opposed to the other areas of acinar epithelium, fostering speculation about the role of estrogen in the development of BPH.[127, 157] The fact that significant alternations occur in the ratio of estrogen to androgen in the serum of aging men has also prompted investigators to study the role of estrogen in BPH.[70, 71, 73, 121, 194] In the human, the localization of the estrogen receptor has long been a controversial issue. This most likely is secondary to the heterogeneity of estrogen-binding sites in prostatic tissue. Multiple binding sites for estrogen have been reported to be present in cytosol as well as nuclear preparations of human prostatic tissues.[51]

Further evidence supporting an additional direct action of estrogen on prostate cells comes from work with the compound estramustine phosphate, a nor-nitrogen mustard carbamate derivative of estradiol-17β-phosphate. Estramustine has been shown to inhibit microtubular assembly and mitotic activity in prostatic carcinoma cell lines DU-145 and PC-3.[75, 167] The mechanism of action of estramustine is not clear, although some evidence suggests that its oncolytic activity may not be attributable to the estrogen moiety or the nitrogen mustard but to a mechanism not yet defined.[174]

Exactly how estrogen exerts its numerous effects on prostatic growth and BPH in man remains to be further clarified. The above recent evidence emphasizes the notion that we will not truly understand the importance of the actions of estrogen and other regulatory hormones involved in prostatic growth until we better clarify and elucidate the cellular events in the regulation of prostate growth.

Prolactin

Prolactin is secreted from the anterior pituitary and is the major hormone responsible for breast enlargement and milk formation in the pregnant female. Its role in the male is not as clearly defined. Grayhack et al were the first to demonstrate prolactin's permissive effect on prostatic growth when they noted its ability to cause increased growth of the lateral lobes of the rat prostate.[64] This has been confirmed by others.[79, 148] Since that time, additional evidence demonstrating a potential role for prolactin in the regulation of prostatic growth has been produced. Patients with BPH have been found to have higher levels of prolactin in serum than do controls.[154] Prolactin receptors have also been demonstrated in prostatic tissue.[7] Prolactin has been shown to stimulate the citric acid production in the rat lateral prostate.[63, 67, 153, 189] This increased citrate production from prostatic epithelial cells has been demonstrated recently in an in vitro model.[56] Lloyd et al demonstrated that prolactin alters androgen uptake and metabolism in the prostate.[115] Recent studies have also shown that the permeability of the prostatic cell membrane to androgen in patients with BPH may be altered in response to prolactin.[53] Like estrogen, the fashion in which prolactin is able to regulate prostatic growth, either alone or in synergism with androgen, will, it is hoped, be clarified as our knowledge of cellular events in this process increases.

Other Hormones Influencing Prostatic Growth

Because prostatic growth occurs in a multihormonal environment, numerous other hormones have been investigated with respect to their possible influence on this growth. These include insulin, growth hormone, thyroid hormones, and adrenocorticotropins. Insulin is secreted from the beta cells in the pancreas and has a major regulatory function in glucose storage and metabolism. Insulin is thought to have a mitogenic effect on growth of the prostate which is similar to that of prolactin. This has been demonstrated in numerous rat models and in vitro models, although evidence in the human is lacking.[6] In vitro experiments involving prostatic epithelial cell cultures have shown the need for insulin in the medium for optimal growth.[141] These experiments have also demonstrated the mitogenic effects of insulin as well as other mitogens such as epidermal growth factor and cholera toxin.[123] Insulin receptors as well have now been characterized in rat prostatic epithelial cells, but not stromal cells.[28]

Growth hormone is considered to be the principal hormone promoting body growth and is involved in the regulation of numerous anabolic processes. Immunocytochemical techniques have detected growth hormone, along with its binding sites in the epithelial and stromal regions of benign and malignant prostate cells.[164, 165] Increased serum concentration of growth hormone has been noted in patients with metastatic prostate cancer.[5, 19] Also, growth hormone stimulates the synthesis of ornithine decarboxylase, which results in the formation of putrescine, the precursor of spermidine, spermine, and other polyamines secreted by prostatic epithelial cells.[1, 149] Whether or not the above evidence signifies that growth hormone has any functional significance in the prostate is unclear at this time.

Although few investigations have looked at the effect of thyroid hormones on prostatic growth, the limited available evidence shows a possible stimulatory effect. In hypophysectomized rats, treatment with thyroxin results in a significant increase in prostate weight.[64] Recently, it has been shown that in rats treated from birth to 25 days of age with a reversible goitrogen (PTU), a significant increase in testicular and accessory sex gland weight, as well as DNA content, was noted with the onset of maturity. This occurred despite the absence of any increase in serum testosterone levels.[37] Although the above information is not conclusive in demonstrating a direct role of thyroid hormones in the elicitation or promotion of prostatic growth, it suggests that an interrelationship exists between the thyroid and prostate with respect to androgen-stimulated prostatic growth.

Evidence also exists that adrenocorticosteroids may influence prostatic growth. Glucocorticoids are able to stimulate prostatic epithelial cells in culture.[123] Administration of cortisol to castrated rats retards cell and weight loss of the prostate.[151] Also, rat and human prostates contain significant amounts of glucocorticoid receptor mRNA.[31] As is the case with the other hormones mentioned, adrenocorticosteroids clearly have some action in prostate cells; their unique contribution to the growth of normal and pathologic prostate cells in vivo has not yet been established.

NONANDROGENIC ROLE OF TESTIS

In man, intact testis and aging are two prerequisites for prostatic growth and subsequent BPH. With our knowledge that orchiectomy results in rapid prostatic involution and that exogenous androgen reactivates prostatic growth, it has long been presumed that the essential role of the testis in the maintenance and promotion of prostatic growth is its production of testosterone. The fact that BPH progresses in aging males at a time when testosterone levels are declining prompts the suggestion that the testis may function in an unknown manner to promote prostate growth. This may be due to a nonandrogenic accessory sex gland–stimulating factor. Evidence for this hypothesis now exists. In 1961, Grayhack demonstrated from an autopsy study that seminal vesicle fluid fructose (an androgen-dependent indicator of seminal vesicle stimulation) showed a progressive profound decrease with age, whereas seminal vesicle weight (a multihormone-dependent indicator of hormonal stimulation) remained constant.[62] These observations support the concept of an effective, at least with regard to weight promotion, accessory sex gland–stimulating substance(s) in the aged male that is not androgen. More recently, in 1985, Grayhack et al demonstrated that the irradiation of testes in dogs with established BPH yielded a decrease in prostate size and the amount of hyperplasia. This contrasted with the BPH in the dogs with intact testes.[68] The level of testosterone was not significantly different in either group, supporting an absence or very limited effect of irradiation on Leydig cell function. These observations strongly suggest that a cellular component in the testis other than the Leydig cells contributes to the regulation of prostatic growth. Recently, Dalton et al and Darras et al have demonstrated an increase in ventral prostate weight, DNA, and protein concentration in rats with intact testes given exogenous DHT or testosterone compared with castrated rats.[43, 44] Once again, this supports the hypothetical secretion of nonandrogenic prostate-stimulating factor from either the testis or the epididymis. An attempt has been made to identify this proposed factor in male seminal plasma. In vitro experiments using human seminal plasma and human benign prostatic epithelial and stromal cells have shown the presence of prostate-stimulating substance(s) in semen. One of the stimulating proteins with a molecular weight of approximately 30 kD was absent from the semen of vasectomized men.[20] Evidence for the existence of a nonandrogenic testicular factor that is able to alter the growth of the androgen-stimulated or maintained prostate is strong but is still being accumulated and is preliminary.

EFFECT OF HORMONES ON A CELLULAR LEVEL: EPITHELIAL-STROMAL CELL INTERACTION

As mentioned earlier, the prostate consists of both stromal and epithelial cells. Over the past 15 years, an abundance of evidence has demonstrated the importance of cellular heterogeneity in the prostate. It is clear that each of these cellular compartments (stroma and epithelium) has unique characteristics with respect to individual biochemistry and function. This compartmental separation was first suspected when the observation was made that castration results in a disproportionate loss of epithelial to stromal cells.[46] Since then, differences have been found in the level of androgen receptors, estrogen receptors, and other hormone receptors and the amount of 5α-reductase activity in the two compartments.[21, 97, 136] Recent evidence supports the notion that the stromal compartment may be the target of androgen and that the resultant trophic mediators produced by the stroma in response to androgen play an important role in the regulation of structural and functional activity of the epithelial cells in the prostate.[41] In this section, we review the evidence supporting this stromal-epithelial relationship and present a working hypothesis regarding the mechanism of action of androgen on the human prostate.

Androgen is a necessary prerequisite and is the single most important mitogenic hormone responsible for prostatic cell proliferation. Exactly how androgen exerts this effect on a cellular level and whether other determinant factors are involved are unclear. The concepts that there exists a delicate epithelial-stromal balance in the prostate and that stroma may mediate the effects of androgen on the epithelial compartment were first introduced by the classic investigations of Cunha and his colleagues. Conducting experiments with the mesenchyma and epithelial tissue from the embryonic urogenital sinus from normal and testicular feminized mice, they demonstrated that (1) the effects of androgens on the epithelial cells in the urogenital sinus are most likely mediated via trophic influences from the stroma and (2) the responsiveness of the prostatic epithelium is likely dependent on the androgen receptor present in the stroma.[39, 40, 42, 101] If the above is indeed true, the relevance as well as role of the androgen receptor in the epithelial cells is unclear and requires further investigation.

In vitro experimentation, using human and rat epithelial-stromal cells grown in tissue culture, also supports the work of Cuhna. Owing to our ability to grow prostatic epithelial cells and stromal cells separately, information regarding the mechanism of action and growth factors begins to emerge. Unlike the effect of androgen in vivo, androgen has no mitogenic action in prostatic epithelial cells in tissue culture.[54, 109] This is also true for the rat prostatic epithelial cells. Under tissue culture conditions, prostatic epithelial cells are able to proliferate without androgen being present in the culture medium. In fact, the addition of androgen in the culture system has no effect on the growth rate of prostatic epithelial cells. The lack of a direct effect of androgen on epithelial cells indicates that androgen itself is not a mitogenic agent to prostatic epithelial cells. This suggests that if androgen is going to have any effect on the prostatic epithelial cells, as demonstrated under in vivo conditions, it must be mediated indirectly through neighboring cells in a paracrine fashion. The most likely candidate for the latter cells should be in the surrounding stromal compartment.

Epidermal growth factor (EGF), on the other hand, is a potent mitogenic agent to prostatic epithelial cells in culture.[54, 123] Evidence also indicates that levels of EGF in the prostate can be stimulated by treatment of the animal with androgen.[77] Recent observations have indicated that prostatic stromal cells can be stimulated by DHT to proliferate, whereas estrogen has a synergistic effect with androgen on proliferation of stromal cells.[170] It remains to be seen whether or not EGF production by stromal cells can be stimulated by androgen in vitro. Fibroblast growth factor (FGF) is another mitogenic agent to the prostate.[134, 168] Transforming growth factor-α (TGF-α) functions as an autocrine growth factor in a human prostate cancer cell line, PC-3.[78] It is unclear at this stage whether TGF-α plays any role in epithelial proliferation in the normal prostate or in BPH.

Although androgen has no direct effect on epithelial proliferation, it does have a direct promoting effect on epithelial differentiation.[54] When normal prostatic epithelial cells are cultured on a layer of extracellular matrix rather than on a plastic surface, they undergo morphologic modification to assume a differentiated morphology and begin to secrete characteristic differentiated proteins—PAP and PSA in the case of the human prostate.[54] Addition of androgen to the culture medium results in a further increase in the production of PAP and PSA by these cells. These observations suggest that androgen has a direct action in the prostatic epithelial cells in promoting differentiation but not proliferation. Addition of secretory materials collected from cultured stromal cells is able to provoke a further increase in the production of PAP and PSA by prostatic epithelial cells, regardless of whether or not androgen is added to the medium. It is interesting to note that transforming growth factor-β (TGF-β) can replace stromal conditioned media to promote production of PAP and PSA by the prostatic epithelial cells. TGF-β by itself is also able to inhibit proliferation of epithelial cells in culture. These observations suggest that TGF-β or the stromal secretory materials are able to act synergistically with androgen to affect epithelial differentiation in the prostate.

Results of recent studies in rat prostate from our laboratory suggest that a small fraction of epithelial cells in the distal tip of the prostatic ductal system are actively undergoing proliferation.[109, 160] The majority of the epithelial cells are in the differentiated state, whereas a small fraction of epithelial cells in the proximal end of the ductal system are actually undergoing programmed cell death. Recognition of the existence of programmed cell death in a normal rat prostatic ductal system has prompted us to postulate that maintenance of epithelial homeostasis in the prostatic ductal system is mediated through distal cell proliferation and proximal cell deterioration. This concept implies a migration of epithelial cells from the distal end toward the proximal end, where they undergo degeneration. The concept of prostatic epithelial homeostasis is important in that an imbalance in either proliferation or degeneration of epithelial cells results in prostatic regression or prostatic growth, as in the case of BPH.

Although depletion of androgen in vivo results in the activation of programmed cell death in the rat prostate, androgen withdrawal in vitro has no effect on epithelial cell survival. However, a high level of TGF-β has been associated with programmed cell death of the prostatic epithelial cells. Thus, it appears that stromal cells also play an important role in programmed cell death of epithelial cells in the proximal segment of the ductal system. Whether or not this inductive effect of the stromal element plays an important role in castration-induced programmed cell death in the prostate remains to be clarified.

Currently, numerous other growth factors and regulatory peptides produced by human or animal cells are either being localized to, or have receptors present in, prostatic tissue. Included among these, aside from those already described, are keratinocyte growth factor (KGF),[17, 140] insulin or insulin-like growth factors I and II,[166] nerve growth factor,[74] somatostatin,[49] inhibin,[155] relaxin,[27] and oxytocin.[2] KGF, a member of the fibroblast growth factor family, is of special interest because of its potent mitogenic activity for epithelial cells; it has thus far not been demonstrated to be mitogenic for fibroblast or endothelial cells. This mitogenic activity has been demonstrated in prostatic epithelial cells in vitro and makes KGF a strong candidate as a mediator of stromal-epithelial interaction and an important paracrine factor in the human prostate. Many of the other proteins listed are under investigation with respect to their ability to stimulate growth and whether they function in an autocrine or paracrine fashion.

In view of the above considerations, androgen action on prostatic epithelial cells seems to be highly complex and dependent on organ or environmental interactions. Current evidence suggests that this interaction is almost certainly with the stroma (Fig. 5–3). The paracrine and autocrine messages that exist in and between epithelial and stromal cells, which are responsible for growth control, seem to be regionalized. We theorize that in the rat prostatic ductal system, cells in the proximal tip, intermediate segment, and distal tip are undergoing different stages of cell death, cellular differentiation, and cell proliferation under the influence and regulation of various growth factors.[105] As more knowledge is gained with respect to the actions and location of various growth factors, such as EGF, KGF, TGF-β, and others, we may be able to further define the stromal-epithelial interactions in various regions of the prostatic ductal system in benign and pathologic conditions. It is important to emphasize that the above-postulated theory, as well as those proposed by others, is based upon current limited knowledge, thus making them speculative and suppositional at best. Further investigation is needed to determine more clearly how the epithelial cells and stromal cells communicate, the importance of the basement membrane and extracellular matrix, and further elucidation of the hormone responsiveness of the individual cells in the prostate. It is hoped that as this additional information is gathered, how androgen and other hormones are able to influence prostatic cell growth and death on a cellular level will become clearer.

SUMMARY

At this time, the endocrine regulation of prostatic growth seems much more complex than previously re-

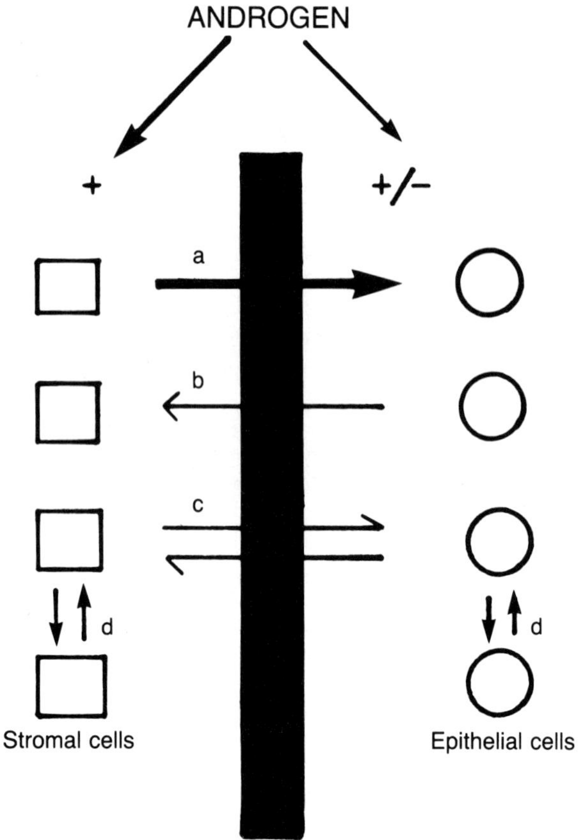

FIGURE 5–3. Postulated stromal-epithelial cell relationships: Androgen stimulates stromal cell proliferation and the production of various growth factors (e.g., epidermal growth factor, transforming growth factor-β, keratinocyte growth factor) involved in the regulation of epithelial growth and proliferation (pathway a). Androgen may also have a direct effect on epithelial cells. Communication between and among stromal and epithelial cells via autocrine and paracrine messengers/growth factors (pathways b, c, and d) is also likely but requires further elucidation.

alized. Our current knowledge indicates that the prostate is critically dependent on androgen for growth. The major androgen in the serum of humans is testosterone, of which the majority is produced by the Leydig cells in the testis. This testosterone is then taken up by prostate cells, where it is converted to DHT by 5α-reductase. Stimulation of prostatic growth and probably BPH depends on this conversion of testosterone to DHT. The stimulatory effect of DHT and, to a lesser extent, other androgens may be further influenced by other hormones such as estrogen and prolactin. Estrogen has both positive and negative effects on prostatic growth, whereas prolactin and other hormones have been found to be mitogens and have synergistic effects on androgen-induced growth. Other factors such as the hypothesized nonandrogenic testicular growth factor have been postulated and may prove to be very important. On the cellular level, it now seems that androgens, and possibly other hormones, are able to exert their proliferative effects on the epithelium in an indirect fashion by their direct stimulation of the stroma and subsequent production of growth factors that promote epithelial cell proliferation. A direct effect of androgen on the epithelial component remains a strong but unproven possibility. Once again, it must be emphasized that the above statements, especially those regarding stromal-epithelial cell interaction, are still speculative at best because of significant gaps in our present knowledge. As additional information is gained regarding the regulation of prostatic growth on a cellular level in both normal and pathologic conditions, we hope to be able to better elucidate how androgens and other hormones influence prostatic growth.

REFERENCES

1. Ablin RJ, Whyard TC: Immunobiological implications of select bioactive molecules in the prostate with a known and unknown target. *In* Farnsworth WE, Ablin R (eds): The Prostate as an Endocrine Gland. Boca Raton, CRC Press, 1990, pp 149–152.
2. Adashi E, Hseuh AJW: Direct inhibition of testicular androgen biosynthesis revealing antigonadal activity of neurohypophysial hormones. Nature 293:650–656, 1981.
3. Anderson KM, Liao S: Selective retention of dihydrotestosterone by prostatic nuclei. Nature 219:277, 1968.
4. Andersson H, Tisell L-E: Morphology of rat prostatic lobes and seminal vesicles after long-term estrogen treatment. Acta Pathol Microbiol Scand 90:441, 1982.
5. Andrews GS: Growth hormone and malignancy. J Clin Pathol 36:935, 1983.
6. Angervall L, Hesselsjo R, Nilsson S, Tissel LE: Action of testosterone on ventral prostate, dorsolateral prostate, coagulating glands, and seminal vesicles of castrated alloxan-diabetic rats. Diabetologia 3:395, 1967.
7. Aragona C, Friesen HG: Specific prolactin binding sites in the prostate and testis of rat. Endocrinology 97:677, 1975.
8. Arai Y: Nature of metaplasia in rat coagulating gland induced by neonatal treatment with estrogen. Endocrinology 86:918, 1970.
9. Arvola I: The hormonal control of the amounts of the tissue components of the prostate. Ann Chir Gynaecol Fenn (Suppl) 50:102, 1961.
10. Aumuller G: Morphologic and endocrine aspects of prostatic function. Prostate 4:195, 1983.
11. Bainborough AR: Squamous metaplasia of prostate following estrogen therapy. J Urol 68:329, 1952.
12. Barrack ER, Berry SJ: DNA synthesis in the canine prostate: Effects of androgen and estrogen treatment. Prostate 10:45–56, 1987.
13. Barrack ER, Bujnovszky P, Walsh PC: Subcellular distribution of androgen receptors in human normal, benign hyperplastic, and malignant prostatic tissues: Characterization of nuclear salt-resistant receptors. Cancer Res 43:1107, 1983.
14. Barrack ER, Coffey DS: The specific binding of estrogens and androgens to the nuclear matrix of sex hormone responsive tissues. J Biol Chem 255:7265, 1980.
15. Berg OA: Effect of stilboesterol on the prostate gland in normal puppies and adult dogs. Acta Endocrinol (Copenh) 27:155–169, 1958.
16. Berry S, Isaacs JT: Comparative aspects of prostatic growth and androgen metabolism with aging in the rat versus the dog. Endocrinology 114:511, 1984.
17. Bottaro DP, Rubin JS, Ron D, et al: Characterization of the receptor for keratinocyte growth factor: Evidence for multiple fibroblast growth factor receptors. J Biol Chem 265:12767–12770, 1990.
18. Brawer MK, Peehl DM, Stamey TA, Bostwick DG: Keratin immunoreactivity in the benign and neoplastic human prostate. Cancer Res 45:3663, 1985.
19. British Prostate Study Group: Evaluation of plasma hormone concentrations in relation to clinical staging in patients with prostate cancer. Br J Cancer 51:382, 1979.
20. Bromberg W, Grayhack JT: Personal communication.
21. Bruchovsky N, Dunstan-Adams E: Regulation of 5α-reductase activity in stroma and epithelium of human prostate. *In* Bruchovsky A, Chapdelaine A, Neumann F (eds): Regulation of Androgen Action. Berlin, Congressdruck R Brückner, 1985, pp 31–35.
22. Bruchovsky N, Lesser B, van Doorn EV, Craven S: Hormonal effects on cell proliferation in rat prostate. Vitam Horm 33:61, 1975.
23. Bruchovsky N, Wilson JD: The conversion of testosterone to 5-androstan 17β-ol-3-one by rat prostate *in vivo* and *in vitro*. J Biol Chem 243:2012, 1968.
24. Bruchovsky N, Wilson JD: The intranuclear binding of testosterone and 5-androstan-17β-ol-one by rat prostate. J Biol Chem 243:5953, 1968.
25. Burrows H: Pathological conditions induced by oestrogenic compounds in the coagulating gland and prostate of the mouse. Am J Cancer 23:490, 1935.
26. Cabot AT: The question of castration for enlarged prostate. Ann Surg 24:265–309, 1896.
27. Cameron DF, Corton GL, Larkin LH: Relaxin-like antigenicity in the armadillo prostate gland. Ann NY Acad Sci 380:231–240, 1982.
28. Carmena MJ, Fernandez-Moreno MD, Prieto JC: Characterization of insulin receptors in isolated epithelial cells of rat ventral prostate: Effect of fasting. Cell Biochem Func 4:19–24, 1986.
29. Carter DB, Yamada K, Harris SE: Developmental aspects of androgen-dependent mRNA from rat ventral prostate using cloned cDNA. Mol Cell Endocrinol 31:199, 1983.
30. Chaisiri N, Pierrepoint CG: Examination of the distribution of estrogen receptor between stromal and epithelial compartments of the canine prostate. Prostate 1:357–366, 1980.
31. Chang C, Kokontis J, Chang CT, Liao S: Cloning and sequence analysis of the rat ventral prostate glucocorticoid receptor cDNA. Nucleic Acids Res 15:9603, 1987.
32. Chen C, Hiipakka RA, Liao S: Prostate alpha protein: Subunit structure, polyamine binding, and inhibition of nuclear chromatin binding of androgen-receptor complex. J Steroid Biochem 11:401, 1979.
33. Chen C, Schilling K, Hiipakka RA, et al: Prostate alpha protein: Isolation and characterization of the polypeptide components and cholesterol binding. J Biol Chem 257:116, 1982.
34. Chung LWK, Coffey DS: Biochemical characterization of prostatic nuclei. II. Relationship between DNA synthesis and protein synthesis. Biochim Biophys Acta 247:584, 1971.
35. Coffey DS: The molecular biology, endocrinology, and physiology of the prostate and seminal vesicles. *In* Walsh PC, Retik AB, Stamey TA, Vaughan ED Jr (eds): Campbell's Urology, 6th ed. Philadelphia, WB Saunders, 1992.
36. Coffey DS, Shimazaki J, Williams-Ashman HG: Polymerization of deoxyribonucleotides in relation to androgen-induced prostatic growth. Arch Biochem Biophys 124:184, 1968.
37. Cooke PS, Meisami E: Early hypothyroidism in rats causes increased adult testis and reproductive organ size but does not change testosterone levels. Endocrinology 129:237–243, 1991.
38. Crawford ED, Eisenberger MA, McLeod DG, et al: A controlled trial of leuprolide with and without flutamide in prostatic carcinoma. N Engl J Med 321:419, 1989.
39. Cunha GR: Androgenic effects upon prostatic epithelium are mediated via trophic influences from stroma. *In* Kimball FA, Buhl AE, Carter DB (eds): New Approaches to the Study of Benign Prostatic Hyperplasia. New York, Alan R. Liss, 1984, p 81.
40. Cunha GR: Tissue interactions between epithelium and mesenchyme of urogenital and integumental origin. Anat Rec 172:529, 1972.
41. Cunha GR, Donjacour AA, Cooke PS, et al: The endocrinology and developmental biology of the prostate. Endocr Rev 8:338–362, 1987.
42. Cunha GR, Lung B: The possible influences of temporal factors in the androgenic responsiveness of urogenital tissue recombinants from wild-type and androgen-insensitive (Tfm) mice. J Exp Zool 205:343, 1978.
43. Dalton DP, Lee C, Huprikar S, et al: Non-androgenic role of testis in enhancing ventral prostate growth in rats. Prostate 16:225–233, 1990.

44. Darras FS, Lee C, Huprikar S, et al: Evidence for a nonandrogenic role of testis and epididymis in androgen-supported growth of the rat ventral prostate. J Urol 148:432–440, 1992.

45. De Jong FH: Inhibin—Its nature, site of production and function. *In* Clarke JR (ed): Oxford Reviews of Reproductive Biology. Oxford, Oxford University Press, 1987, pp 1–54.

46. DeKlerk DP, Coffey DS: Quantitative determination of prostatic epithelial and stromal hyperplasia by a new technique: Biomorphometrics. Invest Urol 16:240–245, 1978.

47. Deming CL, Jenkins RH, Van Wagenen G: Some endocrinological relationships of prostatic hypertrophy: Clinical and experimental studies; Preliminary report. J Urol 33:388–399, 1935.

48. Dermer GB: Basal cell proliferation in benign prostatic hyperplasia. Cancer 41:1857, 1978.

49. Di Sant Agnese PA, de Messey Jensen JL: Somatostatin-like immunoreactive endocrine-paracrine cells in human prostate gland. Arch Pathol Lab Med 108:693–696, 1986.

50. Dorrington JH, Armstrong DT: Follicle stimulating hormone stimulates estradiol-17β synthesis in cultured Sertoli cells. Proc Natl Acad Sci USA 72:2677, 1975.

51. Ekman P, Barrack ER, Greene GL, et al: Estrogen receptors in human prostate: Evidence for multiple binding sites. J Clin Endocrinol Metab 57:166–176, 1983.

52. English HF, Drago JR, Santen RJ: Cellular response to androgen depletion and repletion in the rat ventral prostate: Autoradiography and morphometric analysis. Prostate 7:41, 1985.

53. Farnsworth WE: Prolactin effect on the permeability of benign hyperplastic prostate to testosterone. Prostate 12:222–229, 1988.

54. Fong C-J, Sherwood ER, Sutkowski DM, et al: Reconstituted basement membrane promotes morphological and functional differentiation of primary human prostatic epithelial cells. Prostate 19:221–235, 1991.

55. Forsgren B, Bjork P, Carlstrom K, et al: Purification and distribution of a major protein in rat prostate that binds estramustine, a nitrogen mustard derivative of estradiol-17-β. Proc Natl Acad Sci USA 76:3149, 1979.

56. Franklin RB, Costello LC: Prolactin directly stimulates citrate production and mitochondrial aspartate amino transferase of prostate epithelial cells. Prostate 17:13–18, 1990.

57. Franks LM: Atrophy and hyperplasia in the prostate proper. J Pathol Bacteriol 68:617, 1954.

58. Franks LM: Benign nodular hyperplasia of the prostate: A review. Ann R Coll Surg Engl 14:92–106, 1954.

59. Franks LM: Benign prostatic hyperplasia: Gross and microscopic anatomy. *In* Grayhack JT, Wilson JD, Scherbenske MJ (eds): Benign Prostatic Hyperplasia: NIAMDD Workshop Proceedings, Feb 20–21, 1975. DHEW Publication No (NIH) 76-1113. US Government Printing Office, 1976, pp 63–89.

60. Gardner WU: Estrogens in carcinogenesis. Arch Pathol 27:138, 1939.

61. Geller J, Liu J, Albert JD, et al: Effect of antiandrogen and/or antiestrogen blockage on human prostate epithelial and stromal cell protein synthesis. J Steroid Biochem 25:759–763, 1986.

62. Grayhack JT: Changes with aging in human seminal vesicle fluid fructose concentration and seminal vesicle weight. J Urol 86:142–148, 1961.

63. Grayhack JT: Effect of testosterone-estradiol administration on citric acid and fructose content of the rat prostate. Endocrinology 77:1068–1074, 1965.

64. Grayhack JT, Bunce PL, Kearns JW, Scott WW: Influence of the pituitary on prostatic response to androgen in the rat. Bull Johns Hopkins Hosp 96:154–163, 1955.

65. Grayhack JT, Kozlowski JM: Benign prostatic hyperplasia. *In* Gillenwater JY, Grayhack JT, Howards SS, Duckett JW (eds): Adult and Pediatric Urology, 2nd ed, Vol 2. Chicago, Mosby–Year Book, 1991, pp 1211–1276.

66. Grayhack JT, Kropp KA: Changes with aging in prostatic fluid: Citric acid, acid phosphatase and lactic dehydrogenase concentration in man. J Urol 56:6–11, 1965.

67. Grayhack JT, Lebowitz A: Effect of prolactin on citric acid of lateral lobe of prostate of Sprague-Dawley rats. Invest Urol 5:87–94, 1967.

68. Grayhack JT, Lee C, Brand W: The effect of testicular irradiation on established BPH in the dog: Evidence of a non-steroid testicular factor for BPH maintenance. J Urol 134:1276–1281, 1985.

69. Griffiths J: An enlarged prostate gland eighteen days after bilateral or complete castration. Br Med J 1:579–581, 1895.

70. Griffiths K, Davies P, Eaton CL, et al: Cancer of the prostate: Endocrine factors. *In* Clarke JR (ed): Oxford Reviews of Reproductive Biology, Vol 9. Oxford, Oxford University Press, 1988, pp 192–259.

71. Griffiths K, Davies P, Eaton CL, et al: Oestrogens and the prostate. *In* Khoury S, Chatelain C (eds): Oestrogens and the Prostate. France, Maury-Imprimeur, FIIS et RPG, 1988, pp 308–332.

72. Griffiths K, Davies P, Eaton CL, et al: Endocrine factors in the initiation, diagnosis, and treatment of prostatic cancer. *In* Voigt K-D, Knabbe C (eds): Endocrine Dependent Tumors. New York, Raven Press, 1991, pp 83–129.

73. Griffiths K, Davies P, Harper ME, et al: The etiology and endocrinology of prostatic cancer. *In* Rose D (ed): Endocrinology of Cancer, Vol 2. Boca Raton, CRC Press, 1979, pp 1–55.

74. Harper GP, Barde YA, Burnstock G, et al: Guinea pig prostate is rich source of nerve growth factor. Nature 279:160–162, 1979.

75. Hartley-Asp B: Estramustine-induced mitotic arrest in two human prostatic carcinoma cell lines, DU145 and PC-3. Prostate 5:93–100, 1984.

76. Heyns W, Peeters B, Mous J: Influence of androgens on the concentration of prostatic binding protein (PBP) and its mRNA in rat prostate. Biochem Biophys Res Commun 77:1492, 1977.

77. Hiramatsu M, Kashimata M, Minami N, et al: Androgenic regulation of epidermal growth factor in the mouse ventral prostate. Biochem Int 17:311–317, 1988.

78. Hofer DR, Sherwood ER, Bromberg WD, et al: Autonomous growth of androgen-independent human prostatic carcinoma cells of transforming growth factor α. Cancer Res 51:2780–2785, 1991.

79. Holland JM, Lee C: Effects of pituitary grafts on testosterone stimulated growth of rat prostate. Biol Reprod 22:351–355, 1980.

80. Horton RJ: Androgen hormones and prehormones in young and elderly men. *In* Grayhack JT, Wilson JD, Scherbenske MJ (eds): Benign Prostatic Hyperplasia: NIAMDD Workshop Proceedings, Feb 20–21, 1975. DHEW Publication No (NIH) 76–1113. US Government Printing Office, 1976, pp 183–188.

81. Huggins C, Clark PJ: Quantitative studies on prostatic secretion. II. The effect of castration and of estrogen injection on the normal and on the hyperplastic prostate glands of dogs. J Exp Med 72:747, 1940.

82. Huggins C, Hodges CV: Studies on prostatic cancer. I. The effect of castration, of estrogen and of androgen injection on serum phosphatases in metastatic carcinoma of the prostate. Cancer Res 1:293, 1941.

83. Huggins C, Stevens RA: The effect of castration on benign hypertrophy of the prostate in man. J Urol 43:705–714, 1940.

84. Huggins C, Webster WO: Duality of human prostate in response to estrogen. J Urol 59:258, 1945.

85. Hunter J: Observations in Certain Parts of the Animal Oeconomy. London, 1786.

86. Ichihara I, Kawai N, Heilbronner R, Rohr H: Stereologic and fine-structural studies of prostatic acinar basal cells in the dog. Cell Tissue Res 242:519, 1985.

87. Imperato-McGinley J: Reductase deficiency in man. Prog Cancer Res Ther 31:491, 1984.

88. Imperato-McGinley J, Binienda Z, Arthur A, et al: The development of a male pseudohermaphroditic rat using an inhibitor of the enzyme 5α-reductase. Endocrinology 116:807, 1985.

89. Imperato-McGinley J, Guerrero L, Gautier T, Peterson RE: Steroid 5α-reductase deficiency in man: An inherited form of pseudohermaphroditism. Science 186:1213, 1974.

90. Imperato-McGinley J, Peterson RE, Gautier T: Primary and secondary 5α-reductase deficiency. *In* Serio M, Zanisi M, Motta M, Martini L (eds): Sexual Differentiation: Basic and Clinical Aspects. New York, Raven Press, 1984, p 233.

91. Isaacs JT: Antagonistic effect of androgen on prostatic cell death. Prostate 5:545–557, 1984.

92. Isaacs JT, Coffey DS: Changes in dihydrotestosterone metabolism associated with the development of canine benign hyperplasia. Endocrinology 108:445–453, 1981.

93. Jost A: Problems of fetal endocrinology: The gonadal and hypophyseal hormones. Recent Prog Horm Res 8:379, 1953.

94. Kannan CR: Physiology of testicular function. *In* Essential Endocrinology. New York, Plenum, 1986, pp 291–295.

95. Kannan CR: The pituitary gland. *In* Essential Endocrinology. New York, Plenum, 1986, pp 1–30.

96. King RJB: Structure and function of steroid receptors. J Endocrinol 114:341–349, 1987.

97. Krieg M: Biochemical endocrinology of human prostatic tumours. *In* King RJB, Lippmann ME (eds): Progress in Cancer Research Therapy: Hormones and Cancer 2, Vol 31. New York, Raven Press, 1984, pp 425–440.

98. Krieg M, Bartsch W, Thomsen M, Voigt KD: Androgens and oestrogens: Their interaction with stroma and epithelium of human benign prostatic hyperplasia and normal prostate. J Steroid Biochem 19:155–161, 1983.

99. Labrie F, Dupont A, Belanger A: LHRH agonists and antiandrogens in prostate cancer. *In* Ratliff TL, Catalona WJ (eds): Genitourinary Cancer. Boston, Martinus Nijhoff, 1987, p 157.

100. Lasnitzki I, Franklin HR: The influence of serum on uptake, conversion and action of testosterone in rat prostate glands in organ culture. J Endocrinol 54:333, 1972.

101. Lasnitzki I, Mizuno T: Prostatic induction and interaction of epithelium and mesenchyme from normal wild-type and androgen-insensitive mice with testicular feminization. J Endocrinol 85:423, 1980.

102. Lea OA, Petrusz P, French FS: Prostatein. A major secretory protein of the rat ventral prostate. J Biol Chem 254:6196, 1979.

103. Leav I, Merk FB, Ofner P, et al: Bipotentiality of response to sex hormones of estrogen. Am J Pathol 93:69, 1978.

104. Leav I, Morfin RF, Ofner P, et al: Estrogen and castration-induced effects on canine prostatic fine structure and C19-steroid metabolism. Endocrinology 89:465, 1971.

105. Lee C: Effects of hormones and growth factors on the prostate. International Workshop on BPH, WHO, Paris, June 24–28, 1991.

106. Lee C: Physiology of castration-induced regression in rat prostate. *In* Murphy G, Sandberg AA, Karr JP (eds): The Prostatic Cell: Structure and Function. New York, Alan R. Liss, 1981, pp 145–159.

107. Lee C, Jesik C: Effects of castration, estrogen and androgen administration. *In* Hinman F Jr (ed): Benign Prostatic Hypertrophy. New York, Springer-Verlag, 1983, pp 229–234.

108. Lee C, Prins GS, Henneberry MO, Grayhack JT: Effect of estradiol on the rat prostate in the presence and absence of testosterone and pituitary. J Androl 2:293–299, 1981.

109. Lee C, Sensibar JA, Dudek SM, et al: Prostatic ductal system in rats: Regional variation in morphological and functional activities. Biol Reprod 43:1079–1086, 1990.

110. Lee C, Sherwood ER, Kozlowski JM, Grayhack JT: Role of stromal-epithelial cell interaction in benign prostatic hyperplasia. *In* The Foundation for Prostate Research (ed): Treatment of Benign Prostatic Hyperplasia. Tokyo, Kimbara, 1990, pp 16–26.

111. Lich R Jr, Howerton LW, Amin M: Anatomy and surgical approach to the urogenital tract in the male. *In* Harrison JH, Gittes RF, Perlmutter AD, et al (eds): Campbell's Urology, 4th ed, Philadelphia, WB Saunders, 1978, pp 3–32.

112. Lilja H: A kallikrein-like serine protease in prostatic fluid cleaves the predominant seminal vesicle protein. J Clin Invest 76:1899–1903, 1985.

113. Lilja H, Laurell C-B: The predominant protein in human seminal coagulate. Scand J Clin Lab Invest 45:635–641, 1985.

114. Liu J, Albert JD, Geller J, Faber LE: Effect of tamoxifen on stromal protein synthesis in the human prostate. J Clin Endocrinol Metab 59:710–713, 1984.

115. Lloyd JW, Thomas JA, Mawhinney MG: A difference in the *in vitro* accumulation and metabolism by the rat prostate gland with prolactin. Steroids 22:473, 1973.

116. Lowsley OS: The development of the human prostate gland with reference to the development of other structures at the neck of the urinary bladder. Am J Anat 13:299, 1912.

117. Lowsley OS: The gross anatomy of the human prostate gland and contiguous structures. Surg Gynecol Obstet 20:183–192, 1915.

118. MacDonald PC: Origin of estrogen in men. *In* Grayhack JT, Wilson JD, Scherbenske MJ (eds): Benign Prostatic Hyperplasia: NIAMDD Workshop Proceedings, Feb 20–21, 1975. DHEW Publication No (NIH) 76–1113. US Government Printing Office, 1976, pp 191–192.

119. Mann T: The Biochemistry of Semen and the Male Reproductive Tract, 2nd ed. New York, John Wiley and Sons, 1964.

120. Mao P, Angrist A: The fine structure of the basal cell of human prostate. Lab Invest 15:1768, 1966.

121. Mawhinney MG, Neubauer BL: Actions of estrogen in the male. Invest Urol 16:409, 1979.

122. McConnell JD: Physiologic basis of endocrine therapy for prostatic cancer. Urol Clin North Am 18:1–13, 1991.

123. McKeehan WL, Adams PS, Rosser MP: Direct mitogenic effects of insulin, epidermal growth factor, glucocorticoid, cholera toxin, unknown pituitary factors and possibly prolactin, but not androgen, on normal rat prostate epithelial cells in serum-free, primary cell culture. Cancer Res 44:1998–2010, 1984.

124. McLachlan JA, Newbold RR, Bullock B: Reproductive tract lesions in male mice exposed prenatally to diethylstilbestrol. Science 190:991, 1976.

125. McNeal JE: Anatomy of the prostate—an historical survey of divergent views. Prostate 1:3, 1980.

126. McNeal JE: Developmental and comparative anatomy of the prostate. *In* Grayhack JT, Wilson JD, Scherbenske MJ (eds): Benign Prostatic Hyperplasia: NIAMDD Workshop Proceedings, Feb 20–21, 1975. DHEW Publication No (NIH) 76–1113. US Government Printing Office, 1976, pp 1–16.

127. McNeal JE: Origin and evolution of benign prostatic enlargement. Invest Urol 15:340–345, 1978.

128. McNeal JE: Regional morphology and pathology of the prostate. Am J Clin Pathol 49:347, 1968.

129. McNeal JE: The prostate and prostatic urethra: A morphologic synthesis. J Urol 107:1008–1016, 1972.

130. McNeal JE: The prostate gland: Morphology and pathology. Monogr Urol 4:3–33, 1983.

131. McNeal JE: The zonal anatomy of the prostate. Prostate 2:35, 1981.

132. Merk FB, Ofner P, Kwan PW, et al: Ultrastructural and biochemical expressions of divergent differentiation in prostates of castrated dogs treated with estrogen and androgen. Lab Invest 47:437, 1982.

133. Mobbs BJ, Johnson LE, Connolly JG: Influence of the adrenal gland on prostatic activity in adult rats. J Endocrinol 59:335, 1973.

134. Mydlo JH, Michaeli J, Heston WDW, Fair WR: Expression of basic fibroblast growth factor mRNA in benign prostatic hyperplasia and prostatic carcinoma. Prostate 13:241–247, 1988.

135. Oesterling J, Bilhartz DL, Tindall DJ: Clinically Useful Serum Markers for Adenocarcinoma of the Prostate: Part II—PSA. AUA Update Series, vol 10, lesson 18, 1991.

136. Orlowski J, Bird CE, Clark AF: Androgen 5α-reductase and 3α-hydroxysteroid dehydrogenase activities in ventral prostate epithelial and stromal cells from immature and mature rats. J Endocrinol 99:131–139, 1983.

137. Parker M, Scrace GT: Regulation of protein synthesis in rat ventral prostate: Cell-free translation of mRNA. Biochemistry 76:1580, 1979.

138. Parker MG, Scrace GT, Mainwaring WIP: Testosterone regulates the synthesis of major proteins in rat ventral prostate. Biochem J 170:115, 1978.

139. Parker MG, White R, Williams JG: Cloning and characterization of androgen-dependent mRNA from rat ventral prostate. J Biol Chem 255:6996, 1980.

140. Peehl DM, Stamey TA, Rubin JS: Fibroblast growth factors can replace epidermal growth factor for clonal proliferation of human prostatic epithelial cells. J Urol 145:331A, 1991.

141. Peehl DM, Wong ST, Bazinet M, Stamey TA: *In vitro* studies of human epithelial cells: Attempts to identify distinguishing features of malignant cells. Growth Factors 1:237–250, 1989.

142. Peeters B, Mous J, Rombauts WA, Heyns WJ: Androgen-induced messenger RNA in rat ventral prostate. Translation, partial purification, and preliminary characterization of the mRNAs encoding the components of prostatic binding protein. J Biol Chem 255:7017, 1980.

143. Petrow V: Dihydrotestosterone. *In* Farnsworth WE, Ablin R (eds): The Prostate as an Endocrine Gland. Boca Raton, CRC Press, 1990, pp 3–18.

144. Pousette A, Bjork P, Carlstrom K, et al: On the presence of "prostatic secretion protein" in different species. Acta Chem Scand 34:155, 1980.

145. Price D: Normal development of the prostate and seminal vesicles of the rat with a study of experimental postnatal modifications. Am J Anat 60:79, 1936.

146. Price D, Ortiz E: The relation of age to reactivity in the reproductive system of the rat. Endocrinology 34:215, 1944.

147. Price D, Williams-Ashman HG: The accessory reproductive glands of mammals. *In* Young WC (ed): Sex and Internal Secretions, 3rd ed. Baltimore, Williams & Wilkins, 1961, p 366.

148. Prins GS, Lee C: Influence of prolactin-producing pituitary grafts on the *in vivo* uptake, distribution and disappearance of ^{3}H-testosterone and ^{3}H-dihydrotestosterone by the rat prostate lobes. Endocrinology 110:920–925, 1982.

149. Raina A, Holtta E: The effect of growth hormone on the synthesis and accumulation of polyamines in mammalian tissues. *In* Pecile A, Muller EE (eds): Growth and Growth Hormone. Proceedings of the 2nd International Symposium on Growth Hormones. Amsterdam, Excerpta Medica, 1972, p 143.

150. Rajfer J, Coffey DS: Effects of neonatal steroids on male sex tissues. Invest Urol 17:3, 1979.

151. Rennie PS, Bowden JF, Bruchovsky N, Cheng H: The relationship between inhibition of plasminogen-activator activity and prostatic involution. Biochem J 252:759–764, 1988.

152. Riskand P, Martin J: Functional anatomy of the hypothalamic-anterior pituitary complex. *In* De Groout LJ (ed): Endocrinology. Philadelphia, WB Saunders, 1989, pp 97–107.

153. Rui H, Purvis K: Independent control of citrate production and ornithine decarboxylase by prolactin in the lateral lobe of the rat prostate. Mol Cell Endocrinol 52:91, 1987.

154. Saroff J, Kirdani RY, Chu TM, et al: Measurements of prolactin and androgens in patients with prostatic diseases. Oncology 37:46–52, 1980.

155. Sathe VS, Sheth NA, Phadke MA, et al: Biosynthesis and localization of inhibin in human prostate. Prostate 10:33–43, 1987.

156. Schröder FH: Total androgen suppression in the management of prostatic cancer: A critical review. *In* EORTC Genitourinary Group Monograph 2. Part A: Therapeutic Principles in Metastatic Cancer. New York, Alan R. Liss, 1985, p 307.

157. Schulze H, Barrack ER: Immunocytochemical localization of oestrogen receptors in spontaneous and experimentally induced canine benign prostatic hyperplasia. Prostate 11:145–162, 1987.

158. Schulze H, Isaacs JT, Coffey DS: A critical review of the concept of total androgen ablation in the treatment of prostate cancer. Prog Clin Biol Res 243A:1, 1987.

159. Schulze H, Isaacs J, Senge T: Inability of complete androgen blockade to increase survival of patients with advanced prostatic cancer as compared to standard hormonal therapy. J Urol 137:909, 1987.

160. Sensibar JA, Griswold MD, Sylvester SR, et al: Prostatic ductal system in rats; regional variation in localization of an androgen-repressed gene product, sulfated glycoprotein-2. Endocrinology 128:2091–2102, 1991.

161. Shannon JM, Cunha GR: Autoradiographic localization of androgen binding in the developing mouse prostate. Prostate 4:367, 1983.

162. Shannon JM, Cunha GR, Vanderslice KD: Autoradiographic localization of androgen receptors in the developing urogenital tract and mammary gland. Anat Rec 199:232, 1981.

163. Sheppard H, Tsien WH, Mayer P, Howie N: Metabolism of the accessory sex organs of the immature male rat: Changes in nucleic acid composition and uptake of thymidine-^{3}H induced by castration and methandrostenolone. Biochem Pharmacol 14:41, 1965.

164. Sibley PEC, Harper ME, Joyce BG, et al: The immunocytochemical detection of protein hormones in human prostatic tissues. Prostate 2:175, 1981.

165. Sibley PEC, Harper ME, Peeling WB, Griffiths K: Growth hormone and prostatic tumours: Localization using a monoclonal human growth hormone antibody. J Endocrinol 103:311, 1984.

166. Stahler MS, Panskey B, Budd GC: Immunocytochemical demonstration of insulin or insulin-like immunoreactivity in the rat prostate gland. Prostate 13:189–198, 1988.

167. Stearns ME, Wang M, Tew K, Binder LI: Estramustine binds a MAP-1 like protein to inhibit microtubule assembly *in vitro* and disrupt microtubule organization in DU145 cells. J Cell Biol 107:2647–2656, 1988.

168. Story MT, Livingston B, Beaten L, et al: Cultured human prostate–derived fibroblasts produce a factor that stimulates their growth with properties indistinguishable from basic fibroblast growth factor. Prostate 15:355–365, 1989.

169. Sugimura Y, Cunha GR, Donjacour AA: Morphogenesis of ductal networks in the mouse prostate. Biol Reprod 34:961, 1986.

170. Sutkowski DM, Fong C-J, Sherwood ER, et al: Stromal cells of the human prostate: Initial isolation and characterization. 1992 (in preparation).

171. Swyer GIM: Post-natal growth changes in the human prostate. J Anat 78:130, 1944.

172. Takeda H, Mizuno T, Lasnitzki I: Autoradiographic studies of androgen-binding sites in the rat urogenital sinus and postnatal prostate. J Endocrinol 104:87, 1985.

173. Tenniswood MP, Montpetit ML, Léger JG, et al: Epithelial-stromal interactions and cell death in the prostate. *In* Farnsworth WE, Ablin R (eds): The Prostate as an Endocrine Gland. Boca Raton, CRC Press, 1990, pp 188–198.

174. Tew K, Hartley-Asp B: Cytotoxic properties of estramustine unrelated to alkylating and steroid constituents. Urology 23:28–33, 1984.

175. The LV, Labrie C, Zhao HT, et al: Characterization of cDNAs for human estradiol 17-beta-dehydrogenase and assignment of the gene to chromosome 17: Evidence of two mRNA species with distinct 5′termini in human placenta. Mol Endocrinol 3:1301, 1989.

176. Timms BG, Chandler JA, Sinowatz F: The ultrastructure of basal cells of rat and dog prostate. Cell Tissue Res 173:542, 1976.

177. Tisell LE: Effect of cortisone on the growth of the ventral prostate, the dorsolateral prostate, the coagulating gland and the seminal vesicles in castrated adrenalectomized and in castrated non-adrenalectomized rats. Acta Endocrinol 64:637, 1970.

178. Tisell LE: The growth of the ventral prostate, the dorsolateral prostate, the coagulating glands and the seminal vesicles in castrated adrenalectomized rats injected with oestradiol and/or cortisone. Acta Endocrinol (Copenh) 68:485, 1971.

179. Triche TJ, Harkin CJ: An ultrastructural study of hormonally induced squamous metaplasia in the coagulating gland of the mouse prostate. Lab Invest 25:596, 1971.

180. Tsai YC, Harrison HH, Lee C, et al: Systemic characterization of human prostatic fluid proteins with two dimensional electrophoresis. Clin Chem 30:2026–2030, 1984.

181. Tullner WW: Hormonal factors in the adrenal dependent growth of the rat ventral prostate. *In* Vollmer EP (ed): Biology of the Prostate and Related Tissues. National Cancer Institute Monograph 12. Bethesda, MD, National Cancer Institute, 1963, p 211.

182. Tunn U, Senge Th, Schenck B, Neumann F: Biochemical and histological studies on prostates in castrated dogs after treatment with androstanediol, oestradiol and cyproterone acetate. Acta Endocrinol (Copenh) 91:373–384, 1979.

183. Tunn U, Senge TH, Schenck B, Neumann F: Effects of cyproterone acetate on experimentally induced canine prostatic hyperplasia: A morphological and histological study. Urol Int 35:125–140, 1980.

184. Uke E, Lee C, Grayhack JT: The effect of the cis hydroxyproline on ventral prostatic growth in rats. J Urol 129:171–174, 1983.

185. Van Wagenen G: The effects of oestrin in the urogenital tract of the male monkey. Anat Rec 63:387, 1935.
186. Walsh PC: Human benign prostatic hyperplasia: Etiological considerations. *In* Kimball FA, Buhl AE, Carter DB (eds): New Approaches to the Study of Benign Prostatic Hyperplasia. New York, Alan R. Liss, 1984, p 1.
187. Walsh PC, Gittes RF: Inhibition of extratesticular stimuli to prostatic growth in the castrate rat by antiandrogens. Endocrinology 87:624, 1970.
188. Walsh PC, Hutchins GM, Ewing LL: Tissue content of dihydrotestosterone in human prostatic hyperplasia is not supranormal. J Clin Invest 72:1772, 1983.
189. Walvoord DJ, Resnick MI, Grayhack JT: Effect of testosterone, dihydrotestosterone, estradiol, and prolactin on the weight and citric acid content of the lateral lobe of the rat prostate. Invest Urol 14:60–65, 1976.
190. Wang MC, Papsidero LD, Kuriyama M, et al: Prostate antigen: A new potential marker for prostatic cancer. Prostate 2:89–96, 1981.
191. Welshons WV, Lieberman ME, Gorski J: Nuclear localisation of unoccupied oestrogen receptors. Nature 307:747, 1984.
192. Wendel EF, Brannen GE, Putong PB, Grayhack JT: The effect of orchiectomy and estrogens on benign prostatic hyperplasia. J Urol 108:116–119, 1972.
193. White JW: The results of double castration in hypertrophy of the prostate. Ann Surg 22:1–80, 1895.
194. Wilson JD: The pathogenesis of benign prostatic hyperplasia. Am J Med 68:745, 1980.
195. Wilson JD, Griffin JE, Leshin M, George FW: Role of gonadal hormones in development of the sexual phenotypes. Hum Genet 58:78, 1981.
196. Wilson JD, Lasnitzki I: Dihydrotestosterone formation in fetal tissues of the rabbit and rat. Endocrinology 89:659, 1971.
197. Woodburne RT: Pelvis. *In* Woodburne RT (ed): Essentials in Human Anatomy. New York, Oxford University Press, 1978, pp 479–520.

Chapter 6

IMAGING OF THE PROSTATE

ERIC M. SMITH and MARTIN I. RESNICK

Clinical assessment of the prostate gland is challenging because of the inaccessible location of the gland deep within the pelvis. Traditionally, the only means of diagnosing prostatic disorders was through digital rectal examination, prostatic fluid inspection, serum markers, and surgical exploration. Unfortunately, prostate cancer is the most common malignancy in men, and the limitations of these traditional methods of diagnosing and staging prostate cancer have spurred the development and application of new imaging modalities to assess prostatic disease. Several new noninvasive imaging studies, particularly ultrasonography, computed tomography (CT), and magnetic resonance imaging (MRI), have been developed, and all aid in the evaluation of the prostate; however, all of these new techniques have deficiencies that limit their utility, and no one technique can consistently provide all the information needed by the clinician. In this chapter, imaging of the prostate is reviewed, and the relative merits of the various imaging modalities are examined.

INTRAVENOUS UROGRAPHY AND URETHROGRAPHY

For many years urography and urethrography were the only imaging studies available for prostate evaluation. The kidney-ureter-bladder (KUB) or scout film can demonstrate prostatic calculi, which signify benign prostatic hyperplasia (BPH) if located above the pelvic brim.[80] Osseous metastases from carcinoma may also be visualized on plain films. Most findings on intravenous urography (IVU) due to prostatic disorders are caused by bladder outlet obstruction. Bilateral hydronephrosis is seen in 3 to 6 per cent of patients with prostatism,[90]

and up to one third of patients with prostate cancer present with unilateral or bilateral hydronephrosis.[23] Parenchymal atrophy on IVU may result from such pyelocaliectasis. Tortuous, dilated ureters with elevation of the distal ureter (J-hooking) may also result from severe prostatic enlargement. Bladder findings due to obstruction include increased size, trabeculation, diverticulum formation, a thickened wall, and an elevated postvoid residual; however, postvoid residual is an unreliable sign owing to compensatory detrusor hypertrophy. Many patients with obstruction have no postvoid residual at all,[86] and bladder size as determined by IVU correlates poorly with residuals measured by catheter or ultrasonography.[5] The enlarged prostate often causes a bladder base deformity, an intravesical filling defect, or bladder neck distortion (Fig. 6–1), although these findings are less common in carcinoma than in BPH. A bladder base deformity secondary to prostatic carcinoma is often more irregular than one due to BPH. Urographic assessment of prostate size correlates poorly with prostate weight and resectability.[48]

For many years the routine work-up for BPH included the IVU, but this practice has been increasingly questioned owing to the low yield, risk, and cost of the study. Most investigators do not recommend routine IVU, reserving it instead for men with hematuria, stones, or an atypical history.[1, 72, 90] Similarly, retrograde urethrography and voiding cystourethrography are no longer routinely employed for prostatic evaluation. Retrograde urethrography of advanced prostatic carcinoma typically demonstrates urethral irregularity or an irregular bladder base deformity (Fig. 6–2). Urethrography should be reserved for men with a history of stricture or previous surgery.[80]

The obvious limitations of these contrast studies in evaluating the prostate sparked interest in developing

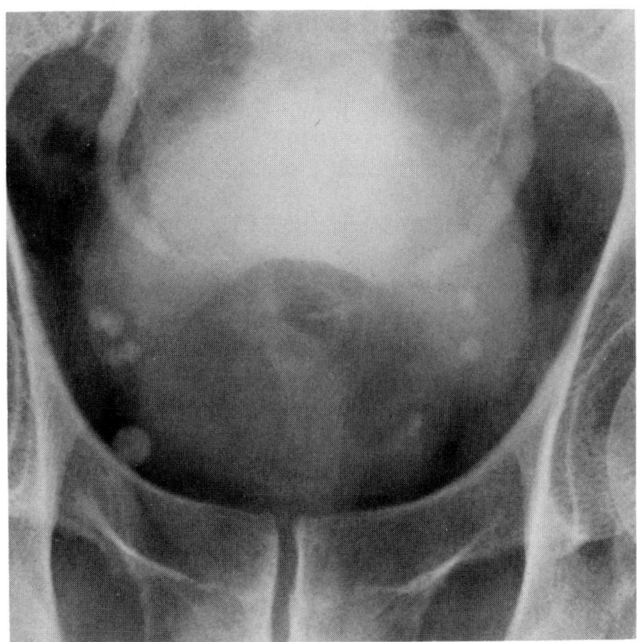

FIGURE 6–1. Intravesical filling defect secondary to prostatic enlargement.

new imaging modalities, and transrectal ultrasonography was the first of these to be widely used.

TRANSRECTAL ULTRASONOGRAPHY

Although the clinical use of ultrasound is a relatively recent phenomenon, the theoretical groundwork was laid in England in World War I, when Paul Langevin developed his method of detecting submerged submarines.[71] Wild and Reid in the 1950s first put ultrasound to medical use, and indeed were the first to propose using a transrectal ultrasonic probe to evaluate the prostate.[95] The medical use of ultrasound then languished until 1968 owing to the poor quality of images obtained with time amplitude echograms; however, the introduction by Watanabe of transrectal B-mode ultrasonography ushered in a new era of prostate imaging.[92] The original chair-mounted probe was replaced by a hand-held probe developed by Boyce et al in 1969,[7] and the first large series of prostate echography was reported by King soon afterwards.[38] The introduction of grey-scale imaging by Boyce and Resnick was a major step toward obtaining clinically useful prostatic images.[65] Further technologic refinements, including high-frequency transducers and real-time imaging, have led to the modern portable ultrasound machine.

A basic understanding of the physics and instrumentation of ultrasound is necessary for its proper use. Acoustic waves are generated from electrical energy via the piezoelectric effect of a transducer and propagated into the tissues. A gel is required as a coupling medium to transmit the acoustic waves from transducer to tissues owing to the markedly different acoustic qualities of air and tissue. Part of the acoustic energy is reflected back

to the transducer after encountering a change in tissue density and is transformed into electrical energy, and an image is generated.[54] Real-time imaging refers to a constantly updated image produced by multiple sequentially driven transducers. The frequency of a transducer affects the resolution of the image obtained, with a higher frequency producing sharper resolution; unfortunately, the higher the frequency the more the signal is attenuated and the less it penetrates tissue.[91] A 7.0-mHz transducer is generally used for the prostate and seminal vesicles. No damage results from the small amount of mechanical energy delivered to the tissues by ultrasonography.[93]

Early transducers used a rotating crystal and could only obtain images perpendicular to the probe known as "transverse" or "axial" views, similar to the horizontal plane of a CT scan. Later, linear array scanners were developed to obtain images in the longitudinal or sagittal plane. Newer mechanical and sector-array scanners can generate images in either plane. Most equipment currently available combines more than one type of transducer into a bimodal probe that can image the prostate in many planes. This has greatly improved the sensitivity of ultrasound prostatic examination.[66] The addition of color Doppler to endorectal ultrasonography to identify internal vasculature and flow may prove to be a valuable technique in the future.[67]

The technique of transrectal ultrasonography is simple. Before the examination, a digital rectal examination should be performed to rule out rectal pathology that may contraindicate probe insertion and to palpate the prostate itself. A cleansing enema is unnecessary for

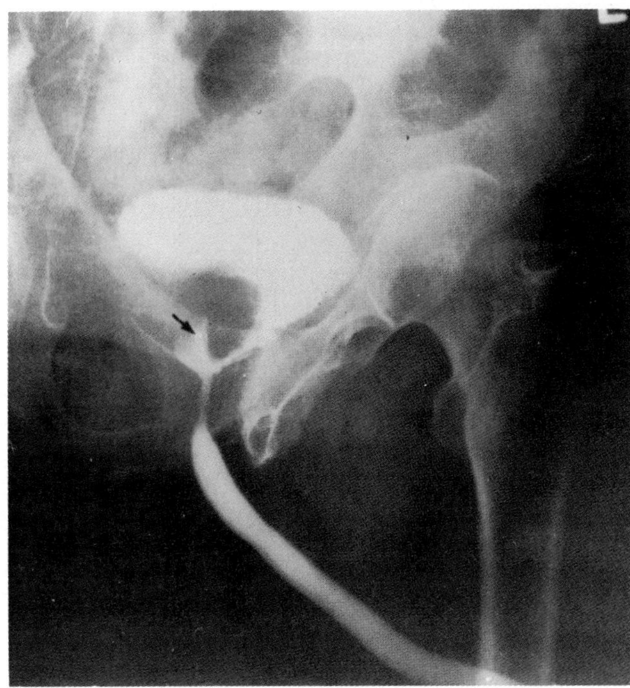

FIGURE 6–2. Irregular filling defect *(arrow)* caused by prostate carcinoma extending into the bladder base. (From Hricak H, Theoni RF: Neoplasms of the prostate gland. *In* Pollack HM [ed]: Clinical Urography. Philadelphia, WB Saunders Co, 1990, p 1390.)

examination alone, although it is recommended for transrectal ultrasound–guided biopsy of the prostate. The position of the patient is the decision of the examiner (e.g., decubitus, lithotomy, knee-chest). Preparation of the probe usually requires placing condoms over the probe in order to use water baths to enhance image quality, although some probes do not require water baths. Careful review of the manufacturer's instructions is necessary because of the variety and variability of instruments available. Although the exact sequence of imaging is unimportant, it is helpful to perform examination in a systematic fashion. Typically, transverse images are obtained at 5-mm intervals beginning at the bladder neck and extending toward the apex. Longitudinal images are then obtained of the midline and the lateral lobes. Appropriately labeled hard copies of images are useful to obtain for future reference.[8a, 93] Only real-time images should be used for interpretation of a study, however.[17]

A clear understanding of the anatomy of the prostate is essential to interpreting sonographic images. The prostate gland lies between the urogenital diaphragm and the bladder outlet. Anteriorly the gland is fixed by the puboprostatic ligaments, and posteriorly lies Denonvillier's fascia. It usually has a cone or chestnut shape and varies in size, averaging 3.4 cm long by 4.4 cm wide and 2.6 cm thick. The urethra passes through the prostate in a straight line except for angulation proximal to the verumontanum. The seminal vesicles lie posterosuperiorly, whereas the ejaculatory ducts enter at the verumontanum. The whole gland is surrounded by a thick fibromuscular capsule.[79a]

The early concept of the prostate as an organ with distinct lobes[79a] has been superseded by the zonal concept of McNeal. He proposed after extensive gross and microscopic dissections that the prostate be divided into distinct glandular and nonglandular regions.[49, 50] The nonglandular fibromuscular stroma is located in the anteromedial portion of the gland, and the glandular regions are divided into the periurethral glands and transition, central, and peripheral zones (Fig. 6–3). Each zone is related to specific segments of the urethra and ejaculatory ducts. The peripheral zone comprises about 75 per cent of the gland in young males and surrounds the urethra along and distal to the verumontanum. It comprises the posterior and lateral portions of the gland. Its glandular architecture consists of small, round acini and its stroma of loosely woven, randomly oriented bundles. Approximately 70 per cent of prostate carcinomas arise there, but BPH does not originate from this area.

The central zone comprises about 25 per cent of the normal prostate, surrounding the ejaculatory ducts throughout their course through the gland. This zone comprises most of the glandular tissue at the base of the gland. Histologically the central zone is characterized by large, irregular acini and tightly arranged muscle fibers. Only about 10 per cent of carcinomas originate in this region, and BPH does not occur here. By contrast, the transition zone is the site of origin of BPH. It is located on both sides of the proximal urethral segment just lateral to the periprostatic sphincter. Although the glandular histology is similar to that of the transition zone, its stroma is more tightly woven. This zone comprises only 5 per cent of the gland in young men, although in adults it may comprise 30 per cent of the prostate and eventually up to 90 per cent. Overall about 20 per cent of carcinomas arise there, and tumors in that region cannot be palpated owing to the overlying peripheral zone. The periurethral glands make up about 1 per cent of glandular tissue and are embedded in the urethral smooth muscle comprising the preprostatic sphincter. BPH arising there causes an enlarged middle lobe.[55, 79a] The nonglandular anterior fibromuscular stroma and periprostatic sphincter are not subject to pathologic change.

Two other aspects of prostate anatomy are important for effective use of ultrasonography. Lee et al described a "trapezoid area" within the peripheral zone bounded by the prostate apex, rectourethralis muscle, membranous urethra, and rectum. The prostatic capsule is thin or absent over this area, and thus carcinoma can easily spread. Similarly, the invaginated extraprostatic space surrounds the ejaculatory ducts as they travel through the central zone, providing an avenue for peripheral zone cancer to travel easily to the seminal vesicles. Carcinoma in both of these areas can be readily detected by ultrasonography, and biopsy for accurate tumor staging can be done.[42]

The appearance of the normal prostate on ultrasonography corresponds to its zonal anatomy (Fig. 6–4). The normal prostate appears as a triangular ellipsoid structure surrounded by a continuous, symmetric surgical capsule. The peripheral zone is arbitrarily deemed isoechoic and is the standard by which the echographic characteristics of other tissues are judged. In the normal prostate the gland has a uniform, homogeneous echo pattern. The posterior portion of the gland appears concave owing to the distortion of the inflated balloon. The apex and midportion are easily visualized, but the base may be difficult to differentiate from the bladder base. The seminal vesicles are seen as paired, slightly hypoechoic structures at the base of the bladder. On longitudinal or sagittal scan the normal prostate has similar acoustic properties, but the gland appears round in the midline (Fig. 6–5). The seminal vesicles are again easily seen.[93] The urethra can also be visualized coursing through the prostate (Fig. 6–6).

Whereas the transverse diameter exceeds the anteroposterior diameter in a normal prostate, the anteroposterior dimension greatly increases in BPH, giving the prostate a rounded appearance (Fig. 6–7). Ultrasonically the capsule is well delineated and may appear thickened owing to compression of the peripheral zone by the enlarging adenoma. The interior of the gland is characterized by multiple fine homogeneous echoes produced by the many small adenomas present and multiple interfaces created by dilated prostatic ducts containing corpora amylacea and microcalculi. There may be areas of hyperechogenicity or hypoechogenicity due to variable areas of hyperplasia and/or inflammation. On longitudinal scan the hyperplastic prostate becomes more

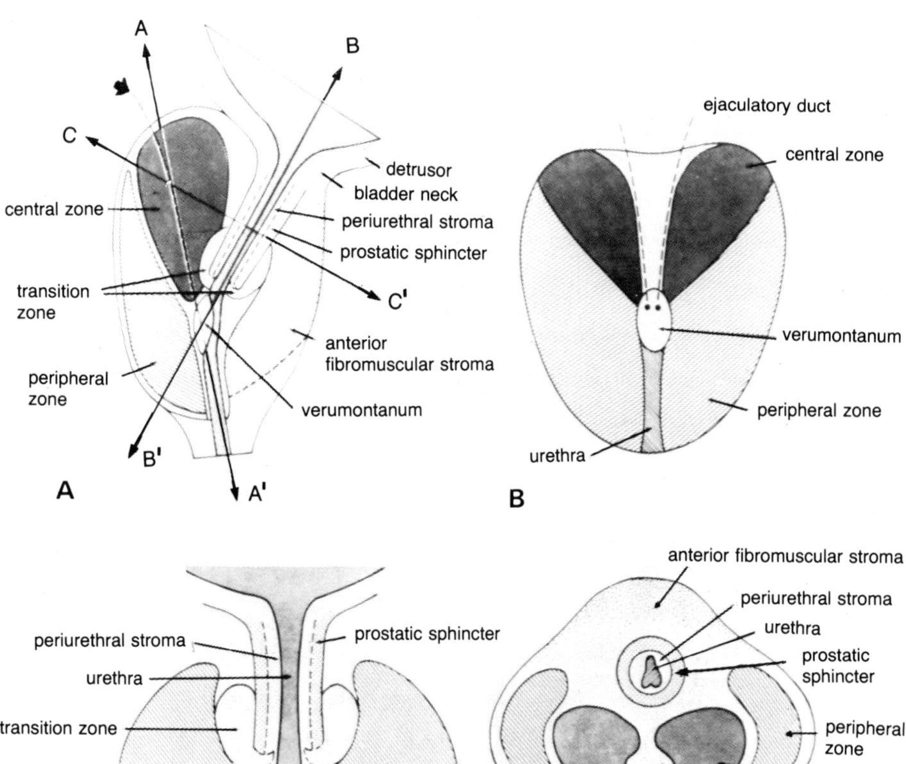

FIGURE 6–3. Internal prostatic architecture. *A,* Midsagittal plane. Open arrow designates course of the ejaculatory ducts. *B,* Coronal section along A-A'. *C,* Oblique coronal section along B-B'. *D,* Transverse section along C-C'. (Redrawn from Resnick MI [ed]: Prostatic Ultrasonography. Philadelphia, BC Decker, 1990, p 37; with permission.)

rounded instead of triangular as it increases in size. The most important characteristic of BPH is that the capsule is well delineated and free of disruption.[54]

Transrectal ultrasonography is infrequently performed on patients with acute prostatitis because of the danger of bacteremia; nevertheless, the gland appears diffusely enlarged and hypoechoic because of inflammation. Prostatic abscesses are usually clearly defined as hypoechoic areas on ultrasonography, and transurethral resection of such abscesses under ultrasound guidance has been

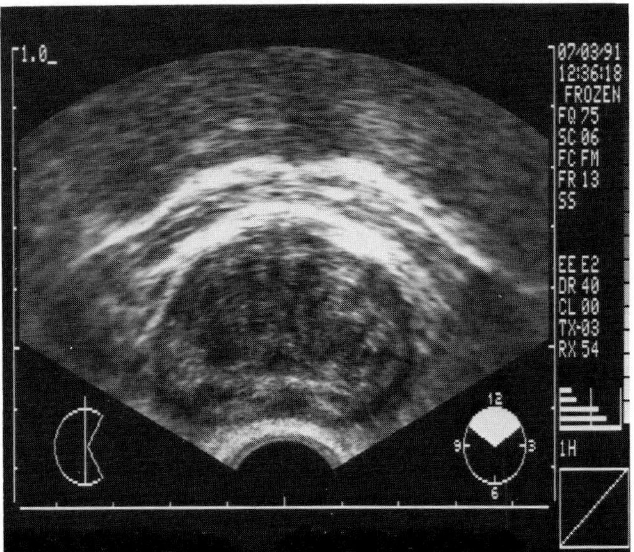

FIGURE 6–4. Transverse transrectal ultrasonogram of normal prostate.

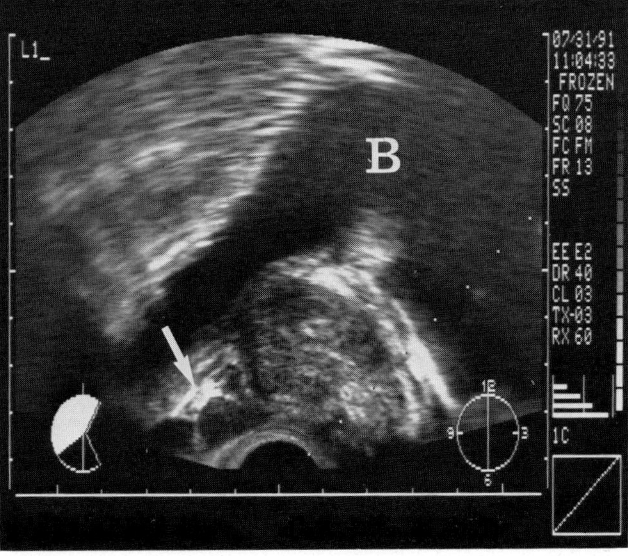

FIGURE 6–5. Longitudinal sonogram of normal prostate and seminal vesicle *(arrow).* B = Bladder.

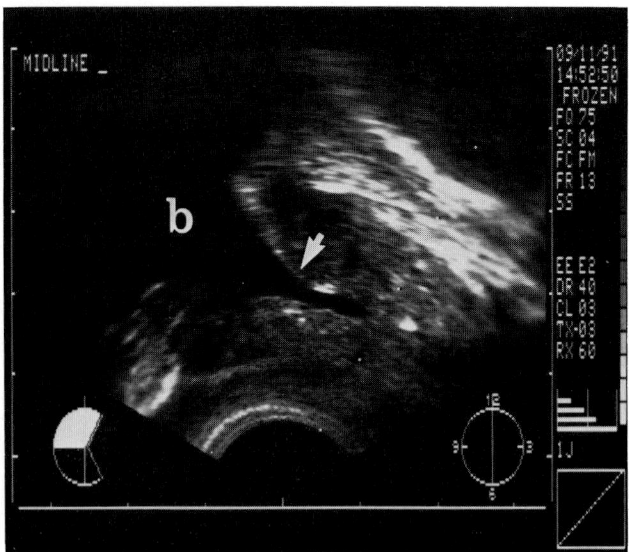

FIGURE 6–6. Longitudinal sonogram demonstrating the urethra *(arrow)*. b = Bladder.

reported.[37] Chronic prostatitis causes diffuse changes, including hyperechoic, symmetric areas extending laterally from the urethra. Prostatitis has no distinct, diagnostic appearance. The variable changes due to chronic inflammation are difficult to distinguish from those of carcinoma, but the capsule should never be disrupted. Ultimately other clinical parameters, such as urinalysis, are more important in the diagnosis of prostatitis. Prostatic calculi appear as clearly defined, highly echogenic areas, often located posteriorly when associated with BPH. Again, unless associated with malignancy, they do not distort the prostatic capsule.[54]

By far the most important application of transrectal ultrasonography is in screening, diagnosing, staging, and monitoring the treatment of prostate carcinoma. In contrast to the homogeneous appearance of the normal gland, the acoustic characteristics of cancer are quite variable. Initial studies using B-mode and early grey-scale technology indicated that carcinoma was hyperechoic.[38, 65] As technology improved, however, many investigators reported that carcinoma could be hyperechoic, isoechoic, hypoechoic, or of mixed echogenicity.[40, 69] Most carcinomas are hypoechoic with irregular margins arising in the peripheral zone (Fig. 6–8). Dahnert et al reported that 76 per cent of prostate cancers in prostatectomy specimens were hypoechoic and 24 per cent isoechoic.[18] Shinohara et al showed that 65 per cent of carcinomas were hypoechoic and 35 per cent isoechoic.[77] The explanation for this variability may be that early carcinomas are of low echogenicity, but as they invade and grow they become more echogenic.[69] Goldstein et al reported that smaller tumors were isoechoic but larger tumors were hypoechoic.[25] Not only is the appearance of carcinoma quite varied, but some carcinomas may not be seen on ultrasonography at all, as shown in patients with normal ultrasound examinations revealing occult carcinoma on prostatectomy performed for benign disease.[62] Adding to the difficulty in determining the nature of a lesion on ultrasonography is the similar hypoechoic appearance of cysts, infarcts, inflammatory conditions, and blood vessels.[93]

The appearance of the prostatic capsule and seminal vesicles can also signify carcinoma. Whereas confined carcinoma has a capsule that is well defined and free of disruption, invasive carcinoma distorts and deforms the continuous, hyperechoic pattern of the capsule (Fig. 6–9). Hypoechoic strands may signify tumor spread into periprostatic fat. Cancer invading the seminal vesicles is visualized as distorted, echogenic areas continuous with tumor involving the gland itself (Fig. 6–10). Invasion of one seminal vesicle only may cause seminal vesicle size and echo asymmetry. Microinvasive capsular disease or

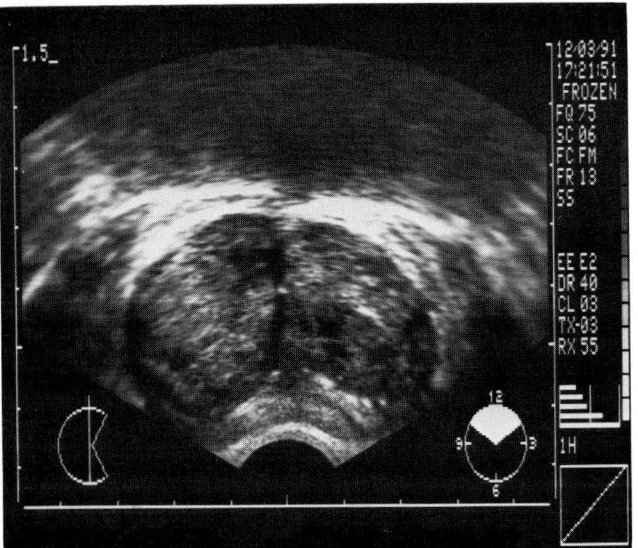

FIGURE 6–7. Transverse transrectal ultrasonogram demonstrating benign prostatic hyperplasia (BPH).

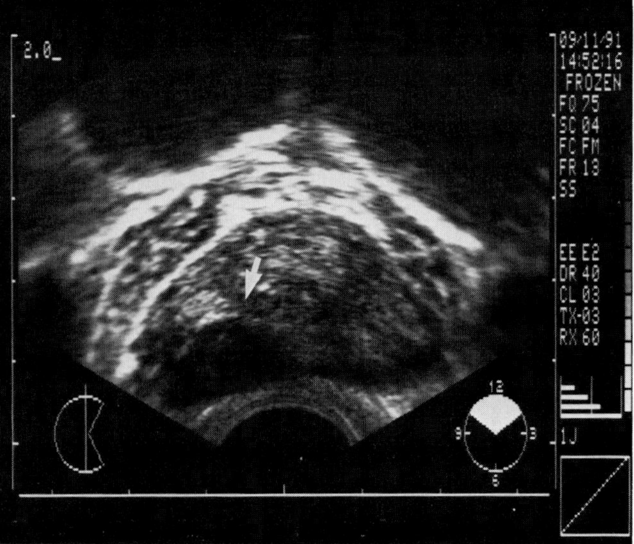

FIGURE 6–8. Transverse transrectal ultrasound scan demonstrating typical hypoechoic area characteristic of prostate carcinoma *(arrow)*.

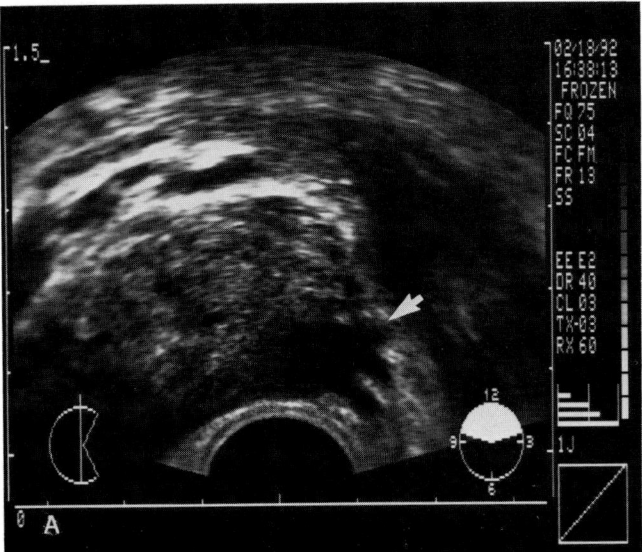

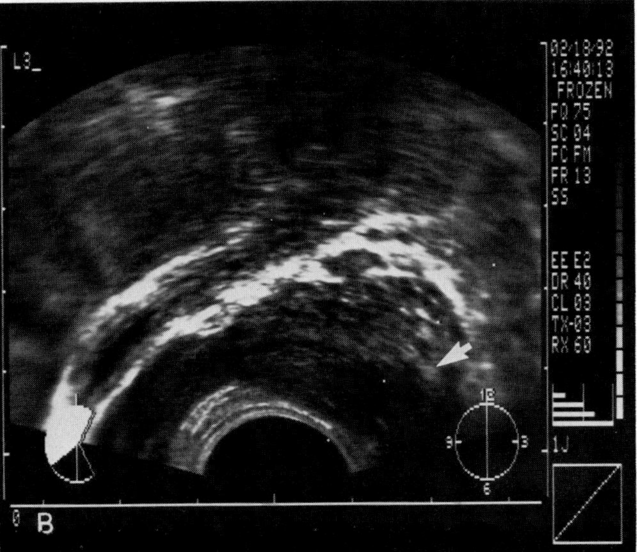

FIGURE 6–9. Prostate cancer. *A,* Transverse image at midprostate shows indistinct boundary echo that is discontinuous on the left side of the gland *(arrow)*. *B,* Sagittal scan of the same patient demonstrating hypoechoic area of cancer *(arrow)*.

microscopic extension into the seminal vesicles cannot be distinguished by ultrasonography.[59]

Although prostate cancer does not have a pathognomonic appearance on ultrasonography, several signs of malignancy are seen with this imaging modality. This has led to the use of ultrasound-guided prostate biopsy by both the transrectal and transperineal routes.[32, 64] An enema and broad-spectrum antibiotic are administered prior to biopsy, and oral antibiotics are usually continued for several days afterwards. Most newer ultrasound instruments feature a needle marker on the screen for accurate needle placement. The development of spring-loaded biopsy guns has further enhanced the diagnostic accuracy of ultrasound-guided needle biopsy. Although ultrasound-guided biopsy has come into widespread use, some controversy remains about whether it is superior to digitally guided biopsies. In one study of 43 patients with negative digitally guided biopsies of palpable nodules, cancer was discovered in 53 per cent using ultrasound-guided biopsy.[30] Others have reported that digitally guided biopsies are just as accurate and that routine ultrasound-guided biopsies are unnecessary.[64] More recently, Hodge et al have shown that random systematic ultrasound-guided biopsies of the prostate, combined with directed biopsies of hypoechoic areas not included in random biopsies, is a highly accurate method of diagnosing prostate cancer.[31] In one study of 44 men with a previously negative systematic digitally guided biopsy, systematic ultrasound-guided biopsies were performed. Only four (9.1 per cent) additional cancers were discovered, and the authors concluded that performing random systematic biopsies was more important than the technique used to guide the biopsy needle.[43] Ultrasonography does offer the advantage of more accurate needle placement for both directed and random biopsies and is recommended especially for biopsy of a palpable nodule if the result of previous digitally guided biopsy is negative. Ultrasound-guided biopsy is also recommended for the palpably normal prostate when other indications of cancer are present, such as an elevated prostate-specific antigen (PSA).[68] In addition to biopsy, ultrasonography may be used to guide radioactive seed implantation.[6] The value of this therapeutic modality remains to be determined.

Whereas the role of ultrasonography in biopsy of the prostate is controversial its role in staging carcinoma is somewhat clearer. Ultrasonography can reveal capsular penetration or seminal vesicle invasion, although microscopic invasion is not seen as noted above. Pontes et al showed that transrectal ultrasonography had a sensitivity of 89 per cent in detecting capsular penetration and 100 per cent in detecting seminal vesicle invasion.[59] A recent series comparing preoperative ultrasonography with 25 pathologic specimens demonstrated a sensitivity of 69 per cent and a specificity of 91 per cent.[29] Digital rectal examination accurately determines stage in only 50 per cent of patients with palpable lesions.[75] The intraprostatic volume of a tumor is an indicator of extracapsular tumor extension, seminal vesicle invasion, and nodal status. In one series of radical prostatectomy specimens, significant capsular penetration was found in 7 per cent of tumors less than 4 cc in volume but was seen in 86 per cent of those larger than 12 cc.[53] Similarly, another series of radical prostatectomy specimens showed seminal vesicle invasion in 6 per cent of tumors less than 4 cc in volume but revealed invasion in 82 per cent of those larger than 12 cc.[88] Lymph node metastases are found in 46 per cent of tumors larger than 12 cc, compared with only 1 per cent of those less than 4 cc.[52]

Ultrasonography can accurately estimate volume of the gland itself,[84] and a variety of methods are used to determine cancer volume, with most based on the maximum transverse diameter of a suspicious lesion. Terris et al performed preoperative volume estimation using several different ultrasound methods on 110 patients undergoing radical prostatectomy and found that preoperative volume estimation correlated poorly with the

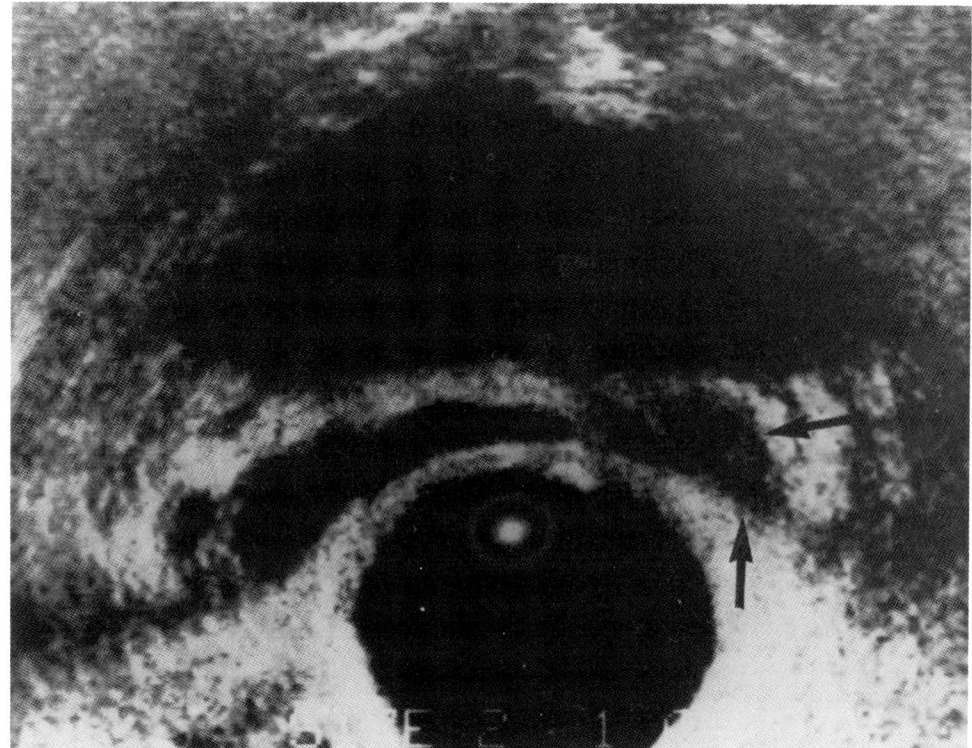

FIGURE 6–10. Transverse transrectal scan demonstrating distortion of the left seminal vesicle secondary to invasive prostate carcinoma *(arrows)*. (From Muldoon L, Resnick MI: Results of ultrasonography of the prostate. Urol Clin North Am 16:697, 1989.)

pathologic specimen. They concluded that although tumor volume is a strong indicator of extraprostatic extension, current sonographic methods used to estimate tumor volume are not accurate enough to base clinical decisions on.[82] Ultrasonography is more accurate than digital rectal examination (DRE). Further studies are needed to fully define the role of ultrasonography in the staging of carcinoma.

Transrectal ultrasonography is also useful in monitoring the response to therapy by serial measurement of prostatic volume.[24] Prostatic size decreases by approximately 30 per cent following either orchiectomy or estrogen therapy.[11] Prostatic size is only slightly reduced in patients who suffer progressive disease within 1 year after castration; moreover, no patient develops distant progression within 1 year if prostatic volume decreases by 50 per cent after treatment. Ultrasonography has also been used to monitor response to chemotherapy or radiation therapy,[22] again by assessing prostatic size, shape, and capsular integrity. Although the decrease in total gland volume is helpful in monitoring response to therapy, the rate of decrease as determined by sequential measurements has not been established as a reliable prognostic indicator.[14] Others have shown that stable disease is difficult to follow with ultrasonography owing to the paucity of local change after radiation therapy.[20] Kabilin et al performed ultrasound-guided biopsies, both directed and random, in 27 men after radiation therapy, and 25 demonstrated cancer. They also correlated these results with PSA and concluded that a rise in PSA was strongly associated with recurrent disease.[35] PSA is a more sensitive indicator of disease progression or recurrence than is ultrasonography and is superior for routine

monitoring of prostate cancer. Ultrasonography is appropriate as an adjunctive imaging modality only.

Finally, the role of transrectal ultrasonography in detection and screening of prostatic carcinoma remains controversial. As noted previously, prostate cancer is the most common malignancy in men, with more than 134,000 new cases diagnosed annually and an autopsy incidence of 30 per cent in men older than 50 years.[21] Up to 75 per cent of these patients have metastatic disease at diagnosis; moreover, up to 80 per cent of patients with nodal involvement die of prostate cancer.[94] These daunting statistics have aroused much interest in the use of ultrasonography as a screening test for cancer.

Several epidemiologic factors influence the use of any screening technique. First, there must be a high enough incidence of the disease in the asymptomatic patient to make screening worthwhile. The age range at highest risk for prostate cancer includes men 40 to 75 years old, and screening should be confined to that group.[61] Second, the aggressiveness of the disease itself needs to be elucidated. Most tumors less than 1 cc in volume do not metastasize,[51] so an ideal screening program would detect occult cancer less than 1 cc in volume. Unfortunately, most prostate cancers remain occult, and Stamey has shown that only 1 of 380 men with prostate cancer dies of this disease.[78] Currently no method exists to differentiate indolent cancers from aggressive ones,[74] although Stamey et al have recently proposed that cancers less than 0.5 cc in volume probably do not attain clinical significance based on the long doubling time of prostate cancer.[79] A screening program should be economically feasible, and with the high incidence of cancer, the cost of screening ultrasonography and biopsy of men at risk has been estimated at well over 7 billion dollars annually.[13] Finally, an appropriate screening test is worthwhile only if there is a cure for the disease. Although radical prostatectomy is curative, the morbidity and mortality of the procedure are high enough that performing it on all men with occult cancer may exceed the morbidity and mortality of prostate cancer itself.

In light of these sobering statistics, let us consider the place of ultrasonography in screening for prostate cancer. A screening test must have high sensitivity, specificity, positive predictive value, and negative predictive value to be effective. A useful screening test for prostate cancer should have a specificity of at least 95 per cent.[85] Older studies show a sensitivity of ultrasonography of 60 to 85 per cent and a specificity of 41 to 79 per cent.[93] More recent studies have demonstrated that ultrasonography can detect cancers that are not palpable. For example, Lee et al screened 784 men with digital rectal examination and transrectal ultrasonography.[41] Digital rectal examination detected 10 tumors, and transrectal ultrasonography detected 20. Other studies have shown that the average calculated tumor volume of cancers detected ultrasonically is 1.8 cm³, compared with 6.0 cm³ by DRE.[27]

Recent work by Cooner et al in defining the role of ultrasonography and PSA in detecting early cancer is enlightening.[17] In their study of 1807 men, DRE alone had a positive predictive value of 36 per cent, and a PSA greater than 4 had a positive predictive value of 35 per cent. If both were abnormal, the positive predictive value was 60 per cent; moreover, abnormal ultrasound results in this scenario only increased the positive predictive value to 62 per cent. Furthermore, if both DRE and PSA were normal, ultrasonography had a positive predictive value of only 2.1 per cent.[17] A limitation of many previous studies of ultrasonography as a screening study is the absence of pathologic correlation; however, a recent study of 51 patients who underwent transrectal ultrasonography prior to radical cystoprostatectomy for bladder cancer showed a specificity of 75 per cent and a sensitivity of 53 per cent for adenocarcinoma of the prostate.[81] Another study correlating ultrasonography with autopsy findings in a random population without a history of prostate cancer demonstrated a sensitivity of 32 per cent and specificity of 64 per cent.[15] In one study of 73 patients with pulmonary malignancies undergoing random systematic ultrasonically guided biopsies, 41 had normal prostates on digital rectal examination. Of these 41 patients, 14 had hypoechoic areas on ultrasonography, but only one yielded cancer on biopsy. The overall specificity of ultrasonography in this study was 69 per cent and sensitivity was 50 per cent.[28] Although ultrasonography alone is not adequate for prostate cancer screening, it may have a role in combination with PSA.[45] Large-scale randomized screening studies to determine the efficacy of DRE, PSA, and ultrasonography have been proposed by the National Institutes of Health in order to resolve this screening dilemma. Until these studies are completed, ultrasonography alone cannot be recommended for screening of prostate cancer.

To summarize, ultrasonography is useful in the staging and biopsy of prostate cancer as well as in monitoring response to therapy; however, the emergence of PSA has cast ultrasonography in a secondary role. Similarly, the use of ultrasonography alone as a screening test cannot be recommended owing to the variable appearance of prostate cancer on ultrasonography. Prostatic ultrasonography can accurately guide biopsy of the gland, and further refinements in technology may ultimately lead to an expansion of its clinical role. The limitations of ultrasonography in imaging the prostate propelled the application of other modalities, particularly CT and MRI, to the prostate.

COMPUTED TOMOGRAPHY OF THE PROSTATE

CT came to the fore in the early 1970s and today is in widespread use throughout the United States. CT scans are produced by measuring the attenuation of radiation in a body slice using a circular scanner array. These data are then transformed and reconstructed into an image using sophisticated computer techniques. The density of tissue on CT scan is assigned a Hounsfield unit, with water assigned a value of zero, air a negative value, and dense body tissue a positive value. Relative contraindications to CT include contrast allergy and pregnancy.[46]

The normal prostate is seen as a homogeneous density on CT scan. Size, density, and gland contour can be shown on CT, and volume can be easily assessed; however, CT cannot delineate the internal architecture of the prostate and often cannot separate normal parenchyma from the capsule.[2, 87] Furthermore, the prostatic margin often cannot be separated from the levator ani or rectum.[19] Because the Hounsfield units for cancer and benign disease overlap, it is impossible to differentiate benign from malignant disease. Benign prostatic hyperplasia may appear as a bladder density. A nodular contour or ragged margin may indicate carcinoma, although neither is pathognomonic for malignancy (Fig. 6–11); moreover, a smooth margin does not exclude carcinoma.[60] CT is unable to reliably differentiate between benign hyperplasia and carcinoma, and indeed between Stages A and B carcinoma.

CT has proved moderately useful for staging prostatic carcinoma. CT can demonstrate extraprostatic extension into adjacent structures (Fig. 6–12) and lymphadenopathy (Fig. 6–13). Unilateral levator ani enlargement or thickening of the rectal wall can signify invasive disease. Visualization of cancer extension into the bladder base or seminal vesicles is not accurate.[34] Hricak et al evaluated the effectiveness of CT in distinguishing between Stages B2 and C in 46 patients with proven carcinoma. In this group clinical staging had an accuracy of 61 per cent, with an understaging rate of 39 per cent. CT was 65 per cent accurate with 19 per cent understaging.[33] Much of the inaccuracy of CT was due to an inability to determine bladder base or seminal vesicle extension (Fig. 6–14). Clearly CT has limited applicability to prostate cancer diagnosis and evaluation of Stage A to C disease.

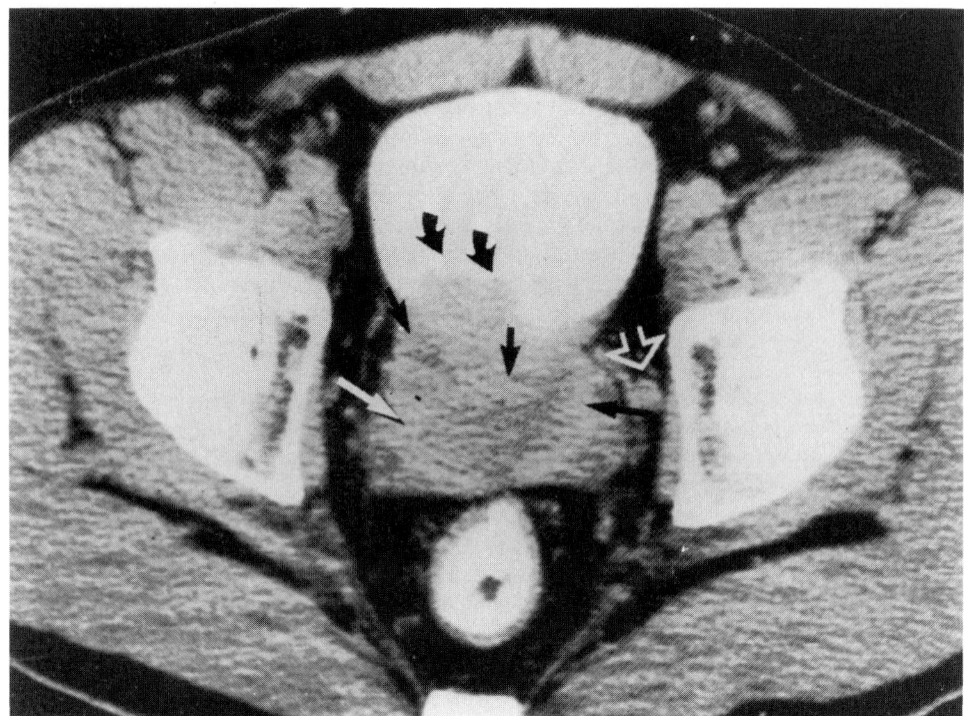

FIGURE 6–11. Enlarged prostate with low attenuation areas *(arrows)* in a patient with prostatic abscess following TURP. Irregular margins *(curved arrows)* extending intravesically are due to carcinoma. Adenopathy *(open arrow)* is seen on the left side. (From Hricak H, Theoni RF: Neoplasms of the prostate gland. *In* Pollack HM [ed]: Clinical Urography. Philadelphia. WB Saunders Co, 1990, p 1392.)

Although CT imaging of localized carcinoma is imprecise, its use in detecting lymphadenopathy is more effective. CT cannot detect micrometastases, and it is unable to delineate the internal architecture of nodes; rather, it detects metastases based on node size, with nodes greater than 1.0 cm considered suspicious and those greater than 1.5 cm considered abnormal, although such enlargement may be secondary to inflammatory disease. Reports of sensitivity vary widely from 25 to 93 per cent, with an overall accuracy of 77 to 93 per cent.[34] Others have shown a CT sensitivity of only 14 per cent in detecting pelvic lymph node metastases.[73] CT scanning can be useful in the evaluation of a patient with a high grade or large tumor or high PSA who is likely to have nodal metastases; however, caution must be exercised to avoid overstaging nodes enlarged because of inflammatory conditions. CT can be used for accurate transperineal iodine-125 prostate implants.[89] CT has also been used for dosage adjustment in external radiation therapy,[26] and in percutaneous drainage of

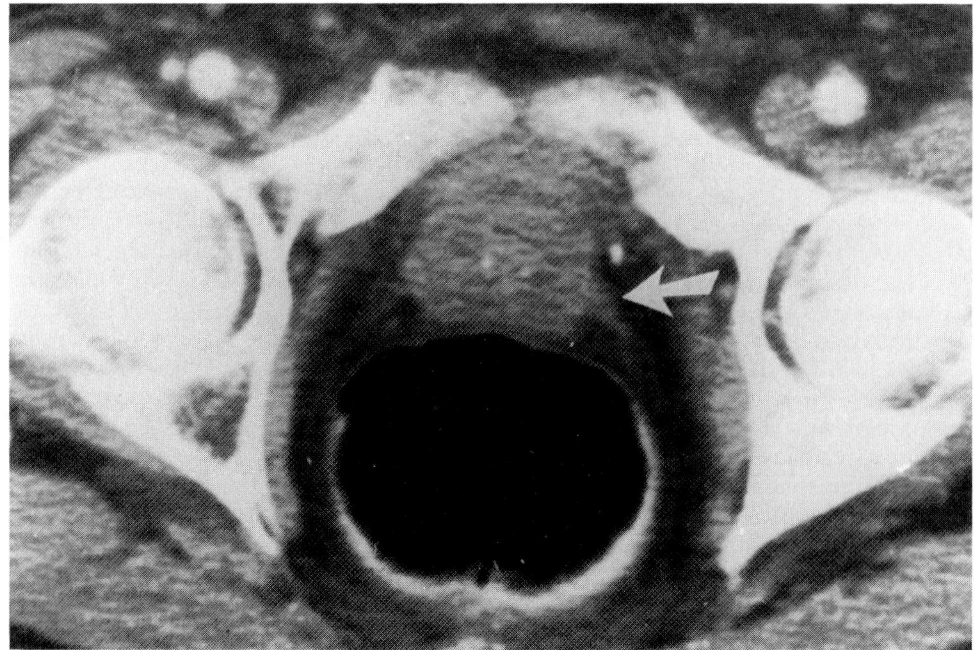

FIGURE 6–12. CT of Stage C prostate carcinoma. Extension of tumor beyond the prostatic capsule *(arrow)* is seen. (From Hricak H, Theoni RF: Neoplasms of the prostate gland. *In* Pollack HM [ed]: Clinical Urography. Philadelphia, WB Saunders Co, 1990, p 1392.)

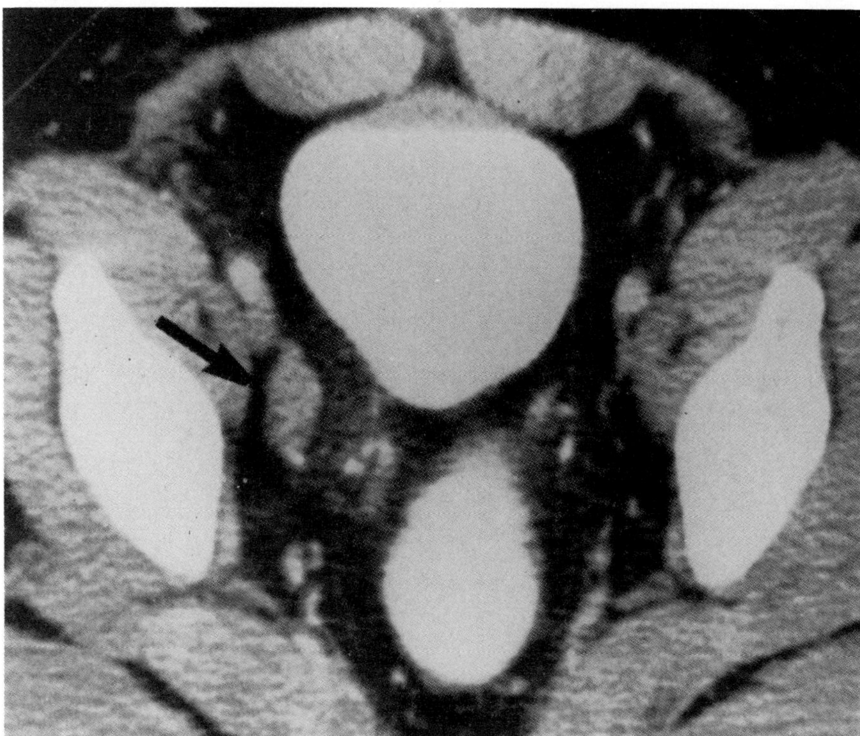

FIGURE 6–13. A lymph node in the right internal iliac chain is seen *(arrow)* in a patient with prostate carcinoma. (From Hricak H, Theoni RF: Neoplasms of the prostate gland. *In* Pollack HM [ed]: Clinical Urography. Philadelphia, WB Saunders Co, 1990, p 1393.)

prostatic abscesses.[36] Finally, CT is useful for evaluation of distant metastases from prostate carcinoma.

The value of imaging the prostate by CT is limited, particularly in the evaluation of localized cancer. Although it may be helpful in evaluation of nodal metastases, its use may be superseded by the widespread acceptance of laparoscopic pelvic lymph node dissection and by new developments in MRI.

MAGNETIC RESONANCE IMAGING OF THE PROSTATE

MRI emerged in 1980 as an outgrowth of the use of nuclear magnetic resonance to study chemical compounds. MRI has several advantages over conventional radiography. It demonstrates differences in magnetic properties and thus can show more contrast than radio-

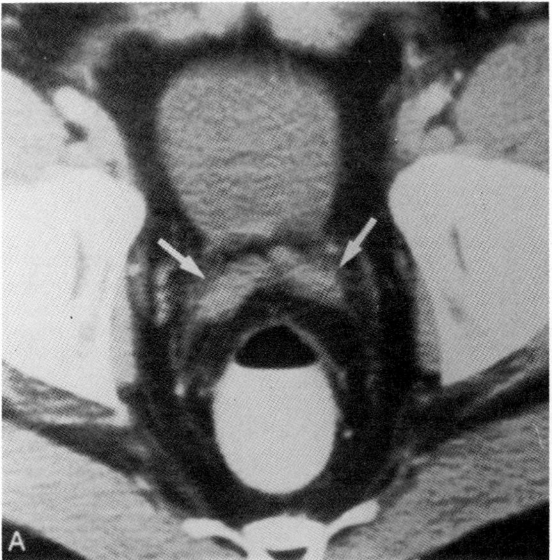

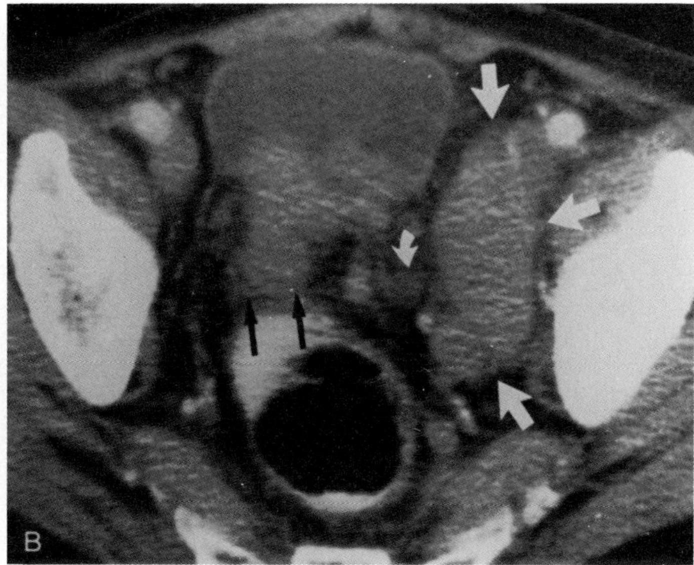

FIGURE 6–14. *A,* Normal seminal vesicles *(arrows). B,* Asymmetry of seminal vesicles in a patient with infiltration of carcinoma into the right seminal vesicle *(black arrows).* Adenopathy *(white arrows)* is seen in the left external iliac chain. Hydroureter *(curved arrow)* is seen on the left. (From Hricak H, Theoni RF: Neoplasms of the prostate gland. *In* Pollack HM [ed]: Clinical Urography. Philadelphia, WB Saunders Co, 1990, p 1393.)

graphic images; moreover, MRI can be used to obtain images in sagittal, coronal, transverse, and/or oblique planes. Furthermore, MRI does not use ionizing radiation, so it is safer than conventional radiography.[39] Contraindications to MRI use include the presence of cerebral aneurysm clips, cardiac pacemakers, and/or other electronic devices (e.g., cochlear implants) inside the body (DA Finelli, personal communication, 1992).[56]

MRI takes advantage of the physical properties of hydrogen nuclei to generate an image. Each hydrogen nucleus contains an odd number of protons and thus generates a minute magnetic field. Each magnetic field can be thought of as a vector force with its own magnitude and direction. They are randomly oriented in the absence of a strong external magnetic field, but when one is applied the nuclei align themselves along the direction of the magnetic field. The nuclei can be oriented in a parallel or antiparallel direction, with each direction signifying a different energy state. Application of radiofrequency pulse makes protons resonate in a higher energy state. When the radiofrequency pulse is terminated, the protons return to a lower energy state and emit a radiofrequency that is received by an antenna. The signal is then processed by a computer to produce an image. The antennae used to transmit and receive these radiofrequencies are referred to as coils, and the closer a coil is to the surface of the object imaged the greater the signal-to-noise ratio is and the greater the resolution obtained. Contrast in MRI depends on tissue proton density, T1, T2, and flow. T1 and T2 refer to the time constants describing the return of excited protons to a baseline energy state after stimulation by a radiofrequency pulse. An MRI pulse sequence can be designed to produce image contrast predominately reflecting proton density, T1, or T2 relaxation. The image produced can thus be varied to

yield more information (DA Finelli, personal communication, 1992).[39]

Surface coils have improved the images obtained with body coils by increasing local signal-to-noise ratios,[47] and newer endorectal surface coils have dramatically improved images even further.[76] T1-weighted images depict the prostate as a homogeneous structure of medium signal intensity without demonstrating intraprostatic anatomic differences (Fig. 6–15). Zonal anatomy is revealed by T2-weighted images, with the peripheral zone appearing as an area of high intensity. The capsule, periprostatic venous plexus, and seminal vesicles can also be visualized. The seminal vesicles have a high-intensity image, whereas the periprostatic venous plexus usually has a lesser intensity (Fig. 6–16). The capsule has a lower signal intensity than the remainder of the gland and should be sharply delineated in the normal prostate.[57]

The promise of MRI lies in its ability to distinguish benign from malignant disease. Benign prostatic hyperplasia usually occurs in the transition zone and causes expansion of this area (Fig. 6–17). The prostate with benign enlargement appears inhomogeneous or nodular on T2-weighted images, but because carcinoma can also occur within the transition zone, body-coil MRI cannot distinguish between the two.[10] Although the normal peripheral zone is homogeneous, with high signal intensity carcinoma appears as an ill-defined defect of lower intensity.[58] Other processes, such as BPH or inflammation, may produce a similar appearance, and the appearance of carcinoma may be highly variable. Early studies have shown that MRI cannot reliably differentiate between benign and malignant processes confined to the gland.[9] In one study the overall sensitivity of MRI in detecting nonpalpable tumors was 58 per cent and specificity was 48 per cent, although it was very sensitive

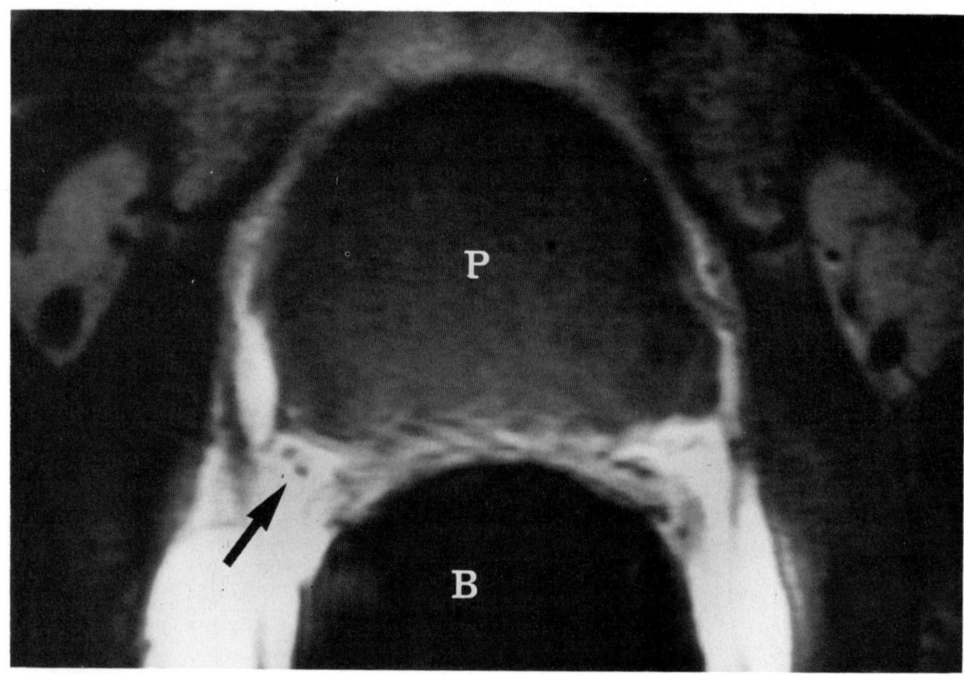

FIGURE 6–15. Normal prostate showing neurovascular bundle *(arrow)*. P = Prostate; B = bladder. T1-weighted image. Endorectal surface coil MRI. TR 500, TE 25; 10-cm FOV; 3-mm slice thickness. (Courtesy of Howard M. Pollack, MD.)

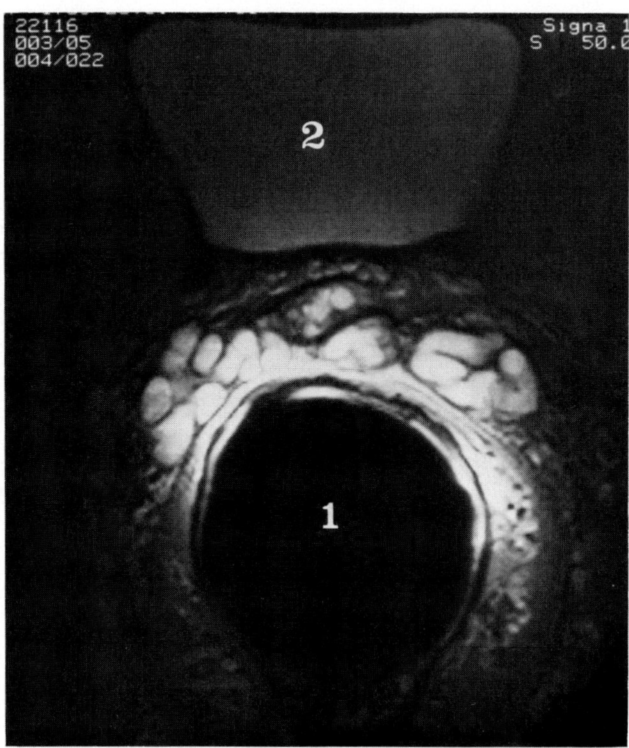

FIGURE 6–16. Normal seminal vesicles. 1 = Endorectal balloon; 2 = bladder. T2-weighted endorectal surface coil MRI. Fast spin echo. TR 4000, TE 100; 1.5 T; 256 × 256 matrix; 10-cm FOV; 4-mm slice thickness. (Courtesy of Howard M. Pollack, MD.)

(85 per cent) in detecting anterior nonpalpable lesions.[12] Endorectal coils may eventually improve resolution enough to make early detection possible.[76]

Although MRI may not reliably reveal intraprostatic malignancy, it demonstrates extraprostatic extension quite readily (Fig. 6–18). Tumor may extend through fat on T1-weighted images or may be seen invading the seminal vesicles on T2-weighted images. Sagittal and coronal images may reveal bladder or rectal invasion. Obliteration of the periprostatic fat by tumor or bladder wall invasion is often signified by an abnormal image intensity. Tempany et al[80a] evaluated invasion of the neurovascular bundle with a body coil and found that MRI had a sensitivity of only 68 per cent and a specificity of 59 per cent. Biondetti et al demonstrated an MRI accuracy of 89 per cent in differentiating Stage B from C or D disease.[4] Others have shown that seminal vesicle involvement is more accurately depicted by MRI than is extracapsular spread, with a sensitivity of detecting nodal metastases of 69 per cent and a specificity of 95 per cent.[3] McSherry et al[53a] examined preoperative staging in 25 patients undergoing radical prostatectomy with blinded DRE, ultrasonography, and MRI. They found a predictive value for tumor confinement of 36 per cent by rectal examination, 37 per cent by ultrasonography, and 30 per cent by MRI, although the results of predicting extracapsular disease were better. They concluded that these methods understage most patients but are fairly specific for extracapsular disease. Rifkin et al conducted a large multi-institutional trial in which 230 patients were staged with ultrasonography, MRI, and surgery. MRI correctly staged 77 per cent of advanced disease and 45 per cent of localized malignancies, and the figures for ultrasonography were not significantly different. Combining the two studies did not improve accuracy. The authors concluded that neither MRI nor ultrasonography was accurate in staging prostate carcinoma because neither detects microscopic spread of disease.[70] Thus, although it is generally accepted that

FIGURE 6–17. Typical biphasic pattern of BPH with Stage B carcinoma of the prostate at 5 and 6 o'clock. 1 = Carcinoma; 2 = BPH. T2-weighted endorectal surface coil MRI. Fast spin echo. TR 4000, TE 100. (Courtesy of Howard M. Pollack, MD.)

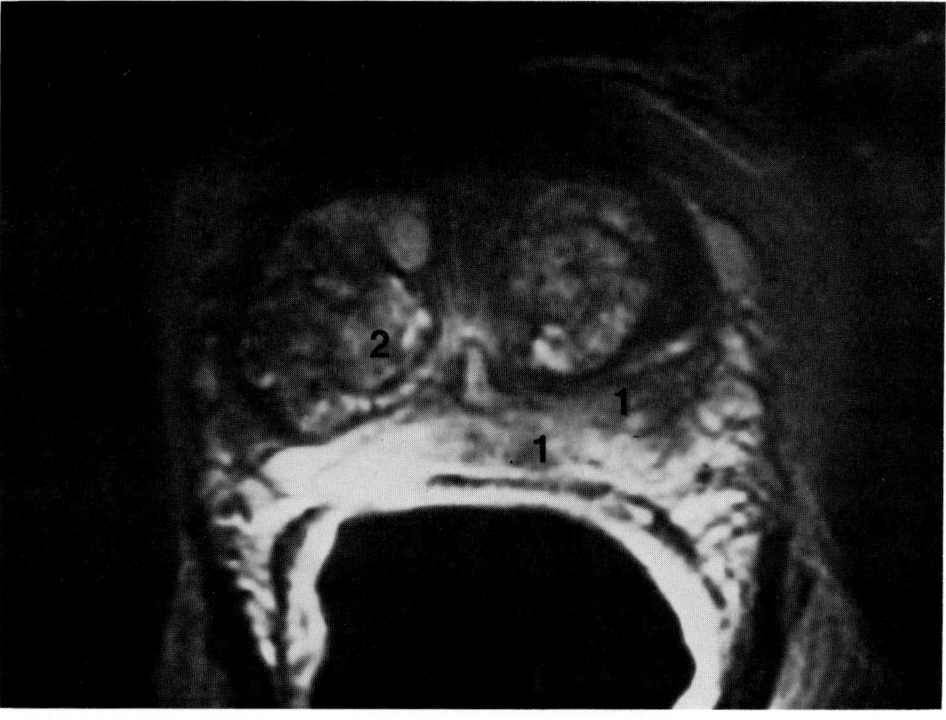

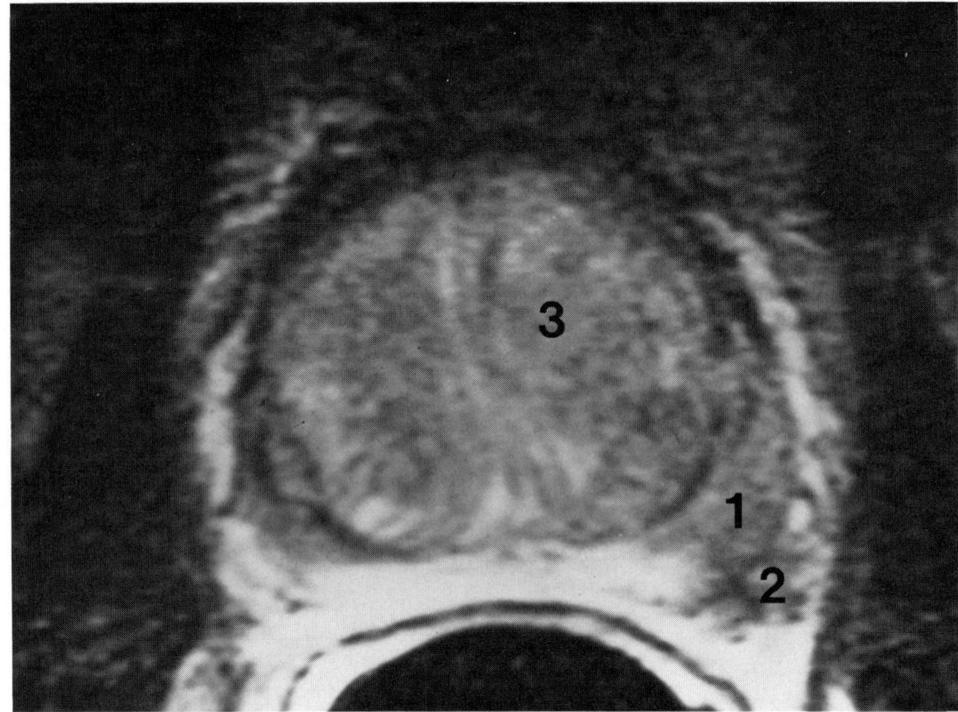

FIGURE 6–18. Stage C carcinoma of the prostate with extension beyond the capsule at 5 o'clock in the area of the neurovascular bundle. Note also large BPH. 1 = Carcinoma; 2 = periprostatic tumor; 3 = BPH. T2-weighted endorectal surface coil MRI. Fast spin echo: TR 4000, TE 100; 1.5 T magnet; 256 × 256 matrix; 2 excitations, 10-cm FOV, 4-mm slice thickness. (Courtesy of Howard M. Pollack, MD.)

MRI is superior to CT in staging prostate carcinoma, its superiority to transrectal ultrasonography has yet to be established. The low accuracy of both MRI and ultrasonography in staging prostate cancer is disappointing. Schnall et al have documented a 16 per cent increase in MRI staging accuracy using endorectal coils, and this technique is promising.[76] Currently, the use of MRI can be recommended only for staging prostate cancer. It does not have a role in screening for prostate cancer owing to its expense, low specificity, and low sensitivity.

SUMMARY

Transrectal ultrasonography, CT, and MRI have all provided new ways to clinically assess the prostate gland; however, the role of each of these is controversial, and none is perfect. Ultrasonography has proved valuable in the staging, monitoring, and biopsy of prostate carcinoma. It cannot currently be recommended as a screening study. MRI has proven more accurate than CT in staging prostate carcinoma, although it is not demonstrably superior to less expensive ultrasound techniques. The role of these imaging modalities may be further altered by the introduction of PSA, laparoscopic lymphadenectomy, and improved imaging technology. Ultimately, a better understanding of prostate cancer itself is needed in order to make best use of these imaging techniques.

REFERENCES

1. Andersen JT, Jacobsen O, Standgaard L: The diagnostic value of intravenous pyelography in infravesical obstruction in males. Scand J Urol Nephrol 12:219, 1978.
2. Arger PH: Computed tomography of the lower urinary tract. Urol Clin North Am 12:677, 1985.
3. Bezzi M, Kressel HY, Allen KS, et al: Prostatic carcinoma: Staging with MR imaging at 1.5 T. Radiology 169:339, 1988.
4. Biondetti PR, Lee JKT, Ling D, Catalona WJ: Clinical stage B prostate carcinoma: Staging with MR imaging. Radiology 162:325, 1987.
5. Birch NC, Hurst G, Doyle PT: Serial residual volumes in men with prostatic hypertrophy. Br J Urol 62:571, 1988.
6. Blasko JC, Rayde H, Grimm PD: Transperineal ultrasound-guided implantation of the prostate: Morbidity and complications. Scand J Urol Nephrol (Suppl) 137:113, 1991.
7. Boyce WH: History of prostatic ultrasonography. *In* Resnick MI (ed): Prostatic Ultrasonography. Philadelphia, BC Decker, 1990, pp 1–16.
8. Boyce WH, McKinney W, Resnick MI, Willard WJ: Ultrasonography as an aid in the diagnosis and management of surgical disease of the pelvis: Special emphasis on the genitourinary system. Ann Surg 184:477, 1976.
8a. Brawer MK: Techniques of examination. *In* Resnick MI (ed): Prostatic Ultrasonography. Philadelphia, BC Decker, 1990, pp 25–32.
9. Bryan JP, Butler HE, Nelson AD, et al: Magnetic resonance imaging of the prostate. AJR 146:543, 1986.
10. Carol CL, Sommer FG, McNeal JE, Stamey TA: The abnormal prostate: MR imaging at 1.5 T with histopathologic correlation. Radiology 165:521, 1987.
11. Carpentier PJ, Schroeder FH, Schmitz PM: Transrectal ultrasonography of the prostate: The prognostic relevance of volume changes under endocrine management. West J Urol 4:159, 1986.
12. Carter HB, Bren RF, Tempany CM, et al: Nonpalpable prostate cancer: Detection with MR imaging. Radiology 178:523, 1991.
13. Chodak GW, Schoenburg HW: Progress and problems in screening for carcinoma of the prostate. World J Surg 13:60, 1989.
14. Clements R, Griffiths GJ, Peeling WB, Edwards AM: Transrectal ultrasound in monitoring response to treatment of prostate disease. Urol Clin North Am 16:735, 1989.
15. Coffield KS, Speights VO, Brawn PN, Riggs MW: Ultrasound detection of prostate cancer in postmortem specimens with histological correlation. J Urol 147:822, 1992.
16. Cooner WH: Anatomy of the prostate as seen by ultrasound. AUA Update Series 9:42, 1990.
17. Cooner WH, Mosely BR, Rutherford CL, et al: Prostate cancer detection in a ultrasonography, digital rectal examination, and prostate specific antigen. J Urol 143:1146, 1990.

18. Dahnert WF, Hamper UM, Eggleston JC, et al: Prostatic evaluation by transrectal sonography with histopathologic correlation: The echogenic appearance of early carcinoma. Radiology 158:97, 1968.
19. Declecq G, Dennis L, Broos J, Appel C: Evaluation of lower urinary tract by computed tomography and transrectal ultrasonography. Comput Tomog 5:153, 1981.
20. Dershaw DD, Scher HI, Smart T: Transrectal sonography of serial evaluation of prostatic malignancy. Urology 36:172, 1990.
21. Frankes LM: Latent carcinoma of the prostate. J Pathol Biol 68:603, 1954.
22. Fujino A, Scardino PJ: Transrectal ultrasonography of prostatic cancer: Its value in staging and monitoring the response to radiotherapy and chemotherapy. J Urol 133:806, 1985.
23. Ganem EJ: The upper urinary tract in advanced prostatic carcinoma. J Urol 78:466, 1957.
24. Gastak SM, Gammelgard J, Holm HH: Transrectal ultrasonic volume determination of the prostate—a preoperative and postoperative study. J Urol 127:1115, 1982.
25. Goldstein LM, Equana S, Scardino PT: Prostate cancer: Echo characteristics, tumor location, and tumor size. *In* Resnick MI (ed): Prostatic Ultrasonography. Philadelphia, BC Decker, 1990, pp 55–72.
26. Gore RM, Ross AA: Value of computerized tomography in interstitial ^{125}I brachytherapy of prostate cancer. Radiology 146:453, 1983.
27. Greene DR, Scardino PT: Transrectal ultrasonography for prostate cancer. PPO Update 4:1, 1990.
28. Hammerer P, Loy V, Dierenger J, Huland H: Prostate cancer in nonurological patients with normal prostate on digital rectal examination. J Urol 147:833, 1992.
29. Hamper UM, Sheth S, Walsh PC, et al: Capsular transgression of prostatic carcinoma: Evaluation with transrectal US with pathological correlation. Radiology 178:791, 1991.
30. Hodge KK, McNeal JE, Stamey TA: Ultrasound guided transrectal core biopsies of the palpably abnormal prostate. J Urol 142:66, 1989.
31. Hodge KK, McNeal JE, Terris MK, Stamey TA: Random systematic versus directed ultrasound guided transrectal core biopsies of the prostate. J Urol 142:71, 1989.
32. Holm HH, Gammelgard J: Ultrasonically guided precise needle placement in the prostate and seminal vesicles. J Urol 125:385, 1981.
33. Hricak H, Dooms GC, Jeffrey RB, et al: Prostatic carcinoma: Staging by clinical assessment, CT, and MRI imaging. Radiology 162:331, 1987.
34. Hricak H, Thoeni R: Neoplasms of the prostate gland. *In* Pollack HM (ed): Clinical Urography. Philadelphia, WB Saunders Co, 1990, pp 1381–1403.
35. Kabalin JN, Hodge KK, McNeal JE, et al: Identification of residual cancer in the prostate following radiation therapy: Role of transrectal ultrasound guided biopsy and prostate specific antigen. J Urol 142:326, 1989.
36. Kadmon D, Ling D, Lee JKT: Percutaneous drainage of prostatic abscesses. J Urol 135:1259, 1986.
37. Kinahan TJ, Goldenberg SL, Azjen SA, et al: Transurethral resection of prostatic abscess under sonographic guidance. Urology 37:475, 1991.
38. King WW, Wilkiemeyer RM, Boyce WH, McKinney WM: Current status of prostatic ultrasonography. JAMA 226:444, 1973.
39. Kressel HY: Magnetic resonance imaging. *In* Walsh PC, Retik AB, Stamey TA, Vaughan ED Jr (eds): Campbell's Urology, 6th ed. Philadelphia, WB Saunders Co, 1992, pp 485–494.
40. Lee F, Gray JM, McCleary RD, et al: Prostatic evaluation by transrectal sonography: Criteria for diagnosis of early carcinoma. Radiology 158:91, 1986.
41. Lee F, Littrup PJ, Torp-Pederson ST, et al: Prostate cancer: Comparison of transrectal US and digital rectal examination for screening. Radiology 168:389, 1988.
42. Lee F, Torp-Pederson ST, Siders DB: Use of transrectal ultrasound in diagnosis, guided biosy, staging, and screening of prostate cancer. Urology 33:S7–12, 1989.
43. Lippmann HR, Ghiatas AA, Sarosdy MF: Systematic transrectal ultrasound guided prostate biopsy after negative digitally guided prostate biopsy. J Urol 147:827, 1992.
44. Lipuma JP, Bryan PJ, Butler HE, Resnick MI: Magnetic resonance imaging of the genitourinary tract. Urol Clin North Am 12:725, 1985.
45. Littrup PJ, Kane RA, Williams CR, et al: Determination of prostate volume with transrectal US for cancer screening. Part I: Comparison with prostate specific antigen assays. Radiology 178:537, 1991.
46. Love L, Churchill RJ: Computed tomography of the urinary tract. *In* Pollack HM (ed): Clinical Urography. Philadelphia, WB Saunders Co, 1990, pp 387–393.
47. Martin JF, Hajek P, Baker L: Inflatable surface coil for MR imaging of the prostate. Radiology 167:268, 1988.
48. McClennan BL: Diagnostic imaging evaluation of benign prostatic hyperplasia. Urol Clin North Am 17:517, 1990.
49. McNeal JE: The prostate and prostatic urethra: A morphological synthesis. J Urol 107:1008, 1972.
50. McNeal JE: The prostate gland. Morphology and pathobiology. Monogr Urol 4:1, 1983.
51. McNeal JE, Bostwick DG, Minduchuk RA, et al: Patterns of progression in prostate cancer. Lancet 1:60, 1986.
52. McNeal JE, Villers AA, Redwine EA, et al: Capsular penetration in prostate cancer. Am J Surg Pathol 14:240, 1990.
53. McNeal JE, Villers AA, Redwine EA, et al: Histologic differentiation, cancer volume, and pelvic lymph node metastases in adenocarcinoma of the prostate. Cancer 66:1225, 1990.
53a. McSherry SA, Levy F, Schiebler ML, et al: Preoperative prediction of pathological tumor volume and stage in clinically localized prostate cancer: Comparison of digital rectal examination, transrectal ultrasonography and magnetic resonance imaging. J Urol 146:85, 1991.
54. Morse RM, Resnick MI: Imaging of the prostate. *In* Paulson DF (ed): Prostatic Disorders. Philadelphia, Lea & Febiger, 1989, pp 28–50.
55. Muldoon LD, Resnick MI: Normal anatomy of the prostate. *In* Resnick MI (ed): Prostatic Ultrasonography. Philadelphia, BC Decker, 1990.
56. New FJ, Rosen BR, Brady TJ: Potential hazards and artifacts of ferromagnetic and nonferromagnetic surgical and dental materials and devices in nuclear magnetic resonance imaging. Radiology 143:139, 1983.
57. Newhouse JH: Clinical use of urinary tract magnetic resonance imaging. Radiol Clin North Am 29:455, 1991.
58. Phillips ME, Kressel HY, Spritzer CE, et al: Prostatic disorders: MR imaging at 1.5 T. Radiology 164:386, 1987.
59. Pontes JE, Eisenkraft S, Watanabe H, et al: Preoperative evaluation of localized prostatic carcinoma by transrectal ultrasonography. J Urol 134:289, 1985.
60. Price JM, Davidson AJ: Computed tomography in the evaluation of the suspected carcinomatous patient. AJR 132:1032, 1979.
61. Resnick MI: Background for screening—epidemiology and cost effectiveness. Prog Clin Biol Res 269:111, 1988.
62. Resnick MI: Evaluation of prostate carcinoma: noninvasive and preoperative techniques. Prostate 1:311, 1980.
63. Resnick MI: Transrectal ultrasound guided versus digitally directed prostatic biosy: A comparative study. J Urol 139:754, 1988.
64. Resnick MI: Ultrasound guided and digitally guided biopsies of the prostate. J Endourol 3:177, 1989.
65. Resnick MI, Willard JW, Boyce WH: Recent progress in ultrasonography of the bladder and prostate. J Urol 117:444, 1977.
66. Rifkin MD: Transrectal prostatic ultrasonography: Comparison of linear array and radial scanners. J Ultrasound Med 4:1, 1985.
67. Rifkin MD, Alexander AA, Helinek TG, Merton DA: Color doppler as an adjunct to prostate ultrasound. Scand J Urol Nephrol (Suppl) 137:85, 1991.
68. Rifkin MD, Alexander AA, Pisarchick J, Matteuci T: Palpable masses in the prostate: Superior accuracy of U.S. guided biopsy compared with accuracy of digitally guided biopsy. Radiology 179:41, 1991.
69. Rifkin MD, Friedland GW, Shortliffe L: Prostatic evaluation by transrectal endosonography: Detection of carcinoma. Radiology 158:85, 1986.
70. Rifkin MD, Zerhouni EA, Gatsonis CA, et al: Comparison of magnetic resonance imaging and ultrasonography in staging

early prostate cancer: Results of a multi-institutional cooperative trial. N Engl J Med 323:621, 1990.

71. Rosenfeld AT, Rigsby CM, Burns PN, Romero R: Ultrasonography of the urinary tract. *In* Pollack HM (ed): Clinical Urography. Philadelphia, WB Saunders Co, 1990, p 319.

72. Sage WM, Kessler R, Sommers LS, Silverman JF: Physician-generated cost containment in transurethral prostatectomy. J Urol 140:311, 1988.

73. Sawczuk IS, deVere White KR, Palmer RG, Olsson C: Sensitivity of computed tomography in evaluation of pelvic lymph node metastases from carcinoma of the bladder and prostate. Urology 21:81, 1983.

74. Scardino PT: Early detection of prostate cancer. Urol Clin North Am 16:635, 1989.

75. Scardino PT, Shinohara K, Wheeler TM, Carter SSC: Staging of prostate cancer: Value of ultrasonography. Urol Clin North Am 16:713, 1989.

76. Schnall MD, Lenkinski RE, Pollack HM, et al: Prostate: MR imaging with an endorectal surface coil. Radiology 172:570, 1989.

77. Shinohara K, Wheeler TM, Scardino PT: The appearance of prostate cancer on transrectal ultrasonography: Correlation of imaging and pathological examinations. J Urol 142:76, 1989.

78. Stamey TA: Cancer of the prostate. Monogr Urol 4:68, 1983.

79. Stamey TA, Frieha FS, McNeal JE, et al: Relationship of tumor volume to clinical significance for treatment of prostate cancer. J Urol 147:303A, 1992.

79a. Sweeney PJ, Resnick MI: The role of ultrasound in prostate cancer. Urol Annu 6:35, 1992.

80. Talner LB: Urinary Obstruction. *In* Pollock HM (ed): Clinical Urography. Philadelphia, WB Saunders Co, 1990, p 1694.

80a. Tempany AC, Rahmouni AD, Epstein JI: Invasion of the neurovascular bundle by prostate cancer: Evaluation with MR imaging. Radiology 181:107, 1991.

81. Terris MK, Frieha FS, McNeal JE, Stamey TA: Efficacy of transrectal ultrasound for identification of clinically undetected prostate cancer. J Urol 146:78, 1991.

82. Terris MK, McNeal JE, Stamey TA: Estimation of prostate cancer volume by transrectal ultrasound imaging. J Urol 147:855, 1992.

83. Terris MK, McNeal JE, Stamey TA: Transrectal ultrasound imaging and in the detection of residual carcinoma in clinical stage A carcinoma of the prostate. J Urol 147:864, 1992.

84. Terris MK, Stamey TA: Determination of prostate volume by transrectal ultrasound. J Urol 145:984, 1991.

85. Thompson IM: Screening for carcinoma of the prostate. AUA Update Series 9:225, 1990.

86. Turner-Warwick R, Whiteside CG, Arnold EP, et al: A urodynamic view of prostatic obstruction and the results of prostatectomy. Br J Urol 45:631, 1973.

87. VanEngecshoven JMA, Kreel L: Computed tomography of the prostate. J Comput Assist Tomog 3:45, 1979.

88. Villers AA, McNeal JE, Redwine EA, et al: Pathogenesis and biological significance of seminal vesicle invasion in prostatic adenocarcinoma. J Urol 143:1183, 1990.

89. Wallner K, Chiu-Tsao S, Jitendra R, et al: An improved method for computerized tomography planned transperineal ^{125}Iodine prostate implants. J Urol 146:90, 1991.

90. Wassermann NF, Lapinte S, Eckmann DR, Rosel PR: Assessment of prostatism: Role of intravenous urography. Radiology 165:831, 1987.

91. Watanabe H: Instrumentation in prostatic ultrasonography. *In* Resnick MI (ed): Prostatic Ultrasonography. Philadelphia, BC Decker, 1990, pp 17–23.

92. Watanabe H, Katoh H: Diagnostic application of the ultrasonography for the prostate. J Urol 59:279, 1968.

93. Waterhouse RC, Resnick MI: The use of transrectal prostatic ultrasonography in the evaluation of patients with prostatic carcinoma. J Urol 141:233, 1989.

94. Whitmore WF: Natural history of low-stage prostatic cancer and the impact of early detection. Urol Clin North Am 17:689, 1990.

95. Wild JJ, Reid JM: Application of echo-ranging techniques to the structure of biopsy tissues. Science 115:226, 1951.

BENIGN PROSTATIC HYPERPLASIA

Chapter 7

ETIOLOGY OF BENIGN PROSTATIC HYPERPLASIA

RUSSELL K. LAWSON

The term *benign prostatic hyperplasia* (BPH) is often used to mean either an enlarged prostate or urinary obstruction. The association between prostate growth and urinary obstruction in aging males seems well established. However, all urologists are aware of the paradox of the patient with a small prostate gland and severe obstruction compared with the man with a large prostate gland and no obstructive voiding symptoms. Until recently, little effort has been made to explain this paradox. Several factors, in addition to prostate growth, appear to cause irritative and obstructive voiding symptoms in older men. Figure 7–1 is a schematic representation of four of these factors and their interrelationship. Prostate growth occurs in the periurethral region of the gland, with outward compression of the outer part of the gland to form a surgical capsule. The surgical capsule resists expansion of this central growth, which produces increased pressure in the inner part of the gland, resulting in increased resistance to urine flow. Alpha-adrenergic nerve tone is another factor that plays an important role in the development of obstructive voiding problems. Smooth muscle fibers in the surgical capsule, fibroadenoma, and bladder neck may all contribute to increased prostatic urethral resistance. Finally, very little is known about possible changes in detrusor function in the aging male that may result in voiding problems. This chapter considers all of these interrelated factors and how they impact on voiding dysfunction in men with BPH.

EMBRYOLOGY

Certain aspects of the embryologic development of the prostate are reviewed because they may play an important role in the genesis of BPH in adult life. The prostate and ejaculatory ducts develop in the embryo from three anlagen: endoderm from the urogenital sinus, mesonephric mesoderm, and mesoderm from the wolffian duct system. For the prostate to develop, the epithelium of the primitive urethra must be primed with androgen before the ductal system develops.[10] A second and equally important factor is the presence of urogenital sinus mesenchyme for the formation of prostatic ducts and acini.[9, 13] A great deal of information regarding the role of urogenital sinus mesenchyme in prostate development has been provided by the elegant work of Cunha and Chung.[8, 11, 12] These investigators have shown that urogenital sinus mesenchyme, but not other embryonic mesenchyme, induces prostate epithelial growth. The fact that the urogenital sinus mesenchyme from fetal mouse can induce prostate growth from a variety of epithelial cells, including mouse bladder cells, has led to speculation that a reawakening of this process is responsible for glandular growth in BPH.[37]

At birth, a regional difference appears to exist in the response of prostate epithelial cells to hormones. The squamous metaplasia caused by maternal estrogen appears to be confined to ducts and acini originating near the wolffian duct system.[7] This functional partition of the gland may be important in the development of BPH because these same cells appear to be involved in early BPH.[21]

SENILE ATROPHY OF THE PROSTATE

A study of 678 prostates obtained at autopsy was published by Moore in 1935.[41] He described the devel-

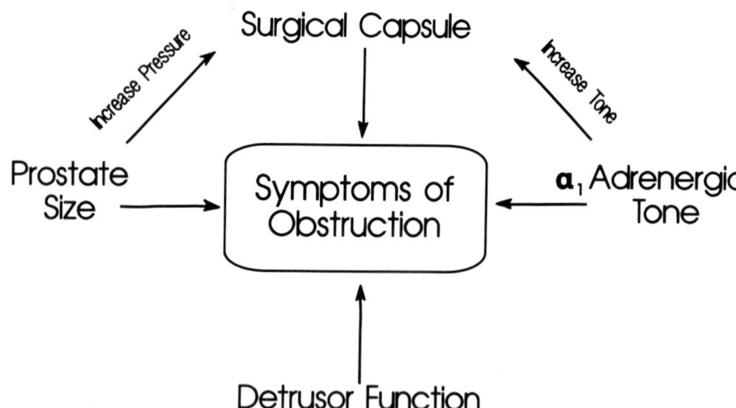

FIGURE 7–1. Schematic representation of the four factors that have impact on the development of obstructive voiding symptoms from BPH.

opment of the prostate from puberty to the involution of the gland in aging men. Involution of the prostate was studied as a histopathologic entity distinct from BPH. By excluding the presence of BPH, carcinoma, and infection in the specimens, he was able to measure size and volume in 129 prostates exhibiting senile atrophy between the third and ninth decades. He was unable to show a statistically significant difference in size in these specimens. Unfortunately, no data are included which indicate the number of cases excluded because of co-existing BPH. A recent study by Watanabe describes the prevalence of BPH and prostate volume in 1121 Japanese men who were part of a large transrectal ultrasound screening program for prostate cancer.[67] He found that when prostate weight is plotted against age, the peak weight occurs at about age 20 and shows a decline to approximately pubertal weight by age 80. A similar study by Mori using ultrasonography to judge prostate weight also demonstrated a decreasing weight with increasing age.[42] Both of these studies fit well with the concept that a significant number of men undergo senile atrophy with little or no superimposed BPH.

Ohnishi followed 16 men with BPH with repeated volume measurements over a period of 7 years.[45] Three of these men demonstrated marked increase in prostate weight, whereas 13 patients showed little change in prostate weight during the observation period. Watanabe states that 20 to 25 per cent of men develop macroscopic BPH, whereas the remaining 75 to 80 per cent of men undergo atrophy and decreasing prostate weight with advancing age.[67] He further found that in the group with BPH, a subset undergoes a rapid increase in prostate weight over a relatively short period of time, and the remainder of men maintain a nearly stable prostate weight. These data are at variance with previously published reports comparing prostate weight with age in men in the United States and may be accounted for by racial differences or the random entry of normal men into the Watanabe study.[65, 67] This work, if confirmed in men in the United States, gives a picture of the natural history of prostate growth very different from current views.

MORPHOGENESIS

BPH begins in the periurethral region of the gland. However, the types of cells involved in the first lesions have not been conclusively established. Motz and Perearneau, in 1905, stated that BPH begins as proliferation of epithelial cells in the periurethral region of the gland.[43] This concept was further extended by Albarran and Halle, who studied 100 prostate specimens and concluded that glandular growth preceded stromal growth in early BPH.[2]

In 1925, Reischauer challenged this concept and presented evidence that the first lesions of BPH are stromal nodules.[52] He further stated that stromal nodules produce a substance that induces the ingrowth of glandular cells and that pure stromal nodules grow only in regions where no glandular cells are present to penetrate them. He concluded that the periurethral glandular cells are involved in BPH because they are in the region where the first stromal nodules form.

The work by Reischauer was confirmed by Demming and LeDuc.[15, 34] An extensive study of autopsy specimens was published in 1943 by Moore, who also concluded that the first lesions of BPH are fibrostromal nodules.[40] Several recent morphologic studies have also found that BPH begins as a stromal proliferation with a secondary ingrowth of glandular tissue.[1, 50] With the exception of recent studies by McNeal, who believes that stromal and glandular elements appear simultaneously, the bulk of evidence supports the thesis that BPH begins as stromal nodules in the periurethral region and that they induce the ingrowth of glandular cells. The question of whether BPH begins as stromal or glandular proliferation is an important one. If the first lesions are stromal, the theory that BPH is caused by hormonal effects on prostate epithelial cells is less tenable.

Quantitative morphometric studies have shown that BPH contains relatively more stromal tissue than glandular tissue compared with normal prostate.[4] This work has recently been confirmed in our laboratory by Shapiro et al.[55] A quantitative morphometric study of electron micrographs from BPH specimens has also been carried out to determine the relative number of organelles (rough endoplasmic reticulum, Golgi apparatus, secretory droplets, lysosomes, mitochondria, and fat droplets) present in stromal and epithelial cells.[3] The stromal cells contain more of these organelles than epithelial cells in BPH. The activation of stromal cells was not seen in normal prostate, suggesting that they are the metabolically active cells in BPH.

The above work on the cell of origin of early BPH and the tissue composition of BPH points to a significant role of glandular/stromal interaction in prostate growth. Until recently, this area of research has received little attention. The finding that the enzyme 5α-reductase, for the conversion of testosterone to dihydrotestosterone (DHT), resides primarily in the stroma is an example of the important interrelationship between stroma and glands in the prostate.[31, 71] Receptors, enzymes, and growth factors may reside in one compartment of the prostate but have a primary effect in another compartment.

The exact location of the first nodules of BPH and the specific epithelial cells that participate in the proliferative response have been the subject of much debate. Jores, in 1894, divided the submucosal glands in the normal prostate into three groups: trigonal, vesicle neck, and periurethral cephalad to the verumontanum.[29] Many investigators believe that these three groups of glands form the glandular component of BPH. However, others have stated that mucosal glands or ductal epithelium are the source of glandular cells in BPH. From a developmental point of view, none of these cells is considered part of the true prostate. Median and subcervical lobe hyperplasia must be derived from the trigonal and subcervical glands described by Jores.[29] Current evidence supports the concept that the glandular compartment of BPH arises from submucosal glands cephalad to the verumontanum.

McNeal has proposed that BPH begins in the region of the prostate which he terms the transition zone.[38] He divides the prostate into three zones: peripheral zone, central zone, and transition zone. The transition zone lies anterior to the peripheral zone and cephalad to the verumontanum. It is best seen microscopically in a coronal section through the prostatic urethra proximal to the verumontanum. The ducts of the transition zone enter the urethra proximal to the ducts of the peripheral zone at the proximal end of the verumontanum. The acini drained by this duct system resemble seminal vesical acini and may be derived from wolffian duct structures rather than from the inductive effect of the mesonephric mesoderm. According to McNeal, the earliest lesions of BPH are proliferation of glandular cells in the transition zone. Further, proliferation of the subcervical and trigonal submucosal glands is a late development in BPH and follows the early lesions seen in the transition zone.

The lateral, median, and subcervical lobes of BPH represent growth of glandular and stromal tissue beginning in the periurethral region with outward compression and distortion of the true prostate. This outward growth produces distinct rings of tissue that can be seen on cross-section. The prostate capsule and the compressed tissue of the true prostate form a surgical capsule surrounding the hyperplastic lobes. A distinct plane of separation can be developed between the adenomatous tissue and the surgical capsule at the time of open prostatectomy.

ROLE OF THE TESTIS IN PROSTATE GROWTH

The role of the testis in prostate development and maintenance of prostate function was first shown by Hunter in 1835.[23] He found that castration of young rats prevents development of the prostate into a normal adult gland. He also determined that orchiectomy in the adult rat results in atrophy of the prostate. The use of bilateral orchiectomy to treat obstructive voiding symptoms from BPH was first proposed by White in 1893.[70] In 1895, Rand reported the results in two patients treated by orchiectomy for BPH and stated that both patients experienced improved voiding following the procedure.[51] In the same year, White reported a series of 111 patients treated by orchiectomy for obstructive BPH and stated that the operation was successful in relieving the obstructive voiding problem.[69] However, the operative mortality in the series was 18 per cent.

Huggins and Stevens in 1940 described the effect of castration on BPH and found the effect to be variable.[21] They noted smaller acinar lumina, fewer papillary infoldings, and decreased epithelial height in the acini of these patients. Interestingly, they also found an increased number of acini per microscopic field, suggesting atrophy of the stroma as well as an effect on the epithelium. In 1972, Wendall et al studied prostate biopsies from men with prostate cancer who were treated with estrogen or by orchiectomy and concluded that the BPH seen in these glands was of lower grade than in men not treated by hormonal therapy.[68] They believe their work supports the concept that androgen is needed to maintain epithelial growth and function in BPH.

Moore reported in 1944 that a group of 28 eunuchs, eunuchoids, and patients with pituitary infantilism showed no evidence of BPH.[39] A second study of 26 eunuchs from China was reported by Jie-ping in 1987.[28] Seven of these men were castrated before puberty, and 18 were castrated between 10 and 26 years of age. The age of castration was not known in one man. The follow-up in these men was 41 to 65 years, and all exhibited nonpalpable (81 per cent) or very small prostates (19 per cent). None of these men had obstructive voiding symptoms. However, 22 (85 per cent) had nocturia 2 to 10 times per night.

Recent work by Grayhack et al suggests that nonsteroidal testicular factor may affect prostate growth.[19] They irradiated the testes of beagle dogs with established BPH with 1500 to 2200 rad as a single dose. Control animals received either no radiation or radiation to the shoulder. This dose of radiation produced major changes in the seminiferous tubules but did not affect the serum levels of testosterone or estradiol. Testicular irradiation resulted in a significant decrease in prostate size and weight, suggesting that a nonandrogenic factor that stimulates prostate growth is elaborated by the testis of aging men.

HORMONES

The role of hormones in the origin of BPH remains controversial. A great deal of research has been done on the effects of various steroid hormones on the prostates of both animals and man without clear-cut evidence that these substances play a direct role in the development of BPH. There is no question that the testis must be present for normal development of the prostate in animals and man. The work of Isaacs has demonstrated the requirement of androgen in the young rat and dog for a normal number of stem cells and amplifying cells to be present in the adult gland.[24] He has shown that the timing of castration in the young of these two species has a direct effect on the maximal gland size that can be achieved when the animals grow to adulthood, a phenomenon termed *imprinting*. The reports discussed earlier indicating reduced prostate growth in eunuchs establish the importance of the testis in normal prostate development in man.[28, 39] The question remains, however, whether the effect of androgen in the adult is simply the maintenance of epithelial cell function or a direct effect on the production of glandular hyperplasia.

The mean serum level of testosterone declines with age, but the mean serum level of DHT remains the same.[49, 62, 64] Earlier work showed no difference in the serum level of testosterone in men with BPH and age-matched controls.[18, 57] However, a recent report by Partin et al has shown a proportional increase in free serum testosterone, estradiol, and estriol with increasing volume of BPH.[46] There are conflicting reports regarding the serum levels of DHT in men with BPH and age-matched controls.[5, 18, 26, 63] The mean serum level of estrogens increases with age, but there is no difference between men with BPH and age-matched controls.[20] There has been much speculation on the possible synergistic effect of estrogen on androgen-induced prostate growth, but no data support this hypothesis in man.

Prostate tissue levels of various hormones have been measured in man, and no differences have been found between patients with BPH and age-matched controls. For a number of years it was thought that BPH contained a higher concentration of DHT than normal tissue, but this turned out to be incorrect.[25] The problem with earlier studies was an erroneous value for DHT in normal tissue caused by improper tissue handling.[66] DHT is found in both the glandular and stromal compartments of BPH. The conversion of testosterone to DHT occurs primarily in the stroma, where the enzyme 5α-reductase is in high concentration.[31] There is also evidence that 5α-reductase is in higher concentration in the stroma of BPH than in normal prostate.[71] At the present time there is no evidence in man to support the thesis that prostate tissue concentrations of steroid hormones play a role in glandular hyperplasia. There is

abundant evidence, dating from the early work of White to the recent work of Walsh, that lowering serum testosterone to castrate levels results in improvement in obstructive voiding symptoms.[48, 69] Peters and Walsh have shown that a modest reduction in prostate size occurs following the administration of a luteinizing hormone–releasing hormone analogue. The decreased serum androgen levels caused by this treatment resulted in atrophy of the glandular compartment of BPH. The 5α-reductase inhibitor finasteride appears to exert its clinical effect by lowering prostate DHT levels.[36] The primary androgen that maintains prostate epithelial cell function is DHT. Blocking the conversion of testosterone to DHT results in glandular atrophy and a decrease in prostate size.

The role of the endocrine system in causing BPH is controversial. Androgen appears to be necessary in the prepubertal period for normal development of the prostate. Androgen is also clearly needed for the maintenance of prostate epithelial cell function. However, evidence of a direct role for androgens in the genesis of glandular hyperplasia is lacking.

GROWTH FACTORS

Deaver suggested in 1922 that prostatic enlargement is due to one or more internal secretions.[14] As mentioned earlier, Reischauer, LeDuc, and others have similarly suggested that substances produced by the prostate stimulate glandular or stromal proliferation.[34, 52] The role of growth factors in the development of BPH has been studied for a number of years, but no definite relationship has been established. The presence of a potent mitogen in the human prostate was first reported from our laboratory in 1979.[27] Subsequent work demonstrated that this mitogen is present in normal human prostate and BPH as well as in carcinoma of the prostate.[33] The mitogen was found to be a member of the heparin-binding growth factor family and was shown to react to antibodies to basic fibroblast growth factor (bFGF).[61] Amino acid sequencing of the growth factor demonstrated homology with the predicted amino acid sequence from the cloned human bFGF gene.[59]

We subsequently demonstrated that bFGF is present in higher concentrations in BPH tissue than in normal adult prostate tissue.[6] Tissue culture studies have shown that human prostate stromal cells produce bFGF and that these same cells respond to bFGF in culture, suggesting an autocrine effect of bFGF on stromal cell proliferation in the intact prostate gland.[60] Peehl and co-workers have found that keratinocyte growth factor (KGF), a member of the heparin-binding growth factor family that is produced by prostate stromal cells, is mitogenic only for prostate epithelial cells.[47] This factor may be a paracrine stimulator of epithelial growth in the intact prostate.

Control of growth induced by these two heparin-binding growth factors may be modulated by transforming growth factor–beta (TGF-β). This factor inhibits the growth of human prostate stromal cells in tissue culture but stimulates the production of bFGF by these cells.[58] Some evidence exists that TGF-β production or release is regulated by testosterone. The interaction of these factors in the prostate may play an important role in both stromal and glandular hyperplasia. A hypothesis that takes into account the role of bFGF, KGF, and TGF-β in normal prostate growth and BPH is shown in Figure 7–2. Many aspects of this hypothesis are currently being studied.

The finding of small stromal nodules in the periurethral region of the prostate as the first histologic evidence of BPH has led us to speculate that macroinjury to the prostatic ducts from voiding, ejaculation, or infection causes stromal proliferation as a healing response.[32] Release of growth factors at the site of injury may result in the formation of primitive mesenchyme with its inductive effect on epithelial growth.

FGF appears to be the primary inducer of mesenchyme in the developing frog embryo.[30] It is interesting to note that human bFGF and frog FGF have 84 per cent amino acid homology, suggesting an important fundamental role of this growth factor in human embryogenesis and mesenchymal growth.[30] Folkman et al have shown that bFGF plays an important role as an angiogenesis factor in wound healing.[16] The primary effect of bFGF—stromal proliferation or angiogenesis—appears to be determined by the anatomic location of the response and the local growth factor milieu.

OTHER HYPOTHESES

Isaacs has proposed the stem cell model to explain BPH (Fig. 7–2).[24] This hypothesis takes into account the involution and growth of established canine BPH seen with castration and androgen replacement. The cell renewal occurs from a population of stem cells and amplifying cells that are not androgen dependent. The set point, or maximum organ size, is determined by the number of stem cells and amplifying cells present in the gland. This number is controlled by androgen from the testis during prostate development. Castration of young rats and dogs prevents development of normal-size prostates following androgen replacement during adulthood. Castration of mature animals causes involution of the gland, with complete restoration of gland size following androgen replacement. The key concept is that in the stable state (zero growth) cell proliferation and cell death are in exact balance, whereas in the hyperplastic prostate cell proliferation exceeds cell death, resulting in organ growth. This hypothesis is attractive because it explains many of the observations made in the canine BPH model. It should be noted that the stem cell model and the growth factor hypothesis are not mutually exclusive because the factors controlling cell proliferation and cell death may be the growth factors that have been identified in human prostate tissue.

McNeal has proposed an embryonic reawakening hypothesis as a cause for BPH.[37] He describes the stromal tissue in BPH as resembling embryonic mesenchyme and suggests that such mesenchyme can induce the growth of adjacent epithelial cells. The inductive effect of urogenital mesenchyme from mouse embryos on epithelial cells of widely different origins to express the prostate epithelial cell phenotype has been well established by Cunha and Chung.[8–13] This work supports the concept that mesenchyme-derived stromal cells in the prostate may, in the aging male, express this embryonic inductive effect on epithelial cells.

PROSTATE CAPSULE

The true prostate capsule and the surgical capsule may play important roles in the production of obstructive voiding symptoms. Ohnishi has provided evidence that as the central part of the prostate undergoes expansile growth, the capsule confines this growth.[44] This results in increased intraprostatic pressure, which causes obstructive voiding symptoms. He has measured the tensile strength of the prostatic capsule in men with BPH and has found that with increasing tensile strength, obstructive voiding symptoms increase. The concept that the degree to which the capsule resists expansion affects voiding symptoms could also explain the paradox of poor correlation of prostate size with the severity of symptoms.

The concept of capsulotomy as a treatment for obstructive voiding symptoms was first reported by Shafik.[54] These patients underwent an external incision of the surgical capsule of the prostate by a suprapubic approach or laparoscopy.[53] Similarly, the beneficial effect of transurethral incision of the prostate may be due primarily to the incision being carried through the prostatic capsule to the periprostatic fat. Both of these procedures

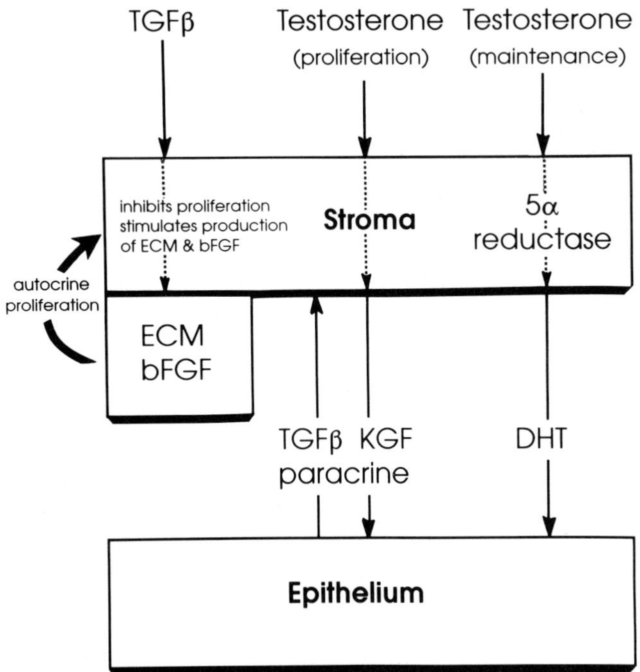

FIGURE 7–2. Schematic representation of the growth factors and their interrelationships that are thought to play a role in stromal and epithelial growth seen in BPH.

decrease intraprostatic pressure by allowing further expansion of the central hyperplastic growth.

ALPHA-ADRENERGIC TONE

A complete discussion of the clinical effects of alpha-adrenergic blockade on obstructive voiding symptoms is found in Chapter 15. However, the role of prostate smooth muscle in causing obstructive voiding symptoms is included in this discussion of the pathogenesis of BPH. Smooth muscle is present in the prostate capsule, hyperplastic stromal nodules, mixed epithelial/stromal nodules, and bladder neck. The tone of the smooth muscle in one or more of these sites appears to have an effect on intraprostatic pressure and obstructive voiding symptoms. The capsule smooth muscle tone as well as connective tissue tensile strength may be important in capsular resistance to expansile growth. Shapiro et al have shown a direct correlation of smooth muscle content of BPH specimens with improvement in urinary flow rates in patients treated with the alpha-blocker terazosin.[56] Changes in normally occurring alpha-adrenergic–mediated smooth muscle tone could also explain the variability in obstructive voiding signs and symptoms seen from hour to hour and day to day in a given patient. The variability in flow rate, residual urine, and obstructive voiding symptoms could easily be accounted for by changes in smooth muscle tone in the prostate.

DETRUSOR FUNCTION

The role of the detrusor muscle in the symptom complex of BPH is poorly understood. The symptoms of BPH are divided into obstructed and irritated voiding problems. Hyperplastic growth, capsule resistance, and smooth muscle tone are all logical effectors of the degree of urinary obstruction but do not have an obvious relationship to irritative voiding symptoms. Some patients have marked improvement in both obstructive and irritative voiding symptoms following prostatectomy for BPH, whereas other patients have persistent irritative voiding symptoms in spite of markedly improved flow rates and reduced or absent residual urine volumes. Changes in bladder smooth muscle function appear to mediate the irritative voiding symptoms of BPH. Unfortunately, very little work has been done in man on the role of the bladder in producing the symptoms of BPH. Recent work using an obstructed rabbit bladder model has provided important new information that may be applicable to the functional bladder changes seen in men with BPH.[35]

REFERENCES

1. Ahluwalia MS, Tandon HD: Nodular hyperplasia of the prostate in North India: An autopsy study. J Urol 93:94–101, 1965.
2. Albarran J, Halle N: Hypertrophie et neoplasies epitheliades de la prostate. Ann Mal Org Gen-Urol 17:113–147, 1900.
3. Bartsch G, Frick J, Ruegg I, et al: Electron microscopic stereo-logical analysis of the normal human prostate and of benign prostatic hyperplasia. J Urol 122:481–486, 1979.
4. Bartsch G, Muller HR, Oberholzer M, Rohr HP: Light microscopic steriological analysis of the normal human prostate and of benign prostatic hyperplasia. J Urol 122:487–491, 1979.
5. Becker H, Kaufmann J, Klosterhalfen H, Voight KD: In vivo uptake and metabolism of ^{3}H-5-α dihydrotestosterone by human benign prostatic hypertrophy. Acta Endocrinol 71:589–599, 1972.
6. Begun FP, Story MT, Jacobs SC, et al: Regional concentration of basic fibroblast growth factor in normal and benign hyperplastic human prostates. J Urol (in press).
7. Brody H, Goldman S: Metaplasia of the epithelium of the prostate glands, utricle and urethra of the fetus and newborn infant. Arch Pathol 29:494–504, 1940.
8. Chung LWK, Cunha GR: Stromal-epithelial interactions: II. Regulation of prostatic growth by embryonic urogenital sinus mesenchyme. Prostate 4:503–511, 1983.
9. Chung LWK, Matsuura J, Rocco AJ, et al: Tissue interactions and prostatic growth: A new mouse model for prostatic hyperplasia. Ann NY Acad Sci 438:394–404, 1984.
10. Cunha GR: The role of androgens in the epithelio-mesenchymal interactions involved in prostatic morphogenesis in embryonic mice. Anat Rec 175:87–96, 1973.
11. Cunha GR: Tissue interactions between epithelium and mesenchyme of urogenital and integumental origin. Anat Rec 172:529–541, 1972.
12. Cunha GR, Fujii H, Neubauer BL, et al: Epithelial-mesenchymal interactions in prostatic development. I. Morphological observations of prostatic induction by urogenital sinus mesenchyme in epithelium of the adult rodent urinary bladder. J Cell Biol 96:1662–1670, 1983.
13. Cunha GR, Lung B: The importance of stroma in morphogenesis and functional activity of urogenital epithelium. In Vitro 15:50–71, 1979.
14. Deaver JB: Enlargement of the prostate, 2nd ed. Philadelphia, P Blakiston's Son & Co, 1992, p 75.
15. Deming CL, Neumann C: Early phases of prostatic hyperplasia. Surg Gynecol Obstet 68:155–160, 1939.
16. Folkman J, Klagsburn M, Sasse J, et al: A heparin-binding angiogenic protein—basic fibroblast growth factor—is stored within basement membrane. Am J Pathol 130:393–400, 1988.
17. Franks LM: Benign nodular hyperplasia of the prostate: A review. Ann R Coll Surg Eng 14:92–106, 1954.
18. Ghanadian R, Lewis JG, Chisholm GD, O'Donoghue EPN: Serum dihydrotestosterone in patients with benign prostatic hypertrophy. Br J Urol 49:541–544, 1977.
19. Grayhack JT, Lee C, Brand W: The effect of testicular irradiation on established BPH in the dog: Evidence of a non-steriodal testicular factor for BPH maintenance. J Urol 134:1276–1281, 1985.
20. Hammond GL, Kontturi M, Vihko P, Vihko R: Serum steroids in normal males and patients with prostatic diseases. Clin Endocrinol 9:113–121, 1978.
21. Huggins C, Stevens RA: The effect of castration on benign hypertrophy of the prostate in man. J Urol 43:705–714, 1940.
22. Huggins C, Webster WO: Duality of human prostate in response to estrogen. J Urol 59:258–266, 1948.
23. Hunter J: On the venereal disease. 4:31, 1786. *In* Works (Ed). London, Palmer, Vol II, 1835.
24. Isaacs JT: Control of cell proliferation and cell death in the normal and neoplastic prostate: A stem cell model. *In* Rogers CH, Coffey DS, Cunha G, (eds): Benign Prostatic Hyperplasia. Washington, DC: U.S. Dept of Health and Human Services. NIH Publication No 87-2881, 1987, pp 85–94.
25. Isaacs JT, Brendler CB, Walsh PC: Changes in the metabolism of dihydrotestosterone in hyperplastic human prostate. J Clin Endocrinol Metabol 56:139–146, 1983.
26. Ishimaru T, Pages L, Horton R: Altered metabolism of androgens in elderly men with benign prostatic hyperplasia. J Clin Endocrinol Metab 45:695–701, 1977.
27. Jacobs SC, Pikna D, Lawson RK: Prostatic osteoblastic factor. Invest Urol 17:195–198, 1979.
28. Jie-ping W, Fang-liu G: The Prostate 41–65 years post-castration: An analysis of 26 eunuchs. Chin Med J 100:271–272, 1987.

29. Jores L: Ueber die hypertrophie des sogenannten mittleren Lappens der Prostata. Virchow's Arch [A] 135:224–247, 1894.
30. Kimelman D, Abraham JA, Haaparanta T, et al: The presence of fibroblast growth factor in the frog egg: Its role as a natural mesoderm inducer. Science 242:1053–1056, 1988.
31. Krieg M, Klotzl G, Kaufmann J, Voigt KD: Stroma of human benign prostatic hyperplasia: Preferential tissue for androgen metabolism and oestrogen binding. Acta Endocrinol 96:422–432, 1981.
32. Lawson RK: Benign prostatic hyperplasia and growth factors. Urologe (A) 29:5–7, 1990.
33. Lawson RK, Story MT, Jacobs SC: A growth factor in extracts of human prostatic tissue. *In* The Prostatic Cell: Structure and Function. New York, Alan R. Liss, 1981, pp 325–336.
34. LeDuc IE: The anatomy of the prostate and the pathology of early benign hypertrophy. J Urol 42:1217–1241, 1939.
35. Levin RM, Longhurst PA, Monson FC, et al: Effect of bladder outlet obstruction on the morphology, physiology, and pharmacology of the bladder. Prostate (Suppl) 3:9–26, 1990.
36. McConnell JD: Medical management of benign prostatic hyperplasia with androgen suppression. Prostate (Suppl) 3:49–59, 1990.
37. McNeal JE: The prostate gland: Morphology and pathobiology. Monographs in Urology, Vol 4, No 1, 1983.
38. McNeal JE: The zonal anatomy of the prostate. Prostate 2:35–49, 1981.
39. Moore RA: Benign hypertrophy and carcinoma of the prostate: Occurrence and experimental production in animals. Surgery 16:152–167, 1944.
40. Moore RA: Benign hypertrophy of the prostate: A morphological study. J Urol 50:680–710, 1943.
41. Moore RA: The evolution and involution of the prostate gland. Am J Pathol 12:599–629, 1935.
42. Mori Y: Measurement of the normal prostatic size by means of transrectal ultrasonotomography. Jpn J Urol 73:767–781, 1982.
43. Motz B, Perearneau: Contribution a l'etude de l'evolution de l'hypertrophie de la prostate. Ann Mal Org Gen-Urin 23:1521, 1905.
44. Ohnishi K: A study of the physical property of the prostate (the second report)—The relationships between dysuria and the strength of the surgical capsule in benign prostatic hypertrophy. J Jpn Urol Assoc 77(9):1388–1399, 1986.
45. Ohnishi K, Watanabe H, Ohe H: Development of benign prostatic hypertrophy estimated from ultrasonic measurement with long-term follow-up. Tohoku J Exp Med 151:51–56, 1987.
46. Partin AW, Oesterling JE, Epstein JI, et al: Influence of age and endocrine factors on the volume of benign prostatic hyperplasia. J Urol 145:405–409, 1991.
47. Peehl DM, Stamey TA, Rubin JS: Fibroblast growth factors can replace epidermal growth factor for clonal proliferation of human prostatic epithelial cells. J Urol 145:475, 1991.
48. Peters CA, Walsh PC: The effect of nafarelin acetate, a luteinizing-hormone-releasing hormone agonist, on benign prostatic hyperplasia. N Engl J Med 317:599–604, 1987.
49. Pirke KM, Doerr P: Age related changes in free plasma testosterone, dihydrotestosterone and oestradiol. Acta Endocrinol 80:171–178, 1975.
50. Pradhan BK, Chandra K: Morphogenesis of nodular hyperplasia—prostate. J Urol 113:210–213, 1975.
51. Rand HW: A contribution to the surgery of the hypertrophied prostate. Ann Surg 22:217–225, 1895.
52. Reischauer F: Die Entstehung der sogenannten prostatahypertrophie. Virchow's Arch [A] 256:357–389, 1925.
53. Shafik A: Closed prostatic commissurotomy: An endoscopic technique for the treatment of benign prostatic hypertrophy. Br J Urol 62:431–433, 1988.
54. Shafik A: Prostatic commissurotomy: A simple technique for the treatment of benign prostatic hypertrophy. Br J Urol 58:157–160, 1986.
55. Shapiro E, Hartanto V, Lepor H: Quantifying the smooth muscle content of the prostate using double-immunoenzymatic staining and color assisted image analysis. J Urol 147:1167–1170, 1992.
56. Shapiro E, Hartanto V, Lepor H: The response to alpha blockade in benign prostatic hyperplasia is related to the percent area density of prostate smooth muscle. Prostate smooth muscle and alpha blockade. Prostate 21:297–308, 1992.
57. Skoldefors H, Blomstedt B, Carlstrom K: Serum hormone levels in benign prostatic hyperplasia. Scand J Urol Nephrol 12:111–114, 1978.
58. Story MT, Baeten LA, Molter MA, Lawson RK: Influence of androgen and transforming growth factor beta on basic fibroblast growth factor levels in human prostate-derived fibroblast cell cultures. J Urol 143:241A, 1990.
59. Story MT, Esch F, Shimasaki S, et al: Amino-terminal sequence of a large form of basic fibroblast growth factor isolated from human benign prostatic hyperplastic tissue. Biochem Biophys Res Comm 142:702–709, 1987.
60. Story MT, Livingston B, Baeten L, et al: Cultured human prostate-derived fibroblasts produce a factor that stimulates their growth with properties indistinguishable from basic fibroblast growth factor. Prostate 15:355–365, 1989.
61. Story MT, Sasse J, Jacobs SC, Lawson RK: Prostatic growth factor: Purification and structural relationship to basic fibroblast growth factor. Biochemistry 26:38–43, 1987.
62. Vermeulen A: Testicular hormonal secretion and aging in males. *In* Grayhack JT, Wilson JD, Scherbenske MD (eds): Benign Prostatic Hyperplasia. Washington DC: US Department of Health, Education and Welfare. (DHEW publication No. (NIH) 76-1113), 1975: 1976. pp 117–182.
63. Vermeulen A, DeSy W: Androgens in patients with benign prostatic hyperplasia before and after prostatectomy. J Clin Endocrinol Metab 43:1250–1254, 1976.
64. Vermeulen A, Rubens R, Verdonck L: Testosterone secretion and metabolism in male senescence. J Clin Endocrinol 34:730–735, 1972.
65. Walsh PC: Human benign prostatic hyperplasia etiological considerations. *In* Kimboll FA, Buhl AE, Carter DB (eds): New Approaches to the Study of Benign Prostatic Hyperplasia. New York, Alan R. Liss, 1984.
66. Walsh PC, Hutchins GM, Ewing LL: Tissue content of dihydrotestosterone in human prostatic hyperplasia is not supranormal. J Clin Invest 72:1772–1777, 1983.
67. Watanabe H: Natural history of benign prostatic hypertrophy. Ultrasound Med Biol 12:567–571, 1986.
68. Wendel EF, Brannen GE, Putong PB, Grayhack JT: The effect of orchiectomy and estrogens on benign prostatic hyperplasia. J Urol 108:116–119, 1972.
69. White JW: The results of double castration in hypertrophy of the prostate. Ann Surg 22:1–80, 1895.
70. White JW: The present position of surgery of the hypertrophied prostate. Ann Surg 18:152, 1893.
71. Wilkin RP, Bruchovsky N, Shnitka TK, et al: Stromal 5-α reductase activity is elevated in benign prostatic hyperplasia. Acta Endocrinol 94:284–288, 1980.

Chapter 8

EPIDEMIOLOGY AND NATURAL HISTORY OF BENIGN PROSTATIC HYPERPLASIA

MICHAEL J. BARRY

EPIDEMIOLOGY OF BENIGN PROSTATIC HYPERPLASIA

Benign prostatic hyperplasia (BPH) is a common condition in older men, both in the United States and worldwide. In the United States, prostatectomy is the second most common major operation, after cataract surgery, performed on Medicare-aged men. In the United States in 1987, approximately 379,000 transurethral and 15,000 open prostatectomies were performed.[47] Furthermore, many men have clinical symptoms attributable to BPH but never have surgery. The frequency of BPH in the US population is the reason that transurethral prostatectomies constituted 38 per cent of the major operations performed by the nation's approximately 7700 urologists in 1986.[54]

Definitions of Occurrence Parameters

The occurrence of a disease like BPH in a population can be described by several parameters.[9] The *incidence* of a condition is the rate of development of new cases in the population over time. The units of incidence are events per person-time. For example, if 10 men out of 1000 develop evidence of BPH over one full year of observation, the incidence rate is 10 per 1000 person-years, or 0.01 per person-year. As the population is followed, more and more men have evidence of BPH over time. The *cumulative incidence* of a disease is the probability of developing the disease over a specified time frame. When incidence rates are constant, the cumulative incidence of the disease can be simply calculated using the formula:[76]

$$CI_t = 1 - e^{-I(t)}$$

For example, if there is a constant incidence of developing BPH of 0.01 case per person-year, then the 5-year probability of developing BPH for men in this population would be:

$$CI_{5\ years} = 1 - e^{-0.01(5)} = 0.049$$

When the incidence rate of a disease is not constant over time, the calculation of cumulative incidence is not as straightforward. The incidence of BPH actually rises sharply with age, requiring that cumulative incidence calculations be based on age-specific incidence rates.

Another occurrence parameter commonly referred to is the *prevalence* of a disease. Prevalence is the proportion of individuals in a population who have the disease at a given point in time. For chronic diseases with low mortality, such as osteoarthritis and BPH, cumulative incidence and prevalence are very similar. However, prevalence and cumulative incidence can be very different. For example, the cumulative incidence of the common cold is very high (almost everyone gets one each year), whereas the prevalence of a cold at any one time is relatively low. Sudden cardiac death, instantly fatal, is a condition with a cumulative incidence but no prevalence!

Epidemiology also involves the search for "occurrence relations" between occurrence parameters and potential "determinants" of those parameters.[69] Incidence rates can be compared for different populations or subpopulations to study these occurrence relations. For example, the incidence of BPH is strongly influenced by age. One study found that the incidence rate of a new clinical diagnosis of BPH was 0.52 per person-year for men aged 65 to 69 and 0.75 per person-year for men aged 70 to 74.[5] A *rate ratio* (frequently called, less accurately, a relative risk or risk ratio) of 0.75/0.52 = 1.44 can be calculated to compare the two rates.

Alternative Definitions of Benign Prostatic Hyperplasia

Fundamental to the study of the epidemiology of a disease is an operational definition of that disease. BPH is a complex disease that can be defined on several levels.[10] First, BPH can be described at the anatomic-pathologic level in terms of a characteristic histopathology.[65] At the physiologic level, BPH can cause bladder outlet obstruction, detectable urodynamically, and secondary physiologic bladder abnormalities, such as uninhibited contractions.[15, 63] Finally, the patient becomes aware of his BPH when these physiologic abnormalities cause urinary symptoms or other complications, such as chronic renal failure due to obstructive uropathy.[72, 79, 80] Studies of the epidemiology of BPH have used different definitions of this condition, from the histologic to the clinical level. A clinical definition of BPH reflects the morbidity of the condition from the patient's perspective.[9, 10] However, urinary symptoms can be caused by other diseases, and a population with clinically defined BPH includes some individuals with other problems.[16]

In recent work, Guess and colleagues[49] found that a similar cumulative incidence of BPH was determined when a clinical definition of BPH was used in one prospective cohort study, compared with findings from previous autopsy studies using a histologic definition of BPH. This important observation supports the use of a well-specified clinical definition of BPH in epidemiologic studies. However, studies using all alternative definitions of BPH are reviewed in this chapter. Because the occurrence of BPH is strongly age dependent, this determinant is discussed along with the basic occurrence parameters of BPH. Then evidence related to other potential determinants is reviewed.

Prevalence of Histologic Benign Prostatic Hyperplasia

A common way to study the prevalence of a disease is to describe the percentage of individuals who have evidence of the condition at autopsy. Five studies of the occurrence of BPH at autopsy have been pooled by Berry and colleagues[13] to describe the prevalence of histologic BPH with increasing age in 1075 men (Fig. 8–1). By age 80, almost 90 per cent of men have histologic evidence of BPH. Although the percentage of men who undergo an autopsy is small, there is no reason to think that men with BPH would preferentially get autopsies; therefore, these estimates are likely reliable ones. The prevalence of histologic BPH at any age serves as an upper limit for the prevalence of clinical BPH. In this same study, data on the weight of prostates at autopsy were used to study the rate of prostatic growth with age. The authors found that the normal adult prostate plateaus at a weight of about 20 grams at age 30. Then the weight remains stable until approximately age 50, when a process of growth is again initiated, so that the average prostatic weight increases to about 35 grams in men in their 80s.

Incidence and Prevalence of Clinical Benign Prostatic Hyperplasia at Different Ages

Data on the occurrence parameters of clinical BPH come from three types of studies: cross-sectional sur-

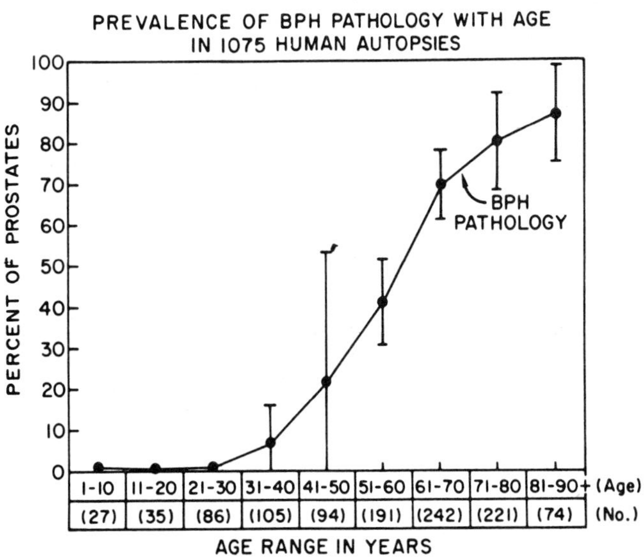

FIGURE 8–1. Age-related increase in prevalence of histologic BPH at autopsy (mean ± standard error of the mean). (From Berry SJ, Coffey DS, Walsh PC, Ewing LL: The development of human benign prostatic hyperplasia with age. J Urol 132:474, © by Williams & Wilkins, 1984; with permission.)

veys, retrospective cohort studies, and prospective cohort studies. The cross-sectional surveys, like autopsy studies, yield data bearing directly on prevalence, whereas the cohort studies can yield incidence *and* prevalence figures.

A number of community-based surveys of urologic symptoms have been conducted in Denmark. Jensen and colleagues[57] examined a group of Danish men over age 50 selected as a random sample from a national population registry. The study defined prostatism as a patient complaint about global voiding problems. Whereas 17 per cent of men had prostatism according to this definition, fully 88 per cent had at least one voiding symptom when asked about urinary symptoms one at a time. Subjects who fit the definition of prostatism had a median objective symptom score of 9 (possible range, 0 to 20), whereas men without prostatism had a median score of 3. Interestingly, peak flow rates adjusted for voided volume were not significantly different in the two groups. Because only 112 of the 200 men randomly selected for study ultimately participated, a bias in response could potentially have had a dramatic influence on the prevalence of prostatism in this study.

More recently, Sommer and colleagues[83] conducted a similar cross-sectional survey of randomly selected Danish men, using a mail questionnaire. Surveys were returned by 382 men (67 per cent of those selected). In the fourth, fifth, sixth, and seventh decades, the percentages of men with a Madsen-Iversen symptom score greater than 9 (the median value for men defined as having prostatism in the Jensen study) were 2 per cent, 7 per cent, 18 per cent, and 23 per cent, respectively. Once again, individual urinary symptoms were quite common. For example, about 70 per cent of men in the seventh decade had daytime frequency (urinating every 3 hours or more often), and 40 per cent had nocturia (twice a night or more). Beier-Holgersen and Bruun[11] found a similarly high prevalence of symptoms in a survey among male residents of Copenhagen in their 60s.

Most recently, Garraway and colleagues[38] have studied the prevalence of BPH among men aged 40 to 79 registered with a general practice in central Scotland. Men whose medical records did not reveal evidence of pre-existing urinary disease were screened with a symptom questionnaire and uroflowmetry (with a 77 per cent response rate). Men with an elevated symptom score or a urinary flow rate less than 15 ml/sec had a determination of prostate volume (and thus weight) by transrectal ultrasonography. Clinical BPH was defined as a prostatic weight over 20 grams in the presence of suggestive symptoms and/or a reduced urinary flow rate. The prevalence of BPH in this population was 14 per cent for men aged 40 to 49, 24 per cent for ages 50 to 59, 43 per cent for ages 60 to 69, and 40 per cent for ages 70 to 79 (these estimates have fairly broad confidence intervals).

Obviously, the threshold for defining the presence of BPH on the basis of symptoms alone makes a large difference in estimates of BPH prevalence from these cross-sectional studies. Even without a uniform definition of BPH, these studies make it clear that urinary symptoms at least suggestive of BPH are extraordinarily common in an older population.

Cohort studies involve assembling groups (cohorts) of patients who are followed over time, either retrospectively or prospectively. Lytton and colleagues[64] performed a retrospective study, assuming that all men living in New Haven, Connecticut, would receive treatment for their prostate disease in three local hospitals. The male population of New Haven was estimated from census data for 1953 to 1961, and the number of prostate operations during those years (with ages of the patients) was obtained from the hospitals. The incidences of surgery for BPH calculated from these data were 0.2 per 1000 patient-years at ages 40 to 49, 1.2 at ages 50 to 59, 5.7 at ages 60 to 69, 10.0 at ages 70 to 79, and 10.9 at age 80 and above.

A caution must be raised about using the rate of prostate surgery as a "proxy" for the incidence rate of clinically significant BPH. Many patients with symptoms of BPH never have surgery. Furthermore, thresholds vary both for referral to a urologist from a primary care physician and for a urologist to recommend prostatectomy. These different thresholds are responsible for up to fourfold variations in prostatectomy rates among small geographic areas defined by hospital catchment areas.[94, 95] Even when states or large parts of states are compared to average out variation among smaller communities, rates of prostate surgery vary 1.7-fold.[22] Finally, even developed countries have remarkably different rates of prostatectomy.[66] To some extent, this variation is facilitated by considerable controversy in the indications for elective prostatectomy among the great majority of men with BPH who have no absolute indications for surgery.[46] This variation makes surgical rates a poor substitute for true incidence rates of BPH.

Several prospective cohort studies address the incidence of BPH as well as the incidence of prostatectomy. The Normative Aging Study is a prospective study of 2280 Boston-area male volunteers, initially with a mean age of 42, who enrolled in a study of normal aging between 1961 and 1970.[33, 43] Men were examined every 5 years until age 52, then every 3 years. The periodic check-ups included questions about urinary symptoms and a digital rectal examination. A clinical diagnosis of BPH was made on the basis of finding an enlarged or abnormally firm prostate, or by a history of urinary symptoms that could not be attributed to some other cause. Obviously, this definition is somewhat subjective. Table 8–1 provides the incidences of both clinical diagnosis of BPH and of prostatectomy in the Normative Aging Study cohort. These incidence data predict that a cohort of 40-year-old men would have a 77 per cent cumulative incidence of a clinical diagnosis of BPH by age 80 and a 29 per cent cumulative incidence of prostatectomy by that age.

The second study is very similar in design. The Baltimore Longitudinal Study of Aging began in 1958 and continuously enrolls new volunteers to replace subjects who leave the study.[5] Subjects are evaluated every 2 years, and the periodic examinations include a questionnaire about urologic symptoms and a digital rectal examination. Of 1057 men who had not had prostatec-

TABLE 8–1. INCIDENCE OF A CLINICAL DIAGNOSIS OF BPH AND PROSTATECTOMY BY AGE IN THE NORMATIVE AGING STUDY COHORT

AGE	INCIDENCE OF CLINICAL BPH (PER 1000 PERSON-YEARS)	INCIDENCE OF PROSTATECTOMY (PER 1000 PERSON-YEARS)
40–49	9.4	0.2
50–59	31.3	4.1
60–69	51.3	12.1
70–87	59.2	19.4

From Glynn RJ, Campion EW, Bouchard GR, Silbert JE: The development of benign prostatic hyperplasia among volunteers in the Normative Aging Study. Am J Epidemiol 121:78, 1985; with permission.

tomy or prostate cancer at baseline, 527 had a clinical diagnosis of BPH and 110 eventually underwent prostatectomy. Table 8–2 gives the age-specific incidences of clinical BPH and prostatectomy for men in this cohort. The results are remarkably similar to findings in the Normative Aging Study cohort. This study also documented that individual symptoms frequently remitted when the same individual was followed over time. For example, of men over 50 reporting hesitancy for the first time, about 27 per cent did not report it at the next examination. Even if hesitancy was reported on two sequential examinations, 19 per cent did not report it on the next examination. Moreover, the age-specific prevalence of BPH defined clinically in this cohort is very similar to the autopsy prevalence of BPH defined histologically.

Age-specific rates of prostatectomy were actually lower among members of the Northern California Kaiser Permanente Medical Care Program, as recently reported by Sidney and colleagues.[81] This study identified 16,219 men at least 40 years old who participated in a multiphasic health check-up in 1971 and 1972. These men were followed forward in the computerized files of the prepaid plan that recorded membership status and surgical procedures performed. The incidence of prostatectomy was approximately 2.5 per 1000 patient-years for men aged 55 to 59, 6 per 1000 patient-years at ages 60 to 64, 9 per 1000 person-years at ages 65 to 69, and 12.5 per 1000 person-years at ages 70 to 74. Whether these lower rates, compared with those of the two previous cohort studies, reflect differences in the patient populations or a higher threshold for performing prostatectomy among the prepaid plan members cannot be discerned from the data available.

Stephenson et al[85] recently reported that prostatectomy rates among residents of Rochester, Minnesota, were closer to the Kaiser Plan rates than the rates in the Boston and Baltimore cohorts. They have also suggested that rates may have been high in the latter two studies as a result of the intensive surveillance cohort members received, including periodic questioning about urinary symptoms and performance of digital prostate examinations. Perhaps examiners recommended further evaluation in situations in which patients would not have sought attention.

Determinants of Benign Prostatic Hyperplasia Occurrence Other Than Age

The dominant determinant of BPH occurrence is age. However, many other factors have been studied as potential determinants of BPH. The cross-sectional study and longitudinal cohort study designs already discussed can be used to study relationships between BPH occurrence and potential determinants. Another useful study design is the case-control study.[52] With this design, cases of BPH and controls without BPH are assembled, and exposure of both cases and controls to a particular determinant is assessed. If the determinant is indeed related to BPH, exposure should be enriched in the histories of BPH patients compared with controls. For example, if being of a particular race were an important determinant of BPH, more cases than controls should be of that race. The exposure odds ratio that can be calculated from case-control data may serve as an estimate of the rate ratio under most circumstances.[68] Case-control studies, although relatively easy to conduct, are notoriously prone to bias, especially in the assembly of cases and controls.[35, 55] Some of these potential biases are highlighted in the discussion of the importance of causal factors for BPH other than age.

Race and Nationality

Two autopsy studies from Charity Hospital in New Orleans in the 1930s raised the question of whether BPH presented at an earlier age in African-American patients.[27, 28] However, these studies may have been biased in terms of different thresholds for hospital admission or for autopsy of patients of different races. Lytton and colleagues,[64] on the other hand, found similar prostatectomy rates among white and African-American men in the New Haven area. More recently, in the study by Sidney et al[81] already discussed, African-Americans and whites had similar rates in a prepaid health plan, where equal access to care for both groups would be expected.

TABLE 8–2. AGE-SPECIFIC INCIDENCE RATES FOR A CLINICAL DIAGNOSIS AND SURGERY FOR BENIGN PROSTATIC HYPERPLASIA

AGE	INCIDENCE OF CLINICAL BPH (PER 1000 PERSON-YEARS)	INCIDENCE OF PROSTATECTOMY (PER 1000 PERSON-YEARS)
40–44	9.5	1.6
45–49	6.6	1.3
50–54	15.8	2.9
55–59	22.8	4.0
60–64	52.9	14.2
65–69	52.3	13.6
70–74	75.0	14.5
75–79	108.0	24.4
80–84	159.0	36.8

From Arrighi HM, Guess HA, Metter EJ, Fozard JL: Symptoms and signs of prostatism as risk factors for prostatectomy. Prostate 16:253. Copyright © 1990. Reprinted by permission of Wiley-Liss, a Division of John Wiley and Sons, Inc.

Studies of BPH in Asian men have been conflicting. A low prevalence of BPH at autopsy was reported from China in the 1930s.[21] Later, Conger[25] found that Japanese- and Chinese-American men had about half the prevalence of BPH of Caucasian men. Fay[34] reported that 16 per cent of men discharged from hospitals in San Francisco with a diagnosis of BPH were Asian-American, compared with 8.3 per cent for all other diagnoses. And Watanabe et al,[93] using a mobile transrectal ultrasound screening unit in Japan, found evidence of BPH in 24 per cent of Japanese men over age 55. Two series from Japan[2, 60] suggest that pathologic evidence of BPH is quite common in Japanese men and is detectable in 80 to 90 per cent of men in their 70s. Finally, the study by Sidney et al[81] revealed a lower rate of prostatectomy in Asian-American than in white men (RR = 0.72), but the difference was not statistically significant (95 per cent confidence interval = 0.49–1.05).

Jewish men in Israel completing a health survey reported symptoms consistent with a prevalence of BPH of 28 per cent for ages 65 to 69, 46 per cent for ages 70 to 75, and 60 per cent for ages over 75.[44] In both the Normative Aging Study[43] and a case-control study by Morrison,[70] Jewish men had an estimated 2.2- to 2.6-fold higher rate of prostatectomy than non-Jewish men. However, in the Normative Aging cohort, being Jewish was *not* associated with a higher incidence of a clinical diagnosis of BPH. This paradoxic finding suggests that Jewish men may have a greater likelihood of coming to the attention of a urologist and undergoing surgery, but not a greater likelihood of developing clinical BPH itself.

An interesting source of data for international comparisons of BPH epidemiology is cause-specific mortality as reported to the World Health Organization.[32, 77, 78] These data have been used to order countries according to reported death rates from BPH. The reported death rates vary considerably, from highs of 20 to 30 per 100,000 men over age 45 in East Germany, Czechoslovakia, and Surinam, to lows of 0.5 to 2.0 per 100,000 in the United States, Japan, Kuwait, Mauritius, Puerto Rico, Honduras, Hong Kong, and Singapore.[32] However, multiple inconsistencies suggest that these data may reflect different recording and reporting practices rather than differences in BPH incidence or the quality of care for this condition. For example, for men over 75, WHO data suggest that death rates from BPH are more than seven times higher in Norway than in the United States. For men in this age group, less frequent occurrence of BPH in the United States is unlikely to explain the difference, because so many American men have clinical evidence of BPH at that age. Furthermore, in data from about the same time period as the WHO mortality statistics are based, rates of prostatectomy were roughly comparable in these two well-developed countries,[66] suggesting that undertreatment should not explain the difference in death rates observed.

In summary, the paucity of well-designed epidemiologic studies makes any firm conclusions about differences in occurrence of BPH based on race or nationality very tenuous.

Dietary Factors

A Japanese case-control study suggested that several dietary habits are associated with BPH.[3] These factors include regular milk consumption, not eating green and yellow vegetables regularly, and not eating pickles at every meal. However, this study made a large number of statistical comparisons between the BPH and control patients. This practice makes it highly likely that some spurious "chance" associations will be found, simply as a result of making multiple comparisons. In addition, no multivariable analyses were performed to define factors that were independently, as opposed to individually, associated with BPH. As a result, the dietary differences might simply have reflected the higher socioeconomic status that was also noted among BPH patients in this study.

Smoking

In a case-control study, men who had surgery for BPH were compared with men admitted to Boston-area hospitals for other diagnoses.[70] In this comparison, smoking was negatively associated with prostatectomy; the estimate of the rate ratio was 0.5. However, no dose-response phenomenon was noted. That is, heavier smoking was not more protective than light smoking. The lack of a dose-response effect tends to weigh against smoking being a true biologic preventive determinant of BPH. Sidney et al,[81] however, also found that current smokers had a lower risk of prostatectomy than did nonsmokers; the relative risk was 0.71 (95 per cent confidence interval = 0.55 to 0.91) in a multivariable model that helps ensure that smoking was independently protective. The nature of the association of smoking and BPH is somewhat clarified by data from the Normative Aging Study.[43] In this study, smoking was negatively associated with prostatectomy (the rate ratio adjusted for age and other risk factors was 0.4, comparing smokers of at least one pack a day with nonsmokers) but not with a clinical diagnosis of BPH. This finding could be explained by a higher threshold for urologists to operate on smokers than nonsmokers, particularly in an era when open, rather than transurethral, prostatectomies were commonly performed and perioperative complications were higher. The failure to identify a dose-response relationship between smoking and BPH in a recent case-control study casts further doubt on these observations.[70a]

Body Habitus

In the Normative Aging Study,[43] a lower body mass index was marginally negatively associated with a clinical diagnosis of BPH. However, because prostate enlargement on digital rectal examination was part of the definition of clinical BPH in this study, a somewhat lower sensitivity of the examination for prostate enlargement in heavier individuals could explain this finding.

Body mass index was also a negative predictor of prostatectomy in the Sidney et al study.[81] Men in the second, third, and fourth quartiles of body mass had progressively lower rates of surgery (RR = 0.95, 0.82, and 0.71, respectively) than men in the leanest quartile.

Sexual History

In general, aspects of the sexual history have not been associated with the development of BPH. However, in the Japanese case-control study by Araki et al,[3] several factors were marginally (and perhaps coincidentally) associated with BPH. These factors were first nocturnal emission before age 20, taking longer than 10 minutes to complete one act of sexual intercourse, and no history of sexual impotence lasting more than 1 month.

Other Diseases

The occurrence of BPH has been positively associated with diabetes and hypertension[18, 74] and negatively associated with liver cirrhosis[12, 86] in older studies. However, men in the Normative Aging Study had careful, periodic measurements of blood pressure and fasting and postprandial blood glucose. In this carefully conducted epidemiologic study, neither of these measurements correlated with the occurrence of clinical BPH or prostatectomy.[43] On the other hand, despite one negative report,[75] the evidence of an inverse relationship between cirrhosis and BPH is relatively strong. In the most recent study, the prevalence of BPH, and particularly epithelial compared with stromal hyperplasia, was considerably lower in cirrhotic men who came to autopsy than in noncirrhotic men.[37] These findings suggest that the hyperestrogenic state of cirrhosis may retard the process of prostatic epithelial hyperplasia. There is a single report of an association between prostate cancer and BPH.[4] However, other studies suggest no association.[48, 50] Furthermore, ratios of cases of prostate cancer to BPH in different countries are highly variable, suggesting no strong relationship between the two diseases.[32, 71, 92]

Medications

In the case-control study by Morrison,[70] users of rauwolfia antihypertensives (reserpine-like drugs) had an estimated rate ratio of 2.2 for BPH surgery compared with nonusers of antihypertensives. However, this finding was barely statistically significant, and again, associations were tested between prostatectomy and many potential determinants. Because reserpine is falling out of favor as an antihypertensive drug, the importance of this association, even if a true causal relationship exists, may be minimal.

Other Factors

In the Japanese case-control study by Araki et al,[3] higher income, educational level, and socioeconomic status were associated with BPH. In contrast, in the Normative Aging Study,[43] socioeconomic status was negatively associated with prostatectomy, although not with a clinical diagnosis of BPH. The Japanese study also suggested an association of BPH with no family history of gastric ulcer or breast cancer, and occupations other than farming, forestry, or fishing. Again, however, some of these associations may be proxies for one another (for example, all the socioeconomic variables may strongly correlate with occupation), and some associations may be chance findings due to the multiple comparison problem.

Ill-defined genetic or environmental factors may be responsible for the finding that BPH occurrence has been observed to vary in different regions of Sudan,[59] and among different ethnic subpopulations of Wales.[7]

Summary

BPH is a common condition, and its occurrence is strongly determined by age. A 40-year-old man has about a 75 per cent chance of developing clinical evidence of BPH by age 80, if evidence of either an enlarged prostate or suggestive urinary symptoms without an alternative explanation are accepted as the definition of clinical BPH. However, from the patient's perspective, this cumulative incidence is an overestimate. Men with an asymptomatic enlargement of the prostate do not feel ill and may not develop urinary symptoms. Even more of these men have only mild symptoms that they do not find very bothersome. For this reason, the cumulative incidence of BPH requiring treatment is much lower.

Surgical rates vary considerably among geographic areas and are a poor proxy for rates of BPH requiring treatment. However, in the Normative Aging Study, projections based on historical Boston-area surgical rates would predict that a cohort of 40-year-old men surviving until age 80 would have about a 30 per cent cumulative incidence of prostatectomy.[43] These projections assume stable surgical rates, however. In fact, age-specific surgical rates in the United States have risen steadily in recent years, as indicated in Table 8–3, suggesting that the actual cumulative incidence for such a cohort assembled today might be even higher. These figures were extracted from National Center for Health Statistics reports on discharges from non-Federal short-stay hospitals[47, 51, 62] and from published statistics of the US Bureau of the Census.[89–91] Because prostatectomies performed in Veterans Administration and military hospitals are not included, these calculated rates are conservative.

No convincing evidence exists that determinants of BPH occurrence other than age are very important, except perhaps smoking (which may be protective). Current evidence suggests that white, African-Ameri-

TABLE 8–3. TOTAL NUMBERS AND RATES OF PROSTATECTOMY OVER 10 YEARS IN THE UNITED STATES

	1978	1983	1987
Number of prostatectomies (thousands)			
Age 45–64	68	79	86
Age ≥65	226	263	307
US male population (millions)			
Age 45–64	21.0	21.2	21.7
Age ≥65	9.8	11.0	11.3
Rate of prostatectomy (per 100,000 man-years)			
Age 45–64	323	373	397
Age ≥65	2310	2438	2713

Data from references 47, 51, 62, 89–91.

can, and Asian men have roughly similar cumulative incidences of BPH with age.

NATURAL HISTORY OF BENIGN PROSTATIC HYPERPLASIA

Natural history refers to the prognosis of a disease over time. Clinicians need to be aware of the natural history of a disease to educate their patients about what the future may hold. Moreover, data on the effectiveness of different treatments can be interpreted only with a knowledge of the untreated natural history of that condition. Comparisons of the course of a disease with and without treatment ultimately let clinicians know whether a given treatment does more good than harm.

Before reviewing the evidence on the natural history of BPH, it is necessary to point out that this data base is extraordinarily sparse in light of the importance of the problem. Given the epidemiologic data already reviewed, a high proportion of the roughly 12 million men over age 65 in the United States must have clinical evidence of BPH, but the natural histories of only a very small number of these men have been reported.

Ideal studies to define the prognosis of a disease follow a cohort of individuals from a well-defined inception point of their illness.[88] In the setting of BPH, building an inception cohort of patients with symptomatic BPH in the community would be highly desirable. Although such studies are under way, no results have yet been reported. Cohorts that define the inception of disease as presentation to a primary care physician or referral to a urologist likely miss a considerable period of natural history of the disease. They must be interpreted cautiously because patients differ in their thresholds to bring symptoms to medical attention, and primary care physicians differ in their threshold for making a referral to a urologist.

Natural History of Benign Prostatic Hyperplasia Symptoms

Again, from the patient's perspective, it is almost exclusively the symptoms of BPH that confer the con-

dition's morbidity.[10] It would be helpful for patients to know whether their BPH symptoms are likely to improve, stabilize, or progress over time, to help make decisions about treatment. Furthermore, the effectiveness of both operative and nonoperative treatments for BPH needs to be measured in terms of the added benefit of the interventions, beyond what improvement can be expected spontaneously.

Several cohort studies have followed a group of patients after presentation with apparent clinical BPH. Clarke[24] described a retrospective series of patients from Peter Bent Brigham Hospital, which included a group of 36 men who had definite BPH without absolute indications for surgery. These men had a mean age of 64. They had had symptoms for an average of 3 years prior to presentation and had records available allowing a mean follow-up of 3.4 years. Over the follow-up period, 25 showed some period of subjective improvement, with the average period of improvement being about 2 years. Ultimately, 12 of these patients underwent a prostatectomy, although the indications were not well specified.

Craigen and colleagues[26] reported on a cohort of 212 patients over age 55 who visited general practitioners in East Anglia with urinary symptoms but who did not eventually prove to have prostate cancer. At presentation, 89 had acute retention and 123 had other urinary symptoms without acute retention. Using a life table analysis to correct for death and loss to follow-up, calculated cumulative incidences of prostatectomy of 60 per cent at 1 year and 80 per cent at 7 years were projected for the men presenting with retention. For men presenting without retention, cumulative incidences of prostatectomy of 35 per cent at 1 year and 45 per cent at 7 years were projected. Unfortunately, the diagnosis of BPH in this study was subjective, and the indications for the operations on cohort members were not specified. No direct information on symptom progression was provided.

Birkhoff and colleagues[14] reported on a small sample of 26 men with prostatism but without absolute indications for surgery, who declined experimental drug treatment and were followed for more than 3 years. Obviously, this small group was highly selected and far from an inception cohort. At the end of 3 years of follow-up, 7 patients (27 per cent) were subjectively improved, 4 (15 per cent) were unchanged, and 15 (58 per cent) were worse. Eventually, 23 of the 26 men underwent a prostatectomy. Individual patients had their symptoms wax and wane considerably over the period of follow-up. However, this small series gives the impression that steady progression of symptoms is the rule for most BPH patients.

Somewhat in contrast to the Birkhoff series is another cohort study reported by Ball and colleagues.[8] They studied 107 patients who were seen at a urology practice in Bristol, England, for symptoms suggesting BPH between 1974 and 1976 and who were not initially treated operatively on unspecified clinical grounds. This cohort had a mean age of 62 at initial evaluation, and 53 had evidence of bladder outflow obstruction on the basis of urodynamic pressure-flow studies. Subjects were contacted 5 years after their initial evaluation to learn their subsequent course. Ten patients (9 per cent) had eventually undergone a prostatectomy. Of the remaining 97, on an overall evaluation of symptoms, 16 (15 per cent of 107) thought that they were worse, 50 (48 per cent) reported that they were about the same, and 31 (29 per cent) thought that they were better. Interestingly, all 10 patients who subsequently had surgery (2 for acute retention and 8 for symptom deterioration) had been classified as urodynamically obstructed at their initial evaluation. This series, closer to an inception cohort than the Birkhoff series, suggests slower symptom progression, with about 70 per cent of patients remaining stable or improving over 5 years of follow-up. However, a substantial number of patients in this series (and other cohorts that are not so thoroughly investigated) may have had suggestive symptoms of BPH but were not demonstrated to have outflow obstruction urodynamically.

The Baltimore Longitudinal Study on Aging provides information on the likelihood of progressing to a prostatectomy depending on the clinical symptoms and signs of BPH identified on periodic study examinations.[5] In this study, age was the dominant predictor of prostatectomy. However, age aside, prostatectomy was more likely in men who reported a change in size and force of their urinary stream or a sensation of incomplete bladder emptying or who were noted to have an enlarged prostate at digital rectal examination. The 464 men showing none of these risk factors had about a 3 per cent chance of eventually undergoing a prostatectomy. With one risk factor present (N = 303), the cumulative incidence was about 9 per cent; with two (N = 178), about 16 per cent; and with all three (N = 112), about 37 per cent. Once again, caution must be used in interpreting these data, because the threshold for recommending surgery was not uniform. These markers may be predictors of urologists recommending surgery to patients, as well as biologic determinants of progressive morbidity from BPH.

Placebo arms of efficacy studies of pharmacologic agents for the treatment of BPH also provide some information on the natural history of BPH.[9, 56] Table 8–4 lists selected studies that included groups of patients randomized to placebo treatment. Most show considerable symptomatic improvement with placebo. This improvement may be attributed to a natural tendency of BPH to improve over at least short intervals, as well as the effect of placebo treatment itself. In general, objective improvement in terms of urine flow rates and residual urine volumes is much less impressive in these trials. Unfortunately, none of these studies is over 1 year in duration, and most last 3 months or less. These data emphasize the importance of using appropriate control groups in the early evaluation of the efficacy of new treatments for BPH.

An important study that should shed new light on the natural history of untreated BPH is a Veterans Administration Cooperative Studies Program randomized trial of transurethral prostatectomy versus a strategy of expectant management (watchful waiting) for men with moderate symptoms of BPH. Enrollment of more than 550 patients is complete, and follow-up is now continuing. Results should become available sometime in 1992. In this study, half the subjects with well-defined symptomatic BPH have been followed carefully symptomatically and urodynamically without initial surgery. Data on the initially untreated arm of this trial should dramatically increase our knowledge of the course and complications of BPH over time.

Progression of Urodynamic Parameters

Even less information is available on the course of basic urodynamic findings over time among BPH patients. In the cohort followed by Ball and colleagues,[8] 64 of the cohort of 107 patients provided a follow-up urinary flow rate after 5 years of watchful waiting. The average peak flow rate fell from 13.1 to 11.9 ml/sec in these individuals over 5 years. Only six of these patients had a fall of greater than 1.2 standard deviations on the Siroky nomogram,[82] thought to represent clear evidence of a within-patient increase in urethral resistance, and only three of these patients actually perceived a diminution in urine flow.

Drach and colleagues[31] have calculated a drop in flow rate for the normal aging population of about 2.1 ml/sec/10 years. Furthermore, this fall seems to be blunted, rather than exaggerated, in patients with baseline low flows due to outlet obstruction.

Acute Urinary Retention

One of the more common complications of BPH is acute urinary retention. In the United States, acute

TABLE 8–4. RESULTS OF PLACEBO ARMS IN SELECTED RANDOMIZED CLINICAL TRIALS OF PHARMACOLOGIC INTERVENTIONS FOR SYMPTOMATIC BENIGN PROSTATIC HYPERPLASIA

REFERENCE	DURATION (WEEKS)	NUMBER (PLACEBO)	RESPONSE		
			Worse	Same	Better
Abrams (1977)[1]	26	29	14%	52%	34%
Geller et al (1979)[39]	20	33	0%	42%	58%
Hedlund et al (1983)[53]	4	20	20%	10%	70%
Resnick et al (1983)[73]	52	22	5%	59%	36%
Carbin et al (1990)[20]	12	27	19%	70%	11%
Kawabe et al (1990)[61]	4	54	2%	42%	56%

Responses are patients' global assessments of symptom change.

retention is the indication for prostatectomy in about 25 to 30 per cent of patients.[36, 67] The incidence of acute retention of urine in men with symptomatic BPH is not entirely clear. In Craigen and co-workers' series,[26] life-table analyses predicted a cumulative incidence of acute retention of 10 per cent over 7 years. Working backwards, using the equation at the beginning of this chapter, this cumulative incidence translates into an incidence rate of 0.015 episodes of retention per person-year. Expressing the rate of acute retention in this manner allows easy comparison with other studies with different periods of follow-up.

In the Birkoff et al series,[14] 9 of between 26 and 53 highly selected patients with BPH developed 10 episodes of acute retention. Because the length of follow-up of each case as well as the exact number at risk is not specified, calculation of an acute retention rate from these data is hazardous. However, this rate might be as high as 0.13 per person-year (assuming that 26 patients had 3 years of follow-up). In the series of Ball and colleagues,[8] the acute retention rate was much lower. Two of 107 patients had acute retention over 5 years. Assuming that the 10 patients who had a prostatectomy did so halfway through the follow-up period, on average, an incidence of acute retention of 0.004 per person-year can be calculated. Even if only the follow-up time of the 53 patients who were considered to be urodynamically obstructed at baseline (this group included all patients who eventually required surgery) is considered, the acute retention rate is still only 0.008 per person-year. These large variations in acute retention rates from reported series project 10-year acute retention rates among men with BPH as low as 4 per cent (using Ball and co-workers' data, including all patients) to as high as 73 per cent (using Birkhoff and co-workers' data)!

Another interesting natural history question is the course of BPH in men who have a first episode of acute retention. Many of these patients undergo a prostatectomy immediately. However, a few series have provided data on the untreated course in these patients. In Craigen and co-workers' series,[26] 55 per cent of patients had a prostatectomy within 3 months of their episode of acute retention, but 20 per cent had not, even 7 years after presentation. A second study followed 59 Danish men who presented to an emergency department with acute retention secondary to BPH.[19] Forty-three of these men (73 per cent) had recurrent acute retention within 1 week. Finally, in the most recent series, 43 of 60 men (72 per cent) with acute urinary retention due to BPH had an unsuccessful voiding trial.[87] The probability of a successful trial did not depend on whether the catheter was removed immediately or after 24 or 48 hours. Bladder volume at the time of catheter insertion was a powerful predictor of the success of the voiding trial: 15 of 34 patients with less than 900 ml had a successful voiding trial, as opposed to 2 of 26 with more than 900 ml. Over the succeeding 6 months of follow-up, none of the 17 men with successful voiding trials had recurrent acute retention. Six had undergone a prostatectomy for severe symptoms, six had minor symptoms, and five were asymptomatic. None of these series indicate whether a longer period of catheter drainage and bladder decompression would result in a higher percentage of successful voiding trials. Such time might be helpful, both to allow recovery of bladder contractility and perhaps to allow edema from any prostatic infarction to resolve.[84]

Chronic Renal Failure Secondary to Obstructive Uropathy

Chronic renal failure due to obstructive uropathy is a feared complication of BPH.[15, 79] Case reports document that this complication can sometimes occur with minimal BPH symptoms.[41, 72] Sometimes, renal insufficiency does not improve with delayed relief of bladder outlet obstruction. The frequency of this complication is not well defined. In one series from Israel,[72] 6 of 345 men coming to prostatectomy had evidence of occult progressive renal damage. These data do not allow an incidence rate to be calculated. No cases of chronic renal failure have been reported in the cohort studies of the natural history of BPH cited in this chapter, but the small number of patients in these series would not allow a low but clinically important rate of this complication to be measured. Research is needed to better estimate this risk and to define optimal monitoring strategies for men with BPH being managed expectantly to detect the early onset of renal deterioration at a reversible stage.

Serious Urinary Tract Infection

Like the risk of chronic renal failure with obstructive uropathy, the risk of urinary tract infection, especially serious upper tract infections and urosepsis, is not well defined. Although the prevalence of bladder outlet obstruction is relatively high among older men with serious urinary tract infection, the probability of serious urinary tract infections in the setting of BPH is probably relatively low. Again, no such cases are reported in the series of BPH patients following a course of expectant management discussed previously.

Bladder Decompensation

Experimental bladder outlet obstruction in animal models leads to rapid hypertrophy of the bladder, with connective tissue deposition.[29, 63] This same histologic picture of dense connective tissue deposition is seen in biopsy samples from trabeculated, chronically obstructed human bladders.[42, 45] However, a recent study suggests that bladder fibrosis seen in older men may be a phenomenon of age and not obstruction, as similar changes are seen in women.[62a] Moreover, about half of men with bladder outlet obstruction demonstrate uninhibited bladder contractions on filling cystometry.[23, 30] Presumably, in many of these men, the development of uninhibited contractions was secondary to the obstruction. These findings raise the question of whether delayed intervention for symptomatic BPH may, in some patients, lead to worse symptomatic outcomes from prostatectomy due to irreversible bladder damage.

Although this "loss-to-cure" theory is reasonable, supporting evidence from clinical research studies has not been forthcoming. The majority of men, even with evidence of severe bladder decompensation, seem to improve after prostatectomy.[40] For example, Jones and colleagues[58] described 32 men with high-pressure chronic retention of urine. These men had residual volumes of 320 to 2690 ml and a mean creatinine clearance of 53 ml/min. Bladder biopsy samples from 23 patients revealed muscular hypertrophy, bladder fibrosis, and a reduced density of acetyl cholinesterase–containing nerve fibers. However, at a mean follow-up of 43 months after prostatectomy, 25 of the 32 patients had a residual volume of less than 200 ml, and the mean creatinine clearance had risen to 82 ml/min. All but one patient had at least an initial improvement in renal function, although three more subsequently deteriorated owing to recurrent obstruction (two from prostate cancer).

Clearly, it is preferable to intervene with definitive relief of obstruction before patients get to this late point in the natural history of BPH. However, the appropriate interval and strategy of periodic monitoring of men with symptomatic BPH have not been well defined. Further research on the natural history of BPH is desperately needed to structure such a clinical policy of watchful waiting.

Summary

Despite the fact that literally millions of elderly men in the United States must be following a largely self-imposed regimen of watchful waiting for symptomatic BPH, the natural history of only a handful of such men is described in the available medical literature. None of these studies is a true inception cohort of men followed from early in the course of their disease. The fact that the 10-year risk of acute retention among these men is projected to be somewhere between 4 per cent and 73 per cent, based on available data from different studies, highlights the uncertainty plaguing this area.

To a large extent, poor knowledge of the natural history of untreated BPH underlies some of the controversy about the indications for intervention in this condition. This controversy in turn has led to three- to four-fold variations in the rate of prostatectomy among small, sometimes adjoining, geographic areas in the United States. Furthermore, the optimal strategy of monitoring men with symptomatic BPH who choose a course of expectant management cannot be defined until this information is available.

REFERENCES

1. Abrams PH: A double-blind trial of the effects of candicidin on patients with benign prostatic hypertrophy. Br J Urol 49:67, 1977.
2. Akimoto M: On the morphologic alteration of the prostate gland on aging. II. A correlative histopathologic study of the latent and manifested nodular hyperplasia of the prostate gland and senile changes of the testis. Jpn J Urol 58:814, 1967.
3. Araki H, Watanabe H, Mishina T, Nakao M: High-risk group for benign prostatic hypertrophy. Prostate 4:253, 1983.
4. Armenian HK, Lilienfeld AM, Diamond EL, Bross ID: Relation between benign prostatic hyperplasia and cancer of the prostate. Lancet 2:115, 1974.
5. Arrighi HM, Guess HA, Metter EJ, Fozard JL: Symptoms and signs of prostatism as risk factors for prostatectomy. Prostate 16:253, 1990.
6. Arrighi HM, Metter EJ, Guess HA, Fozzard JL: Natural history of benign prostatic hyperplasia and risk of prostatectomy: The Baltimore Longitudinal Aging Study. Urology 38:54, 1991.
7. Ashley DJ: Observations on the epidemiology of prostatic hyperplasia in Wales. Br J Urol 38:567, 1966.
8. Ball AJ, Feneley RC, Abrams PH: The natural history of untreated "prostatism." Br J Urol 53:613, 1981.
9. Barry MJ: Epidemiology and natural history of benign prostatic hyperplasia. Urol Clin North Am 17:495, 1990.
10. Barry MJ: Medical outcomes research and benign prostatic hyperplasia. Prostate 3:61, 1990.
11. Beier-Holgersen R, Bruun J: Voiding patterns of men 60 to 70 years old: Population study in an urban population. J Urol 143:531, 1990.
12. Bennett HS, Baggenstoss AH, Butt HR: The testis, breast, and prostate of men who die of cirrhosis of the liver. Am J Clin Pathol 20:814, 1950.
13. Berry SJ, Coffey DS, Walsh PC, Ewing LL: The development of human benign prostatic hyperplasia with age. J Urol 132:474, 1984.
14. Birkhoff JD, Wiederhorn AR, Hamilton ML, Zinsser HH: Natural history of benign prostatic hypertrophy and acute urinary retention. Urology 7:48, 1976.
15. Bishop MC: The dangers of a long urological waiting list. Br J Urol 65:433, 1990.
16. Blaivas JG: Differential diagnosis. *In* Hinman F (ed): Benign Prostatic Hypertrophy. New York, Springer-Verlag, 1983, p 747.
17. Blaivas JG: Multichannel urodynamic studies in men with benign prostatic hyperplasia: Indications and interpretation. Urol Clin North Am 17:543, 1990.
18. Bourke JB, Griffin JP: Hypertension, diabetes mellitus, and blood groups in benign prostatic hypertrophy. Br J Urol 38:18, 1966.
19. Breum L, Klarskov P, Munck LK, et al: Significance of acute urinary retention due to infravesical obstruction. Scand J Urol Nephrol 16:21, 1982.
20. Carbin BE, Larsson B, Lindahl O: Treatment of benign prostatic hyperplasia with phytosterols. J Urol 66:639, 1990.
21. Chang HL: Benign hypertrophy of the prostate. Chin Med J 50:1708, 1936.
22. Chassin MR, Brook RH, Park RE: Variations in the use of medical and surgical services by the Medicare population. N Engl J Med 314:285, 1986.
23. Christensen MM, Bruskewitz RC: Clinical manifestations of benign prostatic hyperplasia and indications for therapeutic intervention. Urol Clin North Am 17:509, 1990.
24. Clarke R: The prostate and the endocrines: A control series. Br J Urol 9:254, 1937.
25. Conger KB: Racial incidence of prostatism in Hawaii: A report of 172 consecutive cases. J Urol 58:444, 1947.
26. Craigen AA, Hickling JB, Saunders CR, Carpenter RG: Natural history of prostatic obstruction: A prospective survey. J R Coll Gen Pract 18:226, 1969.
27. D'Aunoy R, Schenken JR, Burns EL: The relative incidence of hyperplasia of the prostate in the white and colored races in Louisiana. South Med J 32:47, 1939.
28. Derbes VD, Leche SM, Hooker CW: The incidence of benign prostatic hypertrophy among the whites and negroes in New Orleans. J Urol 38:383, 1937.
29. Dixon JS, Gilpin CJ, Gilpin SA, et al: Sequential morphologic changes in the pig detrusor in response to chronic partial urethral obstruction. Br J Urol 64:385, 1989.
30. Dørflinger T, Frimodt-Møller PC, Bruskewitz RC, et al: The significance of uninhibited detrusor contractions in prostatism. J Urol 133:819, 1985.

31. Drach GW, Layton TN, Binard WJ: Male peak urinary flow rate: Relationship to volume voided and age. J Urol 122:210, 1979.

32. Ekman P: BPH epidemiology and risk factors. Prostate (Suppl) 2:23, 1989.

33. Epstein RS, Lydick E, DeLabry L, Vokonas PS: Age-related differences in risk factors for prostatectomy for benign prostatic hyperplasia: The VA Normative Aging Study. Urology 38:59, 1991.

34. Fay R: Prostatic obstruction in Chinese populations. *In* Hinman F (ed): Benign Prostatic Hypertrophy. New York, Springer-Verlag, 1983, p 27.

35. Feinstein AR: Double standards, scientific methods, and epidemiologic research. N Engl J Med 307:1611, 1982.

36. Fowler FJ, Wennberg JE, Timothy RP, et al: Symptom status and quality of life following prostatectomy. JAMA 259:3018, 1988.

37. Frea B, Annoscia S, Stanta G, et al: Correlation between liver cirrhosis and benign prostatic hyperplasia: A morphologic study. Urol Res 15:311, 1987.

38. Garraway WM, Collins GN, Lee RJ: High prevalence of benign prostatic hyperplasia in the community. Lancet 338:469, 1991.

39. Geller J, Nelson CG, Albert JD, Pratt C: Effect of megesterol acetate on uroflow rates in patients with benign prostatic hypertrophy. Urology 14:467, 1979.

40. Ghose RR: Prolonged recovery of renal function after prostatectomy for prostatic outflow obstruction. Br Med J 300:1376, 1990.

41. Ghose RR, Harindra V: Unrecognized high pressure chronic retention of urine presenting with systemic arterial hypertension. Br Med J 298:1626, 1989.

42. Gilpin SA, Gosling JA, Barnard J: Morphological and morphometric studies of the human obstructed, trabeculated urinary bladder. Br J Urol 57:525, 1985.

43. Glynn RJ, Campion EW, Bouchard GR, Silbert JE: The development of benign prostatic hyperplasia among volunteers in the Normative Aging Study. Am J Epidemiol 121:78, 1985.

44. Gofin R: The health status of elderly men: A community study. Public Health 96:345, 1982.

45. Gosling JA, Dixon JS: The structure of trabeculated detrusor smooth muscle in cases of prostatic hypertrophy. Urol Int 35:351, 1980.

46. Graversen PH, Gasser TC, Wasson JH, et al: Controversies about indications for transurethral resection of the prostate. J Urol 141:475, 1989.

47. Graves EJ: Detailed diagnoses and procedures, National Hospital Discharge Survey: 1987. National Center for Health Statistics. Vital Health Stat 13:295, 1989.

48. Greenwald P, Kirmes V, Polan AK, Dick VS: Cancer of the prostate among men with benign prostatic hyperplasia. J Natl Cancer Inst 53:335, 1974.

49. Guess HA, Arrighi HM, Metter EJ, Fozard JL: Cumulative prevalence of prostatism matches the autopsy prevalence of benign prostatic hyperplasia. Prostate 17:241, 1990.

50. Harbitz TB, Haugen OA: Histology of the prostate in elderly men. Acta Pathol Microbiol Scand 80:756, 1972.

51. Haupt BJ: Detailed diagnoses and procedures for patients discharged from short-stay hospitals. DHHS Publ No (PHS) 80-1274, 1978.

52. Hayden GF, Kramer MS, Horwitz RI: The case-control study: A practical review for the clinician. JAMA 247:326, 1982.

53. Hedlund H, Andersson KE, Ek A: Effects of prazosin in patients with benign prostatic obstruction. J Urol 130:275, 1983.

54. Holtgrewe HL, Mebust WK, Dowd JB, et al: Transurethral prostatectomy: Practice aspects of the dominant operation in American urology. J Urol 141:248, 1989.

55. Horwitz RI, Feinstein AR, Harvey MR: Case-control research: Temporal precedence and other problems of the exposure-disease relationship. Arch Intern Med 144:1257, 1984.

56. Isaacs JT: Importance of the natural history of benign prostatic hyperplasia in the evaluation of pharmacologic intervention. Prostate (Suppl) 3:1, 1990.

57. Jensen KM, Jorgensen JB, Mogensen P, et al: Some clinical aspects of uroflowmetry in elderly males. A population survey. Scand J Urol Nephrol 20:93, 1986.

58. Jones DA, Gilpin SA, Holden D, et al: Relationship between bladder morphology and long-term outcome of treatment in patients with high pressure chronic retention of urine. Br J Urol 67:280, 1991.

59. Kambal A: Prostatic obstruction in Sudan. Br J Urol 49:139, 1977.

60. Kato T: Histologic study on hyperplasia of the prostate with special reference to histiogenesis of nodule. Jpn J Urol 58:469, 1967.

61. Kawabe K, Ueno A, Takimoto Y, et al: Use of an alpha$_1$-blocker, YM617, in the treatment of benign prostatic hypertrophy. J Urol 144:908, 1990.

62. Kozak LJ: Detailed diagnoses and procedures for patients discharged from short-stay hospitals. DHHS Publ No (PHS) 85-1743, 1983.

62a. Lepor H, Sunaryadi I, Hartano V, Shapiro E: Quantitative morphometry of the adult human bladder. J Urol 148:414, 1992.

63. Levin RM, Longhurst PA, Monson FC, et al: Effect of bladder outlet obstruction on the morphology, physiology, and pharmacology of the bladder. Prostate (Suppl) 3:9, 1990.

64. Lytton B, Emery JM, Harvard BM: The incidence of benign prostatic obstruction. J Urol 99:639, 1968.

65. McNeal J: Pathology of benign prostatic hyperplasia: Insight into etiology. Urol Clin North Am 17:477, 1990.

66. McPherson K, Wennberg JE, Hovind OB, Clifford P: Small area variations in the use of common surgical procedures: An international comparison of New England, England, and Norway. N Engl J Med 307:1310, 1982.

67. Mebust WK, Holtgrewe HL, Cockett AT, et al: Transurethral prostatectomy: Immediate and postoperative complications: A cooperative study of 13 participating institutions evaluating 3,885 patients. J Urol 141:243, 1989.

68. Miettenen OS: Estimability and estimation in case-referent studies. Am J Epidemiol 103:226, 1976.

69. Miettenen OS: Theoretical Epidemiology. New York, John Wiley & Sons, 1985, p 25.

70. Morrison AS: Prostatic hypertrophy in Greater Boston. J Chron Dis 31:357, 1978.

70a. Morrison AS: Risk factors for surgery for prostatic hypertrophy. Am J Epidemiol 135:974, 1992.

71. Movsas S: Prostatic obstruction in the African and Asiatic. Br J Surg 53:538, 1966.

72. Mukamel E, Nissenkorn I, Boner G, Servadio C: Occult progressive renal damage in the elderly male due to benign prostatic hypertrophy. J Am Geriatr Soc 27:403, 1979.

73. Resnick MI, Jackson JE, Watts L, Boyce WH: Assessment of the antihypercholesterolemic drug, probucol, in benign prostatic hyperplasia. J Urol 129:206, 1983.

74. Roberts HJ: The role of diabetogenic hyperinsulinism in the pathogenesis of prostatic hyperplasia and malignancy. J Am Geriatr Soc 14:795, 1966.

75. Robson MC: The incidence of benign prostatic hyperplasia and prostatic carcinoma in cirrhosis of the liver. J Urol 92:307, 1964.

76. Rothman KJ: Modern Epidemiology. Boston, Little, Brown & Co, 1986, p 31.

77. Rotkin ID: Epidemiology of benign prostatic hypertrophy: Review and speculations. *In* Grayhack JT, Wilson JD, Sherbenske MJ (eds): Benign Prostatic Hyperplasia. DHEW Publ No (NIH) 76-1113. Washington, DC, US Government Printing Office, 1976, p 105.

78. Rotkin ID: Origins, distribution, and risk of benign prostatic hypertrophy. *In* Hinman F (ed): Benign Prostatic Hypertrophy. New York, Springer-Verlag, 1983, p 10.

79. Sachs SH, Aparicio SA, Bevan A, et al: Late renal failure due to prostatic outflow obstruction: A preventable disease. Br Med J 298:156, 1989.

80. Sarmina I, Resnick MI: Obstructive uropathy in patients with benign prostatic hyperplasia. J Urol 141:866, 1989.

81. Sidney S, Quesenberry C, Sudler MC, et al: Risk factors for surgically treated benign prostatic hyperplasia in a prepaid health care plan. Urology 38:513, 1991.

82. Siroky MB, Olsson CA, Krane RJ: The flow-rate nomogram: II. Clinical correlation. J Urol 123:208, 1980.

83. Sommer P, Nielsen KK, Bauer T: Voiding patterns in men evaluated by a questionnaire survey. Br J Urol 65:155, 1990.

84. Spiro LH, Labay G, Orkin LA: Prostatic infarction: Role in acute urinary retention. Urology 3:345, 1974.

85. Stephenson WP, Chute CG, Guess HA, et al: Incidence and outcome of surgery for benign prostatic hyperplasia among residents of Rochester, Minnesota: 1980–1987. Urology 38:532, 1991.

86. Strumpf HH, Wilens SL: Inhibitory effects of portal cirrhosis of liver on prostatic enlargement. Arch Intern Med 91:304, 1953.

87. Taube M, Gajraj H: Trial without catheter following acute retention of urine. Br J Urol 63:180, 1989.

88. Tugwell P: How to read clinical journals III: To learn the clinical course and prognosis of disease. Can Med Assoc J 124:869, 1981.

89. US Bureau of the Census. Statistical Abstract of the United States: 1980 (100th edition). Washington, DC, 1981.

90. US Bureau of the Census. Statistical Abstract of the United States: 1985 (105th edition). Washington, DC, 1986.

91. US Bureau of the Census. Statistical Abstract of the United States: 1990 (109th edition). Washington, DC, 1991.

92. Watanabe H: Natural history of benign prostatic hypertrophy. Ultrasound Med Biol 12:567, 1986.

93. Watanabe H, Ohe H, Inaba T, et al: A mobile mass screening unit for prostatic disease. Prostate 5:559, 1984.

94. Wennberg JE: Dealing with medical practice variations: A proposal for action. Health Affairs 3:6, 1984.

95. Wennberg J, Gittelsohn A: Variations in medical care among small areas. Sci Am 246:120, 1982.

ACKNOWLEDGMENTS: Dr. Barry is a member of the Patient Outcome Research Team for Prostatic Diseases, funded by the Center for Medical Effectiveness Research of the Agency for Health Care Policy and Research (Grant No. HS 06336). He is also a Henry J. Kaiser Family Foundation Faculty Scholar in General Internal Medicine.

Chapter 9

BENIGN PROSTATIC HYPERPLASIA: CLINICAL MANIFESTATIONS AND INDICATIONS FOR INTERVENTION

MORTEN RIEHMANN and REGINALD C. BRUSKEWITZ

ANATOMY AND PATHOANATOMY/PATHOLOGY

The prostate is the largest male sexual accessory gland and the only organ that demonstrates benign neoplasia with increasing age. The prostate can be divided into glandular and nonglandular components.[62] The glandular tissue contains three major zones, which differ histologically and biochemically: the central, transition, and peripheral zones, which comprise approximately 25 per cent, 5 per cent, and 70 per cent of the volume of the normal gland, respectively.[62] The nonglandular prostate is composed of the preprostatic sphincter, striated sphincter, anterior fibromuscular stroma, and prostatic capsule.[62] The preprostatic sphincter is a cylinder of smooth muscle surrounding the proximal segment of the prostatic urethra. Within this sphincter lies the periurethral region, which by volume comprises very little of the gland. It has not been established which zone is best removed, cut, shrunk, heated, or relaxed when benign prostatic hyperplasia (BPH) is treated.

The prostate is histologically composed primarily of epithelium, glandular lumina, and stroma with an epithelium-stroma ratio of 1:2 to 2:3 in the normal gland. With development of BPH, only the transition zone and the periurethral region are sites of hyperplasia.[62, 63] Owing to the angulation of the prostatic urethra, these areas are displaced anteriorly when they are the site of benign neoplasia. In most patients manifesting clinical BPH, the hyperplasia is located within the transition zone.[64] Bartsch et al, Geller, and Lawson state that BPH is primarily a stromal disease.[8, 32, 51] Other authors, however, have stated that BPH is hyperplasia not merely of the stroma but of the epithelium as well.[10, 21, 78] Some suggest that BPH starts as a stromal neoplasia, and this hyperplastic tissue in some way stimulates the epithelial tissue to grow.[51] BPH is a complex pathologic process that varies with age and microscopically reveals a mixture of glandular, cystic, and stromal hyperplasia.

It is not clear at this point whether specific treatments should be aimed at prostates that are predominantly stromal or predominantly glandular. Given the morphologic variability within the gland, it is not clear that the clinician can accurately characterize the individual prostate prior to treatment anyway.

PATHOGENESIS OF BENIGN PROSTATIC HYPERPLASIA

Although some uncertainty exists about whether BPH is primarily a stromal or an epithelial neoplasia, it is evident that one of the contributing factors in BPH is hormonal stimulation.

The crucial influence of the testes in the maintenance of BPH was demonstrated in the 1890s by two investigators, who reported that 80 per cent of patients with BPH improved symptomatically after castration.[17, 93] These reports had little in the way of objective data. Other investigators reported failure of orchiectomy to relieve infravesical obstruction due to BPH. Scott observed that development of BPH was rare when castration was performed before age 30.[82]

Although the testes and aging are essential for the development of BPH, it is not clear which hormone or hormones lead to the disease. 5α-Reductase converts testosterone to dihydrotestosterone (DHT), which is the active intracellular prostatic metabolite. The development and progression of human BPH is mediated by DHT. The observation that the tissue level of this hormone is only slightly elevated in patients with BPH raises questions about whether other causative mechanisms may be at work. The androgen receptor level is elevated in the hyperplastic prostate.[7]

The role of estrogen in the development of BPH is controversial. Coffey and Walsh found that a combination of estrogens and DHT can cause a decrease in the rate of cell death, which could lead to prostate hyperplasia.[21] Estrogen synergizes with 5α-reduced androgens in the experimental induction of BPH in dogs, possibly through an estrogen-induced increase in the level of androgen receptors in the prostate.[90]

McNeal has postulated that localized tissue undergoes changes to the embryonic state which might play a role in nodule genesis.[64, 65] Lawson theorizes that reawakening embryonic tissue may play a role in the pathogenesis of BPH.[51] Several different growth factors have been found in the prostate. Basic fibroblast growth factor (bFGF) is involved in early embryogenesis and is thought to participate, along with other growth factors, in the initiation of stromal hyperplasia.[51]

The pathogenesis of BPH is probably multifactorial. Given the uncertainty surrounding hormones, it is not possible at this point to identify individual patients or prostates that might respond more favorably to hormonal treatment.

NATURAL HISTORY AND EPIDEMIOLOGY

One of the central issues is an epidemiologic characterization of BPH, i.e., how to define BPH progression on histologic, macroscopic, and symptomatic criteria. In papers based on autopsy studies, BPH is normally defined on histologic criteria, which do not necessarily reflect the incidence or prevalence of clinical BPH.

According to Isaacs and Coffey, BPH can be divided into two phases—pathologic and clinical. Although the latter is always preceded by pathologic changes in the prostate, these changes do not invariably lead to clinical manifestations of BPH.[40] Only one half of aging men with gross enlargement of the prostate develop clinical symptoms requiring surgery.[40] Birkhoff estimated that a 50-year-old man has approximately a 25 per cent chance of undergoing a prostatectomy during his lifetime,[12] and Glynn et al stated that 29 per cent of all men are destined to undergo prostatectomy.[34]

Berry et al provided information on growth rate and prevalence of BPH by combining data from 10 autopsy studies with a total of more than 1000 prostates.[10] Autopsy samples indicate that the first signs of BPH are seen in men 31 to 40 years old, with a prevalence of 8 per cent. With advancing age, the prevalence increases progressively so that 50 per cent of men between 51 and 60 years have histologic evidence of BPH, and at age 80 years more than 85 per cent of men have histologic evidence of BPH.[40]

Between the ages of 10 and 20 years, the prostate undergoes the greatest growth and reaches a fully functional state. BPH is associated with continued, slow increases in weight after age 30, and according to Berry et al the disease is probably initiated before age 30.[10] In the Boston Normative Aging Study the cumulative probability that a 40-year-old man will develop BPH was estimated to be 78 per cent.[34]

Ideally, a man destined to have significant clinical manifestations of BPH might be identified in the pathologic preclinical stage and offered effective preventive therapy. Can we identify those men? Are we close to such identification? The answer to both of these important questions is no.

CLINICAL MANIFESTATIONS OF BENIGN PROSTATIC HYPERPLASIA

Symptoms

The symptoms related to infravesical obstruction due to BPH are often referred to as prostatism. These symptoms are very arbitrarily divided into obstructive and irritative.

The *obstructive symptoms* are weak stream, abdominal straining, hesitancy, intermittency, incomplete bladder emptying, and terminal dribbling. The *irritative symptoms* are frequency, nocturia, urgency, urge incontinence, and possibly dysuria.

Other conditions associated with prostatism are acute or chronic urinary tract infection, hematuria, acute urinary retention, chronic retention with or without overflow incontinence, and acute or chronic renal failure.

Urinary Stream

Most males are aware of the "quality" of their urinary stream. With obstruction there usually is a steady, gradual decrease in the force of the stream. The stream can be characterized as normal, variable, weak, and dribbling, and there is often variation with time so that a person with a weak stream for periods of time may report having a subjectively normal flow. The variable tonus of the prostate smooth muscle is postulated to account for this dynamic component of urinary obstruction associated with BPH.

Abdominal Straining

It is generally accepted that some people with prostatism contract the abdominal muscles during voiding to overcome the increased urethral resistance. No correlation between straining and urodynamic or symptomatologic indicators of infravesical obstruction, however, has been shown.[42] A positive correlation between straining and increasing age is found. Straining is probably an individual habit and not a symptom of obstruction.

Hesitancy

In normal men, the time that elapses between the CNS signal to relax the bladder neck and sphincter until the urine flow starts is only a few seconds. Various factors (e.g., stress, the surroundings in which voiding takes place), however, affect this time. This is one of the reasons why voiding is best done in privacy during the urodynamic testing of patients.

Prolonged time from the attempt to initiate micturition to the start of urinary flow is regarded as hesitancy. No specific time interval has been established for what is defined as hesitancy and, in the obstructed male, the delay time may vary from several seconds to minutes. Only the symptoms of hesitancy and slow stream have been correlated with the urodynamic findings of obstruction in men with BPH.[2]

The cause of hesitancy is unclear because it only takes up to about 10 seconds to reach the raised intravesical pressure needed for voiding in a patient with outflow obstruction.

Intermittency

Intermittency is defined as intermittent disruption of the urinary stream during voiding. This is not only seen in patients with BPH but can be caused by urethral strictures, neurologic bladder disorders, and cancer of the prostate as well. The flow curve has a jagged line in patients with intermittency, but the configuration of the curve is nonspecific in diagnosing the origin of the intermittent obstruction.

Incomplete Bladder Emptying

A further desire to void or suprapubic discomfort after voiding is often associated with incomplete bladder emptying in patients with BPH. No statistical correlation, however, is found between preoperative residual volume and urodynamic and cystoscopic findings or symptoms of infravesical obstruction in patients with BPH about to undergo transurethral resection of the prostate (TURP).[15] No correlation is seen between the patient's sensation of bladder emptying and postvoid residual urine volume (PVR),[15] which varies on the same day in patients with BPH.[11] PVR correlates poorly with other signs and symptoms of BPH.

Terminal Dribbling

At the end of voiding, there is a steady decrease in the force of the stream in the obstructed patient and, in some males, the end flow is reduced to dribbling, which

may last for 1 minute or more. Monosymptomatic terminal dribbling is usually not associated with any abnormalities revealed by urodynamics.[88] Terminal dribbling occurs when the detrusor is no longer able to maintain continuous flow, but the pathogenesis is not clear.

Frequency

In evaluating patients' voiding frequency or interval, several factors have to be considered, e.g., fluid intake, habit, medication (especially diuretics), renal and neurologic diseases, and endocrine diseases such as diabetes which might affect bladder function and voided volume. A time interval of about 3 hours between urinations is considered normal.

As mentioned, a decreased time interval between voiding is regarded as one of the irritative symptoms in men with BPH. Some authors find the irritative symptoms associated with uninhibited bladder contractions, but Frimodt-Møller et al did not find such correlation.[2, 5, 31] Cucchi, however, found a correlation between the occurrence of detrusor instability and the degree of obstruction.[24] Speakman et al showed good correlation between the severity and duration of symptoms and the presence of uninhibited bladder contractions.[86, 87]

Nocturia

Nocturia is defined as awakening and voiding because of the desire to void. Voiding once a night is not considered abnormal. The factors predisposing to frequency need to be taken into account when evaluating nocturia, especially intake of fluid and diuretics before going to bed. The examiner should also consider local and systemic diseases, e.g., diabetes, cystitis, and cardiac disorders, with mobilization of edema in the horizontal position.

Urgency and Urge Incontinence

Urgency is a strong desire to void. Urge incontinence is involuntary loss of urine in association with urgency. Often urgency is associated with a premature sensation of bladder fullness. Some investigators believe that patients with high urgency symptom score and high peak urine flow rates require full urodynamic assessment.[86, 87] Frimodt-Møller et al demonstrated significant associations between urge and frequency and nocturia but not between urge and any obstructive symptoms.[31]

Dysuria

Dysuria is defined as a painful voiding—often as a feeling of "passing broken glass" in the penile urethra or a burning sensation during or at the end of micturition. Dysuria is often accompanied by frequency and urgency and is usually related to inflammation of the lower urinary tract caused by urinary tract infection, calculi, carcinoma, or interstitial cystitis. It is doubtful whether dysuria is associated with the symptoms of infravesical obstruction seen in patients with BPH.

Urinary Tract Infection

Symptoms of lower urinary tract infection are pollakiuria, dysuria, suprapubic discomfort and burning, sensation in the pendulous urethra of "passing broken glass" at the end of micturition, and foul-smelling cloudy urine. Significant bacteriuria is usually defined as 10^5 or more colony forming units per milliliter in the urine. Urinary tract infection is often symptomatic with significant bacteriuria. About 30 per cent of patients undergoing prostate surgery have significant bacteriuria preoperatively.[48] Most of these patients have had urinary retention and/or a transurethral catheter.

Although the urethra is often colonized with bacteria, the urinary tract is generally sterile from kidney to bladder neck in normal individuals. The following theoretical considerations may explain the increased incidence of lower urinary tract infections in obstructed patients: decreased periodic "washout" by voiding, higher incidence of transurethral instrumentation, and suppression of local defense mechanisms, probably due to decreased capillary flow in the bladder wall secondary to increased intravesical pressure.

There is no correlation between the amount of PVR and a history of previous urinary tract infection.[15] Bacterial prostatitis may, in fact, be the most common cause of urinary tract infection in men.[66] Prostatitis often occurs during the fifth and sixth decades and is more often seen in diabetics. The patient often complains of recurrent febrile attacks and symptoms of cystitis or pyelonephritis lasting for a couple of days.

Hematuria

Recurrent gross hematuria may arise from dilated veins coursing over the surface of the enlarged, adenomatous gland. These veins can often be seen during cystoscopy. Hematuria in patients with BPH ranges from minor degrees, which are quite common, to recurrent, severe gross hematuria leading to blood clotting and urinary retention.

Urinary Retention

Acute urinary retention in the patient with BPH probably occurs for many reasons. In some people it might be a terminal event of a steadily progressive urinary obstruction, but in other cases it develops suddenly and with more mild antecedent symptoms of prostatism. Craigen et al found that 42 per cent of patients with BPH presented with retention, and one third of these had symptoms of BPH for less than 3

months.[23] In a series of approximately 800 patients undergoing prostate surgery, 10 to 15 per cent presented with acute retention.[58] Birkhoff et al did not find any correlation between the subjective and objective score of prostatism and urinary retention.[13] This finding indicates that retention is not due only to progression of prostatic growth or symptoms.

The exact cause of urinary retention is not known, but increased sympathetic tonus of the prostate, e.g., due to medication with alpha-adrenergic activity, anticholinergics that decrease bladder tonus, or overdistention of the bladder wall, may be involved. Prostatic infarction is another possible mechanism. A mechanical overdistention of the detrusor wall followed by an inability to overcome the urethral resistance has also been proposed. Use of alcohol is a common cause of retention which may be explained by the theory of overdistention and increased sympathetic stimulation.

Renal Failure

One of the most commonly misdiagnosed causes of renal failure is obstructive uropathy.[37] Eighteen per cent of patients undergoing TURP have elevated serum creatinine and/or blood urea nitrogen, but most elevations are mild and due to renal parenchymal or vascular disease and not outlet obstruction with hydronephrosis.[70] Although renal failure is relatively rare in patients with BPH, it is worth noting that uremia can develop with minor urinary symptoms.[73] The World Health Organization believes that 5 per cent of adult male deaths worldwide are due to BPH. In North America and more developed countries, the percentage is far less.

INDICATIONS FOR INTERVENTION

The indications for therapeutic intervention (surgical and nonsurgical) are listed in Table 9–1. Often a patient presents with several of the manifestations of BPH, which makes the decision to proceed with treatment easier. The fact that several choices of treatment exist has to be discussed with the patient. The patient should be informed about advantages, disadvantages, and risks

TABLE 9–1. INDICATIONS FOR INTERVENTION IN BENIGN PROSTATIC HYPERTROPHY

Strong
Urinary retention
Azotemia with hydronephrosis
Severe gross hematuria
Urinary tract infection
Overflow incontinence

Moderate
Symptoms
Pathologic urodynamic findings

Weak
Cystoscopic findings
Prostate size

of each treatment and asked to participate in the selection of treatment. Comorbid disease and patient preference vary from patient to patient, and the urologist must consider these variables when presenting the possibilities for treatment.

Severe mental disturbance and decreased life expectancy because of comorbid disease are the only strong contraindications to surgery. One has to keep in mind that prostatic surgery generally precludes alternative treatment.

The clear-cut indications for intervention as listed in Table 9–1 are relatively easy to define. The moderate and weak indications are more difficult to outline. In a study of nearly 4000 patients, 70 per cent presented with multiple indications.[67]

Urinary Retention

Acute urinary retention constitutes a strong indication for intervention. Breum et al reported that 90 per cent of patients who presented with acute retention required surgery (requirements not further defined) unless they were able to establish a voiding pattern within 1 week.[14] In a study in which patients with acute urinary retention did not immediately undergo prostatectomy, approximately 58 per cent required surgery within 3 months.[23] Urinary retention is associated with a significantly higher postoperative complication rate in patients undergoing TURP.[69] However, urinary retention is not a factor in operative mortality.[69, 70] Initially, urinary retention is treated with catheterization, and in patients with compromised renal function due to infravesical obstruction, the renal function generally improves rapidly when the obstruction is relieved. As mentioned later in this chapter, normalization of renal function prior to intervention decreases the operative risk. In conclusion, acute retention secondary to BPH is a clear indication for prostatectomy in any healthy man who cannot void satisfactorily after retention has been relieved and for whom a precipitating cause such as medication or recent operation can be excluded.

Azotemia

Whereas urinary retention is not associated with a postoperative increase in morbidity or mortality, azotemia is found to be the single most significant factor influencing the morbidity and mortality rates in patients undergoing TURP.[70] Azotemia is a life-threatening illness, and infravesical obstruction due to BPH is a strong indication for surgery.

Hematuria

Minor degrees of hematuria secondary to BPH are relatively common and not per se an indication for surgery. However, recurrent, severe gross hematuria leading to urinary tract blood clotting with urinary retention, anemia, and the need for blood transfusions is a strong indication for surgery. Gross hematuria requires a thorough urinary tract examination. The cause of gross hematuria can be attributed to BPH only when all other possibilities have been excluded.

Urinary Tract Infection

The medical treatment of chronic bacterial prostatitis can be troublesome. Bacterial prostatitis is a known cause of recurrent urinary tract infection and in some "medically resistant" cases prostatectomy is indicated, not only to relieve symptoms but also to prevent urinary tract damage. The infection is often located in the periphery of the gland, and it is important to resect all the infected tissue, including the prostatic calculi, to cure the infection.

Overflow Incontinence

Incontinence is the failure of voluntary control of urination with a constant or intermittent passage of urine. In patients suffering from overflow incontinence, the bladder is usually greatly distended as a result of infravesical obstruction. Often the bladder compliance is increased. Typically, urine dribbles from the urethra when the intravesical pressure rises above the threshold of the urethral resistance owing to the pressure of retained urine.

Because urinary incontinence can be caused by neurologic disorders, cystitis, insufficient urinary sphincter, surgery, bladder hyperreflexia, and infravesical obstruction, any male patient with urinary incontinence should undergo a neurologic and urologic (including urodynamic) examination.

Special Diagnostic Methods and Symptoms

Excretory Urography

In the United States, the majority of urologists perform excretory urography prior to performing prostatic surgery on patients with BPH. Among the upper urinary tract diseases, BPH patients have an increased incidence of hydronephrosis. Impaired renal function is a very important factor leading to increased morbidity and mortality in patients undergoing TURP, but this does not seem to be the case in patients with hydronephrosis and normal renal function undergoing prostatic surgery.[79] Furthermore, excretory urography does not have a significant impact on the management of patients with BPH.[1] Urography or other upper tract imaging in BPH patients should be restricted to patients with symptoms or signs of upper urinary tract disease, hematuria, a history of urinary tract calculi, urinary tract infections, and evidence of renal insufficiency.

Cystoscopy

Cystourethroscopy provides information about possible disorders in the urethra, prostate, bladder neck, and bladder which might be mistaken for BPH or confirms the existence of BPH or obstruction. The procedure can be performed with rigid or flexible instruments.

Findings in patients with BPH-related infravesical obstruction include increased estimated prostatic size and length, obstruction of the prostatic urethra and bladder neck, bladder stones, bladder trabeculation, saccules, and diverticula.

Detrusor opening pressure and urethral resistance are found to correlate significantly with the cystoscopically estimated prostatic weight, prostatic occlusion of the urethra, and the bladder neck–verumontanum distance.[4] Correlation between bladder trabeculation and opening pressure was found in the same study.

Cystoscopy gives valuable information about the site and severity of urinary obstruction.[4] However, this procedure cannot by itself identify which patients require surgery and predict the outcome of surgery, mainly because some men with severe outlet obstruction endoscopically appear normal and vice versa. Cystoscopy is not routinely indicated in the evaluation of BPH.

Prostate Size Determination

Digital palpation is an unreliable method for estimating the size of the prostate,[71, 72] and the size of the gland estimated by this method does not correlate with symptoms.[5] Estimation of prostate weight by simultaneous rectal examination and cystoscopy is found to correlate with resected tissue weight and preoperative obstructive symptoms.[4, 43, 72] Although an enlarged prostate alone in an elderly man is no indication for treatment, it may be of help in the selection of the surgical procedure in the elderly man who also has evidence of significant urinary obstruction. This is discussed in detail later in this chapter.

Urodynamic Testing

Conventional urodynamic investigations for BPH include uroflowmetry, pressure-flow study, and cystometry.

UROFLOWMETRY

Uroflowmetry is the recording of the urinary flow rate—volume per time unit—throughout micturition. This is the most frequently used modality in the documentation of infravesical obstruction. It should be performed in a standardized fashion and in privacy. Also, it should be representative of the patient's usual voiding pattern. The results of uroflowmetry are nonspecific in diagnosing the site of obstruction. The flow curve reflects the interaction between the contracting bladder and outlet resistance and does not differentiate between obstruction and bladder dysfunction. The peak flow rate is generally preferred as the most informative and valuable measurement.

The mean and peak flows depend on intravesical volume, and the peak flow rate is usually reached during the early phase of micturition.[85] In order to use flow rate as an index of outflow obstruction, one has to correct the measured flow rate by intravesical or voided volume. This is done by using so-called flow-rate nomograms, which indicate where the flow rate lies in terms of standard deviations or percentile rank from normal age-matched males. Voided volume has to be at least 150 ml when evaluating peak flows in males.[26]

Patient age as well as volume has to be considered in the evaluation of peak flows. In a random sampling of males in the age range of 50 to 92 years without voiding problems, Jørgensen found a decrease in peak flow from 18.5 ml/sec at age 50 to 6.5 ml/sec at age 80.[46] Beck and Gaudin also found a decrease in peak flow in men with no historical or clinical evidence of urinary obstruction.[9] Not complaining of voiding difficulties, however, is not the same as being free of urinary obstruction.

It is generally accepted that maximal flow rates (Q_{max}) of less than 10 ml/sec are associated with infravesical obstruction, provided that detrusor insufficiency is absent, and that Q_{max} of greater than 15 ml/sec usually excludes urinary obstruction. Patients with Q_{max} between 10 and 15 ml/sec may or may not be obstructed, and further urodynamic testing should be undertaken.[38]

As implied, there are some limitations of uroflowmetry. A poor flow rate could be caused by impaired detrusor contractility as well as infravesical obstruction. Gerstenberg et al found 7 per cent of patients referred for BPH to have high-flow, high-pressure infravesical obstruction, i.e., flow rates greater than 15 ml/sec combined with elevated intravesical pressure during voiding.[33]

There is good evidence, however, that patients with preoperative Q_{max} greater than 15 ml/sec have a lower success rate postoperatively than those with Q_{max} less than 15 ml/sec.[41] It is reasonable to state that in the interpretation of uroflowmetry one has to consider total intravesical or voided volume and to some extent age. Uroflowmetry is a good screening procedure in patients with symptoms of urinary obstruction, but it cannot solely diagnose urinary obstruction. There are no clear guidelines for use of flow testing for selecting patients for treatment.

PRESSURE-FLOW STUDIES

Simultaneous recording of intravesical pressure during voiding gives a rough estimate of the urethral resistance by the relationship P/Q_{max}^2 (P = intravesical pressure). Values greater than 0.6 are normally considered a sign of urinary obstruction. Parameters related to infravesical obstruction are elevated detrusor pressure during flow and peak flow, often in combination with reduced flow. Pressure-flow studies can be used to detect people with high-flow, high-pressure urinary obstruction as well as primary bladder dysfunction without obstruction.

Urethral resistance is related to flow (by definition) and symptoms of urinary obstruction, but it is not useful in predicting which patients will benefit from surgery.[16] Pressure-flow studies cannot be recommended as a screening modality for prostatism because voiding pressure has been found to be of limited predictive value.[42]

CYSTOMETRY

The bladder has two functions—expelling the urine and serving as a reservoir for urine. The ability to expel urine can be estimated by pressure and flow. The reservoir function can be measured by cystometry. By this method, bladder capacity, compliance, and the presence of uninhibited bladder contractions can be studied. The intravesical pressure is measured during filling of the bladder, and a pressure-volume relationship is recorded.

The reservoir function of the bladder is altered with BPH along with pressure and flow. Detrusor instability or uninhibited bladder contractions occur in patients who are not able to suppress increases in intravesical pressure secondary to detrusor contraction between voidings. These contractions can be provoked by a variety of stimuli, such as filling of the bladder. This unstable bladder is graphically characterized by the presence of contractions exceeding 15 cm H_2O. Uninhibited bladder contractions may occur in association with some neurologic diseases and infravesical obstruction, and the incidence is found to increase with age.

Andersen et al[3] found that 53 per cent of healthy elderly males have uninhibited bladder contractions, whereas Jones and Schoenberg[45] found that 11 per cent of older women have uninhibited contractions, suggesting that BPH and not just aging accounts for the majority of uninhibited contractions found in men. Patients with uninhibited detrusor contractions are four times more likely to have a poor postoperative outcome.[87]

The presence of detrusor instability is not related to the degree of urinary obstruction, and the contractions may even arise without any obstruction.[22, 87] Dørflinger et al found that preoperative detrusor contractions were of no predictive value in determining the postoperative outcome.[27]

Symptoms

Symptoms related to BPH represent relative indications for surgical intervention. However, there is a need to objectively evaluate the patient's subjective symptoms. The use of scoring schemes, e.g., as proposed by Madsen and Iversen,[59] minimizes some of the uncertainty about subjective symptoms. A great limitation of scoring schemes has until now been the failure to include a bothersome index and questions dealing with quality of life. For example, a man who feels bothered primarily by getting up each night to void five or six times may not feel any great relief when he postoperatively still has to void five or six times each night, although his total symptom score has been reduced because of the disappearance of terminal dribbling, hesitancy, or other symptoms. Other men might not mind voiding several times each night. What bothers one person might not affect another person to any significant degree in terms of perceived quality of life.

It would be desirable to correlate symptoms with more objective criteria of urinary obstruction, but only hesitancy and slow stream are significantly correlated to urodynamically demonstrated obstruction.[2] Some have regarded these symptoms as more definitive indications for surgical intervention.[60] Irritative symptoms are correlated with uninhibited bladder contractions and not with urinary obstruction,[2, 5] but this is not a consistent finding.[31] Fifty to 60 per cent of patients with BPH preoperatively have uninhibited detrusor contractions, but after surgery the incidence decreases to 20 to 30 per cent.[27]

Conclusions Regarding Urodynamics and Symptoms

The ultimate goal of urodynamic investigations in patients with BPH is that these tests identify patients with infravesical obstruction, and among those, the fraction who would benefit from surgery. Urodynamic studies are performed to confirm the clinical impression but also to evaluate parameters that might alter diagnosis or treatment.

Symptoms, however, correlate poorly with urodynamic findings or urinary obstruction, as only hesitancy and slow stream have been associated with obstruction. This implies the need for an alternate form of objective data confirming infravesical obstruction or other factors, such as detrusor dysfunction unrelated to BPH. Although it is true that patients with peak flows greater than 15 ml/sec have poorer results postoperatively, more than 50 per cent of men with the worst urodynamic combination—high peak flow rate, no elevation of detrusor pressure on pressure flow, and uninhibited bladder contractions—still have a favorable outcome following resection of the prostate. This implies that our schemes for using urodynamics to select patients for treatment leaves much to be desired.

TREATMENT OF PATIENTS WITH BENIGN PROSTATIC HYPERPLASIA AND INDICATIONS FOR EACH PROCEDURE

Transurethral Resection of the Prostate

TURP has, over the last 50 years, become the primary choice of treatment to relieve bladder outlet obstruction and symptoms of prostatism. Approximately 400,000 TURPs are done each year in the United States.[81]

TURP is reported to be a safe and effective procedure for alleviating infravesical obstruction. The mortality rate has been reduced from 2.5 per cent to 0.2 per cent during the last 27 years, and the morbidity is now 18 per cent.[69] More than 80 per cent of patients experience symptomatic relief after TURP.[29, 55]

Fifteen per cent of patients experience no benefit after surgery, and only patients with severe symptoms or acute urinary retention show significant improvement in voiding symptoms *and* quality of life following prostatectomy.[30] Prostatic and urethral reoperations following

TURP are significantly higher in frequency than after open prostatectomy.[80, 92]

In conclusion, there are differing views about the safety and efficacy of TURP. Throughout the United States there is wide variation in the transurethral prostatectomy rates, and there appears to be considerable uncertainty about the indicators for this operation and about which patients are likely to benefit from surgery.[36]

Transurethral Incision of the Prostate

Transurethral incision of the prostate (TUIP) can be performed with various knives, both cold and electrocautery, as well as the standard resectoscope. An Nd-YAG laser has been employed to make urethral or bladder neck incisions or to perform the TULIP procedure.

Compared with TURP, the incision is simple to perform and teach and requires shorter operative time.[57, 74] Shorter operative time minimizes fluid absorption, which may be problematic with TURP. Reduced operative time may decrease postoperative pulmonary and cardiovascular complications.

Transurethral incision of the prostate and bladder neck relieves outflow obstruction, as does TURP among patients randomized to either TUIP or TURP.[19, 28, 50, 57, 74] There are, however, some important differences in the outcome of these two procedures as well as differences in the indications for selecting TUIP or TURP.

Bladder neck contracture is seen in approximately 8 per cent of patients after TURP when it is performed in smaller glands, but very seldom after TUIP.[68, 77, 84] Postresection vesical neck contracture following TURP is generally treated with bladder neck incision as well.[84] Performing prophylactic bladder neck incision in small glands (resectable weight less than 20 grams) in conjunction with TURP reduces the incidence of bladder neck contracture.[49] TUIP is difficult to do effectively and is associated with increased complications in large glands. This suggests that TUIP may be the better operation for smaller glands. TUIP is associated with reduced incidence of retrograde ejaculation compared with TURP, which is an indication for choosing the incision procedure in sexually active or younger men.

With respect to urinary retention, azotemia, and manifestations of infravesical obstruction due to BPH, indications for transurethral incision and resection of the prostate are nearly equal. However, in prostatitis, when the aim is to remove the infected prostate tissue, men with symptomatic BPH and prostate glands with estimated resectable weights greater than 30 grams, and BPH with severe gross hematuria, TURP would be preferable to incision. A disadvantage of TUIP is the potential for missing occult prostatic cancer.

Open Prostatectomy

Open prostatectomy can be performed as a simple perineal, suprapubic, or retropubic prostatectomy. Of all prostatic surgery for benign disease, the perineal prostatectomy is the procedure associated with the highest incidence of impotence; it occurs in about two thirds of the patients.[35, 52] This kind of prostatectomy should be avoided if the patient is potent and sexually active.

Followed over 5 years, patients who had open prostatectomy seemed to do a little better according to global assessment of symptoms than the TURP group.[6] This was, however, a nonmatched, nonrandomized study and the number of patients in the two groups was not equal. In some studies, the decrease in residual urine volume and improvement in peak flow have been significantly better in patients who underwent open prostatectomy than in those who underwent TURP.[83]

The major disadvantages of open prostatectomy are increased incidence of excessive bleeding, wound complications, and longer hospital stay. Very large adenomatous glands (the definition of size limit varies widely among urologists) are considered for open surgery to reduce morbidity.

Balloon Dilatation

Balloon dilatation has been demonstrated to be a simple and safe method. The advantages of this procedure are lower cost than TURP, minimal or no hospitalization, no preclusion of later definitive treatments, and the possibility of performing the procedure under sedation with supplemental analgesia. The procedure is reported to cause neither incontinence nor impotence, and in a study of 50 men, more than 70 per cent were better at a follow-up of 1 to 41 months.[25] After dilatation of 14 patients, McCullough et al[61] reported objective improvement at 2 weeks in terms of peak and mean flow and PVR, but by 3 months no improvement was seen. In a randomized study of TURP versus balloon dilatation, no retrograde ejaculation was apparent in the balloon dilatation group.[47] In a randomized study, no statistically significant difference was seen in improvement of total symptom score or flow rates following balloon dilatation or cystoscopy.[56] The efficacy of balloon dilatation varies considerably from one study to another. Further, does the efficacy not reach the level of TURP?[25] The evaluation of balloon dilatation is hampered by the presence of very few randomized studies.

A positive outcome in patients with very large residual urine volumes, severe symptoms, acute or chronic urinary retention, median lobe hyperplasia, bladder neck contractures, or urethral strictures is less likely. Some or all of these conditions are regarded as relative contraindications.[25, 91]

Prostatic Hyperthermia

Hyperthermia of the prostate has recently been introduced in the treatment of BPH. In the United States it is experimental. Because randomized studies are not available, it is too early to evaluate the outcome of this treatment or to begin offering suggestions about which patients are more likely to respond to this treatment. The procedure is performed either transrectally or transurethrally. Thermotherapy (heating to temperatures greater than 45°C) with simultaneous urethral cooling has been introduced and this procedure may or may not result in outcomes different from those with hyperthermia alone.

Prostate Stents and Coils

Stents and coils placed in the prostatic urethra have been used for the treatment of BPH. They can be temporary or permanent. Nordling et al[76] described an intraprostatic spiral that was inserted under abdominal ultrasonic scanning guidance in "medically unfit" patients. At 3-month follow-up, urinary obstruction was relieved in 41 out of 45 patients, 33 patients voided freely, and 28 of 41 had a satisfactory outcome. Nissenkorn described another temporary stent used as an alternative to an indwelling catheter in patients with urinary retention due to BPH.[75] The permanent stent is another alternative. Williams et al reported that 9 patients treated with this stent voided following the procedure, with peak flows between 10 and 22 ml/sec.[94]

Prostatic stents and coils generally are used in BPH patients with high operative risks and in those who refuse surgery. However, for patients with no evidence of urinary retention or contraindication for surgery, at this point it is difficult to define a precise role for this procedure in the treatment of BPH and to suggest which patients might fare better with this approach.

With this procedure as well, there is the potential for missing occult prostatic cancer. Performing a biopsy of the prostate prior to placing the stent is an option, but a negative finding is no guarantee that the patient does not have prostatic cancer. It is not known whether biopsy, TURP, or radical prostatectomy is significantly complicated by prior stent placement. It might be reasonable to monitor the prostate-specific antigen (PSA) level in patients with prostatic stents. Nothing, however, is reported about how these stents influence the level of PSA.

Little is reported about how these stents influence sexual function. Is antegrade ejaculation preserved? Would these considerations lead to avoidance of these devices in younger and/or sexually active men? At this time these questions cannot be answered.

Medical Treatment

Thus far, pharmacotherapy of patients with BPH has been directed toward relaxation of the prostate smooth muscle fibers and regression of the neoplastic tissue volume (stromal/epithelial). According to Caine, the tone of the prostatic smooth muscle and the physical presence of the hyperplastic tissue account for the dynamic and mechanical components of obstruction, respectively.[18]

The smooth muscle in the adenoma and capsule are rich in alpha-adrenergic receptors in the case of BPH. A variety of alpha-blockers exist, both selective and nonselective. Statistical improvement in urinary flow rates and symptom scores have been shown during therapy with alpha-adrenoreceptor blockade.[54] Until the results of large multicenter, randomized, placebo-controlled studies are published, no definitive conclusion on the role of alpha-adrenoreceptor blockade in the treatment of BPH can be drawn. For the present it is reasonable to offer alpha-blockers to men who have moderate symptoms of BPH and no strong absolute indication for prostatic surgery.[53]

Suppression of androgens can be achieved in a number of different ways, and the current approach is, in general, directed toward drugs that block the synthesis or action of DHT. Peak urinary flow rates improve by approximately 25 per cent, and the volume of the prostate decreases by approximately 30 per cent following androgen suppression.[53] Beneficial clinical and urodynamic effects following androgen suppression cannot match the efficacy of surgical procedures. In this case, a large, multicenter, randomized, placebo-controlled study has been completed. Results from the finasteride study have been reported.[89] No statistically significant regression in total symptom score was seen in patients receiving 1 mg of finasteride daily, whereas statistically significant regression in obstructive as well as irritative symptoms was seen in patients receiving 5 mg of finasteride.[89] At this time it is not possible to determine which patients would benefit from this therapy prior to initiating it. Another concern is selecting the best time for initiation of therapy and determining whether treatment should be administered prophylactically. If so, this poses the question of who should be selected to receive treatment.

Conclusions on Indications for Intervention

When evaluating the results in the treatment of BPH, one has to keep in mind that more than 30 per cent of men with untreated symptomatic BPH experience improvement in subjective symptoms and more than 20 per cent show improvement in objective criteria when followed over a 2.6- to 5-year period.[39]

Symptoms correlate poorly with more objective findings of urinary obstructions. Patients with mild symptoms and peak flows greater than 15 ml/sec seem to have poorer results postoperatively. Only patients with severe symptoms or acute urinary retention show significant improvement in quality of life postoperatively.

When a patient has elected intervention for BPH, the appropriate treatment for the particular patient has to be chosen. The overall physical condition and sexual function of the patient have to be considered as well as prostate size and morphology when making the determination of which treatment is best. Fowler et al[30] concluded that three factors are important when considering surgery for men with BPH: the significance of symptoms to the patient, the probability of positive and negative outcomes, and the significance of these outcomes in that particular patient.

Nonsurgical alternative treatments for BPH appear not to offer the same efficacy as the surgical procedures. The indications for alternative treatments are more weakly defined, partly because the results of multicenter, randomized, placebo-controlled studies are not available for some nonsurgical alternatives.

REFERENCES

1. Abrams PH: Use of the intravenous urogram in diagnosis. *In* Hinman F (ed): Benign Prostatic Hypertrophy. New York, Springer-Verlag, 1983, pp 605–609.
2. Abrams PH, Feneley RCL: The significance of the symptoms associated with bladder outflow obstruction. Urol Int 33:171–174, 1978.
3. Andersen JT, Jacobsen O, Worm-Petersen J, Hald T: Bladder function in healthy elderly males. Scand J Urol Nephrol 12:123–127, 1978.
4. Andersen JT, Nordling J: Prostatism: II. The correlation between cysto-urethroscopic, cystometric and urodynamic findings. Scand J Urol Nephrol 14:23–27, 1980.
5. Andersen JT, Nordling J, Walter S: Prostatism: I. The correlation between symptoms, cystometric and urodynamic findings. Scand J Urol Nephrol 13:229–236, 1979.
6. Ball AJ, Smith PJB: Urodynamic factors in relation to outcome of prostatectomy. Urology 28:256–258, 1986.
7. Barrack ER, Bujnovszky P, Walsh PC: Subcellular distribution of androgen receptors in human normal, benign hyperplastic, and malignant prostatic tissues: Characterization of nuclear salt-resistant receptors. Cancer Res 43:1107–1116, 1983.
8. Bartsch G, Frick J, Ruegg I, et al: Electron microscopic stereological analysis of the normal human prostate and of benign prostatic hyperplasia. J Urol 122:481–486, 1979.
9. Beck AD, Gaudin HJ: The measurement and significance of the urinary flow rate. Aust NZ J Surg 39:99–102, 1969.
10. Berry SJ, Coffey DS, Walsh PC, Ewing LL: The development of human benign prostatic hyperplasia with age. J Urol 132:474–479, 1984.
11. Birch NC, Hurst G, Doyle PT: Serial residual volumes in men with prostatic hypertrophy. Br J Urol 62:571–575, 1988.
12. Birkhoff JD: Natural history of benign prostatic hypertrophy. *In* Hinman F (ed): Benign Prostatic Hypertrophy. New York, Springer-Verlag, 1983, pp 5–9.
13. Birkhoff JD, Wiederhorn AR, Hamilton ML, Zinsser HH: Natural history of benign prostatic hypertrophy and acute urinary retention. Urology 7:48–52, 1976.
14. Breum L, Klarskov P, Munck LK, et al: Significance of acute urinary retention due to infravesical obstruction. Scand J Urol Nephrol 16:21–24, 1982.
15. Bruskewitz RC, Iversen P, Madsen PO: Value of postvoid residual urine determination in evaluation of prostatism. Urology 20:602–604, 1982.
16. Bruskewitz R, Jensen KM-E, Iversen P, Madsen PO: The relevance of minimum urethral resistance in prostatism. J Urol 129:769–771, 1983.
17. Cabot AT: The question of castration for enlarged prostate. Ann Surg 24:265–309, 1896.
18. Caine M: The present role of alpha-adrenergic blockers in the treatment of benign prostatic hypertrophy. J Urol 136:1–4, 1986.
19. Christensen MM, Aagaard J, Madsen PO: Transurethral resection versus transurethral incision of the prostate. A prospective randomized study. Urol Clin North Am 17:621–630, 1990.
20. Coffey DS, Berry SJ, Ewing LL: An overview of current concepts in the study of benign prostatic hyperplasia. *In* Rodgers CH, Coffey DS, Cunha G, et al (eds): Benign Prostatic Hyperplasia, Vol II. Bethesda, MD, 1985, pp 1–13.
21. Coffey DS, Walsh PC: Clinical and experimental studies of benign prostatic hyperplasia. Urol Clin North Am 17:461–475, 1990.
22. Coolsaet B, Blok C: Detrusor properties related to prostatism. Neurourol Urodynamics 5:435–447, 1986.
23. Craigen AA, Hickling JB, Saunders CRG, Carpenter RG: Natural history of prostatic obstruction. J R Coll Gen Practit 18:226–232, 1969.
24. Cucchi A: Detrusor instability and bladder outflow obstruction. Evidence for a correlation between the severity of obstruction and the presence of instability. Br J Urol 61:420–422, 1988.
25. Dowd JB, Smith JJ: Balloon dilatation of the prostate. Urol Clin North Am 17:671–677, 1990.
26. Drach GW, Layton TN, Binard WJ: Male peak urinary flow rate: Relationships to volume voided and age. J Urol 122:210–214, 1979.
27. Dørflinger T, Frimodt-Møller PC, Bruskewitz RC, et al: The significance of uninhibited detrusor contractions in prostatism. J Urol 133:819–821, 1985.
28. Dørflinger T, Øster M, Larsen JF, et al: Transurethral prostatectomy or incision of the prostate in the treatment of prostatism caused by small benign prostates. Scand J Urol Nephrol 104:77–81, 1987.
29. Dørflinger T, England DM, Madsen PO, Bruskewitz RC: Urodynamic and histological correlates of benign prostatic hyperplasia. J Urol 140:1487–1490, 1988.
30. Fowler FJ, Wennberg JE, Timothy RP, et al: Symptom status and quality of life following prostatectomy. JAMA 259:3018–3022, 1988.
31. Frimodt-Møller PC, Jensen KM-E, Iversen P, et al: Analysis of presenting symptoms in prostatism. J Urol 132:272–276, 1984.
32. Geller J: Overview of benign prostatic hypertrophy. Urology (Suppl) 34:57–63, 1989.
33. Gerstenberg TC, Andersen JT, Klarskov P, et al: High flow infravesical obstruction in men: Symptomatology, urodynamics and the results of surgery. J Urol 127:943–945, 1982.
34. Glynn RJ, Campion EW, Bouchard GR, Silbert JE: The development of benign prostatic hyperplasia among volunteers in the normative aging study. Am J Epidemiol 121:78–90, 1985.
35. Gold FM, Hotchkiss RS: Sexual potency following simple prostatectomy. NY State J Med 69:2987–2989, 1969.
36. Graversen PH, Gasser TC, Wasson JH, et al: Controversies about indications for transurethral resection of the prostate. J Urol 141:475–481, 1989.
37. Grossman RA: Oliguria and acute renal failure. Med Clin North Am 65:413–427, 1981.
38. Hald T: High-flow high-pressure obstruction. *In* Hinman F (ed): Benign Prostatic Hypertrophy. New York, Springer-Verlag, 1983, pp 550–552.
39. Isaacs JT: Importance of the natural history of benign prostatic hyperplasia in the evaluation of pharmacologic intervention. Prostate (Suppl) 3:1–7, 1990.
40. Isaacs JT, Coffey DS: Etiology and disease process of benign prostatic hyperplasia. Prostate (Suppl) 2:33–50, 1989.
41. Jensen KM-E: Clinical evaluation of routine urodynamic investigations in prostatism. Neurourol Urodynamics 8:545–578, 1989.
42. Jensen KM-E, Bruskewitz RC, Iversen P, Madsen PO: Predictive value of voiding pressures in benign prostatic hyperplasia. Neurourol Urodynamics 2:117–125, 1983.
43. Jensen KM-E, Bruskewitz RC, Iversen P, Madsen PO: Significance of prostatic weight in prostatism. Urol Int 38:173–178, 1983.
44. Jensen KM-E, Bruskewitz RC, Iversen P, Madsen PO: Abdominal straining in benign prostatic hyperplasia. J Urol 129:44–47, 1983.
45. Jones KW, Schoenberg HW: Comparison of the incidence of bladder hyperreflexia in patients with benign prostatic hypertrophy and age-matched female controls. J Urol 133:425–426, 1985.
46. Jørgensen JB, Jensen KM-E, Bille-Brahe NE, Mogensen P: Uroflowmetry in asymptomatic elderly males. Br J Urol 58:390–395, 1986.
47. Keane PF, Shah JR, O'Donoghue N, Wickham JEA: Resection, incision or balloon dilatation for benign hypertrophy? J Urol 141:254A, 1989.
48. Kiely EA, McCormack T, Cafferkey MT, et al: Study of appro-

priate antibiotic therapy in transurethral prostatectomy. Br J Urol 64:61–65, 1989.
49. Kulb TB, Kamer M, Lingeman JE, Foster RS: Prevention of post-prostatectomy vesical neck contracture by prophylactic vesical neck incision. J Urol 137:230–231, 1987.
50. Larsen EH, Dørflinger T, Gasser TC, et al: Transurethral incision versus transurethral resection of the prostate for the treatment of benign prostatic hypertrophy. A preliminary report. Scand J Urol Nephrol 104:83–86, 1987.
51. Lawson RK: Benign prostatic hyperplasia and growth factors. Urologe 29:5–7, 1990.
52. Lee LW, Malashock EM, Davis NB: Experience with transurethral prostatic resection and perineal prostatectomy in one clinic: A comparative review of 3400 patients. J Urol 80:147–150, 1958.
53. Lepor H: Medical management of benign prostatic hyperplasia. Infect Urol 3–4:52–56, 1991.
54. Lepor H, Knapp-Maloney G, Sunshine H: A dose titration study evaluating terazosin, a selective once-a-day α_1-blocker for the treatment of symptomatic benign prostatic hyperplasia. J Urol 144:1393–1398, 1990.
55. Lepor H, Rigaud G: The efficacy of transurethral resection of the prostate in men with moderate symptoms of prostatism. J Urol 143:533–537, 1990.
56. Lepor H, Sypherd D, Derus J, Machi G: A randomized double-blind study comparing the efficacy of cystoscopy vs. balloon dilatation of the prostate (BDP) in males with symptomatic benign prostatic hyperplasia (BPH). J Urol 145:362A, 1991.
57. Li MK, Ng ASM: Bladder neck resection and transurethral resection of the prostate: A randomized prospective trial. J Urol 138:807–809, 1987.
58. Lytton B, Emery JM, Harvard BM: The incidence of benign prostatic obstruction. J Urol 99:639–645, 1968.
59. Madsen PO, Iversen P: A point system for selecting operative candidates. *In* Hinman F (ed): Benign Prostatic Hypertrophy. New York, Springer-Verlag, 1983, pp 763–765.
60. Martin KW: A discourse on the indications for and the choice of operation. Ann R Coll Surg Engl 52:304–315, 1973.
61. McCullough DL, Herrera M, Harrison LH, Sorrell M: Transurethral balloon dilatation of the prostate (TUBDP)—Alternative to transurethral resection of the prostate. J Urol 141:254A, 1989.
62. McNeal JE: Normal histology of the prostate. Am J Surg Pathol 12:619–633, 1988.
63. McNeal JE: Origin and evolution of benign prostatic enlargement. Invest Urol 15:340–345, 1978.
64. McNeal J: Pathology of benign prostatic hyperplasia. Urol Clin North Am 17:477–493, 1990.
65. McNeal JE: The pathobiology of nodular hyperplasia. *In* Bostwick DG (ed): Pathology of the Prostate. New York, Churchill Livingstone, 1990, pp 31–36.
66. Meares EM, Stamey TA: Bacteriologic localization patterns in bacterial prostatitis and urethritis. Invest Urol 5:492–518, 1968.
67. Mebust WK: Surgical management of benign prostatic obstruction. Urology (Suppl) 32(6):12–15, 1988.
68. Mebust WK: Transurethral incision or resection of the prostate. J Urol 138:852, 1987.
69. Mebust WK, Holtgrewe HL, Cockett ATK, et al: Transurethral prostatectomy: Immediate and postoperative complications. A cooperative study of 13 participating institutions evaluating 3,885 patients. J Urol 141:243–247, 1989.
70. Melchior J, Valk WL, Foret JD, Mebust WK: Transurethral prostatectomy: Computerized analysis of 2,223 consecutive cases. J Urol 112:634–642, 1974.
71. Meyhoff HH, Hald T: Are doctors able to assess prostatic size? Scand J Urol Nephrol 12:219–221, 1978.
72. Meyhoff HH, Ingemann L, Nordling J, Hald T: Accuracy in preoperative estimation of prostatic size. Scand J Urol Nephrol 15:45–51, 1981.
73. Mukamel E, Nissenkorn I, Boner G, Servadio C: Occult progressive renal damage in the elderly male due to benign prostatic hypertrophy. J Am Geriatr Soc 27:403–406, 1979.
74. Nielsen HO: Transurethral prostatotomy versus transurethral prostatectomy in benign prostatic hypertrophy. A prospective randomised study. Br J Urol 61:435–438, 1988.
75. Nissenkorn I: Experience with a new self-retaining intraurethral catheter in patients with urinary retention: A preliminary report. J Urol 142:92–94, 1989.
76. Nordling J, Holm HH, Klarskov P, et al: The intraprostatic spiral: A new device for insertion with the patient under local anesthesia and with ultrasonic guidance with 3 months of followup. J Urol 142:756–758, 1989.
77. Orandi A: Transurethral resection versus transurethral incision of the prostate. Urol Clin North Am 17:601–612, 1990.
78. Pradhan BK, Chandra K: Morphogenesis of nodular hyperplasia-prostate. J Urol 113:210–213, 1975.
79. Roehrborn CG, McConnell JD: Is routine imaging of the urinary tract prior to prostatectomy a justifiable practice? J Urol 145:266A, 1991.
80. Roos NP, Ramsey EW: A population-based study of prostatectomy: Outcomes associated with differing surgical approaches. J Urol 137:1184–1188, 1987.
81. Rutkow IM: Urological operations in the United States: 1979 to 1984. J Urol 135:1206–1208, 1986.
82. Scott WW: What makes the prostate grow. J Urol 70:477–488, 1953.
83. Shah JR, Abrams PH, Feneley RC, Green NA: The influence of prostatic anatomy on the differing results of prostatectomy according to the surgical approach. Br J Urol 51:549–551, 1979.
84. Sikafi Z, Butler MR, Lane V, et al: Bladder neck contracture following prostatectomy. Br J Urol 57:308–310, 1985.
85. Siroky MB: Interpretation of urinary flow rates. Urol Clin North Am 17:537–542, 1990.
86. Speakman MJ, Brading AF, Gilpin CJ, et al: Bladder outflow obstruction—a cause of denervation supersensitivity. J Urol 138:1461–1466, 1987.
87. Speakman MJ, Sethia KK, Fellows GJ, Smith JC: A study of the pathogenesis, urodynamic assessment and outcome of detrusor instability associated with bladder outflow obstruction. Br J Urol 59:40–44, 1987.
88. Stephenson TP, Farrar DJ: Urodynamic study of 15 patients with postmicturition dribble. Urology 9:404–406, 1977.
89. Gormley GJ, Stoner E, Bruskewitz RC, et al: The effect of finasteride in men with benign prostatic hyperplasia. N Engl J Med 327:1185, 1992.
90. Walsh PC: Benign prostatic hyperplasia. *In* Walsh PC, Gittes RF, Perlmutter AD, Stamey TA (eds): Campbell's Urology, 5th ed. Philadelphia, WB Saunders Co, 1986, pp 1248–1265.
91. Wasserman NF, Reddy PK, Zhang G, Berg PA: Experimental treatment of benign prostatic hyperplasia with transurethral balloon dilation of the prostate: Preliminary study in 73 humans. Radiology 177:485–494, 1990.
92. Wennberg JE, Roos N, Sola L, et al: Use of claims data systems to evaluate health care outcomes. JAMA 257:933–936, 1987.
93. White JW: Effects of unilateral castration on the prostate. Ann Surg 21:492, 1895.
94. Williams G, Jager R, McLoughlin J, et al: Use of stents for treating obstruction of urinary outflow in patients unfit for surgery. Br Med J 298:1429, 1989.

EXPERIMENTAL STUDIES ON BLADDER OUTLET OBSTRUCTION

ROBERT M. LEVIN, PENELOPE A. LONGHURST, FREDERICK C. MONSON, NIELS HAUGAARD, and ALAN J. WEIN

Urinary bladder outlet obstruction is a common medical problem. More than 80 per cent of men 50 to 60 years of age and older have various degrees of bladder outlet obstruction secondary to benign prostatic hyperplasia (BPH).[19, 21, 66, 74] Although BPH is the most common cause of outlet obstruction, other causes include carcinoma, sclerosis or fibrosis of the bladder neck, urethral stricture disease, urethral valves, and smooth and striated sphincter dyssynergia.[73]

To understand the effects of outlet obstruction on bladder morphology, physiology, and pharmacology, several animal models of obstruction have been developed using a variety of species including rat, rabbit, guinea pig, and cat. Although there are marked differences in bladder size, capacity, compliance, physiology, and pharmacology among these species, responses to outlet obstruction have many common characteristics. This review is not intended to be a comprehensive treatise on the topic, but it attempts to provide a complete summary of the response of the urinary bladder to partial outlet obstruction. Although the data are taken primarily from the authors' experience using the rabbit model of obstruction, comparisons and contrasts with other species are discussed.

To analyze the effect of outlet obstruction on the bladder, one must have an understanding of normal bladder function and structure.[72–74] Pharmacologically, the bladder can be divided into two sections: bladder body and bladder base.[9, 38] Both the response to autonomic agonists (Fig. 10–1) and the distribution of autonomic receptors (Fig. 10–2) follow this division. Muscarinic receptor density (and the contractile response to

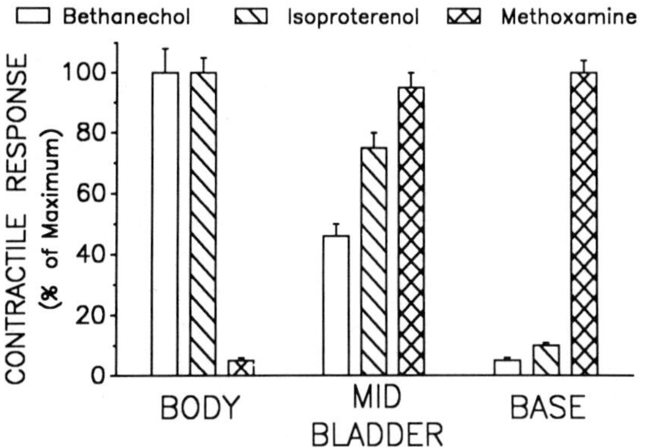

FIGURE 10–1. Response of sequential strips of rabbit urinary bladder to autonomic agonists. Each rabbit was anesthetized with pentobarbital (50 mg/kg) and the urinary bladder removed. The bladder was divided horizontally into the following regions: upper body, lower body, mid-bladder (at the level of the ureteral orifices), upper base, and lower base. Longitudinal strips were obtained from each section and mounted in an isolated water bath containing 30 ml of Tyrode's solution. Each bar represents the mean ± SEM for six to eight individual preparations.

cholinergic stimulation) is greatest in the bladder body and lowest in the bladder base. Similarly, beta-adrenergic receptor density and the response to beta-receptor stimulation (relaxation of bladder smooth muscle) is greatest in the bladder body and lowest in the bladder base; whereas alpha-adrenergic receptor density and the contractile response to alpha stimulation is greatest in the bladder base and lowest in the bladder body. Cho-

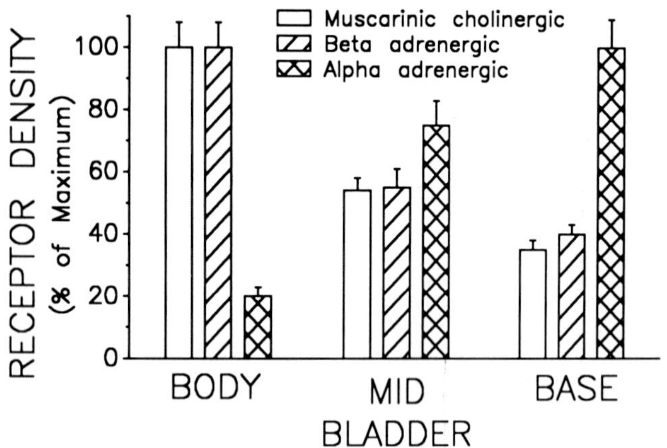

FIGURE 10–2. Autonomic receptor distribution. Each rabbit was anesthetized with pentobarbital (50 mg/kg) and the urinary bladder removed. The bladder was divided horizontally into the following regions: bladder body, mid-bladder (at the level of the ureteral orifices), and bladder base. Each section was frozen and stored under liquid nitrogen and subsequently assayed for muscarinic cholinergic, alpha-adrenergic, and beta-adrenergic receptors by standard radiolig- and binding techniques. Each bar represents the mean ± SEM for six to eight individual preparations.

linergic innervation is dense in both the bladder body and base, whereas adrenergic innervation is dense in the bladder base and sparse in the bladder body (at least in experimental animals).[9, 38]

The two basic functions of the lower urinary tract in mammals are the storage and active expulsion of urine. During bladder filling at physiologic rates, the amount of urine stored increases gradually to relatively large volumes at low intravesical pressures. This phenomenon is related to the passive viscoelastic properties of the bladder. During the filling phase of micturition, sympathetic nerve activity to the bladder increases gradually. Sympathetic activity inhibits excitatory pelvic ganglionic neurotransmission, activates alpha receptors in the bladder base and urethra to cause contraction, and activates beta receptors in the bladder body, resulting in relaxation. As intravesical pressure increases, there is also a gradual increase in somatic reflex stimulation of the external sphincter, which also aids bladder storage.[72–74]

As intravesical pressure increases, sensory nerves are activated and the micturition reflex is induced. The efferent limb of this reflex is the parasympathetic fibers of the sacral pelvic nerves. The organizational center for the micturition reflex is in the brain stem, with both ascending and descending spinal pathways leading to and from this center. Voluntary control of the micturition reflex involves both facilitory and inhibitory centers in higher brain areas.[72–74]

Micturition is accomplished by the coordinated inhibition of the reflexes activated by somatic innervation of the external sphincter, inhibition of the sympathetic nervous system, and activation of the cholinergic inner-

vation of the bladder. There is a graded contractile response to cholinergic (muscarinic) stimulation, with the most superior aspect of the bladder body or dome responding with the strongest contraction and the bladder base and urethra responding with the weakest contraction. The graded contractile response first induces reshaping of the bladder, which includes "funneling" of the relaxed bladder outlet, and then a strong, coordinated contraction of the bladder body causes virtually complete emptying of the bladder. In studies of bladder function in animals, atropine inhibits only a portion of the contractile response to pelvic nerve stimulation (in vivo) or field stimulation (in vitro). Although several putative neurotransmitters have been suggested as mediators of the nonadrenergic, noncholinergic transmission, the most likely candidate is the purinergic neurotranmitter ATP.[3, 6, 37] Although purinergic stimulation has been clearly demonstrated to exist and participate in the micturition response in the rat, rabbit, and cat, conflicting evidence exists as to whether it is functionally significant in pig and human bladders.[5, 59]

The contractile response of the bladder can be divided into two phases: (1) an initial rapid increase in intravesical pressure which shapes the bladder and is associated with the opening of the urethra; and (2) a prolonged period of sustained pressure (plateau phase) during which the bladder is emptied. Figure 10–3 displays the biphasic response of the rabbit whole-bladder preparation to field stimulation.[36, 37] These two phases can be differentiated using both pharmacologic and metabolic indicators, and an understanding of them is important in the study of specific bladder dysfunctions related to ischemia, overdistention, and outlet obstruction.[29, 39, 43] Studies in the experimental animal have demonstrated that purinergic transmission participates only in the initial phasic response to parasympathetic neuronal stim-

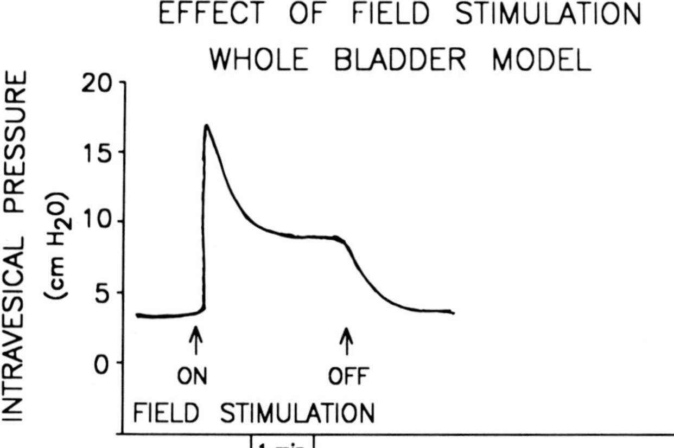

FIGURE 10–3. Biphasic response of the isolated in vitro whole bladder to field stimulation. Each rabbit was anesthetized with pentobarbital (50 mg/kg) and the urinary bladder removed. The bladder was mounted as a whole-organ preparation in an isolated water bath containing 300 ml of Tyrode's solution. This preparation was monitored for both the ability to generate an increase in intravesical pressure and the ability to empty. This figure presents a representative tracing of the effect of field stimulation (80 V, 1 msec, 32 Hz) on intravesical pressure.

MAXIMAL RESPONSE TO VARIOUS AGENTS

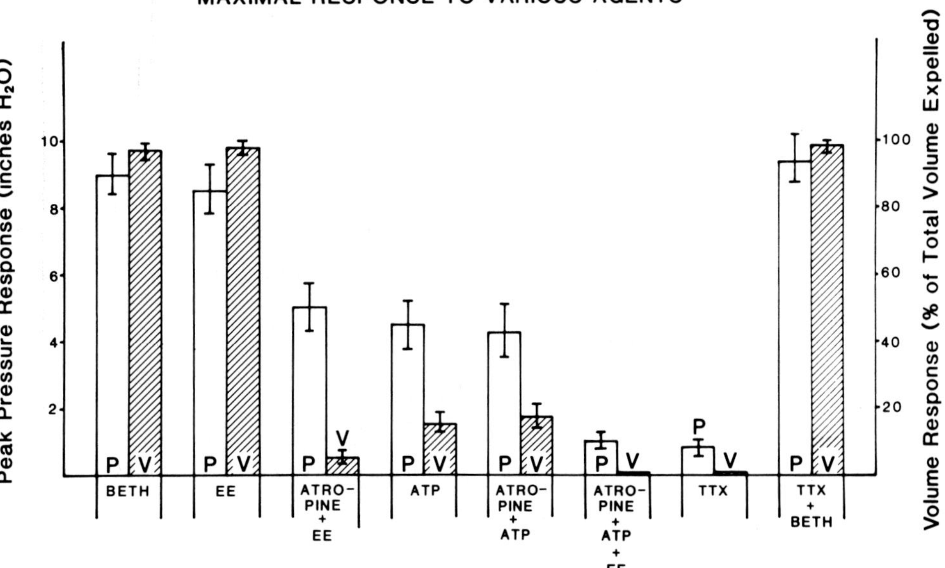

FIGURE 10–4. Pharmacologic response of the isolated whole bladder. Each rabbit was anesthetized with pentobarbital (50 mg/kg) and the urinary bladder removed. The bladder was mounted as a whole-organ preparation in an isolated water bath containing 300 ml of Tyrode's solution. This preparation was monitored for both the ability to generate an increase in intravesical pressure and the ability to empty. Each bar is the mean ± SEM of six to eight individual preparations. BETH = Bethanechol (500 uM); EE = field stimulation (80 V, 1 msec, 32 Hz); TTX = tetrodotoxin.

ulation (in vivo) or field stimulation (in vitro).[37] Figure 10–4 displays several characteristics of bladder pressure generation and emptying. Under normal conditions, bethanechol (muscarinic stimulation) and field stimulation (release of excitatory transmitters) are equally effective at both stimulating an increase in intravesical pressure and emptying the in vitro whole bladder. Although atropine completely inhibits both responses to bethanechol, it inhibits the pressure response to field stimulation by only 50 per cent but emptying by more than 90 per cent. ATP, on the other hand, stimulates only 50 per cent of maximum pressure generation and only 17 per cent of emptying. Preincubation with ATP (desensitization) and atropine inhibits both the pressure and emptying responses to field stimulation (to the same extent as tetrodotoxin).

It is not clear whether relaxation of the urethra during bladder contraction is a purely passive process (mediated by inhibition of alpha-adrenergic–mediated tone) or an active process (mediated by participation of nitric oxide).[8, 32]

Figure 10–5 displays the response of the cat isolated whole-urethra preparation[32] to field stimulation following methoxamine administration. Methoxamine stimulates a sustained increase in intraurethral pressure of more than 20 cm H_2O. Field stimulation (2 to 32 Hz) causes a substantial decrease in intraurethral pressure. There was no significant difference in the magnitude of the response to 2, 4, 8, 16, or 32 Hz. This is similar to the response of rabbit urethral strips described by Dokita et al.[8] If relaxation proves to be a major factor in opening the urethra during bladder emptying, then relative outlet obstruction might be mediated by a decreased function of this inhibitory system.

Experimental studies on outlet obstruction have been performed on a variety of species, including rats,[48, 64, 71] rabbits,[2, 14, 25, 43, 49] guinea pigs,[54] cats,[34] dogs,[55] and pigs.[60] Each species has advantages and disadvantages, and it is unclear which, if any, is most like man. Outlet obstruction is generally produced by the surgical placement of a ligature,[43, 48, 64, 71] cuff,[14, 25, 34] or ring[54, 60] around the urethra. The animal is then allowed to recover and the response to obstruction is studied at various times following surgery.

One of the most striking features of the response of the bladder to experimentally induced outlet obstruction is the speed and magnitude with which the bladder is able to increase its mass (tissue hypertrophy). Figure 10–6 displays the increase in bladder mass in rabbits subjected to severe bladder obstruction.[43] Within 1

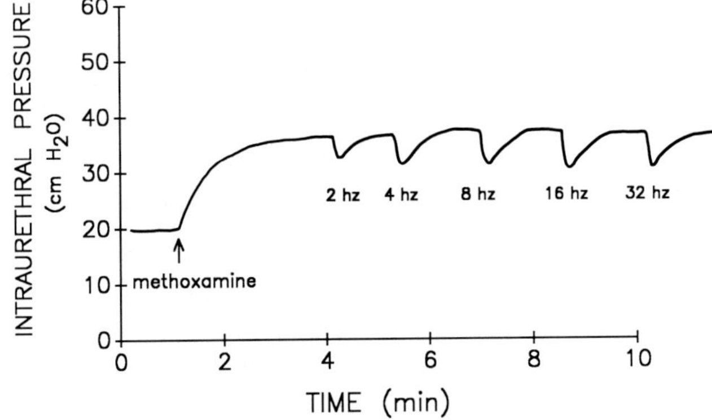

FIGURE 10–5. Effect of field stimulation on the isolated whole cat urethra following methoxamine stimulation. Each cat was anesthetized with pentobarbital (50 mg/kg) and the urethra removed. The urethra was mounted as a whole-organ preparation in an isolated water bath containing 300 ml of Tyrode's solution. Saline was pushed through the urethra using a Harvard syringe pump set at a constant flow rate of 1 ml/min. The minimum pressure required to begin flow through the cat urethra was 20 cm H_2O. Intraurethral pressure was monitored continually.

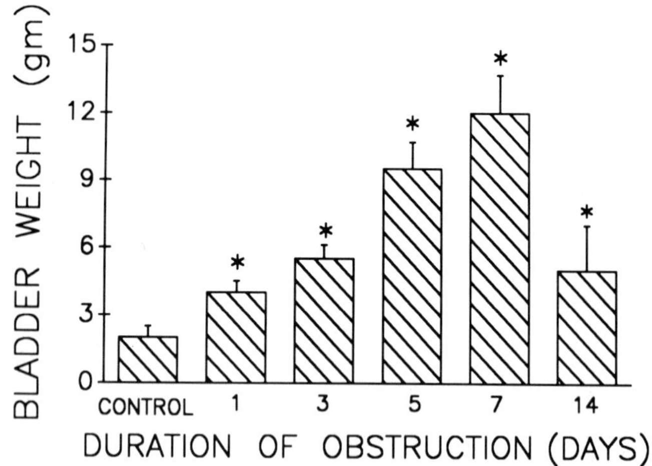

FIGURE 10–6. Effect of outlet obstruction on bladder weight. Each rabbit was anesthetized with pentobarbital (50 mg/kg) and the bladder exposed through a midline incision. The bladder was catheterized with a 10 Fr Foley and a 0 silk ligature was placed snugly around the urethra. The incision was closed and the rabbit allowed to recover for various periods of time. Each bar is the mean ± SEM of six to eight individual preparations.

week, the mass of the rabbit bladder can increase from 1.7 grams to 11 grams. In similar studies in rats, the bladder mass can increase from 56.6 mg (control) to 138 mg after 3 days, 201 mg after 10 days, and 727 mg after 6 weeks.[70] It appears that when the urethra is partially ligated, an initial response of the bladder may be acute overdistention, which signals the rapid and substantial increase in bladder mass. In mild models of outlet obstruction which utilize a "cuff" or ring placed around the urethra, the degree of tissue hypertrophy, or increase in tissue mass, is significantly less than that described in the more severe model, which uses a ligature.[14, 25, 34, 54] Figure 10–7 displays the increase in tissue mass in a mild model of obstruction in rabbits. In this model, there is no initial period of overdistention. Using a jeweler's "jump" ring to create an outlet obstruction in guinea pigs, Mostwin and Brooks reported a modest threefold increase in bladder mass over an 8-week period.[54]

From the point of view of the anatomist, the changes in mass appear to be caused in large part by deposits of collagenous connective tissue,[32, 49, 51, 70, 71] and/or by hypertrophy[2, 15, 17, 18, 48, 49, 60, 70] or hyperplasia[15, 71] in the smooth muscle. Studies of dysfunction generally consider inframuscular changes, which involve increased separation of smooth muscle cells by accumulated collagenous and basement membrane material[2, 12, 49] and neuromuscular[12, 17] and neurosensory changes.[15]

Most of these studies agree that outlet obstruction leads to an increase in bladder mass (bladder hypertrophy), which occurs primarily in the detrusor.[2, 15, 18, 49, 71] Another view is that the increase in bladder mass is a result of significant deposits of connective tissue laid down on the bladder wall. A recently described elastic lamina, which is a normal constituent of the serosa,[51] permits differentiation of this extrinsic layer of connective tissue, because it is deposited between this readily stainable anatomic structure and the mesothelium that lines the peritoneum. According to this latter concept, significant amounts of additional bladder mass are contributed by the serosa, where it is part of the pathologically stimulated bladder wall. Further, Monson et al

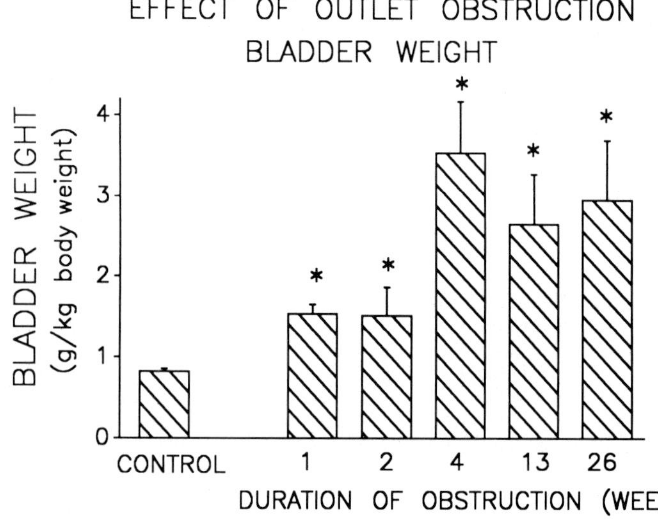

FIGURE 10–7. Effect of mild obstruction on bladder weight. Each rabbit was anesthetized with pentobarbital (50 mg/kg) and the bladder exposed through a midline incision. The bladder was catheterized with a 10 Fr Foley and a latex cuff was placed loosely around the urethra and ligated closed with a 2-0 suture. The incision was closed and the rabbit allowed to recover for various periods of time. Each bar is the mean ± SEM of six to eight individual preparations.

note that this phenomenon appears to be restricted to the part of the serosa associated with the injured bladder and is not observed in (or on) adjacent organs that are also covered by serosa.[51]

Figure 10–8 illustrates the location of this elastic lamina at 1 day after mild obstruction (Fig. 10–8 *A*) and 1 month later (Fig. 10–8*B*). It is apparent that the extrinsic layer of dense fibrous connective tissue becomes a substantial part of the bladder wall even after mild obstruction.[23, 25] The elastic lamina survives as a recognizable (although fragmented) histologic entity until 6 months after obstruction.[23]

In the rabbit and other small laboratory animals, the serosa covers most of the body of the bladder (in contrast to primates) and thus is responsible for a significant contribution to a fibrous response. Also, given the new evidence concerning the plasticity of neural elements in obstructed rat bladders[63] and the apparent independence of at least extramural connective tissue accumulations and contractile dysfunction,[23] there is justification for the suggestion that the functional effects of obstruction are not necessarily all related to structural changes in either muscle or connective tissue.

Elbadawi et al[13] have recently suggested a hypothesis that proposes a sequence of overlapping pathophysiologic structural events following experimental outlet obstruction: (1) the immediate ischemic phase (the first 24 + hours); (2) an adaptive phase (from 3 to 7 days); and (3) a recovery phase (characterized by bladder function recovery at 14 days after obstruction). This model attempts to explain the cyclic degenerative and regenerative structural changes that are observed in the smooth muscle cells of the detrusor. In a recent report,

surgically induced in vivo unilateral ischemia of the bladder of the rabbit demonstrated both the degenerative effects of ischemia on the histology and contractility of the bladder smooth muscle and the surprising regenerative ability of the bladder contractile apparatus.[16]

Elbadawi's theory suggests that the bladder adapts to obstructive damage by an unknown repair mechanism. Steers et al[63] provide evidence of an enriched afferent neural tree in the obstructed bladder. In the short- and long-term obstructed rabbit, Monson et al[51] and Kato et al[23] suggest a consistent functional recovery even though the primary connective tissue deposits, both intrinsic (bladder wall) and extrinsic (serosal), persist for at least 6 months without any substantial change. The ability of the bladder to empty appears to lag far behind the ability of the detrusor to contract in these recovery phenomena.[23]

As described above, ischemia may be an important etiologic factor in the initial response of the bladder to severe outlet obstruction. In a recent light microscopic study of short-term ischemia of the rabbit bladder, morphologic studies 1, 2, and 4 weeks after unilateral ischemia, smooth muscle bundles clearly demonstrate not only the destructive (and degenerative) effects of ischemia but also the regenerative capacity of smooth muscle after collateral circulatory paths are established on the ischemic side of the bladder.[16] Kato et al[23] have reported the functional and structural effects of long-term mild obstruction and have concluded that the mild form of obstruction differs from the severe type by its lack of an initial acute overdistention.

Two terms that have been used for more than a decade in discussions of bladder enlargement are *hypertrophy* and *hyperplasia*. Elbadawi and Meyer[11] have set forth the relevant issues and the parameters of a protocol[50] for morphometry of the detrusor. They note the traditional myth that detrusor hypertrophy is a manifestation of functional compensation and that smooth muscle hyperplasia requires more evidence for proof than has yet been forthcoming. These papers are recommended to the reader who is interested in the quantitative aspects of histologic investigations of bladder pathology, because they cannot be dealt with in any depth here. As a means of emphasizing the potential problems to be faced by those who use the terms *hypertrophy* and *hyperplasia,* we offer a suggestion for the sake of consistency and clarity.

Hypertrophy of a cell requires clear, unequivocal evidence that the volume of the cell has increased. Conclusions that hypertrophy has occurred have generally been based on the assumption that the smooth muscle cell is a uniaxial, bipolar, fusiform cell that is interdigitated in a parallel array with other such cells in fascicles and bundles. Unfortunately, the bladder has no true longitudinal (or circular) layers of smooth muscle that are amenable to this type of morphometric analysis.

Hyperplasia of a cell population requires clear, unequivocal evidence that (1) the cell has entered mitosis with replicated DNA (labeled with some observable marker such as tritium), (2) the cell has divided its DNA between two daughter cells, or (3) the absolute number

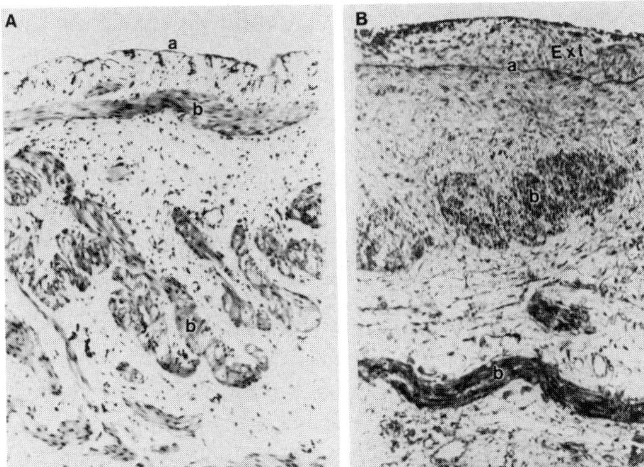

FIGURE 10–8. Effect of obstruction on the serosal lamina of the bladder. Twenty-four hour *(A)* and 1-month *(B)* mild partial outlet obstruction (with Silastic collars) of rabbit urinary bladders. Note the displacement of the elastic lamina of the serosa (a—the dark line on the serosal surface in *A*) after extrinsic connective tissue (Ext in *B*) has been deposited external to the serosal lamina (a in *B*). With respect to the lamina, 24-hour obstructed and normal bladders may be considered identical. Also compare muscle bundles (b in *A* and *B*). Smooth-muscle damage (cell profiles without discernible contents) is evident in both of these specimens. (100 ×, aldehyde fuchsin [elastin] and hematoxylin and eosin.)

of cells has increased. Strongly suggestive evidence of hyperplasia can include evidence that cellular synthesis of DNA increases significantly in a specific population of cells.

In a recent study by Monson et al,[52, 53] evidence is presented that outlet obstruction in rabbits induces a marked activation of the connective tissue elements within the bladder as measured by ^{3}H-thymidine uptake in newly synthesized DNA. At 1 day following obstruction, urothelial incorporation of ^{3}H-thymidine was increased approximately 70-fold with no change in the activity of cellular elements in either connective tissue or muscular compartments. At 3, 5, and 7 days following obstruction, urothelial activity decreased to control levels, whereas both intrinsic and extrinsic connective tissue elements increased substantially. At 14 days, the incorporation of ^{3}H-thymidine declined to near control levels. In general, the incorporation of ^{3}H-thymidine quantitatively matched the rate of increase in bladder mass, and the DNA-synthetic activity was limited to connective tissue elements.

In rats and rabbits, outlet obstruction induces a marked increase in urinary frequency and is associated with a significant decrease in the volume excreted per micturition[64] (urodynamic effects). Figure 10–9 displays representative micturition profiles from control and 1-week obstructed rabbits. The marked increase in frequency and decrease in micturition volume are very apparent (unpublished observation). In addition to changes in voiding frequency and volume, outlet obstruction induces marked increases in voiding pressure.[34, 53, 60] In a study using the isolated whole-bladder preparation from control nonobstructed rabbits, decreasing the outlet diameter by increasing outlet resistance resulted in a threefold increase in voiding pressure, a 60 per cent decrease in the rate of saline expulsion, and a fivefold increase in time required for complete empty-

ing.[35] This study on the effect of increasing the outlet resistance on the in vitro normal bladder is consistent with the alterations in urodynamics observed in the experimental studies.

One of the most controversial topics in the study of outlet obstruction is its effect on contraction and bladder contractile function. Studies on these aspects of bladder function use a variety of methodologies, including tissue strips,[10, 47, 55, 60] bladder rings,[14] in vitro whole-bladder preparations,[2, 43] and in vivo preparations.[48, 49] One of the major problems encountered when comparing contractile data published by different laboratories is that the units used to present data vary considerably. Contractile data from strips can be presented in actual measured units such as grams of tension developed or mNewtons, or it can be normalized to the mass of the isolated strips (i.e., grams of tension per 100 mg wet weight), normalized to the cross-sectional area of the strips (grams/mm^2), or normalized to the maximum response of potassium or itself (per cent of maximum). It is obvious when comparing the response of control versus obstructed strips that conclusions are directly related to the parameters (units) that one measures and the manner in which the data are presented. For example, Mattiasson et al[47] reported that no significant differences were found in the response of isolated strips of obstructed and nonobstructed rat bladders to carbachol when the data were presented as per cent of the response to high potassium, although the response to potassium was decreased by 35 per cent in the obstructed bladders. In the same study, the response of obstructed bladder strips to field stimulation was reduced by 43 per cent and the frequency response curve was shifted significantly to the right (compared with controls).[47] The data were presented directly as mNewtons. If the data had been normalized to either strip mass or cross-sectional area, a significantly greater decrease in the contractile response would have been found. In a study by Ekstrom et al,[10] no decreases in the contractile responses of strips isolated from obstructed rats were found (the data were presented as grams of tension per milligram of tissue). Significant decreases in the contractile responses to cholinergic stimulation and field stimulation have been reported, however, in other studies using rabbits, pigs, and minipigs.[14, 33, 60]

The in vitro whole-bladder preparation has the advantage that one is able to evaluate both the contractile response (as a rise in intravesical pressure) of the bladder as an intact organ and the ability of the bladder to empty. In a severe model of outlet obstruction, the ability of the bladder to empty is reduced to a substantially greater degree than its ability to generate pressure.[43] In addition, the response to field stimulation is reduced to a significantly greater degree than the response to bethanechol (Figs. 10–10 and 10–11), similar to the results described by Mattiasson et al[47] and Speakman et al.[60] The relationship between degree of tissue hypertrophy and contractile dysfunction is presented in Figures 10–12 and 10–13.[23] These data demonstrate that the degree of functional impairment is directly related to the degree of tissue hypertrophy present (and not

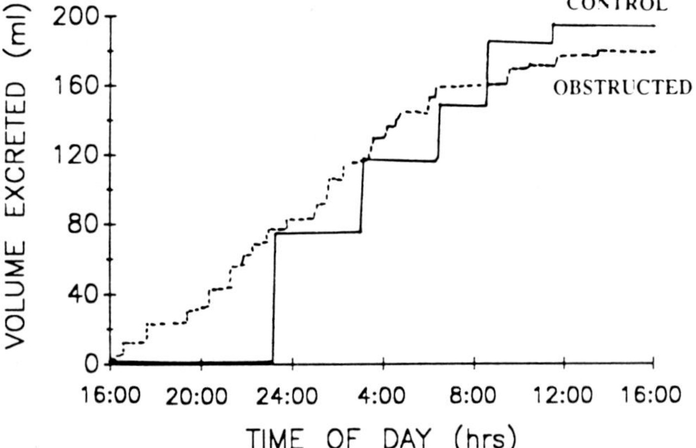

FIGURE 10–9. Micturition pattern for control and obstructed rabbits. Each rabbit was housed in a metabolic cage and the urine collected in a beaker mounted on an OHAUS balance. The weight of the balance was monitored at 5-minute intervals automatically and stored in an IBM-type computer. Thus, 24-hour micturition patterns were generated for each rabbit in the study. The figure presents representative tracings of 24-hour micturition patterns from both a control rabbit and a 7-day obstructed rabbit.

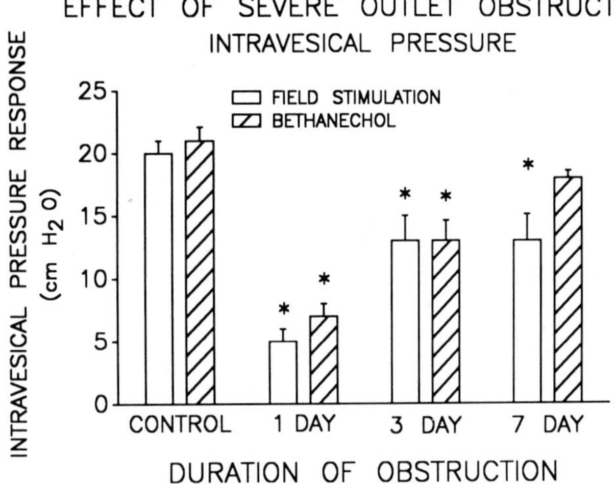

FIGURE 10–10. Effect of severe outlet obstruction on the response to bethanechol and field stimulation: Intravesical pressure. Each rabbit was anesthetized with pentobarbital (50 mg/kg) and the bladder exposed through a midline incision. The bladder was catheterized with a 10 Fr Foley and a 0 silk ligature was placed snugly around the urethra. The incision was closed and the rabbit allowed to recover for various periods of time. Each bar is the mean ± SEM of six to eight individual preparations. Asterisk (*) indicates significant difference from control ($P < 0.05$).

necessarily to duration of obstruction), which in turn is directly related to the degree of obstruction.

As presented above, the ability of the obstructed bladder to empty is reduced to a significantly greater degree than its ability to generate pressure (or generate tension in isolated strips). The ability to empty is directly related to the plateau phase of the contractile response

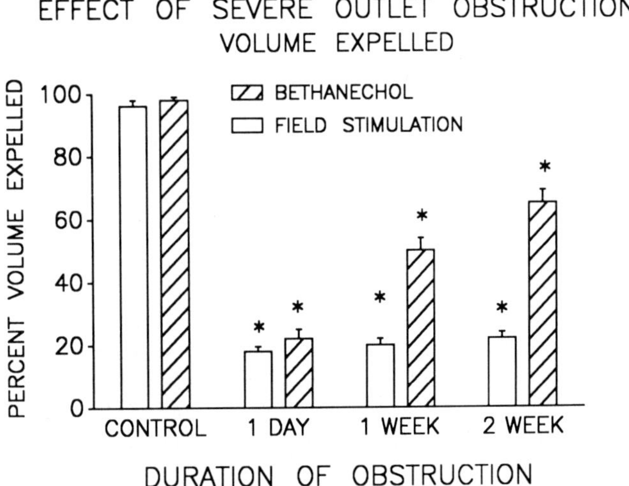

FIGURE 10–11. Effect of severe outlet obstruction on the response to bethanechol and field stimulation: Volume expelled. Each rabbit was anesthetized with pentobarbital (50 mg/kg) and the bladder exposed through a midline incision. The bladder was catheterized with a 10 Fr Foley and a 0 silk ligature was placed snugly around the urethra. The incision was closed and the rabbit allowed to recover for various periods of time. Each bar is the mean ± SEM of six to eight individual preparations. Asterisk (*) indicates significant difference from control ($P < 0.05$).

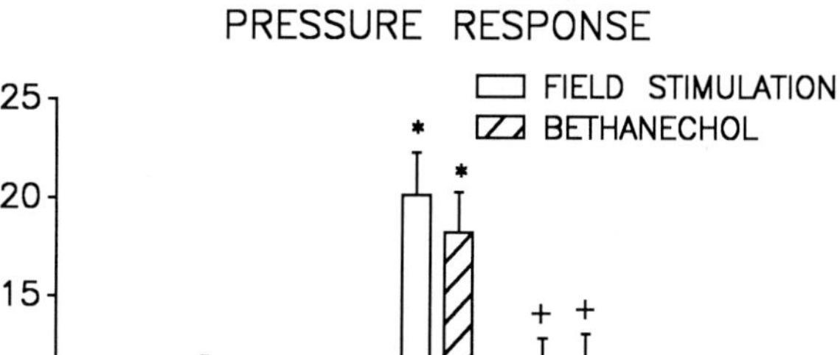

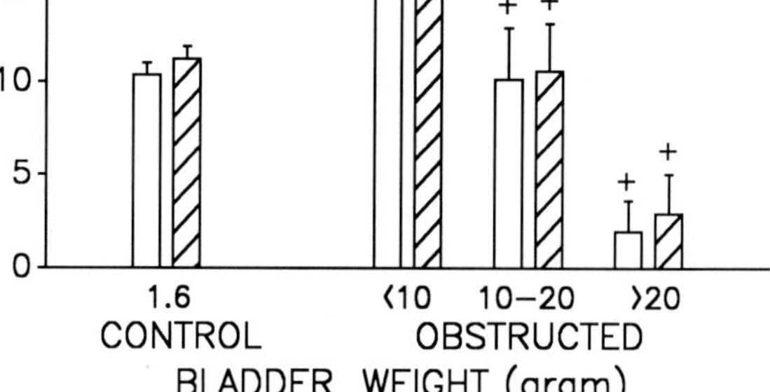

FIGURE 10–12. Chronic effect of mild outlet obstruction on the response to bethanechol and field stimulation: Intravesical pressure. Each rabbit was anesthetized with pentobarbital (50 mg/kg) and the bladder exposed through a midline incision. The bladder was catheterized with a 10 Fr Foley and a latex cuff was placed loosely around the urethra and ligated closed with a 2-0 suture. The incision was closed and the rabbit allowed to recover for various periods of time between 1 and 6 months. Data from all time periods were averaged based on the bladder mass rather than duration of obstruction. Each bar is the mean ± SEM of six to eight individual preparations. Asterisk (*) indicates significant difference from control ($P < 0.05$).

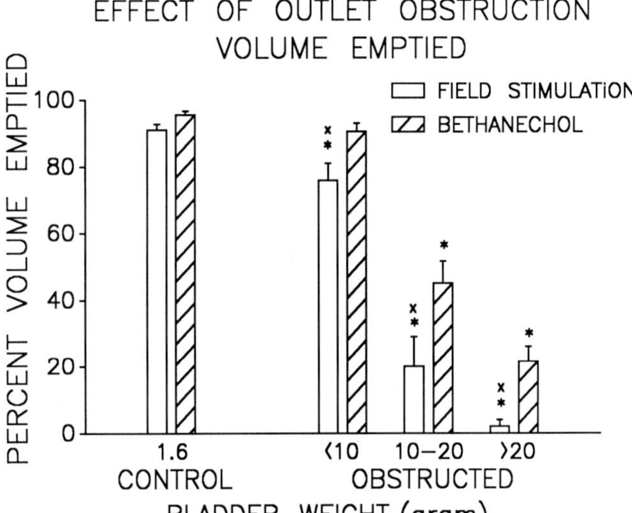

FIGURE 10–13. Chronic effect of mild outlet obstruction on the response to bethanechol and field stimulation: Volume emptied. Each rabbit was anesthetized with pentobarbital (50 mg/kg) and the bladder exposed through a midline incision. The bladder was catheterized with a 10 Fr Foley and a latex cuff was placed loosely around the urethra and ligated closed with a 2-0 suture. The incision was closed and the rabbit allowed to recover for various periods of time between 1 and 6 months. Data from all time periods were averaged based on the bladder mass rather than duration of obstruction. Each bar is the mean ± SEM of six to eight individual preparations. Asterisk (*) indicates significant difference from control; X indicates significant difference from the response to bethanechol ($P < 0.05$).

of the bladder, whereas the pressure response is related primarily to the initial phasic contractile response.[36] Energetically, the initial phasic response appears to be related directly to the intracellular concentration of ATP, whereas the ability to sustain a contraction and empty may be linked to active mitochondrial oxidative phosphorylation. In this regard, mild outlet obstruction results in a significant reduction in mitochondrial respiration (aerobic metabolism), whereas there is an increase in lactate generation (anaerobic metabolism).[24] Further support for the theory that the contractile dysfunction observed in obstruction may be related to decreased mitochondrial function comes from the recent demonstration that the activity of the mitochondrial enzymes malate dehydrogenase and citrate synthase are decreased by 50 per cent, whereas the activity of the cytosolic enzyme creatine kinase is not significantly altered.[20, 31]

Under normal conditions for the rat and rabbit bladder, the maximum contractile response to field stimulation (which acts primarily via the release of neurotransmitters) is approximately the same as the response to direct cholinergic stimulation.[25, 43, 47] Outlet obstruction reduces the response to field stimulation to a significantly greater degree than that to direct cholinergic stimulation.[25, 43, 47, 60] This is consistent with the morphologic demonstration that outlet obstruction induces a specific degeneration of neuronal elements or a partial denervation within the bladder smooth muscle.[12, 47, 60] The loss of functional synapses results in a decrease in the ability of field stimulation to release contractile neurotransmitters and thus reduce the magnitude of the contractile response.

Although considerable evidence exists that obstruction results in a "partial denervation" of the bladder, the development of "denervation supersensitivity" is controversial (see Steers et al[63] for evidence of "innervation supersensitivity").[61, 62] One theory of denervation supersensitivity suggests that receptor density is inversely related to the level of transmitter present. Thus, in conditions in which the level of transmitter is reduced (such as the loss of neuronal synapses), the receptor density increases, which then results in an increased response to exogenously applied agonist. Although some studies report the presence of denervation supersensitivity associated with obstruction,[10, 60] the data are presented normalized to 100 per cent of maximum responses and the ED_{50}s are compared. In addition, neither study correlates changes in response with receptor density, neuronal innervation, or changes in bladder mass. The ability to demonstrate the presence of denervation supersensitivity is significantly affected by the concurrent morphologic changes. Thus, although the denervation that accompanies outlet obstruction may result in increased receptor synthesis, the induced tissue hypertrophy would result in a decreased receptor density and a decreased contractile response.

Consistent with the indirect evidence of end-organ denervation described above is the direct demonstration by Steers et al[61, 62] of marked alterations in the afferent neuronal pathways in rats induced by outlet obstruction. In these nerve-tracing studies using the injection of wheat germ agglutinin–horseradish peroxidase (HRP) into the bladder wall, outlet obstruction was demonstrated to induce a significant hypertrophy of labeled L6 and S1 dorsal root cells, but the mean number of labeled dorsal root ganglion cells was not changed. Furthermore, there was a 60 per cent increase in the area of the labeled afferent terminal field in the intermediolateral region of the L6 to S1 spinal cord.

In addition to the effects on afferent nerve morphology, outlet obstruction induced a significant increase in the tissue level of nerve growth factor. This demonstration by Steers et al[61, 65] indicates that communication between the bladder and its neuronal connections is two way. That is, in addition to the ability of the bladder to respond to alterations in innervation, alterations in bladder function induced by outlet obstruction can influence the central connections to the bladder via local factors such as nerve growth factor.

In line with the above studies, Buttyan et al[4] recently demonstrated that outlet obstruction in rabbits induces rapid and substantial increases in the concentration of a variety of genetic products, including the messenger RNAs (mRNAs) encoding β-actin (a cytostructural element) and basic fibroblast growth factor (bFGF), and a decrease in the concentration of transforming growth factor-β (TGF-β). These changes are consistent in time and magnitude with the increase in bladder mass observed. The increased mRNA for bFGF and associated decrease in TGF-β was associated with an increase in tissue concentration in the bFGF (unpublished observation) and is also consistent with the time course of the increase in ^{3}H-thymidine incorporation in the connective tissue elements within the bladder described earlier.[52, 53]

From these studies, it appears that outlet obstruction initiates a series of (1) actions which begin with acute damage to the bladder (2) as a result of overdistention secondary to the obstruction; (3) this is followed by initial nerve terminal degeneration which initiates a series of gene activations resulting in the synthesis of a variety of local growth factors including nerve growth factor and bFGF, which in turn induces the observed increase in bladder mass and alterations in bladder structure.

Recent studies from several laboratories indicate that in part, the observed alterations in bladder function are directly related to alterations in specific contractile and cytoskeletal proteins.[27, 56, 69] In particular, intermediate-sized filaments (IF), one of the constituents of the cytoplasmic filament, play an important role in the maintenance of cell shape. Vimentin and desmin are proteins that form IFs in mesenchymally derived cells. The concentrations of these proteins are significantly increased in urinary bladder smooth muscle cells in response to obstruction-induced hypertrophy. Interestingly, the increases in total vimentin and desmin are associated with increased amounts of soluble vimentin and desmin. Because this is the fraction that is known to be newly synthesized, this finding indicates that the IFs are important to study in the acute stages of obstruction-induced uropathy.[29, 56, 69]

It is known that the smooth muscle myosin heavy chain exists in two isoforms, SM1 and SM2. Obstruction-induced hypertrophy of the urinary bladder is associated with an alteration of the isoforms of smooth muscle myosin heavy chain and actin isoforms.[29, 56, 69] A recent study carried out by Samuel et al[56] indicates that the ratio of SM1 to SM2 myosin heavy chain shifts from 1:3 to 1:1 following obstruction-induced hypertrophy of the urinary bladder. It is not known how soon after obstruction the shift in the isoforms begins to occur.

The effect of obstruction on tissue biochemistry and metabolism has been the subject of several studies.[25, 43, 70, 71] In both rabbit and rat bladders, RNA (reflecting active protein synthesis) increased significantly at 3 days of obstruction and remained elevated during the period of rapid bladder growth.[43, 71] Although collagen content (per bladder) increased following obstruction, collagen density (per milligram wet weight) significantly decreased in both rat and rabbit models.[43, 70] This is in contrast to histologic studies, which have shown markedly increased connective tissue infiltration in the bladder wall.[12, 14, 49, 51] One of the most striking features of the connective tissue response of the obstructed bladder is the generation of a thick connective tissue sheet extrinsic to the serosal elastin lamina (Fig. 10–7).[51] In metabolic studies, outlet obstruction causes a marked increase in anaerobic metabolism (lactic acid generation) and decreased aerobic metabolism (CO_2 generation).[24]

Clinically, one of the major urologic dysfunctions that often accompany outlet obstruction is the development of involuntary bladder contractions (IVC). IVC can be induced in several animal models of outlet obstruction, including the rat,[45, 46, 64] rabbit,[29] pig,[22, 58, 60] and cat models[26]; hyperreflexia is induced by outlet obstruction.

Under normal conditions, urodynamic evaluation of the rat, rabbit, and pig demonstrate that the bladder fills at low intravesical pressures (with no contractile activity) until a reflex voiding contraction is induced. In the presence of an outlet obstruction, cystometric evaluation demonstrates that spontaneous reflex (nonvoiding) contractions are induced at low intravesical volumes and increase in frequency as the bladder fills. The pig is perhaps the best model to study IVC. The pig can be fully evaluated cystoscopically and urodynamically, and IVCs were observed in 60 to 85 per cent of obstructed pigs.[22, 58] The IVCs were relieved in more than 80 per cent of the pigs following removal of the obstruction.

Similar observations were reported by Malgren in rats.[45, 46] Electrophysiologic studies on the obstructed rats by Steers and de Groat[64] demonstrated that although there were no significant changes in the supraspinal micturition reflex, there was a marked increase in the percentage of rats that showed a short latency spinal reflex. The presence of this spinal reflex could explain the increased presence of spontaneous activity in obstructed rats.

The experimentally produced IVCs have not been characterized pharmacologically to any great extent. In the rat, atropine inhibits the majority of the induced spontaneous activity, but not all, indicating that there are both cholinergic and noncholinergic (or myogenic) components to the hyperreflexia. In rabbits, IVC can be induced by acute distal ligation of the penis. Figure 10–14 displays the development of hyperreflexia upon slow saline infusion into the bladder (in vivo).[26, 29] This hyperreflexia can be completely inhibited by hexamethonium, indicating that the spontaneous contractions are of spinal or supraspinal origin. As in rats, atropine inhibited approximately 90 per cent of the spontaneous activity, indicating that there is a noncholinergic component involved in the spontaneous contractions. In addition, hyperreflexia could be eliminated by treatment of the urethral mucosa with lidocaine, which suggests that hyperreflexia may be initiated by stimulation of urethral efferent receptors.[29]

The cat (unlike the rat, rabbit, guinea pig, and pig) displays spontaneous activity during the normal filling limb of the cystometrogram. Even as an isolated whole-bladder preparation, significant spontaneous contractions are present, demonstrating that the normal cat bladder displays myogenic contractions. There is a marked increase in the myogenic contractions in the obstructed cat bladder (Fig. 10–15).[22, 34]

It is clear that although there are similarities among the various animal models of bladder outlet obstruction, there also are significant differences depending on the species of animal used and the method of producing the outlet obstruction. Although there is probably no single "best" model, the choice of one animal model over another depends on which aspects of outlet obstruction are being studied (e.g., bladder hypertrophy, involuntary bladder contractions, denervation supersensitivity).

Although one of the most important subjects for future investigation is the effect of obstruction on the sensory innervation of the bladder, there is virtually no information on this topic. The following is a brief summary of what is known.

Afferent axons innervating the urinary bladder and urethra are present in parasympathetic pelvic, sympa-

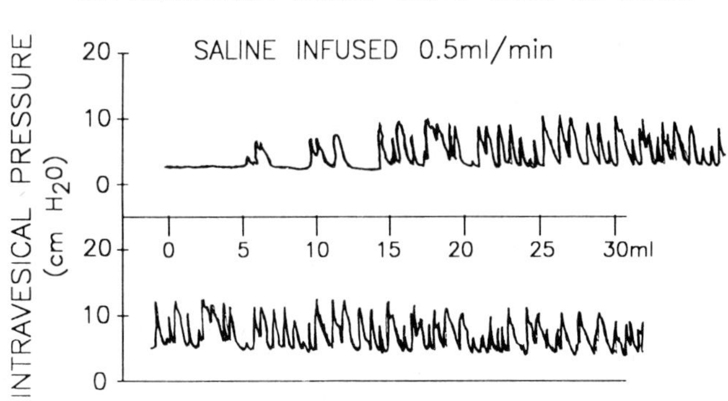

FIGURE 10–14. Effect of urethral ligation on intravesical pressure in the rabbit. Representative tracing of the effect of the development of hyperreflexia following external urethral ligation (under ketamine-xylazine anesthesia).

IN VITRO CYSTOMETRY

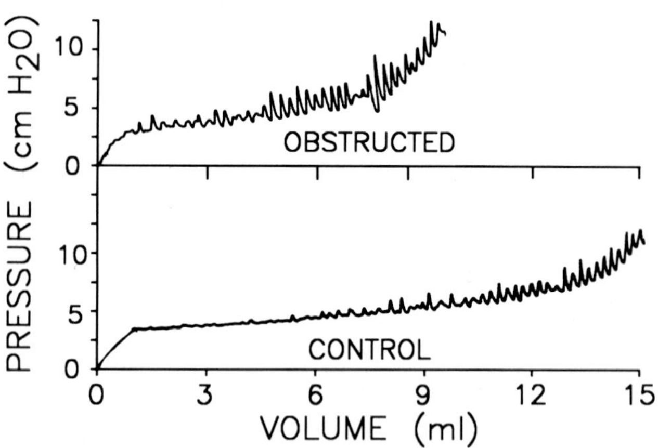

FIGURE 10–15. Effect of obstruction on in vitro cystometry in the cat. Each cat was anesthetized with pentobarbital (50 mg/kg) and the urinary bladder removed. The bladder was mounted as a whole-organ preparation in an isolated water bath containing 300 ml of Tyrode's solution. This preparation was monitored for both the ability to generate an increase in intravesical pressure and the ability to empty. This figure presents a representative tracing of the in vitro cystometrogram of a control and an obstructed cat. Two points should be noted: First, the normal cat bladder displays spontaneous activity that increases as the volume increases. The obstructed bladder displays a greater level of spontaneous activity, both in amplitude of individual spikes and in the frequency of spontaneous contractions.

thetic hypogastric, and somatic pudendal nerves. Small myelinated A δ and unmyelinated C fiber afferents pass through the pelvic nerves to the sacral spinal cord, carrying neuronal impulses from bladder wall tension receptors. The A δ fibers respond to intravesical pressure changes and to noxious stimuli. C fiber afferents, in contrast, do not usually respond to intravesical pressure changes but do respond to mucosal irritation by chemicals.[7]

The chemical capsaicin stimulates transmitter release from sensory nerve endings. Following depletion, desensitization occurs and the neurons can no longer be excited by capsaicin or many other stimuli that activate sensory nerves.[40, 42] A number of different neuropeptides are stored in capsaicin-sensitive afferent nerves. These include substance P, neurokinin A, and calcitonin gene-related peptide. Following capsaicin desensitization, substance P and calcitonin gene-related peptide immunoreactivity are reduced in the rat bladder.[41, 57, 67] In addition, capsaicin pretreatment causes urine retention and increases bladder capacity and mass,[30, 57, 67] effects that mimic those caused by outlet obstruction.

Although the changes seen in bladder function following capsaicin pretreatment are similar to those following outlet obstruction, little is known of the effects of outlet obstruction on sensory nerve function. Andersson et al examined the content and effects of substance P in female rats following 6 weeks of infravesical obstruction.[1] The concentration of substance P was significantly reduced in obstructed bladders compared with controls.

However, because of the increase in mass associated with obstruction, the total content of substance P was significantly greater. There were regional differences in the substance P localization—the lower part of the bladder contained significantly more than the upper portion. Bladder strips from obstructed rats were significantly less sensitive to the contractile effects of substance P than were strips from control rats. Further studies from the same laboratory examined the effects of capsaicin treatment on the development of changes in bladder function associated with obstruction in the rat.[44] Capsaicin treatment, either before or after application of the obstruction, had no effect on the increases in bladder mass. Rats pretreated with capsaicin before obstruction had an increased frequency of micturition compared with obstructed controls. However, there was no obvious micturition contraction, and the volumes excreted were smaller. During cystometry, the micturition volumes and pressures were significantly reduced compared with obstructed controls. Capsaicin treatment had no effect on the development of involuntary bladder contractions. The results, therefore, indicate that intact substance P innervation is not required for the changes in bladder function associated with outlet obstruction and that changes in capsaicin-sensitive sensory nerves are not responsible for the involuntary bladder contractions that accompany cystometry in rats with outlet obstruction.

REFERENCES

1. Andersson PO, Andersson K-E, Fahrenkrug J, et al: Contents and effects of substance P and vasoactive intestinal peptide in the bladder of rats with and without infravesical outlet obstruction. J Urol 140:168–172, 1988.
2. Brent L, Stephens FD: The response of smooth muscle cells in the rabbit urinary bladder to outflow obstruction. Invest Urol 12:494–502, 1975.
3. Burnstock G: Past and current evidence for the purinergic nerve hypothesis. *In* Baer HP, Drummond GI (eds): Physiological and Regulatory Functions of Adenine Nucleotides. New York, Raven, 1979.
4. Buttyan R, Jacobs B, Potter L, Levin RM: Alterations in the genetic activity of the rabbit bladder demonstrates the onset of a tissue remodeling process initiated by partial urethral obstruction. J Urol 145:387A, 1991.
5. Cowan WD, Daniel EE: Human female bladder and its noncholinergic contractile function. Can J Physiol Pharmacol 61:1236–1246, 1983.
6. Dean DM, Downie JW: Contribution of adrenergic and "purinergic" neurotransmission to contraction in rabbit detrusor. J Pharmacol Exp Ther 207:431–445, 1978.
7. de Groat WC: Central neural control of the lower urinary tract. Ciba Foundation Symposium 121 (Neurobiology of Incontinence):27–56, 1990.
8. Dokita S, Morgan M, Wheeler M, et al: N^g nitro-L-arginine inhibits non-adrenergic non-cholinergic (NANC) relaxation in rabbit urethral smooth muscle. FASEB J 5:A1593, 1991.
9. Downie JW, Dean DM, Carro-Ciampi G, Awad SA: A difference in sensitivity to alpha-adrenergic agonists exhibited by detrusor and bladder neck of the rabbit. Can J Physiol Pharmacol 53:525–530, 1975.
10. Ekstrom J, Malmberg L, Wallin A: Transient supersensitivity in the hypertrophied rat urinary bladder. Acta Physiol Scand 126:365–370, 1986.

11. Elbadawi A, Meyer S: Morphometry of the obstructed detrusor: I. Review of the issues. Neurourol Urodynamics 8:163–171, 1989.
12. Elbadawi A, Meyer S, Malkowicz SB, et al: Effects of short-term partial bladder outlet obstruction on the rabbit detrusor: An ultrastructural study. Neurourol Urodynamics 8:89–116, 1989.
13. Elbadawi A, Meyer S, Regnier CH: Role of ischemia in structural changes in the rabbit detrusor following partial bladder outlet obstruction: A working hypothesis and a biomechanical/structural model proposal. Neurourol Urodynamics 8:151–162, 1989.
14. Ghoniem GM, Regnier CH, Biancani P, et al: Effect of vesical outlet obstruction on detrusor contractility and passive properties in rabbits. J Urol 135:1284–1289, 1986.
15. Ghoniem GM, Regnier CH, Susset JG: The importance of the degree of outlet obstruction in detrusor response. Proceedings, 14th Annual Meeting, International Continence Society, Innsbruck, 1984, pp 211–212.
16. Gill HS, Monson FC, Wein AJ, et al: The effects of short-term *in vivo* ischemia on the contractile function of the rabbit urinary bladder. J Urol 139:1350–1354, 1988.
17. Gosling JA, Gilpin SA, Dixon JS, Gilpin CJ: Decrease in the autonomic innervation of human detrusor muscle in outflow obstruction. J Urol 136:501–503, 1986.
18. Goss RJ, Liang MD, Weisholtz SJ, Peltzer TJ: The physiological basis of urinary bladder hypertrophy. Proc Soc Exper Biol Med 142:1332–1335, 1973.
19. Grayhack JT, Kozlowski JM: Benign prostatic hyperplasia. *In* Gillenwater JY, Grayhack JT, Howards SS, Duckett JW (eds): Adult and Pediatric Urology. Chicago: Year Book Medical Publishers, 1987, pp 1062–1126.
20. Haugaard N, Potter LS, Wein AJ, et al: Effect of partial obstruction of the rabbit urinary bladder on malate dehydrogenase and citrate synthase activity. J Urol 147:1391–1393, 1992.
21. Hinman F Jr (ed): Benign Prostatic Hypertrophy. New York, Springer-Verlag, 1983.
22. Jorgensen TM, Djurhuus JC, Jorgensen HS, Sorensen SS: Experimental bladder hyperreflexia in pigs. Urol Res 11:239, 1983.
23. Kato K, Monson FC, Longhurst PA, et al: The functional effects of long-term outlet obstruction on the rabbit urinary bladder. J Urol 143:600–606, 1990.
24. Kato K, Tong-Long Lin A, Haugaard N, et al: Effects of outlet obstruction on glucose metabolism of the rabbit urinary bladder. J Urol 143:844–847, 1990.
25. Kato K, Wein AJ, Kitada S, et al: The functional effect of mild outlet obstruction on the rabbit urinary bladder. J Urol 140:880–884, 1988.
26. Kato K, Wein AJ, Radzinski C, et al: Short term functional effects of bladder outlet obstruction in the cat. J Urol 143:1020–1025, 1990.
27. Kim Y, Samuel M, Levine RM, Chacko S: Alterations of proteins associated with cytoplasmic filaments in obstructed urinary bladder. In press.
28. Kitada S, Kato K, Wein AJ, Levin RM: Experimental models of reflex contractile activity in the rabbit bladder. Neurourol Urodynamics 8:255–262, 1989.
29. Kitada S, Wein AJ, Kato K, Levin RM: Effect of acute complete obstruction on the rabbit urinary bladder. J Urol 141:166–169, 1989.
30. Kudlacz EM, Gerald MC, Wallace LJ: Sensory nerves and urinary bladder function: Effects of diabetes, capsaicin and acrylamide treatment. Gen Pharmacol 20:31–34, 1989.
31. Levin RM, Haugaard N, Levin SS, Wein AJ: Creatine kinase activity in normal and hypertrophied bladder tissue. Mol Cell Biochem 106:143–149, 1991.
32. Levin RM, Hayes L, Eika B, et al: Comparative autonomic response of the cat and rabbit bladder and urethra. J Urol 143:848–852, 1990.
33. Levin RM, High J, Wein AJ: The effect of short-term obstruction on urinary bladder function in the rabbit. J Urol 132:789–791, 1984.
34. Levin R, Kato K, Ruggieri MR, et al: The physiological effect of outlet obstruction in the cat. J Urol 141:335A, 1989.
35. Levin RM, Memberg W, Ruggieri MR, Wein AJ: Functional effects of in-vitro obstruction on the rabbit urinary bladder. J Urol 135:847–851, 1986.
36. Levin RM, Ruggieri MR, Gill HS, et al: Studies on the biphasic nature of urinary bladder contraction and function. Neurourol Urodynamics 6:339–350, 1987.
37. Levin RM, Ruggieri MR, Wein AJ: Functional effects of the purinergic innervation of the rabbit urinary bladder. J Pharmacol Exp Ther 236:452–457, 1986.
38. Levin RM, Shofer F, Wein AJ: Cholinergic, adrenergic, and purinergic response of sequential strips of rabbit urinary bladder. J Pharmacol Exp Ther 212:536–540, 1980.
39. Lin T-L A, Wein AJ, Gill HS, Levin RM: Functional effect of chronic ischemia on the rabbit urinary bladder. Neurourol Urodynamics 7:1–12, 1988.
40. Maggi CA: The role of peptides in the regulation of the micturition reflex: An update. Gen Pharmacol 22:1–24, 1991.
41. Maggi CA, Guiliani S, Santicioli P, et al: Species-related variations in the effects of capsaicin on urinary bladder functions: Relation to bladder content of substance P-like immunoreactivity. NS Arch Pharmacol 336:546–555, 1987.
42. Maggi CA, Meli A: The role of neuropeptides in the regulation of the micturition reflex. J Auton Pharmacol 6:133–162, 1986.
43. Malkowicz SB, Wein AJ, Elbadawi A, et al: Acute biochemical and functional alterations in the partially obstructed rabbit urinary bladder. J Urol 136:1324–1329, 1986.
44. Malmgren A, Andersson PO: The effect of sensory impairment on bladder function in rats with outflow obstruction. Neurourol Urodynamics 9:429–430, 1990.
45. Malmgren A, Sjogren C, Andersson K-E, Andersson PO: Effects of atropine on bladder capacity and instability in rats with bladder hypertrophy. Neurourol Urodynamics 6:331–338, 1987.
46. Malmgren A, Sjogren C, Uvelius B, et al: Cystometrical evaluation of bladder instability in rats with infravesical outflow obstruction. J Urol 137:1291–1294, 1987.
47. Mattiasson A, Ekstrom J, Larsson B, Uvelius B: Changes in the nervous control of the rat urinary bladder induced by outflow obstruction. Neurourol Urodynamics 6:37–45, 1987.
48. Mattiasson A, Uvelius B: Changes in contractile properties in hypertrophic rat urinary bladder. J Urol 128:1340–1342, 1982.
49. Mayo ME, Hinman F: Structure and function of the rabbit bladder altered by chronic obstruction or cystitis. Invest Urol 14:6–9, 1976.
50. Meyer S, Elbadawi A: Morphometry of the obstructed detrusor: II. Principles of a comprehensive protocol. Neurourol Urodynamics 8:173–191, 1989.
51. Monson FC, Goldschmidt MH, Zderic SA, et al: Use of a previously undescribed elastic lamina of the serosa to characterize connective tissue hypertrophy of the rabbit bladder wall following partial outlet obstruction. Neurourol Urodynamics 7:385–396, 1988.
52. Monson FC, McKenna BAW, Wein AJ, Levin RM: Effect of outlet obstruction on ^{3}H-thymidine uptake and metabolism: A radiographic and biochemical study. J Urol 148:158–162, 1992.
53. Monson FC, Wein AJ, McKenna BAW, Levin RM: Preliminary investigation on rabbit urinary bladder hypertrophy using ^{3}H-thymidine and radioautography. Neurourol Urodynamics 9:426–427, 1990.
54. Mostwin JL, Brooks L: A new guinea pig model of urethral obstruction. J Urol 141:335A, 1989.
55. Rohner TJ Jr, Hannigan JD, Sanford EJ: Altered in vitro adrenergic responses of dog detrusor muscle after chronic bladder outlet obstruction. Urology 11:357–361, 1978.
56. Samuel M, Kim Y, Horiuchi KY, et al: Smooth muscle isoform distribution and myosin ATPase in hypertrophied urinary bladder. Biochem Int 26:545–552, 1992.
57. Sharkey KA, Williams RG, Schultzberg M, Dockray GJ: Sensory substance P-innervation of the urinary bladder. Possible site of action of capsaicin in causing urine retention in rats. Neuroscience 10:861–868, 1983.
58. Sibley GNA: An experimental model of detrusor instability in the obstructed pig. Br J Urol 57:292–296, 1985.
59. Sjogren C, Andersson K-E, Husted S, et al: Atropine resistance of transmurally stimulated isolated human bladder muscle. J Urol 128:1368–1371, 1982.

60. Speakman MJ, Brading AF, Gilpin CJ, et al: Bladder outflow obstruction. A cause of denervation supersensitivity. J Urol 138:1461–1466, 1987.
61. Steers WD: Neuroplasticity secondary to infravesical obstruction Neurourol Urodynamics 9:559–561, 1990.
62. Steers WD, Ciambotti J, Erdman S, de Groat WC: Morphological plasticity in efferent pathways to the urinary bladder of the rat following urethral obstruction. J Neurosci 10:1943–1951, 1990.
63. Steers WD, Ciambotti JA, Etzel B, et al: Morphological changes in afferent and efferent neural pathways to the urinary bladder following urethral obstruction in the rat. J Urol 141:323A, 1989.
64. Steers WD, de Groat WC: Effect of bladder outlet obstruction on micturition reflex pathways in the rat. J Urol 140:864–871, 1988.
65. Steers WD, Tuttle J, Creedon D: Hyperplastic and activity-related changes in nerve growth factor in the urinary bladder. J Urol 143:367A, 1990.
66. Sterling AM, Ritter RC, Zinner NR: The physical basis of obstructive uropathy. *In* Hinman F Jr (ed): Benign Prostatic Hypertrophy. New York, Springer-Verlag, 1983, pp 433–442.
67. Su HC, Wharton J, Polak JM, et al: Calcitonin gene-related peptide immunoreactivity in afferent neurons supplying the urinary tract: Combined retrograde tracing and immunohisto-chemistry. Neuroscience 18:727–747, 1986.
68. Tuttle JB, Steers WB, Kolbeck S, Creedon DJ: NGF causes obstruction-induced neural plasticity. J Urol 145:388A, 1991.
69. Uvelius B, Arner A, Malmgren A: Contractile and cytoskeletal proteins in detrusor muscle from obstructed rat and human bladder. Neurol Urodynamics 8:396, 1989.
70. Uvelius B, Mattiasson A: Collagen content in the rat urinary bladder subjected to infravesical outflow obstruction. J Urol 132:587–590, 1984.
71. Uvelius B, Persson L, Mattiasson A: Smooth muscle cell hypertrophy and hyperplasia in the rat detrusor after short-time infravesical outflow obstruction. J Urol 131:173–176, 1984.
72. Wein AJ, Barrett DM: Voiding function and dysfunction. A logical and practical approach. Chicago, Year Book Medical Publishers, 1988.
73. Wein AJ, Levin RM, Barrett DM: Voiding function: Relevant anatomy, physiology, and pharmacology. *In* Gillenwater JY, Grayhack JT, Howards SS, Duckett JD (eds): Adult and Pediatric Urology. Chicago, Year Book Medical Publishers, 1987.
74. Yalla SV, McGuire EJ, Elbadawi A, Blaivas JG (eds): Neurourology and Urodynamics. New York, Macmillan Publishing Co, 1988.

ACKNOWLEDGMENT: Supported in part by grants from the Veterans Administration, NIH Grants RO-1 DK-26508, RO-1 DK 33559, RO-1 DK-39086, and P50-DK-39257.

Chapter 11

THE DIAGNOSIS OF OBSTRUCTIVE UROPATHY

EDWARD J. McGUIRE and WILLIAM D. BELVILLE

NEUROGENIC OBSTRUCTIVE UROPATHY

The simplest example of obstructive uropathy is encountered clinically in patients with areflexic detrusor dysfunction, such as that associated with myelodysplasia or peripheral neuropathy. The detrusor muscle is decentralized, and as it fills it gains pressure. This is unlike a normal bladder, which "accommodates" volume with very little pressure change. Normally the urethral sphincter opens or closes only in response to bladder activity, which is either storage (closed) or micturition (open). These processes are mediated by a very complex neural system, the effect of which is lost when the bladder becomes decentralized. This results in a fixed sphincteric resistance relative to bladder activity. The bladder becomes "obstructed" by the resting function of its sphincter. A 12-year longitudinal study of some 350 myelodysplastic children with decentralized bladder dysfunction at the University of Michigan led to the following observations and conclusions.

The interaction of the bladder with the components of the urethral sphincter, including the bladder neck and smooth and skeletal sphincter, is a relationship determined by the maximum closing pressure of the urethra, a relatively fixed value. Filling the bladder by a suprapubic catheter or a small nonretention urethral catheter finally results in sufficient intravesical pressure to cause leakage. The pressure required to do that determines whether the complications we have traditionally associated with "obstruction" of the bladder by the urethra will occur. These are changes in bladder morphology, including trabeculation, cellule and diverticular formation, symptomatic infection, vesicoureteral reflux, ureteral dilation and loss of function, and finally renal damage and infectious stone formation. These processes are related to elevated bladder pressures during the storage phase of bladder activity, which are in turn directly related to the closing pressure of the outlet. Thus a bladder pressure greater than 40 cm H_2O at the time of leakage has a deleterious effect on compliance, which is proportional to the magnitude of the outlet resistance and the time of the interaction between the bladder and urethra. Compliance improves or does not deteriorate if the outlet resistance is lowered or the bladder is emptied often enough by intermittent catheterization. The degree of damage to compliance is related to the pressure at which the interaction of detrusor and outlet occur and how long that process goes on once the critical interactive pressure of 40 cm H_2O is reached.

The urodynamic diagnosis of obstruction in this circumstance is easy: only the precise determination of the bladder pressure required to drive urine across the sphincter. In order to prove that this is an expression of decentralization, a measure of urethral sphincteric activity (preferably derived from videourodynamics and simultaneous urethral pressure) should be used.

In spinal cord–injured patients, we use identical urodynamic methods involving filling the bladder to determine storage ability, and measurement of the pressure required to drive urine across the reflexly contracting sphincter associated with suprasacral lesions or across the fixed sphincter associated with sacral or infrasacral lesions. As part of a study protocol, we treat reflex vesical activity by immediate institution of anticholinergic agents, and all patients are maintained from the beginning of the study on intermittent catheterization. The overall intent is to maintain intravesical pressures well below 20 cm H_2O. In a mean follow-up period of 60 months, we did not encounter any case of high-pressure, uncontrollable, repetitive detrusor sphincter dyssynergia, a condition that typically develops in patients with spinal cord injury within 1 year of injury. When we elected to use condom catheter drainage in lieu of intermittent catheterization, we did a sphincterotomy sufficient to reduce bladder leak point pressure to a normal range (less than 30 cm H_2O). The overall results in the latter group were identical to those in patients treated by intermittent catheterization. There were no upper tract changes if bladder pressures remained low. These findings in two large groups of patients with neurogenic vesical dysfunction now numbering 475, none of whom have developed upper tract changes in a period of observation which averages 7 years, suggest that the deleterious effects of neurogenic obstructive uropathy are determined by bladder pressure. This large clinical experience allows the inference that the repetitive interaction of bladder and fixed or reflexly elevated sphincteric resistance ultimately exerts an effect on the upper urinary tract by inducing an abnormality of compliance and that there are two methods of treatment: reduction of outlet resistance or prevention of detrusor contractile activity.

ANATOMIC OBSTRUCTIVE UROPATHY

Although prostatic obstruction is the most common cause of obstructive uropathy other than neurogenic causes, other causes include urethral strictures, posterior urethral values, and in women, rarely, some kind of urethral dysfunction usually associated with fibrosis or, more commonly, obstructive uropathy resulting from a prior stress incontinence operation. Because symptoms of bladder instability and irritability, including urge incontinence, frequency, nocturia, and not infrequently a "slow stream," are common before and after stress incontinence operations, the accurate diagnosis of obstructive uropathy is often predicated on some kind of urodynamic testing. Generally this testing includes the determination of residual urine volumes and a cystometrogram demonstrating reflex, high-pressure bladder contractility. These studies do not by themselves establish the diagnosis of obstructive uropathy, which requires evidence of a high-pressure reflex bladder contraction and simultaneous complete relaxation of the external sphincter, and/or a diminished flow rate, or videourodynamic evidence of a significant pressure drop, at midflow across the sphincter-active segment of the urethra superior to the high-pressure zone, which must be relaxed. Despite the common occurrence of uncomfortable bladder symptoms in women, a clear urodynamic diagnosis of obstructive uropathy is rarely made.

PROSTATIC HYPERTROPHY AND OBSTRUCTIVE UROPATHY

The diagnosis of obstructive uropathy is not the same as that of prostatic hypertrophy. It is possible to find patients with very large prostates who do not suffer from obstructive uropathy and others with small or even normal prostates who clearly are obstructed.[3, 10] No one has prospectively evaluated large numbers of patients to determine the relationship between prostatic size, "obstructive" symptoms, and urodynamic findings over long periods of time. At present we are involved in a small longitudinal study of prostatic symptoms, size, and response to treatment. Here we have found too much variability over time in the determination of prostatic volume by ultrasonography, and if ultrasound techniques are unreliable, then rectal examinations are at least as unreliable (Table 11–1).

"Prostatic" symptoms include hesitancy, frequency, urgency, urge incontinence, slowing of the urinary stream, nocturia, interruption of the urinary stream, a feeling of incomplete emptying, dribbling urination, and postvoiding urinary leakage. No symptom, except perhaps in specific circumstances urinary retention, can be exclusively associated with "obstructive uropathy."[13] Even urinary retention is not an absolutely reliable symptom of both prostatic hypertrophy and obstruction, because retention can be related to bladder dysfunction as well as outlet obstruction. Despite difficulty in ascribing obstruction exclusively to prostatic growth in a male patient population, the two processes are often apparently related.[4]

There are two reasons why treatment is undertaken for benign prostatic enlargement: The symptoms are bothersome, and there is a theoretical risk of upper and lower urinary tract damage. We have not yet succeeded in determining by an easily applicable clinical method which patient is obstructed, and which patient, if obstructed, is at risk for the development of urinary retention, upper tract deterioration, renal failure, and/or damage to the bladder, making it dysfunctional and vulnerable to infection or stone formation. It is apparent that we cannot do this simply by determining prostatic size.

Since the Lytton study in the 1960s, which determined the incidence of prostatism requiring surgery in a known patient population served by three hospitals, the American male population has been treated by prostatectomy at an increasing rate.[17, 22] Although the population today is older than that studied by Lytton, and available evidence suggests that microscopic and macroscopic benign prostatic hyperplasia (BPH) are age related, there is no evidence that links morbidity of obstructive uropathy with size of the gland or with age.[5] Clark, for instance, found that subjective, symptomatic improve-

TABLE 11–1. PROSTATIC VOLUME BY ULTRASONOGRAPHY (ANDROGEN INHIBITOR STUDY)*

	N	MEAN INCREASE (%)
Decrease	0	NA
Same	3	NA
Increase 10–20%	12	12
Increase 21–280%	8	97

*N = 23; interval = 6 months.

ment occurred in 25 of 36 patients with a presumed diagnosis of obstructive uropathy due to BPH when followed, and that this improvement lasted a mean 1.9 years.[11] In patients with "severe" prostatism, improvement occurred in 9 of 15 individuals, and this also lasted more than 1 year. Birkhoff et al, in a prospective study, used symptom scores, flow rates, bladder residual volume, renal function, and a determination of prostatic size to monitor the natural history of a group of patients with "prostatism." They found that 8 of 26 subjectively improved at 3 years and 4 of 26 objectively improved.[6] The results of a similar study by Bell and co-workers suggests that at 5 years after a very complete urologic evaluation for "prostatism," only 20 per cent of those thought on the basis of their initial evaluation to be clearly obstructed had undergone surgery. Of the entire symptomatic group, only 10 per cent actually came to surgery.[4]

Patients who did undergo surgery showed a deterioration in urinary flow rates. However, the deterioration was not greater than that demonstrated to occur in both men and women with increasing age and was identical to the rate and magnitude of the decline in peak flow rate recorded by workers at the University of Arizona in "normal" males (those without obstructive prostatism) with aging.[15] These outcome studies, in contrast to the pathologic data demonstrating an increase in the incidence and extent of BPH which occurs in parallel with age, do not show a relationship between age and obstructive uropathy and, by inference, prostate size and obstruction.

That is also true for animal studies in that while we can make the prostate of certain animals grow, the animals do not as a result of that growth suffer from obstructive uropathy.[12] Looking at the available data one could legitimately ask if we have been able to certainly identify in any of the studies of the "natural history" of BPH those patients who actually had the disease *obstructive uropathy* (versus prostatic hypertrophy) and those who did not.

Into this rather confusing situation enters the federal government, concerned about the dollars paid for transurethral resections of the prostate, and the National Institutes of Health, concerned with eliminating renal disease. Recent studies on the outcome of transurethral resection of the prostate (TURP) suggest that this is not as good a procedure as originally thought, and that perhaps a suprapubic prostatectomy is a better operation.[31] Because TURPs are expensive and should be regarded as part of the morbidity associated with BPH, industry and urologists have introduced medical therapy, balloon dilation, hyperthermia, and prostatic stents to avoid TURP. To evaluate any one of these treatment options as well as TURP, or even open surgery, some measure of the effect of the prostate on bladder storage and voiding dynamics is required. It is now reasonably clear that in obstructive BPH, myelodysplasia, and other neurogenic conditions, sustained increases in intravesical pressure induce changes in vesical compliance and that this adverse change is the underlying mechanism whereby upper urinary tract deterioration occurs.[28, 38] This change can result from residual urine volumes,

which put the bladder at the limit of its viscoelastic distensibility, or the repetitive interaction of a contracting bladder and a poorly opening outlet.

This process in BPH, or experimental conditions in animals designed to mimic BPH, takes a long time to develop compared with neurogenic conditions, but clinical studies of patients with upper tract damage related to BPH nevertheless demonstrate that there is always an associated abnormality of vesical compliance.[30] If then we want to measure the risk of a given case of BPH on the upper urinary tract, we could measure bladder compliance and determine the residual urine on several occasions. We could then estimate the mean intravesical pressure during the cycle of bladder activity involving filling and detrusor expulsive activity. We know that sustained bladder pressures above 40 cm H_2O are dangerous, but we know nothing about the effects of more moderate intravesical pressure elevations sustained in conjunction with residual urine accumulation and elevated voiding pressures over long periods of time.

Although traditionally urologists have used radiographic imaging to determine if upper tract abnormalities exist, several studies show these radiographs not to be very cost effective in patients selected for prostatectomy by symptoms.[1] In contrast, however, when sudden retention prompts decompression of the bladder and subsequent operation for prostatism, the incidence of upper tract disease is relatively high, but such patients typically deny prodromal symptoms prior to the onset of severe difficulty with acute urinary retention.[23, 28] Assessment of a potential risk to upper urinary tract function could probably be done by a cystometrogram and a careful determination of bladder compliance, but the evidence of common experience suggests that this would not be useful in patients with "prostatic" symptoms and not easily applicable to those without symptoms, even though the latter large group would presumably contain those few individuals with a potential problem.

If measurement of compliance is not practical even if specific and sensitive, what about measuring intravesical voiding pressure as an index of the degree of prostatic obstruction? Clearly intravesical pressure is related to outlet resistance, both at the time of voiding and with respect to compliance during intravesical urine storage, and this measurement should be a reasonable index of the degree of bladder outlet obstruction.

The few studies of "voiding" pressure that have been done are not definitive. Problems with voiding pressure relate to the relationship between that variable and the bladder outlet, which includes the preprostatic urethra, the prostatic urethra, and the distal, volitional sphincter. As shown by Griffiths and Schaefer, once micturition begins bladder pressure reflects outlet resistance and not the character, strength, or vigor of bladder muscular activity.[18, 32] Therefore, intravesical pressure reflects the amount of outlet resistance offered to the bladder as it tries to push out the urinary stream. We know from pressure flow and voiding urethral pressure profile studies that the normal male bladder faces enough resistance in the optimally open bladder neck and prostatic and

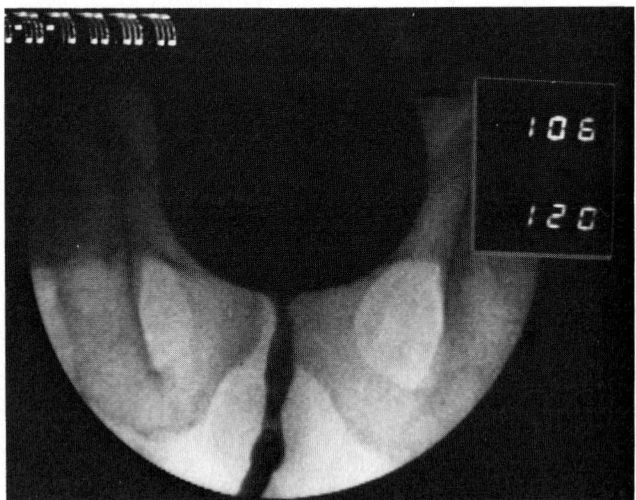

FIGURE 11–1. Midvoiding cystourethrogram from a 22-year-old man with a bulbous urethral stricture related to a straddle injury. The upper pressure (106) is urethral, measured in the proximal bulbous urethra (the marker is just visible), and the lower pressure (120) is measured in the bladder. Allowing 6 cm for height differences in this upright patient between the urethral sensor and that in the bladder, there is 8 cm H_2O stream energy loss across the sphincter-active urethra. The high voiding pressure must be related to a more distal obstruction.

ing of the preprostatic and prostatic urethra, voiding pressures in males above 30 cm H_2O reflect some degree of abnormal outlet resistance.

If we measure a "voiding pressure" of 124 cm H_2O, we know that there is increased outlet resistance, but we are unable to determine by that measurement alone the site or the cause of the increased resistance (Fig. 11–1). It could be that the preprostatic urethra does not open or that the prostatic urethra, compressed and distorted by prostatic hypertrophy, which is in turn held in place by a dense contractile capsule, could be the site of obstruction; but it also might mean only that the patient continued to contract his external sphincter mechanism during the micturition cycle (Fig. 11–2). Without some other data we cannot tell which of these occurred. Because most voiding pressures are recorded with transurethral catheters, it is not difficult to imagine that external sphincter relaxation might be less than perfect. Simple measurement of voiding pressure, then, does not provide a reliable method to diagnose obstructive uropathy associated with prostatic enlargement. If the voiding pressure at the time urine is flowing is normal or less than 30 cm H_2O, then obstructive uropathy is not present, but elevated pressure is not equivalent to obstructive uropathy due to BPH.

distal urethra to require an intravesical pressure of about 20 to 25 cm H_2O to impart sufficient energy to the urinary stream to move it along. Most of the stream energy loss occurs in the area of the membranous urethra.[40] Because normal micturition in its purest form involves total relaxation of the distal or voluntary sphincter concomitant with the bladder contraction and open-

URETHRAL PRESSURE PROFILES

Measurement of the closing pressure exerted along the urethra by the various components of urethral resistance have been described in "normal" individuals, those with prostatic enlargement, and those with obstructive uropathy. Because the interaction of the com-

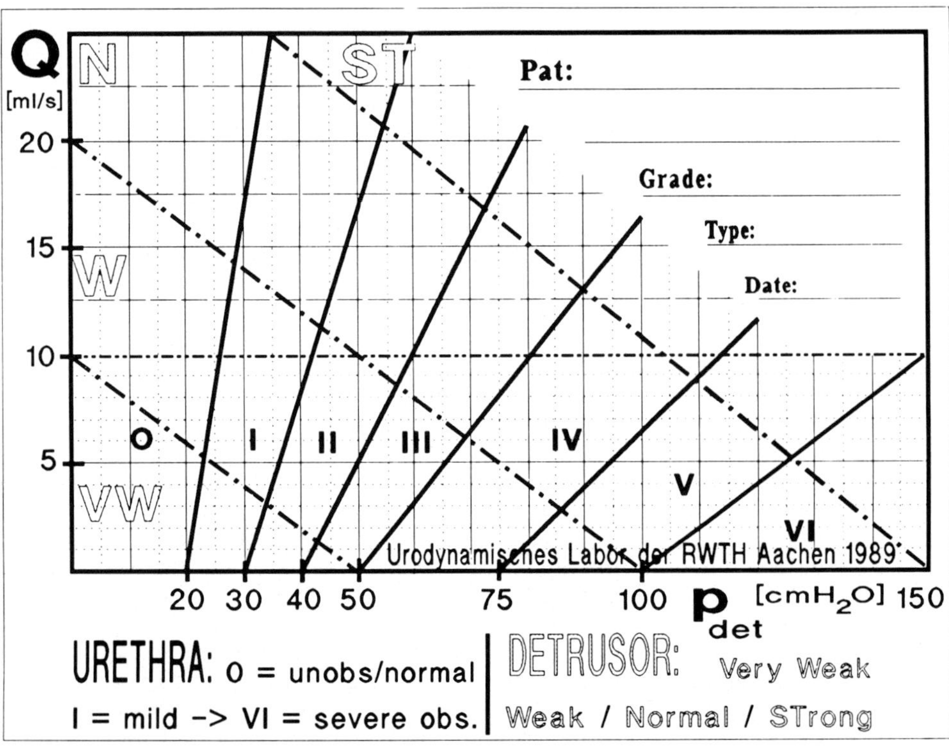

FIGURE 11–2. Pressure-flow plot diagram used by Schaefer in the Aachen Urodynamics Laboratory. A continuous reading of pressure and flow is recorded during micturition. A single point representing the lowest pressure and highest flow is selected and plotted. The position on the diagram indicates the relative obstruction and the strength of the bladder muscle. (Courtesy of Dr. Werner Schaefer, Aachen, Germany.)

ponents of urethral closing pressure and the contracting bladder determines "obstruction," such measurements have to be made *for accuracy* during a bladder contraction, but once the urethra opens and urine flows, an intraurethral pressure-sensing device measures stream energy, or the pressure imparted to the stream by the contracting detrusor, and *not the behavior of the urethra.* Experimental diversion of the urinary stream allows measurement of the pronounced fall in urethral closing pressure which occurs prior to and throughout the detrusor contraction cycle, but that method is not suitable for clinical use. Such studies do show, however, that normally all of the components of urethral closing function cease to operate during micturition, and that even in the absence of a urinary bolus the urethra opens with detrusor contractile activity.

There is no evidence, in clearly defined instances of bladder neck and prostatic obstruction, that an actual increase in intraluminal pressure occurs at the time of a detrusor contraction or that overt dyssynergic activity occurs in the preprostatic or prostatic urethra.[39] Rather, the evidence indicates failure of urethral opening rather than a "hyperclosure," as occurs in patients with spinal cord injury and detrusor sphincter dyssynergia.[25] At rest, prostatic urethral pressures in patients with BPH *and obstruction* are *not* elevated. The effect of prostatic growth on the urethral pressure profile is an increase in the length of the "prostatic urethra." Because the prostatic capsule and stromal musculature are thought to be partly under alpha-adrenergic control, prostatic obstruction of the vesical outlet has been ascribed to persistent alpha-adrenergic tone and an increase in prostatic tissue bulk.[21] The effect of alpha-adrenergic agents on the bladder outlet and/or bladder outlet obstruction have been documented in double-blind controlled studies, but the explanation for those results is not currently available.[2, 8] There is no convincing evidence that alpha-adrenergic tone is influenced by prostatic growth or advancing age. Also, alpha-adrenergic blocking agents have an effect on the preprostatic urethra and the bladder, as well as central neural effects, which in animal studies have been shown to influence distal sphincter resistance. Alpha blocking agents have similar effects in females and prepubertal males. Although stromal hypertrophy clearly occurs in certain cases of BPH, a linkage between that finding and alpha receptors, and pharmacologic therapy by alpha-blocking agents is tenuous. More tissue certainly does not imply increased activity. Moreover, the linkage between urethral behavior and bladder contractile activity is in man and in animals very tightly woven and apparently controlled at the vesical ganglia and distal to that point rather than centrally.[24, 26] Stromal hypertrophy and differences in alpha-adrenergic receptor function or activity may be related, but the explanation of why that should occur is not readily apparent.

FLOW RATES

Beginning with the work of von Garrelts, flow rates have been used to study the work output of the lower urinary tract.[37] Sussett, Siroky et al, and other workers have contributed to our understanding of flow rates and their clinical applicability.[35, 36] Gleason and co-workers measured flow rates and the residual stream energy as a method of determining total detrusor work, in relationship to urethral resistance.[16] Although there is little doubt that calculations of urethral resistance and determination of flow rates have some value, an individual flow rate determination or several flow rate determinations, together with determinations of residual stream energy even if combined with accurate cross-sectional area determinations of the urethra, do not provide conclusive evidence of prostatic obstruction of the vesical outlet, which is the information sought in most cases.

A flow rate is no doubt the product of the interaction of the bladder and urethra, but urologists want to measure this only in terms of the interaction of the prostatic urethra and the bladder. Thus, poor bladder contractility, as well as poor or incomplete external sphincter relaxation, directly interferes with the interpretation of the test on a practical clinical level and renders individual average or peak flow rate values unreliable as a method to prove prostatic obstruction. To use flow rates as a measure of the effect of prostatic growth and prostatic obstruction, all of the other influences on the urethra and bladder must be removed as completely as possible. One method to sidestep this difficulty is to record both bladder pressure and flow at the same time. For further accuracy, a determination of a lack of activity of the external urethral sphincter is helpful. This can be done by an electromyographic determination or by adopting as most reflective of the true detrusor and prostatic urethral relationship that point in micturition at which bladder pressure is lowest and flow rate highest, as suggested by Schaefer, Griffiths, and other workers (Fig. 11–2).[19, 33, 34] Although the latter nearly eliminates external sphincter influences, it does not do so completely. Nevertheless, such measurements make it clear that certain pressure-flow relationships are not compatible with obstructive uropathy. In other words, low-pressure, high-flow rates are clearly not reflective of obstruction, and neither are very low-pressure, low-flow states. It is possible, however, to have normal pressure and low flow in cases of obstruction, and high pressure and low flow related to poor external sphincter relaxation, just as occurs in patients with spinal cord injury. Here, bladder pressures may be very high, flow rates variable but usually poor, and overall detrusor strength or power also poor.

Given the above, even in the best of circumstances, we may—using flow rates, symptom scores, residual urine, and determinations of prostatic size—misidentify from 25 to 50 per cent of patients as suffering from obstructive uropathy related to BPH when in fact they are not obstructed. Adding a placebo effect to any treatment proposed for a group of patients with "BPH" diagnosed by these methods when up to 50 per cent are not obstructed brings on a very fundamental problem.[14] Simply stated, it is nearly impossible to determine whether the treatment actually works. Therefore, sophisticated pressure data are required both to establish that obstructive uropathy actually exists and, more importantly, to determine what a treatment actually does.

An illustration of this phenomenon is contained in the work of Griffiths and associates, who studied the effect of chemical castration on urodynamic parameters in patients with obstructive uropathy associated with prostatic hypertrophy, the latter diagnosis made by careful pressure-flow determinations.[20] During a 12-week treatment period, prostatic size diminished, maximum flow rate increased, residual urine volume fell, but detrusor pressure was unchanged, as was urethral resistance, and only the strength of the detrusor contraction was affected by the treatment. A similar urodynamic study of the effect of alpha blocking agents on BPH and obstructive uropathy demonstrated an increase in detrusor contractile velocity associated with improved flow rates, diminished residual urine, and subjective improvement in symptoms but no change in the bladder outlet at the time of micturition (W. Schaefer, personal communication, 1991). 1-Deamino-(8-D-arginine)-vasopressin (DDAVP), African prune pits, alpha blocking agents, 5-alpha reductase inhibitors, transurethral resection, transurethral incision, balloons, and even castration have *all* been shown to have an effect on symptoms, flow rates, residual urine, retention, and so forth in patients with the presumptive diagnosis of BPH and obstructive uropathy. Because we also know that some 25 to 50 per cent of patients selected for study may not be obstructed by specific urodynamic testing, and considering the enormous placebo effect of instrumentation, it is obvious that despite "improvement" we have no idea what conditions respond or why, nor can we separate "responses" from placebo effects.

As Schaefer pointed out, some individuals who are not urodynamically obstructed prior to TURP get "better" urodynamically after surgery.[33] He attributed this response to the effect of a TURP on voiding by straining, but that is difficult to prove, and for a number of reasons it is unlikely to be the sole explanation. Chalfin and Bradley successfully obliterated unstable detrusor contractility and the uncomfortable symptoms in patients with BPH, not by TURP (which is the usual method) but by the direct injection of a local anesthetic agent into the prostate, suggesting that the prostate by its growth alone may cause uncomfortable symptoms.[9] These findings suggest that we need better methods to describe precisely the conditions we are treating. On a clinical level in 1960, when only 10 per cent of American men came to prostatectomy, perhaps an error rate in diagnosis of 10 to 25 per cent was acceptable. At present, when nearly 30 per cent of American men appear destined for TURP, such a high error rate is less acceptable. Also, we must not forget that pathologic review of all these TURP chips will uncover a sizeable cohort of otherwise nonclinical carcinomas whose treatment may be meddlesome.[29] Given the costs as well as these and other concerns, there has been a recent widespread effort to find alternative treatments for a group of conditions that cannot be accurately identified on clinical grounds alone.

Yalla and co-workers, Blaivas and co-workers, and our own urodynamics laboratory have for many years

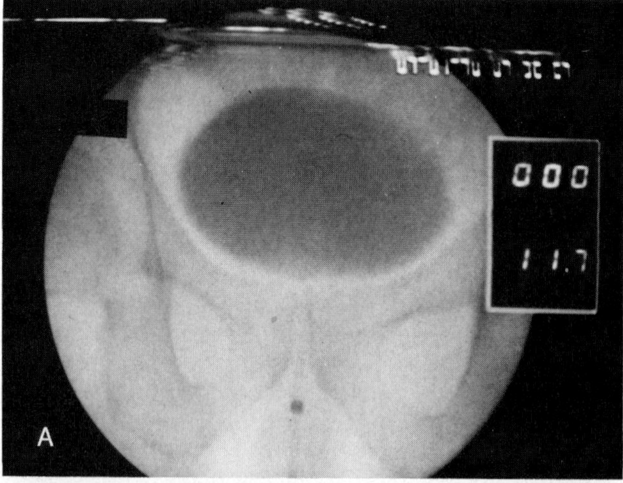

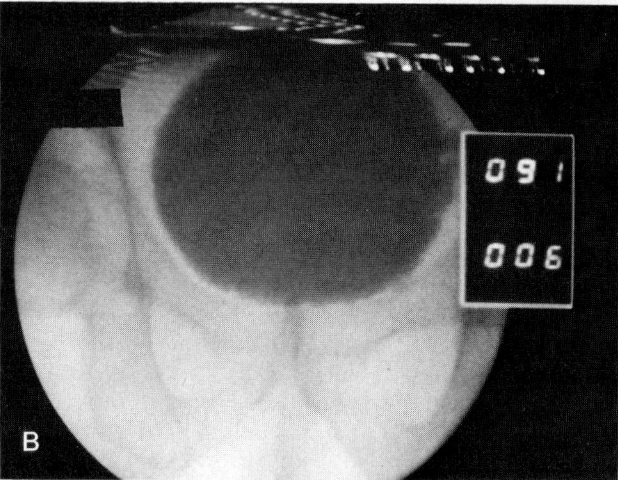

FIGURE 11–3. *A,* Resting cystourethrogram. External sphincter pressure (at marker) is 117; bladder pressure is 0. *B,* "Voiding" study. Bladder pressure is 91; external sphincter pressure is 6. The stream energy loss is at least 79 cm across the proximal and prostatic urethral sphincter. There is prostatic obstruction.

used video multichannel urodynamic evaluation to define the condition "obstructive uropathy."[7, 41] These studies involve measurement of bladder pressure and the characteristics of stream pressure as it crosses the urethra, together with the radiographic and urodynamic determination that full external sphincter relaxation has taken place (Fig. 11–3). These methods at least demonstrate obstructive uropathy and the site of that obstruction. These studies make it obvious that many patients are unable to urinate normally under laboratory conditions in that they often do not completely relax the external sphincter throughout voiding. We use the fluoroscopic picture of the urethra, the voiding pressure, and the pressure drop across the prostatic urethra, but only when the external sphincter is completely relaxed. It is easy to observe the profound effect on voiding pressure that results from external sphincter contractility (Fig. 11–4). Obviously the bladder deals with the totality of urethral resistance, but urologists are interested in (for the diagnosis of BPH *and* bladder outlet obstruction) the interaction of the bladder and the urethra

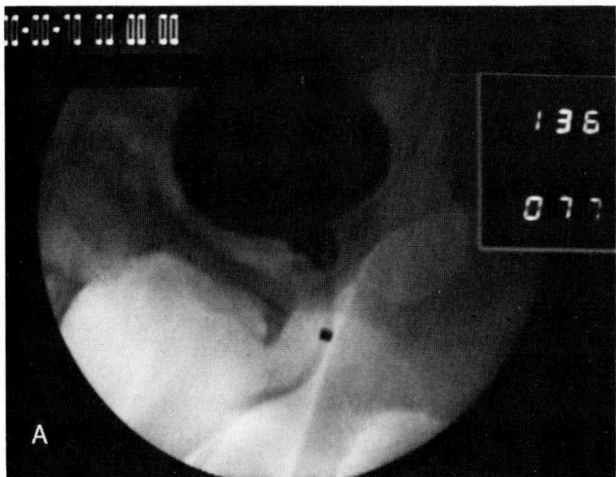

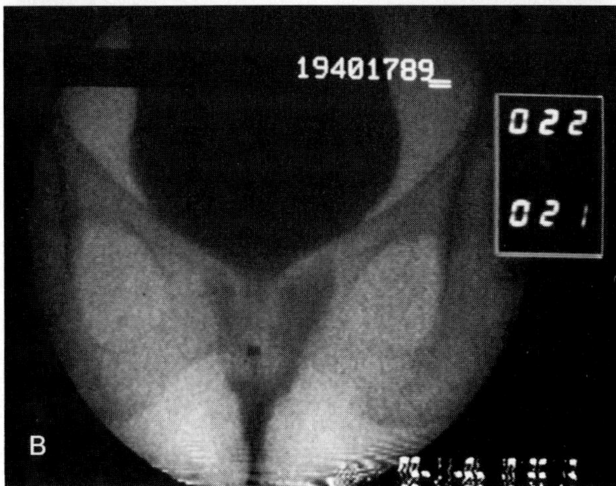

FIGURE 11–4. *A,* Detrusor–external sphincter dyssynergia in a 26-year-old paraplegic man. Note the wide-open prostatic urethra and the hyperclosure of the external sphincter. The external sphincter pressure is 136, and the bladder pressure is 77. *B,* Midvoiding study from a 42-year-old woman with irritative voiding symptoms and urge incontinence following an operation for stress incontinence. There is urethrovaginal reflux. Stream pressure measured at the external sphincter is 21, and bladder pressure is 22. There is no stream energy loss across the urethra. There is no obstruction.

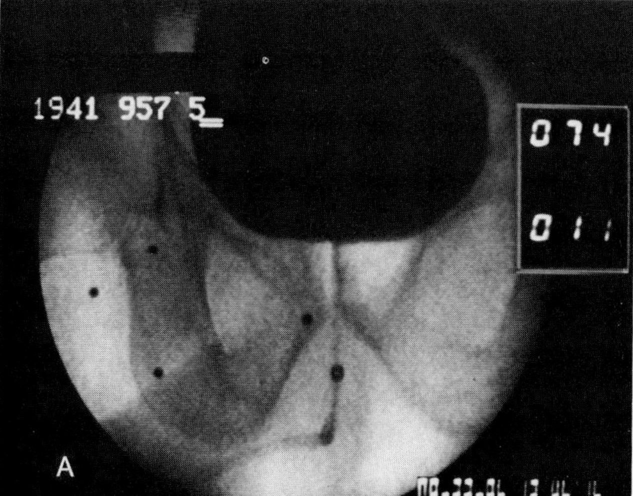

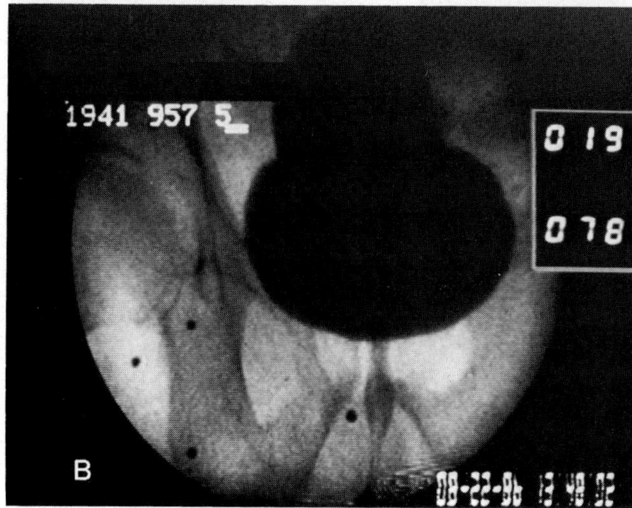

FIGURE 11–5. *A,* Resting cystogram. External sphincter pressure (marked) is 74 and bladder pressure is 11. *B,* Voiding study; external sphincter pressure is 19, and bladder pressure is 78. The bladder neck is narrowed. The mid-prostatic urethra looks normal, but the stream energy loss across the urethra is excessive and indicates obstructive uropathy, superior to the mid-urethral high-pressure zone.

proximal to the external sphincter (Fig. 11–5). For a precise diagnosis, videourodynamics is clearly superior to most other methods. It could be argued that a precise diagnosis is not needed, and that a working clinical diagnosis supplemented by symptom scores and a flow rate is good enough, unless documentation of improvement is required when evaluating some treatment or another. That, however, is simply not valid, because we have no accurate idea what a flow rate or symptom score really measures. Are these data related to "bladder dysfunction," prostate enlargement, or obstructive uropathy? A spontaneous improvement rate of 30 to 60 per cent in patients with "prostatic obstruction" must be taken into account in evaluating any results. Also, the completely identical results recorded after treatment of patients determined to be obstructed by precise pressure/flow studies with alpha blocking agents and testosterone antagonists suggest a common site of action

that is not prostatic. These results showed improved bladder function but no change in the outlet in terms of upstream resistance offered to the bladder when it contracted. Whatever the explanation of these findings, at least one possible explanation is that both agents influence an autonomic receptor in the bladder muscle. Although there is little doubt that we measure effects when we use flow rates and symptom scores, we do not know how these effects are induced, nor can we assume that all of the patients are obstructed, which, in fact, is what we have historically done.

REFERENCES

1. Abrams PH, Roylance J, Finnelly RCL: Excretion urography in the investigation of prostatism. Br J Urol 48:681, 1976.
2. Abrams PH, Shah PJR, Stone R: Bladder outflow obstruction treated with phenoxybenzamine. Br J Urol 54:527, 1982.

3. Ashley DJ: Observations on the epidemiology of prostatic hyperplasia in males. Br J Urol 38:567, 1966.
4. Bell AJ, Finnelly RCL, Abrams PH: The natural history of untreated "prostatism." Br J Urol 53:613, 1981.
5. Berry SJ, Coffey DS, Walsh PC, Ewing LL: The development of human benign prostatic hyperplasia with age. J Urol 132:474, 1984.
6. Birkhoff DD, Wiederhorn AR, Hamilton ML, Zinsser HH: Natural history of benign prostatic hypertrophy and urinary retention. Urology 7:48, 1976.
7. Blaivas JG: Multi-channel urodynamic studies in men with benign prostatic hyperplasia. Urol Clin North Am 17:543, 1990.
8. Caine M, Perlberg S, Metetzk S: A placebo-controlled double blind study of the effect of phenoxybenzamine in benign prostatic obstruction. J Urol 50:551, 1978.
9. Chalfin SA, Bradley WE: Etiology of detrusor hyperreflexia in patients with intravesical obstruction. J Urol 129:938, 1982.
10. Christinsen MM, Bruskewitz RC: Clinical manifestations of benign prostatic hyperplasia and indications for therapeutic interaction. Urol Clin North Am 17:509, 1990.
11. Clark R: The prostate and the endocrines. A control series. Br J Urol 9:254, 1937.
12. Coffey DS, Walsh PC: Clinical and experimental studies of benign prostatic hyperplasia. Urol Clin North Am 17:461, 1990.
13. Craigen AA, Hickling JB, Saunders CRG, Carpenter RG: Natural history of prostatic obstruction. A prospective survey. J Roy Coll Gen Practit 18:226, 1969.
14. Dean GE, Blaivas JG, Kaplan SA: The differential diagnosis of prostatism [abstract]. J Urol 145:2644, 1991.
15. Drach GW, Steinbronn DV: Clinical evaluation of patients with prostatic obstruction: Correlation of flow rates with voided, residual or total bladder volume. J Urol 135:737, 1986.
16. Gleason DM, Bottaccini MR, Reilly RJ: The residual stream energy as a diagnostic index of male urinary outflow obstruction. Invest Urol 10:72, 1972.
17. Glynn RJ, Campion EW, Bouchard GR, Silbert JE: The development of benign prostatic hyperplasia among volunteers in the normative aging study. Am J Epidemiol 121:78, 1985.
18. Griffiths DJ: Urodynamic assessment of bladder function. Br J Urol 49:29, 1977.
19. Griffiths DJ, van Mastrigt R: The routine assessment of detrusor contraction strength. Neurourol Urodynamics 4:77, 1985.
20. Griffiths DJ, van Mastrigt R, Bosh R: Quantification of urethral resistance and bladder function during voiding with special reference to prostatic size reduction on urethral obstruction due to benign prostatic hyperplasia. Neurourol Urodynamics 8:17, 1989.
21. Lepor H, Shapiro E: Characteristics of alpha I adrenergic receptors in human benign prostatic hyperplasia. J Urol 132:226, 1984.
22. Lytton B, Emery JM, Harvard BM: The incidence of benign prostatic obstruction. J Urol 99:639, 1968.
23. Marshall V, Singh M, Blandy JP: Is urography necessary for patients with acute retention of urine before prostatectomy? Br J Urol 46:73, 1974.
24. McGuire EJ, Herlihy EB. Bladder and urethral responses to isolated sacral root stimulation. Invest Urol 16:219, 1978.
25. McGuire EJ, Wagner FM, Weiss RM: Treatment of autonomic dysreflexia with phenoxybenzamine. J Urol 115:53, 1976.
26. McGuire EJ, Wagner F, Weiss RM: Urethral closing pressure after spinal cord injury and its relationship to autonomic dysreflexia. Urol Int 32:97, 1977.
27. McGuire EJ, Weiss RM: Secondary bladder neck obstruction in patients with urethral valves—treatment with phenoxybenzamine. Urology 5:756, 1975.
28. O'Reilly PH, Brooman PJC, Farah NB, Mason GC: High pressure chronic retention, incidence, aetiology and sinister implications. Br J Urol 58:644, 1986.
29. Potosky AL, Kessler L, Gridley G, et al: Rise in prostate cancer incidence associated with increased use of transurethral resection. J Natl Cancer Inst 82:1624, 1990.
30. Radzinski C, McGuire EJ, Smith D, et al: Creation of the feline model of obstructive uropathy. Neurourol Urodynamics 145:859, 1991.
31. Roos NP, Ramsey EW: A population based study of prostatectomy: Outcomes associated with differing surgical approaches. J Urol 137:1184, 1987.
32. Schaefer W: Eine Physiologische Methode Zur Beschreibung der Druch—Flow—Beziehung wahrend der Miktion. Biomedizinisch Technik 21:11, 1976.
33. Schaefer W: Principles and clinical application of advanced urodynamic analysis of voiding function. Urol Clin North Am 17:553, 1990.
34. Schaefer W: Urethral resistance? Urodynamic concepts of physiological and pathological bladder outlet function during voiding. Neurourol Urodynamics 4:161, 1985.
35. Siroky MB, Olsson CA, Krane RJ: The flow rate nomogram II: Clinical correlation. J Urol 123:208, 1980.
36. Sussett JG: Resistance to flow in the lower urinary tract: Clinical application. In Hinman F Jr (ed): Hydrodynamics of Micturition. Springfield, IL, Charles C Thomas, 1981.
37. von Garrelts B: Micturition in the normal male. Acta Chir Scand 144:197, 1957.
38. Wang SC, McGuire EJ, Bloom DA: A bladder pressure management system for myelodysplasia—clinical outcome. J Urol 140:1499, 1988.
39. Woodside JR: Urodynamic evaluation of dysfunctional bladder with obstruction in men. J Urol 124:673, 1980.
40. Yalla SJ: Urethral static pressure profile. In Hinman F Jr (ed): Benign Prostatic Hypertrophy. New York, Springer-Verlag, 1983, pp 576–588.
41. Yalla SV, Waters WB, Snyder H: Urodynamic localization of isolated bladder neck obstruction in men: Studies with micturitional vesicourethral static pressure profiles. J Urol 125:677, 1981.

Chapter 12

CRITERIA FOR ASSESSING OUTCOME FOLLOWING INTERVENTION FOR BENIGN PROSTATIC HYPERPLASIA

ALAN J. WEIN

General Principles

Benign prostatic hyperplasia (BPH) affects approximately 50 per cent of men aged 60.[8] By age 80, some estimates place the incidence at approximately 80 per cent.[19] Lytton et al suggested in 1968 that a 40-year-old man who lived to age 80 had approximately a 10 per cent chance of undergoing prostatectomy. More recently, Glynn et al[22] have suggested a probability three times as high in the United States. Between 400,000 and 450,000 prostatectomies are done yearly for what is originally diagnosed as benign prostatic disease. The total costs (preoperative evaluation, costs of hospitalization, surgical fees, lost productivity time, and treatment of complications or reoperations) account for a significant percentage of the American health care dollar. Add to this fact the recent emphasis on research with regard to the long-term effectiveness and outcome of various medical practices and procedures,[25] the suggestion that overall outcome following transurethral prostatecomy is not as favorable as hitherto assumed,[37] and the suggestion that, except in the case of severe symptoms, prostatectomy may offer far fewer advantages over watchful waiting than previously assumed,[6, 18] and it comes as no surprise that an unnecessary amount of periodical and program space is devoted to the ever-increasing list of alternate strategies for the management of BPH (Table 12–1).

The purpose of this chapter is to discuss general and specific principles for the evaluation of the treatment of BPH. Prospective application of such principles would have doubtless pleased William Heberden, whose experience and common sense prompted the comment, "new medicines and new methods of cure always work miracles for a while."[43]

Initial Considerations

Although an increasing number of clinical trials are of high quality, many still contain deficiencies of design,

TABLE 12–1. TREATMENT OPTIONS FOR BENIGN PROSTATIC HYPERPLASIA

Observation (watchful waiting)

Pharmacologic
  Bulk reducing
    Estrogen
    Luteinizing hormone–releasing hormone agonist
      (LHRH)
    Antiandrogen
    5α-reductase inhibitor
    Aromatase inhibitor
    Growth factor inhibitor
  Tone reducing
    Alpha-1-adrenergic antagonists

Surgical/mechanical
  Urethral stent
  Balloon dilatation
  Probe hypothermia
  Microwave hyperthermia
  Laser prostatotomy (TUIBN-P)
  Diathermy prostatotomy (TUIBN-P)
  Ultrasonic aspiration
  Transurethral resection of the prostate
  Open prostatectomy

conduct, analysis, or presentation of results. These may qualify as only pilot studies, in which a group of selected patients are asked to undergo a new treatment and may be coached as to the results to be expected. The treatment is not compared with either placebo or any other standard or nonstandard treatment except on the basis of historical results, the best of which are generally not chosen. Such a study generally serves only as a preliminary investigation, yielding information as to (1) whether a particular treatment may have some value; (2) if so, over what period of time it should be studied to observe the maximum effect; and (3) what side effects may be expected. Such a study also gives statisticians some idea about how many patients will be required to properly investigate the treatment and compare it with others or with placebo. General criteria for the ideal clinical trial of a drug have long been available[17] and have been applied to BPH.[27, 44] The criteria, equally applied to procedures, include (1) a lack of bias, (2) an adequate number of subjects, (3) appropriate and sensitive methods of evaluation, (4) double-blind conditions with a placebo, and (5) statistical validation.

Bias Elimination

This generally does not constitute a problem. However, unconscious bias can occur, either in the assignment of patients to a particular treatment group or in the assessment of responses. Randomized prospective double-blind studies (see below) virtually eliminate this as a potential problem. If a study is not or cannot be randomized and/or double-blinded, the validity of the results can be considerably increased if the assessments are done by individuals other than those who assigned the patients to the treatment groups or who carried out the treatment.

Sample Size

Three primary considerations are relevant to sample size[20]: (1) the natural history of the condition under study; (2) the magnitude of difference expected as a result of the therapeutic intervention; and (3) the desired level of statistical significance. The theoretical and practical considerations relevant to sample size should be carefully considered with the help of a statistician. Otherwise, a given study may lack the ability to detect clinically important effects of significant magnitude or may overestimate them.

Appropriate and Sensitive Parameters of Evaluation

Ideally, methods of evaluation yield objective data in a form that can be easily analyzed statistically. Subjective data (e.g., symptoms) are generally difficult to quantify and analyze. Most symptoms defy exact quantitation, and it is necessary to attach artificial grades to the severity of various symptoms and analyze changes in these. Although a "symptom score" (see Table 12–3) is a very logical and excellent idea, it is necessary, when dealing with small but statistically significant differences in such scores after treatment, to appreciate exactly what the symptomatic changes have been. Otherwise, the therapeutic efficacy of the treatment under consideration may in fact be overstated. Symptom scores, however, generally do not take into consideration what actually brought the patient to the doctor. Similarly, they do not take into consideration the effects of a given condition and its symptoms or an individual symptom on the patient's activities of daily living or overall quality of life. In other words, it is possible to favorably affect a symptom score without significantly affecting the actual complaint that prompted the patient to seek treatment. It is also possible to favorably affect the symptom responsible for the status change prompting treatment without significantly affecting an overall symptom score. An adequate protocol must also include a method for validating a symptom score. In other words, if symptom status is derived primarily from patient-generated forms, there must be a mechanism to show that these are in fact consistent with what would be obtained by an objective reporter questioning the patient.

Properly chosen urodynamic studies are at first glance an obvious answer for an appropriate and sensitive method of evaluation of a given treatment for BPH. However, there is considerable disagreement about what constitutes appropriate urodynamic criteria by which to measure the response of BPH to treatment. Most workers would agree that flowmetry is the most useful and reliable objective parameter by which to judge the success of treatment of bladder outlet obstruction. However, even relative to flowmetry, considerable disagreements exist as to (1) what constitutes the most significant parameter (mean versus peak flow); (2) what constitutes a significant change; (3) the relationship between rate(s) and volume voided and how to adjust for this statistically; (4) whether flowmetry should be totally noninvasive or in response to a standard filled volume through a catheter; and (5) the consistency of flow parameters in a given individual from one event to another.

Blind, Double-blind, and Placebo-controlled Studies

A prospective randomized double-blind study is the ideal method to determine the clinical efficacy of a therapeutic intervention. Such a protocol virtually eliminates bias and, with an adequate sample size, ensures as much as possible that the results obtained are due to factors other than simple sampling variability. A double-blind study is one in which the subject and the investigator are unaware of the identity of the treatment. This is ideally suited to the comparison of a drug with placebo or with another drug. Unfortunately, it is difficult to use this method for a new invasive therapeutic manipulation. Some interesting ideas have recently surfaced in this area, however, such as inserting a device without activating it (e.g., a balloon catheter or hyperthermia probe).

Ethical considerations obviously pertain to the use of a placebo, particularly if a standard therapy is clearly superior to placebo.[14, 33] However, it has long been recognized, especially in protocols that use subjective criteria for assessment, that "improvement" may occur in up to 35 per cent of placebo-treated patients.[7] This may be a result of true improvement that occurs in accordance with the natural history of the condition, or it may be a result of the placebo effect itself. In general, the placebo effect can be boosted by a very positive, concerned, and enthusiastic attitude on the part of the treating physician, by the length of time spent with the patient, and by an intensive in-hospital type regimen.[7, 33] A patient in such a study must be told that the chances of receiving placebo are 50 per cent and that a placebo is equivalent to no treatment at all. Provided that the patient understands this and consents accordingly, provided that a delay in current accepted treatment is not hazardous to the patient's health, and provided that the risks of the additional studies necessary as a consequence of the protocol are not unpleasant, hazardous, or unacceptable, no ethical problems are raised.[14] Telling the subject that there is a 50 per cent chance of receiving no treatment at all seems to decrease the placebo effect on subjective symptoms and helps to better define the true natural history of the condition under consideration. However, it also seems to decrease the number of patients willing to enter a particular study, especially if it is long term. Unblinded studies, in which both the investigator and the patient know the treatment being received, are certainly easier to perform from the standpoint of patient recruitment, but unconscious bias and placebo effect are both significant problems. Single-blind studies with placebo are those in which only the investigator knows the therapy the subject receives. These are still subject to unconscious (investigator) bias.

In any type of drug study in which placebo is used, it is obvious that its appearance and dosage schedule must be the same as for the drug under consideration. The ideal is to eliminate any other factor that would enable the patient to ascertain whether placebo or medication is being received. Unfortunately, many clinically useful drugs have specific side effects, and it is usually impossible to build into a placebo the potential side effects of the therapeutic agent under consideration without making it something other than an inert compound. Institutional review boards generally require that the side effects of an agent, even in a double-blind placebo-controlled study, be detailed in the consent form. Although it is a perfectly sound ethical consideration, there is a question as to whether patients who receive active drug and develop these side effects are more subject to a placebo effect on the subjective symptoms of the condition under consideration.

Statistical Versus Clinical Significance

Determination of the statistical significance of changes in an objective parameter is generally not a problem in a placebo-controlled study. Existence of a placebo group and the use of a double-blind methodology should eliminate any errors that might otherwise occur because of (1) variability in results of a particular test; (2) improvement that occurs as a result of the natural history of the disease; and (3) statistical sampling. To ensure statistical validity, some mechanism must monitor patient compliance in taking medication or placebo. This generally consists of having the patient record the dosage schedule and return the unused medication at the termination of the study or at various points during the study when evaluation occurs; however, this does not guarantee that the patient has taken the missing drug. If a drug produces a measurable change in serum or in some other status or function, this parameter can be measured to ensure that compliance has occurred.

Subjective variables are difficult to quantify, and many such variables are often graded according to severity and the resultant changes in grade subjected to analysis, either separately or in groups. Unless the changes are marked, this type of analysis has shortcomings. Adjacent categories or grades may exhibit only shades of difference that are not in fact clinically significant. Also missing from this type of analysis is the concept of the most significant symptom, or what caused the patient to come to the physician in the first place. Even more difficult to construct is an index that relates to the overall quality of life, or what effect the symptoms have on the enjoyment or performance of the activities of daily living.

In considering objective changes, the concept of clinical versus statistical significance must also be kept in mind. For instance, an increase in mean flow rate from 4 to 6 ml/sec represents, on average, a statistically significant change, as does a decrease in residual urine from 300 to 200 ml or a decrease in the number of daily episodes of urge incontinence from five to three. However, these changes may not be so clinically significant for a given individual, especially if other forms of therapy are capable of greater improvement. Investigators should point out any differences between statistical improvement and what they consider to be clinically significant improvement. They should also compare these to the results of the gold standard of treatment for that particular entity. Look for both absolute and percentage change. Beware of investigators who prefer to express their data only in terms of percentage rather than absolute values. Such data display, in terms of clinical significance, almost invariably makes treatment effects seem greater than they actually are.

Corollaries

Crossover studies are sometimes used and can be quite informative. Each subject receives one treatment initially and the placebo or alternative treatment during a second period of equal length. The order in which the treatments are given is randomized. This type of design ideally allows each subject to serve as his own control. However, a residual effect from one treatment can influence the effect of the succeeding treatment, and the duration of action of a given therapeutic effect must be considered. If this type of consideration represents a problem, there must be a "washout" period of sufficient duration between the first and second treatment period. A "lead-in" period may likewise be an extremely useful part of a given drug protocol. The lead-in period may simply be a period of baseline data collection without any treatment being administered, or it may include administration of a placebo to all patients, or it may be a combination (this seems ideal) of data collection during a period of no treatment followed by a period of placebo treatment to all patients. Most lead-in periods are 2 to 6 weeks, and the longer the lead-in period, the more information is generated regarding the natural history of the problem being studied and the magnitude of the placebo effect.

Entrance criteria for a study must be broad enough to permit most individuals to enter who actually have the problem being studied. However, the entrance criteria must exclude, as much as possible, patients with a condition that would favorably or unfavorably affect the results of treatment or would produce symptoms that might be confused with those of the disease under consideration. For BPH trials, it is generally agreed that patients with prior prostate surgery, prostatic carcinoma, prostatitis, urethral stricture, bladder neck contracture, bladder stones, neuropathic dysfunction, and infectious or inflammatory disease of the lower urinary tract should be excluded.[19, 27, 44] Likewise, certain categories of patients with various systemic diseases must be excluded, as well as patients who are on, or subsequently placed on, other medications that may affect the clinical result or interact with a study drug. Data collection should be prospectively planned in such a way that all possible relevant variables are included. This permits prospective and retrospective stratification of the treatment group such that if there are subgroups that may especially benefit from treatment, or if there are in fact only certain subgroups that will benefit from treatment, these are readily identifiable.

Drugs must be considered not only according to their pharmacodynamic and pharmacokinetic characteristics but also according to the type of physiologic effect they produce. In other words, if a drug reduces prostatic bulk by producing a metabolic change that begins fairly soon after the onset of medication, but the actual effect on prostatic bulk is exerted through an action on the epithelial component of the prostate that takes 3 to 6 months to become manifest, the study must continue at least for that period, especially if the effect is a gradual and progressive one. For instance, an alpha-1-adrenergic antagonist should exert its effect on flow quite promptly, whereas luteinizing hormone–releasing hormone (LHRH) agonist takes 3 to 6 months or longer for the maximum effect to be seen. A surgical procedure should produce some immediate results, but irritative side effects, which may mask the therapeutic effects, may take some time to resolve. Conversely, the positive effects of a surgical procedure may take months to become noticed, and it may take that long for complications to become manifest as well. Such considerations must determine the minimal length of the study, whereas the maximal length should ideally be capable of detecting tolerance or loss of effect of a drug and recurrence after an invasive procedure.

If a new treatment is being tested for a problem for which others are commonly used, it is of value to the clinician to compare the new modality not only with placebo but also with the "gold standard" of treatment for efficacy, selectivity, side effects, and cost. Finally, if a study is being carried out to determine the therapeutic efficacy of a noninvasive treatment for a condition that is generally treated by an invasive surgical procedure, it is critical to ask if the alternative changes the natural history of the disease as well as the invasive treatment does, and whether invasive treatment is eliminated or simply postponed. Conversely, however, one must be careful to factor into the overall evaluation of a noninvasive versus an invasive treatment the problems suffered by those unfortunate few who develop major side effects following invasive treatment—in the case of prostate surgery, incontinence, impotence, and the need for repeated operations or treatments. In other words, both short- and long-term "average" outcomes should be considered.

CONSIDERATIONS SPECIFIC TO BENIGN PROSTATIC HYPERPLASIA

Symptoms

Many parameters are available for study and evaluation in patients with BPH; few urologists agree on their order of importance in assessing need for treatment and evaluating results of treatment. Consistent with the general principles previously expressed, a consideration of specific measurable variables in patients with BPH is in order, as these constitute the data base for the evaluation of efficacy of any given treatment.

Symptoms have classically formed the initial data base on which to formulate (1) evaluation of potential outlet obstruction; (2) indications for surgery when obstructive BPH is present; and (3) evaluation of results of treatment. Symptoms are generally divided into so-called obstructive and irritative components. Obstructive symptoms occur during the emptying phase and include hesitancy, decreased stream, a feeling of incomplete emptying, straining to void, intermittency, postvoid dribbling, and urinary retention. These symptoms may be characteristic of bladder outlet obstruction or impaired detrusor contractility. Individuals who void frequently in small volumes may also complain of some of these symptoms, simply because of their small voided volume. A patient with involuntary bladder contractions may likewise complain of obstructive symptoms when, after suppressing an involuntary contraction and rushing to the bathroom, he is unable to generate a voluntary contraction even after multiple attempts with straining, leaving him with the sense that he has at least intermittent marked difficulty initiating urination.

Irritative symptoms occur during the filling/storage

TABLE 12–2. SYMPTOM SEVERITY TABLE*

SYMPTOM	0	1	2	3
Nocturia	0	1	2–3	> 4
Daytime frequency	1–4	5–7	8–12	> 13
Hesitancy	< 20%	20–50%	50–99% up to 1 min	100% > 1 min
Intermittency	< 20%	20–50%	50–99% up to 1 min	100% > 1 min
Terminal dribbling	< 20%	20–50%	50–99%	100% or > 1 min or wets clothing
Urgency	0	Occasional	> 50% May rarely lose urine	100% Sometimes loses urine
Impairment of stream	0	Impaired trajectory	Most of time size and force are restricted	Great effort to urinate; interrupts stream
Dysuria	0	Occasional burning	> 50% burning	Frequent and painful burning
Sensation of incomplete voiding	0	Occasional	> 50%	Constant and urgent sensation; no relief on voiding

**Adapted from Boyarsky S, Jones G, Paulson DF, Prout GR Jr: A new look at bladder neck obstruction by the Food and Drug Administration: Guidelines for investigation of benign prostatic hypertrophy. Trans Am Assoc Genitourinary Surg 68:29, 1977; with permission.*

phase of micturition and generally include increased daytime frequency, nocturia, urgency, and incontinence associated with involuntary bladder contractions. However, urgency, urge incontinence, and day and night frequency seem to occur most often in patients with BPH as a result of hyperactivity in response to obstruction. Abrams[2] cites the incidence of detrusor instability in patients with outlet obstruction secondary to prostatism as ranging from 53 to 80 per cent. The high reversal rate of this phenomenon following prostatectomy (45 to 100 per cent) certainly supports this association. Increased day and night frequency may also occur, however, secondary to poor emptying if a significant residual urine remains, resulting in a decreased functional bladder capacity. Urgency may also occur from a bladder that empties very poorly and is almost in "overflow."

Symptom quantitation is difficult, and meaningful comparison of symptoms before and after treatment is even harder. To differentiate therapeutic from placebo effect, it is necessary to have a more exact symptom categorization than simply "better," "improved," "worse," or "no change." Two important facts bear repeating: (1) The natural history of prostatism in some patients is indeed improvement, and (2) there is a substantial placebo effect on subjective symptoms. For instance, Ball et al[5] looked at 107 of 318 original patients with prostatism who did not undergo elective surgery but were followed conservatively (no treatment) for 5 years. Ten of these required surgery, two because of acute retention and eight because of significantly worsening symptoms. Of the remaining 97, 31 considered their symptoms overall "better," whereas 50 considered them the same. Geller et al[21] considered the effect of an antiandrogen, megestrol acetate, on BPH, and included a placebo group. Nineteen of 33 patients indicated that their symptoms were "improved" after 5 months on placebo; 14 experienced no change. Abrams[1] studied the effect of candicidin on BPH in 62 patients awaiting prostatectomy. Of those who completed the study, 45 per cent of the placebo group reported their symptoms "much improved" and an additional 17 per cent reported them "slightly improved"; 38 per cent reported "no change," and none reported worsening over a 6-month period. Using symptom scores, 34 per cent reported improvement, 52 per cent reported no change, and 14 per cent actually worsened.

The concept of a symptom score or severity table for BPH was first developed by an ad hoc group formed by the Food and Drug Administration in 1975; the initial recommendations were published in 1977.[11] Two such symptom score formulations appear in Tables 12–2 and 12–3.[11, 35] Investigators can and have played every game imaginable with such scoring tables, eliminating some symptoms and adding others, changing the weights and definitions of the severity of various symptoms, considering some symptoms separately, or dividing the symp-

TABLE 12–3. SYMPTOM SCORE SHEET*

SYMPTOM	0	1	2	3	4
Stream	Normal	Variable		Weak	Dribbling
Voiding	No strain		Abdominal strain or Crede		
Hesitancy	None			Yes	
Intermittency	None			Yes	
Bladder emptying	Don't know	Variable	Incomplete	Single retention	Repeated retention
Incontinence			Yes (including terminal dribbling)		
Urge	None	Mild	Moderate	Severe (incontinence)	
Nocturia	0–1	2	3–4	> 4	
Diuria	q > 3 h	q 2–3 h	q 1–2 h	q < 1 h	
Total score					

**Adapted from Madsen PO, Iversen P: A point system for selecting operative candidates. In Hinman F Jr (ed): Benign Prostatic Hypertrophy. New York, Springer-Verlag, 1983, pp 763–765; with permission.*

toms into obstructive and irritative groups. For such a formulation to be produced, the patient can simply be asked to check an appropriate blank on a question and answer sheet or fill out a detailed diary and/or answer a series of verbal questions that enable the investigator or a coordinator to generate a symptom score. As mentioned previously, generally no provision is made for considering specifically what actually changed most recently to bring the patient to the physician, what is in fact most annoying to him, what he most wishes corrected or what effect the overall symptom complex, or any one symptom, has on his quality of life, general activities of daily living, or any activity in particular. The American Urological Association has, through its Measurement Committee, begun to formulate indices that address some of these issues (Table 12–4).

Prostate Volume/Size

Size is not necessarily related to obstruction or the symptoms of prostatism, but changes in prostatic size are especially relevant to those types of treatment which nonsurgically reduce prostatic bulk. Digital rectal examination assesses primarily the posterior and lateral portions of the prostate, but such estimation of overall prostatic size is quite subjective, and it is difficult to assign an exact grading system agreed upon by all. Even with the same examiner on different occasions, inconsistent ratings may occur. Endoscopic evaluation of the degree of prostatic enlargement and obstruction is likewise highly subjective, and the reproducibility of estimates varies from examiner to examiner. Bladder neck to veru distance seems to be the only objectively quantifiable parameter that relates to prostatic obstruction, although estimated prostatic weight and degree of lateral lobe occlusion have been cited as others.[4] Certain parameters of urethral pressure profilometry (length and area under the curve) have proved valuable for the preoperative estimation of adenoma weight.[31] Ultrasonography is probably the best and most readily available reproducible form of total prostatic size estimation; Peters and Walsh[36] found an excellent correlation between sonographically estimated and pathologically measured prostatic weight after radical retropubic prostatectomy. Computed tomographic (CT) scanning is an accurate method, but is time consuming, is more expensive than ultrasonography, and involves radiation exposure. Magnetic resonance imaging (MRI) can provide much more elegant images but at a greatly increased cost. MRI may hold the promise of being able to detect differential metabolic or size changes by zone and to distinguish periurethral from peripheral changes and perhaps epithelial from stromal change.

Endoscopic Findings

Endoscopic estimation of prostatic size has previously been mentioned with respect to size evaluation. Endoscopy has some value in excluding other pathologies, but

its other main uses in the evaluation of prostatism are for the observation of trabeculation, itself an almost impossible parameter to reproducibly grade, and for deciding whether an "open" prostatectomy is necessary as opposed to a transurethral resection or incision. Although the prevailing sentiment regarding trabeculation is that it can occur in response to either obstruction, involuntary bladder contractions (probably because of accompanying pseudodyssynergia), or neurologic centralization,[45] Andersen[4] found that trabeculation in patients with prostatism was statistically related only to the urodynamic parameter of opening pressure.

Flowmetry

Significant disagreements exist regarding what constitutes an adequate urodynamic evaluation of prostatism and whether a urodynamically quantifiable definition of obstruction is necessary or desirable. This is not the place for a detailed treatise on the urodynamics of prostatism, but measurable urodynamic parameters exist which can indicate a favorable result, or a lack thereof, in response to treatment of BPH. Of all of these, the general concept of uroflowmetry seems to excite the least controversy. Although diminished flow may be caused by either outlet obstruction or impairment of detrusor contractility, and outlet obstruction may certainly exist in the presence of normal flow, most men with bladder outlet obstruction do have a diminished flow rate and altered flow pattern.[10] Potential problems related to uroflow include the following: (1) Many patients do not or will not void a sufficient volume for accurate measurements; (2) others void with an interrupted stream or with postvoid dribbling, which makes interpretation of the end point of micturition difficult, casting some element of subjectivity into the calculation of average flow rate; (3) some patients are unable to relax sufficiently to void in the same manner as they would in the privacy of their own bathroom; and (4) a considerable discrepancy may exist between the first and subsequent measures of mean and peak flow. Because voiding events are invariably different from point to point in an individual's life, a variety of flow nomograms have been constructed to facilitate comparison of different flow events. Siroky et al[40] developed nomograms (Fig. 12–1) for average and maximum flow rates based upon flow rate measurements in a group of younger men, which were originally collected by Susset et al.[41] According to these data, the average and maximum flow rates depend upon initial bladder volume in a nonlinear fashion. The authors found relatively small variability in a single individual's flow rate over time and further concluded that urinary flow rate, when statistically related to initial bladder volume, could be used to estimate outflow resistance. Among normal men, 97.5 per cent had flow rates consistently greater than -2 standard deviations at all points along the mean nomogram curve for average and maximum flow rate. The authors proposed that such nomograms could therefore be used to identify changes in outflow resistance after medical or

TABLE 12–4. AMERICAN UROLOGICAL ASSOCIATION SYMPTOM INDEX FOR BENIGN PROSTATIC HYPERPLASIA*

A. URINARY SYMPTOMS (SYMPTOM SCORE CRITERIA)	NOT AT ALL	LESS THAN 1 TIME IN 5	LESS THAN HALF THE TIME	ABOUT HALF THE TIME	MORE THAN HALF THE TIME	ALMOST ALWAYS
1. Over the past month or so, how often have you had a sensation of not emptying your bladder completely after you finished urinating?	(0)	(1)	(2)	(3)	(4)	(5)
2. Over the past month or so, how often have you had to urinate again less than 2 hours after you finished urinating?	(0)	(1)	(2)	(3)	(4)	(5)
3. Over the past month or so, how often have you found you stopped and started again several times when you urinated?	(0)	(1)	(2)	(3)	(4)	(5)
4. Over the past month or so, how often have you found it difficult to postpone urination?	(0)	(1)	(2)	(3)	(4)	(5)
5. Over the past month or so, how often have you had a weak urinary stream?	(0)	(1)	(2)	(3)	(4)	(5)
6. Over the past month or so, how often have you had to push or strain to begin urination?	(0)	(1)	(2)	(3)	(4)	(5)

7. Over the last month, how many times did you most typically get up to urinate from the time you went to bed at night until the time you got up in the morning?

(0) none (1) 1 time (2) 2 times (3) 3 times (4) 4 times (5) 5 or more times

AUA Symptom Score = sum of questions A1 to A7 = ________________

B. PROBLEMS DUE TO SYMPTOMS (BOTHER SCORE CRITERIA)	NO PROBLEM	VERY SMALL PROBLEM	SMALL PROBLEM	MEDIUM PROBLEM	BIG PROBLEM
1. Over the past month, how much has a sensation of not emptying your bladder been a problem for you?	(0)	(1)	(2)	(3)	(4)
2. Over the past month, how much has frequent urination during the day been a problem for you?	(0)	(1)	(2)	(3)	(4)
3. Over the past month, how much has getting up at night to urinate been a problem for you?	(0)	(1)	(2)	(3)	(4)
4. Over the past month, how much has stopping and starting when you urinate been a problem for you?	(0)	(1)	(2)	(3)	(4)
5. Over the past month, how much has a need to urinate with little warning been a problem for you?	(0)	(1)	(2)	(3)	(4)
6. Over the past month, how much has impaired size and force of urinary stream been a problem for you?	(0)	(1)	(2)	(3)	(4)
7. Over the past month, how much has having to push or strain to begin urination been a problem for you?	(0)	(1)	(2)	(3)	(4)

AUA Bother Score = sum of questions B1 to B7 = ________________

C. QUALITY OF LIFE DUE TO URINARY PROBLEMS

1. Over the past month, how much physical discomfort did any urinary problems cause you?
   (0) none (1) only a little (2) some (3) a lot
2. Over the past month, how much did you worry about your health because of any urinary problems?
   (0) none (1) only a little (2) some (3) a lot
3. Overall, how bothersome has any trouble with urination been during the past month?
   (0) not at all bothersome (1) bothers me a little (2) bothers me some (3) bothers me a lot
4. If you were to spend the rest of your life with your urinary condition just the way it is now, how would you feel about that?
   (0) delighted (1) pleased (2) mostly satisfied (3) mixed (about equally satisfied/dissatisfied) (4) mostly dissatisfied (5) unhappy (6) terrible
5. Over the past month, how much of the time has any urinary problem kept you from doing the kinds of things you would usually do?
   (0) none of the time (1) a little of the time (2) some of the time (3) most of the time (4) all of the time

Quality of life questions are scored individually.

*From the American Urological Association Measurement Committee (Draft 6-21-91).

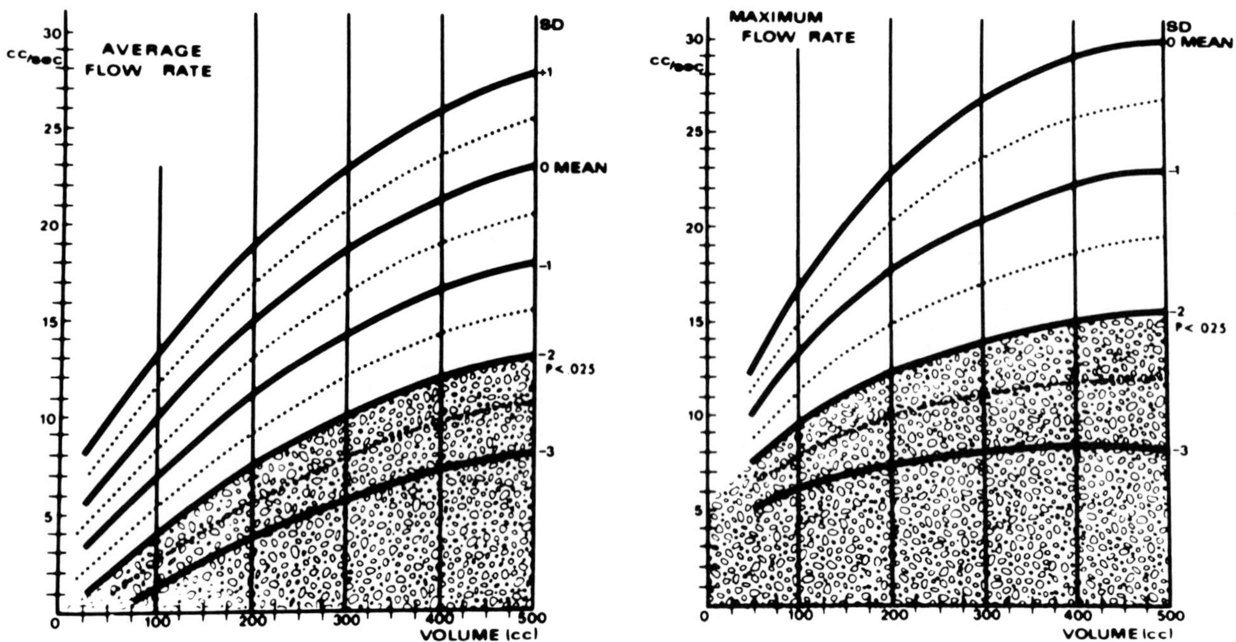

FIGURE 12–1. Flow rate nomograms of Siroky et al[39, 40] relating peak and average flow to intravesical (not voided) volume. The shaded areas represent flow rates highly suggestive of outlet obstruction. (From Siroky MB, Olsson CA, Krane RJ: The flow rate nomogram. I. Development. J Urol 122:665, 1979, © by Williams & Wilkins, 1979; with permission.)

surgical therapy. This is done by simply taking all measurements on one of the nomogram curves back to a standard bladder volume. The authors further concluded that consideration of voided volume rather than initial bladder volume resulted in a gross overestimate of an individual's voiding ability by an average of 2.1 standard deviations, and that the smaller the voided volume compared with the initial bladder volume, the greater the overestimate. Drach et al[16] and Layton and Drach[32] analyzed their flow data somewhat differently. They have stated that the adjusted peak flow rate is the most useful flow parameter to evaluate voiding dysfunction and that this requires consideration of volume voided, rather than total bladder volume, and age. Their adjusted peak flow nomogram for men appears in Figure 12–2. Using this nomogram, an adjusted peak flow rate of less than 16 cc/sec or greater than 1.3 standard deviations below the mean is considered suspicious for bladder outlet obstruction. Although the details of these nomograms differ and the authors' philosophies regarding important parameters likewise differ somewhat, each provides a method for accurately comparing flow events at different times, which, after all, is the most important consideration in comparing flow data before and after treatment for BPH. It should be noted that many nomograms and tables of "acceptable flow rates" are available for various age groups. Some believe that the Siroky nomogram, the most commonly used in this country, overestimates peak and average flow rates for older males and therefore overestimates, according to their 2-standard-deviation rule, the number of older males with bladder outlet obstruction. A recently published set of maximum and average urine flow rates in normal male and female populations, referred to as the

Liverpool nomograms, agree that a certain amount of deterioration in male urinary flow rates occurs with age. As an example for comparison's sake, the Liverpool nomogram in men over the age of 50 sets a maximum urinary flow rate at a voided volume of 300 cc to be 21 cc/sec at the 50th percentile and 11 cc/sec at the 5th percentile. Corresponding average flow rates for these percentiles at this voided volume are 13 cc/sec and 8 cc/sec.[26] It is doubtful that consistency will be achieved among flow nomogram makers. However, one of the systems supported by at least a portion of urodynamicists should be used for comparisons following treatment of BPH.

Residual Urine Volume

If residual urine is present, its reduction is an important parameter in the evaluation of results of treatment of BPH. Most patients with BPH in my practice have a minimal residual urine volume. For many with a significant residual it is impossible to differentiate deficient bladder contractility from outlet obstruction as the primary cause without a pressure-flow study. Most agree that a large residual urine volume reflects at least some bladder dysfunction, but it is difficult to correlate residual urine with either specific symptoms or other urodynamic abnormalities.[12, 28] Insertion of a catheter is the most direct and accurate means of measuring residual urine volume, but, like a filled flow rate, is invasive, causes discomfort, and may introduce infection. Noninvasive methods include isotope scanning and sonography. These are much more expensive and less accurate. Unfortunately for the BPH investigator, there may

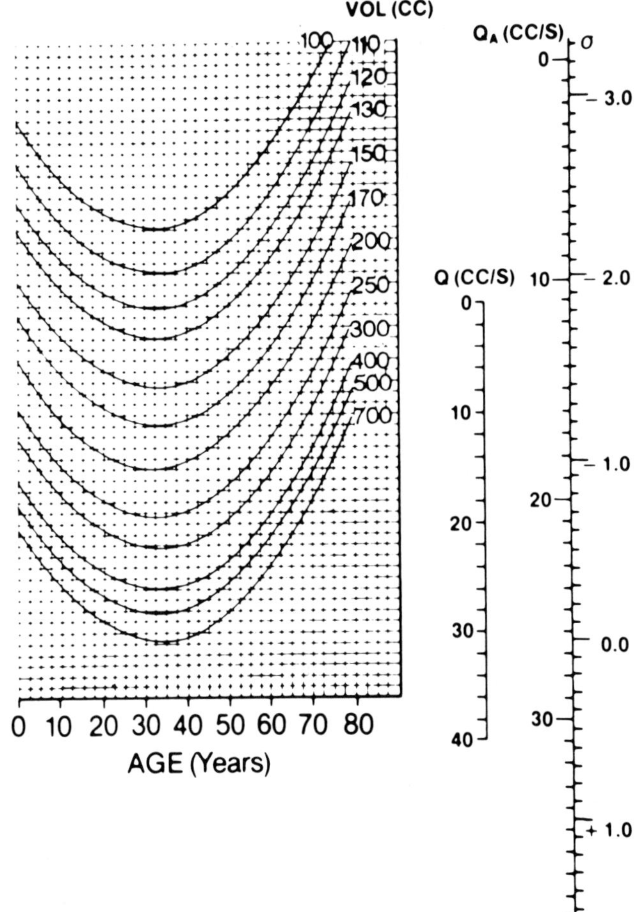

FIGURE 12–2. Flow rate nomogram of Drach et al relating peak flow (Q), age, and voided volume. A perpendicular line is drawn upward from age until it intersects with the curve for volume voided or is between two curves. The right angle line is then extended to the right vertical axis of graph and the point of intersection is marked. The straight edge is used to join this point and the observed peak flow (Q) on the middle scale. Extension of this line intersects with the right scale at a point for adjusted peak flow rate (Q_A) (left side of scale) or for standard deviation (right side of scale). An adjusted Q_A of less than 16 cc/sec or greater than 1.3 standard deviations below the mean is very suspicious for obstruction. (From Drach GW, Laylon T, Bottaccini MR: A method of adjustment of male peak urinary flow rate for varying age and volume voided. J Urol 128:960, 1982, © by Williams & Wilkins, 1982; with permission.)

be a wide variation of residual urine volumes in an individual patient at different times.[9, 12, 28]

Cystometry: Pressure-Flow Studies

Filling cystometry provides information on compliance, the presence and threshold for involuntary bladder contractions, and bladder capacity. Compliance is generally not affected in patients with obstructive BPH, but, as mentioned previously, approximately 50 per cent of such individuals have involuntary bladder contractions. Objective urodynamic documentation of the disappearance of this phenomenon following successful treatment of bladder outlet obstruction is useful, as well as documentation of changes in bladder capacity. However, more important would be changes in concomitant symptoms, such as day and night frequency and urgency.

On a logical basis, bladder outlet obstruction seems to be defined, as Blaivas[10] suggests, by the relationship between flow rate and detrusor contractility. Outlet obstruction is best characterized by a poor flow rate in the presence of a detrusor contraction of adequate force, duration, and speed. With obstruction, detrusor pressure during attempted voiding generally rises, flow rates generally fall, and the shape of the flow curve becomes more plateau-like than parabola-like. There is, however, marked disagreement about the utility of pressure-flow urodynamic measurements in the evaluation of suspected outlet obstruction and in the prediction of the success of treatment, at least by prostatectomy. Articles that best typify those make an excellent case for the use of various types of pressure-flow studies, although some use other mathematical means to further complicate the relationship.[3, 10, 15, 30, 38] Equally forceful arguments against the utility of such measurements are made by Andersen,[4] Bruskewitz et al,[12] and Graversen et al.[23, 24] Recently, Jensen[29] exhaustively reviewed the subject of urodynamic efficacy in the evaluation of elderly males with prostatism. One of the conclusions was that in this group, interpretation of pressure-flow data using the nomogram of Abrams and Griffiths[3] revealed a significantly better subjective outcome of surgery in patients classified as "obstructed" than "unobstructed" (93.1 per cent versus 77.8 per cent). This technique is described in Figure 12–3. Whether such measurements are necessary to evaluate the response of BPH to treatment or how much they add to the evaluation of the efficacy of a drug or procedure is as yet unsettled. Successful treatment of BPH by prostatectomy is generally correlated with a reduction in the detrusor pressure during an increased uroflow. Consideration of the entire pressure-flow plot as described by Abrams and Griffiths[3] may, in fact, prove to be a more accurate and informative way of looking at this relationship. Other still more complicated ways of evaluating simultaneous flow and pressure may narrow further the diagnostic "grey zone" between bladder outlet obstruction and decreased detrusor function and may permit a more precise way of assessing treatment response. It seems fair to say that, at this time, although this type of invasive study may be the most accurate in urodynamically describing response to treatment, it should be the last performed to complete the profile of action of a given drug or procedure on BPH.

Symptomatic Versus Urodynamic Improvement

One final consideration should be mentioned—the seeming dissociation that may occur between symptomatic and urodynamic improvement. This has been most noticeable recently in data concerning balloon dilation and in some studies of new pharmacologic agents. The fact that symptomatic improvement appears to be out of proportion to the amount of urodynamic improve-

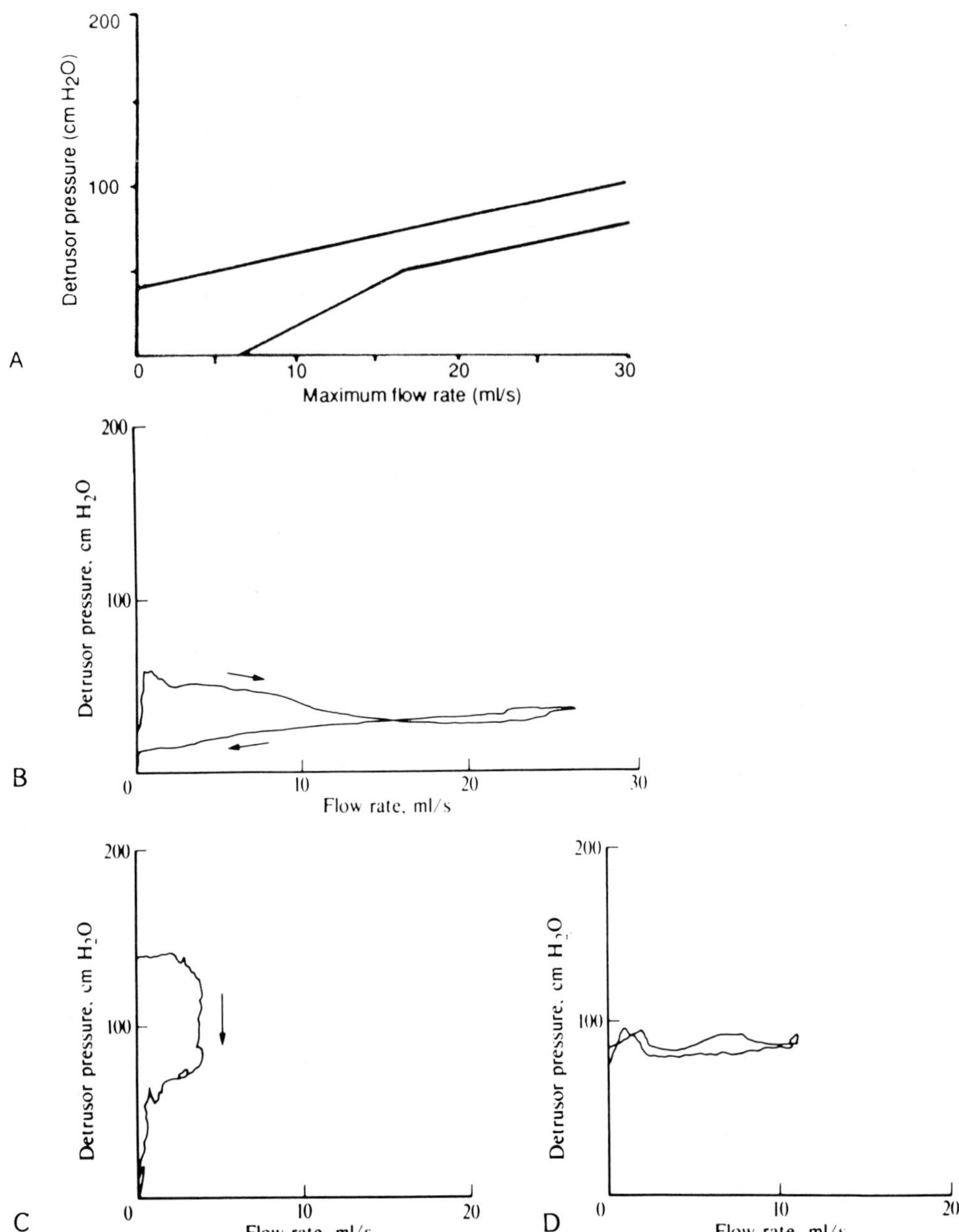

FIGURE 12–3. *A*, Nomogram of maximum flow rate versus detrusor pressure at maximum flow. The two lines divide the figure into three zones—obstructed, equivocal, and unobstructed. A correction of 0.5 second is made for the time lag.[29] By means of X-Y plots it is decided whether patients in the equivocal zone are obstructed. With no obstruction after a fast initial rise in flow rate, the mean slope of the pressure-flow plot is less than 2 cm H_2O/ml/sec and the pressure at the end of voiding less than 40 cm H_2O. Plots with a mean slope greater than 2 cm H_2O/ml/sec and with mean slope less than 2 cm H_2O/ml/sec but with pressure at the end of voiding greater than 40 cm H_2O are classified as obstructed. *B*, X-Y plot indicating no obstruction. Plot is nearly horizontal (mean slope is small) and pressure ahead of voiding is low. *C*, Obstructive X-Y plot. Plot is not horizontal and mean slope (after fast initial rise of flow rate) is large. This plot pattern is often curved so that the mean slope can be only roughly estimated. However, little ambiguity is present because the curvature helps to classify the pattern as obstructive. *D*, Obstructive X-Y plot. Plot is nearly horizontal, but pressure at the end of voiding is high. (From Abrams PH, Griffiths DJ: The assessment of prostatic obstruction from urodynamic measurements and from residual urine. Br J Urol 51:129,1979; with permission.)

ment may, in fact, be assumed to indicate that a given treatment is not equal to the current gold standard of prostatectomy, or that the results will be of shorter duration. However, one important possibility to consider is that the actual symptoms of prostatism have much less to do with urodynamically defined obstruction than we think, and their relief with these other types of treatment has to do more with the correction of some ill-defined mechanism within the prostatic urethra that is not directly related to the amount of mechanical obstruction. Alternatively, it may not be necessary to reduce outlet obstruction by an amount similar to prostatectomy to significantly improve symptoms and prevent bladder and/or upper tract deterioration.

REFERENCES

1. Abrams PH: A double blind trial of the effects of candicidin on patients with benign prostatic hypertrophy. Br J Urol 53:613, 1977.
2. Abrams P: Detrusor instability and bladder outlet obstruction. Neurourol Urodynamics 4:317, 1985.
3. Abrams PH, Griffiths DJ: The assessment of prostatic obstruction from urodynamic measurements and from residual urine. Br J Urol 51:129, 1979.
4. Andersen JT: Prostatism: Clinical, radiologic and urodynamic aspects. Neurourol Urodynamics 1:241, 1982.
5. Ball AJ, Feneley RCL, Abrams PH: The natural history of untreated "prostatism." Br J Urol 53:613, 1981.
6. Barry MJ, Mulley AG, Fowler FJ, Wennberg JW: Watchful waiting versus immediate transurethral resection for symptomatic prostatism: The importance of patients' preferences. JAMA 259:2010, 1988.
7. Benson H, Epstein MD: The placebo effect. JAMA 232:1225, 1976.
8. Berry SJ, Coffey DS, Walsh PC, Ewing LL: The development of human benign prostatic hyperplasia with age. J Urol 132:474, 1984.
9. Birch NC, Hurst G, Doyle PT: Serial residual volumes in men with prostatic hypertrophy. Br J Urol 62:571, 1988.
10. Blaivas JG: Evaluation of bladder outlet obstruction. *In* Paulsen DF (ed): Prostatic Disorders. Philadelphia, Lea & Febiger, 1989, pp 173–192.
11. Boyarsky S, Jones G, Paulson DF, Prout GR Jr: A new look at bladder neck obstruction by the Food and Drug Administration: Guidelines for investigation of benign prostatic hypertrophy. Trans Am Assoc Genitourinary Surg 68:29, 1977.
12. Bruskewitz RC, Iverson P, Madsen PO: Value of postvoid residual urine determination in evaluation of prostatism. Urology 20:602, 1982.
13. Bruskewitz R, Jensen KME, Iversen P, Madsen PO: The relevance of minimum urethral resistance in prostatism. J Urol 129:769, 1983.
14. Claridge M: Assessment of medical treatment. *In* Hinman F Jr (ed): Benign Prostatic Hypertrophy. New York, Springer-Verlag, 1983, pp 308–312.
15. Coolsaet B, Blok C: Detrusor properties related to prostatism. Neurourol Urodynamics 5:435, 1986.
16. Drach GW, Laylon T, Bottaccini MR: A method of adjustment of male peak urinary flow rate for varying age and volume voided. J Urol 128:960, 1982.
17. Fingl E, Woodbury DM: General principles. *In* Goodman LS, Gilman A (eds): The Pharmacologic Basis of Therapeutics. New York, Macmillan, 1975, pp 1–46.
18. Fowler FJ, Wennberg JE, Timothy RP, et al: Symptom status and quality of life following prostatectomy. JAMA 259:3018, 1988.
19. Franks LM: Benign hyperplasia of prostate. Ann R Coll Surg 14:92, 1954.
20. Friedman LM, Furberg CD, DeMetz DL: Fundamentals of Clinical Trials. Boston, John Wright PSG Inc, 1981, pp 69–88.
21. Geller J, Nelson CG, Pilbert JD, Pratt C: Effect of megestrol acetate on uroflow rates in patients with benign prostatic hypertrophy. Urology 14:467, 1979.
22. Glynn RJ, Campion EW, Bouchard GR, Silbert JE: The development of benign prostatic hyperplasia among volunteers in the normative aging study. Am J Epidemiol 121:78, 1985.
23. Graversen PH, Bruskewitz RC, Madsen PO: The predictive value of urodynamic investigations for results following prostatectomy. *In* Paulson DF (ed): Prostatic Disorders. Philadelphia, Lea & Febiger, 1989, pp 232–245.
24. Graversen PH, Gasser TC, Wasson JH et al: Controversies about indications for transurethral resection of the prostate. J Urol 141:475, 1989.
25. Greenfield S: The state of outcome research: Are we on target? N Engl J Med 320:1142, 1989.
26. Haylen BT, Sahby D, Sutherst JR, et al: Maximum and average urine flow rates in normal male and female populations—the Liverpool nomograms. Br J Urol 64:30, 1989.
27. Heyns CF, deKlerk DP: Pharmaceutical management of benign prostatic hyperplasia. *In* Paulson DF (ed): Prostatic Disorders. Philadelphia, Lea & Febiger, 1989, pp 204–231.
28. Hinman F Jr: Residual urine: Measurement and influence in management of obstruction. *In* Hinman F Jr (ed): Benign Prostatic Hypertrophy. New York, Springer-Verlag, 1983, pp 589–596.
29. Jensen KME: Clinical evaluation of routine urodynamic investigations in prostatism. Neurourol Urodynamics 8:545, 1989.
30. Jensen KME, Jorgensen JB, Magnesen P: Urodynamics in prostatism: II. Prognostic value of pressure-flow study combined with stop-flow test. Scand J Urol Nephrol (Suppl)114:72, 1988.
31. Kitada S, Ishisawa N: Urethral pressure profilometry in the prospective assessment for prostatectomy. J Urol 126:89, 1981.
32. Layton TM, Drach GW: Urinary flow rates: Measurement and adjustment. *In* Hinman F Jr (ed): Benign Prostatic Hypertrophy. New York, Springer-Verlag, 1983, pp 524–527.
33. Lebacqz K: Controlled clinical trials: Some ethical issues. Controlled Clinical Trials 1:29, 1979.
34. Lytton B, Emery JM, Howard BM: The incidence of benign prostatic obstruction. J Urol 99:639, 1968.
35. Madsen PO, Iversen P: A point system for selecting operative candidates. *In* Hinman F Jr (ed): Benign Prostatic Hypertrophy. New York, Springer-Verlag, 1983, pp 763–765.
36. Peters CA, Walsh PC: The effect of naferelin acetate, a luteinizing hormone releasing hormone agonist on benign prostatic hyperplasia. N Engl J Med 317:599, 1987.
37. Roos NP, Wennberg JE, Malenda DJ, et al: Mortality and reoperation after open and transurethral resection of the prostate for benign prostatic hyperplasia. N Engl J Med 320:1120, 1989.
38. Schafer W, Rubben H, Noppeney R, Deutz FJ: Obstructed and unobstructed prostatic obstruction: A plea for urodynamic objectivation of bladder outflow obstruction in benign prostatic hyperplasia. World J Urol 6:198, 1989.
39. Siroky MB, Olsson CA, Krane RJ: The flow rate nomogram: I. Development. J Urol 122:665, 1979.
40. Siroky MB, Olsson CA, Krane RJ: The flow rate nomogram: II. Clinical correlations. J Urol 123:208, 1980.
41. Susset JG, Picker P, Kretz M, Jorest R: Critical evaluation of uroflowmeters and analysis of normal curves. J Urol 109:874, 1973.
42. Wein AJ: Where are we: Clinical trials. *In* Zinner NR, Sterling AR (eds): Female Incontinence. New York, Allen R. Liss, 1981, pp 39–43.
43. Wein AJ: Evaluation of treatment response to drugs in benign prostatic hyperplasia. Urol Clin North Am 17:631, 1990.
44. Wein AJ: Principles for evaluation of pharmacologic agents. *In* Hinman F Jr (ed): Benign Prostatic Hypertrophy. New York, Springer-Verlag, 1983, pp 414–418.
45. Wein AJ, Barrett DM: Voiding Function and Dysfunction: A Logical and Practical Approach. Chicago, Year Book Medical Publishers, 1988, pp 278–280.

Chapter 13

TRANSURETHRAL RESECTION OF THE PROSTATE AND TRANSURETHRAL INCISION OF THE PROSTATE

WINSTON K. MEBUST

TRANSURETHRAL RESECTION OF THE PROSTATE

Transurethral resection of the prostate (TURP) for bladder outlet obstruction secondary to benign prostatic hyperplasia (BPH) has been considered to be the gold standard with which other therapeutic modalities are compared. TURP has been associated with good results, both objective and subjective. TURP has been thought to have a minimal mortality rate and an acceptable morbidity rate. However, Roos et al,[63, 64] using insurance claims data, pointed out that the mortality rate at 90 days was 2.5 per cent and the re-resection rate was 2 per cent per year, or 16 per cent at 8 years. In the recent Mebust et al study,[45] the mortality rate at 30 days was 0.2 per cent. The morbidity rate was 18 per cent, and, although the magnitude of the postoperative complications was not reflected in an increased hospital stay, it nevertheless was a significant morbidity rate.

Because of the significant morbidity rate and a suggestion that the long-term mortality and success rates were not as good as had been originally thought, new therapeutic modalities began to evolve. These included alpha-adrenergic blocking agents, hormonal agents, balloon dilatation, and the use of transurethral or transrectal hyperthermia. However, these new modalities must be measured against TURP as to objective and subjective effects upon patients, both immediate and long-term.

In 1989, the United States Congress passed the Omnibus Budget Reconciliation Act, which included the establishment of a new health care department, the Agency for Health Care Policy and Research. This agency was placed within the Department of Health and Human Services, under the Division of Public Health. It was given the mandate by Congress to develop guidelines for medical care and to fund outcomes research. Based upon the large numbers of TURP being performed, their impact on the cost of medical care, an apparent geographic variation in the incidence of TURP, as noted by Wennberg and Gittelsohn,[72] and the development of newer modalities of therapy, it became apparent to the Agency that guidelines were necessary for BPH.

A panel to develop guidelines for the diagnosis and management of BPH had been established by the American Urological Association, but this was impaneled by the new agency and expanded to represent other medical specialties, such as nursing, internal medicine, and radiology. Dr. John McConnell was named chairman and Dr. Claus Roehrborn the facilitator. The committee adopted Dr. David Eddy's[15] methodology of guideline development. Using meta-analysis, the committee was to evaluate existing literature on the diagnosis and treatment of BPH. Expert opinion could be used but would so be identified, when the question at hand could not be addressed by reports in the medical literature. The committee was to take into account the benefits and harms of the diagnostic or therapeutic modalities, consider patient preferences, and evaluate relative costs in writing a practice policy or guideline. Using Dr. Eddy's terminology, a standard would be any procedure, diagnostic or therapeutic, in which the benefits so outweighed the harms that all urologists would do that procedure. A guideline would be established when the benefits outweighed the harms and the majority of patients and physicians would use this procedure but there would be room for exceptions. An option would exist when the harms and benefits were not clearly defined or patient preference was not clearly defined for a given procedure and it was therefore left to the physician and patient to decide whether or not the procedure would be done. Using this terminology, the majority of recommendations would likely be options, followed by guidelines and rarely standards.

The committee reported their recommendations to the Agency for Health Care Policy and Research in October 1992, for subsequent submission to the Department of Health and Human Services for evaluation and implementation.

In this chapter diagnostic procedures, patient evaluation, and outcomes for TURP and transurethral incision of the prostate are reported using individual articles from the literature but also include recommendations of the Agency's BPH Panel.

Historical Review of Transurethral Prostatectomy

The development of transurethral surgery for BPH occurred primarily in the United States. However, Ambroise Paré, in the 16th century, is given credit for doing the first transurethral operation to relieve bladder outlet obstruction.[23] He recognized obstruction from urethral strictures, which he called carnosities. He used a curet and a sharpened hollow sound to shear off these carnosities and relieve obstruction. Sir William Blizard, in 1806, used a double gorget to cut directly into the bladder through the perineum to relieve prostatic obstruction.[52] This surgical approach was associated with significant hemorrhage, infection, incontinence, and operative death and never became widely accepted. In 1830, French surgeons Mercier, Civiale, and D'Etoilles modified the lithotrite so that the narrow blade was sharp. The new instrument was inserted per urethra and the bladder neck incised blindly. Again, because of the complications, this technique was never widely accepted.

In reviewing the development of TURP, Nesbit[51] cited three factors that are important in today's surgical procedure. The first was the development of the incandescent lamp by Edison in 1879. In 1887, Nitze and Leiter independently developed cystoscopes illuminated by the incandescent lamp. The second factor was the development of a high-frequency electrical current that could be used to cut tissue. The high-frequency current was discovered by Hertz in 1888, and in 1908 DeForest's invention of the vacuum tube permitted the development of a continuous high-frequency current. DeForest suggested that the current could be used to cut tissue in surgery. In 1924, Reinholdt Wappler, along with George Wyeth, developed the first practical cutting current instrument. The Wappler family was to have a significant role in the development of instruments for endoscopic

surgery. The McCarthy foroblique telescope, used in TURP, was built by Reinholdt Wappler. Spark gap generators were also being developed at the same time. Bovie of Harvard developed a generator with a heavily damped coagulating current for hemostasis. The two types of currents were put together in one unit by Frederick Wappler in 1931 and marketed as the "complex oscillator" by the American Cystoscope Manufacturers. The third important factor was the concept of a fenestrated tube introduced by Hugh Hampton Young in 1909. He engaged tissue in the fenestration of the tube and blindly sheared off the obstructing tissue with a tubular knife.

In 1926, Bumpus combined the cystoscope with a tubular punch and cauterization for prostate surgery. In 1926, Stern introduced a tungsten wire loop that could be used with a high-frequency current to resect tissue. All these concepts were brought together by McCarthy in 1932, when he introduced his direct-vision resectoscope with a foroblique lens and a wire loop for resection and cauterization of obstructing prostatic tissue.

Debates then raged over the technique of the operation—whether the surgeon should remove just the obstructing tissue or the entire adenoma. Because of the high re-resection rate associated with resecting the obstructing tissue alone, the accepted technique came to be removal of all the adenoma. Surgical technique may be important in explaining the differences in re-resection rates reported in different publications today.

Originally, distilled water was the most common irrigating fluid used. In 1947, Creevy and Webb[13] pointed out the danger of water causing intravascular hemolysis leading to increased morbidity and death rates. Emmett and co-workers,[17] reviewing two large series from the Mayo Clinic in which water or a nonhemolytic solution was used, found a distinct advantage of a nonhemolytic solution in reducing the mortality rate associated with TURP. Currently, studies by Madsen and his associates[40, 57] have pointed out the relationship of fluid absorption to pressure in the prostatic fossa and intravascular absorption during the end of the resection as venous sinuses are exposed.

In the 1970s, the development of a fiberoptic lighting system, together with the Hopkins wide-angle system, significantly improved endoscopic surgery.[34] Previously, the optical system was a series of small lenses placed in a rigid tube. In the Hopkins rod lens system, the air spaces are replaced by solid glass rods and the spacer tubes are shorter and thinner, resulting in minimal obstruction and an increase in the admission of light (Fig. 13–1).

The fiberoptic light system is basically a glass core surrounded by a material of lower refractive index (Fig. 13–2). Light is transmitted from a source through the glass fibers and is trapped and reflected at the inner surface between the primary core and a layer of less refractive material through the flexible core to the endoscope, where it is transmitted into the field.

Modifications in the resectoscope also occurred, such as the constant flow resectoscope described by Iglesias.[35] This permitted resection of the prostate with a relatively low intravesical pressure. The lenses in the optical

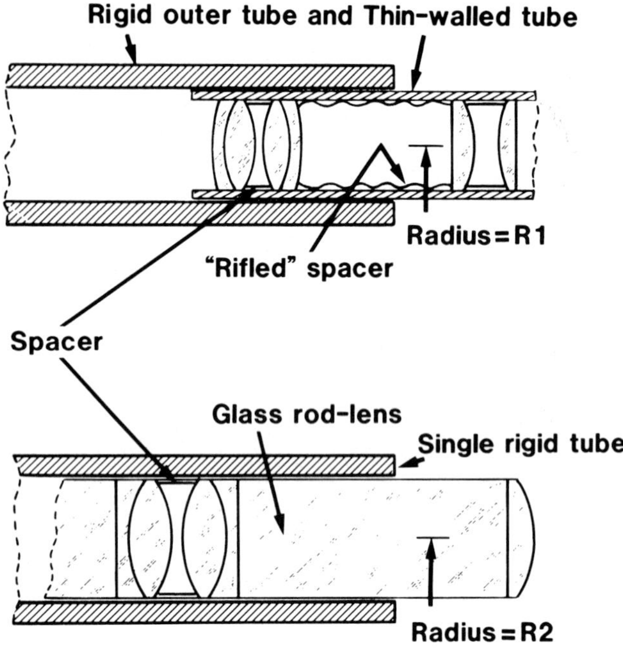

FIGURE 13–1. Traditional endoscope *(above)* had field and relay lens of glass with long air spaces. In the Hopkins lens system *(below)*, the roles of glass and lens are interchanged. The refractive index of glass is higher than that of air, and light transmission is increased. The thin-walled inner tube needed to construct the traditional endoscope is not needed with the glass rod construction. The functional diameter is increased ($R_2 > R_1$), and more light is transmitted in the Hopkins lens system. Modified from H. H. Hopkins. (From Mebust WK, Valk WL: Transurethral prostatectomy. *In* Hinman F Jr [ed]: Benign Prostatic Hypertrophy. New York, Springer-Verlag, 1983; with permission.)

system continue to be improved. The lens system has now been coupled to a television monitor so that the surgeon can operate directly off the monitor without looking through the lens.

Indications for Transurethral Prostatectomy

The indications and patient evaluation for TURP are covered in other chapters. However, certain aspects deserve additional comment.

Lytton et al,[37] in 1968, estimated that the chance of a 40-year-old man having a prostatectomy in his lifetime was approximately 10 per cent. However, Glynn et al,[22] in 1985, raised that estimate to 29 per cent. McPherson et al[44] noted that the incidence of prostatectomy per 100,000 population was 264 in New England, compared with 122 in England. Wennberg and Gittelsohn[72] noted the marked variation in incidence of TURP within the United States. These studies raised the question of whether different criteria were being used to select patients for surgery, not only internationally but also within the United States.

There are very few studies on the natural history of

patients who are seen initially because of modest symptoms of prostatism without absolute indication for intervention (i.e., acute urinary retention). Ball et al,[4] following 97 patients over 5 years, found that the patient symptoms were essentially the same in 52 per cent and worse in only 16.5 per cent. Urodynamic studies revealed little change in that particular group, and only 1.6 per cent developed retention. Conversely, Birkhoff et al,[8] following 26 patients for 3 years, found a 50 to 70 per cent deterioration in the patient's subjective symptoms and 71 per cent deterioration in objective criteria. The development of acute retention was unpredictable.

In the Mebust et al study,[45] 90 per cent of the patients undergoing TURP had symptoms of bladder outlet obstruction or bladder irritability. However, 70 per cent had another indication for surgery as well as symptoms (Table 13–1). Patient symptoms and the degree to which they bother him are an important consideration in whether the patient should have some type of intervention for BPH. Therefore, symptoms should be quantified so that they can be correlated with other parameters, such as flow rate and outcomes of the various interventions used to treat BPH. Currently, two systems are widely used, the Boyarsky[9] system reported in 1977 and the Madsen-Iversen[39] system in 1983. The latter gives more weight to bladder outlet obstructive symptoms.

Michael Barry, Michael O'Leary, and Floyd Fowler, at the request of the American Urological Association, developed a seven-question scoring system that evaluates both obstructive and irritative symptoms. All questions are given equal weight, and the total score possible is 35 points. Unlike the two previous scoring systems, this system was validated as to clarity, test/retest reliability, internal consistency, and criterion validity. This was done by comparing responses of two groups of patients. The BPH group consisted of patients treated by urologists for bladder outlet obstructive symptoms, and a control group consisted of patients ranging from 35 to 50 years of age who had minimal urinary tract

TABLE 13–1. INDICATIONS FOR PROSTATECTOMY AND COMBINATIONS OF OPERATIVE INDICATIONS

INDICATIONS FOR PROSTATECTOMY	NO. (%)
Symptoms of prostatism	3522 (90.7)
Significant residual urine	1336 (34.4)
Urinary retention, acute	1053 (27.1)
Recurrent urinary infection	479 (12.3)
Hematuria	465 (12.0)
Altered urodynamic function	385 (9.9)
Renal insufficiency	176 (4.5)
Bladder stones	116 (3.0)
Combination of operative indications	
Symptoms of prostatism only	1145 (29.5)
Prostatism, residual urine	577 (14.9)
Prostatism, acute retention	372 (9.6)
Prostatism, acute retention and residual urine	217 (5.6)

From Mebust WK, Holtgrewe HL, Cockett ATK, et al: Transurethral prostatectomy: Immediate and postoperative complications. A cooperative study of thirteen participating institutions evaluating 3,885 patients. J Urol 141:243–247, 1989, © by American Urological Assoc., Inc.; with permission.

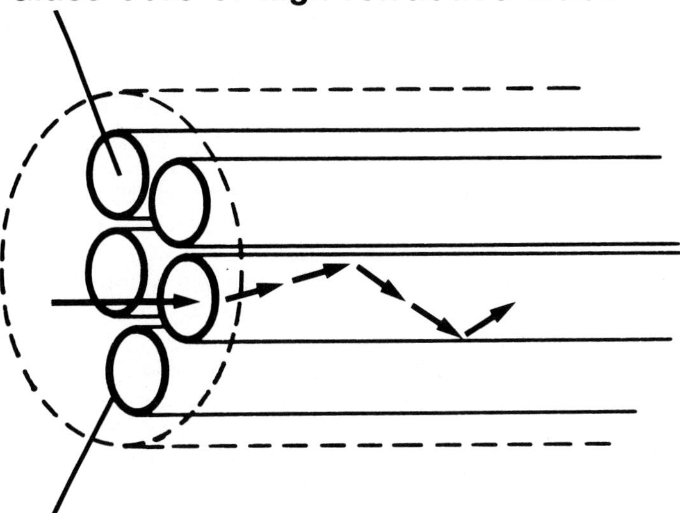

FIGURE 13–2. Glass fibers of high refractive index are surrounded by glass of a low refractive index, which keeps transmitted light trapped within the center core. (From Mebust WK, Valk WL: Transurethral prostatectomy. *In* Hinman F Jr [ed]: Benign Prostatic Hypertrophy. New York, Springer-Verlag, 1983; with permission.)

symptoms of prostatism. Several hundred patients were studied, and it became apparent that this system could differentiate between patients who did and did not have bladder outlet obstructive and irritative symptoms secondary to BPH.

This scoring system was subsequently adopted by the World Health Organization as the international standard in 1991. It was designated the World Health Organization Prostate Symptom Score (WHOPSS). In addition, however, one question was added, reflecting the patient's general overall quality of life with reference to his symptoms of prostatism (Fig. 13–3).

Quantification of patient symptoms now is possible and can be used by the physician in evaluating the

WHOPSS							
	not at all	less than 1 time in 5	less than half the time	about half the time	more than half the time	almost always	
1. Over the past month or so, how often have you had a sensation of not emptying your bladder completely after you finished urinating?	0	1	2	3	4	5	
2. Over the past month or so, how often have you had to urinate again less than two hours after you finished urinating?	0	1	2	3	4	5	
3. Over the past month or so, how often have you found you stopped and started again several times when you urinated?	0	1	2	3	4	5	
4. Over the past month or so, how often have you found it difficult to postpone urination?	0	1	2	3	4	5	
5. Over the past month or so, how often have you had a weak urinary stream?	0	1	2	3	4	5	
6. Over the past month or so, how often have you had to push or strain to begin urination?	0	1	2	3	4	5	
	none	1 time	2 times	3 times	4 times	5 or more times	
7. Over the past month or so, how many times did you most typically get up to urinate from the time you went to bed at night until the time you got up in the morning?	0	1	2	3	4	5	
						Total WHOPSS Score S = ___	
QUALITY OF LIFE DUE TO URINARY SYMPTOMS							
	delighted	pleased	mostly satisfied	mixed about equally satisfied and dissatisfied	mostly dissatisfied	unhappy	terrible
1. If you were to spend the rest of your life with your urinary condition just the way it is now, how would you feel about that?	0	1	2	3	4	5	6
						Quality of Life assessment index L = ___	

FIGURE 13–3. World Health Organization Prostate Symptom Score (WHOPSS). Adopted June 1991.

patient. However, it must be stressed that this is only one parameter used in making the decision about whether or not the patient would need to have some type of intervention for his BPH. Nevertheless, it could be used in stratifying patients by their response to different types of therapy and objective parameters, such as flow rates.

However, certain indications have been accepted as standard indications for intervention by urologists (i.e., acute retention, significant residual urine, hematuria, recurrent infections, and azotemia). In the Mebust et al[45] study, 27 per cent of the patients had acute urinary retention as the primary indication for surgery (Table 13–1). It is impossible to predict which patient, with modest symptoms of prostatism (i.e., symptoms of bladder outlet obstruction and bladder hyperreflexia or irritability), will subsequently develop acute urinary retention.

Residual urine and chronic retention have been considered signs of bladder decompensation in patients with obstructing BPH. However, residual urine can also be secondary to decreased bladder contractility from other disease processes, such as neurogenic disease and the aging process. Furthermore, failure to find residual urine does not mean that the patient does not require surgery.

Hinman,[30] following a series of patients over several years, noted that there seemed to be a gradual increase in residual urine. He suggested that 60 ml might be the indication for intervention. However, a progressive increase in residual urine or chronic urinary retention does not necessarily mean that the patient ultimately develops acute retention.

The amount of residual urine at which surgical intervention should be recommended before bladder changes become irreversible is unknown. In the Mebust et al study,[45] the amount of residual urine considered to be significant was left to the individual investigators, but for 35 per cent of these patients significant residual urine was one of the indications for surgical intervention.

The BPH Panel viewed the measurement of residual urine as an option in which the harms and benefits were not clearly known. It was their position that this is a safety measure to be used in following patients to be sure that they do not develop progressive urinary retention unknown to the urologist and thereby develop irreversible bladder damage.

Recurrent gross hematuria has also been considered an indication for intervention; it occurred in 12 per cent of the patients in the Mebust et al study.[45] The exact pathophysiology of hematuria secondary to BPH is unclear but can lead to significant complications for the patients (i.e., clot urinary retention).

Recurrent preoperative infection has also been considered an absolute indication for intervention. Preoperative infection was found in 12 per cent of patients in the Mebust et al study.[45] However, the incidence was significantly higher in the black population (21 per cent). In contrast, Melchior et al[47] found an incidence of 25 per cent in a study of more than 2000 consecutive cases in which preoperative urinary cultures were done routinely. Conversely, Hasner[27] found an incidence of 8.6 per cent in a smaller series of patients. The source of

infection presumably is the prostate, but its relationship to the presence or absence of residual urine is unclear. Nevertheless, the assumption is that infection related to bladder outlet obstruction will probably recur unless the obstructing prostate is surgically corrected.

Azotemia, which we have defined as a serum creatinine greater than 1.5 mg/dl, is another indication for intervention when the azotemia is secondary to bladder outlet obstruction. Azotemia was found in 4.5 per cent of the patients preoperatively in the American Urological Association (AUA) Cooperative Study.[45] However, patients who have azotemia secondary to bladder outlet obstruction from BPH usually are found to have azotemia at the time they present for consideration for intervention. Azotemia has been associated with an increase in morbidity rate, as these patients are usually anemic and do not tolerate fluid overloads, which can occur during TURP. Furthermore, in patients found to be azotemic at the time they are considered for intervention, the cause of the azotemia may not be completely clear. It could be secondary to another disease process, such as hypertension. A period of catheter drainage (i.e., 10 to 14 days) may be necessary to establish the diagnosis and permit improvement of the renal function prior to surgery.

Preoperative Evaluation

Today, patients are usually admitted on the day of surgery, and their general evaluation must therefore be completed on an outpatient basis. In the AUA Cooperative Study,[45] only 23 per cent of patients did not have significant prior medical problems. The most common problems were pulmonary (14.5 per cent), gastrointestinal (13.2 per cent), myocardial infarction (12.5 per cent), cardiac arrhythmias (12.4 per cent), and renal insufficiency (9.8 per cent).

Prior to this study, the most common cause of death, after TURP, was cardiovascular complications.[33, 47] Patients with renal insufficiency were also noted to be at higher risk. Therefore, it is critically important to evaluate the cardiac, pulmonary, and renal status of patients prior to surgery. A complete blood count, chemistry profile, chest radiogram, and ECG are usual. In the Mebust et al study,[45] 60 per cent of the patients had their upper tracts evaluated. However, the BPH Panel thought that upper tract evaluation should not be done routinely but only in certain circumstances. They found that it was not useful as a screening instrument to identify the patient with incidental renal cell carcinoma. Rather, they believed that indications for upper tract evaluation were hematuria, urinary tract infections, a history of renal calculi, azotemia, or prior urologic surgery. Had these indications been followed, the incidence of upper tract evaluation would be closer to 20 per cent than to 60 per cent, as was found by Mebust et al. Furthermore, the panel thought that intravenous pyelography or ultrasonography should be done at the discretion of the urologist because there would be variations in the patient's clinical status and the availability of imaging techniques. The BPH panel also thought that cystoscopy should not be done routinely in the urologist's office prior to surgery but rather that this could be done at the time of surgery. However, the panel believed that certain situations warranted the use of cystoscopy. This would be when invasive therapy had been recommended, and there was a need to evaluate the size and configuration of the prostate and to rule out other pathology, such as stricture and bladder tumors, in determining the most efficacious invasive therapy.

Urodyamics as a method of preoperative patient evaluation is discussed elsewhere in this book. However, the BPH Panel believed that uroflowmetry was an option for the urologist. It was their opinion that the flow rate, corrected for volume voided, could be useful in selecting patients who would respond better to surgery. They noted that if the maximum (Q_{max}) was less than 15 ml/sec, patients seemed to respond to surgery more objectively than subjectively. It has been the author's opinion that the peak flow rate, Q_{max} corrected for volume, is a useful tool in evaluating patients in whom intervention is being considered. Further, if the patient has a flow rate greater than 15 ml/sec but is severely symptomatic, additional urodynamic testing might be appropriate.

Anesthesia

Sinha and associates[66] reported doing TURPs with local anesthesia. However, most patients are operated on with either a general anesthetic, an epidural, or a subdural spinal block. Nielsen and colleagues[54] noted no difference in blood loss between epidural and general anesthesia. McGowan and Smith[43] evaluated spinal anesthetic versus general anesthetic and found no difference in blood loss, postoperative morbidity, or mortality. However, there was a higher incidence of cardiac arrhythmias with general anesthesia.

Our conclusion is that surgery can be done with either form of anesthesia and that it should be tailored to a particular patient situation.

Perioperative Antibiotics

Preoperative infection should be treated with appropriate antibiotics prior to surgery. However, the role of prophylactic antibiotics remains controversial. Gibbons et al[21] and others found that they did not reduce postoperative infection, but Nielsen et al[55] and others found them to be beneficial.

The length of time during which prophylactic antibiotics should be used in the perioperative period also is not clear. In the Mebust et al study,[45] 61 per cent of the patients were given prophylactic antibiotics and 49 per cent received them beyond 8 days. We believe that the patient should be started on systemic prophylactic antibiotics (e.g., a first-generation cephalosporin) just before surgery. Patients should then be switched to an oral antibiotic (e.g., nitrofurantoin) when intravenous fluids are discontinued. The antibiotics should be continued for 2 to 3 days after the catheter is removed.

Irrigating Fluids

Since Creevy and Webb[13] pointed out the danger of water causing hemolysis, the emphasis has been on using a fluid that is nonhemolytic. Water is certainly less expensive, and surgery can be done safely with it, but today probably 80 per cent of surgeons use a nonhemolytic solution.

In addition to the dangers of hemolysis, there was the concern about the transurethral resection syndrome. This is characterized by mental confusion, nausea, vomiting, hypertension, bradycardia, and visual disturbance.

In the 1950s, several studies were undertaken to determine the amount of fluid absorbed during TURP. Hagstrom,[24] weighing patients preoperatively and postoperatively, calculated that approximately 20 ml/min was absorbed by the patient. However, there appeared to be a wide variation among patients, and it was Oester and Madsen,[57] using a double-isotope technique, who demonstrated that the average was around 1000 ml. Furthermore, one third of the total fluid was absorbed intravenously when the venous sinuses were opened, meaning that most of the fluid was in the periprostatic area. Madsen and Naber[40] demonstrated that the pressure in the prostatic fossa and the amount of fluid absorbed depended upon the height of the fluid above the patient. They noted that when the height of the fluid was changed from 60 to 70 cm, fluid absorption increased more than twofold. They noted that approximately 300 ml/min of fluid was needed for good vision, and this could not be achieved when the fluid was below 60 cm. These observations led to the modification of the surgical technique, such as the Iglesias constant flow resectoscope, the use of a suprapubic catheter, and meticulous and frequent drainage of the bladder when intermittent irrigation is used.

A variety of fluids are used today, such as 1.5 per cent glycine, Cytol (a combination of sorbitol and mannitol), and mannitol. These are not isotonic fluids but rather nonhemolytic; e.g., 1.5 per cent glycine has an osmolarity of approximately 200 mOsm, compared with a normal serum osmolarity of approximately 290 mOsm/kg. Although these fluids do not cause hemolysis, they can be associated with the transurethral resection syndrome.

Harrison and associates[26] pointed out that the transurethral resection syndrome appears to be related to dilutional hyponatremia. Glycine is metabolized to glycolic acid and ammonium, and ammonia intoxication has been suggested as a possible cause of the syndrome.[60] The direct toxic effect of glycine has also been suggested as a possible cause. Glycine is an inhibitor of neurotransmission, and the visual disturbances seen are not the same as one would see with cortical edema. Light perception is usually lost in cortical edema but not usually in the transurethral resection syndrome. Intraocular pressure also has been noted to be unchanged in these patients. O'Donnell[56] suggested that the cause of the transurethral resection syndrome could be absorption of substances from the prostate during the resection. However, correction of the syndrome is quickly achieved with hypertonic saline or diuretics.

Patients usually do not become symptomatic until their serum sodium reaches 125 mEq/L. As noted by Mebust et al,[45] the risk is higher if the gland is larger than 45 grams and the resection exceeds 90 minutes. The incidence of the transurethral resection syndrome in that study was 2 per cent and in 66 per cent of cases, it was corrected simply with diuretics and observation. The relative sodium deficit can be calculated by assuming that 20 per cent of the body weight is extracellular fluid and then calculating the difference between the preoperative and postoperative sodium value. However, this is not a true sodium deficit because the patient is merely overloaded with water. In general, the average patient can be corrected with 200 ml of 3 per cent saline, but this must be given slowly, preferably in several doses, with monitoring of the serum sodium in between.

Cooling the irrigating fluid has been suggested as a means of reducing blood loss.[65] However, others have found no apparent difference in blood loss when the fluid is cooled to 8°C and when warm fluid is used.[72] Allen[2] noted that by using fluid at the ambient temperature, in 1 hour a significant number of patients had a 1°C loss of body temperature and at 2 hours, 2°C, which resulted in significant shivering. To preserve patient comfort, we therefore recommend that the irrigating fluid be warmed and see no apparent problem in increased blood loss.

SURGICAL TECHNIQUE

At the time of surgery, the urethra is calibrated with bougies à boule. The majority of patients calibrate at 28 Fr or greater, but a significant number are smaller.[18] If the distal urethra is inadequate to accommodate the more commonly used 28 Fr urethroscope, a smaller size should be selected. For several years, we have used a 24 Fr resectoscope sheath successfully, even in patients with very large glands.

If the distal urethra is inadequate to accommodate a resectoscope sheath, a perineal urethrostomy may be performed. When one inserts the resectoscope through the more commodious bulbous urethra, the incidence of postoperative urethral stricture is reduced. The technique has been described elsewhere. Basically, a 24 Fr grooved van Buren sound is inserted into the urethra and the perineum tented up. The sound is stabilized with a Conger clamp, and a 2-cm midline incision is made in the bulbous urethra. The cut edges of the urethra are stabilized with stay sutures of 2-0 chromic to facilitate insertion of the resectoscope sheath and subsequently the catheter (Fig. 13–4).

Alternatively, an internal urethrotomy can be done, as advocated by Emmett and associates[18] and Bailey and Shearer.[3] The most common area of narrowing is the postnavicular region. In this circumstance, we prefer to perform a dorsal internal urethrotomy using a curved blade (Fig. 13–5) because a liberal ventral meatotomy often leads to a splattering or errant direction of the urinary stream postoperatively.

Various surgical techniques have been espoused by urologists for removing the prostate adenoma transurethrally. They all use the basic principle that the resection should be done routinely in a step-by-step manner. The resection technique may vary according to the size or configuration of the adenoma but should be based on an orderly plan. Further, all techniques use the principle of resecting ventrally first so that the adenomatous tissue drops down, allowing the surgeon to resect from the top downward rather from the floor upward. However, some surgeons have suggested resecting the floor and the median lobe tissue initially to improve water flow and

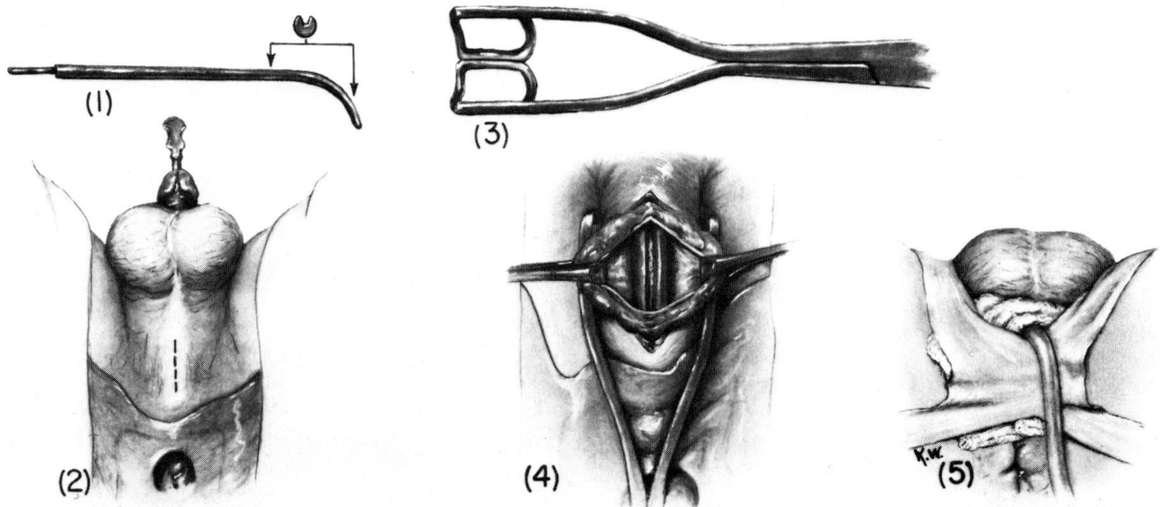

FIGURE 13–4. Grooved sound (1), Conger clamp (3), and technique of perineal urethrotomy (2, 4, 5). (From Mebust WK, Foret JD, Valk WL: Transurethral surgery. *In* Harrison JH, Walsh PC, Perlmutter AD, Gittes RF, Stamey TA [eds]: Campbell's Urology, 4th ed. Philadelphia, WB Saunders Co, 1979, pp 2361–2381.)

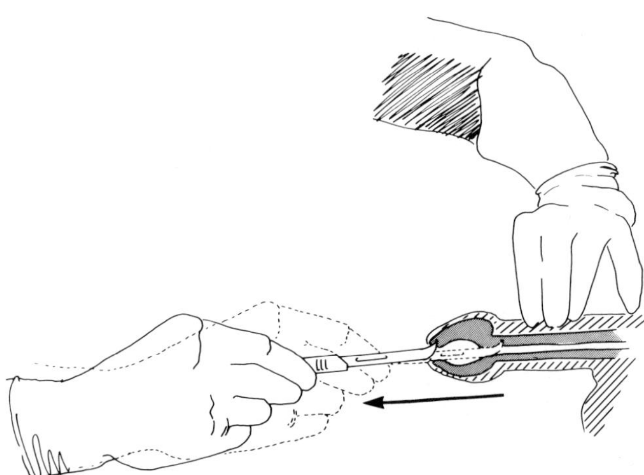

FIGURE 13–5. In doing a dorsal meatotomy, the scalpel with a curved blade is inserted into the urethral meatus beyond the fossa navicularis. The knife is withdrawn parallel to the urethral axis at 12 o'clock. (From Mebust WK: A review of TURP complications and the AUA National Cooperative Study. AUA Update Series 8(24): 186–191, 1989; with permission.)

then proceeding with the ventral resection of the prostate.

As a teaching technique, we often resect one lobe of the prostate, allowing the resident to resect the other. Our standard technique is that described by Nesbit more than 45 years ago.[52] The Nesbit surgical technique is divided into three stages. In the first (Fig. 13–6), the surgeon resects the fibers at the bladder neck and the immediately adjacent prostatic adenoma. Resection is usually begun at 12 o'clock and continued clockwise. At the end of the procedure, if the bladder neck appears to be prominent, we incise it, as recommended by Kulb and co-workers,[36] to reduce the incidence of vesical neck contracture. In the second stage (Fig. 13–7), the adenoma is resected in quadrants. The resectoscope is placed in front of the verumontanum, and the resection begun at the 12 o'clock position so that the lateral lobe tissue falls into the midfossa. The upper or ventral quadrants are resected first. The resection is carried down to the fibers of the surgical capsule. As one resects the lower two quadrants in the floor of the prostate, these fibers become less distinct. The resection is done with an O'Connor rectal shield in place. We use the Iglesias modification of the Nesbit scope so that one hand is free to palpate the depth of resection as the floor tissue is removed. In the third stage (Fig. 13–8), the adenoma is removed immediately proximal to the external sphincter mechanism, preserving the verumontanum. The prostatic apex is concave, and a sweeping motion is used so that the loop is moved from a lateral to a medial direction as it approaches the sphincter. However, Shah and associates[65a] pointed out that 10 to 20 per cent of the prostate projects below the verumontanum. Therefore, it may be necessary to have a small rim of adenoma to avoid sphincter injury.

Turner-Warwick[69] has divided the sphincter mechanism into three areas: the first, immediately adjacent to verumontanum; the second from the verumontanum to the capsule; and the third, beyond the capsule (Fig. 13–9). Injury to the second and third portions of the sphincter can result in significant urinary incontinence. Therefore, we usually begin our resection by placing the resectoscope next to the verumontanum and continue resecting up to the 12 o'clock position, rather than starting at the 12 o'clock position as in the prior two steps.

Intraoperative Modifications and Options and Postoperative Care

In 1975, Iglesias and co-workers[35] introduced the constant-flow resectoscope, suggesting that it would allow a continuous resection, clearer vision, and low intraprostatic fossa pressure with decreased fluid absorption. The surgical time should also be decreased. However, Stephenson and associates[67] compared constant flow and the standard interrupted flow instruments and could find no difference in speed of resection or amount of blood loss or glycine absorption. Similarly, Flechner and Williams[19] found no difference between the two instruments. However, Gellman[20] cautioned that it was important to resect the floor tissue first to improve flow characteristics. At this time, the problem seems to be maintaining a constant inflow and outflow while keeping the pressure low within the prostatic fossa and maintaining good visibility. Therefore, constant-flow irrigation does not appear to have clear-cut advantage over the more standard intermittent irrigation during TURP.

In the early 1970s, Bergman[6] and others[49, 62] suggested that a temporary suprapubic cannula could facilitate

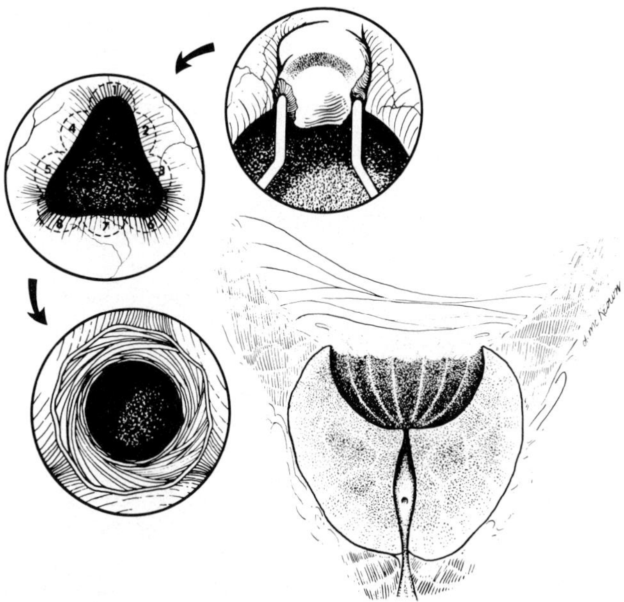

FIGURE 13–6. Nesbit Stage I transurethral prostatectomy. Resection is begun at the bladder neck at the 12 o'clock position. A full-thickness bite with the loop is taken and the resection continued step-wise around the neck bearing the bladder neck fibers. (From Mebust WK, Foret JD, Valk WL: Transurethral surgery. *In* Harrison JH, Walsh PC, Perlmutter AD, Gittes RF, Stamey TA [eds]: Campbell's Urology, 4th ed. Philadelphia, WB Saunders Co, 1979, pp 2361–2381.)

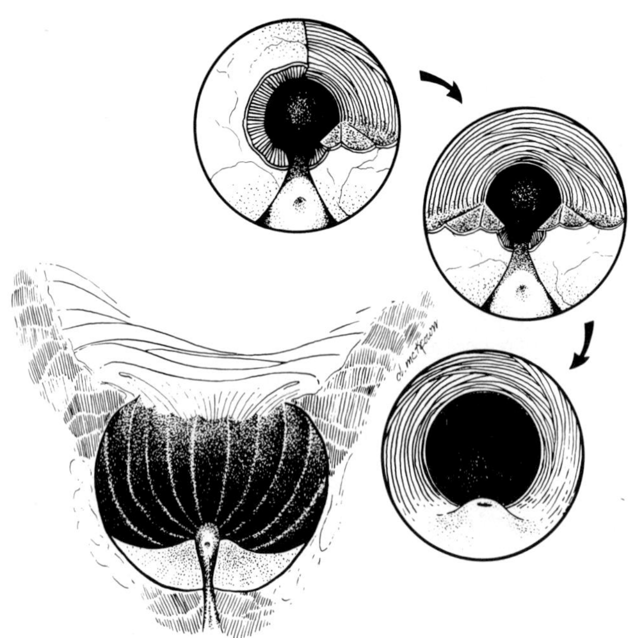

FIGURE 13–7. Nesbit Stage II transurethral prostatectomy. Stepwise resection of the midprostatic fossa in quadrants. The striations of the prostatic capsule are differentiated from the "snowlike" adenoma and limit the depth of resection. (From Mebust WK, Foret JD, Valk WL: Transurethral surgery. *In* Harrison JH, Walsh PC, Perlmutter AD, Gittes RF, Stamey TA [eds]: Campbell's Urology, 4th ed. Philadelphia, WB Saunders Co, 1979, pp 2361–2381.)

TURP by allowing a continuous flow system with reduced absorption of fluids. In 1974, Madsen and Frimodt-Moller[38] reported 577 cases with no problems of fluid absorption but did note a slightly greater blood loss than in conventional TURP. The pressure of the irrigating fluid in the bladder was 8 cm of H_2O and significantly less than the 10 to 15 cm of pelvic venous

pressure. Comparing the suprapubic drainage technique with the Iglesias suction constant flow, Holmquist and co-workers[31] found that the operating time was shorter and the transvesical pressure lower with the former.

During the surgical procedure, a penile erection may occur which can abort surgery unless a perineal urethrostomy is performed. We have found success with ketamine, 0.5 to 0.7 mg/kg, in reducing penile erection. However, others[71] found it not to be successful, and currently we use dilute epinephrine or ephedrine injected directly into the corpora cavernosa.

Vasectomy had previously been recommended as a means to prevent postoperative epididymitis. However, Whitlock and associates[73] found that epididymitis occurred in 5 per cent of patients having a vasectomy and 2 per cent of those who did not. The failure of vasectomy to reduce epididymitis significantly was also found in the Mebust et al study[45] and therefore is not recommended as a routine procedure.

Postoperatively, a 24 Fr catheter is inserted. Some of the newer plastic catheters have an internal diameter equivalent to 24 Fr yet, because of their thin wall, have the external circumference equivalent to an 18 Fr. The catheter is attached to a closed drainage system that incorporates an intermittent or constant irrigation system. We found that constant irrigation using 500 ml/hr of saline significantly reduces the incidence of postoperative clot occlusion. The catheter is then removed as soon as the urine is clear, usually on the first or second postoperative day.

Results

Over the past almost 60 years, there has been a gradual reduction in the mortality rate associated with

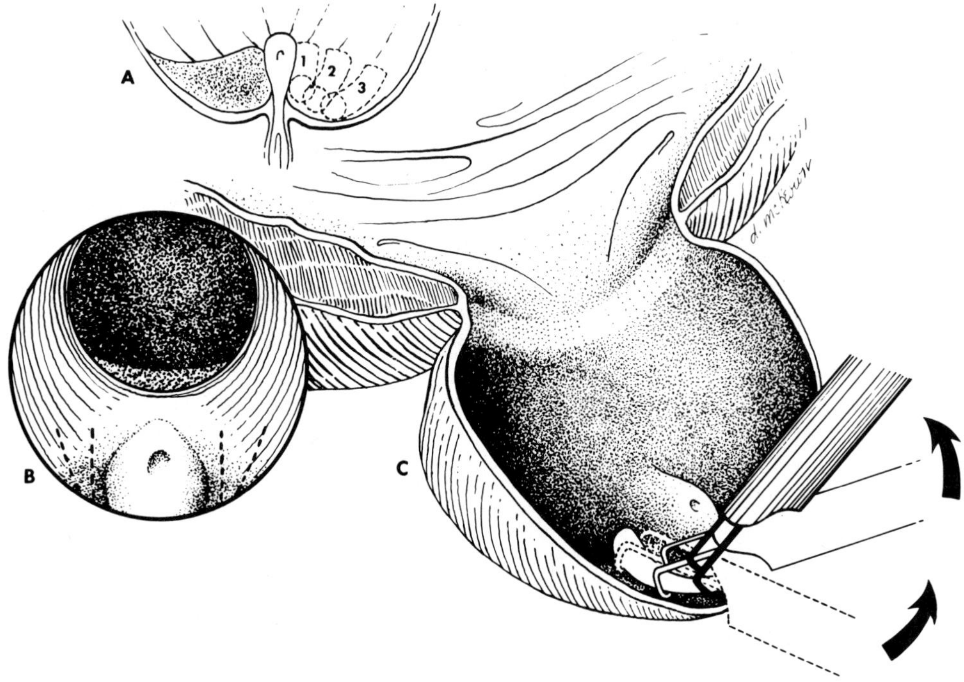

FIGURE 13–8. Stage III transurethral prostatectomy. *A,* Verumontanum is grooved (step I) and the resection carried laterally (steps II and III). *B,* Postresection of the adenoma adjacent to the verumontanum. *C,* Movement of the scope in a lateral to medial direction, emphasizing the concavity of the apical prostatic fossa. (From Mebust WK, Foret JD, Valk WL: Transurethral surgery. *In* Harrison JH, Walsh PC, Perlmutter AD, Gittes RF, Stamey TA [eds]: Campbell's Urology, 4th ed. Philadelphia, WB Saunders Company, 1979, pp 2361–2381.)

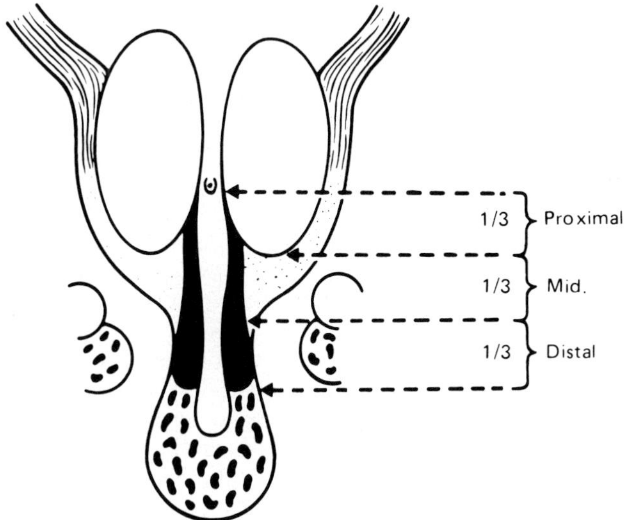

FIGURE 13–9. The distal sphincter mechanism has been divided into three parts by Turner-Warwick: (1) The distal third forms the thickness of the walls of the membranous urethra distal to the apex of the prostatic capsule. (2) The middle third is located within the apex of the prostate capsule. (3) The proximal third extends upward onto the inner surface of the apical prostatic tissue up to the level of the verumontanum. (From Turner-Warwick R: The sphincter mechanisms: Their relation to prostatic enlargement and its treatment. *In* Hinman F Jr [ed]: Benign Prostatic Hypertrophy. New York, Springer-Verlag, 1983; with permission.)

TURP, from 5 per cent in the 1930s[61] to 2.5 per cent in 1962[32] to 1.3 percent in 1974[47] and 0.2 per cent in 1989.[46] Prior to the Mebust et al[45] study, the most common cause of death reported was cardiovascular complications. However, the Mebust et al study found that the most common cause of death was sepsis occurring in patients who were debilitated and had other systemic disease processes.

The morbidity rate in the Mebust et al study[45] was 18 per cent. This was similar to the rates reported in 1962 and 1974. Postoperative complications were defined as any untoward deviation from the expected result, irrespective of the effect of the event. In fact, although the morbidity rate was similar to that in previous studies, the hospital stay was much shorter, suggesting that the events were either less significant or better managed than previously.

The most common problem was failure to void, occurring in 6.5 per cent, half of whom had hypotonic bladders. Postoperative bleeding occurred in 3.9 per cent. Bleeding was defined as need for blood transfusions, but 74 per cent required two units or less of blood. The incidence was higher in patients who had greater than 45 grams of tissue resected (7.5 versus 1.5 per cent) or if the resection time was greater than 90 minutes (7.3 versus 0.2 per cent). Clot retention occurred in 3.3 per cent and infection in 2.3 per cent. Preoperative infection was noted in 11 per cent, and an additional 60 per cent received postoperative antibiotics. The incidence of preoperative infection was certainly less than reported by Chilton and colleagues[11] (20 per cent), Murphy and associates[50] (30 per cent), and Melchior and co-workers[47] (23 per cent). In the last-named

study, all patients had cultures done preoperatively, which was not necessarily the case in the Mebust et al[45] study. Therefore, the incidence of infection preoperatively could have been higher. Nevertheless, the postoperative infection rate, documented by cultures, of 2.3 per cent is similar to the 5 per cent reported by Symes and associates.

In the Mebust et al[45] study, certain risk factors for complications were noted. In patients over age 80, the postoperative morbidity rate was 22.6 per cent, with the most common problems being failure to void and infection. Black men were found to present with acute retention more commonly than white men (44.7 versus 24.7 per cent), had a higher incidence of preoperative infection (21 versus 10 per cent), and had a higher incidence of existing disease, such as stroke. Acute retention, which occurred in 27 per cent of patients, was associated with an increase of postoperative complications, such as infection (4.3 versus 1.5 per cent), failure to void (11 versus 3.6 per cent), and hypotonic bladder (8.4 versus 1.7 per cent).

The Agency for Health Care Policy and Research BPH Panel, in reviewing the literature on transurethral prostatectomy, noted that 87 per cent of patients had improvement of symptoms, 10.5 per cent were unchanged, and 1.9 per cent were worse. The biggest reason for failure to improve symptoms is the persistence or increase of symptoms related to an unstable detrusor (e.g., uninhibited contractions). However, the panel noted that the flow rate increased from 7.9 to 18.2 ml/sec following surgery. Following TURP, the incidence of incontinence was stress (2.2 per cent), urge (2.5 per cent), and total incontinence (0.7 per cent).

The incidence of impotence has been reported to be between 4 and 40 per cent.[25, 33] The BPH Panel found an average incidence report of 13.7 per cent, but having any open surgical procedure was associated with a 5.2 per cent incidence. However, the incidence of 13.7 per cent associated with TURP is lower than for open surgical procedures, such as retropubic prostatectomy (17 per cent), suprapubic prostatectomy (20 per cent), and perineal prostatectomy (32 per cent). In the Mebust et al study,[45] the overall incidence was 3.5 per cent. However, only 1000 patients appeared to have reasonable data to evaluate and, in this subset, the incidence of decreased sexual function was 13 per cent. It is extremely difficult to get good data on erectile impotency secondary to TURP. Critically important in this evaluation are the patient's perception of potency before and after surgery, the presence or absence of an active sexual partner, and general sexual activity of the patient prior to surgery, in that if the patient was having difficulty prior to surgery, in all probability it would get worse. The cause of postoperative impotency is unknown and one can only speculate about possible causes. Nevertheless, impotency is associated with TURP and should be called to the attention of the patient.

Long-term Follow-up

Interestingly, very few data exist on patients followed for several years after TURP. Bruskewitz and associates,[10] in following a series of patients over 3 years, noted at 1 year that patient symptoms were improved in 84 per cent and 10 per cent were approximately the same; at 3 years, 75 per cent remained improved and 13 per cent were the same. The change in symptoms was the development of urge incontinence in those patients several years after surgery. Only one patient among the 84 patients studied required a repeat resection, for an incidence of 2 per cent. However, 10 per cent of patients developed a vesical neck contracture, and all had small prostates preoperatively. There were three late deaths from cancer (3.5 per cent).

Malone and associates[42] reviewed 500 consecutive prostatectomies followed between 5 and 8 years. They noted a significant difference in the 3-year mortality rate between those who presented with acute and chronic retention. The survival rate at 3 years for those with acute retention was 80 per cent, whereas in those with chronic retention it was 65 per cent. Eighty per cent of the patients were asymptomatic. However, those with chronic retention (36 per cent) still had residual symptoms of poor stream, nocturia, and flow rates compatible with a failed detrusor.

Chilton and associates,[11] in studying a large series of patients for 5 years, noted that 4 per cent required re-resection for benign disease during this time. A delayed mortality rate of 0.8 per cent was seen in a group of patients dying from cancer unrelated to the surgery.

Meyhoff and Nordling[48] noted that 90 per cent of their patients were considered to have satisfactory results at 5 years after TURP. Flow rates were improved from preoperative values, although there had been a slight decline in flow rates over the 5-year period. They did, however, note an 8 per cent re-resection rate, but all were patients with essentially small glands, suggesting that these might have been postoperative vesical neck contractures.

Bergman and associates[7] noted a re-resection rate of 2.8 per cent at 5.5 years. Ball and Smith,[5] in following a series of patients, noted that flow rates remained improved postoperatively, but there was a slight decrease over the 5 years that they were followed. Assuming a linear progression, it would take approximately 24 to 30 years to return to preoperative flow rates.

However, Roos and Ramsey[63] found a significant difference in the re-resection rate and late mortality rate following TURP. Using insurance claims data in Manitoba, they noted a re-resection rate of 2 per cent per year, or 16 per cent at 8 years. Information about the initial size of gland requiring repeat resection was not available, nor was the amount of tissue removed at the time of the second resection known. They also noted a mortality rate of 2.5 per cent at 90 days after surgery.

Roos and associates,[64] in a subsequent publication using claims data information from England, Denmark, and Manitoba, Canada, noted that the reoperation rate ranged from 2.7 to 6.7 times greater for TURP than for an open operation. Death rate at 90 days was higher than previously recognized and definitely higher in those who had TURP than in those who had an open prostatectomy. One might assume that the difference in mortality rate was based upon patient selection. However,

Malenka and associates[41] did a careful chart review of the patients in Manitoba, comparing those having TURP with those having an open prostatectomy. The mortality rate seemed to be higher with TURP, and the cause of death most commonly was myocardial infarction in the TURP group. There did not seem to be any differences in the comorbidity factors between the two groups.

This information, based on insurance claims data, is clearly different with respect to long-term mortality and reoperation rate, compared with previous studies that used a chart-review, retrospective analysis. The re-resection rate could be related to the skill of the surgeon or perhaps a higher incidence of vesical neck contracture than had been noted in the other studies. The mortality rate also could have been influenced by many factors, such as the type of hospital in which the surgery was performed, the skill of the surgeon, the size of the gland, the length of operating time, or predisposing cardiovascular problems.

Because of these uncertainties and the significance pointed out by these insurance claims-review studies, a national cooperative prospective study is being undertaken by the American Urological Association and Dr. John Wennberg and his associates at Dartmouth College. They intend to compare watchful waiting, TURP, alpha-adrenergic blockade, and open prostatectomy with reference to the course of the disease, immediate and long-term, following intervention. At this time, five pilot studies are under way, but whether or not the additional 15 centers will be funded to complete the study is not known.

TRANSURETHRAL INCISION OF THE PROSTATE

Historical Review

Transurethral incision of the prostate (TUIP) is not a new procedure. Edwards et al[16] credit Bottini, in 1887, with describing the technique, but Hedlund and Ek[28] credit Guthrie in 1834. Orandi published the first significant series on TUIP in 1973.[58] He credits Aboulken and Steg[1] with calling this concept to the attention of the modern urologist. In 1964, they reported a 75 per cent success rate with divulsion of the prostate to relieve bladder outlet obstruction. Unfortunately, profuse bleeding, incontinence, and infection occurred frequently. It appeared to Orandi that a controlled rupture of the prostatic urethra by endoscopic incisions in predetermined locations eliminates these complications. The procedure seems to be most useful in those who have a small prostate, which has been called a primary vesical neck contracture, median bar, or sclerosis du col, and in those who have obstructive bladder outlet symptoms. Classically, this patient has been a younger man than those undergoing TURP. The advantage of TUIP is that it is quick, technically easier, and associated with less morbidity and less retrograde ejaculation than TURP.

The technique is relatively simple compared with

TURP. It can be done using two incisions, as described by Orandi, or one incision, as described by Christensen and associates.[12] Using a Collings knife, the incision is performed at 5 o'clock and 7 o'clock positions, starting at the ureteral orifice and carrying it to the verumontanum (Fig. 13–10). The incision should be carried deeply so that the deeper portions of the prostatic incision have the fine filaments of the external capsule with occasional protrusion of fat. Care must be taken not to cause undue extravasation or to enter the rectum. The depth of the incision is relatively easy to determine at the bladder neck area. However, as one goes through the floor of the prostate, it may be difficult to determine exactly the depth of the incision. Therefore, a resectoscope loop can be used in this area to give a wider trough and permit more precise, deeper incision. The tissue resected is of course useful for determining whether or not the patient has cancer of the prostate. If this is not done, we recommend a biopsy of the prostate to give relative assurance that the patient does not have an occult carcinoma. Orandi[59] has modified his two-incision technique recently, in which he does not incise the bladder neck but merely limits the incision to the prostatic urethra using two incisions down to the capsule of the prostate.

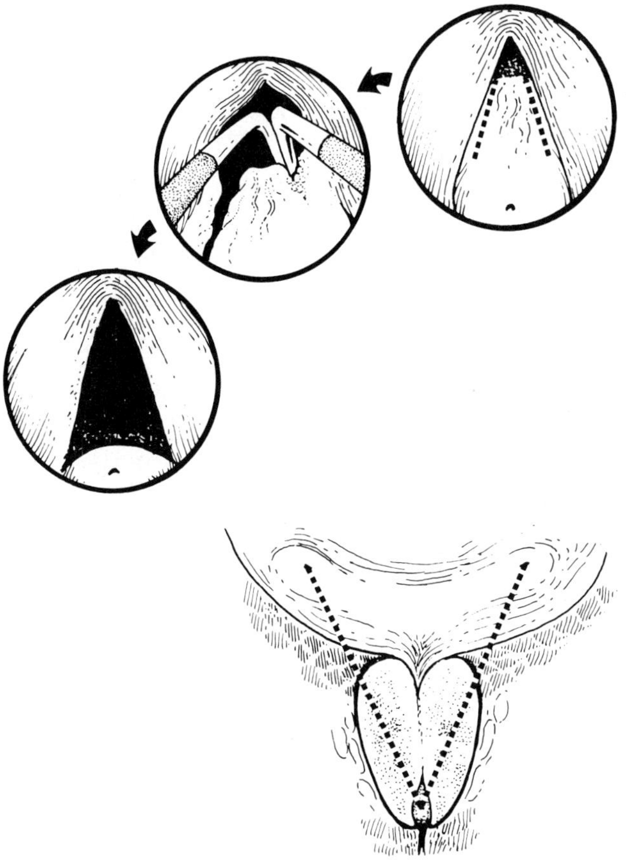

Christensen et al[12] used a single incision at 6 o'clock starting at the interureteric ridge and carried it through the bladder neck and the floor of the prostate to the verumontanum. Conversely, D'Ancona and associates[14] incised the prostatic urethra and bladder neck at the 12 o'clock position. They thought that this incision was simpler to use but did not carry the incision through the prostatic capsule into the periprostatic fat. Our concern is that the 12 o'clock incision, if carried too deeply, might cut into the dorsal vein complex, resulting in excessive bleeding.

Results

The BPH Panel found in their review of literature that 1361 patients had been treated with TUIP and that the peak flow increased from a preoperative value of 7.5 ml/sec to 15.1 ml/sec. The residual urine was improved by 94 per cent, and there was an 80 per cent improvement in patient symptoms. They noted an incidence of stress incontinence of 1.1 per cent and total incontinence of 0.1 per cent. There was a re-treatment rate of 4 per cent.

One advantage of this operation has been allegedly a reduction in the incidence of retrograde ejaculation following transurethral incision of the prostate compared with transurethral resection of the prostate. Following TURP, retrograde ejaculation has been reported in 50 to 95 per cent, but following a transurethral incision of the bladder neck, has been reported in 0 to 37 per cent. Turner-Warwick[69] noted that with one incision, the incidence of retrograde ejaculation was less than 5 per cent, but with two incisions it was 15 per cent. Hedlund and Ek[28] reported no difference between one and two incisions in the incidence of retrograde ejaculation.

There have been a few comparative studies between TURP and TUIP. Nielsen[53] noted that similar results occurred in a group of patients who had small glands and were randomized to either TURP or TUIP. However, there was a better flow rate after TURP (12 ml/sec) than TUIP (9 ml/sec). Helstrom and associates[29] found a better reduction in the maximum bladder pressure flow at maximum voiding with TURP. There was a difference in flow rate favoring TURP, but they did not believe that this was statistically significant.

More recently, Christensen and associates[12] reported a prospective randomized study of 93 patients. Forty-four were randomized to TURP and 49 to TUIP. These patients were followed up to 48 months. They noted an overall subjective improvement in 95 per cent of TURP versus 81 per cent of TUIP patients 3 months after treatment, but there was a gradual decline in subjective improvement over the next 3 to 4 years, so that patient evaluation of success of the operation at 4 years was 64 per cent for TURP and 78 per cent for TUIP. Because of the small number of patients evaluated at that point, there was no statistical difference. They noted a reduction in the symptom score of the patient, but there was

FIGURE 13–10. Transurethral incision of the primary vesical neck obstruction. The incision may be done at the 6 o'clock position or at the 5 and 7 o'clock positions. When performed at the 5 and 7 o'clock positions, the incision is started at the ureteral orifice and extended to the verumontanum. The depth of the incision is enough to expose the filament of structure of the external capsule. (From Mebust WK: A review of TURP complications and the AUA National Cooperative Study. AUA Update Series 8(24): 186–191, 1989; with permission.)

wide variation among patients as to the degree of reduction. There appeared to be greater reduction of obstructive symptoms with both procedures, as opposed to irritative symptoms, but again, no statistical difference was evident. TUIP was associated with a shorter operative time and less blood loss than TURP. The incidence of retrograde ejaculation was 37 per cent with TURP and 13 per cent with TUIP. Again, however, the numbers were not large enough to note a statistically significant difference.

They concluded, from a cost-effectiveness point of view, that TUIP is superior. There was no difference between the two groups in need for further surgery.

SUMMARY

TUIP is an attractive alternative to TURP in patients with smaller glands, such as 20 grams. However, the configuration of the gland is also important in making this decision. It appears to be most useful in patients with the so-called primary vesical neck contracture. If the patient has bilateral lobe hypertrophy, visual obstruction still may remain after the bladder neck is incised. There appears to be no difference between using one or two incisions, as far as outcomes are concerned. One potential disadvantage of TUIP is failure to diagnose occult prostatic carcinoma. Even if a biopsy of the prostate is done with the resectoscope or with a needle, a certain number of patients who have occult carcinoma of the prostate will be missed. Because this operation is usually reserved for younger patients, clinically significant cancer that can be treated with other forms of therapy may be missed. However, it is probably not necessary to do transrectal ultrasonography and preoperative biopsy in patients being considered for TUIP. Rather, these patients should simply be followed with rectal examinations and serum prostate-specific antigen and should undergo biopsy if an abnormality is found. The chance of missing prostate carcinoma in a young man who would benefit from more aggressive therapy is probably less than 5 per cent.

REFERENCES

1. Aboulken P, Steg A: La civulsion de la prostate d'apres 218 observations personneiles. J Urol Nephrol 70:337, 1964.
2. Allen TD: Body temperature changes during prostatic resection as related to the temperature of the irrigating solution. J Urol 110:433–435, 1973.
3. Bailey MJ, Shearer RJ: The role of internal urethrotomy in the prevention of urethral stricture following transurethral resection of prostate. Br J Urol 51:28–31, 1979.
4. Ball AJ, Feneley RCL, Abrams PH: The natural history of untreated prostatism. Br J Urol 53:613, 1981.
5. Ball AJ, Smith PJB: The long-term effects of prostatectomy: A uroflowmetric analysis. J Urol 128:538–540, 1982.
6. Bergman M: Suprapubic drainage in transurethral electroresection. Urologie 10:110–111, 1971.
7. Bergman RT, Turner R, Barnes RW, Hadley HL: Comparative analysis of one thousand consecutive cases of transurethral prostatectomy. J Urol 74:533–548, 1955.
8. Birkhoff JD, Wiederhorn AR, Hamilton ML, Zinsser HH: Natural history of benign prostatic hypertrophy and acute urinary retention. Urology 7:48–52, 1976.
9. Boyarsky S, Jones G, Paulson DF, Prout GR Jr: A new look at bladder neck obstruction by the Food and Drug Administration: Guidelines for investigation of benign prostatic hypertrophy. Trans Am Assoc Genitourin Surg 68:29–32, 1977.
10. Bruskewitz RC, Larsen EH, Madsen PO, et al: 3-Year followup of urinary symptoms after transurethral resection of the prostate. J Urol 136:613–615, 1986.
11. Chilton CP, Morgan RJ, England HR, et al: A critical evaluation of the results of transurethral resection of the prostate. Br J Urol 50:542–546, 1978.
12. Christensen MM, Aagaard J, Madsen PO: Transurethral resection versus transurethral incision of the prostate. Urol Clin North Am 17:621–630, 1990.
13. Creevy CD, Webb EA: A fatal hemolytic reaction following transurethral resection of the prostate gland: A discussion of its prevention and treatment. Surgery 21:56–66, 1947.
14. D'Ancona CAL, Netto NR, Cara AM, Ikari O: Internal urethrotomy of the prostatic urethra or transurethral resection in benign prostatic hyperplasia. J Urol 144:918–920, 1990.
15. Eddy DM: Clinical decision making: From theory to practice— Designing a practice policy standards, guidelines, and options. JAMA 263:3077–3084, 1990
16. Edwards LE, Bucknall TE, Pittam MR, et al: Transurethral resection of the prostate and bladder neck incision: A review of 700 cases. Br J Urol 57:168–171, 1985.
17. Emmett JL, Gilbaugh JH Jr, McLean P: Fluid absorption during transurethral resection: Comparison of mortality and morbidity after irrigation with water and non-hemolytic solutions. J Urol 101:884–889, 1969.
18. Emmett JL, Rous SN, Greene LF, et al: Preliminary internal urethrotomy in 1036 cases to prevent urethral stricture following transurethral resection; caliber of normal adult male urethra. J Urol 89:829, 1963.
19. Flechner SM, Williams RD: Continuous flow and conventional resectoscope methods in transurethral prostatectomy: Comparative study. J Urol 127:257–259, 1982.
20. Gellman AC: Endoscopic prostatectomy with the continuous flow resection technique. Int Surg 65:433–436, 1980.
21. Gibbons RP, Stark RA, Correa RJ Jr, et al: The prophylactic use—or misuse—of antibiotics in transurethral prostatectomy. J Urol 119:381, 1978.
22. Glynn RJ, Campion EW, Bouchard GR, Silbert JE: The development of benign prostatic hyperplasia among volunteers in the normative aging study. Am J Epidemiol 121:78, 1985.
23. Habib NA, Luck RJ: Results of transurethral resection of the benign prostate. Br J Surg Urol 70:218–219, 1983.
24. Hagstrom RS: Studies on fluid absorption during transurethral prostatic resection. J Urol 73:852–859, 1955.
25. Hargreave TB, Stephenson TP: Potency and prostatectomy. Br J Urol 49:683–688, 1977.
26. Harrison RH III, Boren JS, Robison JR: Dilutional hyponatremic shock: Another concept of the transurethral prostatic resection reaction. J Urol 75:95–110, 1956.
27. Hasner E: Prostatic urinary infection. Acta Chir Scand (Suppl) 285:1–40, 1962.
28. Hedlund H, Ek A: Ejaculation and sexual function after endoscopic bladder neck incision. Br J Urol 57:164–167, 1985.
29. Helstrom P, Lukkarinen O, Kontturi M: Bladder neck incision or transurethral electroresection for the treatment of urinary obstruction caused by a small benign prostate. A randomized urodynamic study. Scand J Urol Nephrol 20:187–192, 1986.
30. Hinman F Jr: Residual urine. Measurement and influence in management of obstruction. *In* Hinman F Jr (ed): Benign Prostatic Hypertrophy. New York, Springer-Verlag, 1983, pp 589–596.
31. Holmquist BG, Holm B, Ohlin P: Comparative study of the Iglesias technique and the suprapubic drainage technique for transurethral resection. Br J Urol 51:378–381, 1979.
32. Holtgrewe HL, Mebust WK, Dowd JB, et al: Transurethral prostatectomy: Practice aspects of the dominant operation in American urology. J Urol 141:248–253, 1989.
33. Holtgrewe HL, Valk WL: Factors influencing the mortality and morbidity of transurethral prostatectomy: A study of 2,015 cases. J Urol 87:450–459, 1962.

34. Hopkins HH: Optical principles of the endoscope. *In* Berci G. (ed): Endoscopy. New York, Appleton-Century-Crofts, 1976, pp 3–26.

35. Iglesias JJ, Sporer A, Gellman AC, et al: New Iglesias resectoscope with continuous irrigation, simultaneous suction and low intravesical pressure. J Urol 114:929–933, 1975.

36. Kulb TP, Kamer M, Lingeman JE, et al: Prevention of post-prostatectomy vesical-neck contracture by prophylactic vesical-neck incision. J Urol 137:230–231, 1987.

37. Lytton B, Emery JM, Harvard BM: The incidence of benign prostatic obstruction. J Urol 99:639, 1968.

38. Madsen PO, Frimodt-Moller PC: Transurethral prostatic resection with suprapubic trocar technique. J Urol 132:277–279, 1984.

39. Madsen PO, Iversen P: A point system for selecting operative candidates. *In* Hinman F Jr (ed): Benign Prostatic Hypertrophy. New York, Springer-Verlag, 1983, pp 763–765.

40. Madsen PO, Naber KG: The importance of the pressure in the prostatic fossa and absorption of irrigating fluid during transurethral resection of the prostate. J Urol 109:446–452, 1973.

41. Malenka DJ, Roos N, Fisher ES, et al: Further study of the increased mortality following transurethral prostatectomy: A chart-based analysis. J Urol (in press).

42. Malone PR, Cook A, Edmonson R, et al: Prostatectomy: Patients' perception and long-term follow-up. Br J Urol 61:234–238, 1988.

43. McGowan SW, Smith GFN: Anaesthesia for transurethral prostatectomy: A comparison of spinal intradural analgesia with two methods of general anaesthesia. Anaesthesia 35:847–853, 1980.

44. McPherson K, Wennberg JE, Hovind OB, Clifford P: Small-area variations in the use of common surgical procedures: An international comparison of New England, England, and Norway. N Engl J Med 307:1310–1314, 1982.

45. Mebust WK, Holtgrewe HL, Cockett ATK, et al: Transurethral prostatectomy: Immediate and postoperative complications. A cooperative study of thirteen participating institutions evaluating 3,885 patients. J Urol 141:243–247, 1989.

46. Mebust WK, Valk WL: Transurethral prostatectomy. *In* Hinman F Jr (ed): Benign Prostatic Hypertrophy. New York, Springer-Verlag, 1983, pp 829–846.

47. Melchior J, Valk WL, Foret JD, Mebust WK: Transurethral prostatectomy: Computerized analysis of 2,223 consecutive cases. J Urol 112:634–642, 1974.

48. Meyhoff HH, Nordling J: Long term results of transurethral and transvesical prostatectomy: A randomized study. Scand J Urol Nephrol 20:27–33, 1986.

49. Mosegaard A, Madsen PO: Trocar cystostomy during transurethral prostatic resection. Urology 3:735–740, 1974.

50. Murphy DM, Stassen L, Carr ME, et al: Bacteraemia during prostatectomy and other transurethral operations: Influence of timing of antibiotic administration. J Clin Pathol 37:673–676, 1984.

51. Nesbit RM: A history of transurethral prostatectomy. Rev Mex Urol 35:349–362, 1975.

52. Nesbit RM: Transurethral Prostatectomy. Springfield, IL, Charles C Thomas, 1943.

53. Nielsen HO: Transurethral prostatotomy versus transurethral prostatectomy in benign prostatic hypertrophy: A prospective randomized study. Br J Urol 61:435–438, 1988.

54. Nielsen KK, Andersen K, Asbjorn J, et al: Blood loss in transurethral prostatectomy: Epidural versus general anaesthesia. Int Urol Nephrol 19:287–292, 1987.

55. Nielsen OS, Maigaard S, Frimodt-Moller N, Madsen PO: Prophylactic antibiotics in transurethral prostatectomy. J Urol 126:60–62, 1981.

56. O'Donnell PD: Serum acid phosphatase elevation associated with transurethral resection syndromes. Urology 22:388–390, 1983.

57. Oester A, Madsen PO: Determination of absorption of irrigating fluid during transurethral resection of the prostate by means of radioisotopes. J Urol 102:714–719, 1969.

58. Orandi A: Transurethral incision of the prostate. J Urol 110:229–231, 1973.

59. Orandi A: Transurethral resection versus transurethral incision of the prostate. Urol Clin North Am 17:601–612, 1990.

60. Ovassapian A, Joshi CW, Brunner EA: Visual disturbances: An unusual symptom of transurethral prostatic resection reaction. Anesthesiology 57:332–334, 1982.

61. Perrin P, Barnes R, Hadley H, et al: Forty years of transurethral prostatic resections. J Urol 116:757–758, 1976.

62. Reuter HJ, Jones LW: Physiologic low pressure irrigation for transurethral resection: Suprapubic trochar drainage. J Urol 111:210–212, 1974.

63. Roos NP, Ramsey EW: A population-based study of prostatectomy: Outcomes associated with differing surgical approaches. J Urol 137:1184–1188, 1987.

64. Roos NP, Wennberg JE, Malenka DJ, et al: Mortality and reoperation after open and transurethral resection of the prostate for benign prostatic hyperplasia. Special Article. N Engl J Med 320:1120–1123, 1989.

65. Serrao A, Mallik MK, Jones PA, et al: Hypothermic prostatic resection. Br J Urol 48:685–687, 1976.

65a. Shah PJK, Abrams PH, Feneley RCL, Green NA: The influence of prostatic anatomy and the differing results of prostatectomy according to the surgical approach. Br J Urol 51:549–551, 1979.

66. Sinha B, Haikel G, Lange PH, et al: Transurethral resection of the prostate with local anesthesia in 100 patients. J Urol 135:719–721, 1986.

67. Stephenson TP, Latto P, Bradley D, et al: Comparison between continuous flow and intermittent flow transurethral resection in 40 patients presenting with acute retention. Br J Urol 52:523–525, 1980.

68. Turner-Warwick R: The sphincter mechanisms: Their relation to prostatic enlargement and its treatment. *In* Hinman F Jr (ed): Benign Prostatic Hypertrophy. New York, Springer-Verlag, 1983, pp 809–828.

69. Turner-Warwick R: A urodynamic review of bladder outlet obstruction in the male and its clinical implications. Urol Clin North Am 6:171–192, 1979.

70. Van Arsdalen KN, Chen JW, Vernon Smith MJ: Penile erections complicating transurethral surgery. J Urol 129:374–376, 1983.

71. Walton JK, Rawstron RE: The effect of local hypothermia on blood loss during transurethral resection of the prostate. Br J Urol 53:258–260, 1981.

72. Wennberg JE, Gittelsohn AM: Variations in medical care among small areas. Sci Am 246:120–134, 1982.

73. Whitlock NW, McAninch JW, Stutzman RE: Vasectomy with transurethral resection of prostate. Urology 13:135–138, 1979.

Chapter 14

OPEN PROSTATECTOMY

BERNARD LYTTON

Open surgery for removal of prostatic obstruction began in the 19th century, first as a partial prostatectomy in which obstructing lobes of tissue were removed transvesically during surgery for stones in the bladder. The credit for the first planned procedure belongs to Dr. W. J. Bellfield of Chicago and Mr. McGill of Leeds, England.[1] Dr. Eugene Fuller at The New York Hospital performed a formal enucleation of the prostate in 1895.[3] Following this, the operation became clouded in controversy with regard to priority. Sir Peter Freyer, who practiced at St. Peter's Hospital in London, described his experiences with transvesical prostatic adenectomy and claimed it as his own.[2] It is probable, however, that he heard about the operation from Dr. Ramon Guiteras, who had watched Dr. Fuller perform the procedure. With the perspective of history, these claims become irrelevant. Each of these surgeons made an important contribution to the establishment of open prostatectomy, which at that time carried a significant mortality. The earlier surgeons thought that they were removing the entire prostate, leaving only a capsule of connective tissue. It was not recognized until later that the "capsule" was in fact the compressed remnant of the normal prostate and that only the adenoma was enucleated. A decade or so later, Dr. Hugh Young at Johns Hopkins Hospital in Baltimore used a blindly operated transurethral cold punch to remove obstructing prostatic tissue. The idea was not new, as Dr. Young himself acknowledged when he quoted the description by Dr. August Mercier, who described the use of a cold punch in 1850.

Subsequently, Dr. Young developed the open perineal approach and in 1945, Terrence Millin popularized the retropubic operation.[5] As a precursor to what we are witnessing in all branches of surgery today, an endoscopic method of prostatectomy was developed in the early 1940s by Dr. Theodore H. Davis of North Carolina. This was made possible by the invention of the rod lens telescope. The instrumentation was further developed by Stern and McCarthy, and transurethral resection of the prostate quickly superseded open prostatectomy in the United States. It became accepted in Europe somewhat later, after World War II, when the American experience demonstrated that the mortality and morbidity of prostatectomy were significantly reduced by transurethral resection. With the development of fiberoptic technology, the method became even more firmly established. Evidence has been presented recently that despite a decrease in the immediate postoperative morbidity and mortality with transurethral resection of the prostate (TURP), the long-term survival after this operation is not as good as after an open operation.[6] This difference has been ascribed by some investigators to a higher incidence of co-morbidity in the patients undergoing TURP. However, when these co-morbid factors were applied to the original retrospective studies, the difference persisted. A randomized prospective study is currently being undertaken to clarify this problem.

Open prostatectomy today is generally performed in patients who need to have excision of a bladder diverticulum or open removal of stones that are too large or numerous to be easily removed endoscopically, or when the patient has a gland that is too large to be comfortably resected transurethrally. When the adenoma completely obscures the trigone and ureteral orifices, an open procedure may be preferred. Most urologists are comfortable removing up to 50 to 75 grams of tissue transurethrally. Some more experienced surgeons remove more, but the larger glands take longer to resect and sometimes require a secondary procedure. An open procedure in these cases takes less time, probably has no greater morbidity, and is likely to have a better result. Patients with very large glands are infrequently seen today, as they tend to be treated at an earlier stage in most developed countries.

All of the open procedures are based on the principle of enucleation of the adenoma from the surrounding true prostate, which is compressed to form the surgical capsule. Benign prostatic hyperplasia (BPH) can be likened to a thick-skinned orange; the adenoma that arises from the transitional zone is like the "fruit" that is shelled out from the surrounding "skin," which corresponds to the compressed true prostate.

TRANSVESICAL PROSTATECTOMY

This is probably the most frequently performed open prostatectomy and was the first method to be developed. It was at one time performed as a blind procedure with a small suprapubic incision through which the adenoma was digitally enucleated. No attempt was made at hemostasis in these patients other than the use of a balloon to tamponade the fossa. The bladder was drained with a large suprapubic catheter. The operation was often delayed until the gland "matured" to facilitate the enucleation.

The operation is best performed under direct vision, as it is generally done today. This entails a larger incision that permits better exposure, allows for measures to control bleeding, and enables the surgeon to correct any bladder neck contracture. The patient is supine on the operating table in slight Trendelenburg position with the table broken so as to extend the lumbar spine for better access to the pelvis. A No. 22 Fr Foley catheter is placed in the bladder, which is distended with 200 to 300 ml of saline and the catheter clamped.

The incision may be vertical between the symphysis and umbilicus, with the fascia and muscles being divided in the midline. Alternatively, a Pfannenstiel incision may be made one finger's-breadth above the symphysis. The fascia is divided transversely and reflected off the underlying muscle. The rectus muscles are then separated in the midline. The extraperitoneal perivesical space is easily entered by dividing the anterior perivesical fascia over the lower part of the bladder, which allows the fascia and peritoneum to be swept up off the anterior bladder wall to expose the detrusor and large vessels crossing over its surface.

The anterior wall of the bladder is grasped with two Allis clamps placed 1 cm apart in a relatively avascular area. The bladder wall is tented up and a small incision is made between the clamps to enter the bladder. A sucker is placed through the cystotomy to evacuate the fluid. The bladder incision is enlarged vertically downward for about 6 cm, and a self-retaining retractor is inserted. Any stones or diverticula are removed. The latter are best excised from the inside by pulling the mucosa of the diverticulum inside out so that it can be excised at the neck of the diverticulum. The defect in the muscle is closed with 2-0 chromic sutures.

To improve the exposure, a narrow Deaver retractor may be placed over a sponge to retract the dome and posterior wall of the bladder. The mucosa over the prostate around the internal meatus is circumcised using the cautery with a radius of about 1 cm. The mucosa is reflected off the prostate by blunt dissection. The forefinger is then inserted into the meatus, and the anterior commissure is split down to the capsule by exerting firm pressure anteriorly with the finger. The retractors are removed from the bladder and the plane between the adenoma and capsule is developed digitally on each side. The enucleation is continued posteriorly and around the bladder neck.

Sometimes when the adenoma is large, the urethra can be divided at the apex by pinching it between the thumb and forefinger. If it does not separate easily, the urethra should be divided at the apex of the adenoma with the tip of long curved scissors. It should never be forcibly avulsed, as this may damage the sphincter mechanism in the membranous urethra. The adenoma may be grasped with prostate forceps to facilitate its removal. If it is excessively large, each lobe is removed separately. The fossa should be palpated for residual adenoma that needs to be removed and is then packed with a small sponge to control the bleeding. The bladder neck is inspected and if a posterior shelf is present, it is grasped with an Allis forceps and a wedge excision is performed. Two figure-8 2-0 chromic catgut sutures are placed at the 5 and 7 o'clock positions to control bleeding. The needle should be inserted only a few millimeters proximal to the bladder neck to avoid the ureteric orifices and passed fairly deep into the prostatic fossa so as to include an adequate amount of tissue for hemostasis. The mucosa above the wedge excision should be sutured down into the prostatic fossa over the incised area of the bladder neck.

A No. 22 Fr Foley catheter is inserted through the urethra into the bladder. It is better to delay inflation of the balloon until the bladder has been closed to avoid accidental puncture. If bleeding from the prostatic fossa persists, a circumferential purse-string nylon suture can be placed around the bladder neck with the two ends brought out anteriorly.[4] The two ends are then pulled tight to snug the bladder neck up around the catheter to tamponade the fossa. A No. 26 or 28 Fr suprapubic tube, preferably a Malecot type, is placed through a separate stab incision in the bladder. A 2-0 chromic catgut suture is placed in a figure-8 fashion through the muscle wall, tied below next to the catheter and then around the catheter to make sure that it is not inadvertently pulled out. The bladder mucosa is closed with running 3-0 plain catgut suture and the suture line reinforced by closing the overlying muscle with a running 2-0 chromic catgut suture.

A Penrose or Jackson-Pratt drain is placed in the retropubic space and brought out through a separate stab incision in the right or left lower quadrant. It is preferred to bring the suprapubic tube out through a separate stab incision in the abdominal wall 2 to 3 cm away from the incision. This allows for a more effective closure of the wound and decreases the chances of troublesome superficial wound infection. The rectus muscle is loosely approximated with some interrupted catgut sutures. The fascia is sutured from each end with a running polyglycolic suture, and the free ends are tied in the middle of the wound. The skin is closed with interrupted nylon sutures or clips. The suprapubic tube is secured to the skin with a 2-0 nylon suture. The Foley balloon is inflated with 30 ml of sterile water. Saline should not be used because it sometimes crystallizes in the balloon and may create difficulty in deflation.

The Foley catheter is removed as soon as the urine begins to clear. The suprapubic tube is clamped after 7 days, and if the patient is able to void it is removed. We have experienced little difficulty in spontaneous closure of the suprapubic sinus provided that the tract is created well away from the symphysis pubis. Attachment of the tract to the symphysis prevents retraction and may lead to delayed closure or nonclosure.

RETROPUBIC PROSTATECTOMY

This procedure was first performed in 1908 by Van Stolkum and later popularized by Terrence Millin. The principle of the operation is that the adenoma is removed through an incision in the surgical capsule of the prostate rather than through the bladder. There is therefore no incision of the bladder, obviating suprapubic catheter drainage in most cases, as distention of the bladder by urine or clot does not have the potential for causing disruption. Moreover, the capsular incision allows for a more adequate exposure and inspection of the prostatic fossa to control bleeding. There is an increased risk of intraoperative problems due to injury and bleeding from the retropubic veins.

A Pfannenstiel incision is usually preferred, but a vertical lower midline incision is equally satisfactory. After the rectus and pyramidalis muscles are separated in the midline down to the symphysis, the retropubic space is entered by dividing the transversalis fascia low down and sweeping it upward with the finger. A self-retaining retractor with back blade is inserted to hold back the muscles and retract the bladder. A small sponge is then packed down on each side of the prostate to sweep away the periprostatic fat and to define the lateral limits of the prostate. One or two large superficial retropubic veins are seen crossing over the front of the prostate and are divided between ligatures. This exposes the anterior surface of the prostate just below the bladder neck.

The fatty tissue containing some of the retropubic veins overlying the puboprostatic ligaments can be pushed down and left undisturbed, as it can be a source of troublesome bleeding. Several 2-0 chromic catgut sutures may be placed transversely in the prostatic capsule on either side of the planned line of incision, about 0.5 to 1 cm below the bladder neck, to control bleeding. The capsule is incised transversely (Fig. 14–1) with the electrocautery, making sure that the incision is deep enough to extend through the capsule into the adenoma. It should also extend around to the lateral

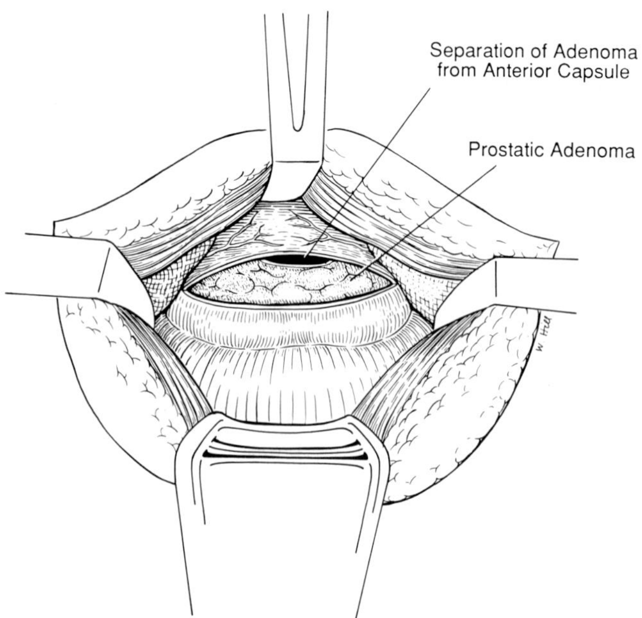

FIGURE 14–1. Retropubic prostatectomy. Incision in the anterior capsule. Separation of the adenoma is begun in the midline as shown. Note sponges placed on each side that help to expose the prostate.

margins of the prostate to provide adequate room for enucleating the adenoma. Too small an incision may lead to uncontrolled tearing of the capsule during the enucleation, making it more difficult to suture the capsule and control bleeding. A lighted sucker is very helpful to aspirate smoke and blood and allow visualization so that an adequate incision can be made. Curved long-handled scissors are used to develop the plane between the anterior capsule and the adenoma. It is best to remove the retractor at this stage. The index finger is then inserted between the surgical capsule and the adenoma to separate the adenoma, and the plane of enucleation is developed anteriorly, laterally, and posteriorly until the urethra is defined. Undue force should not be used with the index finger posteriorly, as this may result in tearing of the capsule into the pararectal space. This part of the enucleation is sometimes facilitated by placing a finger in the rectum to elevate the prostate and provide counterpressure.

It is best to divide the urethra sharply at the apex of the prostate using long scissors. A finger should be placed behind the urethra to localize the site of transection and protect the underlying rectum. The posterior enucleation can then be completed and the gland delivered, with the help of lobe forceps if necessary, in either one or two pieces depending on its size. The retractor is reinserted and the prostatic fossa packed with a small gauze sponge to control bleeding. The prostate is then grasped with Tenaculum forceps and dissected sharply with scissors away from the bladder neck, which is easily identified by its muscle fibers encircling the base of the gland. A bladder neck retractor is used to display the posterior lip, which usually needs to be resected to prevent the development of a bladder neck contracture.

The posterior lip of the bladder neck is grasped with Allis forceps and an appropriate triangular wedge resected. It is not necessary or advisable to cut too far into the trigone, as this tends to produce more postoperative bladder discomfort.

Two figure-8, 2-0 chromic catgut sutures are placed at the 5 and 7 o'clock positions on either side of the wedge resection to control bleeding (Fig. 14–2). It is important when inserting these sutures to use a 3/8-inch curved needle that is inserted into the mucosa only 3 to 4 mm proximal to the bladder neck, taking care to avoid the ureteral orifices. The needle should exit 10 to 15 mm below the bladder neck in the prostatic fossa to provide good purchase and hemostasis. Once sutures have been placed on each side they are used to retract the bladder neck to expose the wedge resection. The mucosa at the edge of the wedge resection is then sutured down to the posterior capsule using interrupted 3-0 chromic catgut sutures. This retrigonizes the raw area, which makes the postoperative course more comfortable and is helpful in controlling bleeding at this site.

The packing in the prostatic fossa is then removed and any obvious bleeding point is either oversewn or lightly fulgurated. A No. 22 or 24 Fr Foley catheter with a 30-ml balloon is placed through the urethra and guided into the bladder. The balloon is not inflated at this stage so as to avoid accidental puncture during suture of the capsule. The bladder neck retractor is inserted and pulled back to define the lateral angles of the incision in the surgical capsule. A 0 chromic catgut suture on a 5/8-inch large needle is placed through the lateral end of the bladder neck and out through the lateral end of the lower lip of the prostatic capsule. A good bite of capsule, approximately 1 cm, should be taken so that

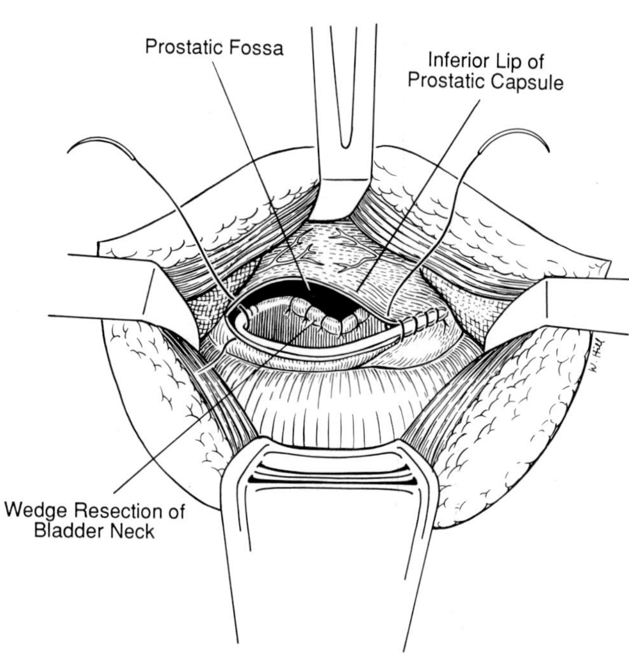

FIGURE 14–3. Retropubic prostatectomy. Capsular closure is begun at each end of the incision. It is important to include bladder mucosa in the proximal capsular sutures.

the suture is tied well below the lateral angle to make it watertight and control bleeding. A similar suture is placed on the other side. The free ends of each tied suture are held in a small clamp and are used to pull the capsule up into the wound to improve the exposure. The two sutures are then run to the midline to close the anterior capsulotomy and are tied together in the midline (Fig. 14–3). It is important to make sure that the mucosal layer of the bladder is included when placing the sutures through the proximal edge of the capsule, because if it is allowed to retract it can be a troublesome source of bleeding in the postoperative period. Once the capsule has been sutured, the Foley balloon is inflated with 30 ml of sterile water, and the bladder is irrigated with warm saline. There should be satisfactory hemostasis at this stage; however, if there is concern about the amount of bleeding, one should not hesitate to insert a small No. 20 or 22 Fr Malecot catheter suprapubically for irrigation and alternative drainage. It is brought out through a separate stab incision away from the wound and can be removed on the fourth or fifth postoperative day without delaying convalescence. A Penrose drain is placed over the suture line and brought out through a separate stab incision lateral to the inferior epigastric vessels and the wound. The fascia is approximated with a running No. 1 PDS (polydioxanone suture) and the skin with staples.

The patient should be given a generous intravenous infusion of 5 per cent dextrose and 0.5 normal saline after the operation—between 125 and 150 ml/hr—to provide an adequate flow of urine. If catheter drainage seems to be impaired, it can often be re-established simply by pushing the catheter further in, away from

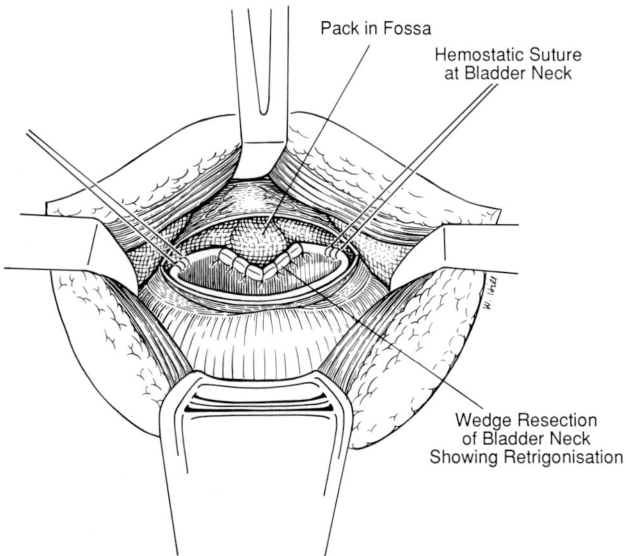

FIGURE 14–2. Retropubic prostatectomy. Enucleation of the adenoma has been completed. Sutures have been placed at the 5 and 7 o'clock positions in the bladder neck to control bleeding. A wedge resection of the bladder neck has been performed.

the clot that forms in the base of the bladder. It is best not to irrigate the bladder postoperatively if possible, as this breaks up the clot and the resultant small pieces are more likely to obstruct the catheter.

In most cases, the drainage is rose colored on the first day and port wine colored on the second day and begins to clear on the third. The catheter is removed when the urinary drainage becomes clear, usually between the third and fifth postoperative day. The short period of catheter drainage that is usually required is one of the advantages of this procedure. Late bladder neck contracture has been reported as a troublesome complication in the first year. This has largely been obviated by performing a routine wedge resection of the bladder neck. The majority of patients have a shorter and more comfortable immediate postoperative course than those undergoing a transvesical procedure. It also tends to be associated with less blood loss intraoperatively.

PERINEAL PROSTATECTOMY

The perineal approach for the enucleation of benign adenomatous hyperplasia is rarely used today. The procedure under direct vision was popularized by Dr. Hugh Hampton Young of Baltimore in 1908, and at the time its most important advantages were that it provided dependent drainage that decreased the incidence of infection and avoided an abdominal incision so that there was less interference with breathing postoperatively. The major disadvantages were the reported 10 per cent incidence of impotence postoperatively, the increased risk of rectal injury intraoperatively, and limited access to the operative site through the perineal incision.

The patient is placed in the exaggerated lithotomy position. This is achieved by hyperflexing the thighs with foot stirrups and placing the sacrum on a small sandbag so that the perineum projects out over the edge of the table and is almost parallel to the floor. In this position, much of the patient's weight is transferred to the shoulders so that shoulder stirrups are required. These must be well padded to prevent any brachial plexus injury. Football players' shoulder pads placed on the patient provide an ideal protection for this purpose.

The incision is an inverted U made between the ischial tuberosities with the apex of the curve over the midportion of the perineum about 3 cm in front of the anus. The lateral ends of the incision should be extended down inside the tuberosities if more access is needed. The incision should not be carried out over the tuberosities because this can be a cause of postoperative pain on sitting. The incision is deepened through the subcutaneous tissues until the ischiorectal fossa on each side can be entered. The inferior skin flap with its subcutaneous tissue, which is retained to preserve its blood supply, is dissected down to expose the central tendon. A No. 24 or 26 Fr curved metal sound is then placed in the urethra with the convexity directed toward the perineal incision. An assistant holds the sound so as to

push the apex of the prostate forward into the wound. The forefinger and middle finger of one hand are then placed in each ischiorectal fossa to pull the rectum downward while gentle traction is exerted on the skin flap with Allis forceps. This places tension on the central tendon and throws it into relief. The tendon is divided sharply in the midline, which allows the transverse perineal muscles to retract upward. This should be a relatively avascular plane, and any bleeding indicates that one is probably in the wrong place.

The anterior rectal wall is exposed and tented up in front of the prostate where it is held by the rectourethralis muscle. The rectourethralis muscle is divided in the midline with scissors just below the transverse perineal muscles to expose the two layers of Denonvilliers' fascia. Once the rectourethralis muscle is divided to expose the apex of the prostate, the space between the two layers of Denonvilliers' fascia can be entered by carefully incising the posterior layer to expose what Young has described as the "pearly gates." This plane can then be entered and developed by blunt dissection with the finger or the back of the scalpel handle. This allows the anterior wall of the rectum to be pushed down to expose the glistening white posterior surface of the prostate. A curved retractor is placed over a small sponge to retract the rectum.

An inverted-U incision is made in the posterior prostatic capsule, with the top of the U about 1 cm below the apex of the prostate. This should be just distal to the verumontanum, which can be felt as a small depression in the capsule posteriorly. This posterior flap, together with the verumontanum, is reflected downward. Enucleation of the adenoma is then begun on each side and around the apex to free the urethra. The anterior portion of the urethra is divided sharply to free the apex of the prostatic adenoma. The adenoma is grasped with lobe forceps and its proximal portion separated from the bladder neck by sharp and blunt dissection. The bladder neck is visualized and a wedge resection is performed if indicated. Hemostatic figure-8, 2-0 chromic catgut sutures are placed at 5 and 7 o'clock positions, with care being taken to avoid the ureteral orifices. The trigonal mucosa is advanced downward over the bladder neck into the prostatic fossa, if possible. All bleeding points are fulgurated or oversewn with 3-0 chromic catgut sutures. A No. 22 Fr Foley catheter with a 30-ml balloon is inserted through the urethra and placed in the bladder with the balloon inflated to 30 ml with distilled water. The capsule is closed with running 2-0 chromic catgut sutures, which are best begun from each lateral end and tied in the middle. A small Penrose drain is placed down to the suture line and brought out through the lateral end of the wound. Subcutaneous tissues are approximated with 3-0 plain catgut sutures, and the skin is closed with interrupted 3-0 nylon sutures, the ends being left long and tied together so as to avoid discomfort of the short ends sticking into the perineum when the patient is sitting. Alternatively, the skin can be closed with a subcutaneous 3-0 plain catgut suture.

The catheter should be retained for at least 3 to 5

days or until the drainage is clear and all perineal drainage has ceased for at least 24 hours. Postoperative problems may include persistent perineal leakage, impotence in a small number of patients, and stress incontinence, which usually recovers after several months.

REFERENCES

1. Bellfield WT: Operations on the enlarged prostate with a tabulated summary of cases. Am J Med Sci 100:439, 1890.
2. Freyer PJ: A new method of performing prostatectomy. Lancet 1:774, 1900.
3. Fuller E: Six successful and successive cases of prostatectomy. J Cutan Genitourin Dis 13:229, 1895.
4. Malament M: Maximal hemostasis in suprapubic prostatectomy. Surg Gynecol Obstet 120:1307, 1965.
5. Millin T: Retropubic prostatectomy: New extravesical technique. Report on 20 cases. Lancet 2:693, 1945.
6. Roos NP, Wennberg JE, Malenka DJ, et al: Mortality and reoperation after open and transurethral resection of the prostate for benign prostatic hyperplasia. N Engl J Med 320:1120, 1989.

Chapter 15

THE ROLE OF ALPHA BLOCKADE IN THE THERAPY OF BENIGN PROSTATIC HYPERPLASIA

HERBERT LEPOR

IS THERE A ROLE FOR NONSURGICAL THERAPY FOR BPH?

Transurethral prostatectomy (TURP) represents the standard therapy for symptomatic benign prostatic hyperplasia (BPH) in the United States. Prostatectomy has become readily accepted for the treatment of symptomatic BPH because the procedure is relatively free of life-threatening complications, and the majority of patients experience symptomatic improvement. TURP gained acceptance among the urologic community without objective prospective or retrospective clinical studies documenting the short- and long-term effectiveness of the procedure. The absence of objective outcomes research presumably was overlooked because there were no other effective treatment alternatives. Historically, academic and practicing urologists did not recognize the importance or feasibility of nonsurgical alternatives for treating BPH. Over the past 5 years, the interest in nonsurgical therapy for BPH has escalated. The quest for a nonsurgical therapy has been motivated by patients seeking to avoid surgery, a federal government seeking to curtail health care expenditures, industry hoping to reap large profits, and a urologic community committed to offering patients the optimal standard of care. Increasing evidence suggests that nonsurgical interventions may be effective for the treatment of selected males with symptomatic BPH. The effectiveness of TURP appears to exceed all nonsurgical therapies currently under investigation.[41] The threshold response resulting in a clinically significant outcome is unknown. Advocates

for medical therapies and minimally invasive surgical therapies often claim that "clinically significant" effectiveness is achieved, whereas morbidity and cost are reduced relative to prostatectomy. Ultimately, guidelines for the management of BPH must be based upon properly designed prospective clinical studies that ascertain relative morbidity, effectiveness, and cost of surgical and nonsurgical therapies. The interest in nonsurgical therapy has prompted efforts to ascertain the morbidity, efficacy, and cost of prostatectomy.

Because nonsurgical therapies are likely to be advocated based upon reduced morbidity, it is pertinent to examine the morbidity associated with TURP. The intraoperative and perioperative morbidity and mortality following TURP have recently been evaluated. Holtgrew et al,[26] under the auspices of the American Urological Association (AUA), conducted a survey designed to clarify the role of TURP in the treatment of BPH. Thirty-five per cent of the practicing urologists in the United States responded to the AUA-sponsored questionnaire. Mebust et al[46] ascertained the morbidity following TURP in a cooperative study involving 3885 consecutive patients selected from 13 institutions representing small group community practices and large multidisciplinary group practices including academic centers. The 13 participating centers reviewed 300 consecutive cases of TURP. The morbidity and mortality of TURP reported in these surveys are summarized in Table 15–1. The complications following TURP are significant. Therefore, the decision to offer prostatectomy must reflect both the potential benefits of intervention and the inherent risks associated with the pro-

TABLE 15–1. MORBIDITY ASSOCIATED WITH TRANSURETHRAL PROSTATECTOMY

	MEBUST ET AL[46] (%)	HOLTGREWE ET AL[26] (%)
Epididymitis	1.2	4.8
Urinary tract infection	2.3	8.4
Impotence	3.5	10.2
Incontinence	0.4	3.3
Transfusion	6.5	10.5
Transurethral resection syndrome	2.0	—
Death	0.2	—

Mebust et al: 3885 consecutive prostatectomies at 13 institutions.
Holtgrewe et al: 35% of practicing American urologists.

cedure. Although surgical and nonsurgical alternatives for the treatment of BPH are not likely to achieve the same degree of efficacy, the relative morbidity of intervention is likely to be a dominant factor favoring the less invasive interventions.

It is generally accepted that TURP is an effective treatment for bladder outlet obstruction secondary to BPH. The most common indication for prostatectomy in the United States is relief of symptoms of prostatism.[46] Approximately 90 per cent of men undergoing prostatectomy have symptoms of prostatism. Other common indications for prostatectomy include significant residual urine (34 per cent), urinary retention (27 per cent), urinary tract infection (12 per cent), hematuria (12 per cent), altered urodynamic function (10 per cent), renal insufficiency (5 per cent), and bladder stones (3 per cent). Approximately 400,000 prostatectomies are performed yearly in the United States.[4] Over the last decade, approximately 3.6 million American men have undergone prostatectomy for symptoms of prostatism, 1.37 million for significant residual urine, 1.08 million for urinary retention, 0.48 million for urinary tract infection, 0.48 million for hematuria, 0.40 million for altered urodynamic function, 0.20 million for renal insufficiency, and 0.1 million for bladder stones. The probability that prostatectomy will relieve urinary retention, reduce postvoid residual, prevent urinary tract infection, reverse renal insufficiency, or prevent bladder stones is unknown. Despite the fact that prostatectomy is one of the most commonly performed operative procedures, the effectiveness of the procedure remains essentially unknown. The paucity of objective clinical data following prostatectomy is striking. Several investigators have ascertained symptom improvement following transurethral prostatectomy.[14, 15, 23, 41, 48, 50] Overall, 20 per cent of patients do not achieve satisfactory resolution of their voiding symptoms following prostatectomy. There are no objective outcome data ascertaining whether TURP improves bladder emptying, reverses renal insufficiency, prevents recurrent urinary tract infections, and relieves acute and chronic urinary retention.

Is there a role for nonsurgical therapy? The intraoperative and perioperative morbidity following pros-

tatectomy are significant. The long-term complication rate associated with prostatectomy has not been critically examined. Approximately 15 per cent of men require reoperation within 8 years.[60] The long-term effectiveness of prostatectomy is unknown. Although prostatectomy is likely to remain the most effective treatment for BPH, the above-mentioned limitations of this procedure provide ample justification to critically evaluate nonsurgical therapies for BPH.

RATIONALE FOR THE USE OF ALPHA-ANTAGONISTS IN BENIGN PROSTATIC HYPERPLASIA

Shapiro et al[55] recently developed a technique for quantifying the cellular elements of the prostate. The technique applies double immunoenzymatic staining and color-assisted computer image analysis. The epithelium and smooth muscle were labeled with rabbit anti-desmin and a mouse anti–human prostatic acid phosphatase (PSAP), respectively. The epithelium, smooth muscle, connective tissue, and glandular lumen stained red, dark brown, light brown, and colorless, respectively, using the double immunoenzymatic staining technique. The thresholds for the color-assisted computer image analysis were set to discriminate the different staining properties of the prostatic cellular elements. The area densities of the cellular elements of the prostate were originally determined from eight transrectal guided biopsy specimens obtained from men with clinical BPH. The area densities of smooth muscle, connective tissue, epithelium, and glandular lumen were 22 ± 4 per cent, 54 ± 4 per cent, 16 ± 6 per cent, and 9 ± 1 per cent, respectively. Overall, the ratio of stroma:epithelium was 4.8:1. Bartsch et al[4] reported that the ratio of stromal:epithelial hyperplasia in BPH is 5:1. Shapiro et al[54] recently reported that mouse anti-actin is a more sensitive label for prostate smooth muscle than rabbit anti-desmin. Double immunoenzymatic staining was performed on 19 transrectal guided biopsy specimens obtained from men with clinical BPH using both mouse anti-actin/rabbit anti–human PSAP and rabbit anti-desmin/mouse anti–human PSAP. The area densities of smooth muscle, connective tissue, epithelium, and glandular lumen in the anti-actin/anti–human PSAP stained tissues were 39 ± 3 per cent, 38 ± 3 per cent, 12 ± 1 per cent, and 11 ± 1 per cent, respectively. The area densities of smooth muscle, connective tissue, epithelium, and glandular lumen in the anti-desmin/anti–human PSAP were 19 ± 2 per cent, 59 ± 2 per cent, 12 ± 1 per cent, and 11 ± 1 per cent, respectively. These morphometric studies demonstrated that BPH is primarily stromal (smooth muscle and connective tissue) hyperplasia and that anti-actin is a more sensitive label of prostatic smooth muscle.

Raz et al[52] were the first investigators to study the physiology and pharmacology of prostate smooth muscle. Their isometric tension studies demonstrated that the rat prostate contracts in the presence of norepinephrine, an adrenergic agonist. Caine and associates subsequently demonstrated that the human prostate adenoma and capsule also contract in the presence of norepinephrine.[11] They recognized the therapeutic implications of pharmacologically altering the tension of prostate smooth muscle in men with symptomatic BPH.[10] In vitro isometric tension studies subsequently demonstrated that the contractile properties of human prostate adenomas are mediated primarily by alpha$_1$ adrenoceptors.[21, 24, 36] Radioligand receptor–binding studies have shown that the human prostate contains a relative abundance of alpha$_1$ adrenoceptors.[20, 42] On the basis of the aforementioned physiologic and pharmacologic observations, alpha$_1$ adrenergic blockers should decrease the resistance along the prostatic urethra by relaxing the smooth muscle component of the prostate. Comparative binding and functional studies of lower genitourinary tissues demonstrated that alpha$_1$ adrenoceptors are sparse in the bladder body and abundant in the bladder base and prostate.[57] Selective alpha$_1$ adrenergic antagonists are therefore ideally suited for the treatment of the dynamic component of bladder outlet obstruction because the resistance along the bladder outlet can be selectively reduced without impairing detrusor contraction.

The proposed mechanism for the efficacy of selective alpha$_1$ blockade in BPH is relaxation of prostatic smooth muscle. It therefore follows that the magnitude of the clinical response to selective alpha$_1$ blockade in BPH should be directly related to the proportion of the hyperplasia that is smooth muscle. Shapiro and Lepor[58] recently examined the relationship between the percentage area density of prostate smooth muscle in the adenoma and the clinical response to terazosin, a selective alpha$_1$ blocker. Prostatic biopsies were obtained under ultrasound guidance from 26 men with clinical BPH prior to initiating terazosin therapy. The dose of terazosin was titrated to 5 mg provided that serious adverse events were not observed. The per cent area density of smooth muscle in the biopsy specimens was quantified using double immunoenzymatic staining and quantitative color-assisted image analysis. A direct relationship between the increase in urinary flow rate and the per cent area density of smooth muscle was observed (Fig. 15–1). The direct relationship between smooth muscle content and clinical response strongly supports the proposed mechanism that the development of bladder outlet obstruction is mediated by prostate smooth muscle tension.

SELECTIVE ALPHA$_1$ BLOCKADE

The autonomic nervous system regulates bodily functions that are not under volitional control. The tension of prostatic smooth muscle is therefore regulated by the autonomic nervous system. The autonomic nervous system is composed of parasympathetic and sympathetic innervation. The distinction between parasympathetic and sympathetic depends solely on the location of the preganglionic cell bodies. Those providing sympathetic and parasympathetic innervation to the pelvic viscera

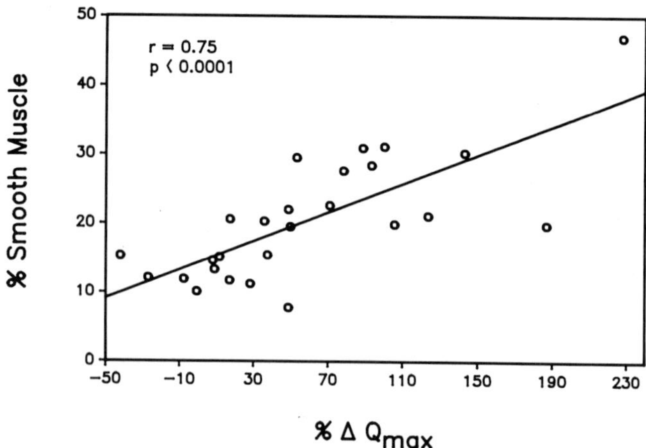

FIGURE 15–1. The relationship between the per cent area density of prostatic smooth muscle and change in peak urinary flow rate ($\%\Delta Q_{max}$) following terazosin therapy is shown for 26 males with clinical BPH. (From Shapiro E, Lepor H: The relationship between histology and clinical response to alpha blockade in men with symptomatic BPH. J Urol 145:265A, © by American Urological Assoc., Inc., 1991; with permission.)

are located in the sacral and thoracolumbar spinal cord, respectively. The terms *parasympathetic/cholinergic* and *sympathetic/adrenergic* are not interchangeable. The distinction between adrenergic and cholinergic innervation depends solely on the neurotransmitter that is released at the postganglionic synapse. The neurotransmitters mediating adrenergic and cholinergic innervation are norepinephrine and acetylcholine, respectively. Norepinephrine binds to adrenergic receptors located on the cell membranes of effector cells such as smooth muscle.

Several subtypes of adrenergic receptors can be pharmacologically distinguished by differential affinities for adrenergic antagonists.[49] The major subtypes of the adrenergic receptor include the alpha and beta receptors.[2] The alpha- and beta-adrenergic receptors have been subclassified as alpha$_1$/alpha$_2$ and beta$_1$/beta$_2$, respectively. Drugs are commercially available to selectively block alpha$_1$, alpha$_2$, beta$_1$, and beta$_2$ adrenoceptors. For example, prazosin and terazosin are selective alpha$_1$ antagonists, whereas yohimbine is a selective alpha$_2$ antagonist. Although norepinephrine represents the neurotransmitter for all adrenergically mediated functions, administration of selective antagonists enhances the specificity and minimizes the morbidity of pharmacologic manipulation of physiologic functions mediated by adrenergic receptors. For example, the tensions of pulmonary and coronary artery smooth muscle are mediated by beta$_1$ and beta$_2$ adrenoceptors, respectively. Selective beta$_1$ antagonists such as terbutaline relieve asthma and chronic obstructive pulmonary disease (COPD) without eliciting tachycardia, whereas selective beta$_2$ antagonists such as propranolol relieve angina without exacerbating COPD.[25]

The principles of selective alpha blockade are also relevant to the treatment of BPH. The human prostate contains an equivalent density of alpha$_1$ and alpha$_2$ adrenoceptors.[20, 56] The tension of prostate smooth muscle is mediated only by the alpha$_1$ adrenoceptor.[21] Nonselective alpha blockers such as phenoxybenzamine antagonize both alpha$_1$ and alpha$_2$ adrenoceptors. The alpha$_2$ blockade associated with nonselective alpha blockers provides no additional efficacy but enhances toxicity.[34] Minneman et al[47] have recently reported the existence of at least two subtypes of the alpha$_1$ adrenoceptor. Pharmacologic studies are currently under way in our laboratory to define which alpha$_1$ adrenoceptor subtype mediates smooth muscle tension. The development of more selective drugs for prostatic alpha$_1$ adrenoceptors is likely to further reduce the toxicity associated with alpha blockade in BPH.

ASSESSING CLINICAL RESPONSE

The ultimate role of alpha blockade and other therapeutic alternatives for BPH must be based upon relative efficacy, morbidity, and cost. The treatment objectives for BPH include amelioration of troublesome symptoms of prostatism, improvement of bladder emptying, reversal of bladder dysfunction, prevention of recurrent urinary tract infection, reversal of renal insufficiency, and alleviation of urinary retention. The ability of therapeutic alternatives to achieve these desired outcomes must be ascertained independently. It is conceivable that a drug therapy may effectively ameliorate symptoms of prostatism without decreasing residual urine or vice versa. Therefore, clinical trials evaluating effectiveness in BPH must define a specific therapeutic objective, identify a cohort of subjects who will benefit from a "favorable" clinical response, utilize standardized and validated outcome measurements, eliminate bias, and enroll an appropriate number of subjects to detect clinically significant changes in the outcome measure.

The most common indication for intervention in subjects with clinical BPH is the relief of urinary symptoms. In order to determine the ability of a treatment to relieve prostatism, the inclusion and exclusion criteria should identify a cohort of men with troublesome symptoms of prostatism secondary to BPH. Ideally, men with other conditions that may masquerade as prostatism, such as diabetes, primary neurogenic disorders, and bladder cancer, must be excluded. An effort should also be made to enroll subjects with bladder outlet obstruction. Unfortunately, no urodynamic parameter reliably discriminates men with prostatism with and without bladder outlet obstruction. Because the enrollment criteria for BPH studies reported in the literature lack uniformity, comparing the relative effectiveness of different therapies based upon a meta-analysis is often misleading.

Several questionnaires have been used to quantify the severity of clinical BPH and ascertain the response to therapy.[6, 44] Although these symptom questionnaires quantified the severity of prostatism, the questionnaires were not validated. The AUA Measurements Subcommittee recently devised and validated a quantitative symptom index in order to standardize the assessment of symptom severity and response to therapy. The World Health Organization recently endorsed the AUA symptom score index and recommended that the index be universally accepted by industry and clinicians. Despite the availability of a validated symptom index, the assessment of symptom improvement must be evaluated using randomized placebo-controlled studies. The variable natural history of prostatism and the very prominent placebo response must be controlled.[28]

Finally, the issue of statistical and clinical significance must be addressed. Although a standard symptom index is available, no consensus currently exists as to what constitutes a clinically significant outcome. A general misconception prevails that the quality and validity of a study depend upon the "number" of subjects enrolled. Increasing the sample size simply reduces the magnitude of a clinical response required to achieve statistically significant outcome. For example, a study can be sufficiently powerful (excessive patient enrollment) to demonstrate that the difference between awakening 1.9 times and 1.8 times at night is statistically significant. Obviously, such a difference is of no clinical significance. Therefore, clinical studies related to symptom improvement in BPH must be appropriately powered and critically interpreted.

No data base related to the ability of any treatment for BPH to reduce residual urine, prevent urinary retention, reverse renal insufficiency, and decrease the incidence of urinary tract infection previously existed. Ultimately, properly designed clinical trials must address the ability of BPH therapies to achieve these treatment outcomes.

ALPHA BLOCKADE IN BENIGN PROSTATIC HYPERPLASIA: SUMMARY OF LITERATURE

Caine et al reported in 1976 that phenoxybenzamine, a nonselective alpha$_1$ blocker, was effective for the treatment of BPH.[10] Over the past 15 years, at least 30 clinical trials evaluating alpha blockade for the treatment of BPH have been documented.[1, 3, 5, 7–10, 12, 13, 16–19, 22, 27, 29–33, 38–40, 43, 45, 51, 53, 59, 61] Most of these studies were deficient in design: sample sizes were small, treatment periods were short, and criteria for enrollment and assessment of efficacy were not well defined. Twenty-seven of the 30 reported clinical trials confirmed Caine's observation that alpha blockers were effective for the treatment of BPH.

The alpha blockers administered in the BPH studies can be subgrouped according to receptor subtype selectivity and duration of half-lives (Table 15–2). Phenoxybenzamine antagonizes alpha$_1$ and alpha$_2$ adrenoceptors, whereas prazosin, alfuzosin, YM617, indoramin, and terazosin are selective alpha$_1$ antagonists. The advantage of the selective alpha$_1$ antagonists is that the incidence and severity of adverse events are far less than with the nonselective alpha blockers. Terazosin represents the only long-acting formulation that has been studied in

TABLE 15–2. SUMMARY OF ALPHA BLOCKERS EVALUATED FOR THE THERAPY OF BENIGN PROSTATIC HYPERPLASIA

Nonselective alpha blockers
Phenoxybenzamine
Selective alpha$_1$ blockers
Prazosin
Alfuzosin
YM617
Indoramin
Selective long-acting alpha$_1$ blockers
Terazosin
Doxazosin

BPH. The longer half-life of terazosin allows for a once-a-day dosing, which is likely to have a favorable impact on compliance. The most common adverse events associated with selective alpha$_1$ blockers include dizziness, lightheadedness, and asthenia. The administration of a once-a-day formulation at bedtime reduces the incidence and severity of dizziness, lightheadedness, and asthenia. Doxazosin is another long-acting selective alpha$_1$ blocker that is currently being investigated for BPH. No data have been published related to the safety and effectiveness of this drug for BPH.

The study designs and outcome assessments for the 30 studies evaluating alpha blocker therapy in BPH are summarized in Tables 15–3 through 15–8. The clinical data base is analyzed separately for the nonselective alpha blockers, selective alpha$_1$ blockers, and selective long-acting alpha$_1$ blockers. A total of 2254 subjects have been enrolled into clinical studies reporting the safety and efficacy of alpha blockade in BPH. Of the 30 studies, 17 (57 per cent) were randomized and placebo-controlled clinical trials. Of the 2254 subjects, 1595 received active drug and 659 placebo.

The definition of effectiveness as it relates to BPH therapy has yet to be established. Because no universally accepted guidelines exist for reporting effectiveness of BPH therapies, the measures used to ascertain outcomes following alpha blockade in the literature are highly variable. The majority of the reported clinical trials excluded subjects with absolute indications for intervention such as urinary retention, urinary tract infection, and renal insufficiency. Therefore, the primary outcome measure addressed by clinical studies was relief of symptoms. Symptom improvement was ascertained using a quantitative symptom index in 9 clinical trials. The subject's self-assessment of improvement was evaluated in 10 clinical trials. Although objective symptom indices were established in the 1970s, the instruments for ascertaining clinical response were only sporadically used in BPH clinical trials. Symptom indices are currently being used routinely to assess symptom improvement. All of the reported clinical experiences evaluating terazosin therapy used the Boyarsky symptom index. Overall, the mean improvement in the total symptom score was 49 per cent. Historically, subjective improvement was often ascertained by the patient's self-assessment of the level of improvement. Subjects either rated the level of improvement (marked, moderate, or slight) or simply indicated whether or not any improvement was observed. A limitation of many of these subjective self-assessments is that "slight" improvement may not represent a clinically significant outcome. The percentages of subjects experiencing any degree of symptom improvement following administration of a nonselective, selective alpha$_1$, or selective long-acting alpha$_1$ blocker were 75 per cent, 82 per cent, and 93 per cent, respectively. The available clinical data base for alpha blockade indicates that symptom improvement is similar for the three groups of alpha blockers.

Uroflowmetry has been used to assess the effectiveness of BPH therapy. Although uroflowmetry may reflect the degree of obstruction along the prostatic urethra, the outcome measure is of limited clinical significance because patients are rarely bothered by a slow urinary stream. Change in maximum urinary flow rate (Q_{max}) was cited in 24 of the alpha-blocker studies reported in the literature. The mean improvement in Q_{max} following administration of nonselective, selective alpha$_1$, and selective long-acting alpha$_1$ blockers was 41 per cent, 47 per cent, and 44 per cent, respectively. The clinical data base for alpha blockers in BPH suggests that the improvement in urinary flow rate is similar for the three groups of alpha blockers.

An important caveat in interpreting effectiveness following alpha blockade relates to the dose dependence of the clinical response. All of the dose-ranging studies with alpha blockers have demonstrated unequivocally that clinical response (improvement in symptom scores and Q_{max}) is dose dependent. The summary of the data base for alpha blockade presented in this chapter does not take into account the relationship between dose and clinical response. The data were not censored according to the appropriateness of the dose. For example, Brooks et al[7] reported one of the only clinical trials demonstrating the lack of efficacy of alpha blockers for the treatment of BPH. The study was intentionally designed to determine the effect of low-dose phenoxybenzamine (10 mg/day). The relative lack of side effects observed in the treatment groups indicated that the failure to demonstrate efficacy was most likely attributable to a dose of phenoxybenzamine insufficient to adequately block the alpha$_1$ adrenoceptor. Lepor et al[43] recently reported a double-blind randomized study comparing placebo and 2, 5, and 10 mg of terazosin. Terazosin was titrated to the predetermined fixed dose provided that adverse events were not observed. Although the improvement in symptom scores of urinary flow rate was dose dependent, the data shown in Table 15–8 reflect the mean improvement for all three treatment groups.

A comprehensive review of all of the reported clinical studies is beyond the scope of this chapter. A detailed review of representative randomized, placebo-controlled studies is presented in the following section in order to illustrate the safety and efficacy of alpha blockers for the therapy of BPH.

RANDOMIZED, PLACEBO-CONTROLLED STUDIES

Phenoxybenzamine

Caine et al[8] reported a placebo-controlled, double-blind study of the effect of phenoxybenzamine on benign

TABLE 15–3. STUDY DESIGN: NONSELECTIVE ALPHA BLOCKERS: PHENOXYBENZAMINE

| REFERENCE | ENROLLMENT | | FOLLOW-UP (weeks) | RANDOMIZED/ PLACEBO | SYMPTOM INDEX | UROFLOWMETRY |
	Total	Active Drug				
Caine et al[10]	9	9	—	No	No	No
Boreham et al[5]	27	27	1	No	No	No
Caine et al[8]	49	24	2	Yes	No	Yes
Gerstenberg et al[19]	9	9	4	No	No	Yes
Caine et al[9]	200	200	—	No	No	Yes
Abrams et al[1]	44	28	4	Yes	No	Yes
Brooks et al[7]	25	15	4	Yes	No	Yes
Ferrie and Patterson[18]	39	21	5	Yes	No	Yes
	402	333		4/8	0/8	6/8

TABLE 15–4. STUDY DESIGN: SELECTIVE ALPHA₁ BLOCKERS

| REFERENCE | ENROLLMENT | | FOLLOW-UP (weeks) | RANDOMIZED/ PLACEBO | SYMPTOM INDEX | UROFLOWMETRY |
	Total	Active Drug				
Prazosin						
LeDuc et al[33]	32	15	4	Yes	No	Yes
Ruutu et al[53]	32	32	4	Yes	No	Yes
Chapple et al[12]	46	22	12	Yes	No	Yes
Yamaguchi et al[61]	146	77	3	Yes	No	Yes
Shimizu et al[59]	16	16	½–6	No	No	Yes
Kirby et al[32]	55	28	4	Yes	No	Yes
Hedlund et al[22]	20	20	4	Yes	No	Yes
Aoki et al[3]	40	40	4	No	No	Yes
Martorana et al[45]	18	18	4	Yes	No	Yes
	405	268		7/9	0/9	9/9
Alfuzosin						
Ramsey et al[51]	31	20	12	Yes	No	Yes
Jardin et al[29]	502	242	26	Yes	Yes	Yes
	533	262		2/2	1/2	2/2
YM617						
Kawabe and Niijima[30]	77	77	2	No	No	Yes
Kawabe et al[31]	231	164	4	Yes	Yes	Yes
	308	241		1/2	1/2	2/2
Indoramin						
Iacovou and Dunn[27]	26	11	8	Yes	No	Yes
Chow et al[13]	121	81	8	Yes	No	Yes
	147	92		2/2	0/2	2/2
	1393	**863**		**12/15**	**2/15**	**15/15**

TABLE 15–5. STUDY DESIGN: SELECTIVE LONG-ACTING ALPHA₁ BLOCKER: TERAZOSIN

| REFERENCE | ENROLLMENT | | FOLLOW-UP (weeks) | RANDOMIZED/ PLACEBO | SYMPTOM INDEX | UROFLOWMETRY |
	Total	Active Drug				
Dunzendorfer[16]	15	15	4	No	Yes	Yes
Lepor[34]	22	22	4	No	Yes	Yes
Lepor et al[38]	39	39	8	No	Yes	Yes
Fabricius et al[17]	52	52	24	No	Yes	Yes
Lepor et al[37]	50	50	4–26	No	Yes	Yes
Lepor et al[39]	29	29	4	No	Yes	Yes
Lepor et al[43]	252	192	12	Yes	Yes	Yes
	459	399		1/7	7/7	7/7

TABLE 15–6. OUTCOME ASSESSMENT: NONSELECTIVE ALPHA BLOCKER: PHENOXYBENZAMINE

REFERENCE	ACTIVE DRUG (N)	Δ Q$_{max}$ (%)	OUTCOME ASSESSMENT Δ Symptom Index (%)	OUTCOME ASSESSMENT Subject Improved (%)	INVESTIGATOR'S ASSESSMENT OF EFFICACY
Caine et al[10]	9	—	—	—	Yes
Boreham et al[5]	27	—	—	—	Yes
Caine et al[8]	24	+88	—	—	Yes
Gerstenberg et al[19]	9	—	—	—	Yes
Caine et al[9]	200	—	—	—	Yes
Abrams et al[1]	28	+43	—	90	Yes
Brooks et al[7]	15	+12	—	60	No
Ferrie and Patterson[18]	21	+22	—	—	No
	333	+41		75	6/8

TABLE 15–7. OUTCOME ASSESSMENT: SELECTIVE LONG-ACTING ALPHA$_1$ BLOCKER: TERAZOSIN

REFERENCE	ACTIVE DRUG (N)	Δ Q$_{max}$ (%)	OUTCOME ASSESSMENT Δ Symptom Index (%)	OUTCOME ASSESSMENT Subject Improved (%)	INVESTIGATOR'S ASSESSMENT OF EFFICACY
Dunzendorfer[16]	15	+31	−48	—	Yes
Lepor[34]	22	+63	−50	89	Yes
Lepor et al[38]	39	+42	−47	91	Yes
Fabricius et al[17]	52	+53	−55	—	Yes
Lepor et al[37]	50	+52	−53	—	Yes
Lepor et al[39]	29	+38	−56	100	Yes
Lepor et al[43]	192	+27	−37	—	Yes
	399	+44	−49	93	7/7

TABLE 15–8. OUTCOME ASSESSMENT: SELECTIVE ALPHA$_1$ BLOCKERS

REFERENCE	ACTIVE DRUG (N)	Δ Q$_{max}$ (%)	OUTCOME ASSESSMENT Δ Symptom Index (%)	OUTCOME ASSESSMENT Subject Improved (%)	INVESTIGATOR'S ASSESSMENT OF EFFICACY
Prazosin					
LeDuc et al[33]	15	+62	—	—	Yes
Ruutu et al[53]	32	+54	—	—	Yes
Chapple et al[12]	22	+34	—	—	Yes
Yamaguchi et al[61]	77	—	—	—	Yes
Shimizu et al[59]	16	+32	—	—	Yes
Kirby et al[32]	28	+59	—	69	Yes
Hedlund et al[22]	20	+41	—	—	Yes
Aoki et al[3]	40	+60	—	95	Yes
Martorana et al[45]	18	+47	—	—	Yes
	268	+49		82	9/9
Alfuzosin					
Ramsey et al[51]	20	—	—		?
Jardin et al[29]	242	+12	—	85	Yes
	262	+12		85	1/2
YM617					
Kawabe and Niijima[30]	77	+22	—	80	Yes
Kawabe et al[31]	164	+31	—	77	Yes
	241	+27		79	2/2
Indoramin					
Iacovou and Dunn[27]	11	+120	—	100	Yes
Chow et al[13]	81	+43		71	Yes
	92	+82		86	2/2
	863	+47		82	14/15

prostatic obstruction. Fifty patients with BPH received 10 mg of phenoxybenzamine or placebo twice a day. The clinical trial lasted only 14 days, and 49 patients completed the trial. The assessment of efficacy was based on improvement in urinary flow rates. The maximum urinary flow in the phenoxybenzamine and placebo groups improved 82 per cent and 30 per cent, respectively. There was a significantly greater improvement in day- and night-time urinary frequency among the phenoxybenzamine-treated patients. The primary limitation of phenoxybenzamine was the incidence and severity of adverse reactions. Eleven patients experienced tiredness, dizziness, impaired ejaculation, nasal stuffiness, or difficulty with visual accommodation. A single adverse reaction was observed in the placebo group. Caine's study unequivocally demonstrated the therapeutic advantage of phenoxybenzamine over placebo. The pitfalls of the study were the failure to establish specific entry parameters, the short duration of the treatment, and the qualitative assessment of symptomatic outcome.

Prazosin

Kirby et al[32] reported a randomized, placebo-controlled study evaluating prazosin for the treatment of prostatic obstruction. Eighty men with BPH between the ages of 50 and 80 years received 2 mg of prazosin or placebo twice a day. Only 55 patients completed the 1-month clinical trial. Assessment of efficacy was based on improvement in urinary flow rates, frequency of micturition, and postvoid residual volume. The peak urinary flow rate improved 59 per cent and 6 per cent in the prazosin- and placebo-treated groups, respectively. The observed improvement in residual urine and voiding frequency in the prazosin-treated group was statistically significant. No adverse reactions were observed in the prazosin-treated group, whereas one subject receiving placebo complained of dizziness and diarrhea. Orthostatic hypotension and erectile or ejaculatory dysfunction were not observed in either the placebo- or prazosin-treated group. Kirby's study demonstrated unequivocally the therapeutic advantage of prazosin over placebo. The pitfalls of the study were the large dropout rate (32 per cent), the short duration of the treatment, the qualitative assessment of symptomatic outcome, and the lack of specific entry criteria.

Terazosin

Lepor et al[43] recently reported the results of a multicenter, Phase III double-blind, parallel-group, randomized, placebo-controlled study of once-a-day administration of terazosin to patients with symptomatic BPH. Three hundred and fourteen patients entered the double-blind treatment with placebo, 2, 5, or 10 mg of terazosin once daily. Statistically significant ($P < 0.05$) decreases from baseline obstructive, irritative, and total symptom scores were observed for all terazosin treatment groups. The 10-mg terazosin treatment group also exhibited significantly greater decreases in irritative and total scores relative to the placebo group. The 5- and 10-mg terazosin treatment groups exhibited a significantly greater decrease in obstructive scores than did the placebo group. The level of improvements in the symptom scores was dose-related. The percentages of patients experiencing a greater than 30 per cent improvement in the total symptom scores for the placebo, 2-, 5-, and 10-mg treatment groups were 38 per cent, 54 per cent, 63 per cent, and 70 per cent, respectively. The percentages of patients experiencing greater than 30 per cent improvement in total symptom score in the 5- and 10-mg treatment groups were significantly greater than for the placebo group.

A statistically significant improvement from baseline was observed in the peak and mean urinary flow rates for all treatment groups. The 10-mg treatment group exhibited a significantly larger increase from baseline in peak and mean urinary flow rates relative to the placebo group. The 5-mg treatment group also exhibited a significantly larger increase in mean urinary flow rate than the placebo group.

The change in urinary flow rate was also a dose-related response. The percentages of patients experiencing a greater than 30 per cent increase in peak urinary flow rate in the placebo, 2-, 5-, and 10-mg treatment groups were 25 per cent, 36 per cent, 35 per cent, and 58 per cent, respectively. A significantly greater proportion of patients in the 10-mg terazosin treatment group exhibited a greater than 30 per cent improvement in peak urinary flow rate than the placebo group.

Overall, the adverse events in the four treatment groups were minor and reversible. Although a higher incidence of asthenia, flu syndrome, and dizziness were observed in the terazosin treatment groups, the differences from placebo were not statistically significant when tested using Fisher's exact test. There was a significantly greater incidence of postural hypotension in the 5-mg terazosin group than in the placebo group. One patient in the 10-mg treatment group developed syncope at the 5-mg dose of terazosin. The incidence of syncope in the 10-mg treatment group was 1 out of 79 (1.3 per cent). The incidence of syncope for all terazosin-treated patients was less than 0.5 per cent.

An effort was made to identify clinical or urodynamic factors that would predict a favorable outcome to terazosin therapy. The relationships between percentage change in total symptom score and peak urinary flow rate with baseline age, prostate size, peak urinary flow rate, mean urinary flow rate, postvoid residual, and total symptom score were examined. No significant association was observed between treatment effect and baseline factors when tested using an analysis of covariance model with terms for baseline factor, treatment groups, and their interaction.

Alfuzosin

Jardin et al[29] recently reported a multicenter randomized, placebo-controlled study comparing alfuzosin, a selective alpha$_1$ blocker, and placebo. Five hundred and eighteen subjects were entered into the study in 32 centers. The patients were randomized to receive placebo or alfuzosin (daily dose of 7.5 or 10 mg). Of the 518 patients, 354 completed the 6-month treatment. The numbers of patient drop-outs at 6 months because of adverse events, lack of cooperation, or loss to follow-up were similar in the two groups. The outcome measures were changes in total Boyarsky symptom score, peak urinary flow rate, and the investigators' and patients' global assessments of therapeutic response. The difference between the decrease in mean total Boyarsky score in the alfuzosin group (from 9.5 to 5.5; 42 per cent decrease) and placebo group (from 9.4 to 6.4; 32 per cent decrease) was statistically significant. Uroflowmetry was evaluable for only 234 patients. The changes in peak urinary flow rate in the placebo and alfuzosin groups were not significantly different (11 per cent increase versus 12 per cent increase). The post-treatment mean urinary flow rates in the placebo and alfuzosin groups were significantly different (6.6 versus 7.5 ml/sec).

The proportion of subjects rating their improvement as good to very good was 50 per cent and 40 per cent in the alfuzosin and placebo groups, respectively. The proportion of subjects judged by the investigators to show good to very good improvement was 61 per cent and 42 per cent in the alfuzosin and placebo groups, respectively. The incidences of dizziness, headache, postural hypotension, asthenia, and impotence were similar in the alfuzosin and placebo groups.

The improvement in urinary flow rate in the alfuzosin-treated group is less than in any other active treatment group reported in the literature. Because a dose-ranging study for alfuzosin has never been reported for BPH, there is no evidence that 7.5 or 10 mg of alfuzosin represents a therapeutic dose. The modest improvement in peak urinary flow rate presumably reflects the selection of a dose of alfuzosin insufficient to achieve adequate inhibition of prostatic alpha$_1$ adrenoceptors. The failure to observe any adverse events attributable to alfuzosin provides further evidence that an inappropriate dose of alfuzosin was selected for the clinical trial.

YM617

YM617 is a selective alpha$_1$ adrenoceptor that is highly selective for prostatic alpha$_1$ adrenoceptor binding sites.[35] Kawabe et al[31] recently reported a multicenter randomized, placebo-controlled study comparing the safety and efficacy of YM617 and placebo in BPH. A total of 270 patients were randomized into four groups: placebo, 0.1 mg, 0.2 mg, and 0.4 mg YM617 once daily. Of the 270 subjects, 231 were evaluable after receiving 2 weeks of placebo and 4 weeks of test drug. The efficacy of YM617 was based upon the change in urinary flow rate, the proportion of subjects experiencing an improvement in obstructive and irritative symptoms, and the patients' self-assessment of improvement. The peak urinary flow rates for the placebo, 0.1-mg, 0.2-mg,

and 0.4-mg groups improved by 12 per cent, 15 per cent, 40 per cent, and 36 per cent, respectively. The changes in peak urinary flow rates for the treatment and placebo groups were not significantly different. The mean urinary flow rate for placebo, 0.1 mg, 0.2 mg, and 0.4 mg improved by 0 per cent, 18 per cent, 27 per cent, and 41 per cent, respectively. The differences between the change in mean urinary flow rates for all treatment groups and placebo were statistically significant.

Unfortunately, a standardized symptom score questionnaire was not used to assess clinical response. The data related to symptom improvement are therefore difficult to interpret. The percentage of patients indicating moderate and marked improvement in the placebo, 0.1-, 0.2-, and 0.4-mg YM617 groups were 10 per cent, 28 per cent, 38 per cent, and 39 per cent, respectively. Adverse events in the placebo, 0.1-, 0.2-, and 0.4-mg YM617 groups were experienced by only 0 per cent, 1 per cent, 3 per cent, and 3 per cent of subjects, respectively.

COMBINATION PHARMACOTHERAPY

The mechanism for bladder outlet obstruction secondary to BPH is related to dynamic and static factors. The dynamic factors are related to prostatic smooth muscle tension, and the static factors are related to the enlarged prostatic adenoma encroaching upon the bladder outlet. Two different pharmacologic strategies have emerged for the treatment of BPH based upon the present concept of bladder outlet obstruction in BPH. Selective alpha$_1$ blockers are directed toward relaxing the prostatic smooth muscle, whereas androgen suppression promotes reduction of prostate volume. Because the presumed mechanisms of action for alpha blockade and androgen suppression are unrelated, it is reasonable to assume that the clinical response following co-administration of these drugs is at least additive. Combination pharmacotherapy for BPH represents an attractive approach to the treatment of BPH.

Lepor and Machi[40] recently reported a pilot open-label study designed to compare selective alpha$_1$ blockade versus the combination of selective alpha$_1$ blockade and androgen suppression. Twenty-nine men received terazosin therapy alone for 1 month and the combination of 5 mg of terazosin and 250 mg of flutamide three times daily for the subsequent 5 months. The efficacy parameters included change in Boyarsky symptom scores, uroflowmetry, and the subjects' self-assessment of symptom improvement. The efficacy parameters were evaluated at 1 month (terazosin alone) and at either 6 months or at the time of early withdrawal from the study (combination therapy). Terazosin alone was associated with statistically significant improvements in total Boyarsky symptom scores (57 per cent decrease) and maximum urinary flow rate (38 per cent increase). Combination therapy resulted in a further reduction of 8 per cent in total symptom scores. Twenty-five per cent of subjects exhibited moderate symptom improvement following the addition of the antiandrogen. The differences in the outcome measures between terazosin alone and combination therapy were not statistically significant. The failure to demonstrate statistical significance is related to the small sample size. The majority of subjects in the pilot combination study developed severe adverse events to flutamide which resulted in either dose reduction or premature withdrawal from the study. The mean reduction of prostate volume observed in the 24 evaluable patients receiving combination therapy was 25 per cent, indicating that adequate androgen suppression was achieved.

The optimal study design for evaluating drug therapy for BPH is a randomized, placebo-controlled study. Lepor has organized a multicenter randomized, placebo-controlled study to compare four treatment groups (placebo, selective alpha$_1$ blockade, androgen suppression, and the combination of selective alpha$_1$ blockade and androgen suppression). Terazosin was selected as the alpha$_1$ blocker because dose-ranging studies have demonstrated the optimal dose. Finasteride was selected for androgen suppression because of its very favorable toxicity profile. A total of 30 Veterans Affairs Medical Centers will enroll 1200 subjects into the above-mentioned study between August 1, 1992 and July 1, 1993. It is anticipated that the active treatment phase of the study will be completed by July 30, 1994. The unique features of the present study are that the relative safety and efficacy of selective alpha$_1$ blockade and androgen suppression will be compared in a similar cohort of subjects using standard outcome measures. The relative efficacy of combination therapy will be compared to that of the individual monotherapies. Conducting the study under the auspices of the Department of Veterans Affairs will increase the likelihood that the study is free of possible bias associated with industry-supported studies.

CONCLUSIONS

There is a definite physiologic and pharmacologic rationale for alpha blockade in the treatment of BPH. The overwhelming majority of clinical studies reported in the literature have confirmed Caine's initial observation that alpha blockade represents effective therapy for BPH. Randomized, placebo-controlled studies have demonstrated that the incidence and severity of adverse events associated with selective alpha$_1$ blockers are typically minor and reversible. The long-acting selective alpha$_1$ blockers such as terazosin, doxazosin, and YM617 are likely to emerge as the preferred alpha blockers because a once-a-day regimen is likely to improve patient compliance and tolerance. The lightheadedness, dizziness, and tiredness associated with selective alpha$_1$ blockade are reduced if the drug is administered prior to bedtime.

The very encouraging clinical data base for selective alpha$_1$ blockers must be cautiously interpreted. The safety of alpha$_1$ blockers assumes that the dose is judiciously titrated and that consideration is given to potential interactions with other cardiovascular medications.

The majority of the alpha blocker clinical trials enrolled subjects with troublesome urinary symptoms lacking absolute indications for intervention. Therefore, the demonstrated effectiveness of selective alpha$_1$ blockers cannot be extrapolated to include the absolute indications for intervention. Approximately 70 per cent of men with symptomatic BPH exhibit a favorable clinical response to selective alpha$_1$ blockade. The clinician must accept that a significant subset of these responders would have improved following administration of a placebo. Unfortunately, there are at present no parameters that identify individuals whose response is placebo mediated. The clinician prescribing selective alpha$_1$ blockers has the assurance that the majority of the observed response is treatment related. The long-term effectiveness and compliance with alpha$_1$ blockade have yet to be unequivocally established. Lepor et al reported that the symptom improvement following terazosin is durable over a period of 24 months. Abbott Laboratories is sponsoring a long-term open-label extension study of those subjects who participated in the randomized, double-blind Phase III studies. Approximately 500 patients are enrolled in the study. The improvement in symptoms has been maintained in more than 150 patients followed for a minimum of 18 months.

The optimal candidate for selective alpha$_1$ blockade has yet to be defined. A reasonable candidate for alpha blocker therapy is the individual with troublesome urinary symptoms that adversely impact upon his quality of life. The potential candidates for selective alpha$_1$ blockade must be counseled that the long-term effectiveness of the drug is unknown and that the treatment option requires a life-time commitment to medical therapy. The man with hypertension and symptomatic BPH represents an optimal candidate for selective alpha$_1$ blockade because it is likely that both conditions can be controlled by a single drug. Often, the degree of bother arising from the symptoms of prostatism is insufficient to justify the inherent risks associated with prostatectomy. In addition, the likelihood of a favorable clinical response is not related to the severity of disease. Therefore, individuals with severe symptoms of prostatism should at least be offered alpha blockade even though the magnitude of the symptoms justifies prostatectomy. It is unreasonable to mandate that alpha blockers be offered prior to prostatectomy because some subjects may be opposed to long-term medical management or may prefer the most definitive form of intervention. The presence of absolute indications for TURP is a relative contraindication for alpha blockade because no data support the efficacy in this subset of patients.

The role of alpha blockade must ultimately be based upon efficacy, safety, and cost. The safety and efficacy have been clearly established in well-controlled studies. The cost of selective alpha$_1$ blockers appears to be very reasonable relative to prostatectomy. A year's supply of terazosin costs approximately $300. A 40-year supply of terazosin is equivalent to the cost of prostatectomy. Alpha blockade results in substantial cost savings relative to prostatectomy provided that the response is durable over decades of follow-up. If the majority of subjects treated with alpha blockers ultimately undergo prostatectomy, then alpha blockers would only add to the cost of treatment of BPH.

It is the author's belief that alpha blockade will emerge as a useful therapy for the treatment of BPH. The public and general medical practitioners are keenly aware of nonsurgical therapies for BPH. Nonsurgical therapy represents an attractive option for many patients with prostatism who desire symptom relief with minimal morbidity. Referring physicians and patients expect the urologist to be familiar with all reasonable treatment options for BPH. Therefore it behooves the urologist to understand the adrenergic pharmacology and physiology of the prostate and at least be familiar with the proper use of selective alpha$_1$ blockers. Urologists must resist the temptation to embrace all new devices and drugs based on preliminary and uncontrolled studies. On the other hand, they must be flexible and respond responsibly to properly designed clinical studies. The urologist may object to any nonsurgical therapy on the basis of the natural history of BPH, issues related to occult prostate cancer, and the superior results achieved with prostatectomy. Unfortunately, few objective data are available related to the outcome of prostatectomy, the natural history of BPH, and the clinical significance of occult prostate cancer. All reasonable issues related to BPH must be discussed with the patient because the patient must ultimately play a pivotal role in selecting therapy, especially when the desired outcome is improvement in the quality of life.

REFERENCES

1. Abrams PH, Shah PJR, Stone R, et al: Bladder outflow obstruction treated with phenoxybenzamine. Br J Urol 50:551, 1978.
2. Ahlquist RR: A study of the adrenergic receptors. Am J Physiol 153:587, 1948.
3. Aoki H, Ohninata T, Tsuzuki M, et al: Clinical studies on the effectiveness of prazosin HCl (Minipress tablets) in the treatment of dysuria accompanying benign prostatic hyperplasia. Urol Int 45 (suppl):18, 1990.
4. Bartsch G, Muller HR, Oberholzer M, et al: Light microscopic stereological analysis of the normal human prostate and of benign prostatic hyperplasia. J Urol 122:487, 1979.
5. Boreham PF, Brainthwaite P, Milewski P, et al: Alpha adrenergic blockers in prostatism. Br J Surg 64:756, 1977.
6. Boyarsky S, Jones G, Paulson DR, et al: A new look at bladder neck obstruction by the Food and Drug Administration regulators: Guidelines for investigation of benign prostatic hypertrophy. Trans Am Assoc Genitourinary Surg 68:29, 1977.
7. Brooks ME, Sidi AA, Hanani Y, et al: Ineffectiveness of phenoxybenzamine in treatment of benign prostatic hypertrophy: A controlled study. Urology 21:474, 1983.
8. Caine M, Perlberg S, Meretyk S: A placebo-controlled double-blind study of the effect of phenoxybenzamine in benign prostatic obstruction. Br J Urol 54:527, 1982.
9. Caine M, Perlberg S, Shapiro A: Phenoxybenzamine for benign prostatic obstruction: A review of 200 cases. Urology 25:542, 1981.
10. Caine M, Pfau A, Perlberg S: A use of alpha adrenergic blockers in benign prostatic obstruction. Br J Urol 48:255, 1976.
11. Caine M, Raz S, Ziegler M: Adrenergic and cholinergic receptors in the human prostate, prostatic capsule, and bladder neck. Br J Urol 27:193, 1975.
12. Chapple CR, Christmas TJ, Milroy EJG: A twelve-week placebo-controlled study of prazosin in the treatment of prostatic obstruction. Urol Int 45(suppl):47, 1990.
13. Chow W, Hahn D, Sandhu D, et al: Multicentre controlled trial of indoramin in the symptomatic relief of benign prostatic hypertrophy. Br J Urol 65:36, 1990.
14. Dorflinger T, England DM, Madsen PO, et al: Urodynamic and histological correlations of benign prostatic hyperplasia. J Urol 140:1487, 1989.
15. Dorflinger T, Oster M, Larsen JF, et al: Transurethral prostatectomy or incision of the prostate in the treatment of prostatism caused by small benign prostates. Scand J Urol Nephrol 104:77, 1987.
16. Dunzendorfer U: Clinical experience: Symptomatic management of BPH with terazosin. Urology 32:27, 1988.
17. Fabricias PG, Weizert P, Dunzendorfer U, et al: Efficacy of once-a-day terazosin in benign prostatic hyperplasia. Prostate 3(suppl):85, 1990.
18. Ferrie BG, Patterson PJ: Phenoxybenzamine in prostatic hypertrophy. A double-blind study. Br J Urol 59:63, 1987.
19. Gerstenberg T, Blaabjerg J, Lykkengaard N, et al: Phenoxybenzamine reduces bladder outlet obstruction in benign prostatic hyperplasia: A urodynamic investigation. Invest Urol 18:29, 1980.
20. Gup DI, Shapiro E, Baumann M, et al: Autonomic receptors in asymptomatic and symptomatic BPH. J Urol 143:179, 1990.
21. Gup DI, Shapiro E, Baumann M, et al: The contractile properties of human prostatic adenomas are unrelated to the development of infravesical obstruction. Prostate 15:105, 1989.
22. Hedlund H, Anderson KE, Ek A: Effects of prazosin in patients with benign prostatic obstruction. J Urol 130:275, 1983.
23. Hellstrom P, Lukkarinen O, Kontturi M: Bladder neck incision or transurethral electroresection for the treatment of urinary obstruction caused by a small prostate. Scand J Urol Nephrol 20:187, 1986.
24. Hieble JP, Caine M, Zalaznik E: In vitro characterization of the alpha-adrenoceptors in human prostate. Eur J Pharmacol 107:111, 1985.
25. Hieble JP, Ruffolo RR Jr: Therapeutic applications of agents interacting with the β-adrenoceptors. *In* Ruffolo RR Jr (ed): β-Adrenoceptors: Molecular Biology, Biochemistry and Pharmacology. Basel, Karger, 1991, pp 210–235.
26. Holtgrewe HL, Mebust WK, Dowd JB, et al: Transurethral prostatectomy: Practice aspects of the dominant operation in American urology. J Urol 141:248, 1989.
27. Iacovou JW, Dunn M: Indoramin—an effective new drug in the management of bladder outflow obstruction. Br J Urol 60:259, 1987.
28. Isaacs JT: Importance of the natural history of benign prostatic hyperplasia in the evaluation of pharmacologic intervention. Prostate 3(suppl):1, 1990.
29. Jardin A, Bensadoun H, DeLauche-Cavallor MC, et al: Alfuzosin for the treatment of benign prostatic hypertrophy. Lancet 1:1457, 1991.
30. Kawabe K, Niijima T: Use of an alpha$_1$ blocker, YM617, in micturition difficulty. Urol Int 42:280, 1987.
31. Kawabe K, Ueno A, Takimoto Y, et al: Use of an alpha$_1$ blocker, YM617, in the treatment of benign prostatic hypertrophy. J Urol 144:908, 1990.
32. Kirby RS, Coppinger SWC, Cocoran MO, et al: Prazosin in the treatment of prostatic obstruction: A placebo-controlled study. Br J Urol 60:136, 1987.
33. LeDuc A, Cariou G, Baron C, et al: A multi-center, double-blind, placebo-controlled trial of the efficacy of prazosin in the treatment of dysuria associated with benign prostatic hypertrophy. Urol Int 45(suppl 1):56, 1990.
34. Lepor H: Nonoperative management of benign prostatic hyperplasia. J Urol 141:1283, 1989.
35. Lepor H, Baumann M, Shapiro E: The stereospecificity of LY253352 for alpha$_1$ adrenoceptor binding sites in the brain and prostate. Br J Pharmacol 95:139, 1988.
36. Lepor H, Gup DI, Baumann M, et al: Laboratory assessment of terazosin and alpha$_1$ blockade in prostatic hyperplasia. Urology 32(suppl):21, 1988.
37. Lepor H, Henry D, Laddu AR: The efficacy and safety of terazosin for the treatment of symptomatic BPH. Prostate 18:345, 1991.
38. Lepor H, Knapp-Maloney G, Sunshine H: An open-label dose

titration study evaluating terazosin for the treatment of symptomatic BPH. J Urol 144:1393, 1990.

39. Lepor H, Knapp-Maloney G, Wozniak-Petrofsky J: The safety and efficacy of terazosin for the treatment of BPH. Int J Clin Pharmacol Therapy Toxicol 27:392, 1989.

40. Lepor H, Machi GM: The combination of terazosin and flutamide for symptomatic BPH. Prostate, 20:89, 1992.

41. Lepor H, Rigaud G: The efficacy of transurethral resection of the prostate in men with moderate symptoms of prostatism. J Urol 143:533, 1990.

42. Lepor H, Shapiro E: Characterization of alpha$_1$ adrenoceptors in human benign prostatic hyperplasia. J Urol 132:1226, 1984.

43. Lepor H, Soloway M, Narayan P, et al: A multicenter fixed dose study of the safety and efficacy of terazosin in the treatment of symptoms of BPH. J Urol 145:1265A, 1991.

44. Madsen PO, Iverson P: A point system for selecting operative candidates. *In* Hinmann F Jr (ed): Benign Prostatic Hypertrophy. New York, Springer-Verlag, 1983, pp 763–766.

45. Martorana G, Gilberti C, Damonte P, et al: The effect of prazosin in benign hypertrophy, a placebo controlled double-blind study. IRCS Med Sci 12:11, 1984.

46. Mebust WK, Holtgrewe HL, Cockett ATK, et al: Transurethral prostatectomy: Immediate and postoperative complications. A cooperative study of 13 participating institutions evaluating 3,885 patients. J Urol 141:243, 1989.

47. Minneman KP, Han C, Abel PW: Comparison of alpha$_1$ adrenergic receptor subtypes distinguished by chloretylclonidine and WB4101. Molec Pharmacol 33:509, 1988.

48. Neal DE, Ramsden PD, Sharples L, et al: Outcome of elective prostatectomy. Br Med J 299:762, 1989.

49. Nichols AJ, Ruffolo RR Jr: Alpha adrenoceptors. *In* Ruffolo RR Jr (ed): β-Adrenoceptors: Molecular Biology, Biochemistry and Pharmacology. Basel, Karger, 1991, pp 1–23.

50. Orandi A: Transurethral incision of prostate compared with transurethral resection of the prostate in 132 matching cases. J Urol 138:810, 1987.

51. Ramsay JWA, Scott GI, Whitfield N: A double-blind controlled trial of new alpha$_1$ blocking drug in the treatment of bladder outflow obstruction. Br J Urol 57:657, 1985.

52. Raz S, Ziegler M, Caine M: Pharmacologic receptors in the prostate. Br J Urol 45:663, 1973.

53. Ruutu ML, Hansson E, Juusela HE, et al: Efficacy and side-effects of prazosin as a symptomatic treatment of benign prostatic obstruction. Scand J Urol Nephrol 25:15, 1991.

54. Shapiro E, Hartanto V, Lepor H: Anti-desmin vs. anti-actin for quantifying the area density of prostate smooth muscle. Prostate 20:259, 1992.

55. Shapiro E, Hartanto V, Lepor H: Quantifying the smooth muscle content of the prostate using double-immunoenzymatic staining and color assisted image analysis. J Urol 147:1167, 1992.

56. Shapiro E, Lepor H: Alpha$_2$ adrenergic receptors in hyperplastic human prostate: Identification and characterization using ^{3}H-rauwolscine. J Urol 135:1038, 1986.

57. Shapiro E, Lepor H: Alpha adrenergic receptors in canine lower genitourinary tissues: Insight into development and function. J Urol 138:979, 1987.

58. Shapiro E, Lepor H: The relationship between histology and clinical response to alpha blockade in men with symptomatic BPH. J Urol 145:265A, 1991.

59. Shimizu K, Nakai K, Imai K, et al: Effects of an alpha$_1$-adrenergic blocker (prazosin HCl) on micturition disturbances associated with benign prostatic hypertrophy. Urol Int 45(suppl 1):40, 1990.

60. Wennberg JE, Roos N, Sola L, et al: Use of claims data systems to evaluate health care outcomes: Mortality and reoperation following prostatectomy. JAMA 257:933, 1987.

61. Yamaguchi O, Shiraiwa M, Kobayashi T, et al: Clinical evaluation of effects of prazosin in patients with benign prostatic obstruction. Urol Int 45(suppl):40, 1990.

Chapter 16

HORMONAL THERAPY IN THE MANAGEMENT OF BENIGN PROSTATIC HYPERPLASIA

DAVID L. BLUESTEIN and JOSEPH E. OESTERLING

Benign prostatic hyperplasia (BPH) refers to a common, nonmalignant enlargement of the prostate that produces clinical symptoms in 30 to 40 per cent of men older than 60 years.[49] Development of BPH is age related. According to an examination of autopsy specimens, the frequency of BPH was 30 per cent in men aged 60 to 69 years and 100 per cent in men older than 90 years.[105] It is estimated that half of all men older than 65 years have some prostatic enlargement, and approximately one third of these men have clinical symptoms of bladder outlet obstruction.[58] Because the population is aging, the number of patients with symptomatic BPH will continue to increase, and the burden of this disease on society will continue to rise.

BPH is a condition characterized by a nodular enlargement of prostatic tissue, resulting in obstruction of the bladder neck and prostatic urethra. This enlargement arises almost exclusively from the small segment of prostatic tissue surrounding the urethra and the preprostatic sphincter.[58] Hence, severe symptoms of obstruction can occur with only a small degree of prostatic enlargement. Histologic studies have documented that BPH is a true hyperplastic process, resulting in increased numbers of both epithelial and stromal cells.[78, 108]

The pathogenesis for the development of BPH has not been fully determined. However, it appears clear that the two major factors necessary for the development of BPH are the presence of the testes and aging. BPH does not occur in men who are castrated before puberty[24, 136, 144]; in fact, it is extremely rare for it to develop in men who undergo castration before the age of 40 years. The only reported case is a man who was castrated at age 28 and underwent a prostatectomy at age 60 because of bladder outlet obstruction.[119] Additional support for the requirement of gonadal hormones in the development of BPH comes from human studies of a Russian sect, the Skoptzys; men in this sect are required to undergo castration at age 35 years as part of an ethnic ritual.[147] These men reportedly do not suffer from BPH and have smaller-than-normal prostates. In a study conducted by Moore[84] in 1944, the prostates of 28 men who had been either castrated or "hypopituitarized" before age 40 years and who had lived to be older than age 55 years were examined post mortem. In this group, he could find no histologic evidence of BPH. In age-matched controls, histologic evidence of BPH was found in more than 50 per cent of the men.

In both the rat and the canine model, BPH can be initiated and augmented with androgenic or androgenic plus estrogenic stimulation. Ehrlichman and his co-workers[37] were able to produce marked prostatic enlargement in castrated rats with atrophic prostates by administering dihydrotestosterone (DHT; 5α-androstan-17β-ol-3-one) or DHT plus 17β-estradiol (1,3,5[10]-estratriene-3,17β-ol). Walsh and Wilson[137] treated castrated beagle dogs with concomitant administration of 17β-estradiol and 3α-androstanediol (5α-androstan-3α,17β-diol), a 5α-reduced androgen. Glandular BPH developed in these dogs. Other investigators observed a similar result when they substituted DHT for the 3α-androstanediol.[32, 85, 132, 133] It should be noted that canine BPH has distinct differences from human BPH. In the dog, the hyperplasia is primarily epithelial and a uniform enlargement is seen. These characteristics are in contrast to the previously described nodular hyperplasia that occurs in men. Additionally, urinary retention rarely occurs in the dog.[58]

The testes secrete both estrogen and testosterone. Testosterone can be irreversibly converted to DHT by the enzyme 5α-reductase. DHT is the most potent human androgen and, in turn, can undergo reversible metabolism to a second androgen, 3α-androstanediol. Testosterone is also the major substrate for the peripheral conversion of androgens to 17β-estradiol by the aromatase enzyme complex. DHT cannot undergo aromatization. Numerous investigators have established that DHT is the major intracellular androgenic metabolite in the prostate.[13, 14] Given the above-described observations, the testes and their hormonal products—androgens and estrogens—appear to be instrumental in the pathogenesis of BPH. Thus, a logical approach for treating BPH and avoiding prostatectomy seems to be elimination of the influence of the testes at one or more points in the chain of hormonal conversions or interactions. Various hormonal manipulations, including castration, luteinizing hormone–releasing hormone (LHRH; GnRH) agonist therapy, 5α-reductase inhibitors, antiandrogens, and antiestrogens, have all been considered in the medical treatment of BPH.

Important factors to consider in evaluation of the responses to the various hormonal interventions include the following:[47] (1) prostatic size, as measured by either transrectal ultrasonography or MRI; (2) peak urinary flow rate, which has been shown to correlate with the cross-sectional diameter of the urethra[18]; (3) symptoms (obstructive and irritative) as determined from standardized questionnaires[74]; and (4) postvoid residual urine volume, which is a product of bladder function and prostatic obstruction. In all studies, the diagnosis of BPH should be clearly established. Misdiagnosis of urethral stricture or neurogenic bladder for BPH almost always produces a lack of clinical response. Prostate cancer must also be excluded because this condition may respond dramatically to hormonal therapy.

ANDROGEN DEPRIVATION THERAPY

Bilateral Orchiectomy

During the past century, it has been known that the symptoms of BPH (prostatism) can be reduced and even eliminated when hormonal therapy is instituted. In 1895, White[141] reported 111 cases in which he performed a bilateral orchiectomy for BPH causing urinary obstruction. He noted improvement of symptoms in 87 per cent of the patients and a palpably smaller prostate in 64 per cent of the patients. White speculated that the lack of response in some men may be due to prostates that are of the "fibrous" type and not the "glandular" variety. One year later, Cabot[16] described 61 men who underwent castration for reduction of enlarged prostates. He found that 84 per cent of the patients had a substantial improvement in ability to urinate, 7 per cent had a moderate improvement, and 10 per cent had no beneficial effect from the castration. The side effects were "uncomfortable flushes of heat" and "hysterical phenomenon." The hysterical reaction that Cabot referred to was likely a consequence of uremia. In 1986, Schroeder and colleagues[112] described the results of bilateral orchiectomy in five patients who were in chronic urinary retention due to benign prostatic enlargement. As determined by transrectal ultrasonography, these patients had a 26 per cent reduction in prostate volume at 3 months of follow-up. By 5 months, all patients were able to urinate spontaneously and none of them required an indwelling catheter.

LHRH Agonists

The use of an LHRH analogue for the treatment of BPH is based on the known physiology of testicular androgen production (Fig. 16–1) and on previous studies in which castration was used as a treatment for BPH. LHRH agonists have an amino acid sequence very similar to the decapeptide LHRH and bind with a high affinity to the LHRH receptor on the plasma membrane of the gonadotropic cells in the anterior pituitary gland. All LHRH analogues have an ethylamide substituted for the carboxy terminal Gly-amide and a D-amino acid substituted at position 6. These agonists have a greater affinity for the LHRH receptor and are more resistant to proteolysis than LHRH.[25] When LHRH agonists are administered daily or as a depot formulation (that is, in a continuous, nonpulsatile manner), they evoke an initial agonist phase of several days to weeks, followed by desensitization (downregulation) and a long-term inhi-

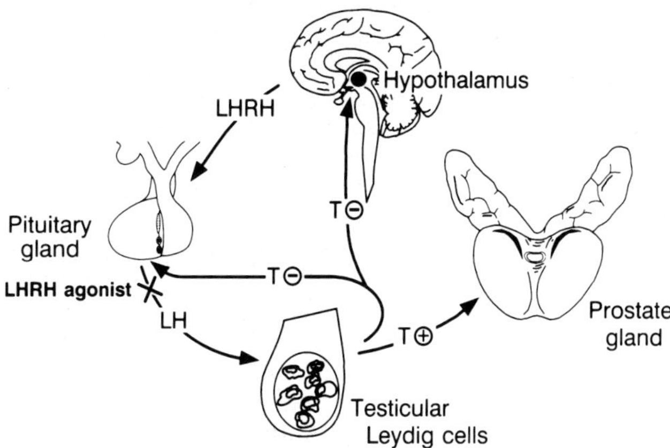

FIGURE 16–1. Hypothalamic-pituitary-gonadal axis. LH = Luteinizing hormone; LHRH = luteinizing hormone–releasing hormone; T = testosterone.

bition of gonadotropin secretion that is virtually complete and selective.[25] What occurs is a progressive decrease in the number of LHRH receptors on the cell surface of the gonadotropic cells. This results in less cellular stimulation and less gonadotropin synthesis and secretion. After approximately 3 to 4 weeks of administration of an LHRH analogue, follicle-stimulating hormone and luteinizing hormone cease to be excreted. Thus, the Leydig cells of the testes fail to be stimulated and the testicular production of testosterone ceases. The serum testosterone concentration decreases to the castration level (50 μg/dl or less).[25] The only source of androgens then is from adrenal production, which accounts for approximately 10 per cent of all androgens in the normal state. In essence, the use of an LHRH agonist produces a medical castration.

The use of LHRH agonists in the treatment of BPH was first investigated in animals in the early 1980s.[1, 35, 92, 135] The first human treated with an LHRH agonist was reported by Schroeder and colleagues in 1986.[112] This patient was in chronic urinary retention and was a poor candidate for a prostatectomy; he also had refused to have a bilateral orchiectomy. The patient was treated with an LHRH analogue (buserelin; 400 μg three times per day) intranasally for 2 months, and within 3 weeks the plasma testosterone value decreased to the castration level. Transrectal ultrasonography revealed a 55 per cent decrease in prostatic size. The patient was urinating freely after 2 months of therapy and did not have a significant postvoid residual urine volume. Gabrilove and co-workers,[45] in 1987, described three patients with BPH who were treated with subcutaneous injection of an LHRH analogue (leuprolide, 1 mg once daily). After 6 months of treatment, prostatic volume, as determined by transrectal ultrasonography, had declined 58 per cent, and the greatest rate of decrease occurred between the second and fifth months of treatment. Serum testosterone, DHT, and 17β-estradiol concentrations decreased to castration levels within 6 weeks after the initiation of treatment and remained at these levels throughout the study. One patient who had acute urinary retention and was managed with a suprapubic cystostomy tube was able to void spontaneously with a minimal postvoid residual urine volume after 5 months of treatment.

More recently, Lukkarinen[72] investigated the effects of an LHRH agonist in 12 men with chronic urinary retention caused by BPH who were in poor medical condition. These patients could not undergo a prostate operation because of the great risk posed by such treatment. The men were given 3.6 mg of a long-acting LHRH analogue subcutaneously monthly for 6 months. All patients acquired a serum testosterone level in the castration range. The mean prostatic volume, as measured by transrectal ultrasonography, decreased by 51 per cent. After 6 months of therapy, 58 per cent of the patients could manage without their indwelling urinary catheter and were satisfied with their ability to urinate. Schlegel and Brendler[111] described six patients with urinary retention resulting from BPH who were not medically able to undergo prostatectomy. These men were treated with daily subcutaneous injections of leuprolide acetate (1 mg) for 6 months. The deaths of three

of the patients during this study affirmed their high operative risk. All patients had a castration level of testosterone during treatment, and all resumed spontaneous voiding within 1 month after starting treatment. One patient, however, continued to catheterize himself at bedtime so that he would not have to get up during the night. The average decline in prostatic size as measured by transrectal ultrasonography was 41 per cent (range, 12 to 70 per cent). Interestingly, the patient with only a 12 per cent reduction in prostatic volume had a dramatic response and the patient who had a 70 per cent reduction in prostatic volume continued to perform intermittent catheterization at bedtime. The clinical results in these patients demonstrate that improvement in voiding does not necessarily correlate with the percentage decline in prostatic volume.

In 1987, Peters and Walsh[103] described nine patients with bladder outlet obstruction due to BPH who were treated with subcutaneous nafarelin acetate (400 μg per day) for 6 months and then followed for 6 months after treatment. Eight patients completed the 6 months of treatment and were followed during the subsequent 6 months. The ninth patient withdrew at 5 months because of mild peripheral edema; the authors considered his evaluation at the time of withdrawal to be his 6-month follow-up. All patients had a reduction in serum testosterone concentration to the castration level by the end of the first month of treatment. After 2 months of not receiving the LHRH agonist, the serum testosterone value returned to the pretreatment level in all men. The mean prostatic size, as determined by transrectal ultrasonography, before initiating treatment was 48 grams. After 4 months of therapy, all patients had a decrease in prostatic size (mean reduction, 24.2 per cent). There was no further decrease during the remaining 2 months of therapy. After treatment had been withheld for 6 months, all of the prostates returned to their pretreatment size.

Morphometric analysis of the prostate biopsy specimens before and at the conclusion of treatment revealed a 21 per cent decline in stromal weight and a 40 per cent decline in the epithelial weight. The variation in DNA content of the prostate with androgen deprivation and restimulation correlated with the change in epithelial weight ($r = 0.77$; $P < 0.05$) but not with the change in stromal weight ($r = 0.23$; $P > 0.3$). A questionnaire was developed to monitor change in obstructive and irritative symptoms. After 6 months of treatment, six (67 per cent) of the patients had a significant improvement in symptom scores; obstructive symptoms improved more than irritative symptoms. The placebo effect, however, was not controlled for in this study. With regard to urinary flow rate, only three of the nine patients (33 per cent) had a peak urinary flow rate of more than 15 ml/sec after 6 months of therapy. There was no significant change in the postvoid residual urine volume after 6 months of treatment.

Gabrilove and colleagues[46] treated 15 men with symptomatic BPH who were poor surgical candidates with 1 mg of subcutaneously administered leuprolide daily. Transrectal ultrasonography of the prostate demonstrated a decrease in prostatic volume of 40 per cent at

4 months and of 46 per cent at 6 months. All patients experienced at least a mild improvement in symptoms, and the obstructive symptoms improved more than the irritative symptoms. Urinary flow rates and postvoid residual urine volumes were not monitored in this study. However, three of the five men (60 per cent) who required urinary catheters before treatment could void well without catheters by the end of treatment. These investigators concluded that LHRH agonist therapy could be effective for a select group of patients with symptomatic BPH who were not surgical candidates.

Bosch and co-workers[8] studied six patients receiving the LHRH agonist buserelin (0.4 mg three times daily intranasally) for 12 weeks. After this period, the mean reduction in prostatic volume, as measured by transrectal ultrasonography, was 29 per cent. After discontinuation of treatment, the prostatic volume returned to near its pretreatment value within 6 to 36 weeks. Urodynamic factors also were assessed in these patients. The peak urinary flow increased, the postvoid residual urine volume decreased, and the frequency of daytime voiding decreased. Although statistically significant, the urodynamic changes were minimal from a clinical viewpoint. These factors returned to pretreatment levels after therapy was withdrawn. No significant correlations were found between changes in prostatic size and any of the urodynamic factors.

In the study by Bianchi and associates,[6] 11 patients with symptomatic BPH who had contraindications to surgical intervention were treated with buserelin. After 6 months of therapy, the mean symptom score decreased significantly ($P < 0.01$). This decrease was primarily the result of improvement in obstructive symptoms rather than irritative symptoms. After 6 months of therapy, the mean prostatic size had decreased by 29 per cent, as measured by transabdominal ultrasonography. There was no significant change in postvoid residual urine volume. As with many of the other investigations, no control group was used.

In a study from Israel in 1991, Matzkin and colleagues[75] investigated the effect of a long-acting LHRH agonist on 20 men with symptomatic BPH. After 6 months of therapy, the men could choose to continue receiving the depot injections or take part in a surveillance-only program for the next 6 months. Of the 20 men, 17 (85 per cent) completed the half year of treatment; of these, 10 (59 per cent) continued treatment for 6 more months and 7 (41 per cent) elected to enter the surveillance-only program. The serum testosterone level declined to castration level in all patients within 1 month and remained at this level for as long as the patient was receiving the LHRH agonist. For those who entered the surveillance-only program, serum testosterone levels returned to pretreatment values within 3 months. Serum estradiol levels decreased by 70 per cent within 1 month of the initiation of treatment, and no changes were noted in serum prolactin levels during the study. By 6 months of therapy, mean prostatic size had declined by 37 per cent. In the surveillance-only group, the prostates had returned to 95 per cent of their original size at the 3-month post-treatment visit. A transient increase in prostatic size (15 per cent) was noted in five patients after 1 month of therapy. This is likely the result of the transient increase in serum testosterone level at the initiation of LHRH agonist therapy. The maximal reduction in prostatic volume was not achieved until after 9 months of therapy. After this time, there was no further reduction in prostatic size.

Peak urinary flow rates improved throughout treatment (9.75 ± 0.5 ml/sec to 11.4 ± 1.1 ml/sec at 6 months of therapy to 15.6 ± 2.9 ml/sec at 12 months). By 6 months of therapy, 35 per cent of the men had achieved a peak flow rate of at least 15 ml/sec. By 3 months after cessation of treatment, the peak flow had returned to near the pretreatment level (10.4 ± 1.5 ml/sec). The postvoid residual urine volume did not decrease significantly in any of the patients during treatment. With regard to symptoms, 10 patients (59 per cent) were considered to have a subjective success; 7 of these also had reached a peak flow of 15 ml/sec or had an increase in peak flow of at least 3 ml/sec. All of the patients who had these benefits continued to have symptomatic and objective improvement for as long as therapy was continued. Overall, 40 per cent had objective and subjective improvement, 27 per cent had objective or subjective improvement, and 33 per cent had no improvement.

Keane and colleagues[63] treated 20 men who had symptomatic BPH with buserelin (0.4 mg intranasally four times daily) for up to 6 months. After 6 months of therapy, there was no significant effect on mean flow rate or mean postvoid residual urine volume. In 65 per cent of the patients, a transurethral resection of the prostate was subsequently performed. Interestingly, all but one of the patients had a predominantly stromal prostate (more than 75 per cent stromal elements) on random pretreatment biopsy. Serum testosterone levels were maintained at the castration level throughout this study. Prostatic tissue levels of DHT and testosterone were significantly reduced in patients taking the drug at the time of operation compared with age-matched controls. Three patients withdrew from the study 4 to 6 weeks before operation. These men had prostatic tissue levels of testosterone and DHT comparable to those in untreated controls. This finding suggests that the effect of buserelin within the prostate is reversible within a relatively brief period.

Forti and co-workers[42] evaluated the effects of the long-acting LHRH analogue goserelin acetate depot on prostatic tissue androgen concentration, 5α-reductase activity, and androgen receptor content in seven men with BPH. The men were treated for 3 months before undergoing prostatectomy. The prostatic tissue concentration of testosterone decreased by 75 per cent and the tissue concentration of DHT and 3α-diol diminished by 90 per cent compared with those in untreated men. Prostatic 5α-reductase activity decreased by 50 per cent, and the mean cytosolic androgen receptor content in the prostatic tissue of the treated patients was significantly lower than that of the untreated men. The decrease in prostatic 5α-reductase activity and the decline in nuclear androgen receptors are most likely due to the decrease in serum androgen levels.[92] The serum testosterone value was at castration levels in all patients within 1 month of the initiation of therapy.

Salerno and colleagues[110] investigated the effect of an LHRH analogue on testosterone, DHT, and 3α-diol levels in human plasma and in prostatic tissue of seven men with BPH. The patients were treated for 3 months with monthly injections of a depot LHRH analogue. Plasma levels of testosterone, DHT, and 3α-diol were reduced to the castration range. The prostatic tissue concentrations of DHT and 3α-diol were reduced by approximately 90 per cent, and the prostatic tissue level of testosterone was diminished about 75 per cent compared with the untreated controls. Hence, DHT, which is the main androgen involved in the pathogenesis of BPH,[144] is reduced by 90 per cent after 3 months of treatment with an LHRH analogue. Thus, the prostatic DHT value appears to be 90 per cent dependent on testicular androgen production.

Side Effects

In the study conducted by Peters and Walsh,[103] all of the patients reported hot flushes, decreased libido, and impotence. Three of the nine patients (33 per cent) complained of a loss of drive and initiative that affected their lives. Sexual activity, however, returned within 4 months after the cessation of treatment. In the study by Gabrilove and colleagues,[46] all 15 men had some hot flushes, decreased libido, and impotence during treatment, but treatment was discontinued early in only 1 patient because of these side effects. Bosch and associates[8] found that all six patients receiving an LHRH agonist experienced hot flushes. This side effect caused one patient to withdraw from the study. All six patients did become impotent. After discontinuation of treatment, all except one regained his normal potency. In the study by Bianchi et al,[6] all of the patients experienced hot flushes. There was little change in libido and potency before or after treatment because of the patients' generalized debilitated state. In the study conducted by Matzkin and co-workers,[75] one patient withdrew from the study after 6 months because of severe hot flushes despite good urologic results. Keane and colleagues[63] reported hot flushes in all patients and severe headaches in 39 per cent. Thus, loss of libido, impotence, and hot flushes are nearly universal side effects of LHRH agonist therapy.

Effect of LHRH Agonist Therapy on Serum Prostate-Specific Antigen

BPH involves both stromal and epithelial elements.[77] Stromal cells are believed to initiate the BPH process.[29] Thereafter, however, stromal-epithelial interactions under the influence of androgens are believed to be responsible for the continued growth of the prostate.[29] Several studies have demonstrated that it is the epithelial rather than the stromal component which is responsive to androgen deprivation.[59, 103, 120]

Prostate-specific antigen (PSA) is a glycoprotein that is produced exclusively by prostatic epithelial cells of all types[93, 121]; it is found in normal, hyperplastic, and malignant prostatic tissue.[43, 138] Serum PSA levels are increased in hyperplastic tissue, prostatic malignancy, and other conditions such as prostatitis and prostatic infarction. Weber and colleagues[139] investigated the relationship of serum PSA to prostatic size and hormonal manipulation. Seven patients with symptomatic BPH were treated with an LHRH agonist (nafarelin acetate) for 6 months and then followed for an additional 6 months. Before the initiation of therapy, the mean serum PSA concentration was 2.95 ± 2.11 ng/ml. After 6 months of therapy, the mean serum PSA value was 0.50 ± 0.39 ng/ml (a reduction of 83 per cent). After 6 months of withholding therapy, the serum PSA levels returned to their pretreatment values. During the treatment and follow-up periods, the serum PSA concentration correlated with (1) the quantity of prostatic epithelium ($P < 0.001$), (2) the serum testosterone level ($P < 0.001$), and (3) prostatic size ($P < 0.05$).

Interestingly, Weber and associates[139] found that the PSA per gram of epithelium did not change significantly after 6 months of therapy (0.43 ± 0.2 ng/ml per gram of epithelium before treatment and 0.48 ± 0.36 ng/ml per gram after treatment). The likely reason that the serum PSA value did not correlate more exactly with prostatic size is that PSA is produced by only the epithelial and not the stromal component. The relative amounts of these two components vary markedly from one prostate to another. For example, the relative amount of epithelium in the prostate in one patient was nearly three times greater than that in another patient in this study. Additionally, the PSA value does not correlate perfectly with the amount of prostatic epithelium. Weber and colleagues speculated that the PSA level may depend not only on the amount of epithelium but also on the architectural integrity of the prostate gland.

In another study of serum PSA levels, Levine and co-workers[67] treated 12 men who had symptomatic BPH with leuprolide for 6 months. There was a steady decline in serum PSA levels, which stabilized after 4 months of therapy. This decline paralleled the decrease in prostatic size as measured by transrectal ultrasonography. The authors stated that the serum testosterone concentration decreased to a low level within 1 month of therapy, but they did not describe the relationship between serum PSA and testosterone. After discontinuation of treatment, prostatic size and serum PSA level gradually increased to pretreatment values. The authors, assuming that the decrease in prostatic size with treatment was due mainly to an involution of prostatic epithelial cells, calculated that the mean serum PSA per gram of prostatic epithelium was 0.35 ng/ml.

The knowledge that only prostatic epithelial cells produce PSA may be helpful in selecting which patients will benefit from medical castration. Patients with a high serum PSA level and a small gland are likely to have a high epithelial-to-stromal ratio and thus would be expected to respond more significantly to LHRH agonist therapy than patients with very large prostates and low serum PSA levels. Any patient who does have a serum PSA value above the reference range, however, must be evaluated for prostate cancer before LHRH agonist therapy is initiated.

Conclusion

LHRH analogues administered either on a daily basis or in a long-acting depot formulation lower a man's serum testosterone and DHT levels to the castration level within 1 month of the initiation of treatment. With lowered levels of circulating androgens, androgenic stimulation to the prostate is diminished, the prostatic epithelium undergoes involution, and prostatic size decreases. The degree of shrinkage varies and is likely a function of the epithelial/stromal composition of the enlarged gland. Glands with a large epithelial component respond more significantly than those with a large stromal component. It is the epithelium and not the stroma which is androgen responsive.[3, 4, 79, 103] Serum PSA concentration, which reflects the ratio of epithelium to stroma in the gland, may be useful in identifying the men most likely to respond to LHRH analogue therapy. Theoretically, men with a high serum PSA concentration and a small prostate gland, with no evidence of prostate cancer, respond most favorably. Overall, 30 to 40 per cent of men with BPH have an improvement in both subjective and objective factors.

The mean reduction in prostatic volume is approximately 30 per cent. As the prostatic enlargement regresses, the patient can urinate more freely because of the diminished bladder outlet resistance. However, symptoms of bladder outlet obstruction may initially worsen in the first 2 to 3 weeks of therapy because of the transient increase in serum androgen levels and the subsequent increase in prostatic size. This effect can be expected to occur in approximately 25 per cent of men receiving LHRH agonist therapy. The increase in prostatic size is modest (15 per cent) but theoretically may be significant enough to cause acute urinary retention in a patient who has nearly complete obstruction before treatment.

The side effects that occur with LHRH agonist therapy can be significant, but they are not known to be life threatening. Hot flushes, decreased libido, and impotence almost always occur. Gynecomastia and headaches can occur also. These adverse effects have caused a small percentage of patients to discontinue treatment. These side effects make patient selection an important issue. LHRH agonist therapy should be limited to elderly, debilitated patients for whom potency is not a concern and who are at high risk with surgical intervention.

Treatment of BPH with an LHRH analogue should be considered a lifetime intervention. Withdrawal of the LHRH agonist causes an increase in serum testosterone and DHT values and a subsequent regrowth of the prostatic tissue. Thus, the patient will be subjected to expensive monthly ($300 to $450) depot injections for the remainder of his life. Three-month depot solutions are currently under investigation and would make the drug more convenient to receive. Although it is not an ideal treatment for BPH, LHRH agonist therapy can be an effective, safe nonsurgical treatment for a select group of men. As more experience is gained in its use, the patient population who would benefit from this therapy will become more clear.

ANTIANDROGENS

Androgens exert their action at the tissue level through high-affinity binding to specific steroid receptors. This in turn stimulates, through a series of complex and not fully understood mechanisms, specific protein biosynthesis.[68–70] DHT is the most potent androgen in terms of stimulating prostatic growth, and it clearly has the highest affinity for the prostatic cell androgen receptor.[142] As discussed previously, the source of circulating androgens is twofold. Testicular androgens constitute approximately 90 per cent of circulating androgens, and adrenal androgens make up the remaining 10 per cent. Bilateral orchiectomy and LHRH agonist therapy to induce androgen deprivation have been studied as possible treatments for BPH. These treatments, however, have no effect on the circulating adrenal androgens.

Several antiandrogenic agents have been reported, but most of these have other hormonal properties that negate their usefulness in the treatment of BPH. Anandron, a true antiandrogen, reduced prostatic weight in the rat.[12, 106] This agent, however, had no significant effect on prostatic weight in men after 2 months of therapy.[34] Oxendolone, an antiandrogen synthesized from dehydroepiandrosterone by C19 demethylation, had beneficial effects in the canine model of BPH.[96, 97] Ostri and colleagues,[99] however, found no benefit with this drug when testing 30 men with symptomatic BPH who received weekly injections for 3 months. These patients had no significant change in prostatic volume, postvoid residual urine volume, or peak urinary flow rate. Flutamide, α,α,α-trifluoro-2-methyl-4'-nitro-m-propionotoluidide (Fig. 16–2), is an orally administered nonsteroidal antiandrogen that is metabolized to a hydroxylated derivative (hydroxyflutamide). It effectively competes with both testosterone and DHT for androgen receptor sites (Fig. 16–3).[128] Flutamide has no antigonadotropic or progestational activity, and thus it does not suppress testosterone levels.[89] In theory, serum testosterone levels may even be increased slightly to compensate for the androgen blockade. Currently, it is approved by the Food and Drug Administration for use

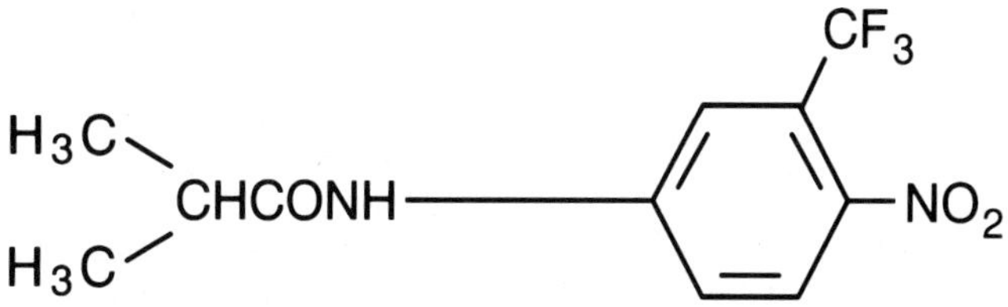

FIGURE 16–2. Chemical structure of flutamide.

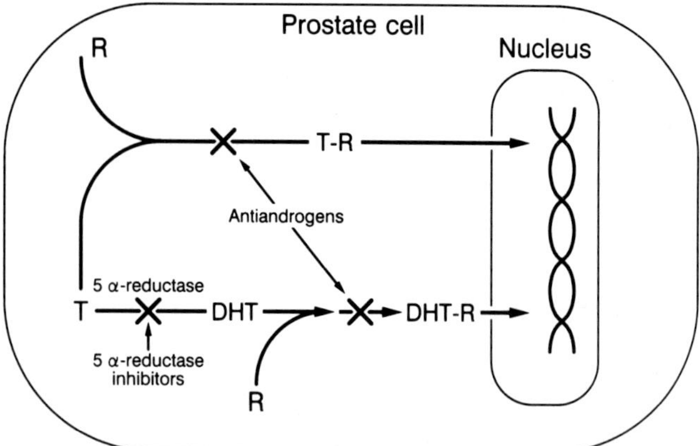

FIGURE 16–3. Mechanisms by which antiandrogens and 5α-reductase inhibitors inhibit prostatic cell activity. DHT = dihydrotestosterone; DHT-R = dihydrotestosterone-receptor complex; R = cytoplasmic receptor for androgens; T = testosterone; T-R = testosterone-receptor complex.

as combination therapy in the management of advanced prostate cancer.

In rats that had undergone orchiectomy, flutamide reduced the rate of prostate DNA synthesis in those concomitantly treated with testosterone propionate.[127] In addition, flutamide inhibited hyperplastic growth of the prostate in rats that had been castrated and were being treated concomitantly with testosterone and DHT.[90] Flutamide also significantly reduced prostatic volume and prostatic epithelial cell height in dogs.[91] BPH returned to baseline status within 2 months after the cessation of therapy. These dogs mated and sired several litters while receiving the flutamide; the findings suggest that spermatogenesis and libido are not impaired by flutamide in the canine model. In the baboon, flutamide shrank the prostate by 66 per cent.[87]

Caine and coinvestigators[17] conducted a double-blind, placebo-controlled human study that examined the effects of flutamide (100 mg three times per day for 12 weeks) on urinary flow rate, residual urine volume, and prostatic size. Although a significant increase in peak urinary flow rate was observed, no significant differences were found between the flutamide-receiving group and the placebo-receiving group in terms of prostatic size and postvoid residual urine volume.

Bonard and co-workers[7] found that flutamide administered over 12 weeks significantly decreased prostatic size, measured as the difference in distance between the bladder neck and verumontanum by transrectal ultrasonography. Stone and colleagues[123, 125] also evaluated the effect of flutamide on prostatic volume, maximal urinary flow rate, and symptoms in men with symptomatic BPH. Prostatic volume decreased by 23 per cent after 3 months of therapy and by 42 per cent at the end of 6 months of therapy; prostatic volume did not change in the placebo-receiving group. Peak urinary flow rates increased by 12 per cent after 3 months of therapy and by 79 per cent after 6 months of therapy. Of note is the fact that only a small number of the patients completed 6 months of therapy. Urinary symptom scores also improved significantly in the flutamide-treated group.

Stone and Clejan,[122] in a subsequent report, described the effect of flutamide on prostatic volume, PSA, and serum testosterone levels in men with BPH. Eleven patients received flutamide (250 mg three times per day) and 11 patients received a placebo. The patients were evaluated after 3 and 6 months of treatment and again at 6 weeks after the therapy was discontinued. After 6 months of treatment, prostatic volume decreased by 35 per cent and serum PSA concentration decreased by 65 per cent. The placebo-receiving group had no change in prostatic volume or serum PSA level. Patients receiving flutamide had a 58 per cent increase in serum testosterone level.

Side Effects

The side effects of flutamide appear to be mild in most cases. In the study by Caine and associates,[17] nipple pain or gynecomastia developed in 47 per cent of the men receiving flutamide, but there were no reports of diminished libido or impotency. In a 1989 study by Stone and co-workers,[123] 49 per cent of the patients experienced gastrointestinal side effects. In 1991, Stone and Clejan[122] described a patient who had to be withdrawn from the study for 2 weeks because of the development of severe diarrhea. Therapy with flutamide was reinitiated and slowly brought back to full dose. Gynecomastia and breast pain are common, occurring in 36 per cent to 54 per cent of patients, but they are mild in most cases. A decrease in potency was described by one patient in each of the studies by Stone and colleagues.[122, 123] There were no reports of decreased libido in either of these investigations. Flutamide also produced significant hepatic toxicity in one patient.[73]

Other Antiandrogens

Cyproterone acetate is a synthetic antiandrogen with progestational activity.[127] By acting as a progestin, it causes a reduction in gonadotropin secretion, which results in lowered serum androgen levels. A severe loss of libido is associated with its use; interestingly, this drug was first developed to suppress sexual activity in sexual deviants.[44]

In 1969, Scott and Wade[120] investigated the use of cyproterone acetate in the treatment of 13 men with BPH in an uncontrolled study. After 15 months of therapy, urinary flow rates improved in 69 per cent of the men and voiding symptoms improved in 85 per cent. Epithelial height, evaluated from needle biopsy specimens, decreased in 72 per cent of the men. Impotence occurred in 27 per cent of the men and led to two men withdrawing from the study. Bosch and colleagues,[8] in 1989, evaluated the effect of cyproterone acetate on prostatic size and urodynamic factors in six men with symptomatic BPH. The subjects received 100 mg orally twice daily for 12 weeks. Prostatic volume decreased approximately 30 per cent, but clinical improvement, as assessed from urinary flow rates, was only minimal.

Regrowth of prostatic tissue occurred after withdrawal of therapy. Hot flushes occurred in 33 per cent of the men, and only one patient retained his potency during the study.

A new pure antiandrogen, Casodex, is currently being investigated. Casodex has been shown to cause a dose-related reduction in ventral prostate and seminal vesicle weights in rats.[44] In the rat, there was also a smaller increase in luteinizing hormone and testosterone levels compared with flutamide-treated rats. In dogs, Casodex induced prostatic atrophy, as determined from histologic appearance.[44] Human clinical studies are currently being conducted to assess the use of Casodex in the treatment of BPH and prostate cancer.

Conclusion

Currently, cyproterone acetate does not appear to have a role in the treatment of BPH. Its progestational properties are associated with significant undesirable side effects. In addition, it has produced liver abnormalities in animal studies and also can induce hepatic neoplasms.[44]

The role of flutamide in the treatment of BPH appears limited at this time. Its distinct advantage over LHRH agonist therapy is that it does not cause impotence or a loss of libido, as universally occurs with LHRH agonist therapy. However, the adverse reactions to this drug are common and troublesome. Gastrointestinal side effects occur in approximately 50 per cent of the patients receiving this drug. Additionally, mild gynecomastia and breast pain occur in 36 to 54 per cent of men. The fact that no patient reported a loss of libido suggests that flutamide is not active in the brain. Given the high incidence of adverse reactions, patient compliance is a serious concern. Additionally, therapy must be lifelong to maintain its effect. Like LHRH agonist therapy, flutamide is expensive, costing approximately $3000 per year.

The concern that flutamide monotherapy may increase gonadotropin secretion, which in turn could increase the serum testosterone to a level that overcomes the androgenic blockade, does not seem to be borne out. According to several studies, androgenic blockade is maintained after 6 months of flutamide monotherapy, as evidenced by decreased prostatic size and lowered serum PSA values despite increased serum testosterone levels. The questions of whether testosterone levels will continue to increase with more prolonged therapy and whether this effect will compromise treatment still need to be evaluated in future investigations.

5α-REDUCTASE INHIBITORS

The intracellular concentrations of androgens within the prostate gland depend on the presence of the numerous prostatic enzymes that regulate steroid interconversions and on the presence of androgen receptors within the prostate cell.[47] DHT, the 5α-reduced metabolite of testosterone, is the biologically active androgen within the prostate. Several elegant experiments have demonstrated that DHT mediates the intracellular action of androgens in the rat prostate.[13, 14]

BPH can be experimentally induced in young normal dogs by treatment with 5α-reduced androgens alone or in combination with 17β-estradiol.[32, 137] In male infants born with a 5α-reductase enzyme deficiency, the prostate is either absent or greatly diminished in size.[81] At birth, male infants with 5α-reductase deficiency have ambiguous genitalia; they have a urogenital sinus with a blind vaginal pouch and a clitoris-like phallus.[81] Their wolffian duct structures, which depend on testosterone rather than DHT, develop normally. However, their urogenital sinus structures, which require DHT rather than testosterone, develop poorly. In adulthood, these individuals have normal or nearly normal muscle mass, libido, potency, and phallus size, but they do not have acne, male-pattern baldness, or normal prostate growth.[81] Genetic studies in these individuals have clearly shown that the biochemical abnormality is a complete or partial deficiency of 5α-reductase activity.[81]

The study of these individuals led to the concept that selective androgenic depletion of DHT may be effective in the treatment or prevention of BPH. It was hypothesized that DHT depletion would selectively interfere with prostatic growth without adversely affecting testosterone-mediated characteristics such as libido and potency. As a result, several inhibitors of the 5α-reductase enzyme were developed. The administration to dogs of 4-MA (N,N-diethyl-4-methyl-3-oxo-4-aza-5α-androstane-17β-carboxamide), a 4-azasteroid with 5α-reductase inhibitor properties, caused a significant decrease in prostatic volume and a decrease in the height of prostate epithelial cells.[10] Other compounds derived from 4-MA also decreased prostatic weight and DHT content in the rat.[11] These agents, however, caused hepatic toxicity and possessed androgen-receptor activity. For these reasons, clinical testing in humans was not pursued. A newer agent developed by Merck Research Laboratories (MK-906; Proscar, finasteride) reduced the prostatic volume of dogs by 64 per cent and caused a significant decrease in DHT levels in the canine prostate.[9] Finasteride, N-(2-methyl-2-propyl)-3-oxo-4-aza-5α-androst-1-ene-17β-carboxamide (Fig. 16–4), was then chosen for human studies.

In phase I clinical studies of finasteride, a single dose caused a significant reduction in the serum levels of DHT in men.[134] A dose of 0.5 mg caused a 65 per cent reduction in plasma DHT levels which persisted for nearly 1 week. Gormley and co-workers[50] administered finasteride in a double-blind, placebo-controlled trial to normal male volunteers at daily doses ranging from 0.04 to 100 mg orally for 10 to 14 days. The men taking between 25 and 100 mg of finasteride daily had a significant reduction in serum DHT levels and a statistically significant increase in serum testosterone levels with doses of 50 and 100 mg. Treatment had no effect on the triglyceride, high-density lipoprotein, low-density lipoprotein, or total cholesterol values. The subjects receiving 0.2 mg and 1.0 mg of finasteride also had significantly lower levels of serum DHT. After therapy

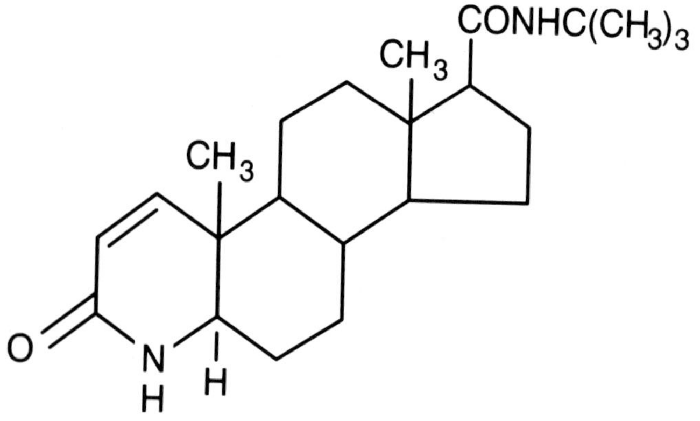

FIGURE 16–4. Chemical structure of finasteride.

was withheld for 2 weeks, DHT returned to pretreatment levels in all of the subjects. McConnell and colleagues[76] in 1989 reported on the effect of finasteride on the intraprostatic testosterone and DHT concentrations. In a placebo-controlled study, the subjects received 50 mg of finasteride daily for 7 days before transurethral resection of the prostate. The prostatic DHT concentration decreased 92 per cent, whereas the prostatic testosterone concentration increased 634 per cent.

The Finasteride Study Group[130] reported the effect of finasteride on serum testosterone and DHT levels, prostatic volume, and urinary flow rates in 67 men with BPH. Serum DHT levels were reduced by 80 per cent at 6 months and remained at that level throughout the 1-year study period. The 16 per cent increase in serum testosterone levels at 1 year was statistically significant but within the normal range for men. There was no significant change in the luteinizing hormone levels. After 6 months and 1 year of therapy, prostatic volumes were reduced by 17 per cent and 19 per cent, respectively, as measured by MRI. After 6 months of therapy, the peak urinary flow rate had increased by a mean of 2.1 ml/sec ($P < 0.05$). At 1 year, the peak urinary flow rate had increased by a mean of 4.0 ml/sec ($P < 0.01$). Approximately 70 per cent of the subjects had an increase of at least 3 ml/sec in peak urinary flow rate after 12 months of therapy. Seven patients (10 per cent) had adverse experiences, but these were not considered to be drug related. This study suggests that finasteride can safely lower serum DHT levels, reduce prostatic size, and improve urinary flow during a 1-year period.

Stoner[126] subsequently reported a multicenter, double-blind, placebo-controlled study of 895 patients with symptomatic BPH. Three hundred patients received placebo, 298 men received 1.0 mg of finasteride daily, and 297 men received 5.0 mg of finasteride daily. These men were followed for 12 months, and response was assessed according to change in (1) prostatic volume, as determined by MRI; (2) peak urinary flow rate; (3) symptom score (obstructive and irritative); and (4) serum PSA value.

Patients treated with either 1.0 mg or 5.0 mg of finasteride had a reduction in serum DHT to castration level at all time points measured. The serum DHT level decreased by 66.5 per cent in the 1.0-mg treatment group and by 70 per cent in the 5.0-mg group. After 12 months of therapy, the testosterone value increased by 7.9 per cent over baseline in the 1.0-mg group and by 9.6 per cent over baseline in the 5.0-mg group. These changes were statistically significant ($P < 0.001$), but the testosterone levels remained within the normal range at all times. All three groups experienced an increase in the serum level of luteinizing hormone at 12 months. The increase was 8.8 per cent in the placebo-receiving group, 14.7 per cent in the 1.0-mg group, and 15.1 per cent in the 5.0-mg group. The difference between the placebo group and the two treatment groups was statistically significant ($P < 0.05$).

There was no change in the serum PSA concentration for the placebo-receiving group. After 12 months of treatment, the serum PSA value was reduced by 48 per cent in the 1.0-mg group and by 50 per cent in the 5.0-mg group ($P < 0.001$ in both groups). The prostatic volume was measured with MRI at 0, 3, 6, and 12 months. At each time point, the decrease in prostatic volume was highly significant compared with the placebo group ($P < 0.001$). After 12 months of therapy, prostatic volume was reduced by 18 per cent in the 1.0-mg group and by 19 per cent in the 5.0-mg group. With regard to bladder outlet obstructive symptoms, 30 per cent of the 1.0-mg group had achieved an increase of 3 ml/sec or more in peak urinary flow at the conclusion of treatment. The increase was at least 3.0 ml/sec in 32 per cent of the 5.0-mg group and in 18 per cent of the placebo group. Symptom scores were determined monthly. The placebo group had improvement in the total symptom score for the first few months, but after month 4 there was a progressive loss of improvement and by month 12 there was a return nearly to baseline. The 5.0-mg group, but not the 1.0-mg cohort, had a statistically significant improvement in obstructive symptom and total symptom scores.

Side Effects

The side effects experienced by the three treatment groups were similar. The only statistically significant differences were the decreased libido and decreased semen volume observed in both finasteride groups ($P < 0.05$). Surprisingly, the 1.0-mg cohort but not the 5.0-mg group had a statistically significant number of men complaining of impotence ($P < 0.05$).

Conclusion

The 5α-reductase inhibitor finasteride appears to have some benefit in the treatment of BPH. Patients receiving this medication have a mean decrease in prostatic volume of approximately 20 per cent and a modest improvement in peak urinary flow rate (2.5 ml/sec) and symptom score (2.5 points). Although the clinical improvement appears only moderate, finasteride has virtually no side effects. The theoretical advantage of decreasing serum DHT levels without decreasing serum testosterone levels appears to be borne out clinically in regard to the untoward effects. The percentage of patients complaining of impotence was approximately 4 per cent. Prostatic volume decreased significantly at 6 months, but there was only a minimal change between 6 and 12 months. Thus, longer-term therapy may not produce much more of a clinical response. Finasteride causes a progressive decrease in the serum PSA concentration, the decline being most marked in the first 3 months of therapy.

The exact role of 5α-reductase inhibitors in the treatment of BPH has yet to be determined. The drug would have to be administered on a lifetime basis, given that the decrease in prostatic volume is reversible within 3 months of discontinuation of the drug. The decrease in serum PSA concentration produced by 5α-reductase inhibitors could significantly alter the usefulness of PSA for detecting early prostate cancer in men receiving the therapy. Because finasteride produced only a moderate improvement in symptoms and urinary flow rate, its greatest role may be in inhibiting the natural progression of the BPH process. Prospective randomized studies with long-term follow-up of a large number of patients will be necessary to document this potential ability of finasteride.

ESTROGEN DEPRIVATION THERAPY

Stromal-Epithelial Interactions

The enlargement of the prostate gland in BPH is due to both glandular and stromal hyperplasia. In humans, light and electron stereologic analysis of normal prostatic tissue compared with BPH tissue has shown that the enlargement in BPH is predominantly the result of stromal hyperplasia.[3, 5] Specific stromal-epithelial interactions are thought to be crucial to the pathogenesis of BPH, and estrogens are thought to have a significant causative or permissive role.[5, 104] In 1925, on the basis of histologic investigations, Reischauer[107] theorized that the stroma induced the glandular component of BPH. Additional studies conducted by Deming and Neumann[33] and by LeDuc[65] supported the early findings of Reischauer. On the basis of his pathologic studies in 1978, McNeal[77] provided evidence to support the role of the prostatic stroma in the induction of human BPH. He deduced that BPH results from a process of glandular budding and branching that is under mesenchymal control; this budding and branching give rise to new alveoli in the periurethral area of the prostate. McNeal thought that this epithelial budding and growth were similar to the glandular morphogenesis that occurs in embryonic tissue as the result of stimulation from the adjacent mesenchymal tissue. He concluded that the stroma in the periurethral transition zone induces the surrounding glands to grow by a process called "reawakening of embryonic properties."

The inductive role of the stroma on the epithelium also has been demonstrated in an animal model (Fig. 16–5) developed by Cunha and Chung.[22, 23, 28, 30, 31, 82, 129] Using the mouse, they showed that embryonic urogenital sinus mesenchyme, the tissue that gives rise to prostatic stroma in adulthood, can induce adult bladder epithelial cells to replicate and form prostate-like glandular structures. The degree of epithelial growth depended on the quantity of mesenchymal tissue present and not on the amount of epithelium. The ability of the mesenchymal tissue to induce adult bladder epithelial cells was found to depend on the hormonal status of the host mouse (that is, induction would not occur in a castrated animal).

Cunha and co-workers[29] used androgen-insensitive mice (Tfm) to further define the hormonal environment necessary for the mesenchyme to induce bladder epithelial cells to undergo prostatic differentiation. Their experiments demonstrated that the stroma is responsive to androgen stimulation and that an intimate interaction between the mesenchyme (stroma) and epithelium is necessary to promote prostatic differentiation and growth. The exact means by which the stroma communicates with the epithelium has not been precisely defined. The basement membrane, extracellular matrix, and nuclear matrix may be involved in the communication between the stroma and the epithelium. These structures have been shown to have such a role in the mammary gland.[66, 88] Other investigators speculate that DHT or various prostatic epithelial growth factors are involved.[20, 21, 27, 100] Additional studies need to be con-

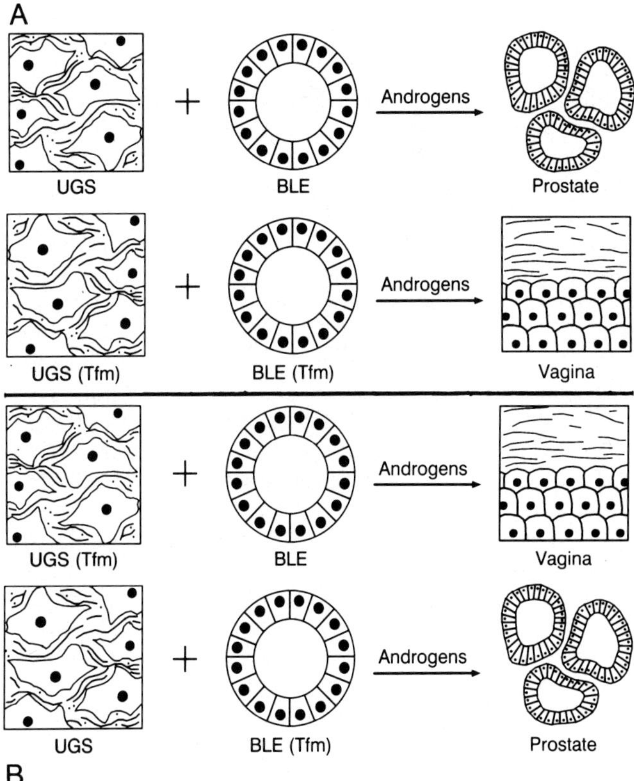

FIGURE 16–5. *A* and *B,* Inductive role of stroma on epithelium: experimental evidence. BLE = bladder epithelium; Tfm = androgen-insensitive mice; UGS = urogenital sinus mesenchyme.

ducted to determine more clearly the mechanism by which the stroma communicates with the overlying epithelium.

Estrogens and BPH

The involvement of estrogens in the pathogenesis of BPH has been theorized for many years. As early as 1935, Burrows[15] suggested that the changes of the prostate in aging men may be due to a relative excess of estrogens. He based this conclusion on pathologic experiments in mice. One year later, Zuckerman[147] postulated that the fibromuscular growth of the prostate was the result of an imbalance favoring an "estrogenic substance" over "the male hormone proper."

As men age, the unbound serum testosterone concentration progressively declines.[148] Meanwhile, the serum free estrone (1,3,5-[10]-estratriene-3-ol-17-one) and 17β-estradiol values remain relatively constant with aging.[56, 148] Consequently, as men age and BPH becomes more prevalent, the serum and intraprostatic ratios of estrogens to androgens increase.[101]

Animal studies have also supported a role for estrogens in the pathogenesis of BPH. Walsh and Wilson,[137] in 1976, examined the role of estradiol and androstanediol in the development of BPH in castrated beagle dogs. They found that androstanediol plus estrogen produced a massive enlargement of the prostate gland, whereas androstanediol alone produced modest enlargement. Other investigators were able to produce prostatic hyperplasia in previously castrated dogs by treatment with DHT plus 17β-estradiol.[32, 85] Additional support for the role of estrogens in the development of BPH comes from biochemical studies that have demonstrated the presence of estrogen receptors in prostatic cells. High-affinity receptors have been isolated in both the cytosol and the nuclei of canine prostatic cells.[19, 36, 57, 131] Moore and co-workers[86] found that treatment of castrated dogs with 17β-estradiol resulted in a 200 per cent increase in the concentration of cytosolic androgen-binding sites. Subsequently, Trachtenberg and colleagues[131] reported that the administration of 3α-androstenediol and 17β-estradiol produced a greater concentration of prostatic androgen receptors than 3α-androstenediol alone in castrated beagle dogs. Taken together, these results suggest that the experimental induction of canine BPH may be due to an estrogen-induced increase in androgen receptors.

In theory, as the number of androgen receptors in the prostatic cell increases, the number of testosterone and DHT complexes within the cell should increase. Through several ill-defined interactions, this process leads to increased DNA transcription, mRNA translation, and subsequent protein biosynthesis. Isaacs and Coffey[61] found that the intraprostatic concentration of DHT was increased in beagle dogs treated with estrogens. Barrack and Berry[2] showed subsequently that this increase in intraprostatic DHT concentration inhibited the rate of cell death. Thus, the administration of estrogens can indirectly enhance prostatic growth by increasing the intraprostatic DHT level, which in turn inhibits cell death.

A positive reaction with immunohistochemical staining for the estrogen receptor has been demonstrated in canine, monkey, and human prostatic tissue.[113, 114, 140] Ekman and co-workers[38] characterized two classes of estradiol-binding sites in the human prostate—high affinity and low affinity—in both normal and BPH tissue. Another finding supporting the role of estrogens in the development of human BPH is that aromatase activity is higher in the periurethral and transition zones of prostates with benign hyperplasia than in the same regions of prostates without benign hyperplasia.[102, 124] This difference suggests that the estrogen concentration should be higher in the periurethral and transition zones of prostates with benign hyperplasia than in normal prostates. Also of significance is the fact that the principal site in the prostate for 5α-reductase activity is the stroma.[26, 143, 144] Hence, the area of the prostate most likely to be under the influence of estrogens is the area where testosterone is reduced to DHT. As discussed previously, DHT is the principal androgen involved in prostatic epithelial growth. From these observations, it can be speculated that estrogens have an influential, although indirect, role in prostatic growth and in the development of BPH.

AROMATASE INHIBITORS

The above-described research led to the concept of developing an antiestrogen therapy for BPH. In the male, the estrogens estrone and 17β-estradiol are produced exclusively by aromatization of androstenedione and testosterone, respectively. This conversion has been demonstrated in the testis, skin, fibroblasts, adipose and muscle tissue, hair follicles, liver, and brain.[40, 41, 60, 71, 83, 109, 115, 116] Stone and co-workers[124] demonstrated that aromatization of androgens to estrogens also occurs in the human prostate. The aromatization of androgens to estrogens is done by the microsomal P450-dependent enzyme system, referred to as aromatase.[55, 98] Thus, an inhibitor of this enzyme system would be an effective antiestrogen therapy (Fig. 16–6).

The first aromatase inhibitor to be developed and investigated extensively was 4-hydroxyandrostenedione (4-OHA; 4-hydroxy-4-androstene-3,17-dione). Habenicht and co-workers[55] studied the effect of androstene-

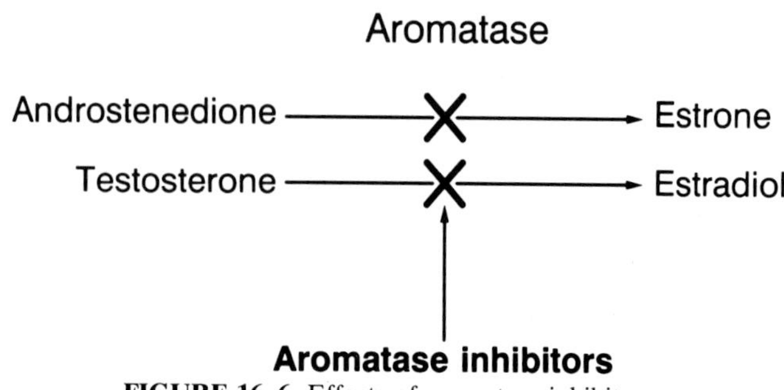

FIGURE 16–6. Effects of aromatase inhibitors.

dione and 4-OHA on castrated beagle dogs. Treatment with androstenedione resulted in BPH characterized only by glandular and stromal hyperplasia. When 4-OHA was added, the estrogen-related effects were antagonized and the hyperplastic effects on the epithelium also were partly inhibited. In another study, Habenicht and El Etreby[54] investigated the effect of an aromatase inhibitor plus an antiandrogen (cyproterone acetate) on the androstenedione-induced changes in the prostates of castrated dogs. The aromatase inhibitor used in this study was 1-methyl-ADD (Atamestane; 1-methyl-androsta-1,4-diene-3,17-dione) (Fig. 16–7). Histologically, the appearance of the prostates treated with 1-methyl-ADD and cyproterone acetate was similar to that of the untreated castrated controls.

In another study, Habenicht and El Etreby[53] examined the effect of cyproterone acetate plus 1-methyl-ADD on the androstenedione-induced prostatic growth in intact beagle dogs. Initially, 1-methyl-ADD alone was administered to the dogs. This antagonized the estrogen-induced effect on the fibromuscular stroma of the prostate. However, it also caused a marked elevation of the serum testosterone and DHT levels, resulting in marked hyperplasia of the glandular component of the prostate. The elevation of serum testosterone and DHT levels is likely due to the lack of negative feedback by estrogens at the level of the anterior pituitary and hypothalamus.[39, 64, 145] The lack of negative feedback by estrogens causes increased production of luteinizing hormone by the anterior pituitary, which stimulates the Leydig cells of the testes to produce more testosterone. When cyproterone acetate was given concomitantly with 1-methyl-ADD, there was complete atrophy of the prostate despite the elevated levels of serum testosterone and DHT. Thus, the best overall treatment of BPH may be an agent that is both antiestrogenic and antiandrogenic.

Juniewicz and associates[62] used a nonsteroidal aromatase inhibitor to treat six intact beagle dogs with naturally occurring BPH. Within 1 week of treatment, the serum luteinizing hormone concentration had increased 500 per cent over that of controls, and it remained elevated during the 6 months of treatment. The serum testosterone concentration increased 1000

per cent after initiation of treatment and remained at that level for the duration of therapy. These increases in the serum luteinizing hormone and testosterone levels were again thought to be due to the lack of negative feedback of estrogens on the hypothalamus and anterior pituitary. Oesterling and colleagues[95] examined these prostates and found no difference in size between the treated and control dogs. The only pathologic difference was that the treated dogs had significantly more prostatic inflammation than the control animals. Thus, aromatase inhibition alone does not appear to be effective in treating spontaneously occurring canine prostatic hyperplasia.

The above-described results cannot be directly applied to humans for two reasons. First, the endocrine system of the dog is not identical to that of the human. Dogs appear to be more sensitive to estrogen deprivation than humans in terms of feedback on the hypothalamus and anterior pituitary.[146] Second, with regard to BPH, the canine prostate consists mainly of epithelium and has very little accompanying stroma, whereas human BPH is predominantly stromal.[3, 5] These differences suggest that aromatase inhibition may be a more effective treatment for BPH in humans than in dogs.

In 1987, Schweikert and Tunn[117] treated 13 men who had complete urinary retention with the weak aromatase inhibitor testolactone. Seven patients (54 per cent) were able to urinate spontaneously after a mean treatment period of 8 weeks. Prostatic volume decreased in all patients. The mean reduction in prostatic volume in those able to micturate was 26 per cent, whereas the mean decrease in those still requiring catheterization was 15 per cent. The serum testosterone concentration was significantly increased in all of the patients, but it remained in the normal range for men. Schweikert and colleagues[118] performed the first clinical investigation of Atamestane (1-methyl-ADD) (Fig. 16–7). Forty-nine men with obstructive BPH received 200 mg three times a day for 3 months. After 3 months of treatment, peak urinary flow had improved slightly and mean residual urine volume had decreased, but these changes were not statistically significant. Prostatic size, as measured by transurethral ultrasonography, decreased by 12 per cent, a difference that was statistically significant. Atamestane was fairly well tolerated; 19 per cent of the patients reported minor adverse experiences. One patient withdrew from the study because of headaches, nausea, and constipation. These initial studies demonstrate that antiestrogen therapy may have some benefit in the treatment of human BPH. Although the changes in peak urinary flow, residual urine volume, and prostatic size were minimal, further investigations appear warranted.

Conclusion

The enlargement of the human prostate gland in BPH is primarily the result of stromal hyperplasia. Additionally, the stroma is believed to induce the glandular component of BPH. Cunha and Chung,[22, 23, 28, 30, 31, 82, 129]

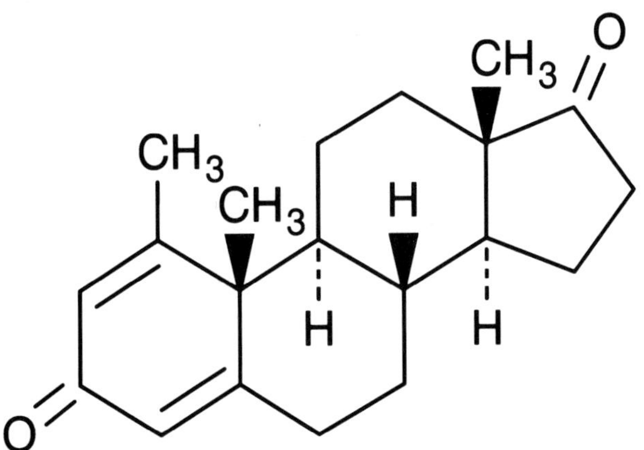

FIGURE 16–7. Chemical structure of Atamestane.

using an animal model, elegantly demonstrated that the stroma is responsive to androgen stimulation and that an intimate interaction between the mesenchyme (stroma) and epithelium is necessary to promote prostatic growth and differentiation.

Estrogens have for many years been theorized to have a role in the pathogenesis of BPH. Animal studies have supported a role for estrogens in the development of BPH. The prostatic enlargement that develops in castrated dogs treated with androgens plus estrogens is more significant than that in dogs treated with androgens alone. Additionally, an estrogen receptor has been identified in canine prostatic cells, and estrogens have been shown to increase the number of androgen receptors in canine prostatic cells. Also, human prostatic estradiol-binding sites have been identified. Aromatase activity has also been shown to be higher in the periurethral and transition zones of prostates with benign hyperplasia than in the same regions of prostates without benign hyperplasia.

These findings lead to speculation that estrogens indirectly induce canine BPH by increasing the number of prostatic-cell androgen receptors. This, in turn, leads to an increased number of androgen-receptor complexes, which result in more cellular stimulation.

In males, 17β-estradiol and estrone are derived exclusively from aromatization of testosterone and androstenedione, respectively, by the aromatase enzyme complex. Thus, serum estrogen concentration could be reduced by inhibiting the aromatase enzyme system. The first widely studied aromatase inhibitor was 4-OHA. In castrated dogs being treated with androstenedione, 4-OHA antagonized the estrogen-related prostatic changes and partly inhibited the glandular hyperplasia. However, when intact dogs were studied with aromatase inhibitor 1-methyl-ADD (Atamestane), the results were different. Because these animals lacked the normal negative feedback of estrogens, markedly elevated serum levels of luteinizing hormone, testosterone, and DHT developed; consequently, prominent glandular hyperplasia developed in these dogs. Thus, aromatase inhibitor monotherapy does not seem to be effective for treating BPH in the canine model.

Because of the differences between humans and dogs in terms of their endocrine systems and prostatic composition, clinical studies were undertaken. Preliminary studies with the weak aromatase inhibitor testolactone and the more potent agent Atamestane demonstrated some benefit in the treatment of human BPH. Patients receiving Atamestane for 3 months had a 12 per cent reduction in prostatic volume and a slight (not statistically significant) improvement in peak urinary flow and postvoid residual urine volume. Currently, a multicenter, double-blind, placebo-controlled study is under way to evaluate Atamestane further. In the future, combination therapies with an antiandrogen and an aromatase inhibitor may warrant investigation once the clinical and safety profiles of aromatase inhibitors are more completely evaluated in humans.

SUMMARY

As the population ages, a natural increase will occur in the number of men afflicted with BPH. Two factors are clearly necessary for the development of BPH: advancing age and the presence of androgens. A 50-year-old man in the United States has a 25 to 35 per cent probability of undergoing prostatectomy for BPH in his lifetime.[94] The morbidity of the various operative procedures for BPH has been estimated to be 15 per cent, and the mortality rate is less than 1 per cent.[48, 80] Transurethral resection of the prostate is the second most common surgical procedure performed in the United States; approximately 400,000 such operations are performed annually.[52] The cost for these procedures is $4.5 billion.[51] With surgical costs increasing, interest in developing nonsurgical treatments for BPH has increased.

The data reviewed above suggest a definite role for androgens and estrogens in the development of BPH and a possible role for androgen deprivation and estrogen deprivation in the treatment of this condition. As early as 1895, Cabot[16] and White[141] recognized that bilateral orchiectomy was a successful treatment for BPH. Later, LHRH agonists were investigated for use in the treatment of BPH. Overall, approximately 30 to 40 per cent of men treated with an LHRH agonist have subjective and objective improvement. Use of an LHRH analogue produces almost universal impotence, loss of libido, and hot flushes. Additionally, this medication has to be continued on a lifetime basis and is very expensive ($4000 to $5000 per year). Given the high cost, significant side effects, and limited success rate of an LHRH agonist, its use in the treatment of BPH appears limited. In the studies reviewed, the patients whose BPH had a predominantly epithelial component responded best. Thus, LHRH agonist therapy should be reserved for debilitated, impotent patients who are at high risk for surgical intervention, refuse orchiectomy, and have a predominantly glandular hyperplastic prostate.

A potential shortcoming of LHRH agonist therapy is the lack of impact on the adrenal androgens. Adrenal androgens constitute approximately 10 per cent of the circulating androgens. Antiandrogens compete with all circulating androgens at the level of the androgen receptor sites. Flutamide, the most extensively studied antiandrogen, seems to have some benefit in the treatment of BPH and some advantages over LHRH agonist therapy. It does not cause impotence and loss of libido, which are universal with LHRH agonist therapy. However, adverse reactions to flutamide are common (primarily gastrointestinal symptoms and gynecomastia), and they have a definite impact on patient compliance. As with LHRH agonist therapy, antiandrogen therapy needs to be continued on a lifetime basis and thus is very expensive ($2000 to $3000 per year). In all of the studies to date, the duration of follow-up has been limited to 1 year. The concern is that prolonged use of flutamide will result in elevated testosterone levels, which will overcome the complete blockade provided by flutamide.

Research has clearly shown that DHT is the primary androgen involved in the pathogenesis of BPH. It was believed that selective inhibition of the formation of DHT without alteration of the serum testosterone concentration would eliminate the side effects of loss of libido and impotency. The enzyme responsible for the conversion of testosterone to DHT is 5α-reductase. The inhibitor of this enzyme most extensively studied to date is finasteride (Proscar). Use of this drug in the treatment of BPH has been shown to have some benefit in terms of (1) decreasing prostatic volume, (2) improving urinary flow rate, and (3) decreasing symptoms. In addition, this agent has virtually no adverse effects. According to the preliminary data, 20 to 30 per cent of men have objective or subjective improvement. This drug may have the greatest benefit in men with early prostatism, in whom it can prevent further progression of the disease process. Clearly, more studies need to be conducted to determine the role of 5α-reductase inhibitors in the treatment of symptomatic BPH.

Recently, interest in estrogen deprivation therapy in the management of BPH has emerged. It has been known for many years that human BPH is composed predominantly of hyperplastic stromal cells rather than epithelial cells. Recently, estrogen receptors in prostatic cells have been identified, and animal studies have shown that estrogen administration can induce BPH. The enzyme complex responsible for the conversion of androgens to estrogens is called aromatase. Overall, monotherapy with an aromatase inhibitor has been shown to be ineffective in the canine model; this lack of response is due to a very sensitive hypothalamic-pituitary-gonadal axis. Lacking the normal negative feedback of estrogens, the anterior pituitary gland secretes increased amounts of luteinizing hormone, which stimulates the Leydig cells of the testes to produce increased amounts of testosterone. Given the differences between men and dogs in terms of their endocrine systems and the pathologic make-up of their prostates in BPH, the animal studies cannot be directly applied to humans. A preliminary study using a weak aromatase inhibitor, testolactone, for the treatment of human BPH revealed some benefit. A preliminary study of the more potent aromatase inhibitor Atamestane also demonstrated some benefit. Currently, a much larger study is being conducted with Atamestane.

Given that human BPH is composed of both stromal and epithelial hyperplastic components and that individuals vary with respect to their relative epithelial-to-stromal ratios, combination therapy with agents that have an impact on both estrogens and androgens may be the treatment of choice. Alternatively, the treatment of choice may be better determined in the future by imaging methods or other means that help determine the relative proportions of epithelial and stromal tissue. Currently, PSA levels can be used as a guide because it is known that only epithelial cells produce PSA.

All androgen-antagonizing therapies lower the serum PSA concentration. This decrease may impair the use of PSA for the detection of early prostate cancer in men receiving these therapies. As of now, the only agent that may soon acquire widespread use is the 5α-reductase inhibitor finasteride. If use of this agent becomes widespread, additional studies will need to be conducted to determine the meaning of serum PSA values in men receiving finasteride.

If hormonal treatment is to be considered successful, the peak urinary flow rate must be significantly improved (to more than 15 ml/sec), a large postvoid residual urine volume must be eliminated, and symptoms (as determined from a standardized questionnaire) must be improved. The clinical response of patients with prostatism who are treated with hormonal therapy varies considerably. This variability can be attributed to several factors: (1) with long-standing bladder outlet obstruction, the bladder itself may become dysfunctional to some degree; (2) each individual prostate has various amounts of stromal and epithelial components; and (3) BPH must be considered a multifactorial disease process.[51] Hormonal therapy may address only one aspect of the disease process.

Currently, no hormonal therapy (androgen or estrogen antagonizing) is as effective as transurethral resection of the prostate in the treatment of symptomatic BPH. As indicated above, some patients respond better than others to this form of medical therapy. Thus, in the future, it will be important to develop the ability to identify which patients are most likely to have a successful outcome with these antiandrogen and antiestrogen treatments.

REFERENCES

1. Auclair C, Stern M, Givner ML: LHRH and analogues as potential therapy for benign prostatic hyperplasia and hormone-dependent cancers. Arch Androl 7:237–244, 1981.
2. Barrack ER, Berry SJ: DNA synthesis in the canine prostate: Effects of androgen and estrogen treatment. Prostate 10:45–56, 1987.
3. Bartsch G, Frick J, Rüegg I, et al: Electron microscopic stereological analysis of the normal human prostate and of benign prostatic hyperplasia. J Urol 122:481–486, 1979.
4. Bartsch G, Keen F, Daxenbichler G, et al: Correlation of biochemical (receptors, endogenous tissue hormones) and quantitative morphologic (stereologic) findings in normal and hyperplastic human prostates. J Urol 137:559–564, 1987.
5. Bartsch G, Müller HR, Oberholzer M, Rohr HP: Light microscopic stereological analysis of the normal human prostate and of benign prostatic hyperplasia. J Urol 122:487–491, 1979.
6. Bianchi S, Gravina G, Podestà A, et al: Treatment of complicated benign prostatic hyperplasia with LHRH-analogues in aged patients. Int J Androl 12:104–109, 1989.
7. Bonard M, de Almeida S, von Niederhäusern W: Placebo-controlled double-blind study in human benign obstructive prostatic hypertrophy with flutamide. Eur Urol 2:24–28, 1976.
8. Bosch RJLH, Griffiths DJ, Blom JHM, Schroeder FH: Treatment of benign prostatic hyperplasia by androgen deprivation: Effects on prostate size and urodynamic parameters. J Urol 141:68–72, 1989.
9. Brooks JR, Berman C, Garnes D, et al: Prostatic effects induced in dogs by chronic or acute oral administration of 5α-reductase inhibitors. Prostate 9:65–75, 1986.
10. Brooks JR, Berman C, Glitzer MS, et al: Effect of a new 5α-reductase inhibitor on size, histologic characteristics, and androgen concentrations of the canine prostate. Prostate 3:35–44, 1982.

11. Brooks JR, Berman C, Primka RL, et al: 5α-Reductase inhibitory and anti-androgenic activities of some 4-azasteroids in the rat. Steroids 47:1, 1986.

12. Brooks JR, Busch RD, Patanelli DJ, Steelman SL: A study of the effects of a new anti-androgen on the hyperplastic dog prostate. Proc Soc Exp Biol Med 143:647–655, 1973.

13. Bruchovsky N, Wilson JD: The conversion of testosterone to 5α-androstan-17β-ol-3-one by rat prostate *in vivo* and *in vitro*. J Biol Chem 243:2012–2021, 1968.

14. Bruchovsky N, Wilson JD: The intranuclear binding of testosterone and 5α-androstan-17β-ol-3-one by rat prostate. J Biol Chem 243:5953–5960, 1968.

15. Burrows H: Pathological conditions induced by oestrogenic compounds in the coagulation gland and prostate of the mouse. Am J Cancer 23:490–512, 1935.

16. Cabot AT: The question of castration for enlarged prostate. Ann Surg 24:265–309, 1896.

17. Caine M, Perlberg S, Gordon R: The treatment of benign prostatic hypertrophy with flutamide (SCH 13521): A placebo-controlled study. J Urol 114:564–568, 1975.

18. Castro JE, Griffiths HLJ: The assessment of patients with benign prostatic hypertrophy. J R Coll Surg Edinb 17:190–194, 1972.

19. Chaisiri N, Valotaire Y, Evens BAJ, Pierrepoint CG: Demonstration of a cytoplasmic receptor protein for oestrogen in the canine prostate gland. J Endocrinol 78:131–139, 1978.

20. Chapdelaine A, Chevalier S: Growth promoting factors for normal canine and human cell in culture. *In* Bruchovsky N, Chapdelaine A, Neumann F (eds): Regulation of Androgen Action. West Berlin, Congressdruck R Bruckner, 1985, p 205.

21. Chaproniere DM, McKeehan WL: Serial culture of single adult human prostatic epithelial cells in serum-free medium containing low calcium and a new growth factor from bovine brain. Cancer Res 46:819–824, 1986.

22. Chung LWK, Cunha GR: Stromal-epithelial interactions: II. Regulation of prostatic growth by embryonic urogenital sinus mesenchyme. Prostate 4:503–511, 1983.

23. Chung LWK, Matsura J, Runner MN: Tissue interactions and prostatic growth. I. Induction of adult mouse prostatic hyperplasia by fetal urogenital sinus implants. Biol Reprod 31:155–163, 1984.

24. Coffey DS, Berry SJ, Ewing LL: An overview of current concepts in the study of benign prostatic hyperplasia. *In* Rodgers CH, Coffey DS, Cunha GR, et al (eds): Benign Prostatic Hyperplasia, Vol 2 (NIH Publication No. 87-2881). Bethesda, MD, National Institutes of Health, 1987, pp 1–13.

25. Conn PM, Crowley WF Jr: Gonadotropin-releasing hormone and its analogues. N Engl J Med 324:93–103, 1991.

26. Cowan RA, Cowan SK, Grant JK, Elder HY: Biochemical investigations of separated epithelium and stroma from benign hyperplastic prostatic tissue. J Endocrinol 74:111–120, 1977.

27. Crabb JW, Armes LG, Carr SA, et al: Complete primary structure of prostatropin, a prostate epithelial cell growth factor. Biochemistry 25:4988–4993, 1986.

28. Cunha GR, Bigsby RM, Cooke PS, Sugimura Y: Stromal-epithelial interactions in adult organs. Cell Diff 17:137–148, 1985.

29. Cunha GR, Chung LWK, Shannon JM, Reese BA: Stromal-epithelial interactions in sex differentiation. Biol Reprod 22:19–42, 1980.

30. Cunha GR, Donjacour AA, Cooke PS, et al: Stromal factors in the development and control of growth in the prostate. *In* Rodgers CH, Coffey DS, Cunha GR, et al (eds): Benign Prostatic Hyperplasia, Vol 2 (NIH Publication No. 87-2881). Bethesda, MD, National Institutes of Health, 1987, pp 15–25.

31. Cunha GR, Fujii H, Neubauer BL, et al: Epithelial-mesenchymal interactions in prostatic development. I. Morphological observations of prostatic induction by urogenital sinus mesenchyme in epithelium of the adult rodent urinary bladder. J Cell Biol 96:1662–1670, 1983.

32. DeKlerk DP, Coffey DS, Ewing LL, et al: Comparison of spontaneous and experimentally induced canine prostatic hyperplasia. J Clin Invest 64:842–849, 1979.

33. Deming CL, Neumann C: Early phases of prostatic hyperplasia. Surg Gynecol Obstet 68:155–160, 1939.

34. de Voogt HJ, Rao BR, Geldof AA, et al: Androgen action blockade does not result in reduction in size but changes histology of the normal human prostate. Prostate 11:305–311, 1987.

35. Dubé JY, Frenette G, Tremblay RR, et al: Involution of spontaneous benign prostatic hyperplasia in the dog under the influence of chronic treatment with a LHRH agonist. Prostate 5:417–423, 1984.

36. Dubé JY, Lesage R, Tremblay RR: Estradiol and progesterone receptors in dog prostate cytosol. J Steroid Biochem 10:459–466, 1979.

37. Ehrlichman RJ, Isaacs JT, Coffey DS: Differences in the effects of estradiol on dihydrotestosterone induced prostatic growth of the castrate dog and rat. Invest Urol 18:466–470, 1981.

38. Ekman P, Barrack ER, Greene GL, et al: Estrogen receptors in human prostate: Evidence for multiple binding sites. J Clin Endocrinol Metab 57:166–176, 1983.

39. Ellinwood WE, Hess DL, Roselli CE, et al: Inhibition of aromatization stimulates luteinizing hormone and testosterone secretion in adult male rhesus monkeys. J Clin Endocrinol Metab 59:1088–1096, 1984.

40. Fishman J, Goto J: Mechanisms of estrogen biosynthesis: Participation of multiple enzyme sites in placental aromatase hydroxylations. J Biol Chem 256:4466–4471, 1981.

41. Folkerd EJ, James VHT: Aromatization of steroids in peripheral tissues. J Steroid Biochem 19:687–690, 1983.

42. Forti G, Salerno R, Moneti G, et al: Three-month treatment with a long-acting gonadotropin-releasing hormone agonist of patients with benign prostatic hyperplasia: Effects on tissue androgen concentration, 5α-reductase activity and androgen receptor content. J Clin Endocrinol Metab 68:461–468, 1989.

43. Frankel AE, Rouse RV, Wang MC, et al: Monoclonal antibodies to a human prostate antigen. Cancer Res 42:3714–3718, 1982.

44. Furr BJA: "Casodex" (ICI 176,334)—a new, pure, peripherally-selective anti-androgen: Preclinical studies. Horm Res 32(Suppl 1):69–76, 1989.

45. Gabrilove JL, Levine AC, Kirschenbaum A, Droller M: Effect of a GNRH analogue (leuprolide) on benign prostatic hypertrophy. J Clin Endocrinol Metab 64:1331–1333, 1987.

46. Gabrilove JL, Levine AC, Kirschenbaum A, Droller M: Effect of long-acting gonadotropin-releasing hormone analog (leuprolide) therapy on prostatic size and symptoms in 15 men with benign prostatic hypertrophy. J Clin Endocrinol Metab 69:629–632, 1989.

47. Geller J: Pathogenesis and medical treatment of benign prostatic hyperplasia. Prostate (Suppl) 2:95–104, 1989.

48. Geller J, Albert J: The effect of aging on the prostate. *In* Korenman SG (ed): Endocrine Aspects of Aging. Amsterdam, Elsevier Biomedical Press, 1982, p 137.

49. Geller J, Bora R, Roberts T, et al: Treatment of benign prostatic hypertrophy with hydroxyprogesterone caproate. JAMA 193:121–128, 1965.

50. Gormley GJ, Rittmaster RS, Gregg H, et al: Dose-response effect of an orally active 5alpha-reductase inhibitor (MK-906) in man [abstract 1225]. 71st Annual Meeting of the Endocrine Society, Seattle, Washington, 1989.

51. Graversen PH, Gasser TC, Wasson JH, et al: Controversies about indications for transurethral resection of the prostate. J Urol 141:475–481, 1989.

52. Graves EJ: Detailed diagnoses and procedures. National Hospital Discharge Survey: 1987. National Center for Health Statistics. Vital Health Stat (13), 100:295, 1989.

53. Habenicht U-F, El Etreby MF: Selective inhibition of androstenedione-induced prostate growth in intact beagle dogs by a combined treatment with the antiandrogen cyproterone acetate and the aromatase inhibitor 1-methyl-androsta-1,4-diene-3,17-dione (1-methyl-ADD). Prostate 14:309–322, 1989.

54. Habenicht U-F, El Etreby MF: Synergic inhibitory effects of the aromatase inhibitor 1-methyl-androsta-1,4-diene-3,17-dione and the antiandrogen cyproterone acetate on androstenedione-induced hyperplastic effects in the prostates of castrated dogs. Prostate 11:133–143, 1987.

55. Habenicht U-F, Schwarz K, Schweikert H-U, et al: Development of a model for the induction of estrogen-related prostatic hyperplasia in the dog and its response to the aromatase inhibitor 4-hydroxy-4-androstene-3,17-dione: Preliminary results. Prostate 8:181–194, 1986.

56. Harman SM, Tsitouras PD: Reproductive hormones in aging men. I. Measurement of sex steroids, basal luteinizing hormone, and Leydig cell response to human chorionic gonadotropin. J Clin Endocrinol Metab 51:35–40, 1980.

57. Hawkins EF, Trachtenberg J, Hicks LL, Walsh PC: Androgen and estrogen receptors in the canine prostate. J Androl 1:234–243, 1980.

58. Hieble JP, Caine M: Etiology of benign prostatic hyperplasia and approaches to its pharmacological management. Fed Proc 45:2601–2603, 1986.

59. Huggins C, Stevens RA: The effect of castration on benign hypertrophy of the prostate in man. J Urol 43:705–714, 1940.

60. Iqbal MJ, Greenway B, Wilkinson ML, et al: Sex-steroid enzymes, aromatase and 5α-reductase in the pancreas: A comparison of normal adult, foetal and malignant tissue. Clin Sci 65:71–75, 1983.

61. Isaacs JT, Coffey DS: Changes in dihydrotestosterone metabolism associated with the development of canine benign prostatic hyperplasia. Endocrinology 108:445–453, 1981.

62. Juniewicz PE, Oesterling JE, Walters JR, et al: Aromatase inhibition in the dog. I. Effect on serum LH, serum testosterone concentrations, testicular secretions and spermatogenesis. J Urol 139:827–831, 1988.

63. Keane PF, Timoney AG, Kiely E, et al: Response of the benign hypertrophied prostate to treatment with an LHRH analogue. Br J Urol 62:163–165, 1988.

64. Krey LC, MacLusky NJ, Davis PG, et al: Different intracellular mechanisms underlie testosterone's suppression of basal and stimulation of cyclic luteinizing hormone release in male and female rats. Endocrinology 110:2159–2167, 1982.

65. LeDuc IE: The anatomy of the prostate and the pathology of early benign hypertrophy. J Urol 42:1217–1241, 1939.

66. Lee EY-HP, Lee W-H, Kaetzel CS, et al: Interaction of mouse mammary epithelial cells with collagen substrata: Regulation of casein gene expression and excretion. Proc Natl Acad Sci USA 82:1419–1423, 1985.

67. Levine AC, Kirschenbaum A, Kaplan P, et al: Serum prostate-antigen levels in patients with benign prostatic hypertrophy treated with leuprolide. Urology 34:10–13, 1989.

68. Liao S: Cellular receptors and mechanisms of action of steroid hormones. Int Rev Cytol 41:87–172, 1975.

69. Liao S, Rossini GP, Hiipakka RA, Chen C: Factors that can control the interaction of the androgen-receptor complex with the genomic structure in the rat prostate. *In* Bresciani F (ed): Perspectives in Steroid Receptor Research. New York, Raven Press, 1980, pp 99–112.

70. Liao S, Tymoczko JL, Casteñeda E, Liang T: Androgen receptors and androgen-dependent initiation of protein synthesis in the prostate. Vit Horm 33:297–317, 1975.

71. Longcope C, Pratt JH, Schneider SH, Fineberg SE: Aromatization of androgens by muscle and adipose tissue *in vivo*. J Clin Endocrinol Metab 46:146–152, 1978.

72. Lukkarinen O: Effect of LH-RH analogue in patients with benign prostatic hyperplasia. Urology 37:92–94, 1991.

73. Lund F, Rasmussen F: Flutamide versus stilboestrol in the management of advanced prostatic cancer: A controlled prospective study. Br J Urol 61:140–142, 1988.

74. Madsen PO, Iversen P: A point system for selecting operative candidates. *In* Hinman F Jr (ed): Benign Prostatic Hypertrophy. New York, Springer-Verlag, 1983, pp 763–765.

75. Matzkin H, Chen J, Lewysohn O, Braf Z: Treatment of benign prostatic hypertrophy by a long-acting gonadotropin-releasing hormone analogue: 1-year experience. J Urol 145:309–312, 1991.

76. McConnell JD, Wilson JD, George FW, et al: An inhibitor of 5α-reductase, MK-906, suppresses prostatic dihydrotestosterone in men with benign prostatic hyperplasia [abstract]. J Urol 141:239A, 1989.

77. McNeal JE: Origin and evolution of benign prostatic enlargement. Invest Urol 15:340–345, 1978.

78. McNeal J: Pathology of benign prostatic hyperplasia: Insight into etiology. Urol Clin North Am 17:477–486, 1990.

79. McNeal JE: The pathobiology of nodular prostatic hyperplasia in the human (BPH pathology in the human). *In* Rodgers CH, Coffey DS, Cunha GR, et al (eds): Benign Prostatic Hyperplasia, Vol 2 (NIH Publication No. 87-2881). Bethesda, MD, National Institutes of Health, 1987, pp 101–108.

80. Mebust WK, Holtgrewe HL, Cockett ATK, et al: Transurethral prostatectomy: Immediate and postoperative complications. A cooperative study of 13 participating institutions evaluating 3,885 patients. J Urol 141:243–247, 1989.

81. Metcalf BW, Levy MA, Holt DA: Inhibitors of steroid 5alpha-reductase in benign prostatic hyperplasia, male pattern baldness and acne. Trends Pharmacol Sci 10:491–495, 1989.

82. Miller GJ, Runner MN, Chung LWK: Tissue interactions and prostatic growth: II. Morphological and biochemical characterization of adult mouse prostatic hyperplasia induced by fetal urogenital sinus implants. Prostate 6:241–253, 1985.

83. Miyairi S, Fishman J: Radiometric analysis of oxidative reactions in aromatization by placental microsomes: Presence of differential isotope effects. J Biol Chem 260:320–325, 1985.

84. Moore RA: Benign hypertrophy and carcinoma of the prostate: Occurrence and experimental production in animals. Surgery 16:152–167, 1944.

85. Moore RJ, Gazak JM, Quebbeman JF, Wilson JD: Concentration of dihydrotestosterone and 3α-androstanediol in naturally occurring and androgen-induced prostatic hyperplasia in the dog. J Clin Invest 64:1003–1010, 1979.

86. Moore RJ, Gazak JM, Wilson JD: Regulation of cytoplasmic dihydrotestosterone binding in dog prostate by 17β-estradiol. J Clin Invest 63:351–357, 1979.

87. Müntzing J, Varkarakis MJ, Yamanaka H, et al: Studies of antiprostatic agents in the baboon. Proc Soc Exp Biol Med 146:849–854, 1974.

88. Nelson WG, Pienta KJ, Barrack ER, Coffey DS: The role of the nuclear matrix in the organization and function of DNA. Annu Rev Biophys Biochem 15:457–475, 1986.

89. Neri R: Pharmacology and pharmacokinetics of flutamide. Urology 34(Suppl):19–21, 1989.

90. Neri RO, Kassem N: Pharmacology and clinical uses of flutamide. *In* Furr BJA, Wakeling AE (eds): Pharmacology and Clinical Uses of Inhibitors of Hormone Secretion and Action. London, Bailliere Tindall, 1987, p 160.

91. Neri RO, Monahan M: Effects of a novel nonsteroidal antiandrogen on canine prostatic hyperplasia. Invest Urol 10:123–130, 1972.

92. Oesterling JE: LHRH agonists: A nonsurgical treatment for benign prostatic hyperplasia. J Androl 12:381–388, 1991.

93. Oesterling JE: Prostate specific antigen: A critical assessment of the most useful tumor marker for adenocarcinoma of the prostate. J Urol 145:907–923, 1991.

94. Oesterling JE: The origin and development of benign prostatic hyperplasia: An age-dependent process. J Androl 12:348–355, 1991.

95. Oesterling JE, Juniewicz PE, Walters JR, et al: Aromatase inhibition in the dog. II. Effect on growth, function, and pathology of the prostate. J Urol 139:832–839, 1988.

96. Okada K, Oishi K, Yoshida O, et al: Study of the effect of an anti-androgen (Oxendolone) on experimentally induced canine prostatic hyperplasia. I. Morphological analysis. Urol Res 16:67–72, 1988.

97. Okada K, Oishi K, Yoshida O, et al: Study of the effect of an anti-androgen (Oxendolone) on experimentally induced canine prostatic hyperplasia. II. Endocrinological analysis. Urol Res 16:73–78, 1988.

98. Osawa Y, Nakamura T, Higashiyama T: Anti-human placenta aromatase and NADPH-cytochrome P-450 reductase antibodies and immunochemical comparison of human, baboon and horse placental estrogen biosynthesis [abstract]. Program and Abstract of 63rd Annual Meeting of the Endocrine Society, June 17–19, 1981, p 156.

99. Ostri P, Swartz R, Meyhoff H-H, et al: Antiandrogenic treatment of benign prostatic hyperplasia: A placebo controlled trial. Urol Res 17:29–33, 1989.

100. Parrish RF, Heston WDW, Pletscher LS, et al: Prostate-derived growth factors. Prog Clin Biol Res 145:181–194, 1984.

101. Partin AW, Oesterling JE, Epstein JI, et al: Influence of age and endocrine factors on the volume of benign prostatic hyperplasia. J Urol 145:405–409, 1991.

102. Perel E, Killinger DW: The metabolism of androstenedione and

testosterone to C_{19} metabolites in normal breast, breast carcinoma and benign prostatic hypertrophy tissue. J Steroid Biochem 19:1135–1139, 1983.

103. Peters CA, Walsh PC: The effect of nafarelin acetate, a luteinizing-hormone-releasing hormone agonist, on benign prostatic hyperplasia. N Engl J Med 317:599–604, 1987.

104. Pirke KM, Doerr P: Age related changes and interrelationships between plasma testosterone, oestradiol and testosterone-binding globulin in normal adult males. Acta Endocrinol 74:792–800, 1973.

105. Randall A, Hinman F Jr: Surgical anatomy of the prostatic lobes. *In* Hinman F Jr (ed): Benign Prostatic Hypertrophy. New York, Springer-Verlag, 1983, pp 672–677.

106. Raynaud JP, Bonne C, Moguilewsky M, et al: The pure antiandrogen RU 23908 (Anandron), a candidate of choice for the combined antihormonal treatment of prostatic cancer: A review. Prostate 5:299–311, 1984.

107. Reischauer F: Die Entstehung der sogenannten Prostatahypertrophie. Virchows Arch Pathol [A] 256:357–389, 1925.

108. Rohr HP, Bartsch G: Human benign prostatic hyperplasia: A stromal disease? New perspectives by quantitative morphology. Urology 16:625–633, 1980.

109. Roselli CE, Resko JA: Androgens regulate brain aromatase activity in adult male rats through a receptor mechanism. Endocrinology 114:2183–2189, 1984.

110. Salerno R, Moneti G, Forti G, et al: Simultaneous determination of testosterone, dihydrotestosterone and 5 alpha-androstan-3 alpha,-17 beta-diol by isotopic dilution mass spectrometry in plasma and prostatic tissue of patients affected by benign prostatic hyperplasia: Effects of 3-month treatment with a GnRH analog. J Androl 9:234–240, 1988.

111. Schlegel PN, Brendler CB: Management of urinary retention due to benign prostatic hyperplasia using luteinizing hormone-releasing hormone agonist. Urology 34:69–72, 1989.

112. Schroeder FH, Westerhof M, Bosch RJLH, Kurth KH: Benign prostatic hyperplasia treated by castration or the LH-RH analogue buserelin: A report on 6 cases. Eur Urol 12:318–321, 1986.

113. Schulze H, Barrack ER: Immunocytochemical localization of estrogen receptors in spontaneous and experimentally induced canine benign prostatic hyperplasia. Prostate 11:145–162, 1987.

114. Schulze H, Claus S: Histological localization of estrogen receptors in normal and diseased human prostates by immunocytochemistry. Prostate 16:331–343, 1990.

115. Schweikert HU: Conversion of androstenedione to estrone in human fibroblasts cultured from prostate, genitals and nongenital skin. Horm Metab Res 11:635–640, 1979.

116. Schweikert HU, Milewich L, Wilson JD: Aromatization of androstenedione by isolated human hairs. J Clin Endocrinol Metab 40:413–417, 1975.

117. Schweikert H-U, Tunn UW: Effects of the aromatase inhibitor testolactone on human benign prostatic hyperplasia. Steroids 50:191–200, 1987.

118. Schweikert HU, Tunn UW, Arnold J, et al: First clinical experience with Atamestane in the treatment of benign prostatic hyperplasia. *In* El Etreby MF, Habenicht U-F, Henderson D, et al (eds): Atamestane: a New Aromatase Inhibitor. Berlin, Diesbach Verlag, 1991, pp 49–51.

119. Scott WW: What makes the prostate grow? J Urol 70:477–488, 1953.

120. Scott WW, Wade JC: Medical treatment of benign nodular prostatic hyperplasia with cyproterone acetate. J Urol 101:81–85, 1969.

121. Sinha AA, Wilson MJ, Gleason DF: Immunoelectron microscopic localization of prostatic-specific antigen in human prostate by the protein A-gold complex. Cancer 60:1288–1293, 1987.

122. Stone NN, Clejan SJ: Response of prostate volume, prostate-specific antigen, and testosterone to flutamide in men with benign prostatic hyperplasia. J Androl 12:376–380, 1991.

123. Stone NN, Clejan S, Ray PS, et al: A double-blind randomized controlled study of the effect of flutamide on benign prostatic hypertrophy: Side effects and hormonal changes [abstract]. J Urol 141:307A, 1989.

124. Stone NN, Fair WR, Fishman J: Estrogen formation in human prostatic tissue from patients with and without benign prostatic hyperplasia. Prostate 9:311–318, 1986.

125. Stone NN, Ray PS, Smith JA, et al: A double-blind randomized controlled study of the effect of flutamide on benign prostatic hypertrophy: Clinical efficacy [abstract]. J Urol 141:240A, 1989.

126. Stoner E: Phase III studies evaluating the 5α-reductase inhibitor process. Annual Meeting of the American Urological Association, Toronto, Ontario, Canada, June 2–6, 1991.

127. Sufrin G, Coffey DS: A new model for studying the effect of drugs on prostatic growth. Invest Urol 11:45–54, 1973.

128. Sufrin G, Coffey DS: Flutamide: Mechanism of action of a new nonsteroidal antiandrogen. Invest Urol 13:429–434, 1976.

129. Sugimura Y, Cunha GR, Bigsby RM: Androgenic induction of DNA synthesis in prostatic glands induced in the urothelium of testicular feminized (Tfm/y) mice. Prostate 9:217–225, 1986.

130. The MK-906 (Finasteride) Study Group: One year experience in the treatment of benign prostatic hyperplasia with finasteride. J Androl 12:372–375, 1991.

131. Trachtenberg J, Hicks LL, Walsh PC: Androgen- and estrogen-receptor content in spontaneous and experimentally induced canine prostatic hyperplasia. J Clin Invest 65:1051–1059, 1980.

132. Tunn U, Senge Th, Schenck B, Neumann F: Biochemical and histological studies on prostates in castrated dogs after treatment with androstanediol, oestradiol and cyproterone acetate. Acta Endocrinol 91:373–384, 1979.

133. Tunn U, Senge T, Schenck B, Neumann F: Effects of cyproterone acetate on experimentally induced canine prostatic hyperplasia: A morphological and histochemical study. Urol Int 35:125–140, 1980.

134. Vermeulen A, Giagulli VA, De Schepper P, et al: Hormonal effects of an orally active 4-azasteroid inhibitor of 5α-reductase in humans. Prostate 14:45–53, 1989.

135. Vickery BH, McRae GI, Bonasch H: Effect of chronic administration of a highly potent LHRH agonist on prostate size and secretory function in geriatric dogs. Prostate 3:123–130, 1982.

136. Walsh PC: Benign prostatic hyperplasia. *In* Walsh PC, Gittes RF, Perlmutter AD, Stamey TA (eds): Campbell's Urology, 5th ed, Vol 2. Philadelphia, WB Saunders Co, 1986, pp 1248–1265.

137. Walsh PC, Wilson JD: The induction of prostatic hypertrophy in the dog with androstanediol. J Clin Invest 57:1093–1097, 1976.

138. Wang MC, Papsidero LD, Kuriyama M, et al: Prostate antigen: A new potential marker for prostatic cancer. Prostate 2:89–96, 1981.

139. Weber JP, Oesterling JE, Peters CA, et al: The influence of reversible androgen deprivation on serum prostate-specific antigen levels in men with benign prostatic hyperplasia. J Urol 141:987–992, 1989.

140. West NB, Roselli CE, Resko JA, et al: Estrogen and progestin receptors and aromatase activity in rhesus monkey prostate. Endocrinology 123:2312–2322, 1988.

141. White JW: The results of double castration in hypertrophy of the prostate. Ann Surg 22:1–80, 1895.

142. Wilbert DM, Griffin JE, Wilson JD: Characterization of the cytosol androgen receptor of the human prostate. J Clin Endocrinol Metab 56:113–120, 1983.

143. Wilkin RP, Bruchovsky N, Shnitka TK, et al: Stromal 5α-reductase activity is elevated in benign prostatic hyperplasia. Acta Endocrinol (Copenh) 94:284–288, 1980.

144. Wilson JD: The pathogenesis of benign prostatic hyperplasia. Am J Med 68:745–756, 1980.

145. Winters SJ, Troen P: Evidence for a role of endogenous estrogen in the hypothalamic control of gonadotropin secretion in men. J Clin Endocrinol Metab 61:842–845, 1985.

146. Worgul TJ, Santen RJ, Saoilik E, et al: Evidence that brain aromatization regulates LH secretion in the male dog. Am Physiol Soc 81:E246, 1987.

147. Zuckerman S: The endocrine control of the prostate. Proc R Soc Med 29 (2):1557–1568, 1936.

148. Zumoff B, Strain GW, Kream J, et al: Age variation of the 24-hour mean plasma concentrations of androgens, estrogens, and gonadotropins in normal adult men. J Clin Endocrinol Metab 54:534–538, 1982.

Chapter 17

BALLOON DILATION/HYPERTHERMIA/ PROSTATIC STENTS FOR BENIGN PROSTATIC HYPERPLASIA

PRATAP K. REDDY

Benign prostatic hyperplasia (BPH) is a normal aging process of men which manifests clinically with the symptom complex of prostatism. Based on the severity of symptoms and the clinical findings associated with BPH, the available treatment options include watchful waiting and transurethral resection of the prostate (TURP). Recently, a wide variety of pharmacologic and procedural treatments have become clinically available or are being clinically tested as suitable treatment options for symptomatic BPH. This chapter details three treatment options, namely, transurethral balloon dilation of the prostate (TUDP), hyperthermia-thermotherapy, and prostatic stent. Transurethral dilation of the prostate has undergone extensive clinical use, and the balloon dilators are approved by the Food and Drug Administration (FDA) for the treatment of BPH. However, hyperthermia and prostate stents are currently under clinical investigation, and instrumentation for these two procedures is not FDA-approved for general use.

TRANSURETHRAL BALLOON DILATION OF THE PROSTATE

TUDP is a recently revived technique for the treatment of symptomatic BPH. Techniques for dilation of the prostate have been in existence for centuries. In the mid-19th century, special metal dilators were developed for the transurethral dilation of the prostate and bladder neck, with several investigators advocating this procedure. Guthrie,[24] in 1830; Civiale,[14] in 1841; Mercier,[42] in 1850; and Kraemer,[35] in 1910, successfully used metal dilators to relieve obstruction from BPH. Hollings-

worth,[26] in 1910, described the procedure of transvesicle anterior commissurotomy of the prostate. During that period, prostatic enucleation was the treatment of choice and carried significant morbidity and mortality. A simpler technique of stretching the bladder neck and prostatic urethra to the size of the index finger through a small suprapubic cystotomy relieved prostatic obstruction and was associated with less morbidity than prostatic enucleation. Otto Franck, in 1938, reported good results using this technique to relieve prostatism.[22] Because this procedure required a cystotomy, its use did not gain popularity over prostatic enucleation. Prostatic dilation was revived when Werner Deisting, in collaboration with Otto Franck, designed a metal prostatic dilator (a modification of the Mercier prostatic dilator) to treat obstruction from BPH (Fig. 17–1). The dilator was introduced transurethrally and was positioned by rectal palpation to prevent injury to the external sphincter. The branches of the dilator were mechanically expanded from 4 to 8 cm in an anteroposterior plane. This resulted in an anterior and posterior commissurotomy and stretching of the prostatic capsule (prostatic ring) without disrupting it. In 1956, Deisting reported excellent results using this dilator to treat 324 patients with BPH.[15] Ninety-five per cent of the patients were cured initially, and long-term results were excellent. At 3, 5, and 8 years follow-up, 83 per cent, 74 per cent, and 48 per cent of the patients, respectively, were free of symptoms.

Dilation of the prostate using Deisting's technique was widely used in Europe in the 1950s and 1960s for treating symptomatic BPH (Table 17–1). Several investigators (Spotoft,[62] Kivioja,[31] Pilgard,[47] Oravisto,[45] and

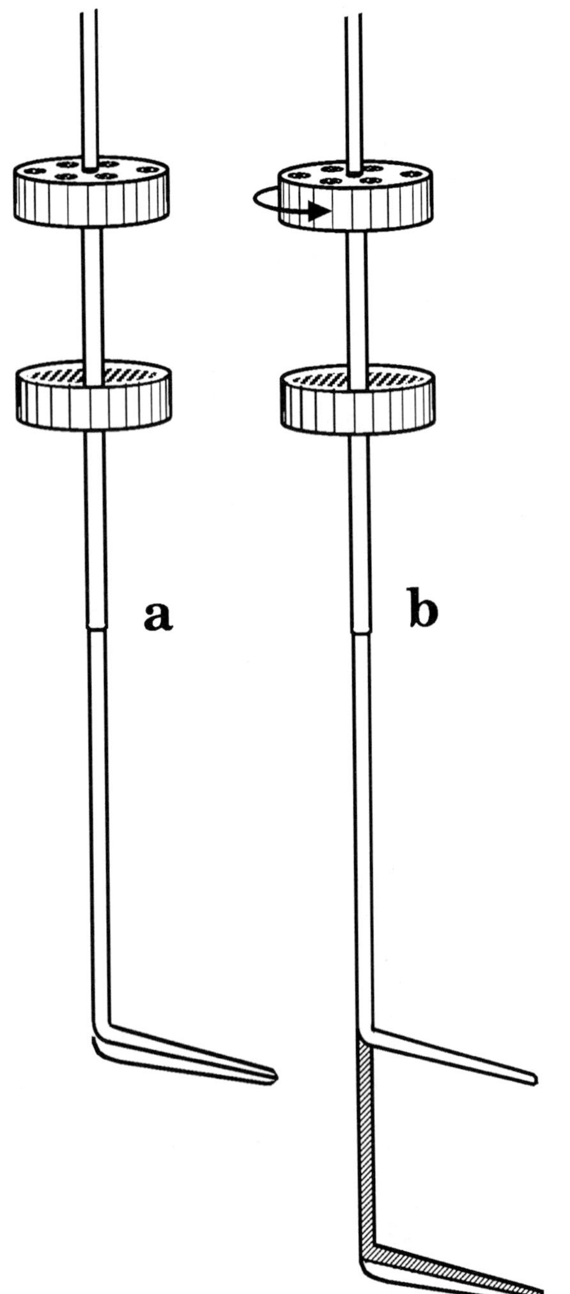

FIGURE 17–1. Deisting prostate dilator. The 24 Fr metal dilator is opened by turning the handwheel.

Backman[6]) reported good results (70 to 90 per cent incidence of relief of symptoms) with this technique and suggested it as an alternative to TURP. Kolberg, however, experienced disappointing results, with only 22 per cent of 55 patients doing well at 1 to 2 years.[34] Also, in 1965, Aalkjaer reported a comparative study of TUDP to TURP and open prostatectomy.[1] One hundred and forty-six dilated patients were compared to 110 TURP or open prostatectomy patients over a 7-year period. Aalkjaer concluded that postoperatively and by 7-year follow-up, open prostatectomy or TURP patients overall experienced significantly far better results than patients with the dilation treatment. However, on closer scrutiny

of Aalkjaer's data, it is evident that patients with smaller obstructing prostates do much better than those with larger prostate glands following TUDP. At 7-year follow-up, only 15 per cent with small prostates required reoperation after TUDP, compared with 60 per cent of patients with large prostate glands who required reoperation after TUDP. This suggests that with proper patient selection, prostatic dilation might have been a suitable treatment option for prostatism. Subsequent to these reports, dilation fell into disfavor. At the same time, great strides were made in the optics and design of the endoscopic instruments and in the diathermy which made TURP the mainstay of the surgical treatment of symptomatic BPH.

Balloon Dilation of the Prostate

Renewal of interest in dilation techniques for treatment of symptomatic BPH relates to advances in balloon catheter technology and the successful use of dilation techniques as an alternative to surgery in the treatment of vascular, biliary, and gastrointestinal strictures. In 1984, Burhenne and associates were the first to report the use of balloon catheters to dilate the prostate to 24 Fr for 30 seconds on 10 male cadavers and demonstrate an increase in the diameter of the prostatic urethra.[8] Burhenne subsequently underwent dilation of his prostate to 24 Fr with relief of prostatism. Quinn and associates performed balloon dilation in six live dogs.[48] In five dogs, they noted that the posterior urethra remained widened for 8 to 23 weeks. Castaneda and colleagues performed balloon dilation of the prostate on 28 dogs using different balloon sizes and dilation times.[11] They concluded that a balloon at least 20 mm (60 Fr) in diameter inflated for 10 minutes was required for satisfactory, long-term patency of the prostatic urethra in dogs.

Fundamentals of Balloon Dilation of the Prostate

Balloon dilation of the prostate is performed by precisely positioning the balloon catheter in the prostatic

TABLE 17–1. RESULTS OF DILATION OF PROSTATE WITH METAL DILATORS

AUTHOR*	NO. OF PATIENTS	SUCCESS RATE (%)			
		0–1 yr	3 yr	5 yr	>7 yr
Deisting, 1956[15]	324	95	93	90	80
Kivioja, 1957[31]	60	71	—	—	—
Kolberg, 1959[34]	55	22	—	—	—
Backman, 1963[6]	133	75	74	—	—
Aboulker and Steg, 1964[2]	218	85	—	—	—
Sandberg and Sandstrom, 1967[58]	150	—	—	58	—
Aalkjaer, 1965[1]	146	84	66	60	55

*Represents reported series with greater than 50 patients.

urethra and inflating it to a predetermined size and period of time in order to cause a commissurotomy or widen the lumen of the prostatic urethra, thereby relieving prostatic obstruction. Dilating the entire prostatic urethra with preservation of the external sphincter is critical to a successful outcome. However, currently, there is a wide variation in the parameters of balloon dilation, namely, balloon size, length of dilation time, balloon pressure, and the role of dilating the bladder neck during prostatic dilation. This is in part due to the evolving catheter technology capable of manufacturing bigger dilating balloons and partly due to the existing balloon catheter designs. It is clear that larger dilating balloons produce better results following dilation. In their clinical trials, Reddy and associates initially used 60 Fr dilating balloons and have since used 75 Fr and 90 Fr balloons.[54] In their current clinical trials using 120 Fr balloon dilators, their preliminary results indicate a better outcome.[52]

Historically, Deisting noted that, using metal dilators, the prostatic urethra required dilation to a diameter of 4 to 8 cm (>120 Fr balloon) to achieve commissurotomy and relaxation of the prostatic capsule.[15] He attributed some of the failures to inadequate dilation of the prostatic urethra. Using fluoroscopy to monitor the process of balloon dilation, Reddy et al[51] have noted that the dilating balloon must be inflated to a pressure of three atmospheres for adequate dilation (fully expanded balloons) to be achieved. This suggests that the prostate can be dilated under low pressure and that the balloon dilators should be able to withstand at least three atmospheres of inflation pressure. Also noted on fluoroscopy was the presence of a constricting band at the level of the bladder neck which was amenable to dilation along with the prostatic urethra. This finding, along with the fact that during TURP and transurethral incision of the prostate (TUIP) the prostatic tissue at the bladder neck is resected or incised, forms the basis for recommending dilation of the bladder neck during prostatic dilation.

Another intriguing aspect of balloon dilation is the length of time the dilation should be maintained. Some investigators have routinely used 10 minutes, whereas others have tried 15 and 20 minutes of dilating time. Existing scientific data suggest that 10 minutes of dilation time is adequate. Castaneda et al concluded that, using similar-sized dilating balloons but different dilation times, dilating the dog's prostatic urethra for 10 minutes resulted in long-term patency of the dog's prostatic urethra.[11] Clinically, it has been observed that during balloon dilation, the balloon pressure drops as the prostatic capsule stretches, requiring periodic inflations to maintain pressure. This process occurs during the first 3 to 5 minutes of dilation, after which no further pressure drops are seen, suggesting completion of the dilation process. Although dilation time of less than 10 minutes may suffice, certainly there appears to be no reason to maintain dilation for longer than 10 minutes.

Balloon Dilators and Techniques

Currently three prostate balloon dilators are commercially available for balloon dilation of the prostate (Table 17–2). The Optilume prostate balloon dilator (American Medical Systems, Minnetonka, MN), the Dowd-II prostate dilator (Meditech, Inc, Watertown, MA), and the TCU dilation catheter (Advanced Surgical Intervention, Inc., San Clemente, CA). The Optilume prostate dilator and the Dowd-II are single-length balloon catheters that can be used under fluoroscopy, cystoscopy, digital guidance, or transrectal ultrasonography (TRUS) for placement. Because the excess length of the balloon is accommodated within the bladder lumen, single-length balloon catheters can be used to dilate prostate glands of varying sizes. Although fluoroscopy, cystoscopy, digital guidance, or TRUS can be used individually or to complement each other, the digital technique of balloon dilation is the most accurate and simplest way to perform balloon dilation of the prostate using the Optilume or Dowd catheter. The TCU dilation catheter comes in different balloon lengths, and the prostatic urethra needs to be premeasured to select the appropriate balloon length. This catheter does not provide for dilation of the bladder neck. The dilation procedure is usually performed under cystoscopic monitoring.

Anesthesia

Balloon dilation of the prostate is a painful procedure and requires some form of anesthetic. Although the prostate gland does not contain many sensory fibers, the prostatic capsule is richly innervated with sensory fibers

TABLE 17–2. PROSTATE BALLOON DILATOR SPECIFICATIONS

	OPTILUME	TCU	DOWD
Dilation balloon length	4 cm	1.5–4 cm	5 cm
Dilation balloon diameter (inflated)	90 Fr	75 Fr	90 Fr
Dilation balloon pressure (atmospheric)	5	3	4
Radiopaque markers	3	1	2
Positioning and monitoring	Digital, endoscopic, fluoroscopic, TRUS*	Cystoscopic, TRUS	Digital, fluoroscopic, endoscopic
Additional features	40 Fr bulbous urethral balloon, positioning collar	15-cc bladder neck balloon	Traction collar, positioning nodule (19 Fr)

*TRUS = transrectal ultrasonography.

from the pelvic plexus that travels along the dorsal lateral aspect of the prostate anterior to the rectum. Dilation of the prostate results in an intense desire to void, which is painful at best. Balloon dilation of the prostate has been performed with the patient under general anesthesia, spinal anesthesia, prostate block, and intravenous analgesia/sedation. The prostate block described by Reddy[49] is a simple procedure that provides adequate local anesthesia of the prostate and enables TUDP to be performed in a clinic or an outpatient setting (Fig. 17–2). In this procedure, 15 to 20 ml of 1 per cent lidocaine solution are injected in the space anterior to the rectal wall between the base of the prostate and the seminal vesicle, to block the prostatic plexus of nerves. After a skin wheal is raised in the perineum, a 22-gauge, 5-inch-long spinal needle is used to access this space. The course of the needle is partially guided with a finger in the rectum. The procedure is performed on both sides. The prostate block, along with topical lidocaine jelly, appears to be adequate to perform TUDP in most cases.

Methodology

The various techniques to perform TUDP using fluoroscopy (Reddy,[54] Dowd and Smith,[19] Castaneda[12]), cystoscopy (Klein et al,[33] Reddy[51]); and TRUS (Sloan[61]) are not described here. The digital technique of performing TUDP using the Optilume prostate dilator (Reddy[50, 51]) is briefly reviewed, as this method is simple, accurate, and probably the easiest way to perform TUDP. All patients undergoing TUDP should have a sterile urine culture and receive prophylactic antibiotics. The procedure is performed in the dorsal lithotomy position. If prostate block or sedation is used, the urethra is anesthetized with 2 per cent xylocaine jelly. An 18 Fr Councill-tipped catheter is used to partially inflate the bladder and to coil a 0.038-inch guidewire within the bladder. The Councill-tipped catheter is removed and the Optilume prostate dilator is advanced into the bladder over the guidewire. A finger is then placed in the rectum to palpate the apex of the prostate. The Optilume prostate dilator is gradually withdrawn until the collar is palpated (Fig. 17–3). This confirms accurate catheter position. Catheter design enables inflation of the fixation balloon below the external sphincter. The dilating balloon is dilated to 90 Fr with an inflation syringe by maintaining the balloon pressure at four atmospheres of pressure. The dilation is maintained for 10 minutes. Bleeding is minimal. Foley catheter drainage is provided for 24 hours.

Mechanism of Dilation of the Prostate

The exact mechanism by which dilation of the prostate causes relief of obstruction is not clearly understood. Several different mechanisms have been considered. Initially, it was thought that dilation of the prostate may cause atrophy of the prostatic adenoma. This was based on the findings that TRUS and MRI studies pre- and

post-TUDP have shown intraprostatic hemorrhage and edema of the prostate gland without any disruption of the prostatic capsule. It was postulated that this could cause thrombosis of the smaller intraprostatic vessels and thereby lead to atrophy of the prostate. Serial MRI studies of the prostate by Johnson et al, however, have not shown this to be true.[28] Moreover, histologic studies of the prostate (in patients who underwent TURP after failed TUDP) do not show any atrophy of the glandular tissue. Retrograde urethrograms performed after TUDP show a definite increase in the lumen of the prostatic urethra. Also, in vitro studies of dilation in explanted human prostate specimens show a definite increase in the lumen of the prostatic urethra as a result of compression of the prostatic tissue. These studies also show a definite stretching of the prostatic capsule without any tears in the capsule. It can therefore be postulated that relief of obstruction results from a mechanical widening of the prostatic urethral lumen as well as a decrease in the resistance to the outflow of urine resulting from stretching of the fibrous ring of the prostate (prostate capsule and surgical capsule).

Deisting, in 1956, suggested that dilation of the prostate resulted in exhaustion of the elasticity of the prostatic capsule and an anterior commissurotomy when the prostate was stretched with metal dilators up to 8 cm (> 120 Fr balloons).[15] It is not clear that commissurotomy or tears in the anterior fibromuscular stroma occur routinely following balloon dilation. This could be due to the inadequate stretching that occurs with currently available balloon dilators (75 to 90 Fr). Balloon dilators of larger size may consistently produce deep tears in the anterior fibromuscular stroma (point of least resistance) and thereby reduce the resistance to the outflow of urine.

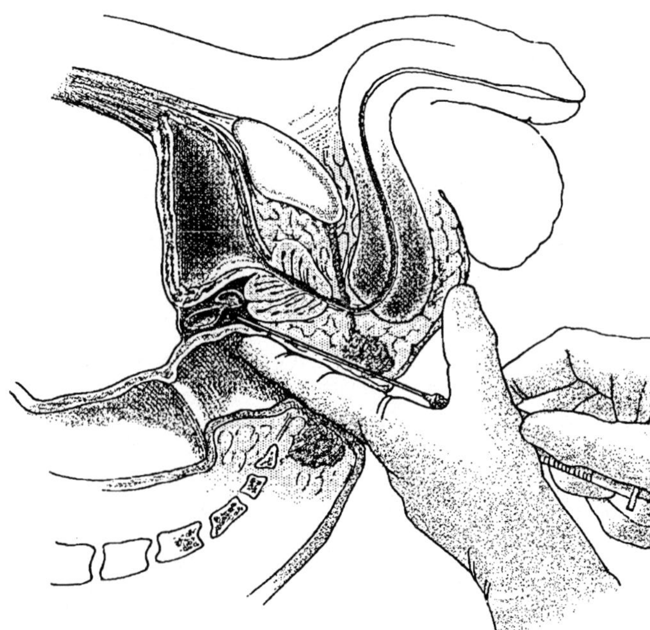

FIGURE 17–2. Prostate block. Shows technique of digitally guided transperineal administration of local anesthetic to the base of the prostate gland.

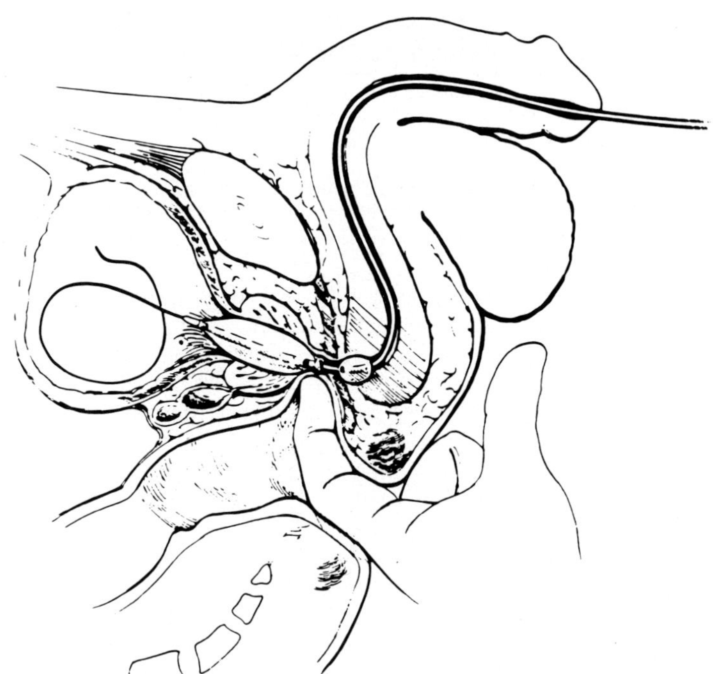

FIGURE 17–3. Digital technique of balloon dilation of the prostate.

Finally, it can be postulated that the process of stretching the prostate could disrupt and bring about changes in the nerve endings in the bladder neck and prostatic urethra which could relieve some of the obstructive and irritative symptoms of BPH.

Results of Transurethal Dilation of the Prostate

Balloon dilation of the prostate has been performed by many investigators using different techniques, balloon sizes, and dilating balloon catheters. Table 17–3 represents some of the larger reported series using TUDP. Overall experience with balloon dilation of the prostate indicates a wide variation of 50 to 80 per cent in the success rate. This wide variation represents a lack of uniform patient selection for TUDP. Earlier studies included patients who now would not be considered for TUDP. It is clear that patients with an enlarged median lobe of the prostate, those with mainly irritative rather than obstructive voiding symptoms, and those with poor bladder function with large residual volumes or in urinary retention are not candidates for TUDP. Patients with chronic urinary retention do not respond, although patients with acute urinary retention may be rendered catheter free following dilation. Wasserman and Reddy,[65a] using the patient selection criteria listed in Tables 17–4 and 17–5, reported excellent results following TUDP in 49 selected patients compared with 42 unselected patients. The selected patient group had a mean symptom score of 14.5, residual urine of 105 ml, and maximum flow rate of 10.7 ml/sec. The unselected patient group had a symptom score of 16.8, residual urine of 249 ml, and maximum flow rate of 7.9 ml/sec. The mean age and prostate size between the two groups were similar. After a mean follow-up of 22 months, statistically significant improvement in symptom score was seen in 80 per cent of the selected patients compared with only 43 per cent of the unselected patients. It is clear that appropriate patient selection for TUDP may produce far better results than the currently published reports indicate. Efficacy of TUDP has been compared with that of standard surgical procedures. Donatucci et al randomized 41 patients to TUDP and TURP and noted a statistically significant decrease in symptom scores in both groups at 6 to 12 months follow-up.[17] The symptom score dropped from 12.5 to 5.1 ($P < 0.01$) in the TURP group and from 14.1 to 7.1 ($P < 0.01$) in the TUDP group. Chiou et al randomized 30 patients to

TABLE 17–3. RESULTS OF DILATION OF PROSTATE WITH BALLOON DILATORS

AUTHOR	NO. OF PATIENTS	SUCCESS (%) <6 Months	SUCCESS (%) >6 Months
Dowd and Smith[19]	50	72	
Goldenberg et al[23]	42	67	
Klein et al[33]	53	64	
Reddy et al[52]	74	70	61 (12 months)
Doughtery et al[18]	55		83 (3–26 months)
Wasserman/ Reddy[65a]	49		80 (6–48 months)
Marks[40]	43		88 (3–24 months)

TABLE 17–4. OPTIMAL CANDIDATE FOR BALLOON DILATION OF PROSTATE

Moderate symptoms of prostatism
Prostate less than 40 grams with predominately lateral lobe obstruction
Residual urine less than 150 ml
Normal bladder function

TABLE 17–5. CONTRAINDICATIONS TO BALLOON DILATION OF PROSTATE

Significant median lobe enlargement
Atonic bladder
Active urinary tract infection
Bacterial prostatitis
Renal failure due to benign prostatic hyperplasia

TUIP and TUDP with a follow-up of 2 to 16 months.[13] They noted success in 87 per cent and 86 per cent, respectively. Kapoor et al performed pressure-flow studies before and 3 months after the procedure in 10 patients undergoing TUDP and compared them with those of 10 patients undergoing TURP.[29] They found that a comparable and significant decrease in bladder pressure and increase in maximum flow rate occurred in both groups.

All these studies indicate that TUDP is effective, based on both subjective and objective criteria, in relieving bladder outlet obstruction from BPH. More recently, improvement in balloon catheter technology has enabled the availability of 120 Fr prostate balloon dilators (American Medical Systems, Minnetonka, MN). Currently, a multicenter clinical trial is under way to test the safety and efficacy of the 120 Fr balloon dilator. Preliminary results indicate that it is safe, and, at 3 months postdilation, more than 90 per cent of patients have noted a significant decrease in symptoms.

Complications of Balloon Dilation of the Prostate

TUDP is a safe procedure. Bleeding is minimal. Mild to moderate hematuria may last 24 to 78 hours. About 5 per cent of the patients undergoing balloon dilation of the prostate may require Foley catheter drainage for longer than 24 hours as a result of prostatic edema. Patients typically resume normal activity in 3 to 5 days. Balloon dilation does not cause any sexual dysfunction, and there is no incidence of impotence following this procedure. The volume of ejaculate varies in the first 3 months following dilation, with both increases and decreases in the quantity being reported. However, by the end of 3 months, all patients had ejaculate volumes comparable to their predilation state (Reddy,[51] Marks[40]). There is no reported incidence of incontinence.

Summary

TUDP by balloon is a safe procedure that can be performed in an outpatient setting. Although different anesthetic agents have been used, the prostate block with or without parenteral analgesia/sedation appears to be adequate. The morbidity of the procedure is minimal, and convalescence is very short. Sexual function is not altered following dilation. Patient selection and proper dilation technique appear to be the hallmarks for a successful outcome. Short-term results indicate a success of over 90 per cent in properly selected patients. Available data suggest a successful outcome lasting at least 2 to 3 years. Long-term studies are pending. Second-stage dilation of the prostate may further prolong relief of symptoms following recurrence. Finally, with the availability of larger balloon dilators, the immediate and long-term efficacy of balloon dilation of the prostate may further improve.

HYPERTHERMIA

Hyperthermia and thermotherapy are other modalities that are being evaluated for the treatment of symptomatic BPH. Hyperthermia as a therapeutic modality has been recognized since ancient times. The beneficial effects of heat in promoting healing have long been recognized. In 1866, Busch first reported the curative effect of hyperthermia on cancer.[9] He noted the complete regression of a sarcoma in a patient following a febrile attack caused by erysipelas infection. In 1917, Rohdenberg noted spontaneous regression of various histologically proven tumors in 192 cases and noted a relationship between fever and tumor regression.[57] Subsequent to this, several investigators have reported the tumoricidal effect of hyperthermia. When the human body temperature was artificially raised to 42 to 45°C, it selectively induced irreversible damage to malignant cells but spared normal cells. Hyperthermia can be delivered to the whole body or to parts of it. In recent years, local hyperthermia has been used alone or in conjunction with radiation therapy or chemotherapy in the treatment of solid tumors that are superficial and accessible. These tumors had to be superficial owing to the limitations of heat application to deep-seated tumors. The fact that the prostate is easily accessible from the rectal cavity led Yerushalmi and colleagues to consider hyperthermia to treat prostate cancer. After successful studies in rabbits using microwave antennae to produce local hyperthermia, Yerushalmi and colleagues used this form of treatment in humans with prostate cancer alone or in conjunction with radiation therapy or hormonal therapy.[67–70] During these clinical studies, they noted that patients with obstructive voiding symptoms had relief of their obstruction. This led to their extending the application of local hyperthermia to treat patients with symptoms of BPH.

Hyperthermia-Thermotherapy Systems and Clinical Trials

Initial clinical trials in the treatment of BPH applied the principles of hyperthermia. The prostate was selectively heated to a temperature of 42 to 45°C. At this temperature, tissue necrosis does not occur. Several hyperthermia sessions lasting 30 to 60 minutes are necessary to produce symptomatic relief of BPH. A later concept is that of thermotherapy, in which the prostate is heated to greater than 45°C in order to produce permanent tissue changes in the prostate. This type of therapy requires a single treatment session and is expected to produce more effective symptomatic relief of BPH. Currently, two hyperthermia systems and one thermotherapy system are under clinical investigation. One hyperthermia system uses a transrectal approach with a directional microwave radiator placed in the rectum and directed toward the prostate. The other is a transurethral approach that uses a symmetrically radiating applicator located within the prostatic urethra. The thermotherapy system uses a transurethral approach to the prostate with surface cooling of the urethra.

The first hyperthermia system clinically used to treat BPH is the Prostathermer (Biodan Medical Systems, Rehovot, Israel). The Prostathermer is a computerized transrectal hyperthermia system. The device consists of a microwave generator (915 mHz), a rectal applicator (directional microwave radiator), and a cooling system for surface cooling and protection of the rectal wall. The rectal applicator has copper-constantan thermocouples to monitor rectal temperature. Similar thermocouples mounted on a transurethral catheter can monitor prostatic urethral temperatures. Using this system, the prostate adenoma can be heated to 42 to 45°C without any thermal injury to the rectum. The treatments are administered in several sessions, with a maximum of two sessions a week. Each session lasts 30 to 60 minutes.

The transurethral system consists of a flexible transurethral applicator operating at 915 mHz (BSD Medical Corporation, Salt Lake City, UT). The applicator is a modified Foley catheter, which ensures easy placement and accurate localization of the prostate (Fig. 17–4). There are two types of applicators, one using three insulated dipole antennae and the other using a single large helical coil antenna.[4] The applicators are equipped with thermosensors to monitor prostatic urethral temperatures. This system appears to maintain prostatic

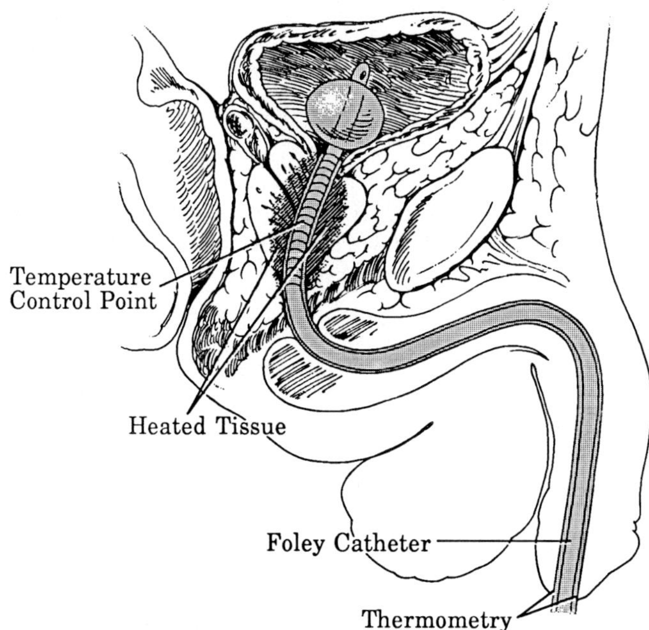

FIGURE 17–4. The transurethral microwave applicator.

tissue temperature in the range of 42 to 45°C in a cylindrically symmetric volume of up to 4 cm in length and a radial penetration of 0.5 cm around the applicator. Surface cooling of the urethra is not required at this temperature range. As with the transrectal system, treatments are administered in several sessions, each session lasting 30 to 60 minutes.

Thermotherapy of the prostate is performed using the system called the Prostatron (Technomed International, Danvers, MA). The system consists of a flexible applicator with microwave antenna that emits at a frequency of 1296 mHz. At this frequency, the applicator is capable of heating the prostatic adenoma to greater than 45°C to cause tissue changes. The applicator also contains a cooling system to prevent any urethral epithelial damage. The position of the applicator is determined by TRUS. Rectal temperatures are monitored by a rectal probe with three thermal sensors at different distances from the anal verge. During the treatments, the power and the cooling system are regulated so that the temperatures never exceed 42.5°C in the rectum and 45°C in the urethra.[10, 16] Owing to the radioactive heating effects of the microwaves, the transitional zone of the prostate attains temperatures above 45°C (47 to 50°C). This type of therapy requires a single session lasting 60 minutes.

Microwave Heating and Effects on Tissue

Microwaves are part of an electromagnetic spectrum with frequency ranging from 300 mHz to 300 gHz. The depth of penetration of the microwaves depends on the frequency; the higher the frequency, the lower the penetration. Microwave heating of the tissue results from polarization of the small molecules in the oscillating electromagnetic field. The maximum heat occurs next to the antenna and decreases exponentially with distance from the source.

The effects of heating with microwaves on the canine prostate using the transrectal system (Biodan) was extensively studied by Leib and colleagues.[37] They found that changes appeared to be time and temperature dependent. Heating at 42.5°C for 1.5 hours was harmless and could be safely repeated with no irreversible changes. However, heating at 42.5°C for 5 hours was associated with definite histologic evidence of tissue damage. Heating the prostate at 44.5°C resulted in severe necrotic damage at 1.5 hours of treatment. In addition, they noted mononuclear inflammatory infiltrations in the interstitium and polymorphonuclear infiltrates in the glandular elements of the prostatic tissue. Using this transrectal microwave hyperthermia system, Yerushalmi performed invasive monitoring of the human prostate and confirmed that a temperature of 42 to 43°C is reached in 10 to 15 minutes after commencement of treatment.[67] Linder et al noted the changes in prostate-specific antigen (PSA) in 18 patients who underwent hyperthermia treatments.[38, 39] Each patient received five treatments lasting 1 hour. They noted no significant difference between pre- and post-treatment PSA levels and concluded that local hyperthermia (41 ± 1.5°C) is atraumatic and does not cause a cytotoxic insult to prostate epithelial tissues.

Lauweryns et al[36] have studied the histologic changes in the prostate after using the transurethral hyperthermia system (BSD Medical Corporation) without cooling. The urethral temperature was constantly maintained at 45°C. Treatments lasted 70 minutes. The histologic changes were periurethral and extended up to 6 mm radially and 4 to 5 cm longitudinally. Acute changes included periurethral edema, parenchymal hemorrhages, and occasional small vessel thrombosis with coagulation necrosis of the smooth muscle. With repeated hyperthermia treatments, these changes were more extensive and deeper. They concluded that repeated treatments resulted in shrinking and retraction of the periurethral prostatic parenchyma due to organizing tissue necrosis and cicatrization.

The histologic changes in the prostate following treatment with the Prostatron were studied by Devonec et al[16] Macroscopically, the urethral mucosa and periurethral tissues were preserved to a depth of 2 to 5 mm from the urethral lumen. The peripheral zone of the prostate and the prostatic capsule were also preserved. The treated zone in between showed tissue changes (Fig. 17–5). Microscopically, the affected areas showed interstitial inflammatory reaction with thrombosis of the small blood vessels, whereas the larger ones were preserved. The normal cellular arrangement of the stroma and acini disappeared. This resulted in shrinking and fibrosis of the affected tissue, thereby decreasing the mechanical obstruction from BPH. Also, possible injury to the alpha-receptor nerve connections in the periurethral area may decrease the dynamic component of obstruction from BPH. Devonec et al[16] have also noted a significant increase in the levels of serum PSA by day seven (as a result of acinar cell damage by heat) to support the histologic findings of tissue damage.

Results of Hyperthermia Treatment

Treatment of BPH using hyperthermia techniques and transurethral microwave thermotherapy has been performed in many centers in Israel, Europe, and the United States. There are wide differences in these reported results as to the criteria used for success, length of follow-up, number of treatment sessions, length of each session, and patient selection. However, common to all studies is the fact that this treatment is easily performed on an outpatient basis with topical anesthesia and minimal morbidity and convalescence. Using the Biodan/BSD system, several investigators have reported 50 to 80 per cent immediate success rate in symptomatic improvement of prostatism (Table 17–6). However, there appears to be minimal or marginal improvement in the urinary flow rates. Strohmaier et al noted disappointing results in 30 patients using the Biodan system and considered it to be an ineffective therapy for BPH.[64] Stawarz and colleagues, in 1991, reported a comparative study of transurethral and transrectal microwave hyper-

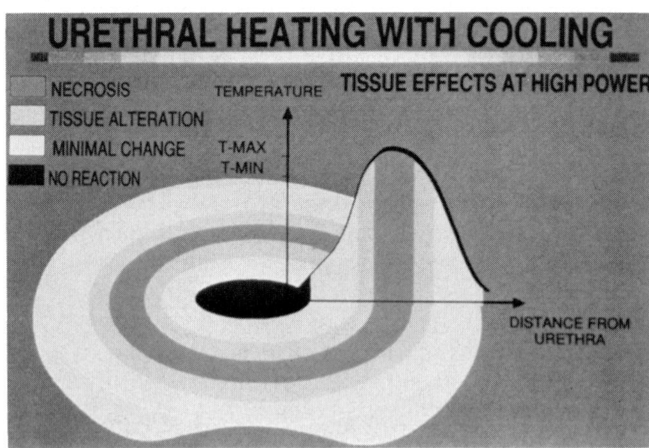

FIGURE 17–5. Tissue changes with thermotherapy. (Courtesy of Technomed International.)

thermia treatments in 36 patients with BPH.[63] They found that in both subjective and objective parameters, major improvement was noted more frequently in the transurethral group than in the transrectal group.

Although thermotherapy has been used recently in clinical trials, available short-term data (Table 17–6) suggest that transurethral microwave thermotherapy may be a more effective therapy than hyperthermia with no increased morbidity.

Complications

The complications following transrectal hyperthermia are reported in a large series of patients from two institutions by Linder et al.[38] Of 435 patients, they noted an overall complication rate of 6.6 per cent. Hematuria occurred in six patients (1.4 per cent), but three of these patients required emergency prostatectomy due to hemorrhage. Other complications included urinary tract infections, rectal pain, urinary retention, and bacteremia. A bothersome complication following thermotherapy is urinary retention in 16 to 20 per cent requiring bladder drainage for 3 to 7 days.[10, 16] Patients also

TABLE 17–6. RESULTS OF HYPERTHERMIA AND THERMOTHERAPY TREATMENTS FOR BENIGN PROSTATIC HYPERPLASIA

		SUCCESS (%)	
AUTHOR	NO. OF PATIENTS	<3 months	> 3 months
Yerushalmi (H)[67]	37(x)	57	47 (6–70 months)
	68	83	72 (6–80 months)
Lindner et al (H)[38, 39]	72(x)	50	40 (12 months)
Servadio et al (H)[60]	124		51 (12 months)
Strohmaier et al (H)[64]	30	7	
Rigatti et al (H)[56]	100	70	
Sapozink (H)[58a]	21	81	
Devonec et al (T)[16]	37	92	
Carter et al (T)[10]	50	70	

x = Patients in urinary retention; H = hyperthermia; T = thermotherapy.

experience an exacerbation of their symptoms for up to 3 weeks.

Summary

Hyperthermia and thermotherapy for BPH are currently under clinical investigation in FDA-approved clinical trials. The treatments appear simple and fairly well tolerated. No anesthesia is required and patients receive treatment as outpatients. The morbidity is low and convalescence short. However, the drawbacks of hyperthermia are the numerous treatment sessions required and the delay before relief of symptoms. Moreover, improvement appears to be more subjective, with lesser changes in the objective parameters of obstruction.

Histopathologic studies of the effects of heat on the human prostate have shown that tissue changes occur to a depth of 6 mm radially around the microwave antenna[36] and that changes in the tissue are time and temperature dependent.[37] This could lead one to speculate that transurethrally delivered hyperthermia treatment may affect the periurethral transitional zone more consistently than the transrectal approach. Clinical reports by Stawarz et al also indicate better resolution of symptoms by the transurethral approach than by the transrectal approach.[63] Hyperthermia, by limiting the temperature in the prostate to less than 45°C, may not bring about changes significant enough to relieve prostatic obstruction. Thermotherapy, on the other hand, raises the intraprostatic temperature to greater than 45°C (47 to 50°C), causing tissue changes, and may therefore be more effective than hyperthermia treatment. Thermotherapy appears to be more promising than hyperthermia treatment in preliminary clinical reports. However, long-term studies and probably comparative studies are needed to prove the safety and efficacy of both hyperthermia and thermotherapy in the treatment for BPH.

PROSTATE STENTS

The use of stents in the prostatic urethra to relieve prostatic obstruction is a relatively new development. Temporary stenting of the stenotic segment following dilatation has been used by urologists for many years. Since the 1970s, the use of stents following balloon angioplasty of strictures in the peripheral arterial system has been investigated. Initially, spiral stents, and more recently, expandable endovascular mesh stents have been shown to be effective in maintaining long-term patency of vascular stenosis, especially in larger blood vessels. This has prompted the use of stents in urology.

The first use of stents in the prostatic urethra to relieve prostatic obstruction was described by Fabian in 1980.[20] He used a metallic spiral stent to maintain patency of the prostatic urethra. Subsequently, other investigators reported favorable results using the spiral stent, especially in patients with urinary retention, as an alternative to indwelling catheters in patients who were not operative candidates. With the availability of endovascular mesh stents, Milroy and colleagues first used them to treat patients with recurrent bulbous urethral strictures.[43] They found long-term patency of the urethral stricture with good resolution of the obstructive symptoms and minor side effects of discomfort for 2 to 3 weeks. They also noted that the stent was completely epithelialized in 4 to 6 months. Favorable experience with this stent in urethral strictures led to the use of the expandable endovascular mesh stents in the prostatic urethra for treating prostatism. At the present time, prostate stents are under clinical investigation in the United States in Internal Review Board–approved clinical trials for use in BPH. The stents are not FDA-approved for general use.

Spiral Stent

Since the original description of the intraprostatic spiral by Fabian,[20] several similar devices have been used. The original intraprostatic spiral was made of stainless steel and was prone to encrustations and urinary tract infections.[21] This spiral stent has since undergone modifications and is currently called the Prostakath (Engineers and Doctors, Copenhagen, Denmark). The Prostakath consists of a surgical-grade stainless steel wire that is designed with spirals at either end and a 2-cm straight segment of wire in between (Fig. 17–6). The wire is coated with 24-karat gold to prevent encrustations. The proximal spiral has multiple loops and traverses the prostatic urethra. The 2-cm segment of the straight wire traverses the external sphincter. The distal spiral has only two loops and is located in the bulbous urethra to prevent proximal migration of the stent. The spiral is 24 Fr in size and comes in lengths of 45, 55, 65, and 75 mm. The prostatic spiral can be placed with the patient under sedation or local anesthesia. A 6 or 7 Fr urethral catheter is passed into the bladder to act as a guide. The Prostakath is mounted on a catheter for introduction and is passed over the ureteral catheter until the tip is thought to be in the bladder, as evidenced by urine appearing in the catheter. The ureteral catheter and the introducing catheter are withdrawn, and the position of the stent is checked endoscopically. Alternatively, the Prostakath can be placed endoscopically with the grasping forceps. Some investigators have used ultrasound guidance to position the stent (Nordling et al).[43a] These spiral stents require changing at least every 6 months. Removal is easily accomplished with the cystoscope and grasping forceps.

FIGURE 17–6. Prostate spiral stent.

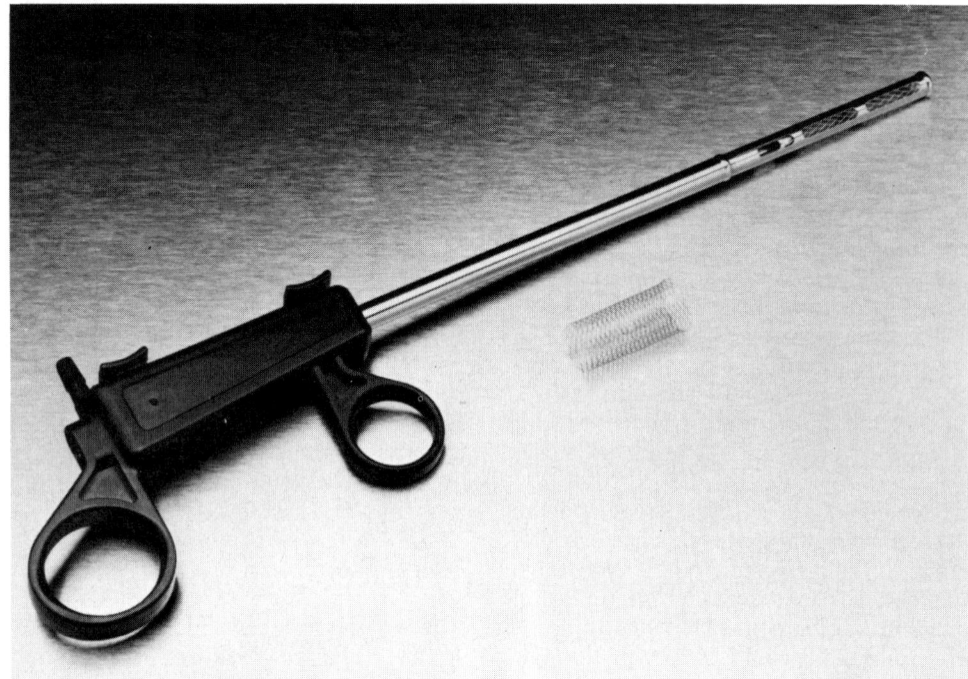

FIGURE 17–7. Prostate stent and deployment tool (Urolume). Note the compressed stent at the distal end of the deployment tool. (Courtesy of American Medical Systems.)

Permanently Implantable Prostate Stents

Currently there are two permanently implantable prostate stents under clinical investigation. The Urolume Wallstent (American Medical Systems, Minnetonka, MN) and the Intra Prostatic Stent (Advanced Surgical Intervention, San Clemente, CA). Both stents are permanently implantable mesh devices designed to undergo epithelialization and become incorporated into the prostatic urethra. The difference between the two stents is in the composition and the slightly different techniques for insertion.

The Urolume is made of a surgical-grade stainless steel alloy that is finely woven into a tubular mesh. The stent is flexible and self-expanding. It is available in 2-, 2.5-, and 3-cm lengths. When fully expanded, the internal lumen of the stent is 42 Fr. The stent comes in a compressed state, mounted at the end of a 21 Fr deployment tool (Fig. 17–7). Placement of the Urolume is performed under anesthesia (general or spinal), prostate block, or sedation. First, the length of the prostatic urethra is measured endoscopically using a 5 Fr ureteral catheter with 1-cm markings. If the length of the prostatic urethra is greater than 3 cm, then two stents are used to cover the length by overlapping the stents by at least 0.5 cm. The stents are positioned endoscopically using the deployment tool from the bladder neck to the verumontanum (Fig. 17–8). Protrusion of the stent beyond these limits is prone to complications and hence calls for immediate repositioning of the stent. The deployment tool has a safety mechanism to confirm accurate positioning before finally releasing the stent, which self-expands to hold the prostatic urethra open.

If postprocedure voiding problems are encountered, a suprapubic tube should be placed temporarily.

The Intra Prostatic Stent is made of titanium and is available in multiple lengths from 1.9 cm to 5.8 cm in 4-mm increments. The stent is not self-expanding and therefore is mounted on a dilating balloon for deployment. When fully expanded, the internal lumen is 33 Fr. Like the Urolume stent, the Intra Prostatic Stent is placed endoscopically using a special delivery system.

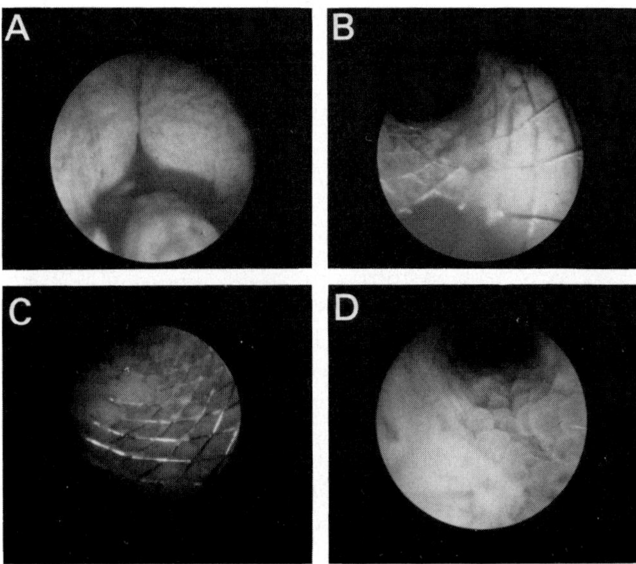

FIGURE 17–8. Endoscopic view of prostate stent in situ. *A,* Preinsertion; *B,* postinsertion; *C,* partial epithelialization at 3 months; *D,* complete epithelialization at 6 months with an open lumen.

The length of the prostatic urethra is measured endoscopically with a calibration catheter. A disposable sheath is passed into the bladder and the appropriate length stent mounted on the delivery tool is passed through the sheath and visually positioned between the bladder neck and verumontanum. Inflating the balloon fully expands the stent. If the stent is malpositioned, it is pushed into the bladder and is removed through the sheath using a special retrieval tool. A new stent can then be placed. As with the Urolume stent, postprocedure urethral catheterization should not be performed for up to 3 months.

Results

The spiral prostate stents have been used mostly as a substitute for long-term indwelling bladder catheters. Yachia noted an 80 per cent immediate success rate in 32 patients who were at high risk for surgery.[66] Harrison and DeSouza reported relief of obstruction in 80 per cent of patients with acute urinary retention, and only 50 per cent in patients with prostatism without retention.[25] Similarly, Vincente et al[65] noted a 74 per cent success rate in 22 patients who had long-term indwelling bladder catheters. The permanently implantable prostate stents also have been used initially in patients who were at risk for surgery and more recently as a treatment alternative for patients with symptomatic BPH. The experience of the various investigators is listed in Table 17–7. Prostatic stents appear to alleviate voiding symptoms in 85 to 100 per cent of the patients in the short period of follow-up (3 to 24 months) available. There appears to be a corresponding improvement in the objective parameters of assessment of obstruction.

Complications of Prostatic Stents

The complications noted by Harrison and DeSouza[25] with the spiral stents include urinary incontinence, migration, hematuria, stricture, and urinary tract infections. Urethral discomfort and irritative voiding symptoms may be present for a few days. Stent migration leading to bladder perforation has been reported by Vincente et al.[65] Yachia noted spontaneous breakage of the stent after 3 months in one patient.[66] Complications following the permanently implantable stents also appear to be minimal. The majority of the complications appear to be in the initial malpositioning of the stent, requiring repositioning. Most patients experience some urethral discomfort and irritative voiding symptoms lasting 1 to 4 weeks. Migration of the stent and urinary tract infections occur less frequently than with the spiral stents.

Summary

Prostate stents are currently under investigation as a treatment alternative for patients with prostatic obstruction. Prostatic spirals appear to be a good alternative for short-term management of prostatic obstruction or for indwelling Foley catheters in long-term management. Insertion and removal of the spiral are simple and can be performed under local anesthesia. Insertion of the permanently implantable prostate stent appears simple. However, removal of the stent is difficult, especially after epithelialization occurs. In the short-term follow-up, permanently implantable stents appear to improve voiding and alleviate symptoms of obstruction. There is concern that continued prostatic enlargement through the mesh stent may cause obstruction in the long term, requiring a surgical procedure. The indwelling stent may complicate a subsequent surgical procedure. Long-term results on the safety and efficacy of these stents will determine their role in the management of BPH.

REFERENCES

1. Aalkjaer V: Transurethral resection/prostatectomy versus dilation treatment in hypertrophy of the prostate II: A comparison of the late results. Urol Int 20:17–22, 1965.
2. Aboulker P, Steg A: La divulsion de la prostate d'apres 218 observations personnelles. J Urol Nephrol 70:337–364, 1964.
3. Abrams P, Gillatt D, Chadwick D: Intraprostatic stent—experience with the ASI stent to treat bladder outflow obstruction. J Urol 145:373A, 1991.
4. Astrahan MA, Ameye F, Oyen R, et al: Interstitial temperature measurements during transurethral microwave hyperthermia. J Urol 145:304–308, 1991.
5. Astrahan M, Imanaka K, Jozsef G, et al: Heating characteristics of a helical microwave applicator for transurethral hyperthermia of benign prostatic hyperplasia. Int J Hyperthermia 7:141–155, 1991.
6. Backman KA: Dilatation of the prostate according to Deisting: Results of follow-up one and two years after the operation. Acta Chir Scand 126:266–274, 1963.
7. Baert L, Ameye F, Willemen P, et al: Transurethral microwave hyperthermia for benign prostatic hyperplasia: Preliminary clinical and pathological results. J Urol 144:1383–1387, 1990.
8. Burhenne HJ, Chisholm RJ, Quenville NF: Prostatic hyperplasia: Radiologic intervention. Radiology 152:655–657, 1984.
9. Busch W: Uber Den Einfluss Welchen Hefgere Erysiplen Zgweilen Auf Organisierte Neubildengen Ausuben. Verhandl Natuth Preuss, Rhein Westphal 23:28–30, 1866.
10. Carter S, Patel A, Reddy P, et al: Single-session transurethral microwave thermotherapy for the treatment of benign prostatic obstruction. J Endourol 5:137–144, 1991.
11. Castaneda F, Lund G, Larson BW, et al: Prostatic urethra: Experimental dilatation in dogs. Radiology 163:645–648, 1987.
12. Castaneda F, Reddy PK, Wasserman N, et al: Benign prostatic hypertrophy: Retrograde transurethral dilation of the prostatic urethra in humans. Radiology 163:649–653, 1987.

TABLE 17–7. RESULTS OF PROSTATE STENTS FOR TREATMENT OF BENIGN PROSTATIC HYPERPLASIA

AUTHOR	STENT TYPE	NO. OF PATIENTS TREATED	SUCCESS (%)
Abrams et al[3]	Intra Prostatic	43	91
Kirby et al[30]	Intra Prostatic	27	89
Parra [46]	Intra Prostatic	14	86
McLoughlin et al[41]	Urolume Wallstent	19	100
Milroy et al[43]	Urolume Wallstent	54	93
Oesterling[44]	Urolume Wallstent	24	100
Reddy[51a]	Urolume Wallstent	14	100

13. Chiou RK, Binard JE, Horan JJ, et al: Current experience of balloon dilatation, transurethral incision, and prostate stent as alternative treatments for benign prostatic hyperplasia. J Urol 145:A707, 1991.

14. Civiale J: Traite Pratique des Maladies des Organes Genito-Urinaire. Paris, 1841 (cited by Edwards L: History of nonsurgical treatment. *In* Hinman F Jr [ed]: Benign Prostatic Hypertrophy. New York, Springer-Verlag, 1983, pp 30–34).

15. Deisting W: Transurethral dilation of the prostate: A new method in the treatment of prostatic hypertrophy. Urol Int 2:158–171, 1956.

16. Devonec M, Berger N, Perrin P: Transurethral microwave heating of the prostate—or from hyperthermia to thermotherapy. J Endourol 5:129–135, 1991.

17. Donatucci CF, Donohue RE, Crawford DE, et al: A randomized community based study of balloon dilatation of the prostate versus transurethral resection. Rocky Mountain Urological Society Study. J Urol 145:A714, 1991.

18. Doughtery JD, Rodan BA, Bean WJ: Balloon dilation of prostatic urethra. Urology 36:203–209, 1990.

19. Dowd JB, Smith JJ III: Balloon dilatation of the prostate. Urol Clin North Am 17:671–677, 1990.

20. Fabian KM: Der interprostatische "partielle catheter" (urologische Spirale). Urology [A] 19:236–238, 1980.

21. Fabricus GB, Matz M, Zepnick H: Die Endourethralspirale—eine Alternative zum Dauerkatheter? Z Arztl Forbild 77:482–485, 1983.

22. Franck O: Die Sprengung des Prostataringes. München Med Wochenschr 21:777–782, 1938.

23. Goldenberg SL, Perez-Marrero R, Lee LM, Emerson L: Endoscopic balloon dilatation of the prostate: Early experience. J Urol 144:83, 1990.

24. Guthrie GJ: On the Anatomy and Diseases of the Urinary Organs. London, 1836 (cited by Edwards L: History of nonsurgical treatment. *In* Hinman F Jr (ed): Benign Prostatic Hypertrophy. New York, Springer-Verlag, 1983, pp 30–34).

25. Harrison NW, DeSouza JV: Prostatic stenting for outflow obstruction. Br J Urol 65:192–196, 1990.

26. Hollingsworth E: Dilatation of the prostatic urethra for the relief of the symptoms of prostatic enlargement. Ann Surg 51:597–599, 1910.

27. Horan JJ, Chiou RK, Binard JE, et al: Balloon dilatation of prostate: A randomized study comparing with transurethral incision of prostate. J Urol 143:281A, 1990.

28. Johnson SD, Kuni CC, et al: MR imaging of patients undergoing prostatic balloon dilation. Radiology 165(P):332, 1987.

29. Kapoor DA, Becher E, Beeth JA, Reddy PK: Urodynamic evaluation of outcome following balloon dilation of prostate versus transurethral resection of prostate. Submitted, J Urol.

30. Kirby R, Lui S, Eardley I, et al: The use of the ASI titanium intraprostatic stent in the treatment of acute retention due to BPH. J Urol 145:389A, 1991.

31. Kivioja O: Dilatatio prostate transurethralis a.m. Deisting: Preliminara resultat fran II kirungiska kliniken. Nord Med 58:1548, 1957.

32. Klein LA: Balloon dilatation of the prostate as compared with transrectal resection of the prostate for treatment of benign prostatic hypertrophy. Urology 9:29–31, 1991.

33. Klein LA: Transurethral cystoscopic balloon dilatation of the prostate. J Endourol 4:183, 1990.

34. Kolberg S: Erfarenheter av Transurethral Prostatadilation Enligt Deisting. Stockholm, Foredrag vid Med risksstamma, 1959.

35. Kraemer F: Ein Eitrag zur Behandlung der Prostata-hypertrophie durch Prostatedehnung. Dtsch Med Wochenschr 36:757–758, 1910.

36. Lauweryns J, Baert L, Vandenhove J, Petrovich Z: Histopathology of prostatic tissue after transurethral hyperthermia. Int J Hyperthermia 7:221–230, 1991.

37. Leib Z, Rothem A, Lev A, Servadio C: Histopathological observations in the canine prostate treated by local microwave hyperthermia. Prostate 8:93–102, 1986.

38. Lindner A, Siegel YI, Korczak D: Serum prostate specific antigen levels during hyperthermia treatment of benign prostatic hyperplasia. J Urol 144:1388–1392, 1990.

39. Lindner A, Siegel YI, Saranga R, et al: Complications in hyperthermia treatment of benign prostatic hyperplasia. J Urol 144:1390–1392, 1990.

40. Marks L: Value of balloon dilation in treatment of youthful patients with prostatism. Urology 39:31, 1992.

41. McLoughlin J, Jager R, Abu PD, et al: The use of prostatic stents in patients with urinary retention who are unfit for surgery. Br J Urol 66:66, 1990.

42. Mercier F: Recherches sur les valvules du col de las vessie. Paris, 1850 (cited by Edwards L: History of nonsurgical treatment. *In* Hinman F Jr (ed): Benign Prostatic Hypertrophy. New York, Springer-Verlag, 1983, pp 30–34).

43. Milroy EJG, Chapple CR, Rickards D: Permanently implanted prostate stent—the Urolume Wallstent. J Urol 145:268A, 1990.

43a. Nordling J, Holm HH, Klarskov, P, et al: The intraprostatic spiral: A new device for insertion with the patient under local anesthesia and with ultrasonic guidance with 3 months of follow up. J Urol 142:756, 1989.

44. Oesterling J: Intraurethral prostatic stents. J Androl 12:423–428, 1991.

45. Oravisto KJ: Indications for Deisting's prostatic dilatation in the treatment of prostatic hypertrophy. Urol Int 11:202–206, 1961.

46. Parra RO: Titanium urethral stent: An alternative to prostatectomy in the high surgical risk patient. J Urol 145:239A, 1991.

47. Pilgard A: Prostatadilatation enligt Deisting: En ny behandlingsmethod for prostatahyertrofi. Svenska Lakartidningen 54:3637–3641, 1957.

48. Quinn SF, Dyer R, Smathers R, et al: Balloon dilation of the prostatic urethra. Radiology 157:57–58, 1985.

49. Reddy PK: A new technique to anesthetize the prostate for transurethral balloon dilation of the prostate gland. Urol Clin North Am 17:55–56, 1990.

50. Reddy PK: Balloon dilation of the prostate: Principles and techniques. J Endourol 5:93–98, 1991.

51. Reddy PK: Role of balloon dilation in the treatment of benign prostatic hyperplasia. Prostate (Suppl III):39–38, 1990.

51a. Reddy PK, Evans R, Eppel S: Prostatic stents in the treatment of benign prostatic hyperplasia. Semin Urol, in press.

52. Reddy PK, McLeod D, Wilson SK, et al: Experience with 120 Fr balloon dilator for transurethral balloon dilation of the prostate for benign prostatic hyperplasia. A multicenter study. Presented at AUA, Washington, DC, 1992.

53. Reddy PK, Wasserman N, Castaneda F, Castaneda-Zuniga WR: Balloon dilation of the prostate for treatment of benign hyperplasia. Urol Clin North Am 15:529–535, 1988.

54. Reddy PK, Wasserman N, Castaneda F, Castaneda-Zuniga WR: Transurethral balloon dilation of the prostate for prostatism: Preliminary report for nonsurgical technique. J Endourol 1:269–273, 1987.

55. Reddy PK, Wasserman N, Sidi AA: Balloon dilatation of the prostate: Can it help the patient with BPH? Contemp Urol Feb/Mar:44–53, 1989.

56. Rigatti P, Guzzoni G, Montorsi F: Local microwave hyperthermia and benign prostatic hyperplasia induced bladder outlet obstruction. *In* Bicher HI (ed): Consensus on Hyperthermia for the 1990s. New York, Plenum Press, 1990, pp 433–437.

57. Rohdenburg GI: Fluctuations in the growth energy of malignant tumours in man, with special reference to spontaneous regression. J Cancer Res 3:193–225, 1917.

58. Sandberg I, Sandstrom B: Dilatation according to Deisting for prostatic hyperplasia. Scand J Urol Nephrol 1:225–226, 1967.

58a. Sapozink MD, Boyd SD, Astrahan MA, et al: Transurethral hyperthermia for benign prostatic hyperplasia: Preliminary clinical results. J Urol 143:944, 1990.

59. Servadio C, Braf Z, Siegel Y, et al: Local thermotherapy of the benign prostate: A 1-year follow-up. Eur Urol 18:169–173, 1990.

60. Servadio C, Leib Z, Lev A: Diseases of prostate treated by local microwave hyperthemia. Urology 30:97–99, 1987.

61. Sloan JB: Prostate balloon dilatation monitored by transrectal ultrasound. Urology 38:20–25, 1991.

62. Spotoft AJ: Hypertrofia prostatae: Transurethral spraengning af prostataringen: Et are erfaring med Deistings metode. Nord Med 55:655–657, 1956.

63. Stawarz B, Szmigielski S, Ogrodnik J, et al: A comparison of transurethral and transrectal microwave hyperthermia in poor surgical risk benign prostatic hyperplasia patients. J Urol 146:353–357, 1991.
64. Strohmaier WL, Bichler K-H, Fluchter SH, Wilbert DM: Local microwave hyperthermia of benign prostatic hyperplasia. J Urol 144:913–917, 1990.
65. Vincente J, Salvador J, Chechile G: Spiral urethral prosthesis as an alternative to surgery in high risk patients with benign prostatic hyperplasia: Prospective study. J Urol 142:1504–1506, 1989.
65a. Wasserman NF, Reddy PK, Zhang G, et al: Transurethral balloon dilatation of the prostatic urethra: Effectiveness in highly selected patients with prostatism. AJR 157:509–512, 1991.
66. Yachia D: Spontaneous breakage of self-retaining intraprostatic stent. J Urol 144:997–998, 1990.
67. Yerushalmi A: Use of local hyperthermia for the treatment of benign prostatic hyperplasia. *In* Bicher HI (ed): Consensus on Hyperthermia for the 1990s. New York, Plenum Press, 1990, pp 167–176.
68. Yerushalmi A, Fishelovitz Y, Singer D, et al: Localized deep microwave hyperthermia in the treatment of poor operative risk patients with benign prostatic hyperplasia. J Urol 133:873–876, 1985.
69. Yerushalmi A, Servadio C, Leib Z, et al: Local hyperthermia for treatment of carcinoma of prostate: A preliminary report. Prostate 6:623, 1982.
70. Yerushalmi A, Shpirer Z, et al: Normal tissue response to localized deep microwave hyperthermia in the rabbit's prostate: A preclinical study. Int J Radiation Oncol Biol Phys 9:77, 1983.

Chapter 18

COMPARATIVE PATHOLOGY OF BENIGN PROSTATIC HYPERPLASIA

JOHN D. STRANDBERG

The pathology of human benign prostatic hyperplasia (BPH) has been studied, described, and classified by many investigators in the past decades, and their findings have been reviewed and summarized by several authors.[26, 27, 41, 53] The morphologic complexity of the disease is evidenced by several classification systems that have been developed over the years and are presented in these and other publications. The purpose of this discussion is briefly to review the pathology of BPH as it is seen and understood in human patients and to compare the human disease with benign proliferative lesions of the prostate which occur in a variety of animal species, both naturally and as the result of experimental manipulations.

Any interspecies comparison of prostatic disease is complicated first and foremost by the great variation in normal gross and microscopic anatomy of the prostate between different species of animals as well as by the diversity of other accessory male sex glands that may also be present. The prostate is the only accessory sex gland that is found in all male mammals, and it is even present in females of a few species such as cottontail rabbits[58] and mastomys (*Praomys* sp.).[73] The prostate in all animals has a relatively constant location and comprises a compound ductular system emptying into the proximal urethra. However, there is considerable interspecies variation in gross organization, histologic composition, and secretory activity of the glands. Price[58] and others have noted the difficulties of interspecies comparisons caused by these marked anatomic, functional, and histologic variations.[52] Furthermore, many animals have seasonal periods of reproductive activity with marked variation in circulating hormone levels, gland weight, and functional activity. Nonetheless, throughout embryologic development the consistent location of the prostatic ducts opening into the proximal urethra is relied upon as an important marker of organ analogy. Just as there is anatomic variability, there is marked species variation in the type and incidence of diseases that affect the prostate. This is especially true of BPH, which is encountered as a common, spontaneous clinical disease in aging males in only two species, humans and dogs. This is one of the major reasons that dogs have been employed in experimental studies of the etiology, pathogenesis, and treatment of BPH, although several authors have cited important differences between canine and human BPH, as noted below. Although they do not evidence clinical or pathologic signs of BPH, several other species of animals develop, both spontaneously and experimentally, prostatic alterations that share some of the basic features seen in the naturally occurring human disease and are thus used to study aspects of prostatic biology and disease. These, too, are included in this presentation.

Despite gross and microscopic differences, prostates in all species share a number of characteristics. They are organs composed of compound tubular or tubuloalveolar glands located at the neck of the bladder with ducts emptying into the proximal urethra. Glands reach full development only in the presence of functional testes and may be contained within the wall of the urethra or project from its external surface in various lobar and lobular patterns. In all species the glands and ducts are lined by two major cell types: secretory cells surrounding an actual or potential lumen and variable numbers of basally located cells of unknown function. This latter cell type has been shown not to be myoepithelium.[64] Transitional epithelial cells may also be found lining ducts near their juncture with the urethra.[18] Depending upon the species, the prostatic secretion may be stored within the glandular lumina or retained in the apical cytoplasm of the secretory cells. This epithelium is surrounded by a basement membrane, which is in turn invested with a connective tissue stroma containing fibroblasts, mast cells, collagen and elastic tissue, smooth muscle cells, blood and lymph vessels, nerves, and ganglia. The relative amount of this stroma as well as its composition and organization varies widely from species to species[18]; as noted below, all these factors are altered in the hyperplastic conditions of the various animal species.

HUMAN BENIGN PROSTATIC HYPERPLASIA

As a disease with recognized long-standing clinical and pathologic importance, BPH is known to cause significant gross alterations to the prostate and the associated urogenital tract, particularly the urinary bladder. The development of histologic alterations is accompanied by increased weight of the affected organ. Berry and co-workers[8] combined data from 10 independent studies and determined that the average weight of prostates was 33 ± 16 grams and that there was an increasing doubling time with age. Between the ages of 31 and 50 years it took an average of 4.5 years for the gland to double in weight; from 51 to 70 years it required 10 years, and after 70 years of age the doubling time was in excess of 100 years. Very large glands weighing more than 100 grams were found in only 4 per cent of men over 70.

This increase in size of the gland is the result of proliferation of epithelial and stromal components, with distortion of normal prostatic architecture and impingement on adjacent structures. BPH does not affect the prostate uniformly. Clinicians and pathologists alike have long recognized that BPH first and most severely involves the prostatic tissue located adjacent to the proximal urethra. This often results in restriction of urine flow and outward compression of peripheral glandular and stromal tissues. The lack of uniformity of the process is evidenced by the formation of nodules and cysts that impinge on the urethra. Traditionally, most glands are examined as cross-sections, and the orientation of the specimens that have been studied has greatly influenced the classification of the disease. It is for this reason that the prostate has been considered to be composed of two major areas, the periurethral and the peripheral zones. McNeal[51–53] stressed the importance of plane of section of the gland to aid in interpretation of lesions and their localization within the prostate. He used an oblique coronal plane of section to encompass the proximal urethra and the prostatic ducts entering into it coupled with a sagittal plane to cope with the angulation of the urethra as is passes through the gland. He used this orientation in reconsidering the anatomy of the lobular pattern of the prostate and pointed out that BPH occurs in a relatively restricted region of the prostate termed the *transitional zone*. This area of the proximal urethra includes the smooth muscle, which surrounds the urethra located anterior to the verumontanum and which is closely associated with glandular elements morphologically indistinguishable from glands found elsewhere in the prostate. BPH arises in this region and comprises both glandular and stromal elements in varying proportions. It was emphasized that there is no observable difference in the epithelium of the area in which BPH develops and that in the peripheral portion of the prostate. However, the stroma of this region is more compact and coarse fibered. The localization of this transitional zone as a site of origin of BPH was supported through the use of microradiographic techniques in demonstrating early lesions near the proximal urethra and proximal to the base of the verumontanum.[33]

All investigators agree that BPH is a proliferative disease in which the glandular enlargement is caused by abnormal proliferation and formation of new ductular and acinar architecture accompanied by stromal proliferation.[18] It has a pleomorphic histologic pattern that corresponds to the nodular, nonuniform gross character. Most nodules occurring in the periurethral or transition zone of the gland reflect proliferation of both stroma and epithelium, and there is evidence of new duct formation (Fig. 18–1). With increasing age, additional prostatic nodules develop; these tend to remain small until about the eighth decade, when they typically undergo an increase in volume. The proliferative changes in the ducts and stroma result in an altered architectural pattern of the ducts and stroma. There is a considerable body of opinion that BPH is primarily a disease in which the stroma reflects the effect of hormonal imbalance, and that the epithelial proliferative changes are secondary to this stromal alteration.[5, 38]

In an extensive early review, Moore noted the terms previously used for this condition: benign hypertrophy, benign enlargement, adenoma, and adenomatous hyperplasia.[55] He preferred the term *nodular hyperplasia.* He conducted an extensive histologic study of approximately 700 prostates, some of which were step-sectioned

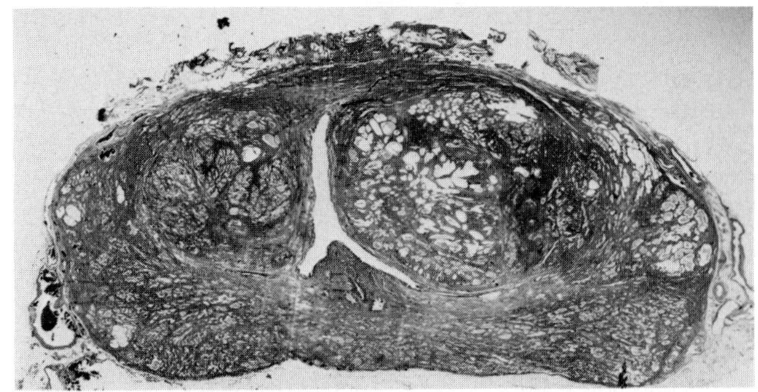

FIGURE 18–1. Prostatic cross-section with well-demarcated nodules of hyperplastic tissue impinging on the urethra and compressing other glandular elements.

and stained by a variety of methods. As in other reports, he described early small periurethral nodules composed of connective tissue; those with perivascular and periductular location were both composed solely of connective tissue, whereas those located within the lobules contained both smooth muscle and glandular elements. In characterizing the alterations it was noted that glandular tissue having the most contact with the areas of proliferating stroma was high and papillary, whereas that oriented away from this stroma was flattened. Rarely was pure epithelial hyperplasia reported. Subsequently, Franks described five types of prostatic nodules based on histologic characteristics and predominant tissue components: (1) stromal (fibrous or fibrovascular), (2) fibromuscular, (3) muscular ("leiomyoma"), (4) fibroadenoma, and (5) fibromyoadenoma.[26] Again, true stromal nodules were found only in subepithelial tissue of the urethra. Glandular elements were observed to vary markedly in amount but were abundant in the most commonly diagnosed category, fibromyoadenoma.

The characteristic nodular pattern seen both grossly and microscopically is the result of localized proliferation of cell types normally present in the region of the gland affected. The stroma consists of smooth muscle, fibroblasts, and collagen. Typical early lesions are predominantly stromal (i.e., smooth muscle) nodules found in the periurethral zones and are generally small, not exceeding 5 mm in diameter (Fig. 18–2). They resemble mesenchyme and are composed of spindle cells with long processes and intercellular reticulin accumulations. Cells may occur in whorls accompanied by small but prominent blood vessels. Mapping studies reveal that these nodules tend to remain small, and it has been postulated that some are scarred areas representing prior infarcts. Many of these nodules contain epithelial elements adjacent to or within the stromal component. Fibromuscular and muscular nodules are composed of demarcated areas of proliferating connective tissue and smooth muscle with or without significant collagen (Fig.

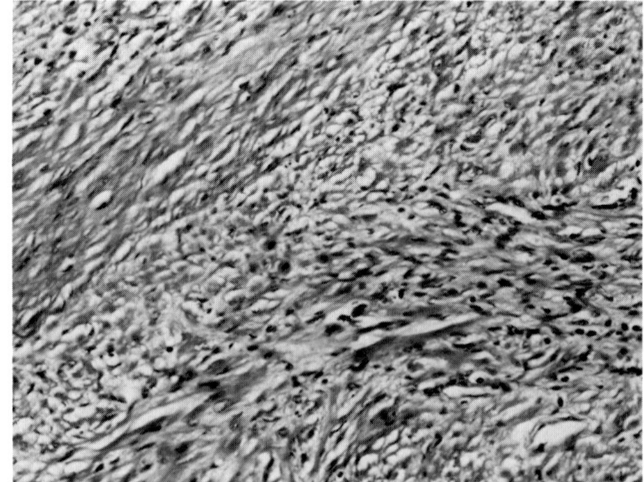

FIGURE 18–3. Interlacing bands of fibroblasts and smooth muscle cells in an area of stromal hyperplasia.

18–3). The epithelial components in these nodules are small. Franks also classified as fibroadenomatous those nodules resembling similar conditions in the breast.[26] These lesions are uncommon and have low secretory epithelium with occasional squamous metaplasia. By far the most common type of BPH is that termed *fibromyoadenomatous* by Franks[26] and is, as indicated by its name, composed of irregularly arranged glandular elements possessing both epithelial and basal cells as well as fibroblasts and smooth muscle cells (Fig. 18–4). These are arranged in nodules of varying size and complexity. The ratios of the individual cell types vary from area to area and from nodule to nodule. Hyperplastic ducts and alveoli are surrounded or divided by the collagen or smooth muscle to form the characteristic nodules. Irregularly shaped alveoli, ducts, papillary formations, and cysts are common (Figs. 18–5 and 18–6).

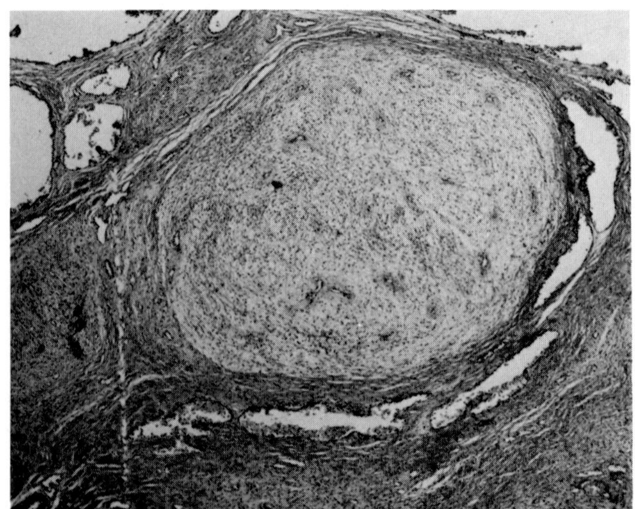

FIGURE 18–2. A small stromal nodule composed of mesenchymal cells with prominent small blood vessels is typical of those found in the periurethral zone.

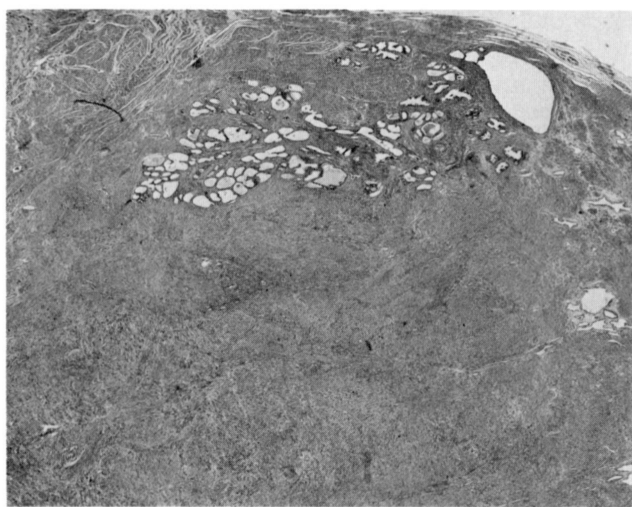

FIGURE 18–4. A relatively large nodule is composed of disorganized fibromuscular connective tissue admixed with pleomorphic glandular elements.

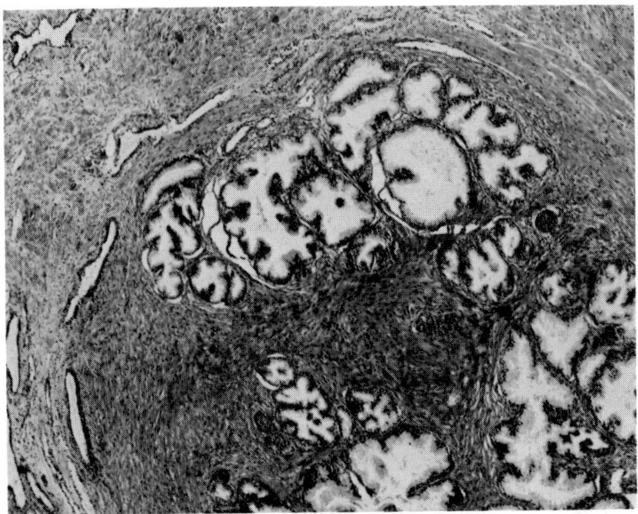

FIGURE 18–5. A nodule of mixed epithelial and stromal components compresses the surrounding prostate, which evidences glandular atrophy.

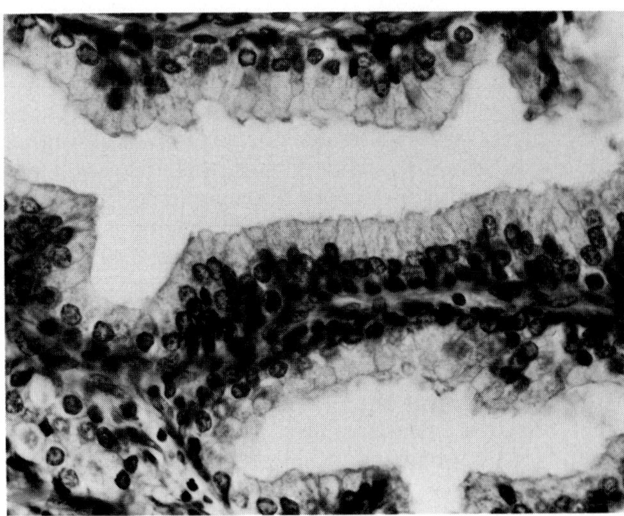

FIGURE 18–7. Both secretory and basal cells can be seen composing the two nuclear layers of the epithelium in hyperplastic foci.

The epithelium is usually well differentiated and ranges from hyperplastic to atrophic. Both cell types that normally line the glands—secretory and basal cells—can be identified, although their ratios may be altered (Fig. 18–7). Epithelial cells surround lumina filled with proteinaceous secretions and range from columnar to squamous with varying amounts of cytoplasm. In addition to secretion, the alveoli often contain corpora amylacea, spherical concretions made up of concentric laminae. As noted, epithelial cells adjacent to the encircling stroma often have more abundant cytoplasm than those toward the center of lobules. The nuclei of epithelial cells are round to oval and normochromatic. The cytoplasm is relatively pale and eosinophilic. Underlying the secretory cells are variable numbers of basal cells whose cytoplasm does not reach the

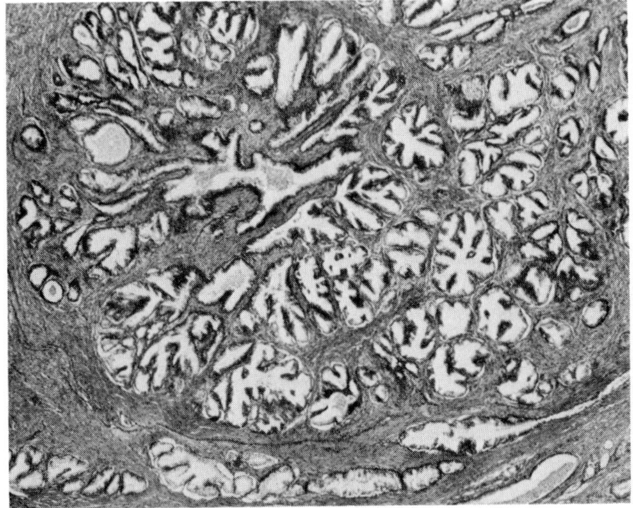

FIGURE 18–6. Hyperplastic nodules may be predominantly epithelial, with formation of new lobules within nodules.

glandular lumen. These cells have essentially normal morphology and appear compressed between the epithelium and the basement membrane. Neither cell population has appreciable mitotic activity. Throughout the affected glands populations of glandular secretory cells outnumber those of basal cells, although basal cells tend to be more numerous in the inner prostatic glands.[27] On the basis of the presence of rare cells with intermediate characteristics, it has been suggested that basal cells are true precursors; alternatively, it has been proposed that they may have a role in the transport of metabolites between the epithelium and the stroma.[48]

Glandular-stromal interactions are recognized as important factors in the development of the pathologic changes of BPH despite the divergence of opinion on which of the two elements is the primary site of the proliferative process.[38] The demonstration of basic fibroblast growth factor (bFGF) as a major growth factor in BPH has added support to other evidence that the stroma may be the primary target organ. Nevertheless, the majority of larger nodules tend to contain prominent glandular elements, and these increase with age along with the extensive proliferation of stroma. The ratio of stroma to glands in prostates of old men with BPH is greater than in normal glandular tissue. The prostatic stroma normally contains several connective tissue elements; the major cell types are fibroblasts and smooth muscle cells which, along with collagen, separate the glandular alveoli within lobules and, in larger bundles, separate the lobules themselves. In BPH, any or all of these components may proliferate and assume abnormal configurations. As noted, small early nodules may be composed entirely of smooth muscle or myxoid elements; these lesions seldom get larger than 0.5 cm in diameter. As the disease progresses there is a substantial increase in stroma separating the glandular elements. This stroma may appear as a diffuse exaggeration of normal interstitium or as more or less well-defined nodular proliferations. Amid the fibrous and muscular elements are numerous blood vessels, nerves (more plentiful near the periphery of the gland), mast cells, and elastic tissue.

Infarction is frequently encountered in BPH (Fig. 18–8). Grayhack and Koslowski reported areas of infarction in up to 25 per cent of large glands; this was associated with squamous metaplasia of glandular elements.[27] Squamous metaplasia of the glandular epithelium is nonspecific, however, and is also encountered with infection, chronic inflammation, and previous surgery. This leads to a common association of squamous metaplasia with chronic irritation. However, squamous metaplasia is also clearly related to hormonal influences and is induced by estrogen administration.

The presence of inflammatory cells in BPH tissues is common; this infiltrate is composed predominantly of mononuclear cells. The significance of this inflammation could reflect either intercurrent infections or immunologic reactions to other unknown stimuli. Recently, it has been proposed that immunologic factors may play an important role in the development of BPH itself.[66] This suggestion was based on finding alterations in the functional populations of mononuclear cells infiltrating hyperplastic compared with normal prostates, and on the demonstration of anti-human leukocyte antigen-DR reactivity in leukocytes and epithelial cells in a high proportion of BPH glands. Prostatic calculi and corpora amylacea are frequently found in prostates of older men. These hyaline structures are formed within the acinar lumina as accretions of protein and mineral around a central nidus of sloughed epithelial cells or other particulate matter.

Atypical hyperplasia and *dysplasia* are terms that have been used to describe epithelial and stromal proliferations that do not fulfill the criteria of neoplasia. Among these are many lesions thought by most investigators to bear some relationship to the development of prostatic carcinoma.[35, 37] There has been considerable discussion on the significance of these lesions, but many investigators have reported a positive correlation of several types of atypical hyperplasia with the presence of prostatic carcinoma. The designation of these lesions as hyperplastic or neoplastic may be problematic, and this topic has been extensively reviewed by Kastendieck and Helpap.[35] The wide range of terminology used to refer to these lesions may be broken into the following three major groups: (1) *Small acinar atypical hyperplasia* includes formation of new glandular elements as a circumscribed area of proliferation of small epithelial cells that resemble prostatic carcinoma in that basal cells are absent and acini are arranged back to back. The central location of this lesion, its association with areas of clear BPH, and a variety of other factors suggest its benign nature. (2) *Cribriform hyperplasia* includes both benign cribriform hyperplasia, considered a special variety of BPH and composed of intraluminal pale secretory cells, and atypical cribriform hyperplasia thought to result from basal cell proliferation and with a less benign significance.[35] (3) *Large cell atypical hyperplasia,* also known as prostatic intraepithelial neoplasia, is believed by many, as the second name indicates, to be a preneoplastic lesion. Areas of large acinar atypical hyperplasia have been frequently noted adjacent to actual carcinomas, and transitions between the two cell populations have been described.

Other unusual variations of BPH include a phyllodes type which mimics cystosarcoma phyllodes of the breast. This possesses atypical hyperplasia of stroma, secretory epithelium, and basal cells, resulting in lesions with elongated ducts and atypical stromal cells.[59] Basal cell hyperplasia by itself has also been reported as an infrequently encountered lesion by Ronnett and Epstein, who showed that cytokeratin staining was of value in differentiating this rare condition from basaloid carcinoma, which it resembles.[61]

Most studies using histochemistry, immunohistochemistry, and receptor localization have demonstrated considerable similarity between BPH and normal prostates and differences between BPH and prostatic carcinoma. One of the earliest and most extensive of these studies was carried out by Brandes, who examined the histochemistry and ultrastructure of human, rat, mouse, and dog prostates.[13] The normal secretory proteins of the prostate, including prostatic acid phosphatase (PAP), prostate-specific antigen (PSA), and beta-microseminoprotein (beta-MSP), were noted to be present in acini and ducts of BPH tissue, but the degree of reactivity was increasingly diminished as the lesions became more undifferentiated.[1] Histochemical studies have revealed no difference between BPH and normal prostate in their content of alkaline phosphatase, located in the walls of blood vessels, and acid phosphatase, nonspecific esterase, beta-glucuronidase, and succinic dehydrogenase, all found in secretory epithelial cells. Several investigators reported the presence of estrogen receptors (ER) in human BPH tissues and cited earlier studies describing ER in both dogs and rats.[22, 36] This localization was believed to support a possible role of estrogen in the development of BPH. Other specialized techniques to differentiate BPH from prostatic carcinoma include sil-

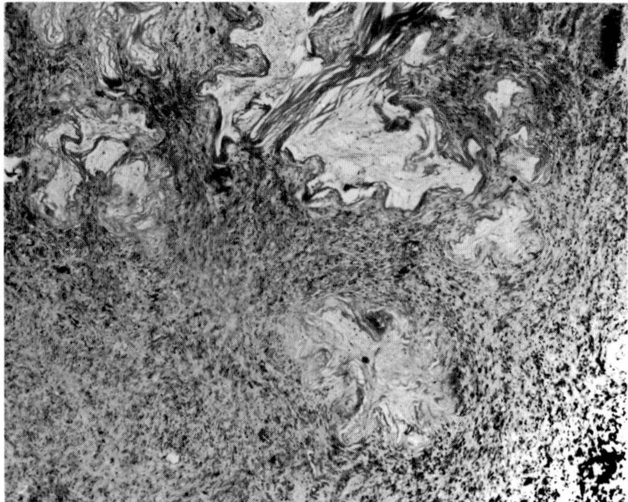

FIGURE 18–8. Human BPH with areas of infarction within a fibromuscular nodule.

ver staining of the nuclear organizing regions; this is based on the fact that these should be increased in malignant conditions. Reports on investigations with both tissue sections and isolated cells revealed lower counts in hyperplastic tissues.[47] These methods raise the possibility of an automated adjunct to histologic diagnosis of prostatic biopsies.

Immunohistochemistry promises to be of increasing help in differentiating BPH from prostatic malignancy by capitalizing on the fact that BPH possesses both epithelial and basal cells, whereas carcinoma has a single epithelial cell population. Attempts to use cytokeratin markers not only to differentiate these two conditions but to explore the significance of atypical hyperplasia show some promise.[28] In an attempt to overcome some of the problems of these methods, a malignant index was developed by Rubenstein and colleagues.[28] This employed several factors, including reactivity to two cytokeratins, epithelial membrane antigen, natural killer (NK) cell activity, PAP, and PSA. This index was elevated both in prostatic carcinoma and, interestingly, in atypical hyperplasia as well.

SPONTANEOUS BENIGN PROSTATIC HYPERPLASIA IN ANIMALS

Dog

The prostate is the only canine accessory sex gland, and dogs are the only animals in which BPH is a significant pathologic problem and one that on occasion produces clinical disease as well. The early work of Wilson and Walsh[71] using the dog as an animal model of BPH has been supplemented and continued by investigators in several laboratories. It is generally agreed that most dogs 6 years and older have gross and microscopic evidence of disease without corresponding testicular changes.[9, 46] The clinical occurrence of this condition in such high incidence in intact male dogs, along with the considerable morphologic similarities to the human condition, have made it a topic of comparative study and experimental manipulation.[16, 17]

Anatomic similarities between the canine and human prostate glands were inferred by Price[58] through studies of embryologic development; she suggested that the dorsocranial portion of the canine prostate is analogous to the human dorsal prostate and that the other regions of the human gland have homologues in the dog as well. At sexual maturity, approximately 1 to 1.5 years, the prostate of a medium-sized dog (beagle) weighs 10 to 15 grams and is approximately the size of a walnut. It surrounds the neck of the bladder, grossly resembling the human gland, and is invested with a capsule of smooth muscle, fibrovascular connective tissue, nerves, and ganglia.

The canine prostate is a compound tubular or tubuloalveolar gland with circumferentially arranged lobules, each with a central ductular system entering the urethra around its entire circumference.[27] The epithelial elements are the predominant component of the fully developed gland and form an arborizing pattern of ducts and alveoli. Unlike the human prostate, the ducts of the periurethral zones in the dog have secretory differentiation. The tubuloalveolar gland is thus secretory throughout its entire course and is lined with columnar epithelial cells with brightly eosinophilic apical cytoplasm. The alveolar spaces contain primary and secondary infoldings of the secretory epithelium. Basally located cells are interposed between and beneath the secretory cells; however, basal cells are much less numerous in the dog than in the human. These basal cells are small with oval nuclei and relatively clear and featureless cytoplasm. In contrast to the human gland, the secretion in the normal canine prostate accumulates within cytoplasmic secretory droplets, and the glandular lumina thus lack obvious secretion. The alveoli are separated by a delicate fibrous connective tissue stroma that blends with the interlobular septa and capsule. The smooth muscle of the capsule appears as a continuation of the tunic surrounding the bladder and urethra. Smooth muscle elements penetrate the surface of the gland and extend into the parenchyma in the interlobular septa. There are also small numbers of smooth muscle cells identifiable within lobules surrounding individual ducts and alveoli. Unlike the human prostate, this muscle is essentially restricted to the outer half of the gland; the region around the urethra is devoid of muscle fibers, and the stroma in this area is composed only of fibroblasts, collagen, and elastic tissue. Occasional mononuclear inflammatory infiltrates are seen in the stroma, especially in the periurethral area.

As noted, much emphasis has been placed on the regional organization of the human prostate in the development of BPH. This raises questions about the possible existence of similar or corresponding lobes of zones in the canine prostate. The existence of regional variations has been observed by the author as well as by Aumüller and colleagues, who noted differences in response to hormonal stimuli between the epithelial cells located in the periurethral zone and those in the more peripheral regions of the prostate.[3] The more peripheral portions of the gland responded to hormones administered to castrated animals, whereas the periurethral epithelial elements showed little or no resumption of secretory activity. Although of considerable interest, this divergent zonal response to the naturally occurring disease remains of uncertain significance. Certainly, in most cases, proliferative changes are found throughout the prostate.

As in human BPH, the role of basal cells remains a topic of interest in the study of proliferative disease of the canine prostate. Basal cells that lack evidence of myofibrils have been considered to be precursors of secretory cells in both the dog and rat.[67] During development, basal cells, as identified by morphology and immunohistochemistry (Laroque, personal communication), are most concentrated at the sites of branch endpoints where glandular proliferation and differentiation are taking place. Increased numbers of basal cells were observed after androstenedione treatment of castrate dogs.[3]

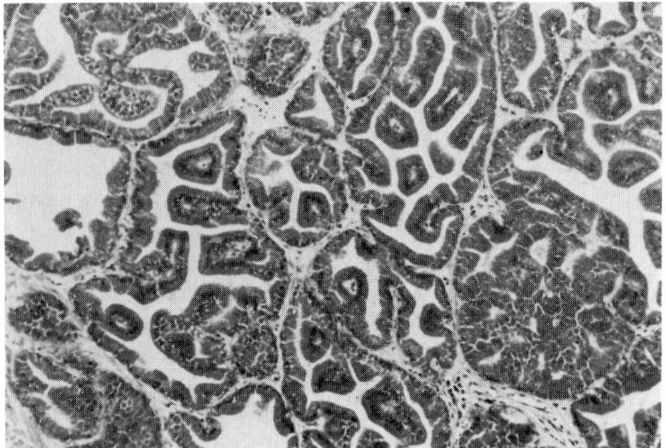

FIGURE 18–9. Glandular hyperplasia of the canine prostate with increased lobular size and epithelial infoldings.

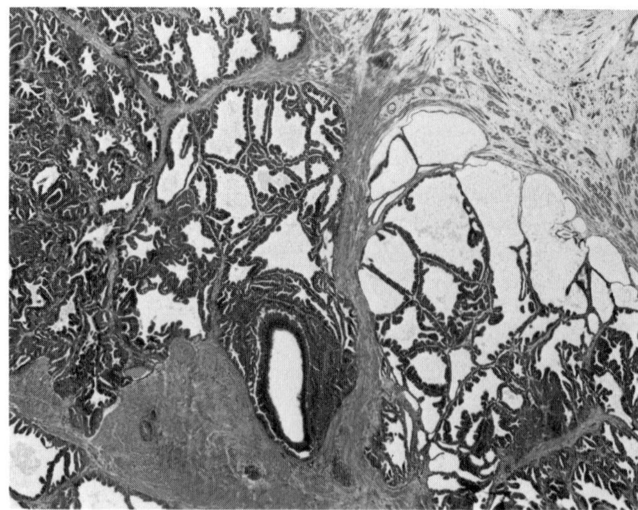

FIGURE 18–11. Canine BPH: Epithelium of varying heights lines cysts and glands.

BPH in the dog was recognized relatively early by veterinary pathologists, and its gross and microscopic characteristics were well documented.[10] It can be separated into two major histologic types: glandular and complex,[14] which appear to develop more or less sequentially with increasing age.[9, 65] In glandular hyperplasia, seen at earlier ages, the most obvious change is in the secretory epithelium, which is often increased in height owing to a greater number of cytoplasmic secretory droplets (Fig. 18–9). Each of the glandular lobules increases in size, and there is more ductular branching throughout the entire gland. The alveoli are larger and have increased cellularity. As a result, the degree of papillary infolding in increased. The stroma may appear less conspicuous because of this glandular proliferation, but total stromal volume is also increased. The epithelial proliferations may form nodules most easily recognized in the periurethral zone but are typically randomly distributed throughout the affected gland.

In complex canine BPH, the form most commonly seen in old dogs, a variety of histologic patterns appear (Fig. 18–10). Nodules of glandular hyperplasia as de-

scribed above are mixed with foci of epithelial atrophy, which may be associated with cystic dilatation of the glands. The cysts are scattered through the gland, although there is some tendency to be more frequent in the periurethral areas, and may be single or involve entire lobules. The epithelium lining the cysts may be attenuated, high and columnar, or mixed (Fig. 18–11). These nodules may be found anywhere in the gland and tend to be somewhat less well circumscribed than those in the human disease. There is both a relative and absolute increase in stromal elements, both smooth muscle and fibrous connective tissue.[46] Chronic inflammation, composed of lymphocytes and plasma cells, is frequently seen and usually located in the stromal bands (Fig. 18–12). Squamous metaplasia of secretory epithelium may occur in inflamed areas.

There continues to be controversy on the similarity of BPH in dogs to the human disease. It is universally

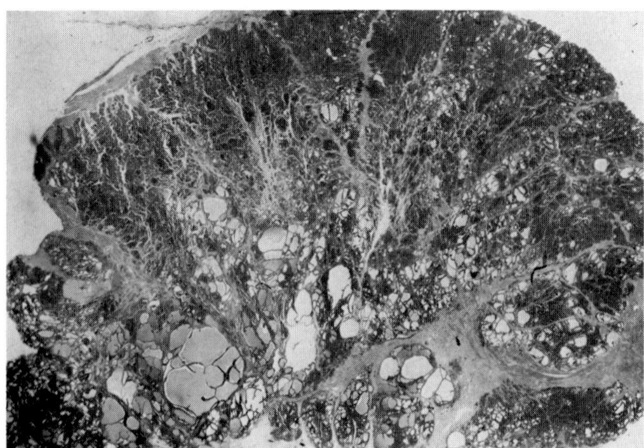

FIGURE 18–10. Hemisection through a canine prostate with complex BPH with irregular collections of cysts and bands of fibromuscular connective tissue.

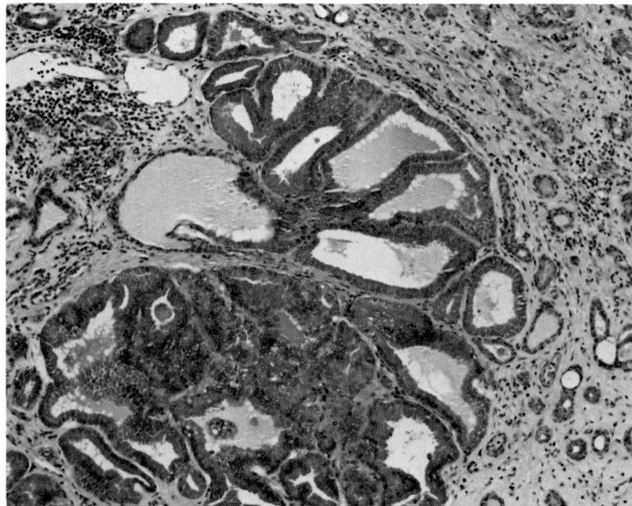

FIGURE 18–12. Canine BPH: A nodule of hyperplastic epithelium lies amid atrophic glands and chronic inflammatory cells.

recognized that both species experience substantial increase in prostatic weight with age. Further, in dogs and men the epithelial and stromal prostatic elements both increase in amount and in a seemingly uncoordinated fashion. Several investigators, including Moore[55] and McNeal,[50] have judged that canine BPH is not comparable to the human disease, citing dissimilarities which include the diffuse nature of the process and "acinar enlargement without budding or generation of new architecture" seen in the canine disease. The predominantly epithelial nature of canine BPH has been cited as a difference from the human disease, although this may merely reflect the relative predominance of epithelium in the canine prostate even in its normal state. The abrupt expansion of pre-existing nodules in human BPH has not been documented in dogs; a more gradual progression has been noted in those instances in which animals have been followed closely, although the subclinical nature of the canine disease in its early stages makes monitoring progression more difficult. Bruengger and co-workers[15] further believe that the dog is a poor model for human BPH because of the assessment of human BPH as "a predominantly stromal hyperplasia with accumulation of connective tissue"—a feature not universally appreciated. Also, canine prostatic smooth muscle is not activated in spontaneous or induced BPH as it is in humans, as documented by electron microscopic morphometry.

ER were found in the transitional epithelium of the subjacent stroma, the periurethral prostatic ducts, and glandular stroma of normal dogs; none was found in the epithelium of normal adults.[63] In contrast, a heterogeneous distribution of ER was found in BPH tissues; their presence was not correlated with any specific cellular pattern. This was at variance with the findings of Laroque (personal communication), who identified ER throughout the glandular epithelium in postpubertal dogs. Such receptors were always present in the stroma. In contrast, androgen receptors were found during prepubertal branching morphogenesis and disappeared as the glands achieved histologic features of mature secretory cells. McEntee and co-workers[49] identified reactivity against human PSA, human prostate-specific acid phosphatase (PSAP), and canine prostatic antigen in tissues from normal dogs and from animals with spontaneous BPH.

Nonhuman Primates

Prostatic hyperplasia in nonhuman primates as a spontaneous entity is uncommonly reported despite their phylogenetic proximity to humans. The fact that, outside zoos and specialized captive breeding and experimental colonies, nonhuman primates rarely achieve old age may be responsible for some underreporting. However, BPH is clearly not a major clinical or pathologic problem in most nonhuman primate species.

As might be anticipated, there is a considerable variation in the normal prostate anatomy between the widely diverse primate species. In an extensive study, Lewis[42] reported two prostatic lobes, which are both morphologically and functionally different in a variety of nonhuman primates; the exceptions were chimpanzees and patas monkeys, in which there was poor separation of lobes. Single-lobed prostates are found in marmosets and orangutans, and the cynomolgus monkey (*Macaca fascicularis*) has poor demarcation of the two lobes of its prostate as well.

Several investigators have questioned the validity of absolute analogies to human structures but have likened the cranial lobe of the rhesus monkey to the human central zone in man and the caudal, which has smaller, round acini, to the peripheral zone of the human gland based on anatomy alone.[52, 58] McNeal opined that the anatomic zone in which human BPH arises is absent in the rhesus and that this might be the reason that the analogous disease is not seen; however, a small zone resembling the human central zone was observed in cynomolgus macaques (*M. fascicularis*). Lewis et al[45] observed that the caudal prostate closely resembles the peripheral zone of the prostate of man from both an anatomic and a biochemical point of view; the cranial lobe is more problematic, having features of both caudal prostate and seminal vesicle. Van Wagenen demonstrated that the cranial lobe of the rhesus prostate had the capacity to coagulate the seminal vesicular secretion.[68]

The histology of most primate prostates reveals an exaggeration of the pattern seen in humans. Essentially all the glandular prostatic tissue of both lobes is dorsal (posterior) to the urethra and the gland does not encircle it. Histologically, both cranial and caudal lobes are composed of acini, forming lobules separated by a prominent fibromuscular stroma. This stroma contains numerous blood vessels and nerves. The alveoli of the caudal lobe are regular in size and outline and lined by pale-staining cuboidal epithelium. Secretion within glandular lumina also stains poorly. Basal cells are inconspicuous in both lobes of the gland. The acini of the cranial lobe are larger and irregular in outline and covered with closely packed columnar epithelial cells with pale eosinophilic cytoplasm. As noted, there is some resemblance of this epithelium to that of the adjacent seminal vesicles. The lightly eosinophilic prostatic secretion is contained within the acini. The stroma is made up of fibroblasts, collagen, and smooth muscle cells and is uniformly distributed throughout the gland, forming a capsule and septa separating glands and acini.

Lewis cited 13 examples of glandular hyperplasia in 100 animals of 12 species with associated fibromuscular stromal proliferation, most commonly in the cranial lobe.[43] In the three species in which it was in the caudal lobe, it resembled the cystic hyperplasia seen in dogs. Although it has been reported in squirrel monkeys (*Saimiri sciureus*)[2] as a nodular growth of epithelial and stromal elements, cystic prostatic hyperplasia or other proliferative lesions are unusual occurrences in New World primates as well.

The author has reviewed prostates from numerous

rhesus monkeys, and several characteristic changes were associated with increasing age. These were found in both lobes and consisted of cystic dilatation of acini with attenuation of the prostatic epithelium. These changes were observed more commonly in the peripheral portion of the anterior lobe. In several instances foci within affected glands contained multifocal proliferative lesions of small basophilic cells which resemble the adenoid basal cell hyperplasia described in humans (Fig. 18–13).[61] Occasional animals demonstrated areas of striking hypercellularity with formation of new ducts lined by deeply basophilic epithelial cells with no evidence of mitotic activity (Fig. 18–14). These were in turn surrounded by a slight increase in areolar stroma. Single or multiple affected areas were encountered, and there was no evidence of local invasion or metastasis. These lesions were interpreted as atypical hyperplasia but were in no way similar to the changes seen in human BPH. McNeal[52] has postulated that nonhuman prostates do not possess a region of the prostate analogous to the periurethral zone in which human BPH develops and that this may be a reason for the lack of this disease in nonhuman primates.

Rodents

Four rodent species have been studied to varying degrees in the investigation of prostatic hyperplasia. The rat and mouse were included in an early review of the general field of animal models by Walsh.[70]

The rat is the rodent in which most of the spontaneous and induced proliferative disease is reported. In order to appreciate these lesions, it is important to be familiar with the normal gross and microscopic anatomy of this relatively complex organ. Rats possess three paired prostatic lobes, which include large ventral glands as well as dorsal and lateral lobes that are sometimes considered together as the dorsolateral prostate. The lobes project from the proximal urethra as distinct anatomic structures that are loosely connected to other

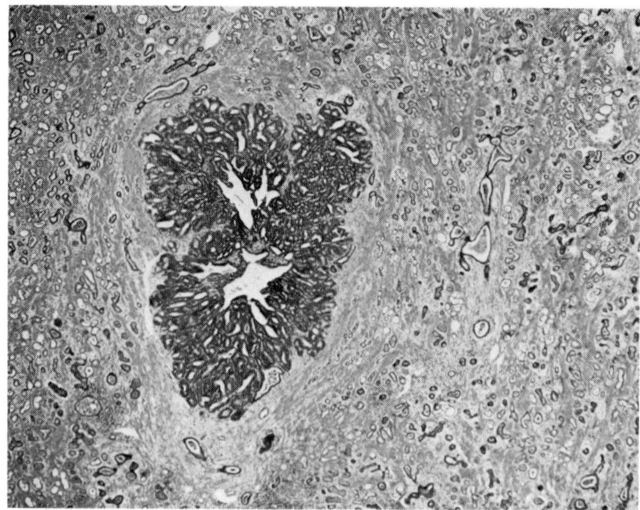

FIGURE 18–14. Rhesus monkey prostate containing a focus of epithelial proliferation surrounded by increased fibromuscular stroma.

adjacent reproductive glands by fibrovascular connective tissue. Each of the lobes is composed of branching tubules lined by secreting epithelial cells with apically placed secretory droplets. There is infolding of the epithelium into the lumen, which is especially prominent in the peripheral portion of the glands. The secretory epithelium is of variable thickness. In general, peripheral tubular epithelium has more abundant apical cytoplasm, whereas epithelium toward the center of the gland is often flattened and cuboidal. Interposed amid these secretory cells are occasional basal cells that lie upon the basement membrane and have little evidence of differentiation. Much of the secretion is accumulated within the glandular lumina, where it appears as a variably eosinophilic, hyaline substance. The rat prostate is principally epithelial, although each of the tubules is invested with a thin coat of smooth muscle and fibrous connective tissue which carries the vascular supply. Evans and Chandler described basal cells and secretory cells in the rat prostate during normal growth as self-replicating cell types with discrete functions as determined by cell-counting methods.[25] Both cell types have long cell cycle times. Differential cytokeratin staining identified basal (RCK 103) and secretory (RCK 53-keratin 18) cells.[69] This study using fluorescent antibody was interpreted as showing that basal cells and secretory epithelial cells are of the same lineage. Basal cells were found to be concentrated in the proximal regions of the ducts.[62] Lee and co-workers emphasized regional variations within lobes of the rat ventral prostate in morphology and in markers of cell death before and after castration.[42] The three regions—proximal, intermediate, and distal—differed from one another not only morphologically but functionally as well. This study found that replicating immature cells were located in the most distal segments, mature and differentiated cells were in the middle, and those undergoing planned cell death were in the proximal ducts. Rouleau and co-workers, on the other hand, localized basal epithelial cells in the proxi-

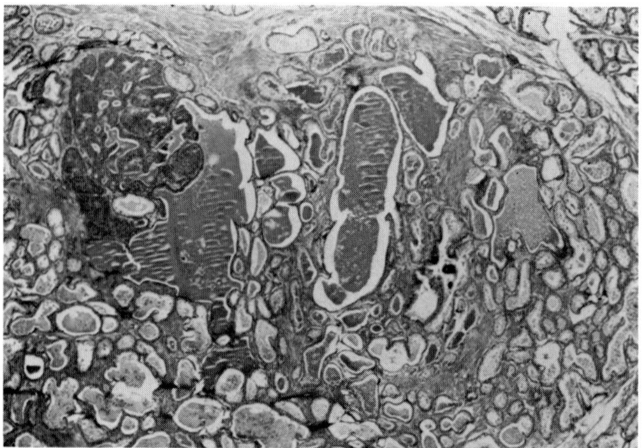

FIGURE 18–13. Anterior lobe of the prostate from an aged rhesus monkey with a focal area of hyperplasia amid mildly cystic glands.

mal portion of the ducts.[62] Both these findings are at variance with another study that showed cellular replication and glandular growth throughout the arborized system of the rat ventral prostate.[4]

The importance of differentiating between the ventral and dorsolateral prostatic lobes in the rat lies in the fact that benign lesions are more common in the ventral prostate and malignancies tend to arise in the dorsolateral portions of the gland.[11] These carcinomas are accompanied by a marked scirrhous response and invasion of surrounding tissues. Metastasis is rarely if ever observed, however.

The hyperplasia of the ventral prostate appears to be part of a process leading to the development of adenomas of the gland; carcinomas of this region are uncommon. In older rats multifocal proliferative lesions of the ventral prostate have been reported; these consist of local epithelial overgrowths within the tubular lumina (Fig. 18–15). These lesions are often considered to be part of a neoplastic progression.[12] The epithelium may assume papillary or cribriform configurations and the individual cells, although atypical, have low mitotic indices and little evidence of nuclear pleomorphism. Secretion within affected tubules appears normal. Squamous metaplasia and focal dysplasia are also seen within some of these areas. In all lobes of the prostate (Fig. 18–16), focal hyperplasia and squamous metaplasia of individual tubules or groups of tubules are common occurrences and have also been shown to be strongly influenced by hormonal stimuli under experimental conditions.[56]

The mouse prostate is organized into lobes extending from the external surface of the urethra similar to the rat, but it lacks lateral lobes and possesses a less well-developed ventral lobe. Mice apparently do not experience spontaneous hyperplastic lesions of the prostate to any appreciable degree.

Several strains of Syrian hamsters have been noted to develop cystic change in the prostate of essentially all animals over 150 days of age. The hamsters of these strains, designated BIO.87.20 and BIO 2.4, differed

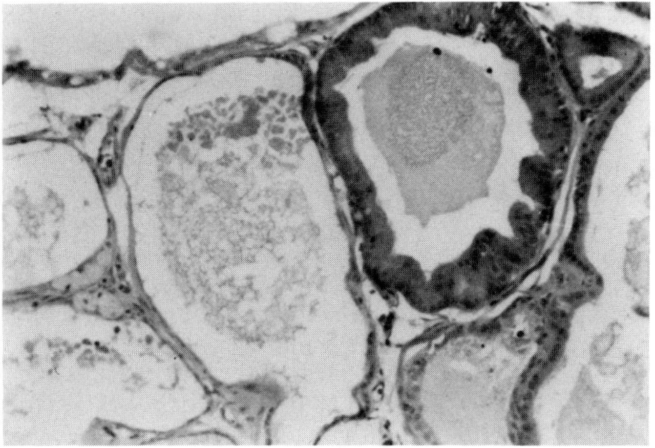

FIGURE 18–15. Ventral prostate from an aged ACI rat showing epithelial hyperplasia of one acinus surrounded by atrophic glands.

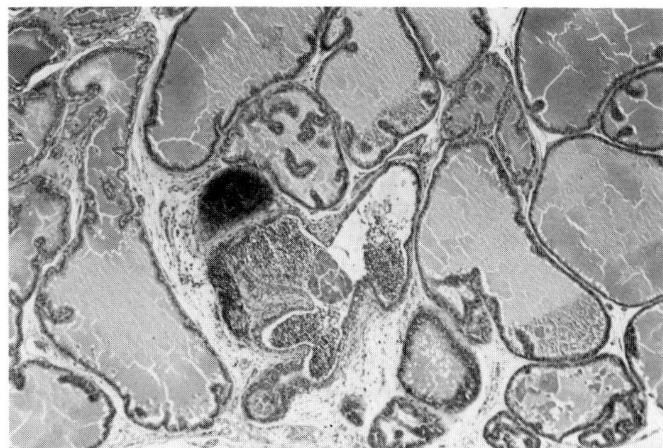

FIGURE 18–16. Lateral prostate of a Lewis rat with focal inflammation of individual acini accompanied by epithelial atrophy and stromal hyperplasia.

from aged hamsters of other strains, in which the condition was not found to occur in life span studies. The pathologic change involved little apparent cellular proliferation and appeared to be principally distention of prostatic tubules with secretion and was found associated with metabolism of cholesterol.[72]

EXPERIMENTAL INDUCTION OF BPH

Dog

The existence of spontaneous prostatic hyperplasia in dogs made them an obvious animal in which to attempt to induce changes that might mimic those in the human disease and thus to elucidate the factors that are important in BPH origin and development. Early studies by Walsh and Wilson[71] reported that prostatic hyperplasia could indeed be induced in castrated dogs through the administration of androgens; the degree of hyperplasia was increased by the simultaneous administration of both androgen and estrogen. The type of androgen that was given also had an effect on the degree of hyperplasia that was achieved. Androstanediol administered along with estrogen was capable of producing prostates that were nearly four times normal weight. The major response was seen in the prostatic epithelium, which showed extensive proliferative and secretory activity. Since these studies, other investigators have also demonstrated that it is relatively easy to produce glandular BPH in dogs through the administration of androgens or combinations of androgen and estrogen to both intact and castrate dogs. The general experience is that the degree of hyperplasia is greater when estrogen is given in conjunction with testosterone and that this proliferative response is even stronger when androstanediol is the androgen.[19, 23]

Experimental replication more typical of canine BPH, the complex form, has met with considerably less success. Grayhack and Kozlowski cite unpublished data that administration of dihydrotestosterone (DHT) to intact dogs results in a significant incidence of induced BPH.[27] It has been shown that testosterone administration to dogs castrated at older ages (6 to 8.5 years) allows development of complex BPH in some animals.[7] However, another feature was seen in these animals, as well as in other studies in which dogs were administered testosterone and androgen and estrogen more than 3 years after castration. Many animals that had undergone such treatment exhibited a differential response between the epithelium of glands surrounding the urethra in the inner third of the gland and those in the outer third. There was evidence of regeneration of secretory activity in the peripherally located tissue, whereas that in the periurethral zone retained a nonsecretory, undifferentiated character. This differential regional phenomenon was also noted by Aumüller and co-workers,[3] who observed that the central or periurethral portion of the gland tends to undergo atrophy after androgen withdrawal or squamous metaplasia after estrogen administration, whereas the peripheral, subcapsular portion of the canine prostate demonstrated secretory activity in the presence of low amounts of androgen. The role of vascular supply to the different regions of the prostate has also been questioned. The regional nature of heightened responsiveness to induction of squamous metaplasia by administration of estradiol was noted by Hohbach, who also observed broadening of the stroma and increased mitosis in basal cells following estrogen administration.[32]

Habenicht and co-workers were able to produce epithelial and stromal proliferation, i.e., androgen- and estrogen-related effects, through treatment of castrated dogs with an aromatizable androgen and the combination of the androgen and an aromatase inhibitor.[31] The estrogenic effects were stromal stimulation and cystic tubular dilatation. DeKlerk and co-workers found it possible to produce glandular hyperplasia in young dogs by administration of both estrogen and an androgen.[19] This was histologically like that seen spontaneously in intact dogs, and in some instances showed extreme proliferation of the secretory epithelium. Further studies based on this observation of the important influence of estrogen failed to prevent BPH development in dogs of approximately 6 years of age through inhibition of endogenous aromatase activity.[57]

When estrogen alone is administered to dogs, several outcomes have been reported. Leav and co-workers found alterations in both epithelial and basal cells after 4 to 6 weeks of treatment of castrated or hypophysectomized dogs.[40] It was believed that the prominent squamous metaplasia seen resulted from basal cell proliferation, whereas the secretory cells underwent both regression and altered differentiation to a type termed estrogen-modified glandular cells. These modified cells had cytoplasmic granules of two types and features suggesting both androgenic and estrogenic influences. This and other evidence have been cited in support of the stimulatory effect of estrogen on prostatic epithelium.[41] Evidence of regional susceptibility of the prostatic epithelium to estrogen administration was reported

by Hohbach, who found it arising most prominently in the dorsolateral regions surrounding the urethra.[32] The possible importance of estrogen in BPH development is suggested by the demonstration of ER in both spontaneous and induced BPH.[63] ER were constantly found in the stroma and urethral tissues; however, in spontaneous disease, heterogeneous distribution in prostatic epithelial cells was observed. It was suggested that the role of estrogen in BPH might be a selective rather than a diffuse one.

The prostatic stroma in dogs, although much less prominent than it is in the human disease, is still an important component of both experimental and naturally occurring BPH. Dense stromal bands tend to be located near the glandular periphery. Morphometric analysis of aging canine prostates demonstrated increase in stromal volume with age in all but the oldest group in a series of beagles ranging from 0.7 to 8.7 years.[74] The absolute stromal volume of glands with BPH averaged approximately twice that of normal animals. Notwithstanding this evidence of proliferation, the smooth muscle in both spontaneous and induced BPH was not shown to exhibit evidence of activation in contrast to smooth muscle from animals treated with estrogen or tamoxifen, an antiestrogen.[15] Inflammation, a common finding in spontaneous BPH in dogs, was found to be associated with administration of an aromatase inhibitor to mature beagles. Diffuse and follicular deposition of lymphocytes was frequent in treated animals and resembled naturally occurring prostatitis. The canine lesions are very much like nonbacterial prostatitis produced in rats by hormonal manipulations noted below. However, they may also represent intercurrent bacterial infections or reactions to foreign antigens or spermatozoa which reflux into the tubules.

Primates

The use of nonhuman primates as experimental subjects for the study of BPH is attractive because of their phylogenetic relationship to humans; this is balanced by the noted anatomic differences in the organs and by the cost and complications of working with animals of these types. In the main, primate-based studies have used three species: rhesus monkeys (*Macaca mulatta*), cynomolgus monkeys (*M. fascicularis*), and baboons (*Papio* species). These species tend to be those used in most other types of primate research, and, as noted earlier, their prostatic morphology resembles that of humans in several ways. Yet, for many reasons, including cost and animal availability, there is a limited number of studies in rhesus monkeys. Lewis reviewed several studies of estrogen administration which consistently produced an increase in stroma with fibromuscular hyperplasia in the utricular area.[43] Morphometric studies of prostates from animals treated with DHT and estrogen as well as with androstanediol plus estrogen showed changes in glandular tissue and stroma, particularly in the caudal lobe, which had similarity to those seen in human BPH.[44] The author has examined prostates from adult rhesus implanted with Silastic capsules containing androgens and estrogen for 13 weeks (P. Juniewicz, unpublished data). These animals exhibited some degree of fibromuscular stromal hyperplasia accompanied by chronic inflammation. However, the nodular and focal changes seen in human BPH were not observed.

Habenicht and co-workers made use of their observation that the cynomolgus monkey possesses a prostate that "seems to be more like the human prostate than that of other primate species."[30] No spontaneous BPH has been identified in this species; however, using androstanedione as an aromatizing substrate for 3 months, estrogenic effects in intact animals were found in marked activation of smooth muscle. This was seen as an increase in the smooth muscle, with the peripheral areas showing especially severe stromal proliferation. No increase in organ weight was observed. In induced BPH in cynomolgus monkeys stromal metachromasia was noted; this is similar to that seen in humans with BPH.[29]

Both glandular and stromal hyperplasia of the prostate were induced in intact adult baboons by the administration of testosterone enanthate for periods of up to 6 months[34]; stromal proliferation similar to that observed in human BPH was especially noticeable in the caudal lobe of the gland in which there was extensive collagen deposition. The degree of epithelial proliferation was striking in some areas, with masses of tightly packed epithelial nuclei in many acini, especially in peripheral areas. In a 1-month study with intact chacma baboons, De Klerk et al noted little response to hormonal stimuli.[20] However, in immature animals there were regional differences in a proliferative response to the administration of androgen and estrogen; the caudal and periurethral portions showed the most stimulatory effect.

Rats

Rats are frequently used in the study of prostate biology. Although spontaneous BPH is an unusual event in rats, the multilobed prostate has proved to be a very useful tool in elucidating the response of different cellular elements, both epithelial and stromal, to hormonal and other stimuli. Studies have focused on the three lobes of the gland, which at times react differently to the same stimuli. These rodent studies have been reviewed by Cunha and co-workers, who outlined current questions in prostate biology, many of which are being explored using rats.[18] Following castration of the rat, the prostate involutes rapidly, with death and atrophy of secretory epithelium and loss of secretion. This is accomplished by a dying back of the prostatic ductular system from the tips of its many branches. Upon subsequent administration of androgen, the regressive changes are reversed, the gland regrows and arborizes, and secretion resumes.

Ehrlichman and co-workers contrasted the response of castrate dogs and rats to administration of testosterone and estrogen.[23] Although this regimen was capable

of producing BPH in dogs, restoration of the rat ventral prostate occurred, but no hyperplasia was produced.

In an attempt to ascertain the role of prostatic basal cells, autoradiography was used to monitor changes in basal and secretory cell populations of the ventral prostate after castration and subsequent testosterone administration.[24] It was found that both populations regressed following castration, but disproportionately and varying regionally within the gland, and that both cell types proliferated with testosterone administration. The role or function of basal cells remains ambiguous. It is certainly possible that, among these cells with rather undistinguished morphology, a subpopulation of true stem cells exists. Regenerating prostate following partial resection demonstrated proliferation and differentiation of basal cells.[6] Alternatively, because both secretory and stem cells can be seen to proliferate, the basal cell could be a fully differentiated cell with as yet unknown function. Cytokeratin markers identified a population of basal cells primarily located in the proximal region of the ducts of the ventral prostate[62]; this location would allow them to remain as a stem cell population after regression of the gland.

In the dorsolateral prostate, both hyperplasia and dysplasia can be induced by the simultaneous administration of testosterone and 17-beta-estradiol.[39] In this study using Noble rats, there was glandular enlargement accompanied by epithelial hyperplasia. Hyperplastic glands also frequently showed dysplastic changes consisting of irregularity in nuclear morphology and cellular enlargement. Acini in hyperplastic foci were composed of closely packed cells that lacked the nuclear abnormalities. It was concluded that estrogen was the major factor in causing the dysplasia, which was amplified by the joint action of estrogen and androgen.

It has been noted that inflammation is a frequent occurrence in both human and canine BPH. Nonbacterial prostatitis in rats has been clearly shown to have an endocrine basis. Severe prostatitis with focal chronic inflammation affecting glands and lobes of the lateral prostate and accompanied by squamous metaplasia of the epithelium, regional proliferation of fibromuscular connective tissue, and filling of the glandular lumina with inflammatory debris has been seen as a spontaneous occurrence. It has been shown that several factors including genetic background, age, and hormonal imbalance all play important roles in this condition.[56, 60]

Mouse

The mouse has gained use as a model for possible mechanisms of BPH induction in studies which have shown that transplantation of urogenital sinus tissue into the prostate of nude mice causes enlargement of the host gland, which depends upon the presence of host androgens.[54] The chimeric glands evidence proliferation of both host and transplanted elements, with pleomorphic glandular elements having morphologic features seen in human BPH occurring predominantly in animals receiving the urogenital sinus transplants, in contrast to those receiving urogenital sinus mesenchyme alone.

Donjacour and Cunha found that branching morphogenesis in neonatal mice is sensitive to but does not require chronic androgen stimulation.[21] Experimental studies of diethylstilbestrol in mice by several investigators resulted in stromal hyperplasia with whorl-like nodules of connective tissue and smooth muscle along with squamous metaplasia. This can be sufficient to cause obstruction to the urinary bladder with subsequent hydroureter and hydronephrosis.[71]

In summary it must be stated that the various natural and experimental animal models of BPH have not provided conditions that fully replicate the human disease. Neither have they allowed us to fully understand the pathogenesis of this disorder. Yet they have shed considerable light on many facets of prostatic biology and pathobiology and continue to point out the importance of the many factors that determine the morphologic and physiologic features of the prostate.

REFERENCES

1. Abrahamsson PA, Lilja H, Falkmer S, Wadstrom LB: Immunohistochemical distribution of the three predominant secretory proteins in the parenchyma of hyperplastic and neoplastic prostate glands. Prostate 12:39–46, 1988.
2. Adams MR, Bond MG: Benign prostatic hyperplasia in a squirrel monkey (*Saimiri scirueus*). Lab Anim Sci 29:674–676, 1979.
3. Aumüller G, Stofft E, Tunn U: Fine structure of the canine prostatic complex. Anat Embryol 160:327–340, 1980.
4. Banerjee PP, Banerjee S, Sprando RL, Zirkin BR: Regional cellular heterogeneity and DNA synthetic activity in rat ventral prostate during postnatal development. Biol Reprod 45:773–782, 1991.
5. Bartsch G, Bruengger A, Schweikert U, et al: Benigne Prostatahyperplasie: Eine stromale Erkrankung. Urologe A 28:321–328, 1989.
6. Bazer GT: Basal cell proliferation and differentiation in regeneration of the rat ventral prostate. Invest Urol 17:470–473, 1980.
7. Berry SJ, Coffey DS, Strandberg JD, Ewing LL: Effect of age, castration and testosterone replacement on the development and restoration of canine benign prostatic hyperplasia. Prostate 9:295–302, 1986.
8. Berry SJ, Coffey DS, Walsh PC, Ewing LL: The development of human benign prostatic hyperplasia with age. J Urol 132:474–479, 1984.
9. Berry SJ, Strandberg JD, Saunders WJ, Coffey DS: The development of canine benign prostatic hyperplasia with age. Prostate 9:363–373, 1986.
10. Bloom F: Hyperplasia. *In* Pathology of the Dog and Cat. Evanston, IL, American Veterinary Publications, 1954, pp 289–295.
11. Boorman GA, Elwell MR, Mitsumori K: Male accessory sex glands, penis, and scrotum. *In* Boorman GA, Eustis SL, Elwell MR, et al (eds): Pathology of the Fischer Rat. San Diego, Academic Press, 1990, pp 419–428.
12. Bosland MC: Hyperplasia, prostate, rat. *In* Jones TC, Mohr U, Hunt RD (eds): Genital System. Berlin, Springer-Verlag, 1987, pp 267–272.
13. Brandes D: The fine structure and histochemistry of prostatic glands in relation to sex hormones. Int Rev Cytol 20:207–276, 1966.
14. Brendler CB, Berry SJ, Ewing LL, et al: Spontaneous benign prostatic hyperplasia in the beagle. J Clin Invest 71:1114–1123, 1983.
15. Bruengger A, Bartsch G, Hollinger BE, et al: Smooth muscle cell of the canine prostate in spontaneous benign hyperplasia, steroid induced hyperplasia and estrogen or tamoxifen treated dogs. J Urol 130:1208–1210, 1983.
16. Coffey DS, DeKlerk DP, Walsh PC: Benign prostatic hyperplasia: Current concepts. Endocrinology 2:495–499, 1976.
17. Coffey DS, DeKlerk DP, Walsh PC: Benign prostatic hyperplasia. *In* James VHT (ed): Endocrinology Proceedings of the V International Congress of Endocrinology, Hamburg, July 18–24, 1976, Vol 2, pp 495–499.
18. Cunha GR, Donjacour AA, Cooke PS, et al: The endocrinology and developmental biology of the prostate. Endocrinol Rev 8:338–362, 1987.
19. DeKlerk DP, Coffey DS, Ewing LL, et al: Comparison of spontaneous and experimentally induced canine prostatic hyperplasia. J Clin Invest 64:842–849, 1979.
20. DeKlerk DP, Human HJ, DeKlerk JN: The effect of 5α-androstane-3α, 17β-diol and 17β-estradiol on the adult and immature chacma baboon prostate. Prostate 7:1–12, 1985.
21. Donjacour AA, Cunha GR: The effect of androgen deprivation on branching morphogenesis in the mouse prostate. Dev Biol 128:1–14, 1988.
22. Donnelly BJ, Lakey WH, McBlain WA: Estrogen receptor in human benign prostatic hyperplasia. J Urol 130:183–187, 1983.
23. Ehrlichman RJ, Isaacs JT, Coffey DS: Differences in the effects of estradiol on dihydrotestosterone induced prostatic growth of the castrate dog and rat. Invest Urol 18:466–470, 1981.
24. English HF, Santen RJ, Isaacs JT: Response of glandular versus basal rat ventral prostatic epithelial cells to androgen withdrawal and replacement. Prostate 11:229–242, 1987.
25. Evans GS, Chandler JA: Cell proliferation studies in rat prostate: I. The proliferative role of basal and secretory epithelial cells during normal growth. Prostate 10:163–178, 1987.
26. Franks LM: Benign prostatic hyperplasia: Gross and microscopic anatomy. *In* Grayhack JT, Wilson JD, Scherbenske MJ (eds): Benign Prostatic Hyperplasia. US Department of Health, Education, and Welfare publication no. (NIH) 76–113, 1976, pp 63–89.
27. Grayhack JT, Kozlowski JM: Benign prostatic hyperplasia. *In* Gillenwater JY, Grayhack JT, Howards SS, Duckett JW (eds): Adult and Pediatric Urology. St. Louis, Mosby-Year Book, 1991, pp 1211–1239.
28. Guinan P, Shaw M, Targonski P, et al: Evaluation of cytokeratin markers to differentiate between benign and malignant prostatic tissue. J Surg Oncol 42:175–180, 1989.
29. Habenicht U-F, El Etreby MF, Lewis R, et al: Induction of metachromasia in experimentally induced hyperplastic/hypertrophic changes in the prostate of the cynomolgus monkey (*Macaca fascicularis*). J Urol 142:1624–1626, 1989.
30. Habenicht U-F, Schwarz K, Neumann F, El Etreby MF: Induction of estrogen-related hyperplastic changes in the prostate of the cynomolgus monkey (*Macaca fascicularis*) by androstenedione and its antagonization by the aromatase inhibitor 1-methylandrostane-1,4-diene,17-dione. Prostate 11:313–326, 1987.
31. Habenicht UF, Schwarz K, Schweikert HU, et al: Development of a model for the induction of estrogen-related prostatic hyperplasia in the dog and its response to the aromatase inhibitor 4-hydroxy-4-androstene-3,17-dione: Preliminary results. Prostate 8:181–194, 1986.
32. Hohbach CH: Ultrastructural and enzyme-histochemical studies of the prostate of the dog under the effect of estradiol. Beitr Pathol 160:260–273, 1990.
33. Jones DR, Parkinson MC, Griffiths GJ, et al: Origin and structure of benign prostatic hyperplasia. Br J Urol 66:506–508, 1990.
34. Karr JP, Untae T, Murphy GP, Sandberg AA: Benign prostatic hyperplasia in the baboon. *In* Kimball FA, Buhl AE, Carter DB (eds): New Approaches to the Study of Benign Prostatic Hyperplasia. New York, Alan R. Liss, 1984, pp 257–289.
35. Kastendieck H, Helpap B: Prostatic "dysplasia/atypical hyperplasia." Urology 34:28–42, 1989.
36. Kirchheim D, Gyökey F, Brandes D, Scott WW: Histochemistry of the normal, hyperplastic, and neoplastic human prostate gland. Invest Urol 1:403–421, 1964.
37. Kovi J, Mostofi FK: Atypical hyperplasia of prostate. Urology 34:23–27, 1989.

38. Lawson RK: Benign prostatic hyperplasia and growth factors. Urologe [A] 29:5–7, 1990.

39. Leav I, Ho SM, Ofner P, et al: Biochemical alterations in sex hormone-induced hyperplasia and dyplasia of the dorsolateral prostates of noble rats. J Natl Cancer Inst 80:1045–1053, 1988.

40. Leav I, Merk FB, Ofner P, et al: Bipotentiality of response to sex hormones by the prostate of castrated or hypophysectomized dogs. Am J Pathol 93:69–89, 1978.

41. Leav I, Ofner P: Proliferative disease of the prostate: Anatomy, pathology and hormone effects. *In* Naftolin F, Hamilton D (eds): Basic Reproductive Medicine. Cambridge MA, MIT Press, 1982, pp 223–289.

42. Lee C, Sensibar JA, Dudek SM, et al: Prostatic ductal system in rats: Regional variation in morphological and functional activities. Biol Reprod 43:1079–1086, 1990.

43. Lewis RW: Benign prostatic hyperplasia in the nonhuman primate. *In* Kimball FA, Buhl AE, Carter DB (eds): New Approaches to the Study of Benign Prostatic Hyperplasia. New York, Alan R. Liss, 1984, pp 235–255.

44. Lewis RW, Dowling KJ, Patterson GM, Goldenberg SF: The nonhuman primate as an animal model for benign prostatic hyperplasia. *In* Rodgers CH, Coffey DS, Cunha G, et al (eds): Benign Prostatic Hyperplasia, Vol II. U.S. Department of Health and Human Services, NIH Publication No. 87-2881, 1987, pp 119–127.

45. Lewis RW, Kim JCS, Irani D, Roberts JA: The prostate of the nonhuman primate: Normal anatomy and pathology. Prostate 2:51–70, 1981.

46. Lowseth LA, Gerlach RF, Gillett NA, Muggenburg BA: Age-related changes in the prostate and testes of the beagle dog. Vet Pathol 27:347–353, 1990.

47. Mamaeva S, Lundgren R, Elfving P, et al: AgNOR staining in benign hyperplasia and carcinoma of the prostate. Prostate 18:155–162, 1991.

48. Mao P, Angrist A: The fine structure of the basal cell of human prostate. Lab Invest 15:1768–1782, 1966.

49. McEntee M, Isaacs W, Smith C: Adenocarcinoma of the canine prostate: Immunohistochemical examination for secretory antigens. Prostate 11:163–170, 1987.

50. McNeal JE: Developmental and comparative anatomy of the prostate. *In* Grayhack JT, Wilson JD, Scherbenske MJ (eds): Benign prostatic hyperplasia: NIAMDD workshop proceedings, Feb 20–21, 1975. US Department of Health, Education, and Welfare, NIH Publication No. 76-113, 1976, pp 1–9.

51. McNeal JE: Normal and pathologic anatomy of prostate. Urology (Suppl) 17:11–16, 1981.

52. McNeal JE: Relationship of the origin of benign prostatic hypertrophy to prostatic structure of man and other mammals. *In* Hinman F Jr (ed): Benign Prostatic Hypertrophy. New York, Springer-Verlag, 1983, pp 152–166.

53. McNeal JE: The prostate gland: Morphology and pathobiology. Monogr Urol 4:3–33, 1983.

54. Miller GJ, Runner MN, Chung WK: Tissue interactions and prostatic growth: II. Morphological and biochemical characterization of adult mouse prostatic hyperplasia by fetal urogenital sinus implants. Prostate 6:241–253, 1985.

55. Moore RA: Benign hypertrophy of the prostate: A morphological study. J Urol 50:680–710, 1943.

56. Naslund MJ, Strandberg JD, Coffey DS: The role of androgens and estrogens in the pathogenesis of experimental nonbacterial prostatitis. J Urol 140:1049–1053, 1988.

57. Oesterling JE, Juniewicz PE, Walters JR, et al: Aromatase inhibition in the dog. II. Effect on growth function, and pathology of the prostate. J Urol 139:832–839, 1988.

58. Price D: Comparative aspects of development and structure in the prostate. Natl Cancer Inst Monogr 12:1–27, 1963.

59. Reese JH, Lombard CM, Krone K, Stamey TA: Phyllodes type of atypical prostatic hyperplasia: A report of 3 new cases. J Urol 138:623–626, 1987.

60. Robinette CL: Sex-hormone-induced inflammation and fibromuscular proliferation in the rat lateral prostate. Prostate 12:271–286, 1988.

61. Ronnett BM, Epstein JI: A case showing sclerosing adenosis and an unusual form of basal cell hyperplasia of the prostate. Am J Surg Pathol 13:866–872, 1989.

62. Rouleau M, Legert J, Tenniswood M: Ductal heterogeneity of cytokeratins, gene expression, and cell death in the rat ventral prostate. Mol Endocrinol 4:2003–2013, 1990.

63. Schulze H, Barrack ER: Immunocytochemical localization of estrogen receptors in spontaneous and experimentally induced canine benign prostatic hyperplasia. Prostate 11:145–162, 1987.

64. Srigley JR, Dardick I, Hartwick RWJ, Klotz L: Basal epithelial cells of human prostate gland are not myoepithelial cells. Am J Pathol 136:957–966, 1990.

65. Strandberg JD, Berry SJ: The pathology of prostatic hyperplasia in the dog. *In* Rodgers CH, Coffey DS, Cunha G, et al (eds): Benign Prostatic Hyperplasia, Vol II. U.S. Department of Health and Human Services, NIH Publication No. 87-2881, 1987, pp 109–117.

66. Theyer G, Kramer G, Assmann I, et al: Phenotypic characterization of infiltrating leukocytes in benign prostatic hyperplasia. Lab Invest 66:96–107, 1992.

67. Timms BG, Chandler JA, Sinowatz F: The ultrastructure of basal cells of rat and dog prostate. Cell Tissue Res 173:543–554, 1976.

68. Van Wagenen G: The coagulating function of the cranial lobe of the prostate gland in the monkey. Anat Rec 66:411–421, 1936.

69. Verhagen APM, Aalders TW, Ramaekers FCS, et al: Differential expression of keratins in the basal and luminal compartments of rat prostatic epithelium during degeneration and regeneration. Prostate 13:25–38, 1988.

70. Walsh PC: Experimental approaches to benign prostatic hypertrophy: Animal models utilizing the dog, rat, and mouse. *In* Grayhack JT, Wilson JD, Scherbenske MJ (eds): Benign Prostatic Hyperplasia. US Department of Health, Education, and Welfare, 1976, pp 215–222.

71. Walsh PC, Wilson JD: The induction of prostatic hypertrophy in the dog with androstanediol. J Clin Invest 57:1093–1097, 1976.

72. Wang GM, Schaffner CP: Effect of candicin and colestipol on the testes and prostate glands of BIO 87.20 hamsters. Invest Urol 14:66–71, 1976.

73. White IA: Accessory sex organs and fluids of the male reproductive tract. *In* Alexander NJ (ed): Animal Models for Research on Contraception and Fertility. Hagerstown, MD, Harper & Row, 1978, pp 105–123.

74. Zirkin BR, Strandberg JD: Quantitative changes in the morphology of the aging canine prostate. Anat Rec 208:207–214, 1984.

PROSTATE CANCER

Chapter 19

HISTOPATHOLOGY OF PROSTATE CANCER

F. K. MOSTOFI, CHARLES J. DAVIS, JR., and ISABELL A. SESTERHENN

This chapter deals with the pathology of malignant tumors of the prostate, including the criteria for pathologic diagnosis, the premalignant lesions, special types of prostate carcinoma (PCa), treatment effects, lesions that simulate PCa, and attempts to improve prognosis. It covers sarcomas of the prostate and carcinomas of the seminal vesicles.

CATEGORIES OF PROSTATIC CARCINOMA

We recognize four categories of PCa.[109]

Latent Carcinoma. PCa may be discovered by the pathologist on postmortem examination of a patient who has had no signs or symptoms referrable to the prostate. These tumors may occur anywhere in the prostate but are usually in the central and peripheral zones and are well differentiated. The frequency of latent carcinoma ranges from 26 to 73 per cent. In a study of latent PCa in six different geographical locations, the International Agency for Research in Cancer found that the incidence of small PCa was the same in all locations, but the incidence of larger PCa varied geographically.[22] It was lowest in Hong Kong and Singapore, intermediate in Israel and Uganda, and high in Germany, Sweden, and Jamaica. These rates correspond to clinical death rates.[131] These observations suggest that either environmental or genetic factors are responsible for clinical

appearance of the tumors. The study of genetic factors may be easier now with newer methods to study molecular genetics.

We have seen a number of latent carcinomas in young men in their 20s, and in one case the tumor was very close to the capsule. What would have happened in this patient had he lived for 10, 20, or 30 years? Information is highly desirable on how these tumors differ from the well-differentiated, clinically discovered PCa's that metastasize and kill the patient.

Incidental Carcinoma. In 6 to 20 per cent of prostatic tissues removed for clinically benign hyperplasia of the prostate (BPH), histologic examination shows PCa. This is the group that is clinically referred to as stage A or T1; and depending on the volume of the tumor, subdivided into A1 or 2 or B1 or 2. This category is located in the periurethral area and is often well differentiated.

The discovery of PCa in transurethral resection (TURP) for BPH raises a number of questions. Would these accidentally discovered PCa's have remained dormant? Should these PCa's be left alone, or do they have the potential for extraprostatic extension and eventual metastasis? The problem is discussed later.

Occult Carcinoma. This is the category in which carcinoma is found in the biopsy of bone or lymph node in a patient who has had no symptoms of prostatic disease. The prostatic origin of these metastatic lesions is demonstrated by elevated serum levels of prostatic acid phosphatase (PAP) and/or prostate-specific antigen (PSA) and confirmed only by a prostatic biopsy.

Clinical Carcinoma. This category includes cases in which digital rectal examination reveals induration, irregularity of the outline, or a nodule. Jewett et al[75] and

---

Hudson and Stout[73] reported that about 50 per cent of these patients had PCa. Measurement of PAP and PSA and ultrasonography are other methods of detection of clinical PCa. These must be confirmed by biopsy.

CRITERIA FOR PATHOLOGIC DIAGNOSIS OF PROSTATIC CARCINOMA

Identification of PCa in its early stage is difficult, if not impossible, because most prostate glands are removed by TURP. Carcinomatous curettings, however, can be distinguished by their usually firm, relatively solid, and frequently distinctive yellow or yellow-orange appearance. The consistency of this tumor is similar to that of scirrhous carcinoma of the breast. In total prostatectomy specimens, the tumor must be at least 5 mm in diameter to be grossly discernible, but its firm or hard consistency is the pathognomonic feature. The tumor may consist of single or multiple nodules, irregular in outline, usually in contact with the capsule, and not sharply demarcated from the surrounding tissue. Many urologists can state with considerable accuracy whether the nodule is surrounded by normal tissue on two or three sides. About one half the carcinomas have a distinct yellow flecking, are firm, and may be granular. Others are gray to white, homogeneous or slightly fibrillar, and hard.

As the tumor grows, the prostate becomes increasingly infiltrated and replaced by carcinoma; eventually it invades the urethra and the trigone anteriorly and the periprostatic tissue posteriorly. The tumor is usually poorly demarcated and merges with adjacent tissue. It usually remains firm but occasionally may be soft with an increasing ratio of epithelial to stromal elements.

The histologic criteria for diagnosis of PCa have been described in detail,[109, 110] but are summarized here. Pathologic diagnosis of PCa is based on nuclear anapla-

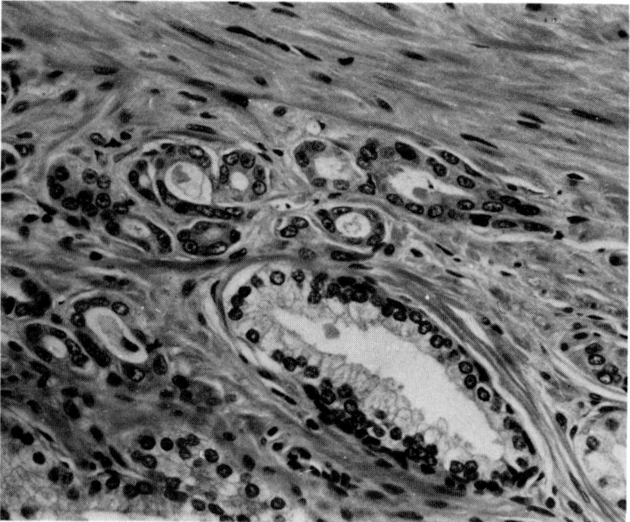

FIGURE 19–1. Prostatic carcinoma showing nuclear anaplasia. The nuclei in the upper portion are vacuolated with prominent nucleoli compared with hyperplastic glands (H & E, original magnification × 160).

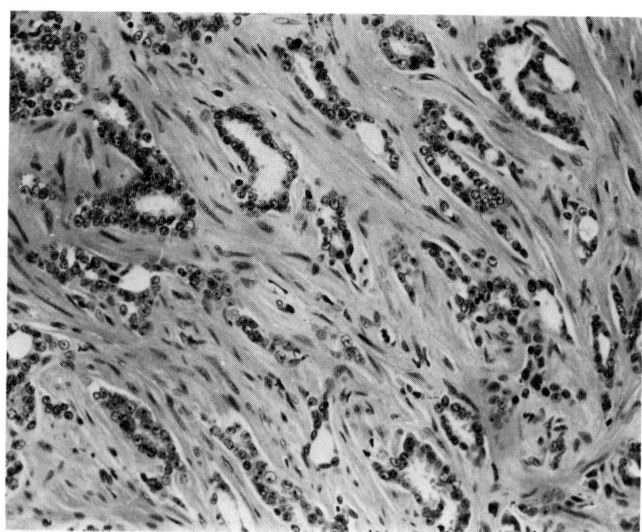

FIGURE 19–2. Prostatic carcinoma showing stromal invasion. Note irregularity and haphazard distribution of acini; pointed edges of acini; and individual cells or clones of cells infiltrating the stroma (H & E, original magnification × 160).

sia, invasion, and architectural disturbances. In most PCa's, the diagnosis of carcinoma is made on the basis of nuclear anaplasia. In the benign prostatic epithelium, the nuclei are round and vesicular. They have one small nucleolus. In PCa, the nuclei are usually larger than those of benign cells. They show some variation in size, shape, and staining but are generally uniform. The chromatin is condensed at the periphery, and there is vacuolization of the nuclei. The presence of a large nucleolus in the secretory cells is recognized as the most important criterion for diagnosis of PCa (Fig. 19–1).

There may be more than one large nucleolus, and the nucleoli may be centrally or peripherally located. Mitotic figures and giant cells are rare, except in high-grade tumors. These changes are easily discernible in low-power microscopic view. Many PCa's show little or no anaplasia and the nucleoli may be small. In such cases, the diagnosis is based on invasion.

Invasion is another important criterion for diagnosis of PCa. The acini of normal and hyperplastic glands are surrounded by a delicate basement membrane. There is often an elastic tissue network demonstrable by electron microscopy[18, 49, 77] and/or by laminin stains[8, 17] surrounding the acini, and the whole is invested by smooth muscle strands. Malignant acini do not have this orderly connective tissue framework. The normal arrangement of elastic tissue is not seen in carcinomatous areas. The earliest sign of invasion is absence of the basal cell layer, but this is not always reliable, as some hyperplastic acini lack a basal cell layer. A break through the basement membrane is an early indication of stromal invasion.

Stromal invasion can be recognized by the loss of acinar-stromal interaction, as evidenced by the distribution of acini, without regard to the regular whorls of smooth muscle fibers (Fig. 19–2), irregularity of the shape of acini (Fig. 19–3), pointed edges of acini, or the presence of outgrowths of individual or groups of neo-

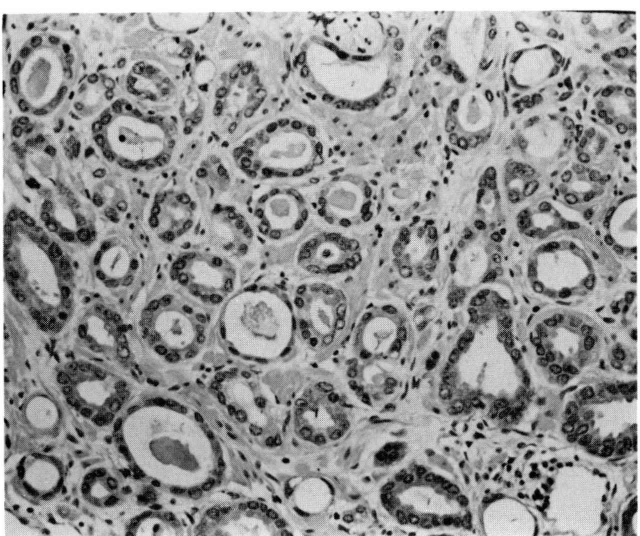

FIGURE 19–3. Prostatic carcinoma showing haphazard distribution and irregularity of outlines of acini and acini lined by a single layer of cells (H & E, original magnification × 100).

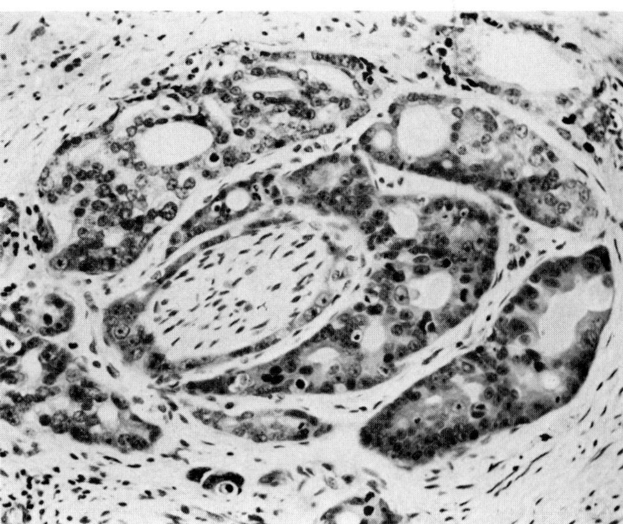

FIGURE 19–5. Prostatic carcinoma showing perineural invasion. Note irregularity of outline and pointed edges of acini (H & E, original magnification × 100).

plastic cells near the acini or scattered in the stroma (Fig. 19–4).

Perineural invasion (Fig. 19–5) has been the indisputable evidence of invasion. Rodin et al have reported that the spaces are not lymphatics but tissue spaces.[123] Byar et al reported that when adequate tissue was available, perineural invasion was found in more than 90 per cent of cases.[24] Mostofi and Price reported that, normally, nerve bundles may be present adjacent to prostatic acini, with only a thin basement membrane separating the two.[110] Byar et al demonstrated that intraprostatic perineural invasion has no clinical significance, but it may proceed to perineural invasion in the periprostatic tissue, and this should be looked for in total prostatectomy specimens.[24]

Vascular and lymphatic invasion is often difficult to recognize in needle biopsies or transurethral (TUR) tissue specimens. This is in part due to cautery or squeeze effect. In contrast to capillaries, which are in intimate relationship to the acini, lymphatics are found only in the stroma.[54] In TUR specimens, invasion of periurethral tissue or the bladder neck can be recognized by the presence of individual neoplastic cells or small acini scattered in the lamina propria, without any relationship to the surface epithelium. In such cases vascular invasion should be looked for and reported.

In needle biopsy, invasion of periprostatic tissue can be recognized by the presence of neoplastic acini in a fibroadipose stroma containing fat cells and nerve tissue. In such cases it is necessary to report the presence of the tumor outside the prostate, as it affects the clinical staging of the tumor and the management of the patient. If the available tissue contains seminal vesicle, invasion of the seminal vesicles should be looked for. Not infrequently, however, in needle biopsy involutional changes in seminal vesicles are misdiagnosed as PCa.

When anaplasia and invasion are absent or problematic, the diagnosis of PCa is based on architectural disturbances. In the normal prostate, the glands radiate from the urethra, and the acini have a characteristic convoluted structure. In the hyperplastic prostate, there is a typical nodular pattern and the radiating arrangement of glands may be lost, but their convoluted pattern is preserved. This is best viewed under low magnification. These features are absent in PCa. Disturbances of the architecture are manifested as haphazard distribution of glands (Fig. 19–6), small and large acini closely packed together (Fig. 19–7), large acini without convolutions (Fig. 19–8), fused glands or glands in glands (Fig. 19–9), or a few glands (Fig. 19–10), but columns and cords or solid sheets (Fig. 19–11). Instead of a double layer of cells lining the acini seen in hyperplastic glands, in PCa there may be a single layer of cells or

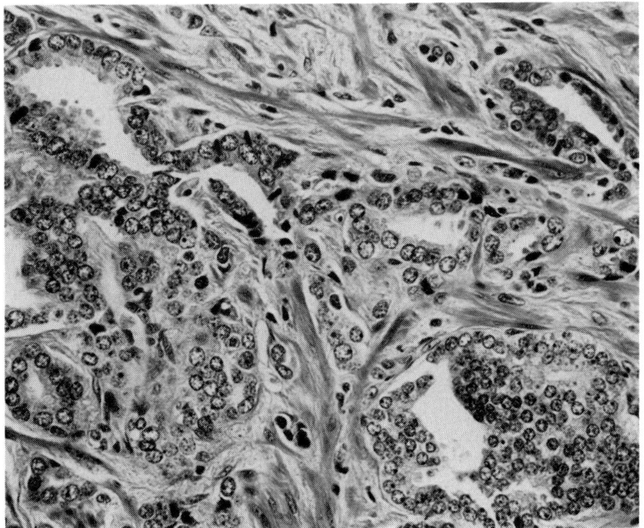

FIGURE 19–4. Prostatic carcinoma showing infiltrating growth by glands and individual cells. Note variation in size of nuclei, nuclear vacuoles, and nucleoli (H & E, original magnification × 100).

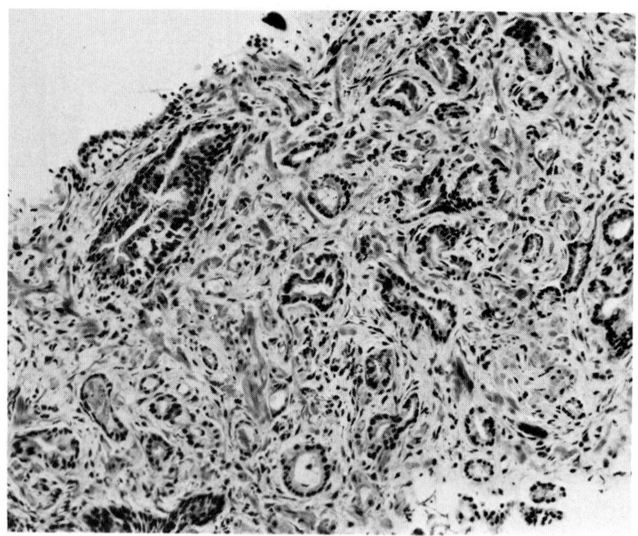

FIGURE 19–6. Prostatic carcinoma showing haphazard dispersion of glands. Note irregularity of outline of acini (H & E, original magnification × 100).

FIGURE 19–7. Prostatic carcinoma showing small and large acini closely packed together. The acini are lined by a single layer of cells. The outlines are irregular (H & E, original magnification × 100).

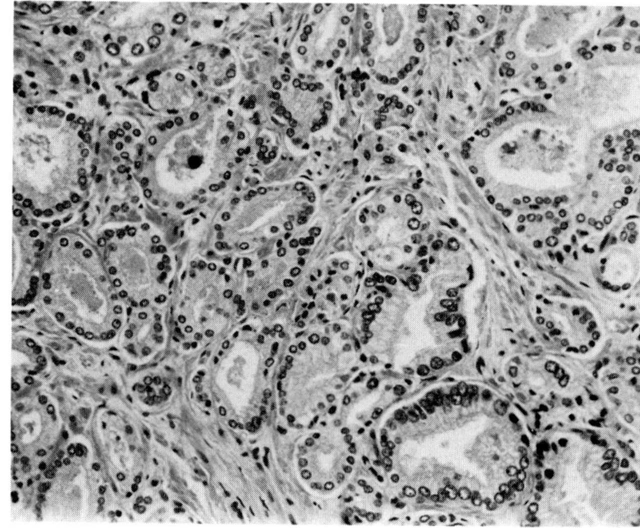

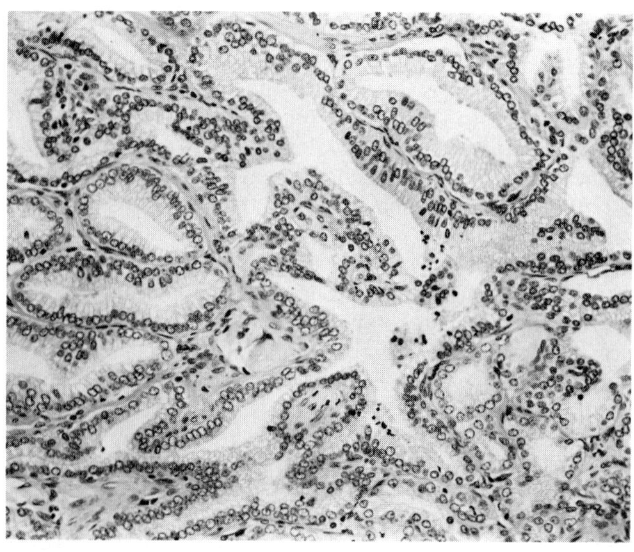

FIGURE 19–8. Prostatic carcinoma showing large acini without convolutions. Many nuclei are vacuolated, and the necleoli are not prominent (H & E, original magnification × 100).

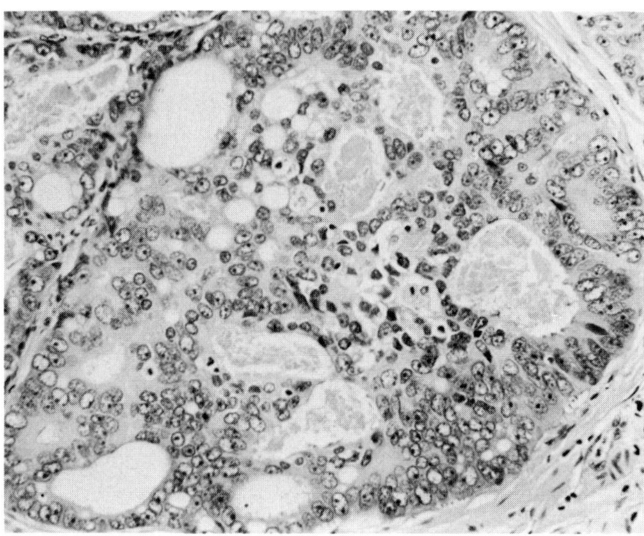

FIGURE 19–9. Prostatic carcinoma showing gland-in-gland growth pattern. The nuclei show moderate variation in size and shape. Many are vacuolated and show large nucleoli. Note absence of basal layer (H & E, original magnification × 100).

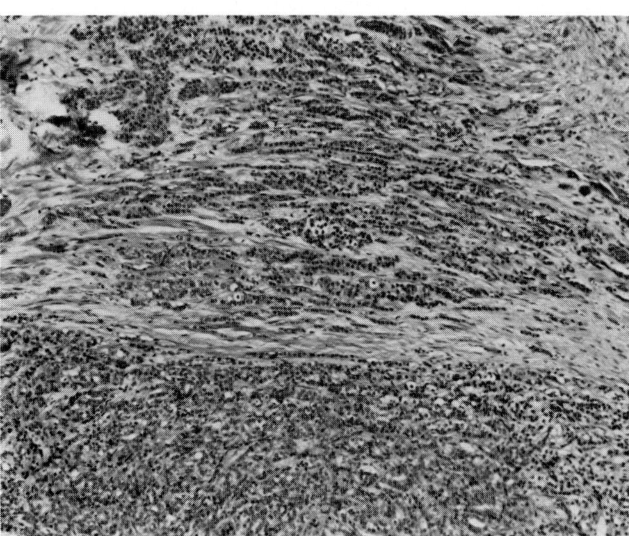

FIGURE 19–11. Undifferentiated prostatic carcinoma consisting of columns and cords and solid sheets (H & E, original magnification × 100).

piling up of cells. Many PCa's show more than one growth pattern, indicating the heterogeneity of PCa.

To be certain about the diagnosis of PCa, we like to see at least one of the three features: disturbed architecture, invasive growth pattern, and/or nuclear anaplasia. We regard nuclear anaplasia, especially large nucleoli in secretory cells, as the most important criterion for diagnosis of PCa. Two additional findings may help in the diagnosis of PCa. Mucin and crystalloids in the lumina of glands should suggest the possibility of PCa. However, both may be seen in benign glands and should not lead to diagnosis of PCa.

CRITERIA FOR CYTOLOGIC DIAGNOSIS OF PROSTATIC CARCINOMA

The classic work of Esposti initiated interest in application of cytology for diagnosis of PCa.[46] Esposti and, more recently, Koss et al[83] and Eble and Angermeier[40] have discussed in detail the cytologic criteria for diagnosis of PCa and the distinction between hyperplasia, atypical hyperplasia, and PCa.

In hyperplasia the typical smear contains epithelial cells arranged in mononuclear cohesive sheets and clusters. The sheets are composed of closely fitting polygonal cells with distinctly outlined cytoplasmic borders, resulting in a "honeycomb" configuration. The small round central nuclei are evenly distributed without crowding or overlapping. The nuclei have fine granular, evenly distributed chromatin with few chromocenters and absent nucleoli or tiny, inconspicuous nucleoli. Other elements are easily recognizable.

Atypical hyperplasia presents cohesive cell nests. The cell borders are somewhat blurred, and the nuclei may become slightly larger and more hyperchromatic. Koss et al[83] emphasize that such sheets are not diagnostic of PCa but must trigger the search for single cancer cells with more classic features—hyperchromatic large nuclei or readily discernible nucleoli. In PCa many cells are either dispersed or arranged in clusters and sheets. The distinction between the two depends on the degree of differentiation. The cell clusters are generally characterized by overlapping of cells, which under low power gives them a thick, crowded, tridimensional appearance. The relationship of the cells within the clusters is disturbed and lacks the orderly "honeycomb" appearance of evenly spaced cells with well-demarcated cell borders seen in hyperplasia. The periphery is often loosely structured, with single cells becoming readily detached during smear preparation. These changes are best studied in single dispersed cells or in small cell clusters. The

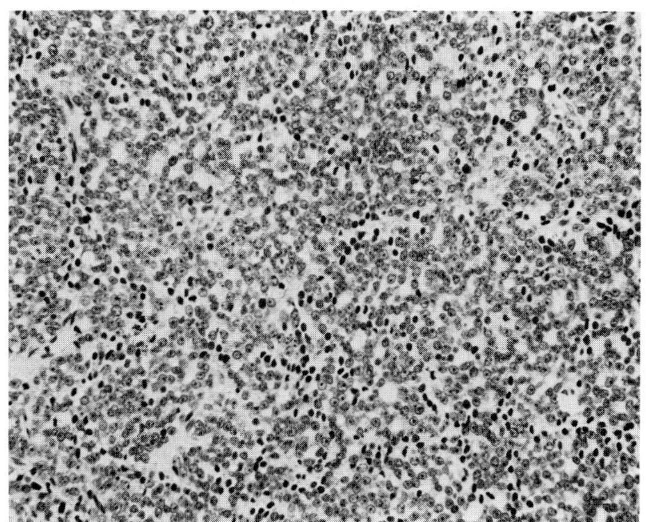

FIGURE 19–10. Poorly differentiated prostatic carcinoma showing sheets of small cells with some gland formation. The nuclei show slight variation in size and shape. The nucleoli are prominent (H & E, original magnification × 100).

presence of enlarged nucleoli is one of the most secure morphologic features of PCa (Fig. 19–12).

Cell Types

In diagnosing PCa, the tendency has been to simply diagnose PCa without any reference to the cell type. By light microscopy, the cytoplasm of a PCa may vary from light-staining to dark or eosinophilic (Fig. 19–13). Kastendieck et al have shown that there may be six different cell types in PCa.[79] These authors did not relate the cell types to behavior or response to treatment.

Sinha et al reported that malignant acini contained numerous columnar secretory cells in untreated, but few treated, prostates.[138] Two distinct basic cells were observed in both groups: type I (light) cells or type II (dark) cells. Type I cells were characterized by round nuclei with many small aggregates of euchromatin, large nucleoli, and electron-lucent cytoplasm. Type II cells had highly pleomorphic nuclei, folded nuclear envelope, sometimes deficient in localized areas, euchromatin, many small aggregates of heterochromatin, large pleomorphic nucleoli, and relatively electron-opaque nucleoplasm. Both cells were invasive. PCa that was or subsequently became refractory to estrogen showed more abundant type II cells than did responsive PCa's. Sinha et al postulated that the type II basal cells, as well as some type I cells, were unresponsive from the outset.[138] These observations have not been confirmed.

Immunochemistry

The advent of specific antibodies against PAP and PSA has enabled demonstration of both enzymes in

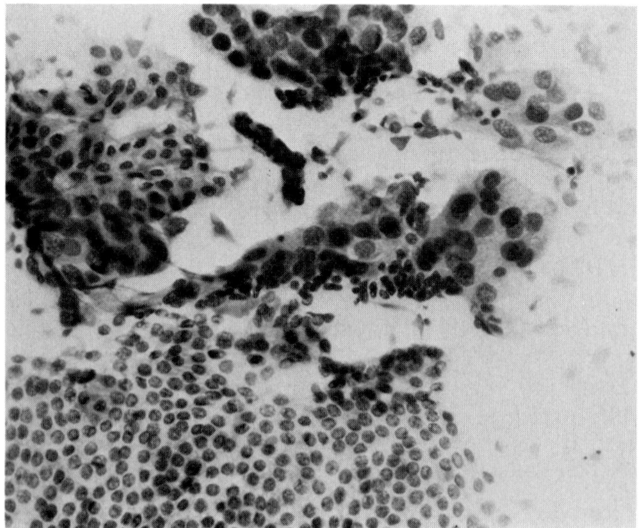

FIGURE 19–12. Prostatic carcinoma and hyperplasia. In the upper half the cells are overlapping, and the nuclei are large and darker staining. At the periphery, the cells are loosely arranged, compared with hyperplasia in the lower half, where the cells are uniform and closely packed. The nuclei are of the same size and shape and vesicular (H & E, original magnification × 150).

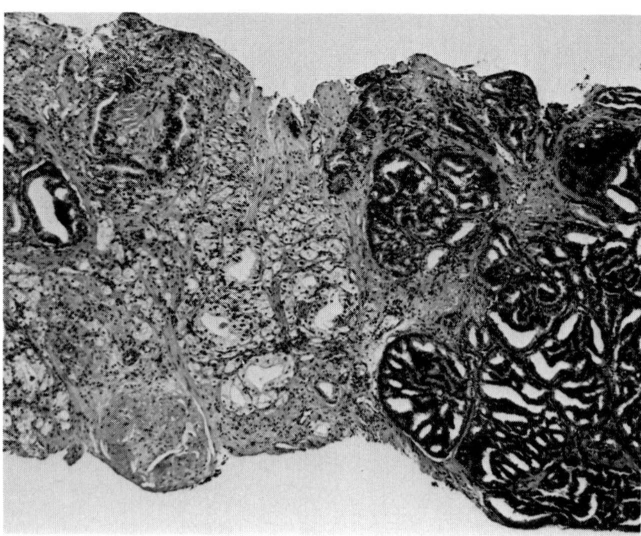

FIGURE 19–13. Prostatic carcinoma showing light and dark staining cells and mixed differentiation, with small acini closely packed in the center and cribriform glands on the sides (H & E, original magnification × 60).

formalin-fixed tissues. In 1936 Gutman and his coworkers described PAP activity at the site of bone metastases from PCa,[65] and later in the serum of patients with metastatic PCa.[64] Thus, PAP became a marker for the detection of metastatic PCa. Huggins and Hodges reported a decrease in serum PAP levels after castration and estrogen therapy.[74] PAP may be elevated in a patient with a large prostate. It is elevated in prostatic infarction, prostatic massage, and prostatitis.

Choe et al were unable to detect positive staining in nonprostatic carcinoma, except for one case of malignant islet cell tumor.[25] Lam et al,[86] Yam et al,[162] and Li et al[87] reported some degree of cross-reactivity expressed by a weakly positive reaction in other organs. Sobin et al reported positive PAP reaction in carcinoids of the rectum.[140] Thus, PAP is of limited value in monitoring progression of metastatic PCa.

Wang et al identified PSA.[156] PSA is a glycoprotein with a molecular weight of 33,000 to 34,000 daltons. It has no subunits but several isomeres. The antigen, as identified, has a pI of 6.9. This is specific for prostatic tissue and PCa.

Sesterhenn et al,[133] using the unlabeled peroxidase-antiperoxidase method,[145] evaluated some 1200 prostates with anti-PAP and anti-PSA in consecutive sections. They reported that in normal and hyperplastic prostates, the prostatic secretory cells lining the prostatic acini, prostatic ducts, and prostatic urethra showed a uniformly strong positive reaction for both PAP and PSA. Transitional epithelium of prostatic ducts and prostatic urethra, the basal cells of prostatic acini, the epithelium of ejaculatory ducts, and the seminal vesicle did not react with either. In well-differentiated PCa, the positive reaction for PAP and PSA was demonstrable in most cells, but the intensity varied. Moderately differentiated tumors revealed a strongly positive reaction in the apical cytoplasm of secretory cells. The reaction was stronger with PAP. Some poorly differentiated PCa's were strongly positive, but a rare tumor was negative for one or the other, and sometimes for both (Figs. 19–14 to 19–16).

Serum levels of PSA are currently being extensively used in the diagnosis and monitoring of patients with PCa. However, it must be noted that the levels of PSA do not always reflect the volume of the tumor.

Murphy reported a new membrane-associated marker defined by a monoclonal antibody called 7E11-C5.[115] He presented a preliminary clinical evaluation and discussed prospects for future development. There is certainly great need for a marker that is truly specific for PCa.

The distribution of keratin expression in PCa depends on the specific subfamily of cytokeratins.[19, 135] In the fetal, infantile, and mature prostates, cytokeratins 5 and 15, recognized by monoclonal antibodies MAB 903 (Enzo Biochemical Company, New York, NY) and MAB 8.12 (Sigma Chemical Company, St. Louis, MO) are expressed in basal cells but not in the luminal secretory cells. In PCa and in benign secretory cells, cytokeratins 8 and 18 are demonstrable. Mammary epithelial membrane antigen is demonstrable in basal cells and some transitional cells of the normal prostate.[139] It is also present in poorly differentiated prostatic acinar carcinomas.

Peanut lectin receptors are demonstrable in most cells of the infant prostate.[11] With maturation, the lectin receptors diminish greatly in number and are predominantly located in basal cells and some secretory cells. Reaction for lectins does not correlate with the presence or intensity of staining for PAP, PSA, or blood group isoantigens. The staining is usually cytoplasmic. Prostatic acinar carcinomas also reveal markedly heterogeneous staining for peanut lectin. The reaction can be seen at the cell surface in a paranuclear "dot" or within the cytoplasm.

Blood group isoantigens can be demonstrated in secretory cells of the prostate as well as in transitional epithelium. The distribution in secretory cells is irregular in normal prostates, indicating a heterogeneous cell population in the normal prostate. CEA is rarely demonstrable in prostatic acinar carcinoma.

Immunoperoxidase staining for *ras* oncogene p21 is a marker that is said to correlate with grade and to have predictive value.[153] BPH did not show any reactivity for *ras* oncogene p21. Reactivity was strongly correlated with nuclear anaplasia but inversely related to glandular differentiation. Viola et al reported immunoreactivity in two of six grade I and four of six grade II tumors, whereas all 17 tumors higher than grade II were invariably positive.[153]

Fan reported an interesting finding.[48] Although only 25 per cent of the cells from the primary lesion expressed *ras* 21 protein, about 90 per cent of the cells from a vertebral metastasis were positive. Wahab and Wright

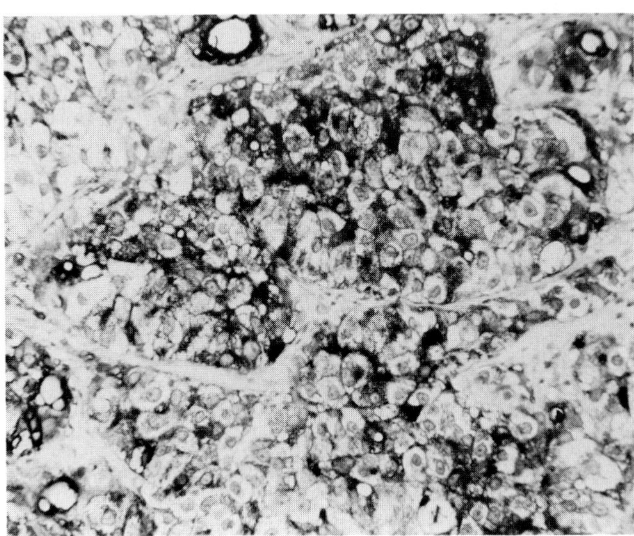

FIGURE 19–15. Same field as Figure 19–14, showing clones of cells with positive reaction for PAP (PAP, original magnification × 100).

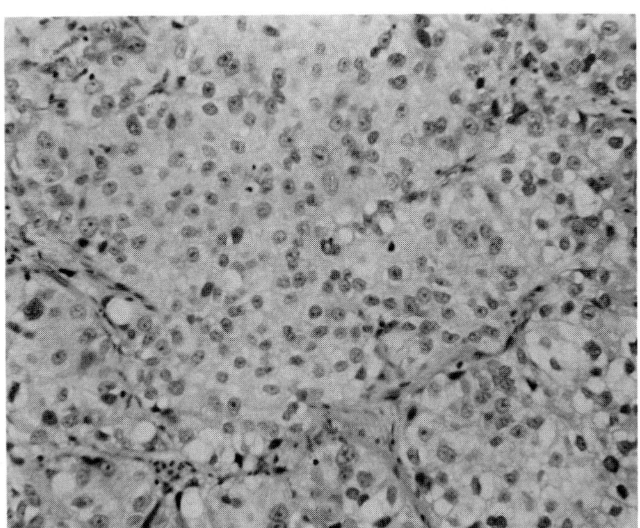

FIGURE 19–14. Undifferentiated prostatic carcinoma. The cytoplasm is pale. The nuclei vary slightly in size and shape. The nucleoli are prominent (H & E, original magnification × 100).

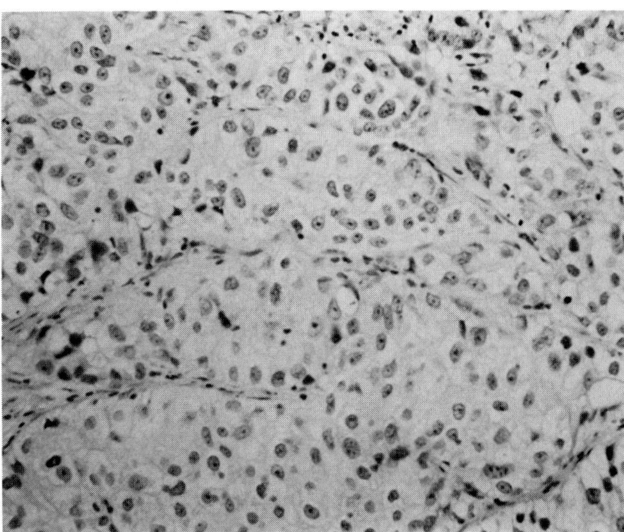

FIGURE 19–16. Same field as Figures 19–14 and 19–15. The cells are negative for PSA. (PSA, original magnification × 100).

reported anti-Leu 7 immunovariability in prostatic epithelial cells.[155] Staining intensity was enhanced, and the percentage of positive cells was higher in BPH and PCa cells but diminished in poorly differentiated PCa. Sheth et al[136] and Doctor et al[38] have found immunoreactor inhibin-like material (ILM) in BPH, where it was localized to the epithelial glandular cells. The intensity of immunoreactivity to ILM decreased from BPH to normal to well-differentiated to poorly differentiated PCa.[38, 136] Brandes has discussed other enzymatic products.[16]

The prostate is a target organ for various receptors.[42, 81, 154, 158, 160] Carcinomas of the prostate respond to hormonal manipulations. Therefore, determinations of androgen receptors are of clinical significance.[1, 42, 120, 124] The presence of estrogen and progesterone receptors, albeit in small numbers, has been identified in cytosols of fresh tissue.[42, 161] Estrogen receptors can be demonstrated by use of fluorescent ligands.[89] Their value and that of other receptors for treatment modalities and prognosis are being explored.[23]

Immunocytochemical studies have revealed that the same PCa cell may produce several different substances, indicative of numerous subsets of cell types. Attempts to correlate the functional status to metastatic potential and metastatic site have been unsuccessful.

Grading of Prostatic Carcinoma

Grading of tumors has been, and continues to be, the pathologist's effort to prognosticate the behavior of tumors. The problems of reproducibility and reliability of grading are well known. The problem is magnified in PCa. PCa's are generally slow-growing tumors. With or without treatment, the patient may live for many years. The tumor presents a wide range of cell types, growth patterns, and degrees of anaplasia. At least 40 grading systems have been proposed but have been found to be unsatisfactory by others.[108]

In an effort to standardize grading systems, Murphy and Whitmore[116] reported that the National Prostatic Cancer Project (NPCP) had recommended that the Gleason system be used with other systems. The Gleason system was proposed in 1966. It recognizes a primary and secondary pattern, and in each, five different patterns. The sum of two constitutes the grade. At the time of NPCP's recommendation, the only reports on the reproducibility, reliability, and utility of the Gleason classification were those of Gleason and associates[58, 60, 61] and Mellinger.[98]

In recommending the Gleason system, Murphy and Whitmore[116] emphasized that the grading systems do not reliably predict the lethal potential of a tumor in an individual patient, nor the responsiveness of an individual to various forms of therapy. They repeatedly cautioned the use of the tumor grade in the individual patient as a basis for treatment decisions. Many urologists, however, have based their treatment on Gleason scores. Gleason 3, 4, and 5 have been regarded as essentially localized tumors, incapable of metastasis.

However, we have seen 50 PCa's with Gleason score 5 or less which showed lymph node metastases without change in the grade of the tumor.

There is considerable literature on the Gleason system, many reports in favor of the system, others against it, and two comprehensive reviews.[62, 106] With one exception,[67] the reports have been on a small number of cases, and none has reported intraobserver or interobserver reproducibility or comparison with any other grading system. Harada et al studied about 1000 cases.[67] They reported that after two tutorials by Gleason, their reproducibility was only 70 per cent. Reproducibility by the same individual on the same slides on two different examinations was 64 per cent for the primary pattern and 44 per cent for the secondary pattern. For the sum of the two, agreement was reached in 38 per cent. According to Murphy and Whitmore,[116] Gleason's own reproducibility was 80 per cent.

Dissatisfaction with the Gleason system has led to modification of the system and proposals for new systems. Pattern 3 has been subdivided into A, B and C, and patterns 4 and 5 into A and B,[60] but the significance of this subdivision is unknown. Four different grading systems have been proposed. All are based on nuclear anaplasia and/or differentiation. In 1975 Mostofi recommended that grading be based on nuclear anaplasia and glandular differentiation. This was accepted by the World Health Organization (WHO) and recommended for international use.[114]

Nuclear anaplasia was defined as variations of nuclear size, shape, and chromatin distribution and the character of the nucleoli. Such variation could be slight (nuclear grade I) (Fig. 19–17), moderate (nuclear grade II) (Fig. 19–18), or marked (nuclear grade III) (Fig. 19–19).

In a study of almost 1000 patients with PCa, Harada et al[67] reported that the death rate for nuclear grade I tumors was 1.24 per cent, for nuclear grade II 4.5 per

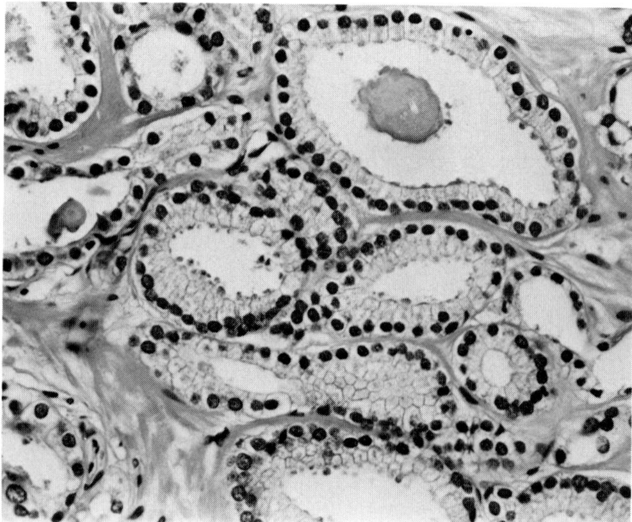

FIGURE 19–17. Prostatic carcinoma, nuclear grade I, showing slight variation in size and shape of glands. Note large and small acini side by side, large acini without convolutions, and acini lined by single layer of cells (H & E, original magnification × 100).

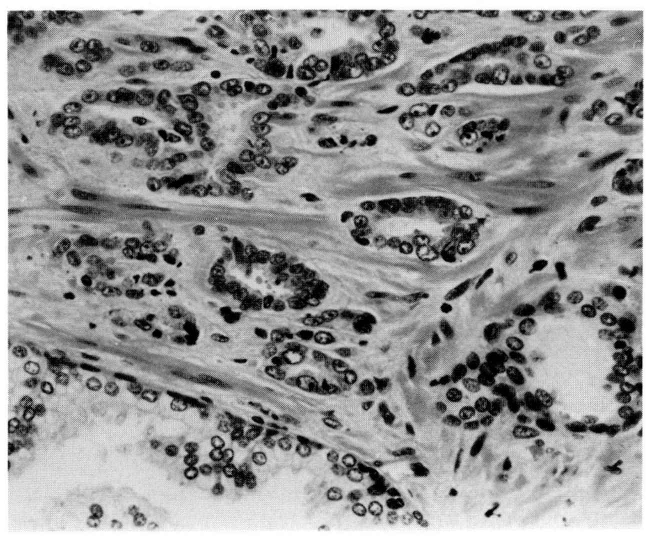

FIGURE 19–18. Prostatic carcinoma, nuclear grade II, showing moderate variation in size and shape of nuclei. Most nuclei have large prominent nucleoli. Note infiltrative growth pattern (H & E, original magnification × 100).

cent, and for nuclear grade III 14.88 per cent. Adding stages (1 to 4) to grades I to III gave the following results: in 191 patients with stage and nuclear grade sum of 2 to 4, the death rate was 0.46 per cent; in 342 with a sum of 5, the death rate was 2.75 per cent; in 357 with a sum of 6, the death rate was 8.53 per cent; in 97 with a sum of 7, the death rate was 25.92 per cent.

Because maturation in the prostate results in the formation of glands, the WHO classification also considers histologic grading based on gland differentiation. Tumors consisting of simple small or simple large glands are considered well differentiated; those with complex glands, fused glands, or glands in glands (cribriform), moderately differentiated; those with few glands, poorly differentiated; and those with columns and cords or solid sheets, undifferentiated.

Harada et al[67] reported that tumors with predominantly simple large or small glands had death rates of 2.67 per cent and 1.18 per cent, respectively. Tumors that consisted primarily of fused glands or glands in glands had rates of 10.4 per cent and 11.1 per cent, respectively. Tumors that consisted principally of columns and cords or solid sheets had a death rate of 18.75 per cent. Expressed numerically, these would be histologic grades 1, 2, 3, and 4, respectively. The two parameters, individually or combined with the clinical stage, have been found to provide good prognostic index.[105, 127, 129, 130]

Schroeder et al[127, 129, 130] evaluated the prognostic significance of 12 histologic and cytologic parameters, correlating each with survival data of 346 patients treated with total prostatectomy. Statistically significant differences in survival rates were found, with only two parameters—glandular differentiation and nuclear anaplasia—confirming the findings of Harada et al.[67]

Boecking et al reported the results of combined histologic grades (degree of differentiation) and cytologic grades (nuclear anaplasia).[13] Four histologic grades and

three nuclear grades were considered. Ratings of 2 and 3 were classified as grade I, 4 and 5 as grade II, and 6 and 7 as grade III. They reported that the prognosis of grade I patients was the same as that of healthy males of the same age. No metastases were seen in grade I patients. The rate of tumor-specific deaths increased with the grade of the tumor. Boecking et al reported that interobserver reproducibility of grading was 91 per cent, where one of the authors graded 100 of the same tumors a month later; his reproducibility for nuclear grade was 75 per cent and for histologic grade was 78 per cent.[13]

Gaeta et al found good correlation between the two parameters and based the final grade on the worse of the two.[55] In 169 cases, six were grade I, with one death. Forty-three were grade II, with 16 deaths. Eighty-three were grade III, with 34 deaths.

Brawn et al proposed a grading system based on differentiation alone.[21] In 84 grade I patients, the 5-year survival rate was 91 per cent; in 75 grade II and III patients, the 5-year survival rate was 60 per cent; for 23 grade IV patients, the 5-year survival rate was 15 per cent. The rate of tumor-specific deaths increased with the grade of the tumor.

Gallee et al compared five grading systems (Broders, Anderson, Mostofi, Gleason, and Mostofi-Schroeder).[56] Grading was performed by five pathologists on 50 prostatectomy specimens. The prognostic impact of the five grading systems (related to both recurrence and death caused by PCa) was judged by the likelihood ratio (LR) test score. For time to recurrence of the Mostofi-Schroeder score, the LR was 6.54 and for the Gleason system it was 1.79. A step-wise procedure demonstrated that the best prognostic performance was reached with the Mostofi-Schroeder and Broders systems used together (with Mostofi-Schroeder weighted 1.5 times larger than Broders).

For time to recurrence the median grading result was

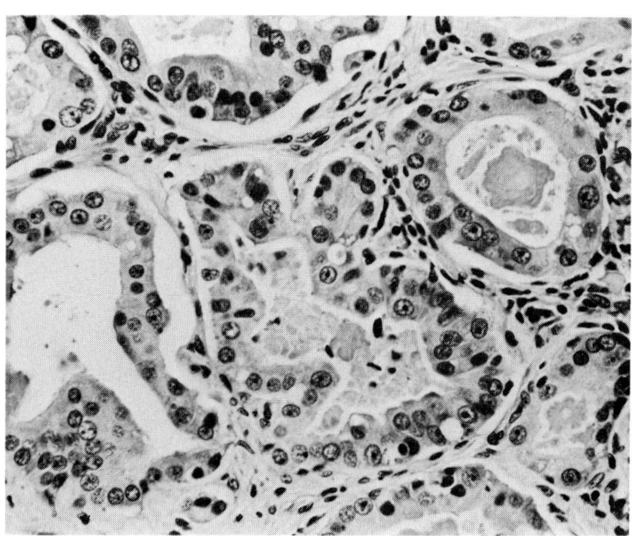

FIGURE 19–19. Prostate cancer, nuclear grade III, showing marked variation in size and shape of nuclei. Most of the nuclei have large nucleoli.

also used, giving results similar to the mean grading result. For time to death from prostatic carcinoma, the LR test scores for all grading systems were relatively low. In this analysis the outcome of the Gleason system showed a minimum of prognostic ability, whereas the Broders and Mostofi-Schroeder systems had a reasonable predictive ability. Because the interobserver variation of the Mostofi-Schroeder system was large, the Broders system is preferable.

The WHO grading system has been adopted by the International Union Against Cancer (UICC)[72] and by the American Joint Committee on Clinical Staging of Tumors.[10] To satisfy this requirement, some centers have labeled Gleason 2, 3, 4, and 5 as well differentiated, Gleason 6, 7 and 8 as moderately differentiated, and 9 and 10 as poorly differentiated. Babaian and Grenow have reported that rearrangement of Gleason scores in three groups did not increase the prognostic impact of the system.[7]

We have presented grading of PCa based entirely on tissue samples. Esposti showed that cytologic grading corresponded well with survival.[46] More recently, Koss et al[83] and Eble and Angermeier have discussed cytologic grading in detail.[40] This system is based primarily on nuclear anaplasia and uses three grades. In grade I tumors the nuclei are slightly enlarged and hyperchromatic, with slight variation in size. A microacinar pattern may be present. In grade II there may be overlapping of cell clusters. The nuclei are enlarged and hyperchromatic with prominent nucleoli. In grade III there is loss of cell cohesiveness and severe nuclear anaplasia and prominent nucleoli. The presence of "rosette-like" structures (see Fig. 19–12) is indicative of glandular differentiation. In addition to the grade of the PCa, the pathologist should comment on the multicentricity, volume, location, and stage of the PCa.

Multicentricity

In a study of 208 total prostatectomy specimens, Byar et al[24] called attention to the multicentricity of PCa's. As many as four or five separate PCa's may be seen in a prostate. The significance of multicentricity is that when a single biopsy is taken, the biopsy may not be representative of all the tumors that are present. Multiple biopsies/biopties would resolve the problem.

Location

Traditionally, it has been known that most PCa's are located in a horseshoe-shaped area in the posterolateral portion of the prostate. This is the area that usually shows atrophy. A number of PCa's occur in the periurethral area and a rare one in the anterior portion.

McNeal has proposed a new anatomic designation for prostate: transition zone, central zone, and peripheral zone.[90] He has indicated that there is a capsule separating transition zone from central zone. Although there is a fibromuscular band in some prostates between the

transition zone and the central zone, most prostates do not show a boundary line between the two. McNeal et al[95] reported that the central zone can be identified by pepsinogen II, but this antibody is not yet commercially available to permit confirmation of McNeal's observations. We have found it difficult to recognize the three zones, particularly the transition zone, in tumor-bearing prostates. From a practical point of view, TUR specimens essentially represent PCa's in the periurethral area (transition zone), whereas needle biopsies represent tumors in the peripheral zone. Obviously, the size of the tumor and the method of surgical approach must be considered in decisions relative to the location of the tumor.

It has been claimed that the transition zone PCa's are essentially nonaggressive tumors. They rarely invade periprostatic tissue, whereas peripheral zone tumors are more aggressive and tend to invade periprostatic tissues. These observations are not surprising because, by their mere location, tumors in the posterolateral portion are likely to invade periprostatic tissue regardless of their size or degree of differentiation. On the other hand, tumors in the periurethral area have a long distance to travel to reach periprostatic areas, but a short distance to invade the prostatic urethra or the bladder neck. The subject will be discussed further.

Volume

It has been recognized for a long time that small tumors are less likely to invade and metastasize than large tumors. In fact, clinical staging of cancers is almost entirely based on the size of the tumor. McNeal has reported that PCa's less than 4 cc in volume appear protected from extensive capsule penetration, positive surgical margins, seminal vesicle invasion, and lymph node metastases.[90] Conversely, PCa's larger than 12 cc in size were a nearly homogeneous group in which all of the adverse determinations tended to be positive. All but two cases of this volume had positive surgical margins, and multiple positive margins were found in one half of the cases. Six of eight positive bladder neck margins were in this group. Positive margins were much less frequent in cancers smaller than 12 cc, and almost all were in this group. At 4 to 12 cc, margins were often in areas of capsule penetration, whereas cancers less than 4 cc had margins produced mainly by surgical incision into the prostate. We have observed seminal vesicle involvement in one and extraprostatic extension in four patients whose tumor volume was less than 1.35 cc. However, large tumors may remain confined to the prostate without periprostatic extension, seminal vesicle involvement, or lymph node metastases.

Prostatic Capsule

A number of references in the literature discuss the importance of the prostatic capsule and its role in progression of PCa. The existence of a distinct prostatic capsule has been questioned. Ayala et al, studying cross-sections of whole-organ sections of the prostatectomy specimen, reported that the capsule was made up of a band of concentrically placed fibromuscular tissue that was an inseparable component of the prostatic stroma.[5] The space was sparse in glandular elements, particularly in the anterior portion, and the outer fibromuscular layer was no longer present. They concluded that the prostate does not have a true capsule, but only an outer fibromuscular band. Thus, this is the structure that is referred to as the capsule.

Byar et al[24] reported on the stages of capsular involvement; the tumor may extend to the capsule (20 per cent), it may invade but not penetrate the capsule (35 per cent), or it may penetrate the capsule or through the capsule (16 per cent). Penetration of the capsule is a late phenomenon and is indicative of a poor prognosis.

PATHOLOGIC STAGING

There are two different clinical staging systems: the ABCD system used in many clinics in the United States, the TNM system proposed by the International Union Against Cancer (UICC)[72] and adopted by the American Joint Committee on Clinical Stage Classification (AJC).[10] Stage A is applied to PCa found in tissues removed for BPH; stage B to tumors confined to the prostate; stage C to tumors that have extended outside the prostate; and stage D to metastatic tumor. Each is further subdivided into 1, 2, or 3. In essence, these are clinical estimates of the local status of the PCa.

A new TNM system has been proposed.[128] The primary tumor is categorized as T1, T2, T3, or T4, depending on local extension, and each is further divided into two or three categories. In this classification, lymph node metastasis is categorized as N and distant metastasis as M, both with numerical subcategories.[128] Pathologic staging is based on the clinical staging, and it is designated pT. The following stages are recognized:

pTX—Primary tumor cannot be assessed.

pTO—No evidence of primary tumor.

pT1—Clinically inapparent tumor, not palpable or visible by imaging.

pT1a—Tumor an incidental histologic finding in 5 per cent or less of tissue resected.

pT1b—Tumor an incidental histologic finding in more than 5 per cent of tissue resected.

pT1c—Tumor identified by needle biopsy (e.g., because of elevated serum PSA).

pT2—Tumor is confined within the prostate.

pT2a—Tumor involves half of the lobe or less.

pT2b—Tumor involves more than half of a lobe, but not both lobes.

pT2c—Tumor involves both lobes.

pT3—Tumor extends through the prostate capsule.

pT3a—Unilateral extracapsular extension.

pT3b—Bilateral extracapsular extension.

pT3c—Tumor invades seminal vesicles(s).

pT4—Tumor is fixed or invades adjacent structures other than seminal vesicles.

pT4a—Tumor invades bladder neck and/or external sphincter and/or rectum.

pT4b—Tumor invades levator muscles and/or is fixed to the pelvic wall.

A similar system is used for regional lymph node metastases.

Pathologic staging can best be done in total prostatectomy specimens, but the urologist often desires staging of biopsy/biopty specimens because it affects the clinical management of the patient. In the ABCD system, if the tumor is found in three pieces or less, if it constitutes less than 5 per cent of the tissue, and if it is low grade, it is classified a stage A1. If it is in more than three pieces or constitutes more than 5 per cent of the tissue or is high grade, it is A2. Correa et al reported that 8 per cent of stage A1 tumors showed progression but no deaths, compared with 63 per cent recurrence and 25 per cent deaths in stage A2 tumors.[28] If the biopsy/biopty is taken from both sides, the urologist desires information on whether the tumor is confined to one side (B1) or if it is present on both sides (B2).

Stage A1 (T1a) tumors have generally been regarded as insignificant and not requiring further treatment. Epstein et al reported on 94 stage A tumors with a follow-up of up to 18 years.[45] Twenty-six patients died of unrelated causes in less than 4 years without progression. Eighteen died between 4 and 18 years after diagnosis without evidence of progression. Forty-two patients remained free of progression at 8 to 18 years. Eight showed progression, indicating that some stage A low-grade tumors have the potential to progress. The transformation rate is variable but has been calculated to take roughly 7 years.[159]

In a later study, Epstein et al reported that 18 of 21 patients who had prostatectomy for stage A tumors had residual tumor.[44] In 13 of these the residual tumor was small, 5 had substantial residual tumors, and only 3 had no tumor. This observation suggests that the available tissues on which the diagnoses of stage A were made were not true representations. Soloway and Altwein have reported that a repeat TUR in incidental PCa offers little information and may complicate subsequent therapy, e.g., radical prostatectomy.[141]

In needle biopsies/biopties Dhom[32] suggested three groups—group 1 tumors constituting less than 10 per cent of the tissue; group 2 tumors constituting more than 10 per cent but less than 100 per cent; and group 3 constituting 100 per cent of the tissue. These three features—multicentricity, location, and volume—are best detected by proper examination of total prostatectomy specimens.

EXAMINATION OF PATHOLOGIC TISSUES

Because clinical diagnosis and management of the patients with PCa depend to such a large extent on pathologic diagnosis, standardization of pathologic processing and reporting of the tissue becomes imperative.

Biopsy/Biopty Tissues. The tissue obtained by biopsy/biopty can be fixed and embedded routinely, but the sections should not exceed 5 mm in thickness. In small pieces of tissue, understandably, pathologists desire several levels of the tissue. It is advisable to mount these on different slides so that extra sections of the biopty are available if a second opinion is necessary, or if the patient is to be transferred to another center for definitive treatment.

Transurethral Tissues. Ideally, all the tissues should be embedded and examined. However, in most laboratories limitation of resources makes this ideal unattainable. The tissue should be weighed, and pieces that are granular and/or dry should be selected for sectioning. At least four cassettes should be sent through, and the remaining tissue saved. If the examined sections show PCa, additional sections should be examined.

Total Prostatectomy Specimens. The specimen should be weighed and measured. To maintain shape, the specimen should be suspended by the seminal vesicles in adequate amounts of buffered formalin. Different colored ink should be used for the left and right halves and corresponding adnexal structures. We use black ink for the anterior midline and left lateral margins. Step-serial sections should be cut at 2.5 mm. Thinner sections are difficult to embed, and sections thicker than 3 mm miss small tumors and may not be comparable to NMR levels.

Three-dimensional computerized reconstruction of the sections is the easiest method to provide accurate and reliable information about the multicentricity, location, and volume of the tumor and the location and relationship of premalignant foci to the PCa. The advantage of three-dimensional computerized reconstruction is that the specimen can be viewed from several angles to give better information about the position and location of the tumors and correlation with imaging findings.

If facilities are not available for large sections, the slices may be cut into four pieces, labeled, and sectioned. Ideally, all sections should be examined, but if facilities are missing, the section from the posterolateral area (particularly the apex) should be sent through.

CYTOLOGY SPECIMENS

Esposti must be credited with renewal of interest in needle aspiration cytology use in PCa.[46] The introduction of the Franzen 22-gauge needle has facilitated and popularized the application of the procedure in PCa.[53]

Esposti,[46] Koss et al,[83] and Eble and Angermeier[46] have discussed in detail the proper method of obtaining cytologic samples, their preparation and interpretation. All three require training and experience, especially the interpretation. Mohler et al have demonstrated that the 22-gauge needle secures not only cytologic samples but tissue for histologic study.[101]

CORRELATION OF BIOPSY/BIOPTY WITH TOTAL PROSTATECTOMY SPECIMENS

A suspicious digital rectal examination or an ultrasound-detected hypoechoic area may lead to pathologic diagnosis of PCa. The patient may then be subjected to radiation therapy or total prostatectomy. If the latter, routine pathologic examination may not show any PCa. In such cases, more detailed examination of the total prostatectomy specimen, including the site of the biopsy/biopty and, as stated earlier, step-section of the specimen at 2.5-mm intervals must be carried out. Any tumor less than 3 mm may not be found in routine sections. We have seen a number of cases in which total prostatectomy specimens showed only a PCa that was less than a single low-power view. These prostates usually show areas of premalignant change.

PREMALIGNANT LESIONS

The subject has received considerable attention recently, probably because of the introduction of ultrasonography in the examination of the prostate. Epithelial and glandular abnormalities in cancer-bearing prostates have been known for a long time and variously designated. These generally fall into two categories, those in which there is anaplasia of intra-acinar secretory epithelium and those in which there is new gland formation. These two distinct categories are often confused.

In the first category the changes are confined to intra-acinar secretory cells, but there is no new gland formation. This category has been variously designated as precancerous lesion,[33, 51, 91, 100, 104, 110, 118, 122] hyperplasia with malignant change,[107, 110] carcinoma in situ,[146, 151] dysplasia,[79] intraductal dysplasia with three grades,[94] ductal acinar dysplasia with three grades,[92] large acinar atypical hyperplasia,[85] and prostatic intraepithelial neoplasia.[14]

As in the bladder and the cervix, the term *dysplasia* has caused much confusion. It was originally introduced into the prostatic vocabulary by Kastendieck et al.[79] They subsequently dropped the term (1980). McNeal and Bostwick resurrected the term and divided it into three grades.[94] Bostwick and Brawer, using the same criteria, definitions, and grading, substituted prostatic intraepithelial neoplasia with three grades.[14] Kastendieck and Helpap have reviewed the situation in detail.[80] Drago et al[39] reported that the International Conference sponsored by the American Cancer Society recommended that the term *dysplasia* be dropped and that *prostatic intraepithelial neoplasia* (PIN) be used for these lesions and graded high and low grade, the former including grades 2 and 3 of Bostwick and Brawer and low grade for PIN 1.

We have difficulty in recognizing low-grade PIN unless it is concomitant with low-grade PCa. We limit the diagnosis of PIN to lesions in which the intra-acinar cells are identical to those of PCa cells, except that the cells are still inside the acini.

PIN, as defined by us, has a characteristic appearance (Figs. 19–20 and 19–21). The area stands out as a group of pre-existing, generally large acini or ducts that are more cellular than the adjacent hyperplastic glands. The cells are usually large. There is generally intra-acinar growth of cells, resulting in piling up of the epithelium. Occasionally, however, the lining cells may be one or two layers thick. The characteristic feature is the change in the nuclei. They are large and may vary in shape. The nuclei are vacuolated and contain one or more large nucleoli. Viewed by themselves, the cells are indistinguishable from nuclear grade 2 or 3 PCa, but in PIN, by definition, the changes are confined to the acini or ducts. The basal layer may be continuous or discontinuous.

PIN, as defined by us, stands out in the section as a cellular area, usually with large acini. It is characterized as an intra-acinar proliferation of secretory cells that show nuclear anaplasia. The neoplastic secretory cells are indistinguishable from PCa cells and show varying degrees of nuclear anaplasia, similar to those seen in PCa. The involved secretory cells are partly or completely surrounded by a layer of basal cells and/or intact basement membranes. There is no new gland formation.

PIN, as thus defined, is closely associated with invasive PCa, either next to it or elsewhere in the prostate. Kovi and Mostofi[85] reported that in patients under the age of 60, the association of PIN with invasive PCa was 87 per cent. The prevalence of PIN in cancerous glands decreased with age. In step sections and three-dimensional reconstruction, we have demonstrated that PIN is located in the peripheral zone in 68.8 per cent of cases. In 2.6 per cent, it occurred in the inner zone, and in 28.6 per cent it was evenly distributed and associated closely with PCa, but it occurred elsewhere in the

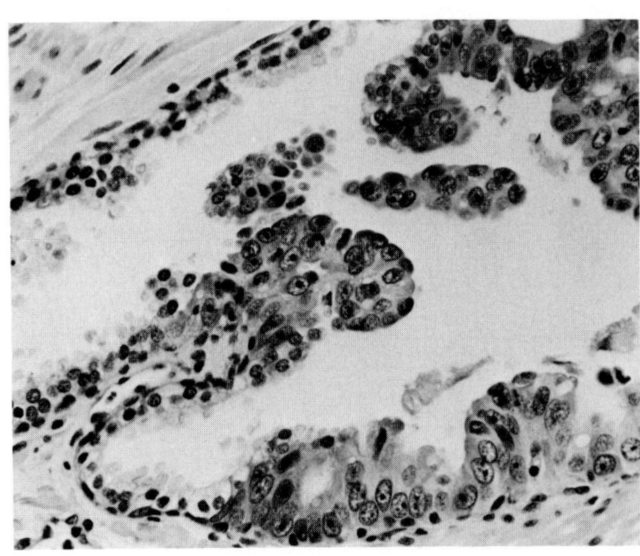

FIGURE 19–21. Prostatic intraepithelial neoplasia. Benign secretory cells alternating with markedly anaplastic cells. Compared with hyperplasia, the nuclei are large and contain large nucleoli (H & E, original magnification × 160).

prostate as well. This distribution corresponds to that of PCa.

In most cases the immunopathologic reactions of PIN are identical to the accompanying PCa. The proliferation rate of the PIN, as determined by ³H thymidine,[69] and study of nucleolar organizing regions (AGNORs) show that PIN is close to PCa.[119, 132]

The relationship of PIN to prostatic carcinoma involves their frequent association, identical location, cytologic resemblance, immunopathologic reactions, and proliferation rate. These observations indicate that PIN is a preinvasive stage of some PCa's—a carcinoma in situ. However, the natural history of PIN and whether all PINs progress to invasive PCa are unknown. There is certainly need for research in this area.

The second category of premalignant changes is variously designated as atypical hyperplasia[4, 57, 69, 84, 102, 110, 146] or atypical adenomatous hyperplasia.[9] These refer to aggregations of small glands lined by a single layer of secretory cells (i.e., absence of basal cell layer). In such cases, the differential diagnosis is small acinar PCa or microacinar hyperplasia. When the glands are closely aggregated with no suggestion of stromal dispersion, which characterizes infiltrating PCa, and the individual cells are completely normal in appearance, we classify the group as microacinar hyperplasia. When there is any doubt about whether or not either of the two features (invasive dispersion and/or nuclear anaplasia) is present, the lesion is classified as atypical glands (Fig. 19–22). This category probably is a precursor of small acinar well-differentiated PCa, with which it is often confused.

Brawn introduced the term *adenosis*, which he defined as a dysplastic glandular proliferation containing (1) mild nuclear pleomorphism of the prostate gland and/or (2) atypia of the growth pattern of the prostate gland.[20] A mild degree of nuclear pleomorphism, including nu-

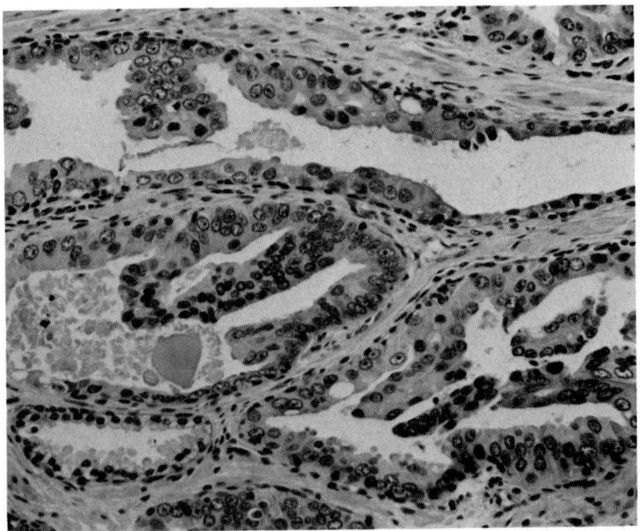

FIGURE 19–20. Prostatic intraepithelial neoplasia. The acini have preserved basal cells. The secretory epithelium shows moderate anaplasia. There is piling up of epithelium with papillary formation in the lumen. Note that in one area the acini are lined by atrophic epithelium (H & E, original magnification × 100).

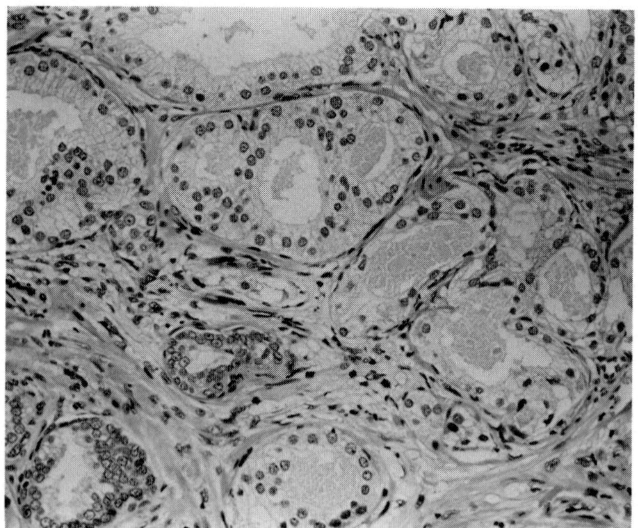

FIGURE 19–22. Atypical glands consisting of small and cribriform acini. The nuclei show some variation in size and shape but no nucleoli or vacuolization (H & E, original magnification × 100).

cleoli, has been regarded as adenosis when the pleomorphism is confined to circumscribed collections of glands. An infiltrating pattern of prostate glands is accepted as adenosis when the infiltrating glands are lined by columnar cells with benign nuclei. In practice, the term *adenosis* seems to be applied to any lesion that presents some difficulty to the pathologist and ranges from well-differentiated PCa to hyperplasia. We do not use the term.

In neither prostatic intraepithelial neoplasia nor atypical glands, "atypical adenomatous hyperplasia," do we know the interval between the discovery of these lesions and development of a clinical PCa. Whenever either PIN or atypical glands are seen in a needle biopsy or TUR specimen, additional sections should be studied to find possible PCa, and the urologist should be alerted that the patient may have PCa elsewhere or may develop it later. Careful follow-up of those below the age of 60 is indicated.

TREATMENT EFFECTS

Various nonsurgical modalities are used in treating PCa. A great deal is known about their pathology.[52, 110]

Estrogen Therapy. In responding cells, the nuclei are reduced in size by about 50 per cent, condensation of chromatin and pyknosis of nuclei are seen, and the nucleoli are lost or very small. Vacuolization of cytoplasm is an early finding. Coalescence of vacuoles results in rupture of the cell membrane (Fig. 19–23). PAP and PSA may be seen in the cells. The non-neoplastic portion shows atrophy of glandular epithelium, squamous metaplasia of the ducts, and varying degrees of hyperplasia of basal cells. Stromal fibrosis is present.

Radiation Therapy. The nuclei are enlarged, chromatin is clumped, and nuclei are pyknotic and sometimes bizarre. The cytoplasm shows vacuolization and

rupture of cell membranes (Fig. 19–24).[82] The tumor-free portions show atrophy of secretory epithelium, squamous metaplasia, and nuclear atypia. There may be multinucleated bizarre cells. The stroma may show degeneration of smooth muscle cells, edema, proliferation of fibroblasts, and hyalinization.[82]

The effects of radiation on the cytoplasm and DNA may be direct or indirect. A radiated cell may divide one or more times before all progeny have lost the capacity to divide. The cell may suffer no damage or may die. It may survive but be unable to divide or may produce unusual forms.

Alken et al provided a comprehensive study of tissue alterations.[3] Alken performed biopsies on patients receiving treatment, and these biopsies were studied by Dhom and Drego.[35] Their classic work, confirmed by Helpap[71] and Boecking and Auffermann,[12] has clarified the situation. Mostofi et al have called attention to the development of squamous and sarcomatoid carcinomas after prolonged treatment.[111]

Histologic changes after antiandrogen therapy essentially are similar to radiation changes. There may be massive tumor cell loss, but some areas may show little or no change (Fig. 19–25*A* and *B*).

It is sometimes difficult for a pathologist to be certain about the viability and biologic potential of treated PCa, especially after radiation therapy. An ultrasound-directed rebiopsy some months later usually resolves the problem.

Siders and Lee reported that ultrasound-guided biopsies of hypoechoic areas of 125 PCa patients treated by definitive radiation revealed that 71.2 per cent had persistent carcinoma.[137] They reported change in DNA ploidy and grade. Following radiation therapy, 30.6 per cent of pretreatment diploid tumors were found to be aneuploid after treatment. Similarly, there was a 24 per cent increase in the number of poorly differentiated tumors following therapy. They observed that a number

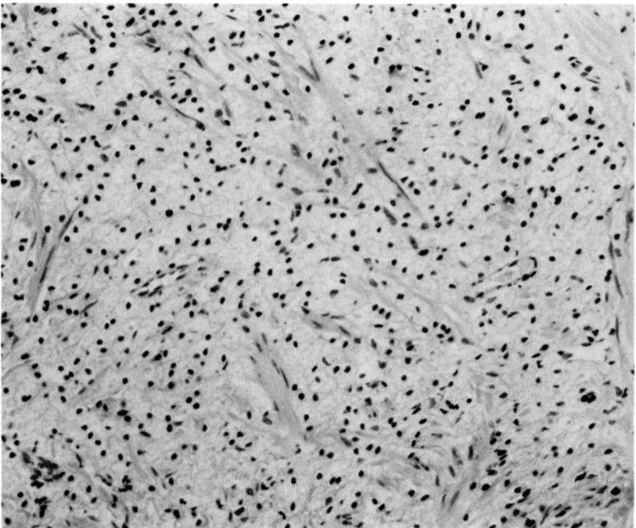

FIGURE 19–23. Estrogen-treated prostatic carcinoma showing vacuolization of cytoplasm, loss of cell borders, and pyknosis of nuclei (H & E, original magnification × 100).

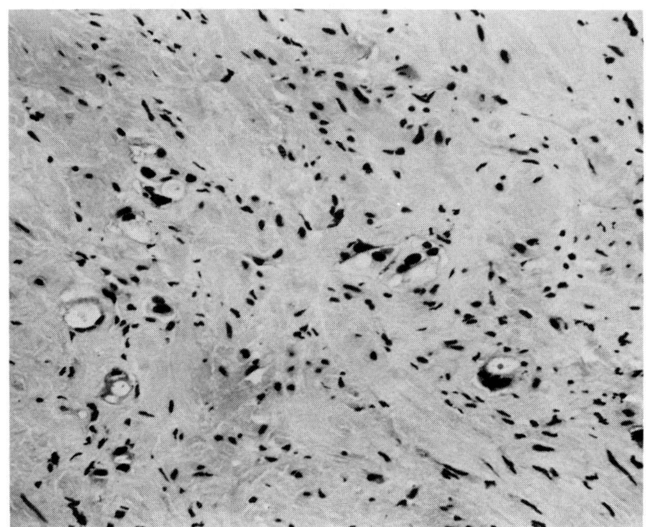

FIGURE 19–24. Irradiated prostatic carcinoma showing tumor cells with vacuolated cytoplasm, loss of cell borders, and pyknotic and bizarre nuclei (H & E, original magnification × 100).

of patients with persistent postradiation carcinoma, but with clinically localized disease, may be cured by subsequent surgery. Salvage radical prostatectomy found localized cancer in 16 of 20 patients. They claimed that transrectal ultrasonography for early detecting and staging was crucial for patient selection for definitive salvage therapy. The final outcome in this group was not reported.

SPECIAL TYPES OF PROSTATIC CARCINOMA

As mentioned earlier, PCa presents several growth patterns. One pattern deserves discussion, as it has been the source of some confusion.

Small Acinar PCa. This type of PCa has been the subject of misinterpretation and confusion with certain hyperplasias. The subject has been discussed in detail by Kovi[84] and Srigley.[142]

In small acinar PCa the glands are uniformly small, round, or slightly ovoid. They are lined by a single layer of high cuboidal or low columnar cells. The basal layer is absent. The cytoplasm varies from pale and finely vacuolated to granular or eosinophilic or amphophilic. In most cases, the nuclei are fairly uniform, but there may be some variation in size and shape of nuclei. The nuclei may be vacuolated and show large nucleoli (Fig. 19–26). However, the nuclei may be hyperchromatic without any apparent nucleolus. The glands have an infiltrating growth pattern splitting the fibromuscular stroma. They have no relationship to a duct. The histologic features of microacinar hyperplasia and PCa are discussed later.

Endometrioid Carcinoma. Melicow and Pachter[96] and Melicow and Tannenbaum[97] described endometrioid PCa. Two categories were identified. In one, the glands are lined by tall columnar epithelium with vacuolated

cytoplasm and single or double layers of nuclei (Fig. 19–27). In the other, the cells are cuboidal, often piled, and the cytoplasm is granular. We have seen this papillary growth pattern elsewhere in the prostate in cystic areas. The "endometrioid pattern" is almost invariably associated with typical PCa, and the cells react positively with PAP and PSA. We consider this tumor to be a different growth pattern of PCa.

Mucinous Adenocarcinoma. Some luminal mucin is present in many PCa's, but rarely the tumor may consist entirely of mucinous adenocarcinoma (Fig. 19–28), raising the possibility of secondary carcinoma. The true nature of the lesion can be readily identified by PAP and PSA, both of which are positive.

Transitional and Squamous Cell Carcinoma. Rarely, a prostatic biopsy may reveal a transitional or squamous cell carcinoma. Before such cell types can be accepted as a primary PCa, a clinically undetected carcinoma in situ or an infiltrating carcinoma of the bladder neck

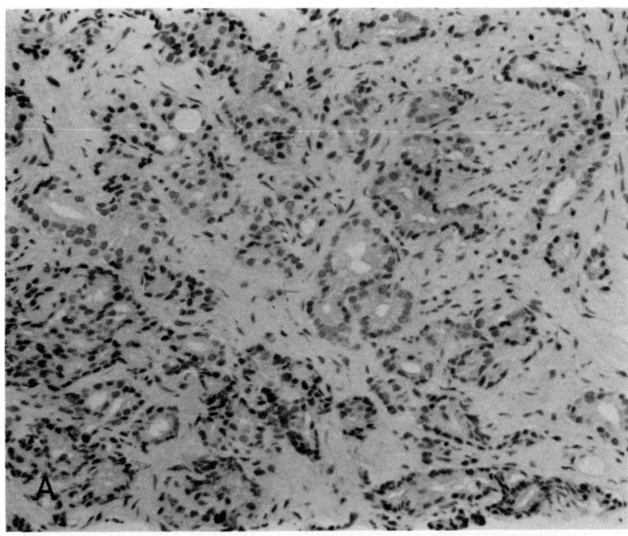
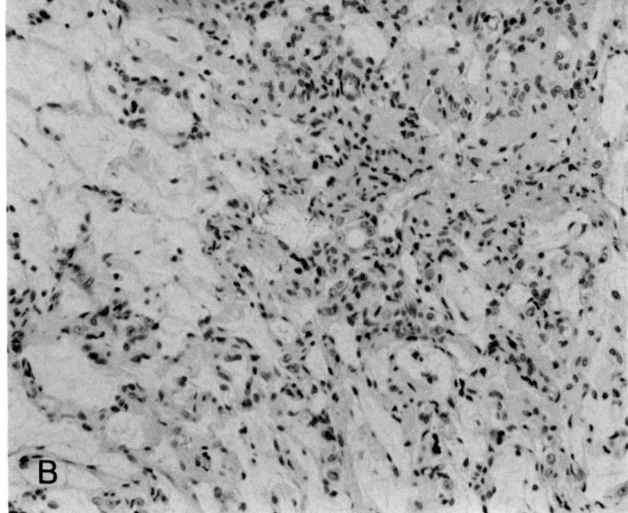

FIGURE 19–25. *A,* Well-differentiated and moderately differentiated prostatic carcinoma. This is prior to treatment (H & E, original magnification × 100). *B,* Antiandrogen therapy changes consisting of massive necrosis of the neoplastic cells. Note persistence of viable cells (H & E, original magnification × 100).

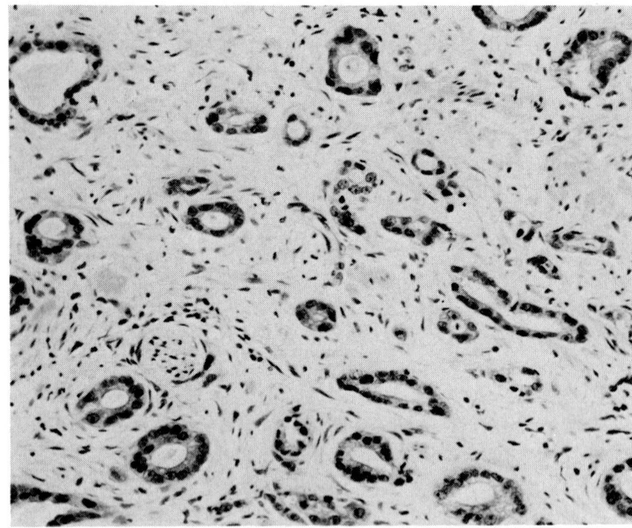

FIGURE 19–26. Microacinar prostatic carcinoma showing dispersion of small acini. Several large acini are seen. Note pointed edges of acini (H & E, original magnification × 100).

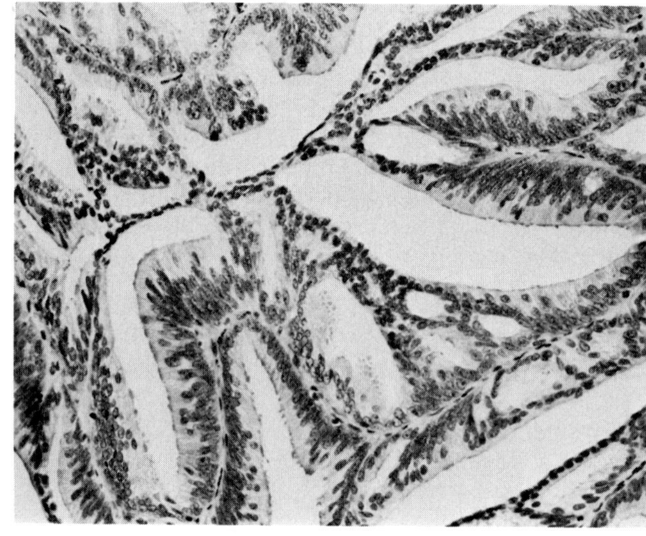

FIGURE 19–27. "Endometrioid carcinoma" showing large acini lined by columnar epithelial cells with basal nuclei (H & E, original magnification × 100).

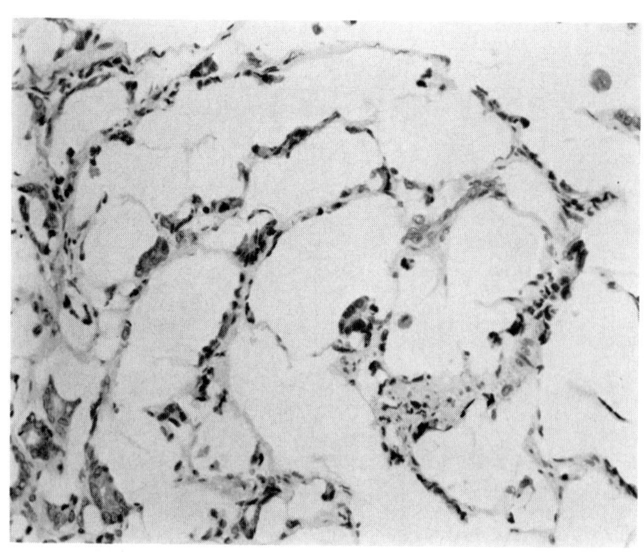

FIGURE 19–28. Mucinous prostatic carcinoma showing groups of tumor cells and lakes of mucin (H & E, original magnification × 100).

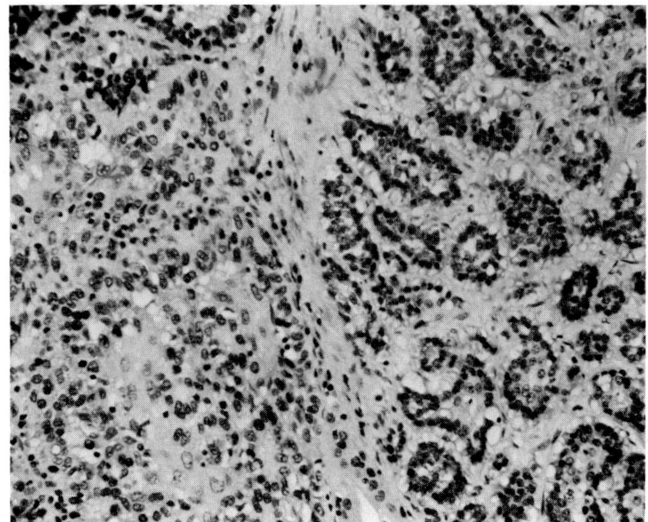

FIGURE 19–29. Basal cell carcinoma. On the right side the tumor mimics basal cell hyperplasia. On the left side the tumor consists of sheets of primitive tumor cells (H & E, original magnification × 100).

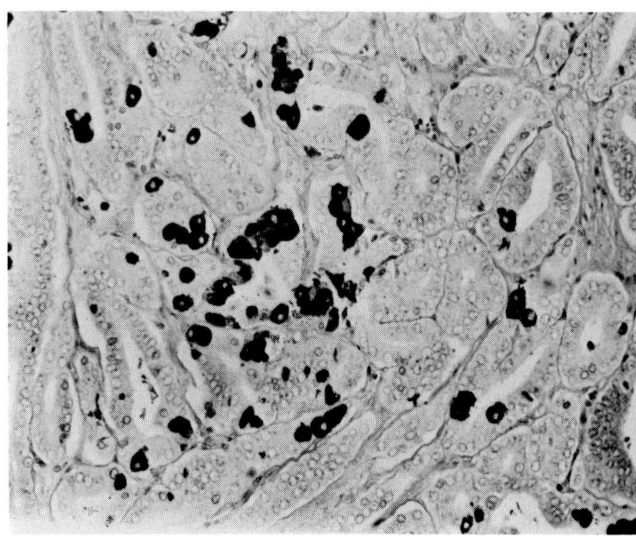

FIGURE 19–31. Same field as Figure 19–30, showing a number of tumor cells with positive silver staining (silver stain, original magnification × 100).

should be ruled out. Such tumors have a tendency to grow along the prostatic ducts from the prostatic urethra deep into the posterior lobe and be mistaken initially for a PCa.

Basal Cell Carcinoma. A rare variant of carcinoma is derived from basal cells and, histologically, it shows the typical pattern of basal cell hyperplasia, plus solid sheets of poorly differentiated cells with mitoses and tumor necrosis (Fig. 19–29). There may be focal areas of squamous, transitional, and acinar differentiation. If these features are equivocal, recognition of basal cell carcinoma can be made by extraprostatic invasion by the tumor.

Adenoid Cystic Carcinoma. Most, if not all, the reported cases of adenoid cystic carcinoma are variants of basal cell hyperplasia. If there is no anaplasia of cells,

there is associated basal cell hyperplasia, and the lesion is intraprostatic, it is not adenoid cystic carcinoma. To date, we have not seen a true case of adenoid cystic PCa.

Neuroendocrine Tumors. A prostatic tumor may show a few endocrine cells or may consist entirely of carcinoid cells (Figs. 19–30 and 19–31) or small oat cell–like tumors (Fig. 19–32).[1, 23, 29, 37, 154, 157] These tumors are capable of producing many endocrine and other substances. Neuroendocrine substances demonstrated in PCa cells are serotonin, neuron-specific enolase, chromogranin, thyroid-stimulating hormones, adrenocorticotropic hormone, calcitonin, and others. In all such cases, PAP and PSA are valuable in determining prostatic origin of the tumor. Recognition of neuroendocrine cells may be clinically important, because resistance to treat-

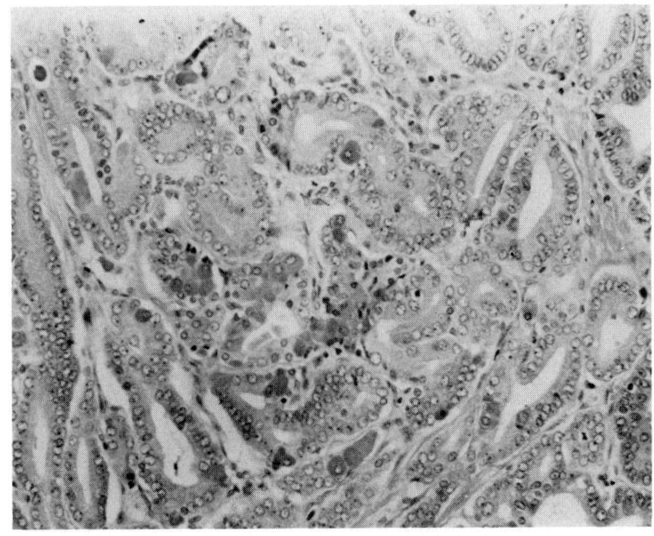

FIGURE 19–30. Prostatic carcinoma showing isolated endocrine cells with dark granular cytoplasm (H & E, original magnification × 100).

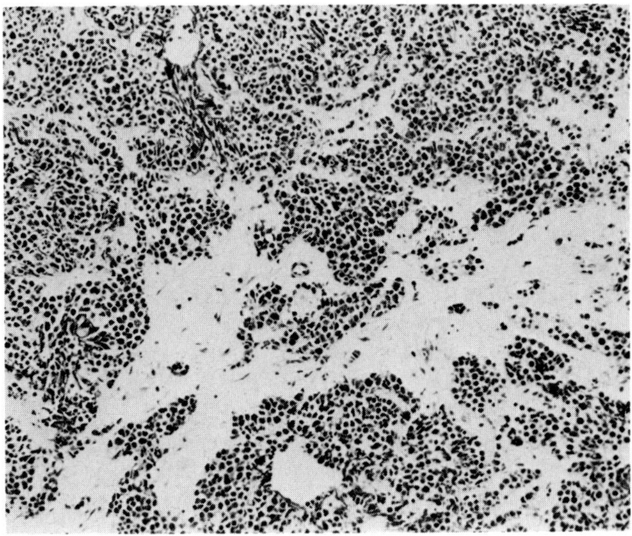

FIGURE 19–32. Prostatic carcinoma, small cell types (H & E, original magnification × 100).

ment may be due to the presence of these cells. It should be noted that neuroendocrine activity is not limited to oat cell tumors but may be present in hexagonal cells.

Cohen et al have reported that of 22 stage B patients, 4 died of the disease.[27] Three of them were positive for neuroendocrine cells. Of 20 stage C patients, 5 died of the disease, and all 5 were positive for neuroendocrine cells. Of 48 patients with stage D disease, 37 died of tumors; 34 of them were positive for neuroendocrine cells. They claimed that this prognostic factor was significantly superior to the Gleason grading system. The findings have not been confirmed yet; however, because these cells have a paracrine function, the observation of Cohen et al seems to have considerable merit.

PITFALLS IN PATHOLOGIC DIAGNOSIS OF PROSTATIC CARCINOMA

A number of benign lesions may simulate PCa.[15, 35, 110, 112, 113, 163] These may be intraprostatic or extraprostatic. Intraprostatic lesions include atrophy, variants of hyperplasia, inflammatory lesions, and iatrogenic changes. Extraprostatic structures include seminal vesicles, Cowper's gland, and nephrogenic adenoma.

Intraprostatic Lesions

Atrophy is the most frequently misdiagnosed benign lesion of the prostate. Two types of atrophy have been described, simple atrophy and sclerosing atrophy. In simple atrophy the glands are small and have a lobular arrangement around a collapsed duct. They are lined by a single layer of epithelium. The nuclei are small and darkly staining. The cells have very little cytoplasm (Fig. 19–33). The nuclei appear close together as in a string of pearls. The fibromuscular stroma shows some atrophy. In sclerosing atrophy, the stroma shows sclerosis.

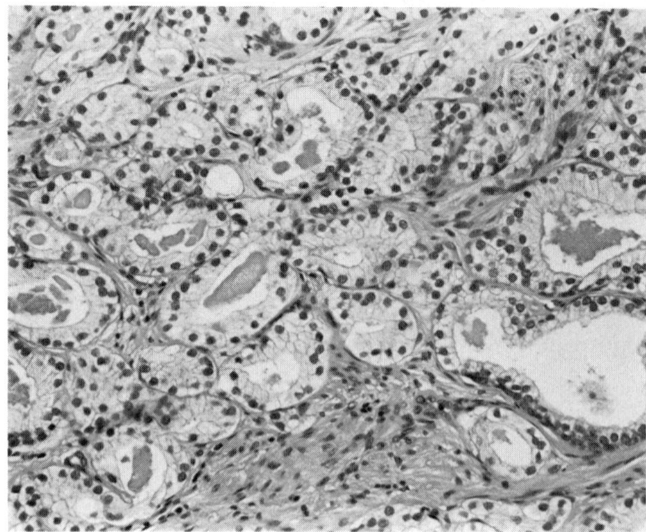

FIGURE 19–34. Microacinar hyperplasia: small acini lined by normal secretory cells with small regular nuclei without any anaplasia. The acini are closely packed (H & E, original magnification × 100).

In contrast, in PCa the epithelial cells usually have considerable cytoplasm, the nuclei are larger, and the chromatin distribution is coarse. The nuclei are vacuolated and there may be a prominent nucleolus.

Variants of Hyperplasia

Florid glandular hyperplasia is usually nodular and consists of large numbers of simple or complex glands with little intervening stroma. In addition to large numbers of closely packed glands, the basal layer is absent in some of the glands. However, the nuclei are small and uniform and the nucleoli are either absent or small.

Microacinar hyperplasia (Fig. 19–34) consists of simple small glands, which are frequently located at the

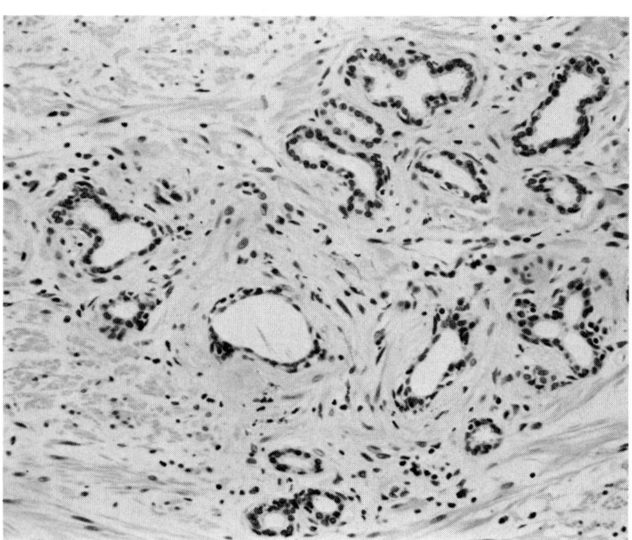

FIGURE 19–33. Atrophy of prostate showing collapsed acini lined by a layer of small cells with small dark-staining nuclei (H & E, original magnification × 100).

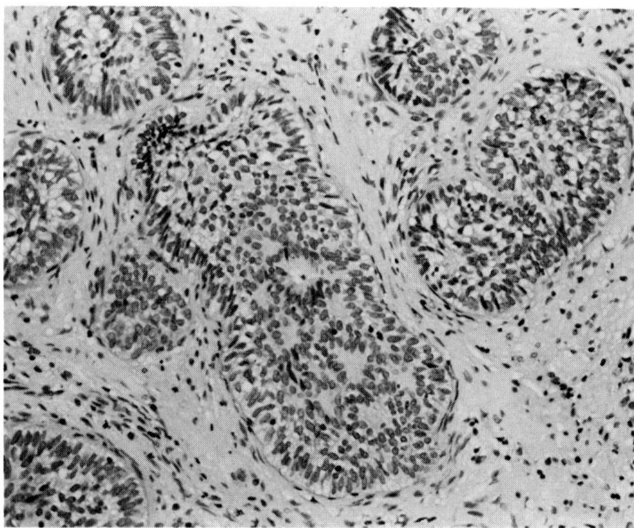

FIGURE 19–35. Basal cell hyperplasia with minimal focal secretory differentiation (H & E, original magnification × 100).

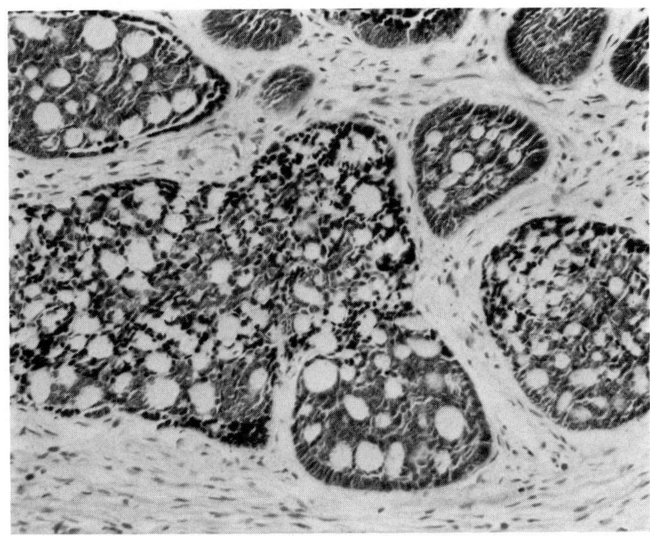

FIGURE 19–36. Basal cell hyperplasia with adenoid cystic pattern (H & E, original magnification × 100).

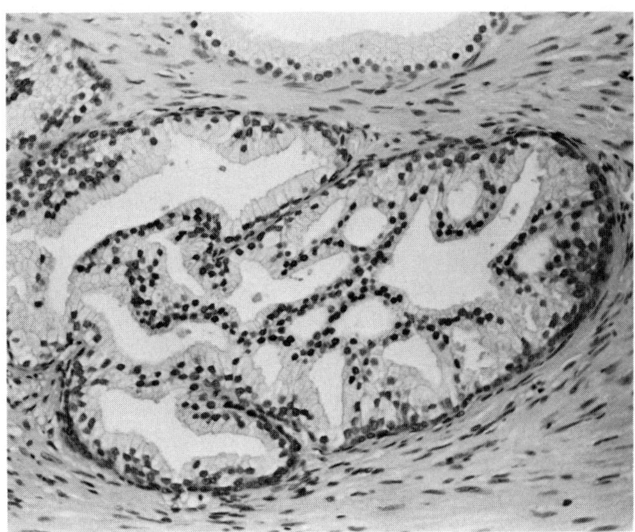

FIGURE 19–37. Cribriform hyperplasia with gland-in-gland growth. The cells are benign (H & E, original magnification × 100).

periphery of evolving hyperplastic nodules but may comprise the whole nodule. If it surrounds a duct, it has been referred to as lobular hyperplasia. The presence of small, closely packed acini lined by a single layer of cells suggests PCa, but no nuclear anaplasia or dispersion of glands is seen.

Basal cell hyperplasia (Fig. 19–35), also referred to as fetalization of the prostate or basal cell adenoma, is an incidental finding in hyperplastic prostates. Three categories are recognized: single or multiple acini occurring in aggregates, focally or diffusely. The cell nests can form acini (with lumina) or appear as solid nests. In most basal cell hyperplasias, there is usually some secretory differentiation of luminal cells, best demonstrated by PAP and PSA stains. The basal cells stain with cytokeratin 5 and 15, recognized by monoclonal antibodies MAB 903 (Enzo Biochemical Company, New York, NY) and MAB 8.12 (Sigma Chemical Company, St. Louis, MO). Occasionally, squamous change may be seen in the center of small nests. In some cases the basal cells form anastomosing cords one or two cell layers thick; others form masses surrounding circular spaces. This group has a lobular pattern and may be misinterpreted as "adenoid cystic carcinoma" (Fig. 19–36). In all categories of basal cell hyperplasia, the cells are small and of uniform size, with no evidence of anaplasia. Small nucleoli may be present in basal cells and occasional mitoses. Another distinguishing feature of basal cell hyperplasia is that the cell nests have a regular outline, and the basement membrane is intact and may be hyalinized. The stroma is usually hyperplastic.

Cribriform hyperplasia shows a gland-in-gland growth pattern (Fig. 19–37). In contrast to cribriform carcinoma, there is often a layer of hyperplastic basal cells. The cells and the nuclei are uniform, the nucleoli are small, and the nuclei in the center are identical to those at the periphery. A delicate fibrovascular stroma may be detected between the glands. The surrounding stroma

is hyperplastic, and there is usually associated basal cell hyperplasia. In cribriform PCa the basal layer is absent, the nuclei may become pyknotic toward the center, the nucleoli are prominent, and there is associated glandular carcinoma elsewhere.

Fibroglandular nodule (sclerosing adenosis) consists of hyperplastic stroma with small, irregularly distributed glands, which are often surrounded by a thick basement membrane (Fig. 19–38).

In postatrophic hyperplasia there is a typical pattern of lobular distribution and a number of typically atrophic glands, but other glands may have considerably more cytoplasm and active nuclei.

Reactive hyperplasia is a reparative process encountered in acute and chronic prostatitis. The residual duct has a cribriform appearance admixed with inflammatory

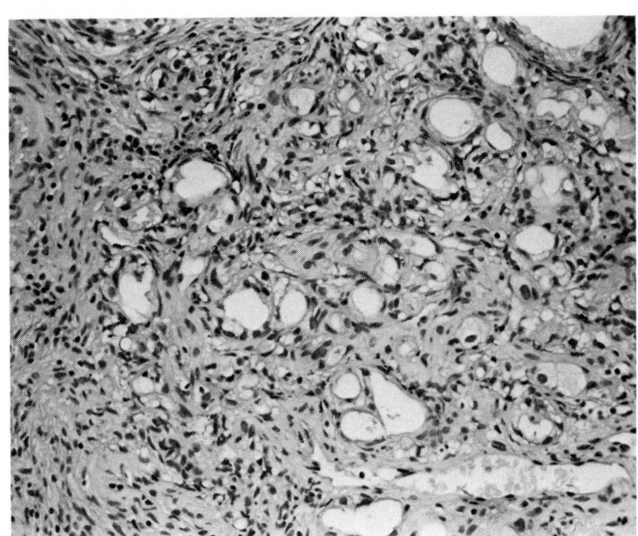

FIGURE 19–38. Fibroglandular nodule with cellular stroma associated with glands of varying sizes (H & E, original magnification × 100).

cells. The appearance and the massive inflammatory infiltrate should lead to the correct diagnosis.

Papillary hyperplasia is most frequently seen in prostatic urethra. It appears as a villous adenoma or polypoid hyperplasia. The proliferating cells are columnar and generally associated with recognizable basal cells. The nuclei are totally bland. The distinction from papillary carcinoma rests entirely on nuclear appearance.

Ejaculatory ducts show the same changes as seminal vesicles and are discussed with them.

Inflammatory lesions may also simulate PCa. The massive lymphocytic infiltration, especially if lymphocytes are surrounded by a halo (Fig. 19–39), may simulate undifferentiated PCa. In contrast to undifferentiated PCa, the infiltrate in chronic prostatitis is pleomorphic and associated with necrosis of acini and the ducts. No acinar structures are seen; PAP, PSA, and mucin stains are negative; and the cells react positively with leukocytic common antigen.

Iatrogenic Changes

The most frequent of these is cautery effect on PCa, prostatic hyperplasia, and normal prostate. The cells become elongated and hyperchromatic, simulating transitional cell carcinoma. Additional sections and careful examination reveal the true nature of the findings. Histologic changes in treated PCa and prostate have been discussed.

Extraprostatic Lesions

Involutional changes may occur in seminal vesicles. The mucosal outfoldings of seminal vesicles mimic closely packed acini. The presence of hyperchromatic nuclei is often confusing. Careful examination reveals

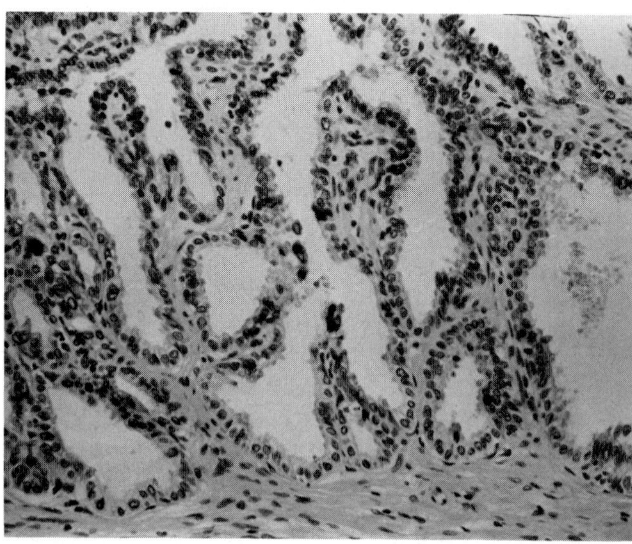

FIGURE 19–40. Involutional changes in seminal vesicles. Large hyperchromatic nuclei in luminal cells (H & E, original magnification × 100).

the organoid pattern of seminal vesicles, as well as lipofuscin pigment in the cytoplasm. Large hyperchromatic nuclei are usually present but are confined to luminal cells (Fig. 19–40). The presence of seminal vesicles in TURP or biopsy is the second most frequent cause of misdiagnosis after prostatic glandular atrophy.

Cowper's gland consists of small, regular, round acini lined by low columnar mucin-containing epithelium surrounding a central duct. The nuclei are small and regular and lack anaplasia (Fig. 19–41).

Nephrogenic adenoma seen in TURP usually occurs in proximity to the mucosa. It consists of tubular structures of varying sizes lined by cuboidal, flat, or hobnail cells. The nuclei are small and round. The stroma is edematous with varying amounts of inflammatory cells. If PCa is suspected, PAP and PSA reveal its true nature.

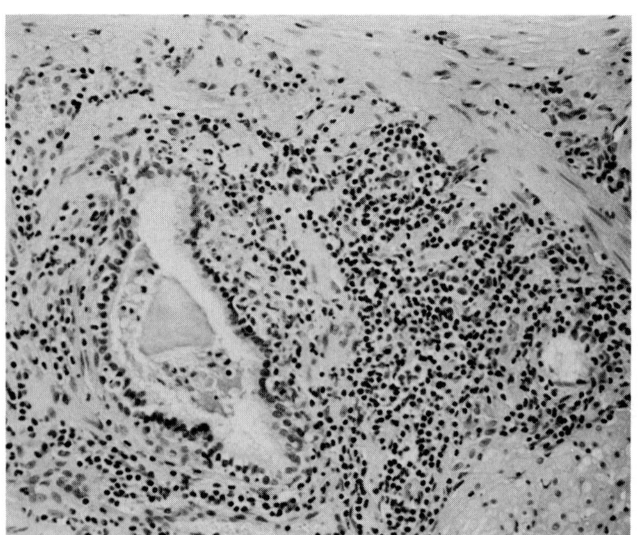

FIGURE 19–39. Chronic prostatitis with invasive lymphocytic infiltration mimicking undifferentiated prostatic carcinoma. Note the involvement of acini (H & E, original magnification × 100).

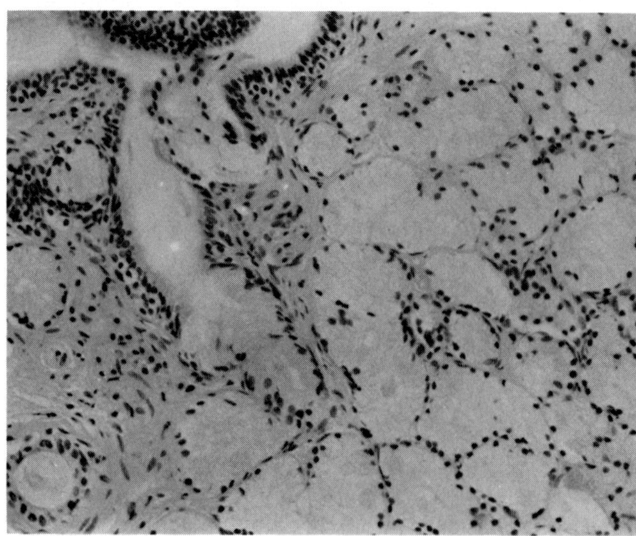

FIGURE 19–41. Cowper's gland. Benign mucinous glands and related duct (H & E, original magnification × 100).

Miscellaneous Findings

Occasionally, nerve fibers may be in intimate contact with benign glands. Such glands do not show anaplasia and the glands are not inside the perineural membrane.

Skeletal muscle is an integral part of the lateral lobes and the base of the prostate and may be present in transurethral specimens or biopsy. The presence of benign or neoplastic glands in the midst of skeletal muscle should not be interpreted as extraprostatic extension. Normal prostatic glands may rarely be found in periprostatic fat, bladder, and urethra. Such structures indicate ectopic prostatic glands.

Squamous metaplasia associated with infarction is sometimes confusing because of pleomorphism of nuclei, but the presence of old or recent hemorrhage and ischemic necrosis and scarring are indicative of the true nature of the lesion. Mucinous metaplasia of prostatic glands is rare.

ATTEMPTS TO IMPROVE PROGNOSTIC CAPABILITIES

Grading and staging have been, and continue to be, the standard methods of prognostication. In the prostate, these have been of limited value. In recent years considerable effort has been committed to improve prognostic capabilities. Among these may be mentioned DNA analysis, determination of proliferation phase (S-phase), morphometry, cell motility, image analysis, hybridization, tissue culture, animal model studies of xenograft in hairless and transgenic mice, Dunning carcinoma, and studies of chromosomes. The discussion is limited to DNA analysis, morphometry, and chromosomal studies.

DNA analysis can be done by Feulgen stain or flow cytometry. It is now well established that flow cytometry can offer additional prognostic information. Prostatic tumors have been subdivided into diploid, tetraploid, aneuploid, and nonaneuploid.[2, 31, 50, 63, 121, 144, 149, 150] Tribukait's classic work[148–150] is discussed in detail, as it has been confirmed by others.

In fine-needle aspirations of benign prostates and untreated PCa, Tribukait has demonstrated a relationship of DNA flow cytometry to histologic grade. In 806 benign prostates, 93 per cent were diploid, 6 per cent were tetraploid aneuploid, and 1 per cent were nonetraploid aneuploid. In 139 atypias, 84 per cent were diploid, 12 per cent were tetraploid aneuploid, and 4 per cent were nonetraploid aneuploid. In 344 well-differentiated tumors, 58 per cent were diploid, 32 per cent were tetraploid aneuploid, 7 per cent were nonetraploid aneuploid, and 3 per cent had multiple cell lines. In 386 moderately differentiated tumors, 29 per cent were diploid, 37 per cent were tetraploid aneuploid, 28 per cent were nonetraploid aneuploid, and 6 per cent showed multiple cell lines. In 136 poorly differentiated tumors, 10 per cent were diploid, 23 per cent were tetraploid, 41 per cent were nonetraploid aneuploid, and 26 per cent showed multiple cell lines. Four-

year survival decreased from more than 95 per cent for patients with initially diploid tumors to about 25 per cent for patients with tumors containing several aneuploid cell populations. Survival of patients with tetraploid tumors and tumors with one nontetraploid aneuploid cell population was about 80 per cent and 40 per cent, respectively.[148, 149] Tribukait noted that changes in ploidy may occur with time.[150] Repeated fine-needle aspirations of 199 untreated patients during a mean observation time of 20 months revealed ploidy changes of diploid and tetraploid tumors at an annual rate of about 9 per cent. He reported that metastatic potential evaluated by bone scans and confirmed by radiographic examination varied with ploidy. In 419 patients studied at admission, distant metastases were found in 7 per cent of patients with diploid tumors, in 17 per cent with tetraploid tumors, in 25 per cent with aneuploid tumors, and in 52 per cent with tumors containing multiple aneuploid cell lines.

He reported that diploid tumors were most common in stage T1 but rare in stage T4. Tetraploid tumors increased to maximum values in stage T2 and T3. Nonetraploid aneuploid tumors, with one or more than one aneuploid cell population, were rare in T1 lesions but increased from 17 per cent in T2 to about 60 per cent in T4 tumors.

Adolfsson et al selected 167 patients with untreated grades 1 and 2 low-stage PCa for close surveillance without treatment.[2] Eleven failed follow-up, and in another 11, the records were incomplete. Thus, they had 146 patients with a median age of 68 years. Initially, 69 had diploid tumors, 68 tetraploid, and 9 nontetraploid aneuploid tumors. Because the course of the 9 did not differ from the course of those with tetraploid tumors, they were grouped together. Seventy-one per cent were grade 1 and 67 per cent were T2. During a median observation of 50 months, 99 patients remained untreated and 57 received treatment because of either rapid local progression or development of metastasis. Of the 146 patients observed, 77 had locally progressive disease and 10 had metastases while still untreated. Of patients with metastatic disease, 2 had initially diploid and 8 had nondiploid tumors. Of special interest is their observation that (a) patients with low-grade, low-stage tumors, DNA diploid, did in fact have local progression and occasionally metastases when left untreated and (b) slightly more than 50 per cent of DNA diploid tumor patients had tumor progression after 5 years.

Deitch and deVere-White observed that DNA flow cytometry offered additional prognostic information for PCa.[30] However, for individual patients, this added information may have limited value because approximately 15 per cent of those with diploid tumors experience disease progression within 5 years, compared with those with nondiploid disease, once PCa becomes disseminated. They reported that DNA flow cytometry can be used to predict tumor volume.

Falkmer has clarified the advantages and disadvantages of flow cytometry and compared them to those of image DNA cytometry.[47] The main advantage of flow cytometry is that resolution on the x-axis of the histogram is high owing to the high degree of sensitivity to quantification of the DNA amount by means of microfluorometry. The coefficient of low DNA cytometry histogram peaks is low when fresh specimens of PCa are investigated. The reproducibility of a flow DNA histogram for neoplastic cells is under poor control because cell suspensions of solid tumors with more than one cell component and different amounts of cell debris are likely to give rise to flow cytometry DNA histograms of a compound character.

Flow cytometry has other serious disadvantages. It provides no possibility for simultaneous cytodiagnostic identification of analyzed cells. Another disadvantage is that neuroendocrine cells are lost in the analysis.

Calculation of nuclei in the S-phase of the cell cycle from DNA histograms can give valuable information regarding the proliferation rate. Because samples of PCa do not consist of 100 per cent neoplastic cells, the overwhelming amounts of total cell mass in a tumor nodule often comprise stromal cells, normal epithelial cells, inflammatory cells, and other non-neoplastic elements. In PCa the estimated fraction of genuinely neoplastic cells can vary from 10 per cent to 90 per cent in many typical specimens analyzed. Consequently, in such a situation an accurate calculation of an S-phase fraction in tumors with a flow cytometry DNA histogram of diploid types is almost impossible to perform. The coordinate axis of histograms on which the highest resolution is present is the x-axis.

The main advantage of image DNA cytometry is that analysis is done on histopathologically or cytodiagnostically identified neoplastic cells and nuclei. Nuclear DNA content can be assessed in selected nests of neoplastic parenchyma or in small foci of premalignant lesions, avoiding all other non-neoplastic elements or artifacts.

In contrast to flow cytometry DNA histograms, the y-axis of image cytometry DNA histograms is consequently not superimposed by values from non-neoplastic cells, cellular debris, or cellular triplets or doublets. Another advantage is the possibility of repeating the same assessment in other laboratories and with simultaneous documentation of cells measured.

The main disadvantages are that the number of cells rapidly analyzed is only 100 to 500, statistical confidences are low, and there is a subjective component in image DNA cytometry. However, this can be reduced by means of computerized evaluation technique. Falkmer has recommended that the results of DNA assessment using flow cytometry and image analysis be combined and both correlated with results of histopathologic assessments and clinical data.[47]

PCa has a low proliferation rate, which is difficult to detect by flow cytometrically determined S-phase. Mention has already been made of the work of Helpap. Using ^{3}H thymidine, Helpap compared the labeling index of typical hyperplasia, atypical hyperplasia, and PCa.[69] Poorly differentiated PCa had a labeling index of 0.2 to 2.4 per cent, whereas cribriform PCa had a labeling index of 0.4 to 5.7 per cent.

Another method of determining proliferation rate is by in vivo injection of bromodeoxyuridine.[117] Nucleolar organizing regions (NORs) have also been used for determination of proliferation rate. NORs are special areas in chromosomes 13, 14, 15, 21, and 22 identified as the sites of ribosomal DNA genes (rDNA). They have a distinct nucleoprotein structure that is used in their identification. NORs can be demonstrated in paraffin-embedded tissues by the use of colloidal silver stains, referred to as argyrophilic aggregates (AG-NORs).[66, 119] They are useful histologic markers of cell proliferation, because they have been found to correlate with flow cytometrically derived S-phase activity and with immunoreactivity of cells with monoclonal antibody KI-67. Measurements of projected AGNOR areas show substantial differences between prostatic hyperplasia and PCa and slight but significant differences between PIN and PCa.[132]

Using morphometry, Tannenbaum et al measured the nucleolar surface area.[147] In patients with no evidence of disease 3 or more years after radical prostatectomy, the initial biopsy demonstrated nucleolar surface areas that averaged 1.28 μm^2 (range 0.60 to 2.27 μm^2). With a single exception in 52 patients, progression of the disease was always accompanied by a nucleolar surface area measuring larger than 2.40 μm^2.

Diamond et al reported that the mean nuclear roundness factor for all malignant prostatic cells was 1.059, compared with a mean nuclear roundness factor for all normal epithelial nuclei of 1.034.[36] Comparing tumors that had metastasized with tumors of patients who were alive and well 14 years later, they found a mean nuclear roundness factor of 1.069 for the former and 1.047 for the latter. The mean roundness factor of the normal nuclei was identified for the two groups. Clark has reported that usefulness of the nuclear roundness factor is limited to low-grade tumors, and it is not reliably applicable to needle biopsies.[26]

Diploid tumors by flow cytometry may not be diploid by karyotypic analysis. They may be aneuploid by in situ hybridization and use of a panel of chromosome probes on cell suspensions or smears.[152]

It has long been known that chromosomal aberrations are the cause of change from normal to malignant growth. However, mechanical difficulties in chromosome preparations have prevented testing the theory in solid tumors. The studies have been especially difficult in PCa because PCa is a slow-growing tumor, and in tissue cultures it has been difficult to simultaneously avoid overgrowth of stromal cells. Various techniques have been employed. Abnormalities have been reported involving chromosomes 7 and 10. The reader is referred to the overviews of chromosome study by Sandberg,[125] Heim and Mitelman,[68] and Lundgren et al.[88]

We have used a different approach to the problem.[132] In our attempt to eliminate the difficulties of culturing the tumor cells or mincing the tumor to study the cells, we have developed a protocol to identify numerical aberrations of chromosomes in routinely fixed paraffin-embedded tissue sections, utilizing in situ hybridochemistry with biotinylated DNA probes specific for the alpha satellite regions of various chromosomes. To date, we have studied six prostates. We have found that in four of the six, there was either a gain or loss of chromosome material. In one of four cases, a single aberration involved trisomy 17. In one of the cases there was monosomy for chromosomes 10 and 17. The number of cases, whether using cultures, cell suspension, or our method, is too small to draw any conclusions, but the potential of facilitating chromosome studies on prostate cancer is most exciting.

SARCOMAS

Sarcomas of the prostate constitute less than 0.1 per cent of all malignant prostate tumors. They may occur at any age, but 30 per cent develop during the first decade of life and 75 per cent before the age of 40, but they may also occur in older patients.

Rhabdomyosarcoma is most commonly found in children. In a study of the Registry cases, Enzinger and Weiss reported that of 558 rhabdomyosarcomas, 190 were in the genitourinary tract and retroperitoneum and 15 were in the prostate.[43] When the tumor involves the bladder, it has a grapelike configuration, but in the prostate itself, it is a grayish-white, nonencapsulated mass. The majority of the tumors consist of embryonal rhabdomyosarcomas. Enzinger and Weiss[43] described the histology in detail, which is briefly summarized here.

Embryonal rhabdomyosarcoma is the most common type. Considerable variation in cellularity may be seen with less cellular, loosely textured, myxoid areas alternating with hypercellular and densely packed areas, with varying numbers of scattered rhabdomyoblasts. The least differentiated tumors consist of small round or oval cells with hyperchromatic nuclei and indistinct cytoplasm. Better-differentiated forms have many rhabdomyoblasts with eosinophilia and deeply staining stringy or fibrillar cytoplasm (Fig. 19–42). Cross-striations are rare and are found most readily in spindle- and strap-

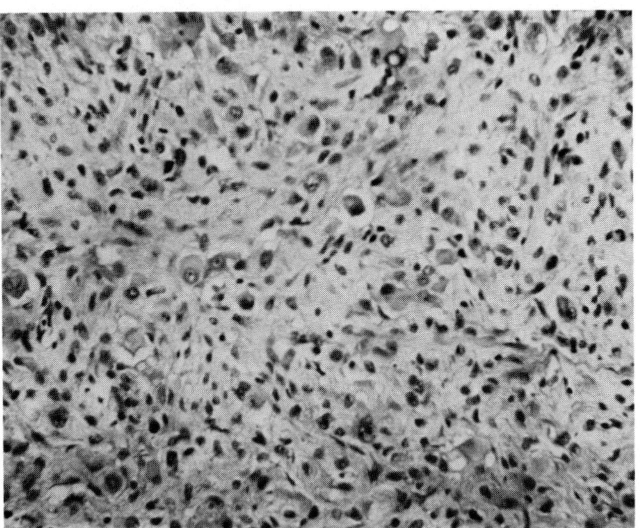

FIGURE 19–42. Embryonal rhabdomyosarcoma showing immature cells and many rhabdomyoblasts with considerable amount of cytoplasm (H & E, original magnification × 100).

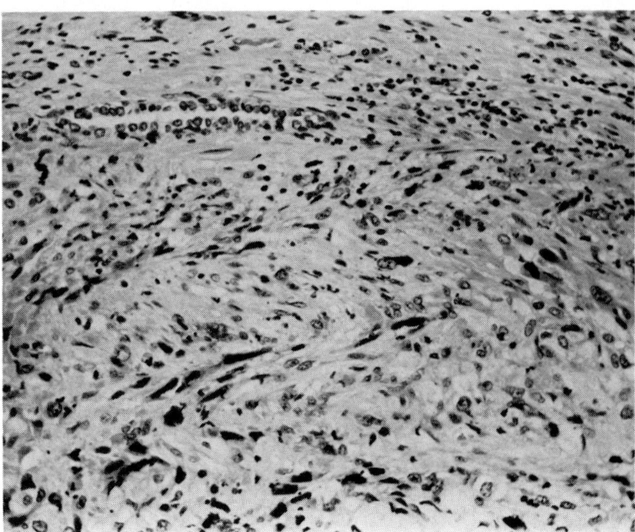

FIGURE 19–43. Leiomyosarcoma of prostate showing fascicles of spindle-shaped cells with hyperchromatic nuclei (H & E, original magnification × 100).

shaped rhabdomyoblasts. Masson stains and demonstration of myoglobin are helpful in difficult cases. Foci of immature cartilage or osseous tissue may be present.

Two other types may be seen—the alveolar and the pleomorphic. The former is composed of ill-defined aggregates of poorly differentiated round or oval tumor cells that frequently show loss of cellular cohesion and formation of irregular alveolar spaces.

Leiomyosarcomas constitute about 25 per cent of prostate sarcomas. They usually occur in older patients, although some cases have been reported in children. Leiomyosarcomas are usually large tumors infiltrating the prostate and periprostatic tissue. The tumor is soft in consistency, simulating BPH. Histologically, the tumor consists of interlacing bands of spindle-shaped cells with a more or less eosinophilic cytoplasm. The nuclei are cigar shaped and vesicular. They show varying degrees of anaplasia and mitotic activity (Fig. 19–43).

Generally speaking, the diagnosis of leiomyosarcoma is based on increased mitotic activity. However, some of the leiomyosarcomas of the prostate may have low mitotic activity, making it difficult to distinguish the lesion from a cellular leiomyoma. In such cases, more representative examination of the specimen is desirable. The differentiation between low-grade leiomyosarcoma and stromal hyperplasia is sometimes difficult, but a trichrome stain may be helpful. Leiomyosarcoma cells are usually thinner and more interlacing. Both leiomyosarcoma and rhabdomyosarcoma give a positive reaction for desmin and actin.

Stromal sarcomas are undifferentiated, highly malignant spindle-cell tumors that do not react with any myogenous stains (Fig. 19–44).

CARCINOSARCOMA

To make a diagnosis of carcinosarcoma, there must be definite carcinomatous and sarcomatous elements. Desmoplastic reaction of the stroma is seen in some

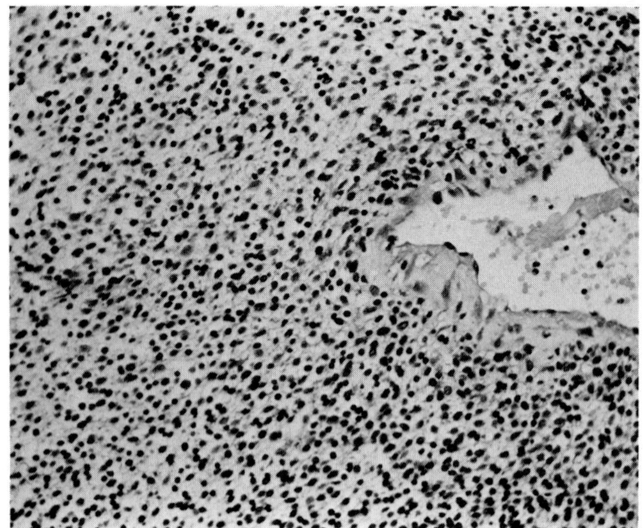

FIGURE 19–44. Stromal sarcoma of prostate showing undifferentiated small neoplastic tumor cells (H & E, original magnification × 100).

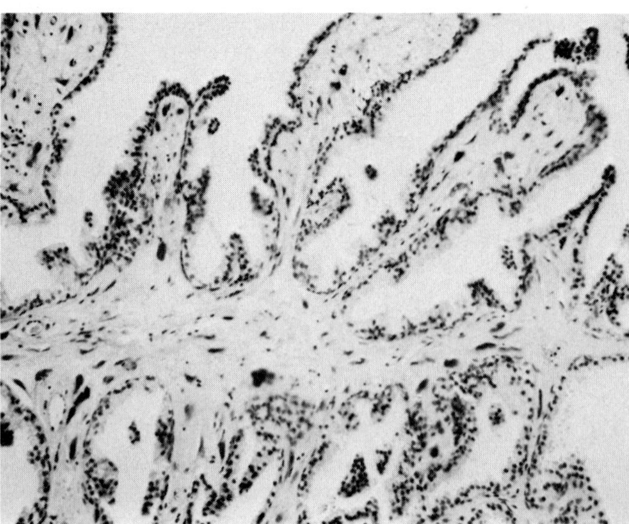

FIGURE 19–45. Phylloides tumor showing large dilated convoluted acini and bizarre-shaped stromal cells (H & E, original magnification × 70).

prostatic carcinomas, usually following estrogen therapy. Sometimes it is severe enough to lead to a diagnosis of sarcoma. Chondroblastic or osteoblastic areas may be present. There is concern in such cases about whether it is a carcinoma with spindle-cell areas and chondro-osteoblastic metaplasia or a true carcinosarcoma. Each tumor must be evaluated by the extent and type of its noncarcinomatous elements and their relationship. If progressive stages can be demonstrated from carcinoma to spindle cells, if there seems to be a stroma for both components, and if the cells are undifferentiated, it is probably a rare spindle-cell carcinoma. We believe that most tumors designated carcinosarcomas represent spindle-cell carcinoma or desmoplastic reaction of the stroma. We designate as carcinosarcoma only lesions that contain definite neoplastic cartilage or bone.

OTHER TUMORS

In malignant lymphoma, the cells are uniform, and they infiltrate between individual muscle bundles with apparent compression and atrophy of the muscle and acini. In leukemic involvement of the prostate, the vascular channels contain many lymphocytes. Malignant melanoma is rarely seen in the prostate, and it may be primary there, but a secondary melanoma should be ruled out. Liposarcoma and malignant fibrous histiocytoma are extremely rare and pathologic curiosities.

PHYLLOIDES TUMOR (CYSTOSARCOMA PHYLLOIDES)

This is an unusual tumor that is seen mostly in the female breast but may rarely be encountered in the prostate. The characteristic finding in both organs is a

stromal proliferation, which in the prostate often has bizarre nuclei. The accompanying glandular component shows varying degrees of epithelial hyperplasia. The glands are often cystic, enlarged, and distorted by the stromal component (Figs. 19–45 and 19–46). If not completely excised, the tumor frequently recurs.

Occasionally, the stromal element is very cellular with increased mitotic activity, indistinguishable from fibrosarcoma. In such cases, the patient is likely to develop metastases, but these may be delayed.

As in its counterpart, the breast, it may be difficult to predict the ultimate outcome. Therefore, the term phylloides tumor appears to be more appropriate than cystosarcoma phylloides.

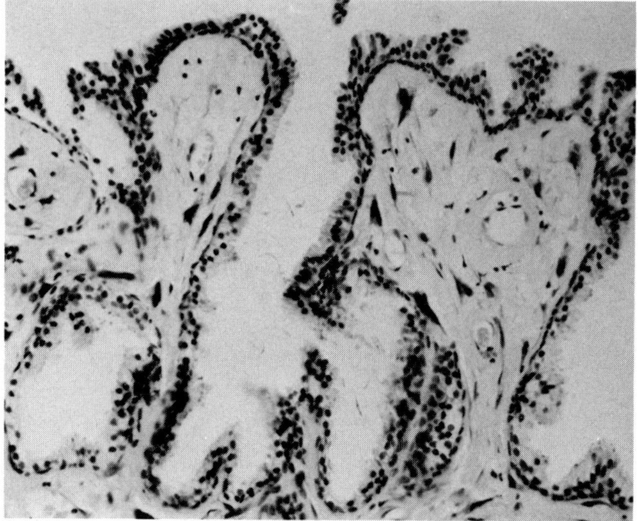

FIGURE 19–46. Same field as Figure 19–45, showing phylloides tumor. Higher power (H & E, original magnification × 100).

MALIGNANT LESIONS OF THE SEMINAL VESICLES

This tumor occurs most often in patients over 50 years of age, but we have seen it in a young patient with associated anomalies of the genitourinary tract. In confirmed cases, the tumor involves primarily seminal vesicles, with secondary spread to the prostate and the other seminal vesicle. The tumor is often large and may measure 10 to 15 cm in diameter.

Histologically, the tumor consists of a papillary adenocarcinoma, but it may be a mixture of adenocarcinoma and undifferentiated carcinoma. The cells are columnar, and with clear cytoplasm there may be lipofuscin pigment, but this is not characteristic, as it can be seen in some prostatic carcinomas as well. The cells form papillary and acinar structures. Involutional changes in seminal vesicles, described earlier, are frequently misdiagnosed as carcinoma.

REFERENCES

1. Abrahamsson PA, Wadstrom LB, Alumets J, et al: Peptide-hormone and serotonin-immunoreactive tumor cells in carcinoma of the prostate. Pathol Res Pract 182:298–307, 1987.
2. Adolfsson J, Ronstrom L, Hedlund P, et al: The prognostic value of modal deoxyribonucleic acid in low grade, low stage, untreated prostatic cancer. J Urol 144:1404–1409, 1990.
3. Alken CE, Dhom G, Hohbach M, et al: Therapie des Prostata Carcinoma und Verlaufskontrolle. Urologe A 11:216–220, 1972.
4. Andrews GS: Latent carcinoma of the prostate. J Clin Pathol 2:197–208, 1949.
5. Ayala AG, Ro JY, Babaian R, Grignon DJ: The prostate capsule. Does it exist? Its importance in the staging and treatment of prostatic carcinoma. Am J Surg Pathol 13:21–27, 1989.
6. Azzopardi JG, Evans DJ: Argentaffin cells in prostate carcinoma: Differentiation from lipofuscin and melanin in prostatic epithelium. J Pathol 4:247–251, 1971.
7. Babaian RJ, Grenow WA: Reliability of Gleason grading system in comparing prostatic biopsies with total prostatectomy specimens. Urology 25:564–568, 1985.
8. Bankhoff H, Wernert N, Dhom G, Remberger N: Basement membrane in fetal, adult, normal, hyperplastic, and neoplastic prostate. Virch Arch [A] 418:375–381, 1991.
9. Baron E, Angrist A: Incidence of occult adenocarcinoma of the prostate after fifty years of age. Arch Pathol 32:787–793, 1941.
10. Beahrs GH, Henson DE, Hutter RVP, Meyers MH: American Joint Committee on Cancer: Manual for Staging of Cancer. Philadelphia, JB Lippincott, 1988.
11. Bischof W, Aumuller G: Age dependent changes in the carbohydrate pattern of human prostatic epithelium as determined by peroxidase labeled lectins. Prostate 3:507–513, 1982.
12. Boecking A, Auffermann W: Cytological grading of therapy-induced tumor regression in prostatic carcinoma: Proposal of a new system. Diagn Cytopathol 3:108–111, 1987.
13. Boecking A, Kiehn J, Heinzel-Wach M: Combined histological grading of prostatic carcinoma. Cancer 50:288–294, 1982.
14. Bostwick DG, Brawer MK: Prostatic intra-epithelial neoplasia and early invasion in prostate cancer. Cancer 59:788–794, 1987.
15. Bostwick DG, Srigley JR: Premalignant lesions. *In* Bostwick DG (ed): Pathology of the Prostate. New York, Churchill Livingstone, 1990, pp 48–54.
16. Brandes D: Prostate carcinoma. *In* Hill GS (ed): Uropathology, Vol 2. New York, Churchill Livingstone, 1989, pp 1239–1249.
17. Brandes D, Kirchheim D: Histochemistry of the prostate. *In* Tannenbaum M (ed): Urologic Pathology: The Prostate. Philadelphia, Lea & Febiger, 1977, pp 1235–1249.
18. Brandes D, Kirchheim D, Scott WW: Ultrastructure of human prostate, normal and neoplastic. Lab Invest 13:1541–1560, 1964.
19. Brawer MK, Peehl DM, Stamey TA, Bostwick DG: Keratin immunoreaction in benign and neoplastic human prostate. Cancer Res 45:3663–3667, 1985.
20. Brawn PN: Adenosis of the prostate: A dysplastic lesion that can be confused with adenocarcinoma. Cancer 49:826–833, 1982.
21. Brawn PN, Ayala AA, Eschenbach AC, et al: Histologic grading study of prostatic adenocarcinoma: Development of a new system and comparison with other methods. Cancer 49:113–120, 1982.
22. Breslow N, Chan CW, Dhom G, et al: Latent carcinoma of prostate at autopsy in seven areas. Int J Cancer 20:680–688, 1977.
23. Brolin JAE: Steroid receptor assays in human benign and malignant prostates based on biochemical, immunohistochemical and immunocytochemical technique. Berlin, Springer-Verlag, 1992, pp 1–68.
24. Byar DP, Mostofi FK: VA Cooperative Urological Research Group: Carcinoma of the prostate: Prognostic evaluation of certain pathological features in 208 radical prostatectomies. Cancer 30:5–13, 1972.
25. Choe BK, Pontes JE, McDonald J, Rose NR: Purification and characterization of human prostatic acid phosphatase prepa-
26. Clark TD: Nuclear roundness factor: A quantitative approach to grading in prostate carcinoma, reliability of needle biopsy tissue and effect of tumor stage on usefulness. Prostate 10:199–206, 1987.
27. Cohen RS, Glezerson G, Haltezee Z: Neuroendocrine cells: A new prognostic parameter in prostatic cancer. Br J Urol 68:258–262, 1991.
28. Correa RJ Jr, Anderson RG, Gibbons RP, Mason JT: Latent carcinoma of the prostate. Why the controversy? J Urol 111:644–646, 1974.
29. Dauge MC, Delmas V: A.P.U.D. type endocrine tumour of the prostate: Incidence and prognosis in association with adenocarcinoma. *In* Murphy GP, Khoury S, Kuss R, et al (eds): Progress in Clinical and Biological Medicine. New York, Alan R. Liss, 1986, pp 529–531.
30. Deitch AD, deVere-White RW: Flow cytometry as a predictive modality in prostatic cancer. Hum Pathol 23:352–359, 1992.
31. deVere-White RW, Deitch AD, Tesluk H, et al: Prognosis in disseminated prostatic cancer as related to tumor ploidy and differentiation. World J Urol 8:47–50, 1990.
32. Dhom G: Classification and grading of prostatic carcinoma. Rec Results Cancer Res 60:14–26, 1977.
33. Dhom G: Frische neoplastische Veraandrungen der Prostata. Verh Dtsch Ges Pathol 63:218–231, 1979.
34. Dhom G: Histopathology of prostatic carcinoma. Diagnosis and differential diagnosis. Pathol Res Pract 179:277–283, 1985.
35. Dhom G, Drago FS: Therapy of prostatic cancer and histopathologic follow-up. Prostate 3:531–542, 1982.
36. Diamond DA, Berry SJ, Jewett HJ, et al: A new method to assess metastatic potential of human prostate cancer: Relative nuclear roundness. J Urol 128:729–734, 1982.
37. di Sant Agnese PA, de Mesy Jenson KL: Neuroendocrine differentiation in prostatic carcinoma. Human Pathol 18:849–856, 1987.
38. Doctor VM, Sheth AR, Simha MM, et al: Studies on immunocytochemical localization of inhibin-like material in human prostatic carcinoma: Comparison of its distribution in normal, benign and malignant prostates. Br J Cancer 53:547–554, 1986.
39. Drago JR, Mostofi FK, Lee F: Introductory remarks and workshop summary. Urology 34(Suppl):2–3, 1987.
40. Eble JN, Angermeier PA: The role of fine needle aspiration and needle core biopsies in the diagnosis of primary prostatic carcinoma. Hum Pathol 23:249–257, 1992.
41. Ekman P, Barrack ER, Burjnovsky P, Walsh PC: Steroid receptor profiles on subcellular fractions of different human prostatic tissues [abstract]. J Urol 131:121A, 1984.

42. Ekman P, Barrack ER, Walsh PC: Simultaneous measurement of progesterone and androgen receptors in human prostate. A microassay. J Clin Endocrinol 55:1089–1099, 1982.

43. Enzinger FM, Weiss S: Rhabdomyosarcoma of the genitourinary tract and retroperitoneum. *In* Soft Tissue Tumors. St Louis, CV Mosby Co, 1983, pp 341–371.

44. Epstein JI, Cho KA, Quinn PD: Relationship of severe dysplasia to stage A (incidental) adenocarcinoma. Cancer 65:2321–2327, 1990.

45. Epstein JI, Paul G, Eggleston JC, Walsh PC: Prognosis of untreated stage A1 prostate carcinoma: A study of 94 cases with extended follow-up. J Urol 136:837–839, 1986.

46. Esposti PI: Cytologic diagnosis of prostatic tumors with the aid of transrectal aspiration biopsy: A critical review of 1,110 cases and a report of morphologic and cytochemical studies. Acta Cytol 10:182–186, 1966.

47. Falkmer UG: Methodologic sources of errors in image and flow cytometry DNA assessments of the malignancy potential of prostatic carcinoma. Hum Pathol 23:360–367, 1992.

48. Fan K: Heterogeneous subpopulations of human prostatic adenocarcinoma cells: Potential usefulness of p21 protein as a predictor for bone metastasis. J Urol 139:318–322, 1988.

49. Fisher ER, Sieracki JC: Ultrastructure of human normal and neoplastic prostate. Pathol Ann 5:1–26, 1970.

50. Frankfurt OS, Chin JL, Englander LS, et al: Relationship between DNA ploidy, glandular differentiation and tumor spread in human prostate cancer. Cancer Res 45:1418–1423, 1985.

51. Franks LM: Atrophy and hyperplasia in the prostate proper. J Pathol Bacteriol 68:617–621, 1954.

52. Franks LM: Estrogen-treated prostatic cancer. Cancer 13:490–501, 1960.

53. Franzen S, Giertz G, Zajicek J: Cytological diagnosis of prostatic tumors by transrectal aspiration biopsy. A preliminary report. Br J Urol 32:193–196, 1960.

54. Furusato M, Mostofi FK: Intraprostatic lymphatics in man, light and ultrastructural observations. Prostate 1:15–23, 1980.

55. Gaeta JF, Asirwatham JE, Miller G, Murphy GP: Histological grading of primary prostatic cancer: A new approach to an old problem. J Urol 123:689–693, 1980.

56. Gallee MPW, Ten Kate FJW, Mulder GH: Histological grading of prostate carcinoma in prostatectomy specimens. A comparison of prognostic accuracy of five grading systems. Br J Urol 65:368–375, 1990.

57. Gleason DF: Atypical hyperplasia, benign hyperplasia and well differentiated adenocarcinoma. Am J Surg Pathol 9(Suppl):53–67, 1985.

58. Gleason DF: Classification of prostatic carcinomas. Cancer Chemother Rep 50:125–128, 1966.

59. Gleason DF: Gleason grading system. *In* Bostwick DG (ed): Pathology of the Prostate. New York, Churchill Livingstone, 1990, pp 83–93.

60. Gleason DF: The Veterans Administration Cooperative Urologic Research Group. Histologic grading and clinical staging of prostatic carcinoma. *In* Tannenbaum M (ed): Urologic Pathology: The Prostate. Philadelphia, Lea & Febiger, 1977, pp 171–174.

61. Gleason DF, Mellinger GT: The Veterans Administration Cooperative Urological Research Group: Prediction of prognosis for prostatic adenocarcinoma and combined histological grading and clinical staging. J Urol 111:58–64, 1974.

62. Grayhack JT, Assimos DG: Prognostic significance of tumor grade and stage in patients with carcinoma of the prostate. Prostate 4:13–33, 1983.

63. Greene DR, Taylor SR, Wheeler TM, Scardino PT: DNA/ploidy analysis of incidental and early clinical cancer. J Urol (Suppl) Abstr 746, 1991.

64. Gutman EB, Robinson JN: Determination of serum "acid" phosphatase activity in differentiating skeletal metastasis secondary to prostatic carcinoma from Paget's disease of bone. Am J Cancer 38:103–108, 1940.

65. Gutman EB, Sproul EE, Gutman AB: Significance of increased phosphatase activity of bone at the site of osteolytic metastases secondary to carcinoma of prostate gland. Am J Cancer 28:485–495, 1936.

66. Hansen AB, Ostergard B: Nucleolar organizing regions in hyperplastic and neoplastic prostatic tissue. Virchow Arch(A) 417:9–13, 1990.

67. Harada M, Mostofi FK, Corle DK, et al: Preliminary studies of histological prognosis in cancer of the prostate. Cancer Treat Rep 61:223–225, 1977.

68. Heim S, Mitelman F: Cancer cytogenetics. New York, Alan R. Liss, 1987, p 240.

69. Helpap B: The biologic significance of atypical hyperplasia of the prostate. Virchows Arch(A) 387:307–317, 1980.

70. Helpap B: Preneoplasien der Prostata. Extracta Urol 6:287–317, 1983.

71. Helpap B: Treated prostatic carcinoma: Histologic, immunochemical and cell kinetic studies. Appl Pathol 3:230–241, 1985.

72. Hermanek P, Sobin LH: UICC TNM Classification of Malignant Tumours. Berlin, Springer-Verlag, 1987, pp 141–144.

73. Hudson PB, Stout AP: Prostatic cancer: Comparison of physical examination and biopsy for detection of curable cancer. NY State J Med 66:351–355, 1966.

74. Huggins C, Hodges CV: Studies on prostate cancer: The effect of castration, or estrogen and of androgen injection on serum phosphatase in metastatic carcinoma of the prostate. Cancer Res 1:293–297, 1941.

75. Jewett HJ, Bridge RW, Gray SR Jr, Shelley WM: The palpable nodule of prostate cancer: Results of 15 years after radical excision. JAMA 203:403–405, 1968.

76. Kastendieck H: Correlations between atypical primary hyperplasia and carcinoma of the prostate. Pathol Res Pract 169:366–387, 1980.

77. Kastendieck H: Ultrastructural Pathology of the Human Prostate Gland. Stuttgart, Gustav Fischer Verlag, 1977, pp 10–47.

78. Kastendieck H, Altenahr E: Cyto- and histomorphogenesis of the prostate carcinoma. A comparative light and electron microscopic study. Virchow's Arch [A] 370:207–224, 1976.

79. Kastendieck H, Altenahr E, Husselmann H, Pressel M: Carcinoma and dysplastic lesions of the prostate. Z Krebs Forsch 88:33–54, 1976.

80. Kastendieck H, Helpap B: Prostatic dysplasia/atypical hyperplasia: Terminology, histopathology, pathobiology and significance. Urology (Suppl) 34:28–42, 1989.

81. Keenan EJ, Ramsey EE, Kemp ED: The role of prolactin in the growth of the prostate gland. *In* Murphy GP, Sandberg AA, Karr JP (eds): The Prostate Cell. Structure and Function, Part B. New York, Alan R. Liss, 1981, pp 9–18.

82. Kiesling VP, Friedman HI, McAninch JW, et al: The ultrastructural changes of prostatic adenocarcinoma following external beam radiation therapy. J Urol 122:633–639, 1979.

83. Koss LG, Woyke S, Schriber K, et al: Thin needle aspiration biopsy of the prostate. Urol Clin North Am 11:237–251, 1984.

84. Kovi J: Microscopic differential diagnosis of small acinar adenocarcinoma of prostate. Pathol Ann 20:157–196, 1985.

85. Kovi J, Mostofi FK, Heshmat MY, Enterline JP: Large acinar atypical hyperplasia and carcinoma of the prostate. Cancer 61:555–561, 1988.

86. Lam MKW, Yam LT, Wilbur HJ, et al: Comparison of acid phosphatase isoenzymes of human seminal fluid, prostate and leukocytes. Clin Chem 25:1285–1289, 1979.

87. Li CY, Lam MKW, Yam LT: Immunohistochemical diagnosis of prostatic cancer with metastases. Cancer 46:706–712, 1980.

88. Lundgren R, Kristopherson U, Heim S, et al: Multiple structured chromosome rearrangements including del(7q) and del(10q) in an adenocarcinoma of the prostate and cancer cytogen. Cytogenetics 35:103–108, 1988.

89. Martin PM, Magdelenat HP, Benyahia B, et al: New approaches for visualizing inherently fluorescent ligands and image intensification. Cancer Res 43:4956–4965, 1983.

90. McNeal JE: Cancer volume and site of origin of adenocarcinoma in the prostate. Relationship to local and distant spread. Hum Pathol 23:258–266, 1992.

91. McNeal JE: Morphogenesis of prostatic carcinoma. Cancer 18:1659–1666, 1965.

92. McNeal JE: Significance of duct acinar dysplasia in prostatic carcinoma. Prostate 13:91–102, 1988.

93. McNeal JE: The prostate and prostatic urethra: A morphological synthesis. J Urol 107:1008–1016, 1972.

94. McNeal JE, Bostwick DG: Intraductal dysplasia: A premalignant lesion of the prostate. Hum Pathol 17:64–71, 1976.

95. McNeal JE, Leav I, Alroy J, Skutelsky E: Differential lectin staining of central and peripheral zones of prostate and alterations in dysplasia. Am J Clin Pathol 89:41–48, 1988.

96. Melicow MM, Pachter MR: Endometrioid carcinoma of prostatic utricle (uterus masculinus). Cancer 20:1715–1722, 1967.

97. Melicow MM, Tannenbaum M: Endometrioid carcinoma of uterus masculinus (prostatic utricle): Report of six cases. J Urol 106:892–902, 1971.

98. Mellinger GT: Prognosis of prostatic carcinoma. *In* Grundmann E, Valusieck W (eds): Tumors of Male Genital System. Berlin, Springer-Verlag, 1977, pp 171–198.

99. Mendelsohn G, Maksem J: Divergent differentiation in neoplasms: Pathologic, biologic, and clinical considerations. Pathol Ann 21 (Part I):91–119, 1986.

100. Miller A, Seljelid B: Cellular atypia of the prostate. Scand J Urol Nephrol 5:17–21, 1971.

101. Mohler JI, Erozan YS, Walsh PC: Fine needle core and aspiration biopsy: A new method for diagnosis of prostatic carcinoma. Cancer 63:1846–1855, 1989.

102. Moore RA: Benign hypertrophy of the prostate. A morphologic study. J Urol 50:680–710, 1943.

103. Moore RA: The evolution and involution of the prostate gland. Am J Pathol 12:599–624, 1936.

104. Moore RA: The morphology of small prostatic carcinoma. J Urol 33:224–234, 1935.

105. Mostofi FK: Grading of prostatic carcinoma. Cancer Chemother Rep 59:111–117, 1975.

106. Mostofi FK: Grading of prostatic carcinoma—current status. *In* Bruce A, Trachtenberg J (ed): Adenocarcinoma of the Prostate. New York, Springer-Verlag, 1987, pp 29–46.

107. Mostofi FK: Precancerous lesions of the prostate. *In* Carter RL (ed): Precancerous States. London, Oxford University Press, 1984, pp 303–310.

108. Mostofi FK: Problems in grading carcinoma of prostate. Semin Oncology 3:161–169, 1976.

109. Mostofi FK, Davis CJ Jr: Male reproductive system. *In* Kissane M (ed): Anderson's Pathology, 9th ed. St. Louis, CV Mosby, 1990, pp 907–915.

110. Mostofi FK, Price EB Jr: Tumors of Male Genital System (Fascicle 8). Atlas of Tumor Pathology, 2nd Series. Washington, DC, Armed Forces Institute of Pathology, 1973, pp 236–338.

111. Mostofi FK, Sesterhenn IA, Davis CJ Jr: Can pathology predict response? Role of classic methods and modern techniques. EORTC Genitourinary Group Monograph 10-Urologic Oncology: Reconstructive Surgery Organ Conservation and Restoration of Function, 1991, pp 237–248.

112. Mostofi FK, Sesterhenn IA, Davis CJ Jr: Progress in pathology of carcinoma of prostate. Progr Clin Biolog Res 243A:445–475, 1987.

113. Mostofi FK, Sesterhenn IA, Davis CJ Jr: Prostatic carcinoma. Problems in interpretation of prostatic biopsies. Hum Pathol 23:223–241, 1992.

114. Mostofi FK, Sesterhenn IA, Sobin LH: Histological Typing of Prostate Tumours. Geneva, World Health Organization, 1980, pp 17–21.

115. Murphy GP: Lucy Wortham James Basic Research Award. Markers of prostatic carcinoma. Arch Surg 127:1404–1427, 1991.

116. Murphy GP, Whitmore WF: A report of the workshops on the current status of the histologic grading of prostate cancer. Cancer 44:1490–1494, 1979.

117. Nemoto R, Hattori K, Uchida K, et al: S-phase fraction of human prostate adenocarcinoma studied with in vivo bromo-deoxy-uridine labeling. Cancer 66:509–514, 1990.

118. Oyasu B, Bahnson RR, Norwels K, Garnet JE: Cytological atypia in prostate gland: Frequency, distribution and possible relevance to carcinoma. J Urol 135:959–962, 1986.

119. Ploton D, Menager M, Joannesson P: Improvement in the staining and in visualization of the argyrophilic proteins of the nucleolar organizing region at the optical level. Histochem J 18:5–14, 1986.

120. Pousette A, Borgstom E, Hogberg B, Gustafsson JA: Analysis of the androgen receptor in needle biopsies from human prostatic tissue. *In* Murphy GP, Sandberg AA, Karr JP (eds): The Prostatic Cell Structure and Function, Part B. New York, Alan R. Liss, 1981, pp 299–311.

121. Reber MW, Bart RS: Flow cytometry of solid tumors. *In* Melamed MR, Mendesohn ML: Flow Cytometry and Sorting. New York, Wiley & Liss, 1990, pp 745–754.

122. Rich AR: On the frequency of the occurrence of occult carcinoma of the prostate. J Urol 33:215–223, 1935.

123. Rodin AE, Larson DL, Roberts DK: Nature of perineural space invaded by prostate carcinoma. Cancer 20:1771–1779, 1967.

124. Sadi VS, Walsh PC, Barrack ER: Image analysis of androgen receptor (AR) immunostaining in metastatic prostate cancer. Greater heterogeneity of hormonal therapy. J Urol (Suppl) 145, Abstr 730, 1991.

125. Sandberg AA: The Chromosomes in Human Cancer and Leukemia. New York, Elsevier, 1991, pp 823–827.

126. Schroeder FH, Belt HE: Carcinoma of the prostate: A study of 213 prostates with stage C tumors treated by total perineal prostatectomy. J Urol 144:257–261, 1975.

127. Schroeder FH, Bloom JH, Hop WC, Mostofi FK: Grading of prostatic cancer: The prognostic significance of the presence of multiple architectural patterns. Prostate 6:403–415, 1985.

128. Schroeder FH, Hermanek P, Denis L, et al: The TNM classification of prostatic cancer. Prostate Suppl 4:129–139, 1992.

129. Schroeder FH, Hop WC, Bloom JH, Mostofi FK: Grading of prostate carcinoma, I. Analysis of the prognostic significance of single characteristics. Prostate 6:81–100, 1985.

130. Schroeder FH, Hop WC, Bloom JH, Mostofi FK: Grading of prostatic carcinoma. Multivariant analysis of prognostic parameters. Prostate 7:13–20, 1985.

131. Segi M, Kurihara M: Cancer mortality for selected sites in 24 countries. Tokyo, Japan Cancer Society 1972, No 6, p 81.

132. Sesterhenn IA, Becker RL, Avallone FA, et al: Image analysis of nucleoli and nucleolar organizing regions in prostatic, hyperplasia, intraepithelial neoplasia and prostatic carcinoma. J Urogen Pathol 1:61–74, 1991.

133. Sesterhenn IA, Mostofi FK, Davis CJ Jr: Immunopathology in prostate and bladder tumors. *In* Russo J (ed): Immunocytochemistry in Tumor Diagnosis. Boston, Martinus Nijhoff Publishing, 1985, pp 337–350.

134. Sesterhenn IA, Mostofi FK, Davis CJ Jr, van Dekken H: Numerical chromosomal aberrations in interphase nuclei of genitourinary tumors by in situ hybridochemistry. Lab Invest 64, Abstr 298, 1991.

135. Sherwood FR, Theyer G, Steiner G, et al: Differential expression of specific cytokeratin polypeptides in the basal and luminal epithelium of the human prostate. Prostate 18:303–314, 1991.

136. Sheth NA, Doctor VM, Sheth AR: Cellular immunolocalization of inhibin-like peptide in human benign prostatic hyperplasia. Arch Androl 14:155–159, 1985.

137. Siders DB, Lee F: Histologic changes of irradiated prostatic carcinoma diagnosed by transrectal ultrasound. Hum Pathol 23:344–351, 1992.

138. Sinha AA, Blackard CE, Seal U: A critical analysis of tumor morphology and hormone treatments in the untreated and estrogen treated response and refractory human prostatic carcinoma. Cancer 40:2836–2850, 1977.

139. Sloane JP, Omerod MG: Distribution of epithelial membrane antigen in normal and neoplastic tissues and its value in diagnostic tumor pathology. Cancer 47:1786–1795, 1981.

140. Sobin LH, Hjermstad BM, Sesterhenn IA, Helwig E: Prostatic acid phosphatase activity in carcinoid tumors. Cancer 58:136–138, 1986.

141. Soloway MS, Altwein JE: The management of incidental T1a G1 prostatic cancer. Prostate Suppl 4:149–151, 1992.

142. Srigley JR: Small acinar patterns in the prostate gland with emphasis on atypical adenomatous hyperplasia and small acinar carcinoma. Semin Diag Pathol 5:254–272, 1988.

143. Srigley J, King S, Van Nostrand AWP, Robinette M: The "preneoplastic" prostate: A giant section whole organ study of 72 radical prostatectomies. Lab Invest 54:61A (Abstr 359), 1986.

144. Stephenson RA, James BC, Gay H, et al: Flow cytometry of prostatic cancer: Relationship of DNA contact to survival. Cancer Res 47:2505–2507, 1987.
145. Sterberger LA, Hardy PH, Cuculis JJ, Meyer HG: The unlabeled antibody enzyme method of immunohistochemistry. Preparation and properties of soluble antigen-antibody complex (horseradish peroxidase, anti horseradish peroxidase) and its use in identification of spirochetes. J Histochem Cytochem 18:315–333, 1970.
146. Tannenbaum M: Differential diagnosis in uropathology: Carcinoma in situ of prostate gland. Urology 5:143–146, 1975.
147. Tannenbaum M, Tannenbaum S, DeSanctis PN, Olsson CA: Prognostic significance of nucleolar surface area in prostatic cancer. Urology 19:546–551, 1982.
148. Tribukait B: DNA flow cytometry in carcinoma of the prostate for diagnosis, prognosis and study of tumor biology. Acta Oncol 30:187–192, 1991.
149. Tribukait B: Flow cytometry in assessing the clinical aggressiveness of genitourinary neoplasms. World J Urol 5:108–122, 1987.
150. Tribukait B: Rapid flow cytometry of prostatic fine needle aspiration biopsies. In Karr JP, Coffey DS, Gardner W (eds): Prognostic Cytometry and Cytopathology of Prostatic Cancer. New York, Elsevier, 1989, pp 236–242.
151. Ullman AS, Ross OA: Hyperplasia atypism and carcinoma in situ of prostatic periurethral glands. Am J Clin Pathol 47:497–504, 1967.
152. van Dekken H, Pizzolo JG, Reuter VE, Melamed MR: Cytogenetic analysis of human solid tumors by in situ hybridization with a set of 12 chromosome specific DNA probes. Cytogenet Cell Genet 54:103–107, 1990.
153. Viola MV, Fromowitz F, Oravez S, et al: Expression of ras oncogene p21 in prostate cancer. N Engl J Med 314:133–137, 1986.
154. Vuitch MF, Mendelsohn G: Relationship of ectopic ACTH production to tumor differentiation. A morphologic and immunohistochemical study of prostatic carcinoma with Cushing's syndrome. Cancer 47:296–299, 1981.
155. Wahab ZA, Wright GL Jr: Monoclonal antibody (antibody Leu 7) directed against natural killer cells reacts with normal benign and malignant prostate tissues. Int J Cancer 36:667–683, 1985.
156. Wang MC, Papsidero LD, Kuriyama M, et al: Purification of a human prostate specific antigen: A new potential marker for prostatic cancer. Prostate 2:89–96, 1981.
157. Weaver MS, Fadi W, Abdul Karim FW, et al: Paneth cell–like change in the prostate gland. Am J Surg Pathol 16:62–68, 1992.
158. Weber MM. Polypeptide hormones and the prostate. Am J Surg Pathol 16:63–88, 1992.
159. Whittemore AS, Keller JB, Betenson R: Low grade latent prostate cancer volume: Predictors of clinical cancer incidence. J Natl Cancer Inst 83:1231–1235, 1991.
160. Witorsch RJ: Visualization of prolactin binding sites in prostate tissue. Am J Surg Pathol 16:89–113, 1992.
161. Wolf RM, Schneider SL, Englander LS, et al: Progesterone and estrogen receptor analysis of prostatic cancer and benign prostatic hyperplasia using sucrose density gradient centrifugation techniques. J Urol 131 (Abstr 70), 1984.
162. Yam LT, Janckilla AJ, Lam WKW, Li CY: Immunohistochemistry of prostatic acid phosphatase. Prostate 2:97–107, 1981.
163. Young RH: Pseudoneoplastic lesions of the prostate gland. Pathol Annu 23:105–128, 1988.

Chapter 20

EPIDEMIOLOGY AND NATURAL HISTORY OF PROSTATE CANCER

FRANK P. BEGUN

There is a saying that the only things that you can count on in life are death and taxes. However, for men a third inevitability probably should be added, that of prostate cancer. The epidemiology of prostate cancer is still poorly understood. This stems in part from the fact that little is known about the specific causes of the disease. In addition, the natural history of prostate cancer is extremely variable and has not been well studied. Prostate cancer is the most common neoplasm diagnosed in men in the United States and accounts for 20 per cent of all newly diagnosed cancers.[108] It is also the second most common cause of male cancer deaths in the United States, accounting for approximately 11 per cent of these.[105, 106, 108] Prostate cancer is the only cancer that exists with no peak age of occurrence. It is rarely found in men younger than 40 years old. However, there seems to be a steady increase in the incidence and prevalence with increasing age. Most prostate cancer exists as histologic, latent, or occult disease. These terms are often used synonymously, and all describe a form of prostate cancer that never becomes clinically evident and is found incidentally at the time of prostate surgery or autopsy. Prostate cancer would clearly be the most common cancer if all men with this form of the disease were accurately diagnosed and included in the epidemiologic data.

Unfortunately, the only known prerequisites for the development of prostate cancer are increasing age, a male karyotype, and androgen stimulation. This presents a major dilemma, because it will become critical to understand the epidemiologic factors that are involved as our ability to diagnose prostate cancer increases. In addition, logical approaches to diagnosis and treatment demand a knowledge of the natural history and biologic behavior of the different forms of the disease. This chapter attempts to address some of these issues and questions.

EPIDEMIOLOGY

Definitions

Several terms need to be defined before embarking on a discussion of the epidemiology of prostate cancer. *Incidence* refers to the risk of developing prostate cancer during a specific time period. This represents the number of new cases diagnosed and is usually expressed per 100,000 men. *Prevalence*, on the other hand, refers to the number of men who actually have the disease during a given period of time. This is the total number of cases in existence during that time frame. The true prevalence of prostate cancer is unknown because most men have the incidental form of the disease and are, by definition, undiagnosed. Age adjustment is often carried out to express the incidence or prevalence in terms of population age. *Mortality rate* is the number of deaths per unit population per year and *disease-specific mortality rate* refers to the actual number of deaths due to prostate cancer.

The incidence of prostate cancer appears to be increasing in the population. Silverberg and Lubera observed that the incidence of prostate cancer, in 1975, for white men and black men was 6.1 per cent and 7.2 per cent, respectively. Corresponding figures in 1986 demonstrated an 8.7 per cent and a 9.4 per cent incidence in the two populations.[107] However, this may have reflected an increased ability to detect prostate cancer with new diagnostic modalities such as prostate ultrasonography and prostate-specific antigen (PSA). In addition, screening programs, newer biopsy techniques, and an increased awareness of the disease, causing more men to seek evaluation, may also have accounted for this increase. A similar increase in the prostate cancer mortality rate has also been noted. In 1975, there was a 2 per cent and a 2.6 per cent probability of dying of prostate cancer in the white and black populations. This rose to 2.6 per cent and 4.3 per cent, respectively, by 1985.[107, 121] Interestingly, this increased mortality rate demonstrated a proportionally smaller rise compared with the increased incidence noted above. This has prompted speculation that this is a result of improved survival due to better treatment methods. However, what this more likely represented is better detection and recording of the occult forms of the disease.

Race

Much of the epidemiologic work that has been carried out has been directed toward an evaluation of the differences in the incidence of prostate cancer in men of various ethnic and racial backgrounds. One observation, which has been consistent throughout these studies, is that the prevalence of histologic disease found in autopsy specimens is similar for the different geographic regions and different ethnic groups studied.[1, 15, 56–58] However, the incidence of clinically evident disease and the disease-specific mortality rates show wide regional variations. The highest incidence of prostate cancer in Caucasian populations occurs in Scandinavia, and there is a 220-fold difference in the incidence of clinical prostate cancer between Swedish and Honduran men.[30, 104] The overall US incidence is approximately equal to that of northern Europe.[30] Lower rates have been noted in southern Europe and South America, and the lowest rates in the world occur in Eastern Europe and Asia.[56, 107, 125]

Studies of racial differences in the United States have shown that blacks have a significantly higher risk of developing prostate cancer. In addition, US blacks seem to have an increased mortality rate and appear to present with more advanced stages of the disease at the time of diagnosis.[70, 84] However, when properly controlled for stage, grade, and type of treatment, there may be no difference in the behavior of prostate cancer in the black population.[70]

Migration Studies

Migration studies have provided insight into the discrepancy between the latent and clinical forms of prostate cancer with respect to incidence and prevalence. Relocation of men from areas with a low incidence to areas with a high incidence of clinical prostate cancer results in an increase in the disease with each successive generation. This is true for Asian and black Americans compared with native Asians and Africans. Studies of

African men and their US counterparts shows a sixfold greater incidence of progressive prostate cancer in the US black population, yet no differences in the histologic form of the disease were found.[58] Studies of Japanese men migrating to Hawaii or to the US mainland show a low incidence of clinical disease in the native Japanese populations and the first-generation immigrants. However, the incidence of diagnosed cancer and the mortality rate increase with successive generations.[1, 30, 52, 56, 125] A 10-fold increase in prostate cancer has been noted in Asian immigrants to Hawaii. However, this remains below the rate observed in the corresponding Caucasian population.[101] Similar data have been reported for European populations and Mexican-Americans.[80, 111] Unfortunately, no studies of population migration from high-incidence areas to low-incidence areas have been carried out, and it is not known whether a reverse phenomenon occurs.

The above data suggest that environmental factors may be responsible for these differences. Unidentified factors may result in the transformation of prostate cancer from an indolent to a biologically active form. Carter and associates have suggested that multiple factors may be necessary to change a normal prostate epithelial cell into a prostate cancer cell with the biologic potential to grow and metastasize.[21] In addition, genetic factors may affect the individual cell's susceptibility to these environmental stimuli; therefore, the development of prostate cancer may be the result of a complex series of interactions between inherent and extrinsic factors.

Religion

The highest prostate cancer mortality rate has been found in US Protestants. Catholics appear to have an intermediate death rate, and Jews have the lowest.[56, 121] This may be due to the Eastern European origin of most US Jews.[125] It is interesting that Mormons, with their particular lifestyle, have shown a decreased mortality rate related to several cancers, but similar differences have not been noted with respect to prostate cancer.[31, 32, 72, 119] This is not a uniform observation because California Mormons have been shown to have a decreased mortality rate and Utah Mormons to have a higher mortality rate than age-matched US controls.[32] The significance of this remains unclear. Data from these studies also suggest that smoking has no direct association with and carries no increased risk for the development of progressive prostate cancer.

Environmental Factors

This is probably one of the most intriguing topics related to the epidemiology of prostate cancer, especially when the previously discussed migration data are considered. Unfortunately, it is impossible to study, on an individual basis, all of the external factors that may play a role in the development of prostate cancer. In addition, no single factor or group of factors have been conclusively shown to inpart a greater risk for the development of progressive disease. It has often been assumed that industrial and chemical substances can act as promoters of neoplastic change. Support for this comes from the fact that men residing in urban environments appear to have a slightly increased risk for the development of cancer and an increase in the mortality rate.[11] Exposure to chemical substances, industrial waste products, and air pollutants may account for this.

A number of different occupations appear to carry a greater risk for the development of prostate cancer. These include printers, painters, rubber workers, textile workers, mechanics, loggers, ship fitters, people employed in drug and chemical industry, and farmers. In addition, car salesmen, bookkeepers, janitors, shipping and receiving clerks, and people employed in the personnel services also appear to be at greater risk.[34, 121, 122] Some of these industries involve direct or indirect exposure to various chemicals and toxins. Clearly, printers, painters, rubber workers, and drug and chemical workers fall into this category. In addition, farmers may be at increased risk because of exposure to substances contained in fertilizers, pesticides, and herbicides. Why people with occupations such as bookkeeping or those involved in sales or personnel services would be at greater risk remains unclear. Obviously, no single factor or group of factors has been identified that accounts for the increased incidence of prostate cancer observed in men employed in these very diverse fields.

Blair and Fraumeni observed that regional variations occur within the United States.[11] There appears to be an increased mortality rate in the Midwest and North Central States. In addition, two clusters of counties, with the highest prostate cancer mortality rates, were found in New England and the North Midwest section of the country. Interestingly, there were high proportions of men employed in the printing industry in these two areas. Several studies have noted an increased mortality rate with increasing socioeconomic status.[11, 119] However, other studies have shown either higher rate of prostate cancer in lower socioeconomic classes or no correlation.[11, 35, 47]

Trace Elements and Heavy Metals

Zinc is a trace element found in increased concentration in prostatic secretions. The exact role that zinc plays in prostate function is not known. Although there have been no well-controlled studies evaluating the relationship of zinc to prostate cancer, decreased zinc levels have been noted in prostate cancer patients.[60] Cadmium is a heavy metal found in industrial environments. There is a possible association between prostate cancer and exposure to cadmium because increased levels have been found in patients with prostate cancer.[34, 60] However, other studies have failed to show an association, and no conclusions can be drawn from the available data.[64, 96, 121]

Familial Factors

Familial tendencies toward the development of prostate cancer have been reported.[18, 78] Interestingly, an increased risk of prostate cancer has also been noted in relatives of people with colon cancer and women with breast cancer.[11, 114] Although no specific HLA haplotype has been found to be associated with the development of progressive prostate cancer, men with blood type A seem to have an increased risk.[7] Several studies have been demonstrated a threefold to fourfold increase in the incidence and/or disease-specific mortality rate in first-order relatives of men with the disease.[79, 100, 124] This appeared to be especially true when the cancers occurred in younger men.[18, 79]

The specific factors that contribute to the development of the biologically active form of prostate cancer are unknown and may represent a perfect example of the complex interplay between "nature and nurture." In other words, some men may have prostate epithelial cells with a preprogrammed genetic disposition to carcinogenic transformation. However, exposure to multiple environmental factors may be necessary prior to the emergence of neoplastic clones. Genetic factors may also act by modulating the individual cell's susceptibility to these external influences. Still other promotional factors may be required to change these cells from a latent or inactive form to a biologically active state with the ability to grow and metastasize.

Diet

There has been much controversy concerning the relationship of dietary factors to prostate cancer. Many studies appear to indicate a strong correlation between fat consumption and the emergence of clinical prostate cancer.[11, 20, 62] The increase in the incidence and mortality of prostate cancer appears to parallel increased fat consumption in the US population.[39, 40] Not surprisingly, areas in the United States with the highest consumption of dairy products and red meat appear to demonstrate the highest age-adjusted prostate cancer mortality rates.[11, 53] Fat may directly modulate the normal prostate or prostate cancer cell or may act in a permissive fashion to increase its susceptibility to additional stimulation. Dietary fat may also act as a promoter of prostate cancer by affecting the cellular hormonal milieu. Pollard and Luckert observed that fat appears to reduce the time necessary for the induction of prostate cancer in response to testosterone stimulation in certain strains of rats.[94] Another way that fat consumption may contribute to the development of prostate cancer relates to the absorption of vitamin A. Increased circulating levels of beta-carotene seem to depend on vitamin A intake and have been associated with a decreased incidence of certain neoplasms.[9, 92] However, although some studies have demonstrated a decreased risk, others have shown an increased risk of prostate cancer development related to increased vitamin A consumption.[43, 50, 63, 88] Obviously, no conclusions can be drawn from these conflicting observations.

Increased consumption of tofu and rice appears to be associated with a decreased incidence of prostate cancer and may account for some of the differences noted in Asian and Asian-American populations.[102] The consumption of increased quantities of refined carbohydrates has also been implicated as a causative factor. The above data may provide some explanation for the observed differences in the rates of prostate cancer noted in migrating populations. Men moving to the United States may consume a more "Western diet," and this may partially account for the greater incidence of clinical prostate cancer found in these groups than in age-matched populations in their countries of origin.[61, 62, 69]

Benign Prostatic Hyperplasia

The evidence that benign prostatic hyperplasia (BPH) is related to prostate cancer is inconclusive. There probably is no direct relationship, and there has been no direct evidence that the development of BPH leads to prostate cancer. Most prostate cancer occurs in the peripheral zone of the gland, separate from those regions that give rise to BPH. However, recent data from McNeal et al suggest that Stage A cancers may be located primarily in the anterior portion of the gland and invade the fibromuscular stroma and BPH nodules.[77] This may not necessarily indicate an etiologic relationship but may merely represent a coincidental finding. Armenian and associates observed that BPH patients had approximately a fourfold to fivefold greater likelihood of developing prostate cancer.[3] However, their study was flawed because half of the data was obtained from clinical and not pathologic observations. Other histologic studies of prostatectomy specimens have failed to demonstrate an increased risk of prostate cancer in BPH patients.[44] The only definite association that seems to exist between BPH and prostate cancer is their mutual requirement of androgen stimulation.

Hormonal Factors

As mentioned above, one of the few things that is known about the prostate is that androgens are necessary for the growth and development of normal, benign hyperplastic, and neoplastic prostate cells. Eunuchs who are castrated prior to puberty are at minimal risk for the development of prostate cancer.[25] However, the exact role that androgens play in the carcinogenic process is unclear. They may function as initiators of the neoplastic process, or they may serve a facilitary role by maintaining the normal prostatic epithelium or prostatic carcinoma cells. Studies have been conflicting as to whether testosterone levels are increased or decreased in patients with prostate cancer.[29, 37, 46, 79] Glantz has suggested that the decreased number of occult prostate cancers, found in autopsy specimens of patients with

cirrhosis of the liver, is secondary to decreased circulating testosterone or increased circulating estrogen levels.[38] Lower rates of clinical prostate cancer have also been reported in men with alcoholic cirrhosis.[71] Estrogens probably do not play a direct role but may act by inhibiting luteinizing hormone release and ultimately resulting in a decrease in androgen levels.

Paradoxically, serum testosterone concentrations appear to decrease with age, whereas the incidence of prostate cancer increases. A possible explanation relates to the fact that although testosterone levels are decreasing, they still may remain within the normal physiologic range. In addition, subnormal values may be adequate to stimulate or at least maintain prostate cancer cells. Another explanation may be that the carcinogenic events that require or involve androgen stimulation occur years before the actual emergence of the prostate cancer clones. Other evidence for the relationship of hormones to prostate cancer has come from the Noble rat model. Estrogen and testosterone stimulation have resulted in the development of prostate cancers in certain strains of these animals.[87]

In summary, no consistent pattern of hormone levels has been observed in prostate cancer patients. Most data fail to demonstrate any statistically significant correlation between circulating testosterone levels and the risk of developing either the occult or progressive form of the disease. Androgens may merely serve to maintain the prostate epithelium, or they may increase the individual cell's susceptibility to the external inductive factors involved in the neoplastic process. They may also maintain the carcinoma cells once neoplastic transformation has occurred.

Sexual Activity

The data concerning sexual activity and its relationship to prostate cancer are vague. Several studies have shown an increased risk of prostate cancer in men who have engaged in early and frequent sexual activity. The possible association of prostate cancer with early sexual activity may provide some insight into the role played by androgens.[2] Previous exposure to sexually transmitted diseases and an increased number of sexual partners seem to carry greater risk.[100, 112] Heshmat et al demonstrated similar curves in the incidence of gonococcal infections and prostate cancer deaths with a 45-year delay.[51] It has also been suggested that increased fertility, an increased number of children, extramarital sexual activity, and sexual relationships with prostitutes may confer a greater risk of prostate cancer development.[2, 100, 112] However, there are no consistent data and no well-controlled studies to support these allegations. In fact, Rotkin observed an increased risk of prostate cancer with decreased sexual activity.[97] Other studies have shown an increased risk in men who were celibate or never married.[95, 100] Wynder et al found no correlation between the risk of prostate cancer and marital status or number of children.[125]

Viruses

Viruses have been implicated as promoters of neoplastic transformation. A number of DNA viruses have been postulated to play a role in the development of prostate cancer.[5, 68, 91] Type II herpes simplex viruses have been found on electron micrographic evaluations of human prostate cancer cells.[22] Anti–herpes simplex type II immunoglobins were found more often in patients with prostate cancer than in those with BPH.[5] Cytomegalovirus (CMV) has been found in human semen.[68] However, when human prostate cancer tissue was tested, only 2 of 34 specimens were found to express CMV antigens.[99] Several RNA viruses have also been suggested as causative agents because RNA particles and viral core material have been found in prostate cancer tissue.[74, 89] Reverse transcriptase activity has also been demonstrated in human prostate cancer tissue and may provide indirect evidence concerning the role of RNA viruses.[36] The presence of the H-*ras* oncogene p21 antigen in prostate cancer tissue provides additional evidence in support of a viral cause. This protein was not found in the prostatic tissue of normal and BPH glands but was found in prostate cancer specimens. The antigen appeared to occur with greater frequency as the grade of the prostate cancer increased. All high Gleason grade cancers were found to be positive, whereas only two of six prostates with well-differentiated lesions expressed the p21 protein.[117]

Conclusions

Although many factors may influence the development and subsequent growth of prostate cancer, no specific entity has been identified that clearly puts men at greater risk. Data from migration studies clearly suggest that environmental and dietary factors may play a key role, not necessarily in the initial development of prostate cancer, but rather in the alteration of the disease to a more biologically active form. Clearly, much more work needs to be carried out to identify the variables involved and to determine their exact contribution to the neoplastic process. This strategy may enable clinicians to structure interventions aimed at reducing the risk of the development of prostate cancer. In addition, better methods for detection may result in earlier treatment and a reduction in the historically high disease-specific mortality rates.

NATURAL HISTORY

Background

The natural history of prostate cancer is an extremely complex issue. The only thing that is known with any degree of certainty is that prostate cancer must start out as localized disease during the initial phases of its development. Although this may seem like an extremely simplistic statement, the fact remains that very little is known about the growth and development of early prostate cancer. Very few studies exist that have followed patients with untreated prostate cancer. Similarly, randomized prospective evaluations of the various treatments for prostate cancer, using untreated controls, are not available owing to moral and ethical considerations. Most early-stage disease is treated either surgically or with radiation therapy. What information is available comes from a handful of studies that have followed "untreated" patients for variable periods of time. However, most of these patients have received some form of palliative treatment at some point during the course of their disease. Therefore, the term *natural history* is really a misnomer. The true natural history of a cancer represents the behavior of the tumor from the time of cellular transformation, resulting in the emergence of neoplastic cells, to the time of the demise of the untreated host.[120] Most of what we know about the growth and progression of prostate cancer must be inferred from the available indirect data. Similarly, the early natural history of the disease is unknown because diagnosis always occurs at some point after these initial events take place.

Three key issues arise with respect to the natural history of prostate cancer. First, what are the factors and events that lead to malignant transformation? Second, when and why does the transformation from occult to clinically evident disease occur? Finally, what is the natural history of untreated prostate cancer? The biologic potential and the natural history of each individual prostate cancer are probably the end result of a number of factors. These include certain intrinsic properties that may be genetically predetermined. In addition, various extrinsic carcinogenic influences may cause an alteration in the genetic composition of these cells, resulting in transformation to a more malignant form. In addition, there are a number of poorly understood tumor-host factors that may influence the growth and development of prostate cancer cell populations.[120] Last, environmental factors influence the growth and development of prostate cancer as discussed in the previous epidemiology section. The fact is that the vast majority of men with prostate cancer have a clinically silent form of the disease. Some of these patients develop a biologically active form that eventually progresses and becomes metastatic if left untreated. One of the most significant shortcomings in prostate cancer diagnosis is that it is impossible to predict into which category an individual patient will fall. A review of these issues and a discussion of the available data concerning the behavior of various stages of the disease are the subjects of this section.

Theories

Two different theories pertaining to the development and progression of prostate cancer are widely held. One hypothesis, set forth by Stamey, holds that when histologic or occult prostate cancer is detected, all the cells have already completed all the steps necessary to produce fully malignant and biologically active tumors.[110]

Therefore, all that is necessary for the cancer cell population to progress and metastasize is sufficient time for the tumor to double and increase in volume.[76] Furthermore, the histologic form of the disease is merely prostate cancer that is found in the early stages of development and progression. In other words, when it is diagnosed in an 80 year old, it signifies that the disease had its onset late in the patient's life. McNeal and Stamey have observed that prostate cancer doubling is a relatively slow process compared with that of other cancers.[76, 110] They have postulated that it takes approximately 10 years from neoplastic transformation to the development of a tumor with a volume of 1 cc. If the above theory is correct, then time should be the sole controlling factor and the clinical manifestation of prostate cancer should be the same in various populations, assuming that the incidence of histologic disease and the life expectancies of the populations are similar.[21] However, although the prevalence of histologic cancer in the various world populations is very similar, clear-cut differences exist in the prevalence of clinical disease. This holds true for US and Japanese men, whose respective populations have demonstrated similar life expectancies. These observations appear to contradict the above hypothesis.

A second theory suggests that not all histologically diagnosed tumors have undergone all the transformational steps necessary to produce clinically evident cancers. Additional events may be necessary before continued growth and progression can occur.[21] If this is true, then occult or histologic disease can occur at any age and remain inactive for indefinite periods of time. These tumors may eventually undergo additional transformations that result in a more biologically active form. Carter and associates have analyzed epidemiologic data derived from studies of prostate cancer in native Japanese, migratory Japanese, and native US populations.[21] Their analysis served as the basis for the proposal that a multistep process is necessary in the transformation of a normal prostate cell to a malignant prostate cancer cell. Their data also support the fact that a similar number of steps are necessary in Japanese and American men to complete this malignant transformation. The reason for the difference in the incidence of clinically manifest prostate cancer in the two populations may be that the probability of one or more of the transforming steps occurring is less in Japan than in the United States. This again implies the role of environmental influences. Their data also suggest that histologic prostate cancer and clinical prostate cancer are different forms of the disease and not the same disease at different points on a time continuum. It has been postulated that the above data could have been prejudiced by better cancer screening and detection in the US population. However, Japanese screening studies using transrectal ultrasonography (TRUS) have failed to demonstrate significant differences in the occurrence of prostate cancer in men older than 55 years, compared with their US counterparts.[21, 118]

The above questions are critical with respect to the diagnosis and treatment of prostate cancer. If Stamey's theory is valid, then the detection of all prostate cancer is critical. This is especially true in younger men because it is only a matter of time before the cancer grows and progresses to the point of the development of metastatic disease. However, if the alternative theory is true, then identification of the factors that contribute to the neoplastic transformation process would be the first step in the development of strategies that might delay or even halt the carcinogenic process.

Determinants of Tumor Growth and Malignant Potential

The detection of early-stage prostate cancer has increased as a result of diagnostic modalities such as TRUS and PSA. In addition, screening programs and mass media coverage have heightened the public's awareness and have resulted in more men seeking evaluation. One of the caveats of early detection is to diagnose the disease before it progresses to a metastatic form. Therefore, the ultimate goal of any screening or detection program should be to reduce cancer-specific mortality. However, the number of clinically evident prostate cancers represents only a small fraction of the total number of men with the disease. Therefore, the key question may not be who has prostate cancer but rather, of those who do have the disease, who is at risk for tumor growth and progression? It seems logical that any variable that can help to predict the biologic behavior of an individual case of prostate cancer would be of great benefit to clinicians.

Age may play a role in the natural history of prostate cancer because the incidence of the disease increases with age. However, several investigators have suggested that younger men may present with more advanced and biologically aggressive cancer at the time of diagnosis.[54] However, this may be artifactual and may relate to the smaller number of Stage A cancers diagnosed in the younger age cohorts. Conditions such as BPH, hematuria, or urinary tract infections are less likely to occur in younger men, and fewer of these patients present for urologic evaluation. Consequently, fewer incidentally diagnosed early stage tumors are found, resulting in a falsely elevated proportion of the more advanced cancers. In addition, the fact that younger patients are at risk for disease progression for a longer period of time may make it appear that prostate cancer is more lethal, when it actually is not. In fact, younger patients with Stage B tumors had better survival rates than patients over 50 years of age. This may have been due to the fact that a greater number of young patients underwent radical prostatectomy than did their older counterparts.[54]

A number of features about prostate cancer cells may be indicators of their biologic behavior. Tumor stage and tumor grade have been shown to be related to the growth rate and metastatic potential of prostate cancer.[28, 67, 76, 90] However, the interrelationship between these parameters is extremely complex. Patients with high-grade tumors (Gleason score 8 to 10) have a very high percentage of positive pelvic lymph nodes at the time of surgical staging. This is in contrast to patients with low-grade tumors (Gleason score 2 to 4), who rarely have lymphatic involvement.[67, 90] It has also been shown that the chance of understaging increases as the stage of the tumor increases.[83] Therefore, the likelihood of pelvic lymph node metastasis seems to follow reasonably well with the clinical stage as well as the pathologic grade of the primary tumor. However, in other studies the relationship between tumor stage, tumor grade, and lymph node metastases is not as clear. Smith and Middleton demonstrated that approximately one third of patients with high-grade but low-stage prostate cancers had metastatic disease. Similarly, only one half of those patients with low-grade but Stage C prostate cancer had metastases.[109]

Nuclear roundness has also been evaluated as a predictor of the biologic behavior of prostate cancer. Well-differentiated tumor cell populations appear to have round and uniform nuclei, whereas those of poorly differentiated cancer cells appear more variable and pleomorphic. An accurate correlation between the degree of nuclear roundness and the clinical course of patients with Stage B prostate cancer following radical prostatectomy has been reported.[27] Tumor ploidy has also been proposed as a means of predicting the behavior of various prostate cancers. Techniques such as flow cytometry lend themselves to evaluation of fresh biopsy specimens or fixed paraffin-embedded tissues. A predominantly diploid or tetraploid cancer cell population seems to be associated with a better prognosis and a greater responsiveness to androgen ablation.[113] Other studies have demonstrated a direct correlation between ploidy and tumor grade, stage, progression, and survival.[12, 85, 115, 123] However, one problem with the use of these various techniques relates to the methods used to obtain tissue. Cancer cell populations are often extremely heterogeneous, and the use of needle biopsy techniques may result in significant inaccuracies due to sampling errors. Therefore, it is difficult to draw conclusions about the biologic potential of a tumor when only a small number of the cells in the population are being evaluated.

Similarly, the heterogeneity of the cancer cell population can also be reflected in differing rates of cell growth and division. Theoretically, the biologic activity of a tumor should reflect the characteristics of the individual cells that comprise it. However, the growth and metastatic potential of a tumor and ultimately the prognosis and host survival may reflect the behavior of only a small fraction of the cancer cells within the population. This may depend on a number of factors, including cell cycle time, cell death rate, and the number of cells actually involved in the process of cell division at a given time. These factors may be highly variable and may change during the natural history of the tumor. This is especially important when considering the growth rate of a specific cancer. The emergence of more biologically active clones of cells may change the tumor population characteristics and lead to more rapid growth and metastasis.

The metastatic potential of prostate cancer cells may be related to growth rate, but this is certainly not the sole determinant. Additional factors such as cell motility, cell membrane characteristics, and cell-cell and cell–extracellular matrix interactions probably contribute to the individual cell's ability to metastasize. Epithelial and stromal interactions may play a key role in the modulation the cancer cell's behavior. These interactions may involve one of a number of growth factors. Basic fibroblast growth factor (bFGF) has been implicated in the carcinogenic process.[41, 42] It is unknown whether bFGF plays a role in human prostate cancer. Higher concentrations of bFGF have been found in neoplastic glands.[86] Work in our laboratory has been aimed at trying to determine whether there are differences in the concentrations of bFGF in the latent and biologically active forms of prostate cancer. Unfortunately, very preliminary data have failed to show significant differences in prostate cancers of various stages and grades.

Growth and Metastatic Patterns of Prostate Cancer

Knowledge of the routes of growth and the spread of prostate cancer is important when considering methods of diagnosis and treatment. Early growth usually takes place within the gland, with local extension and lymphatic or hematogenous spread occurring later in the course of the disease. Growth within the gland can be unifocal or multicentric and homogeneous or heterogeneous. Pericapsular extension seems to occur in one of two ways. The tumor may encroach upon the capsule and displace it to the point where penetration and extraprostatic spread occurs. Alternately, cells may invade directly through the tissue planes. This probably represents a more malignant and biologically aggressive form of the disease. Once capsular violation has occurred, the periprostatic tissues, seminal vesicles, bladder neck, and ureters may become involved via direct extension of the tumor. Rectal extension is a rare occurrence. This is thought to be due to the fact that the Denonvilliers' fascia acts as a deterrent to metastatic spread. Ureteral involvement is usually a late manifestation of the disease and may be diagnosed only when renal insufficiency or anuria occurs.

Other routes of spread involve lymphatic and hematogenous channels. The most common site of initial lymph node involvement is the obturator nodes.[75] Other lymph node groups involved, in order of decreasing frequency, are the hypogastric, external iliac, presacral, presciatic, common iliac, inguinal, periaortic, mediastinal, and supraclavicular.[75, 98] Lymphatic progression usually occurs in a sequential fashion, but "skip" lesions may occur in 5 per cent of patients. This is characterized by involvement of more distant groups without evidence of disease in the obturator or hypogastric nodes.[75] Interestingly, the pathologic pattern found in lymph node metastases can be different from that of the primary tumor in up to 25 per cent of patients.[66] This is not surprising when cancer cell population heterogeneity and biopsy sampling error are considered.

Osseous metastases usually follow lymphatic spread but can occur without obvious nodal involvement. The axial skeleton appears to be most often involved. The reason for this predilection is unknown. One theory has postulated that spread to the skeletal structures occurs via Batson's venous plexus.[8] In addition, the lymphatic drainage of the prostate may somehow predispose to cancer cells reaching these structures. However, there may be organ-specific conditions or factors that result in a preferential environment that favors prostate cancer cell growth in the large central skeletal elements. The most common sights of involvement, in decreasing order, are the ilium, ischium, lumbosacral spine, thoracic spine, ribs, and femur.[16]

Visceral metastases usually occur in the very late stages of the disease and are often clinically silent. Autopsy studies have revealed that metastases in the lungs, liver, adrenals, and kidneys occur most often.[98]

Premalignant Lesions

Recently, a number of histologic patterns have been identified in prostate tissue that are thought to represent premalignant changes.[14, 16] The most widely accepted term for these entities is *prostatic intraepithelial neoplasia* (PIN). It has been postulated that PIN represents a stage of neoplastic transformation intermediate between dysplasia and overt carcinoma. It may also be the forerunner of, or the common pathway leading to, the latent and progressive forms of the disease. PIN is characterized by epithelial cellular proliferation leading to "crowding" and the eventual disruption of the normal basal cell architecture.[14]

Evidence for the association between PIN and prostate cancer comes from histologic evaluations. PIN most often occurs in the peripheral zone of the gland, the site where most prostate cancer arises.[14, 116] The frequency of PIN has been shown to be higher in prostates with carcinoma.[116] In addition, the cytologic characteristics of PIN are almost identical to those of prostate cancer.[14] PIN also seems to occur in association with invasive carcinoma, and the degree of atypia seems to increase with closer proximity to the cancer.

These observations have led to the hypothesis that PIN represents a field change phenomenon similar to that observed in bladder cancer. Actual evidence that PIN gives rise to carcinoma is lacking because available diagnostic methods do not allow serial evaluation of individual lesions. Therefore, PIN may merely represent a concurrent or coincidental disease entity. However, the fact that PIN may be a precursor or an intermediate form of prostate cancer lends further support to the multistep theory discussed in previous sections.

Stage A Prostate Cancer

A major problem that exists when discussing Stage A prostate cancer is the fact that no standard criteria are available for the differentiation between Stage A1 and A2 disease. Attempts have been made to identify dif-

ferences in the prognosis and metastatic potential between these two forms, but studies have been hampered by the lack of standard definition. Past data have shown that approximately 8 to 10 per cent of patients with Stage A1 prostate cancer develop progressive disease and 2 per cent die of cancer within 5 to 10 years.[19, 24, 49] More recently, Epstein et al demonstrated that 16 per cent of patients with well-differentiated A1 lesions progress after 8 years or longer.[33] A1 lesions have been shown to have a 10-year mortality rate of less than 5 per cent whereas 25 per cent of patients with A2 lesions die within the same time period.[103] Lymphatic involvement is rare for true Stage A1 cancer. Men with untreated well-differentiated Stage A tumors appear to have a normal 15-year life expectancy, whereas patients with untreated high-grade tumors demonstrate a normal 10-year but a decreased 15-year survival.[48] Thirty per cent of patients with Stage A2 disease develop distant metastases and 20 per cent die within 5 to 10 years.[19, 24, 49] However, these patients may have understaged C or D lesions that were not truly localized cancers at the time of diagnosis.

Cantrell et al followed 82 patients for a minimum of 4 years or until disease progression.[19] Those patients with a Gleason score of 4 or less showed no disease progression, and only 2 per cent progressed if less than 5 per cent of the total prostate was involved. This was compared with a 32 per cent progression rate if greater than 5 per cent of the gland was neoplastic. In addition, if the Gleason score was greater than 4, 17 per cent eventually developed progressive disease. Epstein et al followed 94 patients with untreated Stage A1 prostate cancer. This was defined as a Gleason score of 7 or less with no more than 5 per cent of the gland involved. Eight patients developed disease progression within 8 years and six of these eight patients ultimately died of their prostate cancer.[33] Blute et al followed 23 untreated patients with Stage A prostate cancer for a minimum of 10 years. They found that the 10-year survival was the same as in age-matched controls. Two of 8 patients with A2 disease and 4 of 15 patients with A1 disease had progression at a mean follow-up of 11.5 years.[13]

Approximately 25 per cent of "A2" prostate cancers have already spread to regional nodes at the time of diagnosis.[28] A2 lesions may be more biologically active, with a greater metastatic potential, than their Stage A1 or B1 counterparts. Patients with suspected A2 disease must be carefully evaluated for the presence of lymphatic involvement because this clearly alters prognosis and treatment options.

Stage B Prostate Cancer

The natural history of Stage B disease is less well known owing to the fact that most patients undergo some form of curative treatment. Studies of men with Stage B lesions treated with transurethral resection (TURP) and/or hormonal therapy have reported 5- and 10-year survivals of 53 to 60 per cent and 34 to 40 per cent, respectively.[23, 82] Other investigators have analyzed the course of untreated patients and have found 5-year survivals of 71 to 90 per cent and 10-year survivals of 55 to 58 per cent. In addition, between 20 and 28 per cent of patients with Stage B disease live up to 15 years after diagnosis.[6, 59, 73]

Hanash et al evaluated the natural history of men with more advanced Stage B cancer treated with TURP. Eighty-five per cent of the 129 patients in their study had B2/B3 lesions. They reported a 5-year, 10-year, and 15-year survival of 19 per cent, 4 per cent, and 1 per cent, respectively.[48] Approximately 25 per cent of patients with B1 lesions develop metastasis and 28 per cent die within 5 years.[23] In patients with B2 disease, approximately 80 per cent develop metastases and 70 per cent die within 5 to 10 years.[48] It is unclear from these studies whether the poorer prognosis observed in men with higher Stage B disease is due strictly to greater tumor volume. An alternate explanation relates to the correlation between tumor stage and tumor grade. These hypotheses are not mutually exclusive, and certainly additional factors are involved.

Finally, Whitmore studies 75 Stage B patients who remained untreated for at least 1 year following diagnosis.[120] This study is very difficult to interpret because most of the men eventually underwent some form of treatment, including I-125 seed implantation, TURP, and hormonal manipulation. The median survival was found to be 216 months for patients with B1 lesions, 138 months for B2 lesions, and 197 months for B3 lesions. Fifteen-year survival rates for Stage B1, B2, and B3 cancers were 67 per cent, 42 per cent, and 67 per cent, respectively. Of the 75 patients, only 11 died of prostate cancer, and several were lost to follow-up, representing a possible total prostate cancer mortality rate of 24 per cent.

Stage C/D Prostate Cancer

The data on Stage C disease are even more discouraging. Approximately 60 per cent of patients with untreated Stage C cancer progress over a 5-year period, with 50 per cent developing metastases and 75 per cent dying within 10 years.[10, 16] Eighty-five per cent of patients with D1 disease progress or develop distant metastases within 5 years. Most die of metastatic disease within 3 years of the time of diagnosis. Fifty per cent of patients with D2 disease die within 3 years, 80 per cent within 5 years, and 90 per cent within 10 years.[4, 10, 26, 45, 66, 81, 93] Surprisingly, 10 per cent of these patients are still alive 10 years after the diagnosis of metastatic cancer was made. This may reflect the effects of hormonal manipulation. However, it may also represent a subset of patients with very slowly progressive disease.

Conclusions

It appears clear, from the above discussion, that prostate cancer is an extremely complex disease about which more is unknown than known. The more information that we uncover concerning its epidemiology and natural history, the more questions appear to arise. One of the key issues seems to be our inability to predict the biologic behavior of any given tumor. Because most patients with prostate cancer have a nonclinical form of the disease, this creates a dilemma concerning the best diagnostic and treatment approach for these men. This is especially critical in light of the fact that digital rectal examination, PSA, prostate ultrasonography, and needle biopsy techniques have improved our ability to find prostate cancer. With new diagnostic modalities, our ability to detect these cancers will certainly improve.

The philosophy behind early detection is based on the fact that every cancer must be confined to the prostate gland at some time in its development. Therefore, the goal of early detection is to identify lesions prior to progression, when they are still potentially curable. A critical question that bears directly on these issues is whether or not the precise point of neoplastic change or transformation to a metastatic state can be identified. Some investigators have suggested that this can be done solely on the basis of tumor volume. On the other hand, transformation of prostate cells to adenocarcinoma cells is a multistep process occurring over variable periods of time. Therefore, the traditional view that the metastatic potential of prostate cancer depends on grade, volume, and stage may not be entirely correct.

The true end-point of any type of cancer diagnostic and treatment plan should be prevention of disease progression and, more importantly, reduction of the disease-specific mortality rate. It remains to be seen whether the earlier detection of prostate cancer, in greater numbers of men, will accomplish these goals. A means of identifying the factors that determine or control the biologic activity of this disease might improve our ability to predict which patients actually need or would benefit from treatment. This dilemma was probably best summed up by Whitmore when he asked, "Is cure necessary in those in whom it may possible, and is cure possible in those in whom it is necessary?"[120] Until more is known about the epidemiology and natural history of prostate cancer, this question will remain central to the scientists and clinicians studying this disease.

REFERENCES

1. Akazaki K, Stemmermann GN: Comparative study of latent carcinoma of the prostate among Japanese in Japan and Hawaii. J Natl Cancer Inst 50:1137, 1973.
2. Armenian HK, Lilienfeld AM, Diamond EL, et al: Epidemiologic characterics of patients with prostatic neoplasms. Am J Epdiemiol 10:47, 1975.
3. Armenian HK, Lilienfeld AM, Diamond EL, et al: Relationship between benign prostatic hyperplasia and cancer of the prostate: A prospective and retrospective study. Lancet 2:115, 1974.
4. Bagshaw MD: Radiation therapy of prostatic carcinoma. *In* Crawford ED, Borden TA (eds): Genitourinary Cancer Surgery. Philadelphia, Lea & Febiger, 1982, pp 405–411.
5. Baker LH, Mebust WK, Chin TDY, et al: The relationship of

herpesvirus to carcinoma of the prostate. J Urol 125:370–374, 1981.

6. Barnes R, Hirst A, Rosenquist R: Early carcinoma of the prostate. Comparison of stages A and B. J Urol 115:404, 1976.

7. Barry JM, Goldstein A, Hubbard M: Human leukocyte A and B antigens in patients with prostatic adenocarcinoma. J Urol 124:847, 1980.

8. Batson OV: The function of the vertebral veins and their role in the spread of metastases. Ann Surg 112:138, 1940.

9. Bertram JS, Kolonel LN, Meyskins FL Jr: Rationale and strategies for chemoprevention of cancer in humans. Cancer Res 47:3021, 1987.

10. Blackard CE, Byar DP, Jordan WP Jr, et al: Orchiectomy for advanced prostate carcinoma: A reevaluation. Urology 1:553, 1973.

11. Blair A, Fraumeni JF Jr: Geographic patterns of prostate cancer in the United States. J Natl Cancer Inst 61:1379, 1978.

12. Blute ML, Nativo O, Zincke H, et al: Pattern of failure after radical retropubic prostatectomy for clinically and pathologically localized adenocarcinoma of the prostate. Influence of tumor deoxyribonucleic acid ploidy. J Urol 142:1262, 1989.

13. Blute ML, Zincke H, Farrow GM: Long-term follow-up of young patients with stage A adenocarcinoma of the prostate. J Urol 136:840, 1986.

14. Brauer M: Implications of premalignant lesions in the prostate. Cont Urol 2:62, 1990.

15. Breslow N, Chan CW, Dhom G, et al: Latent carcinoma of prostate of autopsy in seven areas. Int J Cancer 20:680, 1977.

16. Byar DP: The Veterans Administration Cooperative Urological Research Group's studies of cancer of the prostate. Cancer 32:1126, 1973.

17. Byar DP, Corle DK: Veterans Administration Cooperative Urological Research Group: VACURG randomized trial of radical prostatectomy for stages I and II prostate cancer. Urology 17(Suppl):7, 1981.

18. Cannon L, Bishop DT, Skolnick M, et al: Genetic epidemiology of prostate cancer in the Utah Mormon genealogy. Cancer Surv 1:47, 1982.

19. Cantrell BB, De Klerk DP, Eggleston JC, et al: Pathologic factors that influence prognosis in stage A prostate cancer: The influence of extent versus grade. J Urol 125:516, 1981.

20. Carroll KK, Kohr HT: Dietary fat in relation to tumorigenesis. Prog Biochem Pharmacol 10:308–353, 1975.

21. Carter HB, Piantadosi S, Isaacs JT: Clinical evidence for and implications of the multistep development of prostate cancer. J Urol 143:742, 1990.

22. Centifano YM, Kaufman HE, Zam ZS, et al: Herpesvirus particles in prostate carcinoma cells. J Virol 12:1608, 1973.

23. Cook GB, Watson FR: Twenty single nodules of prostate cancer not treated by total prostatectomy. J Urol 100:672, 1968.

24. Correa RJ Jr, Anderson RG, Gibbons RP, Mason JT: Latent carcinoma of the prostate—Why the controversy? J Urol 111:644, 1974.

25. Deaver JB: Etiology and predetermining factors of benign prostatic hypertrophy. *In* Enlargement of the Prostate: Its History, Anatomy, Etiology, Pathology, Clinical Causes, Symptoms, Diagnosis, Prognosis, Treatment, Technique of Operations and After-treatment. Philadelphia, Blakiston, 1922.

26. de Vere-White R, Babaian RK, Feldman M: Adjunctive therapy with interstitial irradiation for prostate cancer. Urology 19:395, 1982.

27. Diamond DA, Berry SJ, Jewett HJ, et al: A new method to assess metastatic potential of human prostate cancer: Relative nuclear roundness. J Urol 128:729, 1982.

28. Donohue RE, Mani JH, Whitesel JA, et al: Pelvic lymph node dissection: Guide to patient management in clinically locally confined adenocarcinoma of the prostate. Urology 20:559, 1982.

29. Drafta D, Proca E, Zamfir V, et al: Decreased steroids in benign prostatic hypertrophy and carcinoma of the prostate. J Steroid Biochem 17:689, 1982.

30. Dunn JE: Cancer epidemiology in populations of the United States. Cancer Res 35:3240, 1975.

31. Enstrom JE: Cancer and total mortality among active Mormons. Cancer 42:1943, 1978.

32. Enstrom JE: Cancer mortality among Mormons in California during 1968–1975. J Natl Cancer Inst 65:1073, 1980.

33. Epstein JI, Paull G, Eggleston JC, Walsh PC: Prognosis of untreated stage A1 prostatic carcinoma: A study of 94 cases with extended followup. J Urol 136:837, 1986.

34. Ernster VL, Selvin S, Brown SM, et al: Occupation and prostate cancer. A review and retrospective analysis based on death certificates in two California counties. J Occup Med 21:175, 1979.

35. Ernster VL, Winkelstein W, Selvin S Jr, et al: Race, socioeconomic status, and prostatic cancer. Cancer Treat Rep 61:187, 1977.

36. Farnsworth WE: Human prostatic reverse transcriptase and RNA-virus. Urol Res 1:106, 1973.

37. Ghanadian R, Puah CM, O'Donoghue EPN: Serum testosterone and dihydrotestosterone in carcinoma of the prostate. Br J Cancer 39:696, 1979.

38. Glantz GM: Cirrhosis and carcinoma of the prostate gland. J Urol 91:291, 1964.

39. Gordon T, Crittenden M, Haenszel W: Cancer mortality trends in the United States, 1930–1955: End results and mortality trends in cancer. Natl Cancer Inst Monogr 6:1, 1961.

40. Gortner WA: Nutrition in the United States, 1900 to 1974. Cancer Res 35:3246, 1975.

41. Gospodarowicz D, Ferrara N, Schweigerer L, Neufeld G: Structural characterization and biological functions of fibroblast growth factor. Endocrine Rev 8:95, 1987.

42. Gospodarowicz D, Neufeld G, Schweigerer L: Fibroblast growth factor. Mol Cell Endocrinol 46:187, 1986.

43. Graham S, Harighey B, Marshall J, et al: Diet in the epidemiology of prostate cancer. J Natl Cancer Inst 70:687, 1983.

44. Greenwald P, Kirmss V, Polan AK, et al: Cancer of the prostate among men with benign prostatic hyperplasia. J Natl Cancer Inst 53:335, 1974.

45. Grossman HB, Batata H, Hilaris B, Whitmore WF Jr: 125-I implantation for carcinoma of the prostate: Further followup of first 100 cases. Urology 20:591, 1982.

46. Habib FK: Evaluation of androgen metabolism studies in human prostate cancer: Correlation with zinc level. Prevent Med 9:650, 1980.

47. Hakky SI, Chisholm GD, Skeet RG: Social class and carcinoma of the prostate. Br J Urol 51:393, 1979.

48. Hanash KA, Utz D, Cook EN, et al: Carcinoma of the prostate: A 15 year follow up. J Urol 107:450, 1972.

49. Heaney JA, Chang HC, Daly JJ, Prout GR Jr: Prognosis of clinically undiagnosed prostatic carcinoma and influence of endocrine therapy. J Urol 118:283, 1977.

50. Heshmat MY, Kaul L, Kovi J, et al: Nutrition and prostate cancer: A case-control study. Prostate 67:7, 1985.

51. Heshmat MY, Kovi J, Herson J, et al: Epidemiologic association between gonorrhea and prostatic carconoma. Urology 6:457, 1975.

52. Holnszel W, Kurihoro M: Studies of Japanese migrants. J Natl Cancer Inst 40:43, 1968.

53. Howell MA: Diet as an etiological factor in the development of cancers of the colon and rectum. J Chron Dis 28:67, 1975.

54. Huben R, Mettlin C, Natarajan N, et al: Carcinoma of prostate in men less than fifty years old: Data from American College of Surgeons' National Survey. Urology 20:585, 1982.

55. Hutchison GB: Etiology and prevention of prostatic cancer. Cancer Chemother Rep 59:57, 1975.

56. Hutchison GB: Epidemiology of prostate cancer. Semin Oncol 3:151, 1976.

57. Hutchison GB: Incidence and etiology of prostate cancer. Urology 17(Suppl):4, 1981.

58. Jackson MA, Ahluwalia BS, Herson J, et al: Characterization of prostatic carcinoma among blacks: A continuation report. Cancer Treat Rep 61:167, 1977.

59. Johansson JE, Andersson SO, Krusemo UB, et al: Natural history of localized prostate cancer. Lancet 1:799, 1989.

60. Kipling MD, Waterhouse JAH: Cadmium and prostatic carcinoma. Lancet 1:730, 1967.

61. Kolonel LN: Cancer patterns of four ethnic groups in Hawaii. J Natl Cancer Inst 65:1127, 1980.

62. Kolonel LN, Hankin JH, Lee J, et al: Nutrient intakes in relation to cancer incidence in Hawaii. Br J Cancer 44:332, 1981.

63. Kolonel LN, Hinds MW, Nomura AMY, et al: Relationship of dietary vitamin A and ascorbic acid intake to the risk for cancers of the lung, bladder, and prostate in Hawaii. Natl Cancer Inst Monogr 69:137, 1985.

64. Kolonel L, Winkelstein W Jr: Cadmium and prostatic carcinoma. Lancet 2:566, 1977.

65. Kramer SA, Cline WA Jr, Farnham R, et al: Angiography in the staging of prostatic cancer. Prostate 2:433, 1981.

66. Kramer SA, Farnham R, Glenn JF, et al: Comparative morphology of primary and secondary deposits of prostatic adenocarcinoma. Cancer 48:271, 1981.

67. Kramer SA, Spahr J, Brendler CB, et al: Experience with Gleason's histopathologic grading in prostate cancer. J Urol 124:223, 1980.

68. Lange DJ, Kummer JF, Hartley DP: Cytomegalovirus in semen: Persistence and demonstration in extracellular fluids. N Engl J Med 291:121–123, 1974.

69. Lea AJ: Neoplasms and environmental factors. Ann R Coll Surg 41:432, 1967.

70. Levine RL, Wilchinsky M: Adenocarcinoma of the prostate: A comparison of the disease in blacks versus whites. J Urol 121:761, 1979.

71. Lloyd CW, Williams RH: Endocrine changes associated with Laennec's cirrhosis of the liver. Am J Med 4:315, 1948.

72. Lyon JL, Garner JW, Klauber MK, Smart CR: Low cancer incidence and mortality in Utah. Cancer 39:2608, 1977.

73. Madsen PO, Graversen PH, Gasser TC, et al: Treatment of localized prostatic cancer: Radical prostatectomy versus placebo: A 15-year followup. Scand J Urol Nephrol 110:95, 1988.

74. McCombs RM: Role of oncornaviruses in carcinoma of the prostate. Cancer Treat Rep 61:131, 1977.

75. McLaughlin AP, Saltzstein SL, McCullough DL, et al: Prostatic carcinoma: Incidence and location of unsuspected lymphatic metastases. J Urol 115:89, 1976.

76. McNeal JE, Bostwick DG, Kindrachuk RA, et al: Patterns of progression in prostate cancer. Lancet 1:60, 1986.

77. McNeal JE, Price HM, Redwine EA, et al: Stage A versus stage B adenocarcinoma of the prostate: Morphological comparison and biological significance. J Urol 139:61, 1988.

78. Meikle AW, Smith JA, West DW: Familial factors affecting prostatic cancer risk and plasma sex-steroid levels. Prostate 6:121, 1985.

79. Meikle AW, Stanish WM: Familial prostatic cancer risk and low testosterone. J Clin Endocrinol Metab 54:1104, 1982.

80. Menck HR, Henderson BE, Pike MC, et al: Cancer incidence in the Mexican-American. J Natl Cancer Inst 55:531, 1975.

81. Morales P, Golimbu M: The therapeutic role of pelvic lymphadenectomy in prostate cancer. Urol Clin North Am 7:623, 1980.

82. Moskovitz B, Nitecki S, Levin DR: Cancer of the prostate. Is there a need for aggressive treatment? Urol Int 42:49, 1987.

83. Murphy GP, Beckley S, Brady MF, et al: Treatment of newly diagnosed metastatic prostate cancer patients with chemotherapy agents in combination with hormones versus hormones alone. Cancer 51:1264, 1983.

84. Murphy GP, Natarajan N, Pontes JE, et al: The national survey of prostate cancer in the United States by the American College of Surgeons. J Urol 127:928, 1982.

85. Nativ O, Winkler HZ, Rax Y, et al: Stage C prostatic adenocarcinoma: Flow cytometric nuclear DNA ploidy analysis. Mayo Clin Proc 64:911, 1989.

86. Nishi N, Matuo Y, Kunitomi K, et al: Comparative analysis of growth factors in normal and pathologic human prostates. Prostate 13:39, 1988.

87. Noble RL: The development of prostatic adenocarcinoma in Nb rats following prolonged sex hormone administration. Cancer Res 27:1929, 1977.

88. Ohno Y, Yoshida O, Oishi K, et al: Dietary β-carotene and cancer of the prostate: A case-control study in Kyoto, Japan. Cancer Res 48:1331, 1988.

89. Ohtsuki Y, Seman G, Dmochowski L, et al: Brief communication: Virus-like particles in a case of human prostate carcinoma. J Natl Cancer Inst 58:1493, 1977.

90. Paulson DF: The prognostic role of lymphadenectomy in adenocarcinoma of the prostate. Urol Clin North Am 7:615, 1980.

91. Paulson DF, Rabson AS, Fraley EE: Viral neoplastic transformation of hamster prostate tissue in vitro. Science 159:200, 1968.

92. Peto R, Doll R, Buckley JD, et al: Can beta-carotene materially reduce human cancer rates? Nature 290:201, 1981.

93. Pilepich MV, Perez CA, Bauer W: Prognostic parameters in radiotherapeutic management of localized carcinoma of the prostate. J Urol 124:485, 1980.

94. Pollard M, Luckert PH: Promotional effects of testoterone and dietary fat on prostate carcinogenesis in genetically susceptible rats. Prostate 6:1, 1985.

95. Ross RK, Deapen DM, Casagrande JT, et al: A cohort study of mortality from cancer of the prostate in Catholic priests. Br J Cancer 43:233, 1981.

96. Ross RK, McCurtis JW, Henderson BE, et al: Descriptive epidemiology of testicular and prostatic cancer in Los Angeles. Br J Cancer 39:284, 1979.

97. Rotkin ID: Studies in the epidemiology of prostatic cancer: Expanded sampling. Cancer Treat Rep 61:173, 1977.

98. Saitoh H, Hida M, Shimbo T, et al: Metastatic patterns of prostate cancer-correlation between sites and number of organs involved. Cancer 54:3078, 1984.

99. Sanford EJ, Geder L, Laychock A, et al: Evidence for the association of cytomegalovirus with carcinoma of the prostate. J Urol 118:789, 1977.

100. Schuman LM, Mandel J, Blackard C, et al: Preliminary report. Cancer Treat Rep 61:181, 1977.

101. SEER Program: Cancer incidence and mortality in the United States, 1973-1981. *In* Horm JW, Asire AJ, Young JL, et al (eds): NIH Publication No 85–1837, 1984.

102. Severson RK, Normura AMY, Grove JS, et al: A prospective study of demographics, diet, and prostate cancer among men of Japanese ancestry in Hawaii. Cancer Res 49:1857, 1989.

103. Sheldon CA, Williams RD, Fraley EE: Incidental carcinoma of the prostate: A review of the literature and critical reappraisal of classification. J Urol 124:626, 1980.

104. Silverberg E: Cancer statistics, 1980. CA 30:23, 1980.

105. Silverberg E, Boring CC, Squires TS: Cancer statistics. CA 40:9, 1990.

106. Silverberg E, Lubera JA: A review of American Cancer Society estimates of cancer cases and deaths. CA 33:2, 1983.

107. Silverberg E, Lubera JA: A review of American Cancer Society: Estimate of cancer cases and deaths. CA 36:9, 1986.

108. Silverberg E, Lubera JA: Cancer statistics. CA 38:5, 1988.

109. Smith JA Jr, Middleton RG: Pelvic lymph node metastasis from prostatic cancer: Influence of tumor grade and stage. American Urological Association Abstract No. 238, 1982.

110. Stamey TA: Cancer of the prostate: An analysis of some important contributions and dilemmas. Monogr Urol 3:67, 1982.

111. Staszewski J, Haenszel W: Cancer mortality among the Polish-born in the United States. J Natl Cancer Inst 35:291, 1965.

112. Steele R, Lees REM, Kraus AS, et al: Sexual factors in the epidemiology of cancer of the prostate. J Chron Dis 24:29, 1971.

113. Tavares AS, Costa J, Maia JC: Correlation between ploidy and prognosis in prostatic carcinoma. J Urol 109:676, 1973.

114. Thiessen EU: Concerning a familial association between breast cancer and both prostatic and uterine malignancies. Cancer 34:1102, 1974.

115. Tribukait B: Rapid-flow cytometry of prostatic fine needle aspiration biopsies. *In* Karr JP, Coffey DS, Gardner W Jr (eds): Prognostic Prostatic Cytometry and Cytopathology of Prostate Cancer. New York, Elsevier Science Publishing, 1989, pp 236–242.

116. Troncoso P, Babaian RJ, Ro JY, et al: Prostatic intraepithelial neoplasia and invasive prostatic adenocarcinoma in cystoprostatectomy speciments. Urology 34(Suppl):52, 1989.

117. Viola MV, Fromowitz F, Oravez S, et al: Expression of ras oncogene p21 in prostate cancer. N Engl J Med 314:133, 1986.

118. Watanabe H, Ohe H, Inaba T: A mobile mass screening unit for prostatic disease. Prostate 5:559, 1984.

119. West D, Powell J: Prostate cancer in Utah. Am J Epidemiol 110:359, 1979.

120. Whitmore WF Jr: Natural history of low-stage prostatic cancer and the impact of early detection. Urol Clin North Am J 17:689, 1990.
121. Winkelstein W Jr, Ernster VL: Epidemiology and etiology. *In* Murphy GP (ed): Prostatic Cancer. Littleton, MA: PSG Publishing Company, 1979, pp 1–17.
122. Winkelstein W Jr, Kantor S: Prostatic cancer: Relationship to suspended particulate air pollution. Am J Public Health 59:1134, 1969.
123. Winkler HZ, Rainwater LM, Myers RP, et al: Stage D1 prostatic adenocarcinoma: Significance of nuclear DNA ploidy patterns studied by flow cytometry. Mayo Clin Proc 63:103, 1988.
124. Woolf CM: An investigation of the familial aspect of carcinoma of the prostate. Cancer 13:739, 1960.
125. Wynder EL, Mabuchi K, Whitmore WF Jr: Epidemiology of cancer of the prostate. Cancer 28:344, 1971.
126. Zhang P, Cheng S, Zhou Y: General survey to detect prostatic disease in 1,165 aged males over 60. Chinese J Geriatr 3:99, 1984.
127. Zincke H: Extended experience with surgical treatment of stage D1 adenocarcinoma of prostate: Significance influences of immediate adjuvant hormonal treatment (orchiectomy) on outcome. Urology 33:27, 1989.

STAGING, CLINICAL MANIFESTATIONS, AND INDICATIONS FOR INTERVENTION IN PROSTATE CANCER

PAUL C. PETERS

STAGING

Staging refers to the extent of a cancer within the human body. Clinical staging refers to the extent of the disease as determined by preoperative assessment by means of laboratory tests, including biopsy and physical examination of the patient. Pathologic staging refers to the histologically determined extent of the disease within the patient's body. Pathologic staging is done by assessment of the surgically removed tissues and organs and often exceeds the clinical estimation of the extent of the disease process. In the case of a patient with prostate cancer, this is exemplified by finding a microscopically positive node at surgery when preoperative assessment by ploidy, prostate-specific antigen (PSA), bone scan, physical examination, and acid phosphatase gave no clue that such extension was present and what was thought to be a clinical Stage A or B patient is really a Stage D1 patient.

CLINICAL STAGING OF CANCER OF THE PROSTATE

Once the diagnosis of carcinoma of the prostate is established by microscopic evaluation of tissue, clinical staging proceeds. It is important from the standpoint of prognosis and application of appropriate treatment to ascertain preoperatively whether localized or metastatic disease is present. The rectal examination may be positive for pelvic fixation but is examiner dependent and

can seldom stand alone as the only diagnostic modality needed. Rectal examination has a detection rate of 1.5 to 2.2 per cent[4] as a screening test for prostate cancer and even less value as a sole predictor of metastatic disease. Transrectal ultrasonography (TRUS) is helpful, but some prostate carcinomas are isoechoic and their extent cannot be determined by TRUS. TRUS does not evaluate pelvic nodes that may harbor microscopic disease. One can image the seminal vesicles entering the prostate, and a biopty gun biopsy of this area may show that Stage C disease is already present, i.e., seminal vesicle involvement. Accuracy of determining seminal vesicle involvement is 77 to 85 per cent by TRUS-guided biopsy.

CT can cause one to suspect pelvic or distant node involvement, but tissue confirmation is necessary. However, CT with controlled needle biopsy or aspiration of an enlarged node may spare a patient an unnecessary exploration and open biopsy. MRI is more expensive than TRUS but enjoys a slight advantage over TRUS in staging the extent of disease in and around the prostate (75 to 65 per cent), except for the TRUS biopty gun in detecting seminal vesicle involvement. MRI has no advantage over CT in diagnosing lymph node involvement in the pelvis.

PSA, a protein with a molecular weight of approximately 33,000 daltons, is secreted by prostate cells. If benign prostatic hypertrophy (BPH) cells secrete x amount, prostate cancer cells secrete 10x. PSA provides about a 60 per cent accuracy in predicting whether local or metastatic disease is present. Stamey has reported that a PSA greater than 40 ng/ml is associated with 63 per cent node-positive disease.[15] As a staging modality used alone, PSA finds its greatest use in predicting persistent disease in the post–radical prostatectomy patient. The current value in our laboratory for zero PSA is 0.05 ± 1 ng/ml (Hybritech method); any rise above this value following prostatectomy suggests that prostate cancer cells are still present in the patient. The half-life of PSA is approximately 3.5 days. Bone scanning with technetium-99 monodiphosphate (MDP) has about a 98 per cent accuracy (2 per cent false positives) in detecting metastases to bone. In our experience, about 25 per cent of patients exhibit metastases to soft tissue first instead of bone.

Benson has proposed the use of PSA density (PSAD), which is the ratio of serum PSA to the volume of the prostate as measured by TRUS. As noted above, prostate cancer produces a higher level of serum PSA per unit volume than does BPH. In a study by Benson, mean PSA values for BPH were 3.7 ± 3.3 ng/ml, whereas prostate cancer values were 24.4 ± 36.9 ng/ml.[1, 2] PSAD for BPH was 0.044 and for cancer 0.58. PSAD may find its best use in strengthening suspicion for prostate cancer in patients with PSA values between 4 and 10 ng/ml, as PSA already enjoys a 96 per cent specificity when the PSA is greater than 10 ng/ml. The detection rate for the presence of cancer with an abnormal digital rectal examination (DRE) and a PSA greater than 10 ng/ml is 72 per cent.

PATHOLOGIC STAGING

For staging, the author currently uses a modification of a classification proposed by Jewett (Table 21–1). Stage A refers to nonpalpable disease localized to less than 5 per cent of the gland (Stage A1). Stage A2 disease refers to a carcinoma diffusely spread to both sides of the gland and occupying more than 5 per cent of the gland but still nonpalpable. Stage B may be defined as palpable disease by rectal examination. Stage B0 refers to a palpable nodule that one encounters in perhaps 5 to 7 per cent of patients and represents the extent of the disease in the patient and is less than 1.5 cm in diameter. Such cases, still rare in our overall experience with carcinoma of the prostate, have a most favorable prognosis. Stage B1 refers to an area of involvement greater than 1.5 cm in diameter but con-

fined to one lobe. Stage B2 refers to disease involving both lobes (often 5 to 6 cm in diameter) but with no palpable or microscopic evidence of extension beyond the capsule of the prostate. Stage C disease refers to a lesion that has spread beyond the anatomic capsule of the prostate into the periprostatic fat or into the adjacent seminal vesicles. Often this extension is not detected clinically or by ultrasound-controlled biopsy and is found only when the surgical specimen is examined after a radical prostatectomy. Stage D disease is characterized by extension of the prostatic carcinoma into an adjacent visceral organ such as the bladder or the rectum or to the regional lymph nodes. Patients who have metastases only to the adjacent obturator or internal iliac nodes are said to have Stage D1 disease, whereas individuals having extension above the pelvis to distant visceral organs such as the liver or lungs are said to have Stage D2 disease, as are those with metastases to bone or distant (outside the true pelvis) nodes, i.e., supraclavicular or para-aortic nodes. The unique ability of prostate carcinoma to extend to the cranium via the paravertebral plexus of Batson connecting with the pelvic venous plexus has long been noted. Lytton has suggested that the pattern of random distribution of metastases may be explained by the cells obtaining access to the circulation and being distributed by the beating heart.[12] Jacobs has suggested bone structure to explain the frequency of involvement in bone, particularly the lumbar spine and pelvis, by metastatic carcinoma of the prostate.[10]

Staging the extent of the disease process is important to select the proper mode of treatment for the patient. Curative forms of therapy are applied to localized disease, i.e., surgery, external beam radiation therapy, and, occasionally, interstitial therapy. Systemic therapy is used when metastatic disease is present, i.e., hormonal therapy or chemotherapy. Such systemic therapy is usually palliative.

Several tests are now available for preoperative clinical staging. Among them are rectal examination, prostatic acid phosphatase (PAP) serum enzyme method, radioimmunoassay of PAP, isotope (technetium-99) bone scan combined with radiographic magnified views over suspicious "hot" areas, serum PSA, CT of the soft tissues of the pelvis, and MRI of the pelvis and soft tissues. Each of these tests has a unique usefulness in

TABLE 21–1. STAGING OF PROSTATE CANCER

STAGES	MODIFIED JEWETT STAGING	TNM CLASSIFICATION
Stage A1	Nonpalpable involving <5% of gland by volume	T1a—Three foci or less
Stage A2	Diffuse, both sides of gland multicentric, >5% of gland, nonpalpable	T1b—More than three foci
B0 or Stage B1 nodule	Palpable, occupying <1.5 cm circumscribed nodule to palpation	No comparable
Stage B1	Palpable, not circumscribed occupying one lobe, <1.5 cm in size	T2A—Palpable
Stage B2	Palpable, occupies two lobes >1.5 cm in size	T2B—Palpable
Stage C	Extracapsular extension to seminal vesicles, bladder neck, or periprostatic fat seminal vesicle positive = C2	T3—Not fixed
Stage D1	Regional pelvic node; positive obturator or internal iliac or external node in true pelvis. Hydronephrosis secondary to outlet obstruction	N1—Single node 2 cm or less

detecting the presence of or delineating the extent of a carcinoma of the prostate in a given individual. Cost effectiveness demands careful selection for each specific case. A general preoperative screen given a positive biopsy includes a DRE, a PSA determination (sometimes two or three), a serum PAP measurement, and an isotope bone scan before going to lymphadenectomy and then definitive surgery or radiation therapy for attempted cure.

Value of Individual Tests in the Staging of Carcinoma of the Prostate

The DRE remains a valuable part of the urologist's evaluation of the prostate. Who has not sat for 20 or 30 minutes discussing the minutiae of the voiding history with a patient only to step next door for the DRE and find a fixed prostate with direct extension to the pelvic wall? Similarly, a patient with a normal PSA is found to have an obvious area of induration in the prostate which proves positive for carcinoma on needle biopsy. One can often get a good idea of the local extent of the disease by DRE. It is the author's experience that the pathologic extent is at least as great as predicted by the DRE and usually more extensive. One should palpate the prostate after the patient has just emptied his bladder and should try to move the prostate from side to side and superiorly and inferiorly as well. Inability to do this may indicate extensive local disease.

CLINICAL MANIFESTATIONS

Localized disease is often asymptomatic. The major symptom produced by a still localized cancer of the prostate is *an acute onset* of *obstructive* symptoms regardless of age. As the carcinoma extends from the outer to the inner prostate, less mobility of the lateral lobe during micturition occurs. The brain interprets this as an obstruction. This may be quite subtle at first; the patient may be aware of a difference in his voiding pattern which he interprets as a slight degree of obstruction. Flow rates remain in the 10 to 15 ml/sec range. DRE may be normal and the PSA slightly elevated (in the 5 to 6.5 range). If the PSA is normal, the lesion may be missed. If carcinoma is present, however, the obstructive symptoms may progress and the patient will present in acute retention within 18 to 20 months. In our Parkland experience (1960 to 1969), 42 per cent of the patients with carcinoma of the prostate presented in acute retention. In a lifetime series reported by Dr. John Hand, 43 per cent of his 109 patients with carcinoma presented in acute retention.[9]

Localized carcinoma of the prostate may present as an area of induration (over 5 to 10 per cent of the time) or as a palpable prostate nodule. Thirty-three to 50 per cent of these nodules prove on biopsy to contain carcinoma. Even with a normal PSA, a study of 34 of 39 radical prostatectomy specimens done by us in 1991 revealed the carcinoma to be more extensive than judged by preoperative studies including PSA, serum PAP, bone scan, and DRE even when the carcinoma presented as an area of induration. Thus, at our institution we are not operating on early cancer of the prostate as defined by pathologic extent. Persistent painless microhematuria may be the only clue to the presence of a carcinoma of the prostate, particularly a ductal transitional cell cancer. PSA is of little help, as is also true of ultrasonography in early cases. Urine cytology may give a clue, as well as fine-needle aspiration and systematic biopsy of the base, mid-portion, and apical areas of the gland. Persistent perineal pain and sciatic pain radiating into the buttock or thigh posteriorly are usually associated with extension beyond the prostate rather than localized disease.

ADVANCED DISEASE

This, too, may be asymptomatic even when bony metastases are present. Patients may present with constipation or even later obstructive bowel symptoms when the lesion protrudes into the rectum, compressing the passage and requiring differentiation from a ring lesion of primary colon or rectal cancer. Weight loss, neurogenic bowel dysfunction, and a whole range of motor and sensory neurologic complaints, including paraplegia, sciatica, and lumbar nerve root pain, may be present from metastases that cause spinal cord or nerve root compression. Myelophthisic anemia from marrow replacement may lead to diagnosis by marrow biopsy even if the prostate is normal by rectal palpation. PSA and biopty gun use provide confirmation of the origin of the disease. The patient may complain of a diffuse arthritis when extensive bone disease is present, or pain emanating from an isolated bony metastasis may be the first clue to the presence of metastatic prostate carcinoma. Acid and alkaline phosphatase enzymes reach their highest levels in patients with bone disease. Lumbar spine and pelvis are involved in 75 per cent of patients with metastases to bone. Some believe that a nutrient factor is present in the bone (NGF). Lytton suggests that the pattern of metastasis depends on a random distribution of cells in the circulation by the beating heart.[12]

INDICATIONS FOR INTERVENTION

Localized Disease

Channel Transurethral Resection of the Prostate

Currently, patients presenting with Stage D disease and retention are offered castration or castration and Eulexin (flutamide) 250 mg every 8 hours. If they are unable to void well within 3 months of this initial therapy, they are offered transurethral resection of the prostate (TURP). Approximately 70 per cent of patients are able to void satisfactorily in 6 to 8 weeks after castration and androgen blockade with flutamide; about 30 per cent require the so-called channel TURP. At the time of surgery, the operator resects enough tissue to allow the patient to void, sparing tissue distally near the prostate apex in an effort to prevent incontinence. Such patients may become incontinent later if the sphincter becomes involved with the progression of the carcinoma. How much should one resect in such cases? I believe one should resect enough tissue so that if the resectoscope is placed at the level of the verumontanum, one can see the opening into the bladder and no tissue falling into the circle visualized at the bladder neck. The channel TURP requires repeating in 30 per cent of our cases if the patient survives 5 years.

If one has made the diagnosis of localized disease, alternatives for therapy must be discussed with the patient. I admit a bias for selecting radical prostatectomy after negative lymphadenectomy. Survival figures for external beam therapy compared with radical prostatectomy are similar at 10 years, but note was not made of whether the patients are alive or alive with no evidence of disease, and staging as judged by current methods was not complete; i.e., no lymphadenectomy as done today was carried out in these patients. Survival rates are as follows:

	5 Years	10 Years	15 Years
Jewett (no lymph node dissection)	92%	70%	29%
Bagshaw (no extracapsular extension)	93%	76%	21%
Barnes (orchiectomy only)	—	—	33%

Walsh and Jewett have subsequently reported that no patient in the Jewett series survived 15 years if the disease was at least Stage B2 and extraprostatic extension was observed pathologically.[16] Fifteen-year data are not available in patients selected for radical prostatectomy after negative lymphadenectomy using current methods of selection. Middleton has recently surveyed a group of patients who had radical prostatectomy (usually by the perineal route) after negative lymphadenectomy and permanent slides of the nodes and reports a 59 per cent 10-year survival.[13] Clearly, late failures occur because unrecognized metastases are present at the time of surgery.

I prefer radical prostatectomy after negative lymphadenectomy because I have seen recurrence or activation of the primary lesion in the prostate years after completion of radiation therapy which does not occur after radical prostatectomy, although local recurrence in the prostate bed is well known. Failures due to unrecognized metastatic disease present at the time of external beam therapy or surgery occur in either case, numbering 15 per cent in my experience. I do not expect this to be modified significantly by PSA testing, as many of these patients have a normal PSA of less than 4.0 ng/ml (Hybritech) at the time of their original treatment (radiation therapy or surgery) for cure. Paulson et al have reported a higher local failure rate for radiation therapy

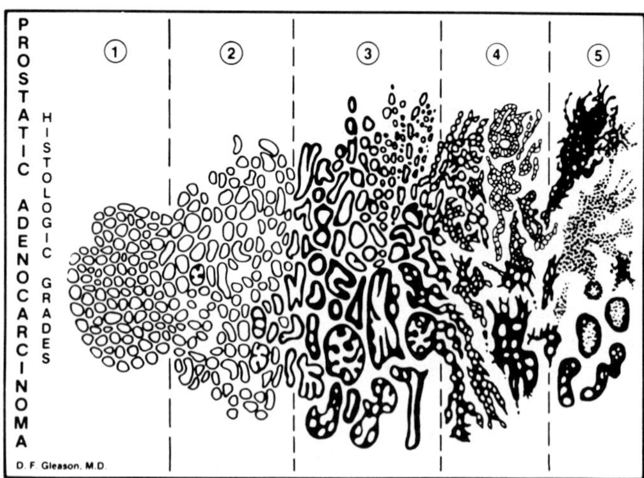

FIGURE 21–1. Simplified drawing of Gleason system. It has good inter- and intraobserver reproducibility. It is based on a pattern rather than individual cellular changes. (From Epstein JI: Pathological considerations for the practicing urologist. *In* Cancer of the Prostate: Current and Future Directions. Philadelphia, CoMed Communications, 1989, p 14; with permission.)

than surgery in patients staged pathologically by lymphadenectomy prior to treatment and then randomized to one of the two treatment groups.[14]

Radical Salvage Prostatectomy

Patients who were originally selected for external beam radiation therapy in our experience show evidence of local failure more than twice as often as do individuals who originally had retropubic or perineal surgery. Paulson et al have reported a similar experience.[14] PSA testing is allowing earlier identification of these failures. If the disease is found to be active, i.e., positive biopsy and rising PSA, and provided that bone scan, MRI, and serum PAP remain negative, salvage prostatectomy may be considered. Goldstone et al have reported on a series of 25 such patients.[8] Complication rates are higher, but in carefully selected cases an acceptable elimination of cancer is obtained. Rectal injury occurred in 5 of 25 patients, potency was present in 15 patients preoperatively, and 3 patients exhibited some penile turgor postoperatively. Eight of 15 patients remained incontinent. None who was incontinent at 10 months postoperatively regained continence without further treatment, i.e., artificial sphincter. Positive margins were present in 8 and seminal vesicle invasion in 7, and 10 cases were confined to the prostate.

GRADING OF PROSTATE CANCER

Grading combined with staging is of some use to the urologist in helping to assess prognosis for survival in a given patient. We use the Gleason grading system (Figs. 21–1 and 21–2). Gleason and Mellinger, in studying

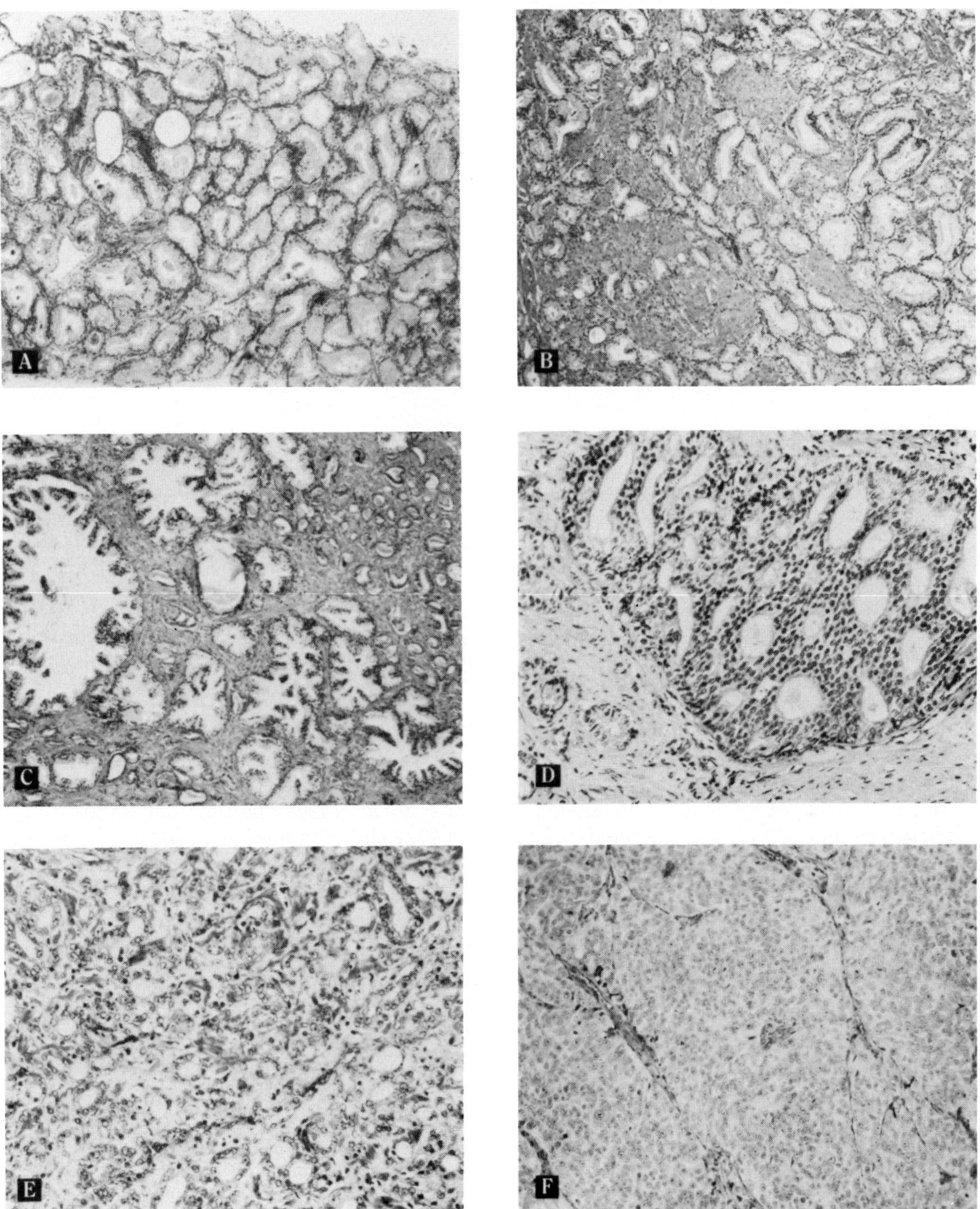

FIGURE 21–2. Gleason grading system. *A*, Gleason grade 1 tumor is composed of a circumscribed nodule of uniform, single, separate, closely-packed glands (original magnification ×100). *B*, In Gleason grade 2, although the tumor is still fairly circumscribed, at the edge of the tumor nodule there can be minimal extension by neoplastic glands into the surrounding non-neoplastic prostate. The glands in grade 2 are still single and separate, yet are more loosely arranged and not quite as uniform as in grade 1 (original magnification ×50). *C*, Grade 3 tumor infiltrates in and among the non-neoplastic prostate with the glands having marked variation in size and shape. Many of the glands are smaller than those seen in grade 1 or 2 tumor (original magnification ×120). *D*, Smoothly circumscribed cribriform nodules of tumor are also classified as grade 3 (original magnification ×90). *E*, In Gleason grade 4 tumor, the glands are no longer single and separate as seen in grades 1 through 3, and they are composed of fused glands with ragged infiltrating edges (original magnification ×160). *F*, The Gleason grade 5 tumor shows no glandular differentiation with either solid masses of cells, individually infiltrating cells, or nests of tumor with central necrosis (original magnification ×80). (From Epstein JI: Pathological considerations for the practicing urologist. *In* Cancer of the Prostate: Current and Future Directions. Philadelphia, CoMed Communications, 1989, p 12; with permission.)

TABLE 21–2. HISTOLOGIC PATTERNS OF ADENOCARCINOMA OF THE PROSTATE (see Fig. 21–1)*

PATTERN	MARGINS OF TUMOR AREAS	GLAND PATTERN	GLAND SIZE	GLAND DISTRIBUTION	STROMAL INVASION
1	Well defined	Single, separate, round	Medium	Closely packed	Minimal, expansile
2	Less definite	Single, separate, rounded, but more variable	Medium	Spaced up to one gland diameter, average	Mild, in larger stromal planes
3	Poorly defined *or*	Single, separate, more irregular	Small, medium, or large	Spaced more than one gland diameter, rarely packed	Moderate, in larger or smaller stromal planes
3	Poorly defined	Rounded masses of cribriform or papillary epithelium	Medium or large	Rounded masses with smooth sharp edges	Expansile masses
4	Ragged, infiltrating	Fused glandular masses or "hypernephroid"	Small	Fused in ragged masses	Marked, through smaller planes
5	Ragged, infiltrating *or*	Almost absent; few tiny glands or signet ring cells	Small	Ragged anaplastic masses of epithelium	Severe, between stromal fibers or destructive
5	Poorly defined	Few small lumina in rounded masses of solid epithelium; central necrosis?	Small	Rounded masses and cords with smooth, sharp edges	Expansile masses

*From Gleason DF: Veterans Administration Cooperative Urological Research Group: Histologic grading in clinical staging of prostatic carcinoma. *In* Urologic Pathology: The Prostate. Edited by M. Tannenbaum. Philadelphia, Lea & Febiger, 1977. Used with permission.

microscopic sections at low power (40 ×) made from the prostates of individuals undergoing prostatectomy, noted that there were at least two patterns of cell arrangement in a given case, a predominant pattern and a less frequent, or minority, pattern (Table 21–2).[7] They assigned a number of 1 to 5 (according to degree of differentiation and stromal reaction) to each of the two patterns, listing the predominant pattern first. Thus, a given cancer might be given the number 2 if the predominant pattern was well differentiated, and a number 5 if the minority pattern were less well differentiated, giving a Gleason score of 7 (2 + 5). It was soon found that nodal metastases were infrequent in patients having a Gleason score of 2, 3, or 4 and present in a high percentage in patients having a Gleason score of 7, 8, or 9. Whether one uses the Gleason, Gaeta, or Mostofi grading system, the major problem with each of them is failure to offer accurate prognosis for the given patient with an intermediate-grade tumor, i.e., Gleason 5 or 6.[7]

In a given prostate cancer, many variations in the genetic make-up and morphology exist. This heterogeneity makes it difficult to assess prognosis based on grade alone. An overall assessment of the patient, age, Gleason score, markers such as PSA, and oncogene content must all be taken into account. No grading system can stand alone in offering precise prognosis in an individual patient even though the course of an undifferentiated (Gleason score 9) neoplasm is usually progressive.

The association of prostatic intraepithelial hyperplasia (PIN), formerly atypical hyperplasia, although not diagnostic of cancer and not helpful in prognosis, alerts one to the presence of associated cancer or the possible impending development of cancer. PIN is demonstrated in the peripheral zone of the prostate, where a majority of invasive cancers start. PIN is associated with elevated levels of PSA. Also, octahedral crystals in areas of PIN acini are seen, further increasing the suspicion of cancer. These stain eosinophilic on hematoxylin and eosin stain, are seen in the lumina of the gland, and are associated with the presence of cancer elsewhere in the prostate. They are protein, not amyloid or PSA. They have not been seen in BPH or other benign diseases of the prostate.[11]

As noted above, despite the limits of grading in assessing the prognosis of an individual patient, it is of some use combined with other features and does give clinicians a basis for comparison when discussing their individual experiences.

REFERENCES

1. Benson MD, Whang IS, Olsson CA, et al: The use of prostate specific antigen density to enhance the predictive value of intermediate levels of serum prostate specific antigen. J Urol 147:817–821, 1992.
2. Benson MC, Whang IS, Pantuck A, et al: A means of distinguishing benign prostatic hypertrophy and prostate cancer. J Urol 147:815–816, 1992.
3. Brawer MK, Rennels MA, Nagel RB, et al: Prostate intraepithelial neoplasia: A lesion that may be confused with cancer on prostate ultrasound. J Urol 142:1510–1512, 1989.
4. Catalona WJ, Smith DS, Ratliff TL, et al: Measurement of prostate-specific antigen in serum as a screening test for prostate cancer. N Engl J Med 324:1156, 1991.
5. Elder JS, Jewett HJ, Walsh PC: Radical perineal prostatectomy for clinical Stage B$_2$ carcinoma of the prostate. J Urol 127:706, 1982.
6. Epstein JI: Pathological considerations for the practicing urologist. *In* Wein AJ, Malkowicz SB (eds): Cancer of the Prostate, Current Practice, Future Directions. Philadelphia, CoMed Communications, 1989, p 15.
7. Gleason DF, Mellinger GT, and the Veterans Administration Cooperative Urological Research Group: Prediction of prog-

nosis for prostatic adenocarcinoma by combined histological grading and clinical staging. J Urol 111:58, 1974.
8. Goldstone LM, Scardino PT, and the Veterans Administration Cooperative Urological Research Goup: Salvage radical prostatectomy. *In* Cantini M, et al: Controversies in Prostate Cancer Management. Philadelphia, JB Lippincott, 1990, pp 447–460.
9. Hand JR: Analysis of factors influencing the survival of 109 men treated conservatively for carcinoma of the prostate. Trans Am Assoc Genitourinary Surg 65:97, 99, 1973.
10. Jacobs SC: Spread of prostate cancer to bone. Urology 21:337, 1983.
11. Jensen PE, Gardner WA Jr, Piserchia PV: Prostatic crystalloids: Association with adenocarcionoma. Prostate 1:25–30, 1980.
12. Lytton B: The role of the vertebral veins in the dissemination of prostate carcinoma. J Urol 126:753, 1981.
13. Middleton RW: Survival data following radical prostatectomy. Presented to joint meeting with Texas Genitourinary Surgeons, Salt Lake City, UT, Feb. 28, 1992.
14. Paulson DF, Lin GH, Hinshaw W, Stephani S: Radical surgery vs. radiotherapy for adenocarcinoma of the prostate. J Urol 128:502, 1982.
15. Stamey TA: Prostate specific antigen as a serum marker for adenocarcinoma of the prostate. N Engl J Med 317:909, 1987.
16. Walsh PC, Jewett HJ: Radical surgery for prostate cancer. Cancer 45:1906, 1980.

Chapter 22

THE ROLE OF TUMOR MARKERS IN THE DIAGNOSIS AND TREATMENT OF PROSTATE CANCER

WILLIAM J. ELLIS and MICHAEL K. BRAWER

Historically, tumor markers have enhanced our understanding of the natural history of neoplasms and allowed evaluation of the efficacy of therapeutic maneuvers. In the first half of the century, Charles Huggins won the Nobel Prize for his work incorporating acid phosphatase as a marker to monitor the effect of hormonal therapy on prostatic carcinoma. More recently, the discovery of prostate-specific antigen (PSA) has led to a flurry of activity defining the use of this marker in prostatic disease. In this chapter we review the current status of tumor markers in the detection, staging, and monitoring of prostate carcinoma.

PROSTATIC ACID PHOSPHATASE

The acid phosphatases are a group of enzymes that hydrolyze phosphate esters under acidic conditions. Acid phosphatase activity is found in many different human tissues but was first described in 1924 by Martland in the cytoplasm of erythrocytes.[76] In 1935 Kutscher and Wolbergs reported elevated concentrations of acid phosphatase in human ejaculate and prostate tissue.[62] Gutman and associates at Columbia were responsible for much of the early knowledge of acid phosphatase in prostatic disease. In 1936 they described high acid phosphatase activity not only in the normal prostate gland, but in prostate cancer and bony metastases of prostate

cancer.[47] This elevation of acid phosphatase activity was not noted in other neoplastic bony lesions or in Paget's disease. Shortly thereafter, Gutman and Gutman as well as Barringer and Woodard reported increased acid phosphatase activity in the serum of patients with metastatic prostate cancer.[4, 46] Robinson and the Gutmans followed up this report with a report of acid phosphatase activity in 44 patients with prostate cancer.[96] They found normal levels in all patients with clinically localized disease. Sixteen of 19 patients with elevated acid phosphatase levels had roentgenographic evidence of metastases, and marked increases in acid phosphatase activity were associated with new or increasing metastatic lesions. This relationship between acid phosphatase and prostatic carcinoma was used by Huggins and Hodges to monitor the effect of hormonal manipulation on metastatic prostate cancer.[56] Huggins went on to win the Nobel Prize, and the clinical application of the acid phosphatase as a tumor marker was firmly established.

Biochemistry

Acid phosphatase is produced by the glandular epithelial cells of the prostatic acini, which concentrate the acid phosphatase into lysosomes and secretory vacuoles. The secretory vacuoles are then transported to the apical cell membrane, where their contents are excreted into the glandular lumen. Acid phosphatase levels in the prostatic fluid are from 50 to 100 times higher than those found in the serum.[19] At birth, acid phosphatase levels

Supported in part by a Merit Review Grant from the Veterans Affairs Administration.

in the prostate are less than 1 per cent of adult values.[45] The function of acid phosphatase, either within the prostatic epithelial cell or as a component of the seminal fluid, is not known.

The acid phosphatases consist of at least five different isoenzymes. Isoenzyme 2, which has a molecular weight of 100,000 daltons and consists of two identical subunits, has been found predominantly in the prostate and thus is called prostatic acid phosphatase (PAP).[49] However, this isoenzyme is also found in the spleen, pancreas, and granulocytes.[100] Immunologic techniques can identify the enzyme in the liver, brain, lung, testicle, bladder, heart, skeletal muscle, spleen, vas deferens, and platelets.[49]

Immunohistochemistry

Immunohistochemical preparations localize PAP to the luminal cells of the prostate. Glands of cloacogenic origin, including the periurethral glands in both genders and anal glands in men, have shown staining with PAP.[59, 92] Both benign and malignant glandular epithelium may also stain, including pancreatic islet cells, rectal carcinoid tumors, breast carcinomas, and renal tubular epithelium.[49] Despite these exceptions, the strong immunopositivity of prostate carcinoma for antibody directed against acid phosphatase makes this an excellent immunohistochemical marker for identifying prostate carcinoma in cases of carcinoma of unknown primary.[5, 68]

Assays

The enzymatic assays for acid phosphatase measure the hydrolysis of an added substrate under appropriate acidic conditions. This phenomenon can be quite nonspecific. The common approaches to improving the specificity of this assay involve the use of substrates specific for PAP or the use of specific inhibitors of PAP. The initial studies of PAP by Gutman and Gutman used the disodium monophenyl phosphate substrate, as previously described by King and Armstrong.[46, 60] However, this substrate lacked specificity for the prostatic fraction of acid phosphatase. Erythrocytes produce one of the major non-PAPs.[49] Abul-Fadl and King noted that L-tartrate produces 95 per cent inhibition of PAP activity while having no effect on erythrocyte acid phosphatase activity.[1] Unfortunately, this inhibition is not specific. Acid phosphatase from the bone, spleen, liver, platelets, and kidney is inhibited to some degree by L-tartrate. Formalin has also been used as a selective inhibitor of erythrocyte acid phosphatase which does not affect PAP.[1] Other substrates for the measurement of acid phosphatase activity include beta-glycerophosphate, para-nitrophenyl phosphate, phenolphthalein phosphate, thymolphthalein monophosphate, beta-naphthyl phosphate, and alpha-naphthyl phosphate. Of these substrates, the thymolphthalein monophosphate substrate is thought to be most specific for the prostatic fraction of acid phosphatase.[19, 98]

There are basically two types of immunologic assays for PAP. Foti and colleagues have described the standard-type radioimmunoassay for the detection of PAP.[39] Polyclonal antibodies are produced from rabbits immunized with PAP. Competitive binding between the patient's antigen and radiolabeled antigen added in known quantities is used to determine the level of patient antigen present. The Tandem-R PAP (Hybritech, Inc., San Diego, CA) is an immunoradiometric "sandwich" assay that uses two mouse monoclonal antibodies which recognize two different epitopes on the PAP molecule.[31] The first fixed antibody extracts the antigen from the serum, whereas the second radiolabeled antibody permits labeling of the extracted antigen.

Enzyme immunoassays involve techniques whereby the antigen is extracted from the serum using polyclonal or monoclonal antibodies.[49] A phosphate substrate is then added, and the enzymatic activity of the isolated acid phosphatase is recorded. A variation of this technique is counterimmunoelectrophoresis as developed by Chu.[22] This technique involves the electrophoresis of serum against the antibody, which fixes the serum in a precipitant line. The enzymatic activity of this precipitant line is then determined.

In the laboratory, the sensitivity and specificity of immunologic techniques for determining PAP level appear to be greater than for the enzymatic techniques. However, in clinical settings the immunologic techniques do not appear to have any advantage over the enzymatic techniques, and, in fact, enzymatic assays may actually have more clinical usefulness.

Clinical Considerations in Acid Phosphatase Measurements

As previously described, acid phosphatases are produced by a number of nonprostatic cells within the body. It follows then that acid phosphatase activity can be elevated by nonprostatic disorders. Granulocytes possess the prostatic isoenzyme of acid phosphatase.[63] Serum acid phosphatase levels can be elevated in acute granulocytic leukemia, myeloproliferative disease, and acute lymphoblastic leukemia. Solid malignancies have also been found to elevate serum acid phosphatase levels, including tumors of the stomach, lung, breast, and pancreas, as well as rectal carcinoid tumors.[49]

Diseases of the bones may elevate enzymatic determinations of serum acid phosphatase. The most common of these disorders encountered is Paget's disease.[97] Interestingly, although Paget's disease elevates acid phosphatase determinations by the enzymatic method, the immunologic determinations of PAP remain normal. Other bony abnormalities, including osteogenesis imperfecta, osteoporosis, and primary hyperthyroidism, may also elevate serum acid phosphatase as determined by enzymatic techniques.[49]

Gaucher's disease is an autosomal recessive disorder of glucocerebroside metabolism which commonly involves the liver, spleen, and bones. The enzymatic determination of acid phosphatase is generally elevated

TABLE 22–1. SERUM ACID PHOSPHATASE VERSUS CLINICAL STAGE

	ASSAY TYPE	PER CENT ABNORMAL BY STAGE		
		OC	C	D
Foti et al (1977)[39]	E	14	29	60
Cooper et al (1978)[26]	E	9	46	
Bruce et al (1980)[16]	E	9	17	73
Murphy et al (1979)[80]	E	11	17	51
Van Cangh et al (1982)[120]	E	21	31	78
Foti et al (1977)[39]	I	60	71	92
Cooper et al (1978)[26]	I	43	94	
Bruce et al (1981)[17]	I	22	24	78
Murphy et al (1979)[80]	I	36	49	69
Van Cangh et al (1982)[120]	I	21	54	89

E = Enzymatic assay; I = immunologic assay; OC = organ-confined

in this condition.[29, 97] Other conditions that can elevate enzymatic acid phosphatase determination include thromboembolic disorders, thrombocytosis, jaundice, and diabetes mellitis.[49]

Acid phosphatase levels can vary tremendously depending on techniques of specimen handling. Serum should be rapidly separated from the clot in the blood. This prevents false elevation of acid phosphatase levels from acid phosphatase present in erythrocytes, leukocytes, and platelets. Maximum stability of acid phosphatase occurs at a pH of 6.2.[50] Serum samples should therefore be buffered with citrate or acetate buffers. These should be stored on ice and run within a few hours.

PAP values can vary markedly throughout the day. Doe and Mellinger described a circadian pattern of PAP secretion with the peak serum concentration occurring at 2:00 P.M. and the nadir occurring at 11:00 P.M.[33] Subsequent studies have confirmed the marked variations in PAP levels.[13, 75, 85] However, these studies have been unable to define a clear circadian pattern to the PAP secretion. Schifman et al noted the variability in PAP levels to be as much as 70 per cent.[101]

PAP is rapidly eliminated from the serum with a first half-life of 0.5 to 2.5 hours.[125, 127] The protein-bound fraction is eliminated with a half-life of 11 days.[125]

A number of investigators have studied the effect of prostatic manipulation on serum acid phosphatase levels. After simple digital rectal examination, most have found little change in serum acid phosphatase levels. We recorded acid phosphatase levels in 18 men at 5 and 30 minutes after a standard digital rectal examination.[12] None of the 18 men showed evidence of increased serum acid phosphatase levels. However, after prostate massage, between 10 and 60 per cent of patients had elevations in serum acid phosphatase.[49] It appears that the more traumatic prostate massage is capable of releasing acid phosphatase into the serum.

Surgical procedures may also elevate serum PAP. Simple catheterization and cystoscopy may elevate the acid phosphatase, especially in larger glands.[44] More traumatic procedures such as prostate needle biopsy, transurethral resection of the prostate, and open prostatectomy are associated with much higher elevations in acid phosphatase levels.[49]

Prostatic infarction causes an acute release of acid phosphatase into the serum. Howard and Fraley reviewed 96 open prostatectomies and noted that the 8 patients with elevated acid phosphatase levels preoperatively were the only patients with evidence of prostatic infarction in the histologic specimen.[53] Subsequent studies have confirmed these findings.[103, 123] Bacterial prostatitis can be associated with elevations in serum acid phosphatase levels.[120] Urinary retention has also been reported to cause change in elevations in serum acid phosphatase.[17, 24] However, this elevation may be due to coexisting prostatic infarct or prostatitis.

Acid Phosphatase in the Diagnosis of Prostate Cancer

Serum PAP is a much less sensitive and specific marker of prostatic carcinoma than is PSA. The exact role of PAP in the diagnosis and staging of prostate carcinoma is difficult to deduce through comparison of published reports. Not only are there a wide variety of immunologic and enzymatic assays available for determination of acid phosphatase levels, but many of the studies use clinical rather than pathologic staging.

Elevations of enzymatic acid phosphatase are not generally useful for detecting clinically localized disease (Table 22–1). For example, whereas 10 to 15 per cent of patients with clinically localized disease have elevations in enzymatic acid phosphatase, 50 to 75 per cent of patients with metastatic disease show elevation of enzymatic acid phosphatase. The subsequent development of immunologic assays for acid phosphatase improved the sensitivity of acid phosphatase in the detection of local disease. Table 22–1 also summarizes the results of several studies evaluating immunologic assays for acid phosphatase.

The introduction of immunologic assays for acid phosphatase with their improved sensitivity in detecting clinically localized disease resulted in a surge of enthusiasm for the use of acid phosphatase in screening for prostate cancer. Several subsequent screening investigations were performed. Cooper screened 6320 men with a radioimmunoassay for PAP and found 62 carcinomas.[27] Vihko and colleagues found five unsuspected carcinomas in 771 men.[124] Fleishman and associates attempted to assess the false-positive rate of the immunoassay for PAP.[37] They screened 295 men and noted 17 who had palpably benign prostates with an abnormal PAP. None of these 17 patients was found to have evidence of carcinoma in their simple prostatectomy specimens. Likewise, Fair and associates studied 349 men who underwent simple prostatectomy and found no statistical difference in the PAP values by radioimmunoassay in the 16 patients with Stage A carcinoma and those without cancer.[35]

The initial report of Foti and associates was reevaluated by Watson and Tang.[39, 131] Based on the assumption that the prevalence of prostatic carcinoma in the United States is 35 per 100,000 (the 1964 incidence of clinical carcinoma of the prostate), they predicted that, with the sensitivity and specificity reported by Foti, only 1 of 244 men screened who had a positive test would indeed have prostatic carcinoma. This report, coupled with the results of the above studies, tempered the enthusiasm for serologic prostate cancer screening.

Acid Phosphatase and Staging of Prostate Cancer

The concept of elevated acid phosphatase levels in patients without detectable metastatic disease as an indicator of extracapsular spread is an old one. In 1951 Nesbitt and Baum reviewed 1150 cases of prostate carcinoma.[84] They noted that 20 per cent of prostate cancer patients without evidence of metastatic disease had elevations in serum acid phosphatase. They also noted that these patients had a much higher likelihood of death from prostate carcinoma than did those with normal acid phosphatase levels. They concluded that the acid phosphatase elevation implied the presence of occult metastatic disease.

More recently, other groups have confirmed the ability of elevated enzymatic acid phosphatase levels to predict more extensive disease. Whitesel performed pelvic lymphadenectomy on 343 patients with carcinoma of the prostate.[134] Of the 25 patients who had persistently elevated enzymatic acid phosphatase preoperatively, 15 had positive nodes and 10 had negative nodes at the time of lymphadenectomy. Of the 10 patients who had negative lymphadenectomies with elevated acid phosphatase, 5 of 7 patients followed for 2 years or more developed metastatic disease. They concluded from this study that elevated enzymatic acid phosphatase values in the absence of other evidence of metastatic disease indicates occult metastatic disease. Whitesel and colleagues applied the term D0 to describe this condition. Unfortunately, in this study the majority of patients were treated with radiation therapy or hormonal ablation. Therefore, the possibility that the late development of metastatic disease was from the remaining primary tumor cannot be ruled out.

Pontes et al had reported 20 patients with clinically localized prostate carcinoma and elevated acid phosphatase levels by the Roy method.[93] In all 20 cases the patients were found to have tumor involving the lymph nodes at time of exploration. Bahnson and Catalona performed a retrospective review of 100 consecutive patients with clinically localized prostate carcinoma who had preoperative serum acid phosphatase values determined by the Roy method prior to radical prostatectomy.[3] Five of the six patients with elevated acid phosphatase levels preoperatively had pathologic evidence of extracapsular tumor extension. The one patient without pathologic upstaging had a persistently elevated acid phosphatase postoperatively. The Johns Hopkins group reported that none of 275 patients in their series who underwent bilateral pelvic lymphadenectomy and radical prostatectomy had organ-confined disease if their preoperative acid phosphatase determination by the Roy technique was elevated.[88] The M. D. Anderson Hospital group reviewed 217 consecutive extended pelvic lymphadenectomies.[77] All 18 patients with elevated enzymatic acid phosphatase values using thymolphthalein as the substrate were found to have positive lymph nodes. These studies indicate that enzymatic acid phosphatase determinations using the thymolphthalein substrate provide valuable staging information to the urologist. Elevations of this analyte strongly suggest the presence of extracapsular disease.

PROSTATE-SPECIFIC ANTIGEN

The discovery of PSA has been responsible for many of the recent advances in our understanding of prostate cancer biology. In most respects PSA is the best marker for prostate cancer, and, indeed, this test is probably the best tumor marker available today. The introduction of this assay into clinical practice has revolutionized the way prostate cancer patients are monitored, especially after their disease has been treated. The utility of PSA as an immunohistochemical marker is well established. The value of this analyte in the early detection and staging of prostate cancer is undergoing extensive evaluation.

History

In 1971 Hara et al described an antigen they found in human seminal plasma which they called gamma-seminoprotein.[48] Li and Beling subsequently isolated two antigens from human seminal plasma.[69] One of these antigens, called semen E-1 antigen, was the same protein previously described by Hara and associates. They determined this protein to have a molecular weight of approximately 31,000 daltons. Sensabaugh isolated and provided a detailed characterization of the semen-specific protein in human seminal plasma which he called P-30.[102] His group later proposed that the presence of P-30 could be used as evidence of rape.[42]

In 1979 Wang et al at Roswell Park reported the identification of an antigen specific to prostate tissue which they had isolated.[130] Using antiserum to this antigen, they were able to detect the presence of this

TABLE 22–2. PROSTATE-SPECIFIC ANTIGEN IMMUNOHISTOCHEMISTRY

AUTHOR	PRIMARY CAP*	METASTATIC CAP	IRRADIATED CAP	OTHER†
Nadji et al (1981)[83]	73/73	49/49		0/78
Stein et al (1982)[114]	13/15			
Vernon and Williams (1983)[121]	30/30		5/5	
Ford et al (1985)[38]	63/65	16/17		0/13
Brawer et al (1989)[10]			33/33	
Sohlberg et al (1990)[107]	23/23			
TOTAL	202/206	65/66	38/38	0/91

*Prostate carcinoma
†Nonprostate carcinoma

antigen in normal, benign hyperplastic, and malignant prostate tissues. The antigen was not detected in nonprostatic tissues. They first suggested the term *prostate-specific antigen* to describe this protein. They determined the molecular weight of this antigen to be 33,000 to 34,000 daltons without subunits; the isoelectric point was observed to be 6.9. In further studies, Wang and associates found PSA in seminal plasma to be identical to that purified from prostate tissue.[129] Recent studies have confirmed identity between PSA, P-30, gamma-seminoprotein, and semen E-1 antigen.[41]

When the Roswell Park group examined the serum from patients with advanced prostate cancer, only 17 of 219 patients (8 per cent) were found to have detectable PSA in their serum by the relatively crude technology of rocket electrophoresis.[90] This assay could not detect PSA levels below 500 ng/ml. Owing to this poor analytic sensitivity, PSA was not detected in the serum of normal men in the study. Subsequently, when a more sensitive ELISA assay for PSA was developed, PSA could be detected in the serum of all men with prostates.[61] In addition, PSA levels were elevated in benign prostatic hyperplasia (BPH) and in prostate cancer.

Biochemistry

PSA is a 34-kilodalton neutral serine protease of the kallikrein family produced by epithelial cells of prostatic origin. The protein is present in the cytoplasm of prostatic epithelial cells and is secreted apically by luminal cells into the prostatic acini. Sinha and colleagues have elegantly demonstrated the ultrastructural localization of PSA in rough endoplasmic reticulum and cytoplasmic vesicles and granules using immunogold techniques.[105] This enzyme is not produced by other cells within the prostate, including the basal cells, or by cells within the seminal vesicles.[89] PSA production appears to be regulated by the androgen receptor, as PSA mRNA can be induced by androgens and inhibited by androgen receptor blockade in the LNCaP model.[135]

Functionally, PSA is involved in the liquefaction of the seminal coagulum.[66, 72] Specifically, PSA has been shown to act on a group of high molecular weight seminal vesicle proteins, commonly referred to as seminal vesicle antigen.

Structurally, PSA is a 240-amino acid glycoprotein monomer. The isoelectric points of various isoforms of the molecule range from 6.8 to 7.2.[128] The amino acid sequence has been elucidated.[132] The gene coding for PSA has been identified on chromosome 19q13, where it is closely linked to the gene of another protease, human glandular kallikrein-1.[116] Studies indicate there is an 82 per cent homology between the genes for PSA and kallikrein-1.[95]

Immunohistochemistry

As noted above, the specificity of PSA for epithelial cells of prostatic origin makes this marker extremely useful for immunohistochemical analysis. One case report describes apparent ectopic benign prostate glands labeling immunohistochemically with antibodies to PSA.[14] Recently a report from Japan noted that polyclonal antibodies against PSA demonstrated immunoreactivity with 11 of 25 perianal glands in men and 6 of 26 periurethral glands in both sexes.[59] Similar staining in the female periurethral glands had been noted previously.[92] In addition, anti-PSA staining has been detected in normal Skene's glands and in a Skene's gland tumor.[108, 118]

Despite these rare cases of apparent nonspecific anti-PSA staining, PSA remains an excellent marker for immunohistochemical analysis of tumors of unknown origin.[38, 117] Several studies have previously evaluated the staining of primary, metastatic, and irradiated prostate cancer with PSA antibodies (Table 22–2). Nearly all of these tumors show immunoreactivity with PSA antibodies. Of note is the observation of persistent positive immunohistochemical staining in all of the irradiated prostates studied in these series. Prostatic carcinoma tends to be heterogeneous. Some cells within a given tumor stain more intensely than others, and some apparently do not elaborate PSA at all. In general, as the grade of a tumor increases, the intensity of the immunohistochemical staining tends to decrease and more cells are devoid of labeling.[38] BPH stains more intensely than prostatic intraepithelial neoplasia (a putative premalignant lesion) or carcinoma.[107]

A technique related to immunohistochemistry is in situ hybridization. The Mayo Clinic group showed that in situ hybridization with PSA mRNA localizes PSA production to epithelial cells in a pattern similar to that revealed by immunohistochemical techniques.[94]

Assays

As the clinical utility of serum PSA emerged, numerous assays for the measurement of PSA were developed. The assays most commonly used in the United States are the Tandem-R and Tandem-E (Hybritech, Inc., San Diego, CA) and the Pros-Check (Yang Laboratories, Bellevue, WA). The Hybritech and Yang assays use different methodologies to assess the level of PSA in the serum and report different values for the same specimen.

The Tandem-R assay is an immunoradiometric "sandwich" assay. The assay uses two mouse monoclonal antibodies to different epitopes on the PSA molecule. One antibody is fixed in a solid phase to a bead and extracts the PSA from the serum. The second anti-PSA antibody is radiolabeled and binds to the now fixed PSA antigen. The analytic sensitivity for this assay is 0.1 to 0.2 ng/ml.[21, 52] The clinical sensitivity, meaning the lowest serum level that can reliably be distinguished from a true "0" reading, has been reported to range from 0.1 to 0.6 ng/ml.[21, 34, 54] Each laboratory must independently determine the low end detectability for the assay. One drawback of the Tandem-R assay is a hook effect, which is found in high PSA levels (5,000 to 10,000 ng/ml).[81, 119] PSA concentrations this high tend to be read at approximately one order of magnitude lower than the true value. This is an aberration of the one-step double-antibody assay. If high serum PSA levels are suspected, the serum should be run in dilutions. Alternatively, running the assay in two steps eliminates this hook effect.

The Tandem-E assay is an immunoenzymatic "sandwich" assay. This assay also uses two mouse anti-PSA monoclonal antibodies. However, in this method, the second antibody is labeled with alkaline phosphatase rather than with a radioactive isotope. Activity of this labeling enzyme, rather than radioactivity, is then measured. The analytic and clinical sensitivities of this assay are the same as those for the Tandem-R assay.[86] The major advantage of this assay is that no radioactivity is used. This has advantages with respect to radioactive materials and the costs of laboratory operation.

The Pros-Check assay is a conventional radioimmunoassay that uses polyclonal rabbit anti-PSA antibodies. The analytic sensitivity of this assay is 0.1 to 0.2 ng/ml.[21, 52] The clinical sensitivity has been reported to be 0.2 to 0.3 ng/ml.[52, 70] No hook effect is noted with this assay at high serum PSA levels. One potential disadvantage is the inherent instability of polyclonal antibody generation.

The two assays have been compared by Chan et al and Hortin et al. PSA levels obtained with the Pros-Check assay are from 1.4 to 1.8 times higher than those obtained with the Tandem-R assay on the same specimen.[21, 52] Nevertheless, both apparently measure the same analyte because the correlation between the two assays was found to be between 0.95 and 0.99. The Stanford group has recently shown that the difference in the assays is due to differences in the standards supplied with the kits.[43] When common standards are substituted for those in the kits, results obtained with the two assays are nearly identical.

Recently, Scandinavian researchers have drawn attention to the complexes formed in the serum between PSA and protease inhibitors.[115] The major protease inhibitor binding with PSA is alpha$_1$-antichymotrypsin. The resulting complex, which has a molecular weight of 100,000 daltons, accounted for 41 to 100 per cent of the PSA immunoreactivity by the Tandem-R assay. Other protease inhibitors accounted for little PSA binding. A higher percentage of the serum PSA was found in the complexed form in patients with higher PSA levels. In addition, sera from prostate cancer patients had a higher proportion of PSA complexed with alpha$_1$-antichymotrypsin than sera from BPH patients with similar PSA levels.

Other PSA assays are currently in development. The IMX assay (Abbott Laboratories, Abbott Park, IL) is an immunoradiometric "sandwich" assay. This assay uses a mouse monoclonal antibody in the solid phase and a radiolabeled goat anti-mouse polyclonal antibody. The assay is being promoted as an "ultrasensitive" assay. The analytic sensitivity of this assay is 0.03 ng/ml; the clinical sensitivity is between 0.6 and 0.10 ng/ml.[122]

Prostate-Specific Antigen in the Normal Population

Many tumor markers, such as alpha-fetoprotein, carcinoembryonic antigen, and beta-hCG in the male, are substances produced by cells in the process of aberrant differentiation or reversion to fetal differentiation. These so-called oncofetoproteins are not normally produced in measurable quantities by normal adult cells. Thus the presence of these markers in the serum of a patient is likely to indicate the presence of disease. In contrast, PSA is produced in large quantities by normal prostate epithelial cells. Thus, normal men without prostatic disease have detectable levels of PSA in their serum. Further confounding the situation is the fact that BPH, which is associated with elevations in PSA levels, is present in the majority of men over age 50. Finally, subclinical prostatic carcinoma is extremely prevalent. For example, autopsy studies have shown carcinoma to be present in more than 30 per cent of men over the age of 50.[51] Thus, the problem in constructing a normal range for PSA becomes obvious. Without histologic examination of a man's prostate, it is not possible to exclude prostatic disease.

Tissue levels of PSA are similar per gram of tissue in BPH, prostate cancer, and normal prostate tissue.[15] However, individual prostate cancer cells often produce less PSA than the epithelial cells of BPH or normal glands.[107] Also, PSA expression in prostate cancer tends to decrease as the Gleason grade rises.[91] It appears that elevations of PSA concentrations in prostate pathology are not related solely to the total amount of PSA being produced. Rather, in prostatic disease the prostate appears to be made "leaky," allowing egress of PSA to the lymphatics or capillaries. Several possible explanations for this phenomenon exist. These include disruption of the normal basement membrane and basal cell layer surrounding prostatic acini, allowing leakage of the PSA into serum; obstruction of prostatic ducts due to carcinoma, causing increased back-pressure and leakage of PSA from acini; and loss of cell polarity with dedifferentiation and resultant basal as well as apical secretion of PSA.[19]

As mentioned above, it is impossible to establish a "normal" population of men to define the normal prostatic markers. However, the "normal" distribution of PSA levels within populations of men without clinical evidence of prostatic disease has been defined by several investigators. The manufacturer's suggested reference range (mean + 2 SD) for the Tandem-R assay is less than 4.0 ng/ml.[82] Chan et al defined the reference range (mean + 3 SD) for normal men over 40 years old as 2.8 ng/ml, whereas the same reference range for men under 40 years old was 2.0 ng/ml.[21] Ercole et al found a similar reference range (mean + 2 SD) from 207 normal men over 40 years of age to be less than 4.0 ng/ml.[34] For normal men under 40 years of age, all of whom had PSA values less than 4.0 ng/ml, the reference range was 1.8 ng/ml. This is likely explained by the lack of prostate pathology in this group. Catalona and colleagues evaluated 1653 men aged 50 years or older without a history of prostate cancer or prostatitis using the Tandem-R assay.[20] Serum PSA levels were noted to be less than 4.0 ng/ml in 1516 (92 per cent), between 4.0 and 9.9 ng/ml in 107 (6 per cent), and 10.0 ng/ml or greater in 30 (2 per cent). We found similar levels of PSA in a study of 1249 men over the age of 50. Of these patients, 1062 (85 per cent) had serum PSA levels less than 4.0 ng/ml, 149 (12 per cent) had levels between 4.1 and 10.0 ng/ml, and 38 (3 per cent) had levels greater than 10.0 ng/ml.[7] A trend of increasing PSA values with increasing age was also noted, as shown in Table 22–3.

Chan and associates also defined the reference range for the Pros-Check assay using the same specimens they used to determine the reference range for the Tandem-R assay.[21] They determined the upper limit of normal for the Pros-Check PSA to be less than 3.0 ng/ml for patients less than 40 years of age and 4.2 ng/ml for patients greater than 40 years of age. Stamey et al evaluated 157 "normal" men between 21 and 76 years of age to determine the reference range for the Pros-Check assay.[112] They defined the normal range for PSA as 0 to 2.5 ng/ml.

Clinical Considerations in Prostate-Specific Antigen Measurements

In several important clinical aspects, PSA exhibits much less variability as a tumor marker than does PAP. With the possible exception of the periurethral glands, PSA is not produced by tissues of nonprostatic origin. Therefore, changes in the serum levels of this antigen reflect changes in the prostate alone.

PSA appears to be less susceptible to diurnal variation, which can produce large differences in intraindividual PAP assessment. Dejter et al monitored for 24 hours three groups of 10 men each with either BPH, prostate cancer, or normal glands.[32] They noted no circadian variability in either PSA or PAP values. The mean variability was 18 per cent for PSA, compared with 51 per cent for PAP. Schifman et al looked at morning and afternoon blood specimens collected from 10 individuals with prostate cancer over a 3-day period.[101] The mean intraindividual coefficients of variation (CV) for enzymatic and immunologic acid phosphatase determinations were 23.8 per cent and 21.5 per cent, respectively. On the other hand, the mean CV for intraindividual PSA determinations was only 6.2 per cent. Maatman monitored serum PSA levels every 4 hours for a 24-hour period in eight patients with stage D prostate cancer.[74] He found the average CV in intraindividual PSA levels to be within 7.6 per cent of the mean. These data suggest that the timing of the phlebotomy for PSA determination is relatively unimportant.

The ambulatory status of a patient does appear to be a significant factor with respect to PSA levels. Stamey et al reported that PSA levels dropped an average of 18 per cent after 24 hours of hospitalization.[112] The cause of this decrease is unclear. However, it is recommended that all PSA levels be drawn on an ambulatory basis.

PSA serum samples are also considerably more stable than PAP serum samples. Schifman and associates assessed analyte stability by allowing serum samples to stand at room temperature for 24 hours.[101] PSA concentrations decreased a mean of 3.1 per cent, whereas PAP concentrations decreased a mean of 15.2 per cent. Hybritech recommends that sera be frozen at $-20°C$ within 24 hours of collection, but Simm and Gleeson found serum PSA (Tandem-R) to be stable for up to 14 days when stored at 4°C.[104] Repeat freeze-thaw cycles were noted to increase assay variability.

The route by which PSA is eliminated from the serum is unclear. Hepatic metabolism is the probable mechanism. PSA is detectable in the urine of normal men but not in the urine of men with ileal conduits.[58] Urinary PSA is probably the result of secretion of PSA into the prostatic urethra, and renal excretion of this analyte apparently does not take place.

By monitoring serum PSA levels after radical prostatectomy, Stamey et al were able to show that elimination of PSA from the serum follows a two-compartment model.[112] During the first 6 hours after operation the serum levels decrease, with an average half-life of 12 hours. However, after 12 hours the elimination half-life

TABLE 22–3. PROSTATE-SPECIFIC ANTIGEN VERSUS AGE

AGE (years)	NO. (%)	MEAN (ng/ml)	MEDIAN (ng/ml)	SD (ng/ml)
50–59	222 (17.8)	1.62	1.0	6.5
60–69	600 (48.0)	2.7	3.8	1.4
70–79	365 (29.2)	3.1	5.0	1.7
>79	62 (5.0)	8.8	11.9	2.2
TOTALS	1249	2.9	2.2	10.4

TABLE 22–4. SERUM PROSTATE-SPECIFIC ANTIGEN IN PATIENTS WITH HISTOLOGICALLY CONFIRMED BENIGN PROSTATIC HYPERPLASIA

AUTHOR	ASSAY	PSA >2.5 (%)	PSA >4.0 (%)	PSA >10.0 (%)
Ercole et al (1987)[34]	Tandem-R		75 (21)	10 (3)
Ferro et al (1987)[36]	Tandem-R			13 (33)
Hudson et al (1989)[54]	Tandem-R		35 (21)	3 (2)
Stamey et al (1987)[112]	Pros-Check	70 (88)		

was 2.2 ± 0.8 days. For practical purposes the initial, more rapid elimination can be ignored. Oesterling et al evaluated PSA levels in 30 patients on postoperative days two through ten.[88] Their group calculated the half-life of PSA elimination to be 3.2 ± 0.1 days. These half-life calculations allow one to predict that up to 3 weeks may be necessary for PSA levels to reach their new baseline following extirpative surgery.

The effect of digital rectal examination (DRE) on PSA levels is controversial. Using the Yang assay, Stamey et al noted that both PSA and PAP serum levels were increased by 1.5 to 2 times 1 minute after prostate massage.[112] In contrast, Brawer et al noted no change in PSA or PAP levels measured by the Tandem-R technique in 26 men monitored 5 and 30 minutes following standard DRE.[12] Yaun and Catalona also noted no elevation of serum PSA in 43 men evaluated immediately before and at 5- and 10-minute intervals after DRE.[136] One of 20 patients was noted to have an elevation of PSA after prostatic massage, whereas transrectal ultrasonography (TRUS) caused PSA elevations in 3 of 36 patients. Finally, Crawford et al reported no significant change in PSA levels in 1420 men after DRE performed as part of a national prostate screening protocol.[28] The reason for the discrepancy between Stamey's data and those of the others is unclear. It is doubtful that these differences could be explained by the use of a polyclonal rather than a monoclonal assay. More likely they are due to differences in the practitioner's examination technique and reflect prostatic trauma incurred during prostatic massage compared with a "standard" DRE. Overall, these data support the validity of serum PSA values drawn after a "standard" DRE.

Following transperineal needle biopsies of the prostate, Stamey showed that PSA levels increased by 57 times.[112] The Mayo Clinic group found that 5 to 21 (median 14.5) days were required for PSA values to stabilize in 19 men undergoing TRUS-guided needle biopsy of the prostate.[87] The Washington University group noted that transrectal needle biopsy using the spring-loaded biopsy gun caused PSA elevations in 89 of 100 men.[136] In addition, PSA elevations persisted for more than 2 weeks in 27 of the 89 men. We recently studied 127 men following TRUS-guided sextant prostate needle biopsies with the Biopty gun needle (unpublished observations). We observed a 20 per cent or greater elevation in PSA level present in 15 per cent of patients 28 days after their procedure. These data reaffirm the importance of drawing PSA levels prior to prostate needle biopsy. Values drawn even several weeks after prostate needle biopsy may reflect spurious elevation of the baseline value. After prostate needle biopsy, PSA levels do not necessarily fall to baseline levels with a half-life of 2 to 3 days. Significant disruptions of the normal glandular architecture, local inflammation, and fistula formation may allow PSA to "leak" into the serum for weeks or months, giving spuriously elevated PSA levels.

Prostate-Specific Antigen in Nonmalignant Prostatic Disorders

Because PSA is produced by both benign and malignant prostatic epithelial cells, it follows that elevations in serum PSA can occur in nonmalignant conditions. Trauma, inflammation, and proliferation are all processes that can cause increased leakage of PSA into the serum. The inflammatory response appears to allow leakage of PSA back across the basement membrane into the circulation. Patients with acute bacterial prostatitis may have significant elevations in their PSA levels.[30] Prostate infarction may cause dramatic elevations in acid phosphatase levels in men with BPH.[123] Elevations of PSA in this setting have not been studied. However, it is assumed that PSA would be markedly elevated as well. Acute urinary retention is associated with elevations of serum PSA.[2] Retention is often caused by prostatic inflammation or infarction. These factors may account for the elevations in PSA seen in this setting.

Prostate-Specific Antigen and Benign Prostatic Hyperplasia

The majority of men at risk for developing prostate cancer have histologic evidence of BPH. Several groups have shown that PSA levels can be elevated in patients with BPH alone (Table 22–4). The contribution of this benign hyperplastic tissue must be taken into account when interpreting serum PSA values.

Stamey compared pre- and postoperative PSA levels in 7 men undergoing simple retropubic prostatectomy and 90 men undergoing transurethral resection of the prostate (TURP) for BPH.[112] In the group undergoing simple retropubic prostatectomy, the values ranged from 9.5 to 44 (mean 24) ng/ml. Between 34 and 146 (mean 89) grams of hyperplastic tissue were removed from these prostates. Three weeks after the prostatectomy, serum PSA values were 1.7 ng/ml or less in all 7 patients. In the group of TURP patients, preoperative serum PSA levels decreased from 0.3 to 37 (mean 7.9) ng/ml to 6.7 ng/ml or less (mean 1.3 ng/ml). PSA levels were elevated (greater than 2.5 ng/ml by Pros-Check assay) in 86 per cent of the patients preoperatively. The contribution of BPH in the two groups was calculated to be 0.29 ng/ml per gram of tissue in the retropubic prostatectomy group and 0.31 ng/ml per gram of tissue in the TURP group.

Morphometric analyses of radical retropubic prosta-

TABLE 22–5. PROSTATE-SPECIFIC ANTIGEN AND PATHOLOGIC STAGE (% PSA >10.0 ng/ml)

			INVASION METASTASES		
AUTHOR	ASSAY	ORGAN CONFINED	CAPSULAR PENETRATION	SEMINAL VESICLE	LYMPH NODE
Ercole et al (1987)[34]	Tandem-R	7	32	100	71
Hudson et al (1989)[54]	Tandem-R	11	5	0	100
Oesterling et al (1988)[88]	Tandem-R	10	20	61	71
Stamey et al (1987)[112]	Pros-Check		82	95	100

tectomy specimens have been unable to correlate the volume of BPH present with serum PSA levels preoperatively.[91, 111] Stamey has suggested that PSA from cancer in these specimens masks the elevation of serum PSA due to BPH.

Weber et al studied serum PSA in men with clinical BPH being treated with the luteinizing hormone–releasing hormone agonist nafarelin.[133] They found in patients with BPH that the best correlation exists between PSA and epithelial weight, not between PSA and prostate size. They also noted a threefold variation in the epithelial contribution to total prostatic weight. This variation in BPH histology may account for differences in the serum PSA contributions per gram of BPH tissue.

Brawer et al evaluated prostatic tissue removed from 81 men who underwent either TURP or simple open prostatectomy for presumed benign disease.[11] All tissue was sectioned and examined for prostatic pathology. Preoperatively 36 of the 81 men were known to have PSA levels greater than 4.0 ng/ml. Of these patients with elevated PSA levels, 11 were found to have adenocarcinoma of the prostate, 13 had prostatic intraepithelial neoplasia (PIN, a putative premalignant change), and 11 had evidence of acute inflammation. Of the 26 patients with BPH with or without chronic inflammation, only one had a PSA elevated above 4.0 ng/ml. These data suggest that BPH alone rarely elevates PSA above 4.0 ng/ml by the Tandem-R method.

Prostate-Specific Antigen and Prostatic Intraepithelial Neoplasia

PIN fulfills the majority of requirements for a premalignant change in the human prostate. PIN bears similar morphology to invasive carcinoma, with the cells demonstrating moderate to severe cytologic atypia. In the highest grade of PIN, the cells cannot be differentiated from those of cancer. Unlike carcinoma, PIN has a basal cell layer present, but this may be disrupted.[6] In addition, PIN occurs with a greater degree of severity and extent in organs harboring invasive carcinoma as opposed to those without, has both spatial and zonal relationship to invasive carcinoma, and shares a number of phenotypic similarities to prostate cancer, as demonstrated by a variety of probes and immunohistochemical techniques.

The disruption of the basal cell layer suggests the potential for easier egress of PSA from the luminal cell layer to the prostatic capillaries. As noted above, in the

investigation comparing serum PSA and simple prostatectomy histology, we observed that 13 of 25 men (52 per cent) with PIN had PSA above the 4.0 ng/ml cutoff.[11] Similarly, 71 per cent of the patients with invasive carcinoma and 69 per cent with acute inflammation had elevated PSA. Only 1 of 26 men with BPH alone or BPH associated with chronic inflammation was noted to have a PSA greater than 4.0 ng/ml.

More recently, we performed a study in which men with PIN on prostate needle biopsy underwent repeat ultrasound-guided prostatic needle biopsy. A strong correlation was found between PIN grade on the initial biopsy and subsequent carcinoma. Whereas 2 of 11 patients with PIN grade 1 initially had carcinoma (18 per cent), all 10 patients with grade 2 or 3 PIN were demonstrated to have invasive carcinoma on the repeat biopsy.[8] Sixteen of these patients had PSA determination prior to the second biopsy. The PSA was greater than 4.0 ng/ml in 14 per cent of the patients with grade 1 in the initial biopsy, compared with 57 per cent of those with PIN grade 2 or 3. Moreover, whereas no man who had negative biopsies on the repeat examination had a PSA greater than 4.0 ng/ml, 56 per cent of the men with carcinoma had a PSA greater than 4.0 ng/ml before repeat biopsy.

We conclude that PIN may be associated with elevated PSA and that this may have clinical importance. The well-recognized spatial relationship between PIN and prostatic carcinoma and the fact that there is much higher incidence of PIN in glands with invasive carcinoma suggest that the elevated PSA may be related to "missed" carcinoma on the initial biopsy or TURP specimen. Clearly this was the explanation in the majority of patients who underwent repeat prostate needle biopsy shortly after an index biopsy that showed PIN. Nevertheless, the association of PIN with PSA and with carcinoma suggests the importance of these correlations.

The Role of Prostate-Specific Antigen in Prostate Cancer Staging

PSA provides the clinician with additional information to use in the preoperative staging of prostate cancer patients. Several series have evaluated the relationship between PSA and pathologic stage (Table 22–5). These studies have all shown a correlation between prostate cancer pathologic stage and serum PSA levels for the groups of patients studied.

The Stanford group evaluated radical prostatectomy

specimens with morphometric analysis and determined that PSA levels in the serum corresponded to tumor volume in the prostatectomy specimens.[112] They calculated a serum value of 3.5 ng/ml/cc of cancer in the specimen (Pros-Check assay). The Johns Hopkins group has reaffirmed the positive correlation between tumor volume and serum PSA.[91]

The data in Table 22–5 show an overall correlation between pathologic stage and PSA. However, for an individual patient, serum PSA is a poor predictor of pathologic stage. As the reader can see from Figure 22–1, there is a wide distribution of PSA levels for a given pathologic stage.

There are several explanations for the poor predictive value of PSA in the individual patient. The Johns Hopkins group has shown that there is an inverse correlation between PSA levels and Gleason score when the tumors are controlled for size.[91] This would allow larger, more poorly differentiated tumors to secrete less PSA than smaller, better differentiated tumors. An alternative explanation is that the BPH contribution to serum PSA is an interfering factor. However, most of these studies have shown that the contribution from BPH is minimal in relation to the contribution from the prostate cancer. Finally, there is likely variability in the size of primary tumors at the time they metastasize.

A problem common to many of these studies is that at least some of the serum PSA levels were drawn after the diagnosis of cancer was made (i.e., preoperatively in the hospital). As Stamey has demonstrated, PSA falls significantly during hospitalization.[112] In addition, these previous reports on PSA and staging did not control for the timing of prostate biopsy or other significant prostate manipulations. As discussed previously, several studies have shown that a significant percentage of patients have persistent elevation of the serum PSA after biopsy.[87, 112, 136]

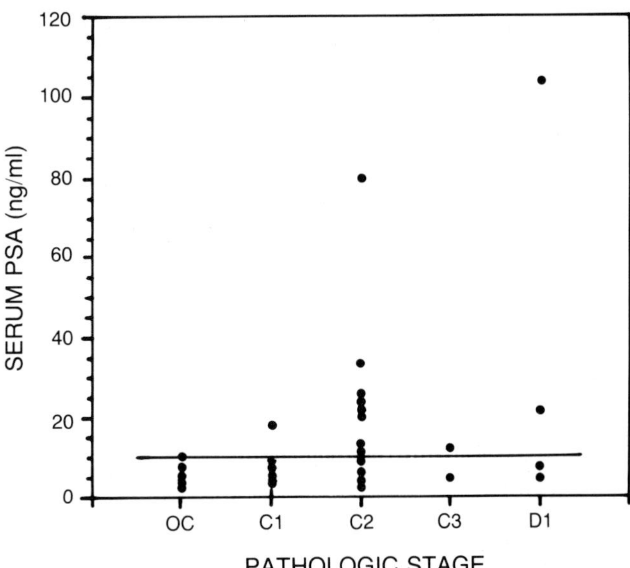

FIGURE 22–2. Serum PSA versus pathologic stage when values are obtained before prostate needle biopsy. OC = Organ-confined; C1 = capsular invasion; C2 = positive margin; C3 = seminal vesicle invasion; D1 = lymph node metastases.

The recent screening study by Catalona and associates supports the hypothesis that elevated prebiopsy PSA as determined by the Hybritech assay is an ominous sign.[20] In this report, 15 of the 16 men with prebiopsy serum PSA levels greater than 10.0 ng/ml who underwent surgery for clinically localized prostate cancer had evidence of extraprostatic spread of their tumors.

In a nonscreening series shown in Figure 22–2, we have noted that none of the 14 tumors found in men with prebiopsy PSA greater than 10.0 ng/ml were organ confined on pathologic examination (unpublished observations). Comparison of Figure 22–2 with Figure 22–1 shows a much better correlation between serum PSA and stage when the PSA value is determined before biopsy. However, 30 to 50 per cent of patients with serum PSA levels above 10.0 ng/ml have no detectable prostate carcinoma by systematic biopsy.[7, 20] Therefore, to assume that all men with prebiopsy PSA values of 10.0 ng/ml or more have extraprostatic spread of prostate cancer would be illogical, as there is no detectable prostate cancer of any stage in many of these patients.

The Mayo Clinic group recently evaluated the relationship of radionuclide bone scans with serum PSA determinations in the evaluation of newly diagnosed untreated prostate cancer patients.[23] They found that only 1 of 306 patients with a serum PSA level of 20.0 ng/ml or less had a positive bone scan. The negative predictive value of the serum PSA of less than 20.0 ng/ml was 99.7 per cent. PSA was more reliable and accurate than local clinical stage, tumor grade, acid phosphatase, or PAP in predicting bone scan findings. This study estimates the probability of a positive bone scan with a serum PSA of 10.0 ng/ml or less at 1.4 per cent. Based on these findings, these authors no longer obtain radionuclide bone scans on newly diagnosed untreated patients with serum PSA values of less than

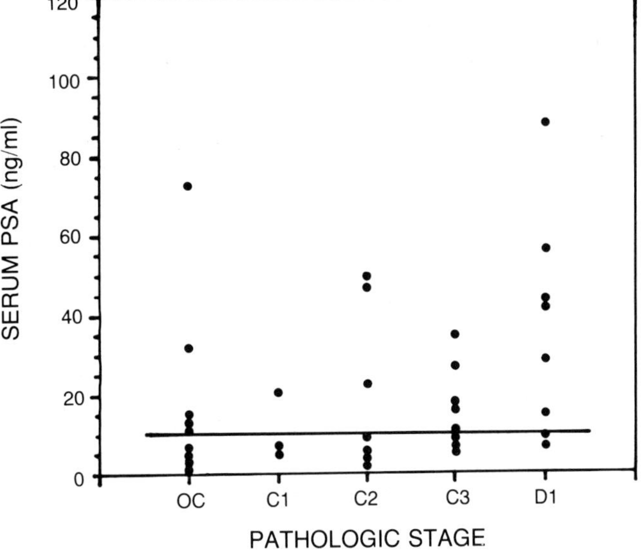

FIGURE 22–1. Serum PSA versus pathologic stage when values are obtained preoperatively. OC = Organ-confined; C1 = capsular invasion; C2 = positive margin; C3 = seminal vesicle invasion; D1 = lymph node metastases.

TABLE 22–6. PROSTATE-SPECIFIC ANTIGEN STAGING IN SCREENING POPULATION

AUTHOR	PSA (ng/ml)	BENIGN (%)	ORGAN-CONFINED TUMOR (%)*	C + D (%)*
Catalona et al (1991)[20]	4.0–9.9	66/85 (78)	10/17 (59)	7/17 (44)
	10.0+	9/27 (33)	1/16 (6)	15/16 (94)
Brawer et al (1992)[7]	4.0–9.9	64/87 (74)	9/12 (75)	3/12 (25)
	10.0+	9/18 (50)		4/4 (100)

*Includes only tumors with pathologic staging

10.0 ng/ml. In addition to the rare patient whose metastatic disease is missed with such an approach, this protocol eliminates the potential benefit of a baseline scan with which to compare future scans for any changes. Nonetheless, the staggering economic savings of such an approach may warrant its implementation.

The Role of Prostate-Specific Antigen in the Detection of Prostate Cancer

As previously discussed, the fact that PSA is produced by both benign and malignant cells within the prostate complicates the use of this marker in the early detection of prostate cancer. The data from large screening studies have recently become available. Catalona and associates recently conducted a screening study of 1653 men using Tandem-R PSA as the initial test to identify subjects for further evaluation.[20] Six per cent of the patients had PSA levels between 4.0 and 9.9 ng/ml, and 2 per cent had levels greater than 10.0 ng/ml. In the group with PSA levels between 4.0 and 9.9 ng/ml, 22 per cent were found to have prostate cancer at the time of TRUS-guided needle biopsy. At the time of prostatectomy, 59 per cent of these patients had tumors confined to the prostate. In contrast, carcinoma was found in 67 per cent of the patients with PSA levels greater than 10.0 ng/ml. However, only 6 per cent of these patients had organ confinement of their tumors. Overall, serum PSA level was a better predictor of prostate cancer than either TRUS or DRE.

As depicted in Table 22–6, we noted similar findings in our screening evaluation of 1249 men.[7] In this study, patients with an abnormal Tandem-R PSA (greater than 4.0 ng/ml) were further evaluated with DRE, TRUS, and six systematic prostate biopsies. Twenty-seven per cent of patients with a PSA between 4.1 and 10.0 ng/ml were found to have carcinoma, whereas 50 per cent of men with PSA greater than 10.0 ng/ml showed histologic evidence of carcinoma. All four patients with PSA level greater than 10.0 ng/ml who were surgically explored had evidence of extracapsular disease. In the group with preoperative PSA levels of 4.1 to 10.0 ng/ml, 9 of 12 (75 per cent) had organ-confined disease. It should be noted in this study that for 8 of the 32 carcinomas detected the patients had no abnormality noted on rectal examination. Furthermore, four additional carcinomas were found in patients with only asymmetry on DRE. Thus, 37 per cent of the carcinomas may have been missed on a routine DRE.

Many screening studies have attempted to combine serum PSA with TRUS and DRE in order to improve the sensitivity and specificity of the screening process. Lee and associates studied the additional predictive value of DRE and PSA in 250 men with hypoechoic lesions on TRUS.[67] The chance of a positive biopsy was 41 per cent with abnormal TRUS alone, 52 per cent with both abnormal TRUS and PSA (greater than 2.6 ng/ml, Pros-Check), and 71 per cent with abnormal TRUS, PSA, and DRE.

Cooner et al evaluated 1807 men in a urologic practice with serum PSA, DRE, and TRUS.[25] All patients with hypoechoic lesions of the prostate were biopsied. Elevated PSA or abnormal DRE alone gave a 35 per cent chance of a positive biopsy. Abnormal PSA and DRE resulted in a 60 per cent positive predictive value, whereas abnormal PSA and the presence of a hypoechoic lesion on TRUS predicted cancer in 48 per cent of patients. If all three tests were abnormal, cancer was detected 62 per cent of the time.

The major disappointment in using PSA alone as a screening test is that, pathologically, a high percentage of the tumors detected extend beyond the prostatic capsule. This may reflect the initial evaluation of a screening cohort in which all stages of disease may be represented. Subsequent evaluation of this cohort is anticipated to result in a higher percentage of organ-confined disease being detected.

Clearly, PSA measurements alone are inadequate as an early detection test. Indeed, if one looks at several series of radical prostatectomy patients, a significant percentage of patients have serum PSA levels of less than 4.0 ng/ml preoperatively, as measured by the Tandem-R assay (Table 22–7). Likewise, of 500 men

TABLE 22–7. PREOPERATIVE PROSTATE-SPECIFIC ANTIGEN AND RADICAL PROSTATECTOMY

AUTHOR	ASSAY	NO.	PER CENT PSA > 2.8 ng/ml	4.0 ng/ml	10.0 ng/ml
Lange et al (1989)[64]	Tandem-R	100	84	71	41
Partin et al (1990)[91]	Tandem-R	350	71	43	
Hudson et al (1989)[54]	Tandem-R	41		85	29
Brawer et al (1989)[8]	Tandem-R	60	80	78	30
TOTAL	Tandem-R	551	75	55	29
Stamey et al (1989)[109–111]	Pros-Check	102	91		

recently undergoing ultrasound-guided systematic random prostate biopsies in our institution, carcinoma was detected in 127 (25 per cent) (unpublished data). Thirty-nine per cent of the cancers were found in men with a Tandem-R PSA less than 4.0 ng/ml. New efforts are being directed at this group of patients. Serial PSA measurements may be of value in this group. PSA density, correlating serum PSA values with prostate gland size, may also improve screening accuracy.

Prostate-Specific Antigen in Monitoring Response to Treatment

Because PSA is secreted in proportion to tumor volume, potentially the greatest use of PSA is to monitor response to treatment. This test should allow for earlier detection of treatment failures. In addition, the introduction of this marker should allow for better comparison of different treatment modalities for prostate cancer.

Radical Prostatectomy Patients

After a radical prostatectomy with organ-confined disease, there should be no prostate tissue left in the body. Theoretically, postoperative PSA levels should decrease to the undetectable range. Given the half-life of PSA of between 2.2 and 3.2 days, this level should be attained by 3 weeks postoperatively. The presence of a persistently detectable serum PSA level is suggestive of residual disease.

The Stanford group noted that no patient who had detectable serum PSA levels (Pros-Check) 3 weeks following radical prostatectomy subsequently had a decrease in their PSA to undetectable levels without adjuvant therapy.[111] Furthermore, they noted that no patient with pelvic lymph node metastases reached undetectable PSA levels without adjuvant therapy. The Johns Hopkins investigators noted that no patient with an undetectable PSA level had clinical evidence of recurrent disease following radical prostatectomy.[18] Conversely, all patients with clinically detectable distant recurrence had elevated PSA levels postoperatively.

PSA is more sensitive than DRE in detecting local recurrences after radical prostatectomy. Lightner and associates biopsied the urethrovesical anastomoses of 57 patients with PSA (Tandem-R) greater than 0.4 ng/ml but no other evidence of persistent disease.[71] Prostate carcinoma was found in the anastomotic biopsies of 42 per cent of the patients. In contrast, no anastomotic biopsies revealed carcinoma in a control group of 30 patients with PSA values less than 0.4 ng/ml. Rectal examination revealed a similar spectrum of findings whether patients were grouped according to PSA values or biopsy results.

Hudson and associates monitored postoperative PSA values in 93 patients after radical prostatectomy.[54] Eighty-six had undetectable PSA levels postoperatively. Seven of the 86 (8.1 per cent) had a subsequent rise in PSA values to a mean of 70.6 ng/ml during the first year of follow-up. Forty-seven followed for less than 1 year and 32 followed for 12 to 33 months have persistently undetectable PSA values and no evidence of recurrence. Similarly, Lange et al reported that 33 of 36 patients (92 per cent) whose PSA levels decreased to less than 0.2 ng/ml 2 to 3 months postoperatively remained without evidence of disease 6 to 70 months afterwards.[64] All 16 patients with PSA levels greater than 0.4 ng/ml had subsequent progression of their disease. These studies indicate that the majority of patients who achieve undetectable serum PSA values postoperatively remain without evidence of recurrence. These preliminary findings need to be confirmed with long-term studies.

The UCLA group has reported PSA values in a group of 230 men followed for a median 48 months after radical retropubic prostatectomy with pathological T1–3, N0, M0 disease.[113] All patients followed with serial PSA values who developed recurrent disease had elevations of PSA prior to clinical recurrence. Forty-one of 175 patients with current PSA levels and no clinical evidence of progression had elevations of their PSA levels, suggesting disease recurrence. Clinical disease-free survival at 5 and 10 years was 82 per cent and 72 per cent, respectively. If detectable serum PSA is considered evidence of recurrence, these values drop to 62 per cent and 41 per cent, respectively. These data indicate that elevations in serum PSA antedate clinical recurrence.

In the follow-up of the asymptomatic patient with stable serum PSA values, bone scans are likely not necessary. Lange and associates have shown that PSA elevations can be detected in cases of recurrence from 12 to 24 months before disease recurrence is detected on bone scan.[64]

In the group of patients who have persistently elevated PSA values after radical prostatectomy without other evidence of disease, it is hypothesized that a large percentage may have low-volume disease localized to the pelvis. Lange and associates treated 29 patients who had negative bone scans and CT scans with adjuvant pelvic radiation therapy.[65] In 82 per cent PSA levels decreased by more than 50 per cent, including 43 per cent in whom values decreased to undetectable levels by 6 months after treatment. The Washington University group evaluated adjuvant radiation in a similar group of radical prostatectomy patients.[55] In 9 of 21 patients (43 per cent) PSA levels decreased to undetectable levels. However, 3 of these 9 patients subsequently developed increasing PSA levels.

The Stanford group has reported the results of adjuvant radiation therapy in 25 patients after radical prostatectomy.[73] PSA levels in 12 of the patients never normalized after prostatectomy, and they underwent radiation therapy when they regained continence. Only 1 of these 12 has had a durable response (including an undetectable PSA) to the radiation treatment. In contrast, 7 of 13 patients with a delayed increase in PSA after surgery have maintained undetectable PSA levels at a median of 18 months after initiation of radiation therapy. These patients with delayed elevation of PSA after radical prostatectomy may represent a subgroup of patients who are better responders to adjuvant radiation therapy. The long-term durability of these responses remains to be validated.

In the future, development of supersensitive PSA assays will allow the identification of patients with persistent disease at an earlier point in time. However, whether this early detection of residual disease will result in a therapeutic advantage with currently available treatments is unclear.

Prostate-Specific Antigen After Primary Radiation Therapy

The use of PSA as a marker of prostate carcinoma may provide invaluable information in studies comparing the relative merits of radiation therapy and radical surgery for localized prostate cancer. Serum PSA levels have been estimated to decrease with a half-life of 1 month following radiation therapy.[78] The Stanford group has published the largest series of patients who have undergone radiation therapy and had monitoring of their PSA levels.[109] They followed 183 patients for a mean of 61 months after completion of the radiation therapy. These patients represented all stages, although the majority had clinically localized disease. Following radiation therapy, 11 per cent of the patients had reductions in their PSA levels to undetectable levels. Another 25 per cent of the patients were within the normal range (0 to 2.5 ng/ml, Pros-Check). In the remaining 65 per cent of patients, PSA levels remained elevated. During the first year after radiation therapy, PSA levels were decreasing in 82 per cent of the patients. However, these levels continued to decline after 1 year in only 8 per cent of the patients. In fact, in 51 per cent of the patients PSA levels were increasing after the first year. Hudson et al noted that only 3 of 18 patients who appeared to be free of tumor clinically after radiation therapy had undetectable PSA values following radiation.[54] Thirty-nine per cent of these patients had Tandem-R PSA values of 4.0 ng/ml or greater.

Russell et al studied 143 men who received external beam irradiation, either photon or fast neutron, for clinically localized prostate cancer with a median follow-up of 27 months.[99] They noted that the chance of complete response (normalization of PSA with no tumor detectable by radiographic studies or DRE) was associated with the pretreatment PSA values. Patients with pretreatment PSA values less than four times the normal value had an 82 per cent chance of complete response, whereas pretreatment PSA values greater than four times normal were associated with only a 30 per cent chance of complete response. The time to normalization of PSA also appears to be important. Ninety-four per cent of men with normalization of PSA within 6 months have remained complete responders, compared with 8 per cent of men with persistently elevated PSA values at 6 months.

Kabalin performed TRUS-guided sextant biopsies on 27 men following external beam radiation therapy.[57] In this investigation, 25 of 27 patients had persistent carcinoma detected on biopsy. All four patients with normal PSA levels (less than 2.5 ng/ml), including one patient with an undetectable PSA, had positive biopsies, suggesting that PSA levels may underestimate the incidence of persistent tumor. Also of note in this study was the fact that 20 of 22 men with normal DRE had positive prostate needle biopsy. Thus, serum PSA values may be a much more accurate method of monitoring treatment efficacy in the patient treated with radiation therapy than the traditional DRE.

Prostate-Specific Antigen and Hormonal Therapy

In cases of metastatic prostate cancer, one of the standard criteria for response to therapy has been the decrease in acid phosphatase. Greater than 50 per cent decrease in acid phosphatase level is considered indicative of a partial response.[106] Such formal criteria have not been set for the use of PSA in monitoring prostate cancer. However, PSA undoubtedly will be used in the future as an objective end-point in prostate cancer clinical trials.

Ercole and associates monitored PSA levels in 49 patients with Stage D2 disease who subsequently received endocrine therapy.[34] Patients were evaluated with National Prostatic Cancer Project response criteria.[106] In the 31 patients who achieved a favorable response to hormonal therapy, the median PSA value decreased from 85 to 2.1 ng/ml. In contrast, in the 18 patients with an unfavorable response to endocrine therapy, the median PSA value decreased from 160 to 155 ng/ml. Sixty-six per cent of those patients who showed a favorable response to hormonal therapy also showed normalization of their PSA values during treatment. Hudson et al observed a similar phenomenon.[54] They noted that 13 of 14 patients without active disease after hormonal therapy had PSA values of less than 10.0 ng/ml. In contrast, 16 of 18 patients with active Stage D2 disease after hormonal therapy had PSA values of greater than 10.0 ng/ml.

The Stanford group also evaluated Stage D2 prostate cancer patients following treatment with antiandrogen therapy.[110] They noted that 9 per cent of their patients had a subsequent decrease in PSA values to undetectable levels. Twenty-two per cent of patients had PSA values within the normal range. The PSA nadir was reached within 5 months in 9 of 11 patients followed with several PSA values at frequent intervals after initiation of therapy. After 6 months, 21 of 29 patients (72 per cent) were noted to have increasing PSA values.

Miller and associates evaluated the predictive value of PSA levels in 51 patients with metastatic prostate cancer who received hormonal therapy.[79] The group of patients with normalization of their PSA values within 6 months of the initiation of therapy showed a survival advantage over the group that did not achieve normal PSA values. There were no statistically significant differences in pretreatment PSA values in the two groups. Gillatt et al reported similar findings in 136 men with metastatic prostate cancer treated with hormonal therapy.[40] They noted that PSA levels at 3 and 6 months, but not pretreatment PSA, were significantly related to survival.

SUMMARY

For more than 50 years acid phosphatase has been one of the most valuable tools in the urologist's armamentarium of tests in the diagnosis, staging, and monitoring of prostatic carcinoma. In the past several years, PSA, which is a superior analyte in most respects, has replaced acid phosphatase as a laboratory test for prostate cancer. PSA is a more stable compound, exhibits less diurnal variability, and is more specific for prostate epithelial cells.

Despite these shortcomings relative to PSA, acid phosphatase retains a role in the management of prostate carcinoma. PAP remains a valuable immunohistochemical marker for prostate cancer. For reasons that are not entirely clear, despite their apparent superiority in the laboratory, currently available immunoassays for PAP appear to be less useful clinically than the more specific enzymatic assays. Neither PAP assay has sufficient diagnostic accuracy for prostate cancer to be useful in screening studies. However, enzymatic acid phosphatase determinations, especially when the thymolphthalein substrate is used, provide unique information in the staging of prostate carcinoma. Elevations of PAP by this technique should make the clinician extremely suspicious that the patient has extracapsular disease.

PSA, which is produced by the normal prostate to liquefy the seminal coagulum, has become one of the most useful tumor markers yet discovered for any neoplasm. This analyte has provided new insights into the efficacy of current therapeutic options for prostate carcinoma. Treatment failures are detected by rising PSA levels long before they are evidenced clinically.

The performance characteristics of PSA have increased interest in prostate screening. Studies have shown that an increased number of prostate cancers can be detected by screening populations with serum PSA. To date, however, a survival advantage for those patients screened has yet to be demonstrated. Because of the relatively slow progression of this tumor, even at high stage, resolution of the questions surrounding prostate cancer screening likely will not be forthcoming for years.

Serum PSA values correlate closely with prostate tumor burden. For groups of patients, serum PSA values also correlate with stage. Unfortunately, for an individual patient with prostate cancer, pathologic stage cannot be accurately predicted by serum PSA values.

The future for tumor markers in prostate carcinoma is exciting. The development of new and more sensitive PSA assays will allow for earlier detection of treatment failures after radical prostatectomy. Answers will be provided to questions of screening and therapeutic efficacy. Undoubtedly, with time new markers will be developed which will complement PSA and PAP in the management of prostatic carcinoma.

REFERENCES

1. Abul-Fadl MAM, King EJ: Properties of acid phosphatases of erythrocytes and of the human prostate gland. Biochem J 45:51, 1949.
2. Armitage TG, Cooper EH, Newling WW, et al: The value of the measurement of serum prostate specific antigen in patients with benign prostatic hyperplasia and untreated prostate cancer. Br J Urol 62:584, 1988.
3. Bahnson RR, Catalona WJ: Adverse implications of acid phosphatase levels in the upper range of normal. J Urol 137:427, 1976.
4. Barringer BS, Woodard HQ: Prostatic carcinoma with extensive intraprostatic calcification. Trans Am Assoc Genitourinary Surg 31:363, 1938.
5. Bentz MS, Cohen C, Demers LM, Budgeon LR: Immunohistochemical demonstrations of prostatic origin of metastases. Urology 19:584, 1982.
6. Bostwick DM, Brawer MK: Prostatic intraepithelial neoplasia (PIN) and early invasion in prostatic cancer. Cancer 59:788, 1987.
7. Brawer MK, Chetner MP, Beatie J, et al: Screening for prostatic carcinoma with prostate specific antigen. J Urol 147:841, 1992.
8. Brawer MK, Lange PH: Prostate-specific antigen: Its role in early detection, staging, and monitoring of prostatic carcinoma. J Endourol 3:227, 1989.
9. Brawer MK, Nagle MD, Bigler SA, et al: Significance of prostatic intraepithelial neoplasia on prostate needle biopsy. Urology 38:103, 1991.
10. Brawer MK, Nagle RB, Pitta W, et al: Keratin immunoreactivity as an aid to the diagnosis of persistent adenocarcinoma in irradiated human prostates. Cancer 63:454, 1989.
11. Brawer MK, Rennels MA, Nagle RB, et al: Serum prostate-specific antigen and prostate pathology in men having simple prostatectomy. Am J Clin Pathol 92:760, 1989.
12. Brawer MK, Schifman RB, Ahmann FR, et al: The effect of digital rectal examination on serum levels of prostate-specific antigen. Arch Pathol Lab Med 112:1110, 1988.
13. Brenckman WD Jr, Lastinger LB, Sedor F: Unpredictable fluctuations in serum acid phosphatase activity in prostatic cancer. JAMA 245:2501, 1981.
14. Bromberg WD, Kozlowski JM, Oyasu R: Prostate-type gland in the epididymis. J Urol 145:1273, 1991.
15. Bruce AW, Choe BK: Tumor markers in prostatic disease. *In* Bruce AW, Trachtenberg J (eds): Adenocarcinoma of the Prostate. New York, Springer-Verlag, 1987, pp 196–219.
16. Bruce AW, Mahan DE, Belville WD: The role of the radioimmunoassay for prostatic acid phosphatase in prostatic carcinoma. Urol Clin North Am 7:645, 1980.
17. Bruce AW, Mahan DE, Sullivan LD, Goldenberg L: The significance of prostatic acid phosphatase in adenocarcinoma of the prostate. J Urol 125:357, 1981.
18. Carter HB, Partin AW, Oesterling JE, et al: The use of prostate-specific antigen in the management of patients with prostate cancer: The Johns Hopkins experience. *In* Catalona WJ, Coffey DS, Karr JP (eds): Clinical Aspects of Prostate Cancer. New York, Elsevier Science Publishing Co, 1989, pp 247–254.
19. Catalona WJ: Prostate Cancer. Orlando, FL, Grune & Stratton, 1984, pp 57–83.
20. Catalona WJ, Smith DS, Ratliff TL, et al: Measurement of prostate-specific antigen in serum as a screening test for prostate cancer. N Engl J Med 324:1156, 1991.
21. Chan DW, Bruzek DJ, Oesterling JE, et al: Prostate-specific antigen as a marker for prostatic cancer: A monoclonal and a polyclonal immunoassay compared. Clin Chem 33:1916, 1987.
22. Chu TM, Wang MC, Scott WW, et al: Immunochemical detection of serum prostatic acid phosphatase: Methodology and clinical evaluation. Invest Urol 15:319, 1978.
23. Chybowski FM, Larson Keller JJ, Bergstralh EJ, Oesterling JE: Predicting radionuclide bone scan findings in patients with newly diagnosed, untreated prostate cancer: Prostate specific antigen is superior to all other clinical parameters. J Urol 145:313, 1991.
24. Collier D St. J, Pain JA: Acute and chronic retention of urine:

Relevance of raised serum prostatic acid phosphatase levels: A prospective study. Urology 27:34, 1986.

25. Cooner WH, Mosley BR, Rutherford CL Jr, et al: Prostate cancer detection in a clinical urological practice by ultrasonography, digital rectal examination and prostate specific antigen. J Urol 143:1146, 1990.

26. Cooper JF, Foti AG, Herschman HH, Finkle W: A solid phase radioimmunoassay for prostatic acid phosphatase. J Urol 119:388, 1978.

27. Cooper JF: The radioimmunochemical measurement of prostatic acid phosphatase: Current state of the art. Urol Clin North Am 7:653, 1980.

28. Crawford ED, Schutz M, Clejan S, et al: The effect of digital rectal examination on prostate specific antigen. J Urol 145:398A, 1991.

29. Crocker AC, Landing BH: Phosphatase studies in Gaucher's disease. Metabolism 9:341, 1960.

30. Dalton DL: Elevated serum prostate-specific antigen due to acute bacterial prostatitis. Urology 33:465, 1989.

31. Davies SM, Gochman N: Evaluation of a monoclonal antibody-based immunoradiometric assay for prostatic acid phosphatase. Am J Clin Pathol 79:114, 1983.

32. Dejter SW Jr, Martin JS, McPherson RA, Lynch JH: Daily variability in human serum prostate-specific antigen and prostatic acid phosphatase: A comparative evaluation. Urology 32:288, 1988.

33. Doe RP, Mellinger GT: Circadian variation of serum acid phosphatase in prostatic cancer. Metabolism 13:455, 1964.

34. Ercole CJ, Lange PH, Mathisen M, et al: Prostate specific antigen and prostatic acid phosphatase in the monitoring and staging of patients with prostatic cancer. J Urol 138:1181, 1987.

35. Fair WR, Heston WDW, Kadmon D, et al: Prostatic cancer, acid phosphatase, creatinine kinase-BB and race: A prospective study. J Urol 128:735, 1982.

36. Ferro MA, Barnes I, Roberts JBM, Smith PJB: Tumour markers in prostatic carcinoma: A comparison of prostate-specific antigen with acid phosphatase. Br J Urol 60:69, 1987.

37. Fleischman J, Catalona WJ, Fair WR, et al: Lack of value of radioimmunoassay for prostatic acid phosphatase as a screening test for prostatic cancer in patients with obstructive prostatic hyperplasia. J Urol 129:312, 1983.

38. Ford TF, Butcher DM, Masters JRW, Parkinson MC: Immunocytochemical localisation of prostate-specific antigen: Specificity and application to clinical practice. Br J Urol 57:50, 1985.

39. Foti AG, Cooper JF, Herschman H, et al: Detection of prostatic cancer by solid-phase radioimmunoassay of serum prostatic acid phosphatase. N Engl J Med 297:1357, 1977.

40. Gillatt D, Gingell C, Smith PJB: Serum prostate specific antigen for the assessment of response to hormonal therapy. J Urol 143:207A, 1990.

41. Graves HCB, Kamarei M, Stamey TA: Identity of prostate specific antigen and the semen protein P30 purified by a rapid chromatography technique. J Urol 144:1510, 1990.

42. Graves HCB, Sensabaugh GF, Blake RT: Postcoital detection of male-specific semen protein. Application to the investigation of rape. N Engl J Med 312:338, 1985.

43. Graves HCB, Wehner N, Stamey TA: Comparison of a polyclonal and monoclonal immunoassay for PSA: Need for an international antigen standard. J Urol 144:1516, 1990.

44. Greene FT, Thompson IM: The effects of various manipulations on serum phosphatase levels in benign disease. J Urol 112:232, 1974.

45. Gutman AB, Gutman EB: "Acid" phosphatase activity of the serum of normal human subjects. Proc Soc Exp Biol Med 38:470, 1938.

46. Gutman AB, Gutman EB: An "acid" phosphatase occurring in the serum of patients with metastasizing carcinoma of the prostate gland. J Clin Invest 17:473, 1938.

47. Gutman EB, Sproul EE, Gutman AB: Significance of increased phosphatase activity of bone at the site of osteoplastic metastases secondary to carcinoma of the prostate gland. Am J Cancer 28:485, 1936.

48. Hara M, Inorre T, Fukuyama T: Some physico-chemical characteristics of gamma-seminoprotein, an antigenic component specific for human seminal plasma. Jpn J Legal Med 25:322, 1971.

49. Heller JE: Prostatic acid phosphatase: Its current clinical status. J Urol 137:1091, 1987.

50. Henneberry MO, Engel G, Grayhack JT: Acid phosphatase. Urol Clin North Am 6:629, 1979.

51. Holund B: Latent prostatic carcinoma in a consecutive autopsy series. Scand J Urol Nephrol 14:29, 1980.

52. Hortin GL, Bahnson RR, Daft M, et al: Differences in values obtained with 2 assays of prostate specific antigen. J Urol 139:762, 1988.

53. Howard PJ Jr, Fraley EE: Elevation of the acid phosphatase in benign prostatic disease. J Urol 94:687, 1965.

54. Hudson MA, Bahnson RR, Catalona WJ: Clinical use of prostate specific antigen in patients with prostate cancer. J Urol 142:1011, 1989.

55. Hudson MA, Catalona WJ: Effect of adjuvant radiation therapy on prostate specific antigen following radical prostatectomy. J Urol 143:1174, 1990.

56. Huggins C, Hodges CV: Studies on prostatic cancer: The effect of castration, of estrogen and of androgen injection on serum phosphatases in metastatic carcinoma of the prostate. Cancer Res 1:293, 1941.

57. Kabalin JN, Hodge KK, McNeal JE, et al: Identification of residual cancer in the prostate following radiation therapy: Role of transrectal ultrasound guided biopsy and prostate specific antigen. J Urol 142:326, 1989.

58. Kabalin JN, Hornberger JC: Prostate-specific antigen is not excreted by human kidney or eliminated by routine hemodialysis. Urology 37:308, 1991.

59. Kamoshida S, Tsutsumi Y: Extraprostatic localization of prostatic acid phosphatase and prostate-specific antigen: Distribution in cloacogenic glandular epithelium and sex-dependent expression in human anal gland. Hum Pathol 21:1108, 1990.

60. King EJ, Armstrong AR: Convenient method for determining serum and bile phosphatase activity. Can Med Assoc J 31:376, 1934.

61. Kuriyama M, Wang MC, Papsidero LD, et al: Quantitation of prostate-specific antigen in serum by a sensitive enzyme immunoassay. Cancer Res 40:4658, 1980.

62. Kutscher W, Wolbergs H: Prostate phosphatase. Hoppe-Seylers Zeitschr Physiol Chem 236:237, 1935.

63. Lam WKW, Yam LT, Wilbur HJ, et al: Comparison of acid phosphatase isoenzymes of human seminal fluid, prostate, and leukocytes. Clin Chem 25:1285, 1979.

64. Lange PH, Ercole CJ, Lightner DJ, et al: The value of serum prostate specific antigen determinations before and after radical prostatectomy. J Urol 141:873, 1989.

65. Lange PH, Lightner DJ, Medini E, et al: The effect of radiation therapy after radical prostatectomy in patients with elevated prostate specific antigen levels. J Urol 144:927, 1990.

66. Lee C, Keefer M, Zhao ZW, et al: Demonstration of the role of prostate-specific antigen in semen liquefaction by two-dimensional electrophoresis. J Androl 10:432, 1989.

67. Lee F, Torp-Pedersen ST, Littrup PJ, et al: Hypoechoic lesions of the prostate: Clinical relevance of tumor size, digital rectal examination, and prostate-specific antigen. Radiology 170:29, 1989.

68. Li CY, Lam WKW, Yam LT: Immunohistochemical diagnosis of prostatic cancer with metastasis. Cancer 46:706, 1980.

69. Li TS, Beling CG: Isolation and characterization of two specific antigens of human seminal plasma. Fertil Steril 24:134, 1973.

70. Liedtke RJ, Batjer JD: Measurement of prostate-specific antigen by radioimmunoassay. Clin Chem 30:649, 1984.

71. Lightner DJ, Lange PH, Reddy PK, Moore L: Prostate specific antigen and local recurrence after radical prostatectomy. J Urol 144:921, 1990.

72. Lilja H, Laurell CB: The predominant protein in human seminal coagulate. Scand J Clin Lab Invest 45:635, 1985.

73. Link P, Freiha FS, Stamey TA: Adjuvant radiation therapy in patients with detectable prostate specific antigen following radical prostatectomy. J Urol 145:532, 1991.

74. Maatman TJ: The role of prostate specific antigen as a tumor marker in men with advanced adenocarcinoma of the prostate. J Urol 141:1378, 1989.

75. Maatman TJ, Gupta MK, Montie JE: The role of serum prostatic acid phosphatase as a tumor marker in men with advanced adenocarcinoma of the prostate. J Urol 132:58, 1984.

76. Martland M, Hansman FS, Robison R: The phosphoric-esterase of blood. Biochem J 18:1152, 1924.

77. McDowell GC II, Johnson JW, Tenney DM, Johnson DE: Pelvic lymphadenectomy for staging clinically localized prostate cancer. Urology 35:476, 1990.

78. Meek AG, Park TL, Oberman E, Wielopolski L: A prospective study of prostate specific antigen levels in patients receiving radiotherapy for localized carcinoma of the prostate. Int J Radiat Oncol Biol Phys 75:1982, 1990.

79. Miller JI, Ahmann FR, Drach GW, Bottaccini MR: Serum PSA levels predict duration of remission and survival post hormone therapy of metastatic prostate cancer. J Urol 145:384A, 1991.

80. Murphy GP, Chu TM, Karr JP: Prostatic acid phosphatase—the developing experience. Clin Biochem 12:226, 1979.

81. Myrtle JF: More on "hook effects" in immunometric assays for prostate-specific antigen. Clin Chem 35:2154, 1989.

82. Myrtle JF, Klimley PG, Ivor LP, Brun JF: Clinical utility of prostate-specific antigen (PSA) in the management of prostate cancer. Adv Cancer Diag, Hybritech, Inc, 1986.

83. Nadji M, Tabei SZ, Castro A, et al: Prostatic-specific antigen: An immunohistologic marker for prostatic neoplasms. Cancer 48:1229, 1981.

84. Nesbitt RM, Baum WB: Serum phosphatase determination in diagnosis of prostatic cancer: A review of 1,150 cases. JAMA, 145:1321, 1951.

85. Nissenkorn I, Mickey DD, Miller DB, Soloway MS: Circadian and day-to-day variation of prostatic acid phosphatase. J Urol 127:1122, 1982.

86. Oesterling JE: Prostate specific antigen: A critical assessment of the most useful tumor marker for adenocarcinoma of the prostate. J Urol 145:907, 1991.

87. Oesterling JE, Bergstralh EJ: Prostate-specific antigen (PSA) following prostate biopsy (Bx) and transurethral resection of the prostate (TURP): Length of time necessary to achieve a stable value. J Urol 145:251A, 1991.

88. Oesterling JE, Chan DW, Epstein JI, et al: Prostate specific antigen in the preoperative and postoperative evaluation of localized prostatic cancer treated with radical prostatectomy. J Urol 139:766, 1988.

89. Papsidero LD, Kuriyama M, Wang MC, et al: Prostate antigen: A marker for human prostate epithelial cells. J Natl Cancer Inst 66:37, 1981.

90. Papsidero LD, Wang MC, Valenzuela LA, et al: A prostate antigen in sera of prostatic cancer patients. Cancer Res 40:2428, 1980.

91. Partin AW, Carter HB, Chan DW, et al: Prostate specific antigen in the staging of localized prostate cancer: Influence of tumor differentiation, tumor volume and benign hyperplasia. J Urol 143:747, 1990.

92. Pollen JJ, Dreilinger A: Immunohistochemical identification of prostatic acid phosphatase and prostate specific antigen in female periurethral glands. Urology 23:303, 1984.

93. Pontes JE, Choe BK, Rose NR, et al: Clinical evaluation of immunological methods for detection of serum prostatic acid phosphatase. J Urol 126:363, 1981.

94. Qui S-D, Young CY-F, Bilhartz DL, et al: In situ hybridization of prostate-specific antigen in human prostate. J Urol 144:1550, 1990.

95. Riegman PHJ, Vlietstra RJ, van der Korpert JAGM, et al: Characterization of the prostate specific antigen gene: A novel human kallikrein-like gene. Biochem Biophys Res Comm 159:95, 1989.

96. Robinson JN, Gutman EB, Gutman AB: Clinical significance of increased serum "acid" phosphatase in patients with bone metastases secondary to prostatic carcinoma. J Urol 42:602, 1939.

97. Romas NA, Hsu KC, Tomashefsky P, Tannenbaum M: Counterimmunoelectrophoresis for detection of human prostatic acid phosphatase. Urology 12:79, 1978.

98. Roy AV, Brower ME, Hayden JE: Sodium thymolphthalein monophosphatase: A new acid phosphatase substrate with greater specificity for the prostate enzyme in serum. Clin Chem 17:1093, 1971.

99. Russell KJ, Dunatov C, Hafermann MD, et al: Prostate specific antigen in the management of patients with localized adenocarcinoma of the prostate treated with primary radiation therapy. J Urol 146:1046, 1991.

100. Schacht MJ, Garnett JE, Grayhack JT: Biochemical markers in prostatic cancer. Urol Clin North Am 11:253, 1984.

101. Schifman RB, Ahmann FR, Elvick A, et al: Analytical and physiological characteristics of prostate-specific antigen and prostatic acid phosphatase in serum compared. Clin Chem 33:2086, 1987.

102. Sensabaugh GF: Isolation and characterization of a semen-specific protein from human seminal plasma: A potential new marker for semen identification. J Forensic Sci 23:106, 1978.

103. Silber I, Rosai J, Cordonnier JJ: The incidence of elevated acid phosphatase in prostatic infarction. J Urol 103:765, 1970.

104. Simm B, Gleeson M: Storage conditions for serum for estimating prostate-specific antigen. Clin Chem 37:113, 1991.

105. Sinha AA, Wilson MJ, Gleason DF: Immunoelectron microscopic localization of prostatic-specific antigen in human prostate by the protein A–gold complex. Cancer 60:1288, 1987.

106. Slack NH, Murphy GP, Participants in the National Prostatic Cancer Project: Criteria for evaluating patient responses to treatment modalities for prostatic cancer. Urol Clin North Am 11:337, 1984.

107. Sohlberg OE, Bigler SA, Brawer MK: Prostate specific antigen immunohistochemistry in prostatic intraepithelial neoplasia. J Urol 143:202A, 1990.

108. Spencer JR, Brodin AG, Ignatoff JM: Clear cell adenocarcinoma of the urethra: Evidence for origin within paraurethral ducts. J Urol 143:122, 1990.

109. Stamey TA, Kabalin JN, Ferrari M: Prostate specific antigen in the diagnosis and treatment of adenocarcinoma of the prostate. III. Radiation treated patients. J Urol 141:1084, 1989.

110. Stamey TA, Kabalin JN, Ferrari M, Yang N: Prostate specific antigen in the diagnosis and treatment of adenocarcinoma of the prostate. IV. Anti-androgen treated patients. J Urol 141:1088, 1989.

111. Stamey TA, Kabalin JN, McNeal JE, et al: Prostate specific antigen in the diagnosis and treatment of adenocarcinoma of the prostate. II. Radical prostatectomy treated patients. J Urol 141:1076, 1989.

112. Stamey TA, Yang N, Hay AR, et al: Prostate-specific antigen as a serum marker for adenocarcinoma of the prostate. N Engl J Med 317:909, 1987.

113. Stein A, deKernion JB, Smith RB, et al: Post radical prostatectomy PSA levels in patients with organ confined and locally extensive prostate cancer. J Urol 147:942, 1992.

114. Stein BS, Petersen RO, Vangore S, Kendall AR: Immunoperoxidase localization of prostate-specific antigen. Am J Surg Pathol 6:553, 1982.

115. Stenman U, Leinonen J, Alfthan H, et al: A complex between prostate-specific antigen and α_1-antichymotrypsin is the major form of prostate-specific antigen in serum of patients with prostatic cancer: Assay of the complex improves clinical sensitivity for cancer. Cancer Res 51:222, 1991.

116. Sutherland GR, Baker E, Hyland VJ, et al: Human prostate-specific antigen (APS) is a member of the glandular kallikrein gene family at 19q13. Cytogenet Cell Genet 48:205, 1988.

117. Tell DT, Khoury JM, Taylor HG, Veasey SP: Atypical metastasis from prostate cancer. JAMA 253:3574, 1985.

118. Tepper SL, Jagirdar J, Heath D, Geller SA: Homology between the female paraurethral (Skene's) glands and the prostate. Immunohistochemical demonstration. Arch Pathol Lab Med 108:423, 1984.

119. Vaidya HC, Wolf BA, Garrett N, et al: Extremely high values of prostate specific antigen in patients with adenocarcinoma of the prostate: Demonstration of the "hook effect." Clin Chem 34:2152, 1988.

120. Van Cangh PJ, Opsomer R, De Nayer P: Serum prostatic acid phosphatase determination in prostatic diseases: A critical comparison of an enzymatic and a radioimmunologic assay. J Urol 128:1212, 1982.

121. Vernon SE, Williams WD: Pre-treatment and post-treatment evaluation of prostatic adenocarcinoma for prostate specific antigen. J Urol 130:95, 1983.

122. Vessella RL, Noteboom J, Lange PH: Clinical trial of an ultra-sensitive prostate specific antigen (PSA) immunoassay. Clin Chem 37:1026, 1991.

123. Vihko P, Kontturi M: Transient high serum prostate specific acid phosphatase measured by radioimmunoassay in prostatic infarction. Scand J Urol Nephrol 15:213, 1981.

124. Vihko P, Kontturi M, Lukkarinen O, et al: Screening for carcinoma of the prostate. Rectal examination, and enzymatic and radioimmunologic measurements of serum acid phosphatase compared. Cancer 56:173, 1985.

125. Vihko P, Schroeder FH, Lukkarinen O, Vihko R: Secretion into and elimination from blood circulation of prostate specific acid phosphatase, measured by radioimmunoassay. J Urol 128:202, 1982.

126. Wadström J, Huber P, Rutishauser G: Elevation of serum prostatic acid phosphatase levels after prostatic massage. Urology 24:550, 1984.

127. Wadström J, Wenk M, Huber P: Serum half life of prostatic acid phosphatase. Urol Res 13:131, 1985.

128. Wang MC, Kuriyama M, Papsidero LD, et al: Prostate antigen of human cancer patients. *In* Busch H, Yeoman LC (eds): Methods in Cancer Research XIX. New York, Academic Press, 1982, pp 179–197.

129. Wang MC, Valenzuela LA, Murphy GP, Chu TM: A simplified purification procedure for human prostate antigen. Oncology 39:1, 1982.

130. Wang MC, Valenzuela LA, Murphy GP, Chu TM: Purification of a human prostate specific antigen. Invest Urol 17:159, 1979.

131. Watson RA, Tang DB: The predictive value of prostatic acid phosphatase as a screening test for prostatic cancer. N Engl J Med 303:497, 1980.

132. Watt KWK, Lee PJ, M'Timkulu T, et al: Human prostate-specific antigen: Structural and functional similarity with serine proteases. Proc Natl Acad Sci 83:3166, 1986.

133. Weber JP, Oesterling JE, Peters CA, et al: The influence of reversible androgen deprivation on serum prostate-specific antigen levels in men with benign prostatic hyperplasia. J Urol 141:987, 1989.

134. Whitesel JA, Donohue RE, Mani JH, et al: Acid phosphatase: Its influence on the management of carcinoma of the prostate. J Urol 131:70, 1984.

135. Young CY-F, Montgomery BT, Andrews PE, et al: Hormonal regulation of prostate-specific antigen messenger RNA in human prostatic adenocarcinoma cell line LNCaP. Can Res 51:3748, 1991.

136. Yuan JJ, Catalona WJ: Effect of digital rectal examination, prostate massage, transrectal ultrasonography and needle biopsy of the prostate on serum prostate specific antigen levels. J Urol 145:213A, 1991.

Chapter 23

SCREENING FOR PROSTATE CANCER

SAMUEL T. THOMPSON and MARTIN I. RESNICK

Screening for a specific disease can be defined as examining an asymptomatic population in order to identify them as being likely or unlikely to have the preclinical phase of that disease, with the intent of identifying patients early so that successful treatment can be instituted. An important component of this definition is that treatment of the disease, for instance a malignancy, positively influences survival, i.e., reduces mortality. Screening procedures may be used to establish the prevalence of a disease without any disease control objectives such as the recent human immunodeficiency virus (HIV) testing of different populations, be they armed forces recruits or emergency room patients. The sole information-gathering objective of this type of approach is not true screening.

The history of screening has its roots in the case-finding activity of the Middle Ages and was used to control infectious diseases before any other meaningful therapy was available. The objective of case finding was to interrupt the transmission of an infectious disease. The leper colonies of antiquity were instituted with this objective in mind, and the more recent isolation techniques used for tuberculosis were effective in their day. With the advent of highly effective treatment for many infectious diseases, case finding, or screening, has been applied to the early detection of many diseases in order to intervene and affect morbidity and mortality.

Screening for congenital defects in children was initiated at the beginning of this century. The Association for the Prevention and Relief of Heart Disease (later, the American Heart Association) was formed in 1915 with one of its stated goals being early detection of heart defects. School children were examined for heart defects as a response to an association report.[1] Congenital dislocation of the hip is another example of a disease that can be detected by a screening test during physical examination of the newborn, in which treatment greatly affects later disability.[17]

Studies of the pathology and cytology of cancer of the cervix have been the source of many fundamental ideas in the realm of cancer screening. *Diagnosis of Uterine Cancer by the Vaginal Smear*, by Papanicolaou and Traut, was published in 1943 and introduced the "Pap" test as the first cancer screening test.[48] It has now become an extension of the routine physical examination in women. This work led to the enormous increase in cancer screening activities of the past three decades, and the influence of this work extends to screening for many chronic diseases.

The search for asymptomatic disorders has now become a routine feature of medical care. Gone is the time when the practice of medicine concerned a small number of ill patients, for now large numbers of well persons are given recommendations about when certain screening tests should be administered in an attempt to detect various diseases during their early, asymptomatic phases. The goal of this chapter is to define the fundamentals of an effective screening program and review the current state of knowledge regarding screening for prostate cancer.

CHARACTERISTICS OF A SCREENING PROGRAM

The overall objective of a screening test is to lower morbidity and mortality of a population by detecting and treating patients with the preclinical stage of a disease.[41] For this objective to be met, both the screening test and the disease process must meet certain requirements.

The Neoplasm

A neoplasm must meet several requirements for screening to be effective. First, it must pass through a preclinical phase during which it is detectable but undiagnosed, and, second, early treatment must offer some advantage over later treatment.[10] Third, the neoplasm must represent a serious health risk as measured by mortality and lost productivity in the population.

A neoplasm must pass through a detectable preclinical stage in order for a screening program to be effective. The preclinical stage is that time period in the natural history of the neoplasm when detection by a screening test is possible but symptoms have not yet developed. The preclinical stage begins when the pathologic process is first present, which, with our present state of knowledge, is ill defined. Signs that can be detected by screening tests such as bleeding, a mass, or biochemical changes develop later and more gradually in the disease process. The preclinical stage ends when the symptomatic person seeks medical attention.

Obviously, there is no point in screening for a disease if treatment cannot influence the outcome independently of when symptoms develop. The comparatively long duration of the preclinical phase of chronic versus acute diseases is one reason that screening is directed almost exclusively at chronic conditions. Early detection and treatment of a large number of patients are feasible when the preclinical phase is long. If the preclinical phase is short, almost continous rescreening of a patient population would be necessary to affect mortality.

It is also recognized that there is frequently variation in the length of the preclinical phase within a particular disease; therefore, cases may progress slowly or rapidly, and specific signs might present at different points in that preclinical phase. Because of such variation, a group of patients with preclinical disease will include a distribution of manifestations.

There is no point to a screening program if early treatment is not helpful in controlling a disease process. Neoplasms are treated most effectively in their early stages and in this regard lend themselves to screening programs. The successes achieved thus far in treating breast and cervical cancer are due in part to treating an earlier stage of the disease and thus improving survival.[13, 56] It is important to recognize that the treatment of these detected localized stages must be effective in improving survival for screening programs to be successful. It is also important to emphasize that the neoplasm which is the subject of the screening program must represent a serious health risk to justify the morbidity and expense of screening.

The Test

The screening test itself must be able to differentiate a population into those with preclinical disease and those without it. Many pitfalls must be avoided with screening tests, for screening errors can stem from the test itself or its interpretation.

There usually is an inherent variability in the screening test itself. For example, a Pap smear cytology specimen may not include malignant cells that were present on the cervix, or a screening chest radiograph, because of poor technique, may not detect a mass that is present and otherwise detectable. In this fashion incorrect performance of the screening test affects its usefulness.

Another important measure of a screening test is its reliability. The reliability of a test is its ability to yield the same result, positive or negative, on repeated application in a person with a given level of disease. The reliability gives no information on the correctness of the test, but rather depends on the variability in the measurement of the test and the manifestation of the disease on which the test is based. Reliability, often termed interobserver or intraobserver variability, is one of the preliminary assessments of a screening test.

The interpretation of a screening test, or assignment of positive or negative result, can lead to important errors in a screening program. The manifestation on which a screening test is based is often found in patients without the disease and conversely can be absent in those with the disease. Occult blood in the stool occurs in patients with colon tumors as well as those with diverticulitis or other benign bowel diseases, and some patients with colon tumors may not, at the time of collection, have occult blood in the stool. Sensitivity and specificity measure the ability of a test to correctly identify diseased and nondiseased people. Fundamental to their definition is a diagnostic test to which the screening test can be compared.

The ability of a test to diagnose the preclinical stage of a disease is referred to as the *sensitivity* of the test. Sensitivity is defined as the proportion of cases with a positive screening test among all cases of preclinical disease as defined by a diagnostic test.

$$\text{Sensitivity} = \frac{\text{No. Positive Tests}}{\text{No. True Positive} + \text{No. False Negative}}$$

There are certain problems with applying this definition rigorously. First, the gold standard diagnostic test for many neoplasms is often a surgical procedure that cannot be applied to an asymptomatic population, and therefore the true prevalence of the preclinical stage of a disease may not be known with accuracy. Second, the diagnostic test is subject to error itself, and one diagnostic procedure may be more sensitive than another. A given screening test may appear more sensitive if compared with a relatively insensitive diagnostic test. Therefore, any estimate of sensitivity should be regarded as the sensitivity of one test (the screening test) relative to another (the diagnostic test) rather than as a value with absolute meaning. Despite these limitations, the concept of sensitivity is a basic and necessary measure of a screening test.

The *specificity* of a test is its ability to distinguish as negative those people who do not have the disease.

$$\text{Specificity} = \frac{\text{No. Negative Tests}}{\text{No. True Negative} + \text{No. False Positive}}$$

As a corollary to sensitivity, specificity depends on the ability to distinguish a person who does not have the disease and is frequently determined by a negative diagnostic test with the same attendant invasiveness or may depend on long-term follow-up to ensure that the disease does not develop. Screening involves testing a large number of people who do not have the target disease; thus specificity, or the ability of a test to distinguish those people without the disease, is an important measure of the screening test.

For screening to be successful, a test is needed that has a high sensitivity and specificity. Tests with low sensitivity fail to detect the disease in a significant number of people and convey a false sense of security concerning the absence of disease. Low specificity leads to a large number of positive diagnostic tests, with the additional morbidity and cost, in people who will ultimately be found not to have the disease. In using a screening test with low specificity, there is the additional psychological effect of initially misdiagnosing a large number of people with a disease they do not have.

For any screening program to be effective at reducing morbidity and mortality, a substantial proportion of cases must be detected during the preclinical phase with enough lead time for treatment to be more effective than it would be if the disease were not detected early. A case that is detected by screening experiences lead time from detection up to the time at which diagnosis would have occurred without screening.[28] Such a patient would not have had symptoms during the lead time interval, and without screening the existence of the disease would not be known. If lead time is insufficient, cases will not be treated in time to retard or stop their ultimate progression. Sensitivity is the property of a test which enables cases to be detected early. Lead time is the property of the disease which allows the screening test diagnosis and effective treatment to be implemented.

Positive predictive value is the probability that the disease is in fact present given a positive test result; similarly, the *negative predictive value* is the probability that the disease is absent given a negative test result.

Positive Predictive Value =
$$\frac{\text{No. Positive Tests}}{\text{No. True Positive + No. False Positive}}$$

Negative Predictive Value =
$$\frac{\text{No. Negative Tests}}{\text{No. True Negative + No. False Negative}}$$

These calculations are based on sensitivity, specificity, and prevalence of the disease in the population to be screened and are helpful in evaluating the value of a test from a statistical standpoint. Neither sensitivity nor specificity relates to the prevalence of the disease; therefore, misinformation can result when these measures are used alone in evaluating a screening test.

For a test with a given sensitivity and specificity, the predictive value increases with the prevalence of the disease. Therefore, the predictive value of a screening program can be increased by restricting the program to those people with a relatively high prevalence of preclinical disease, i.e., a high-risk group, or by screening at longer intervals to maintain the prevalence of preclinical disease at a higher level in a population. Either approach must be balanced against the overall loss of the effectiveness of a screening program by restricting its use to a high-risk population and longer screening intervals.

In prostate cancer, the age of patients is a good method of selecting a high-risk group. Few would disagree that 30-year-old men should not be screened for carcinoma of the prostate. Screening of 365 men between the ages of 40 and 49 at Brooke Army Medical Center by digital rectal examination revealed no detectable cases of prostatic carcinoma.[63] Additionally, men older than 80 years should not be screened because of the lack of effective treatment in this age group. The important question is which age range should be included. It is important to choose an age range that includes the preclinical phase of the cancer, and the upper limits of the age range should be in a group of patients who would be amenable to treatment if the disease is detected. On the basis of these assumptions, an age range from 50 to 75 years would be reasonable for the detection and treatment of the preclinical phase of prostate cancer.

A high positive predictive value suggests that a reasonably high proportion of the costs of a program are in fact being expended for the detection of the disease during its preclinical phase. A low positive predictive value suggests that a high proportion of the costs are being wasted on the detection and diagnostic evaluation of false positives, people who have positive screening test but not the disease. A low predictive value is more likely to be the result of poor specificity than poor sensitivity. It is the specificity that determines the number of false positives. False positives are derived from people without the disease, who constitute the vast majority of people tested in a screening program. Although the proportion of false positives may be low, even a small loss of specificity can lead to a large increase in their absolute number and a large decline in predictive value.

Cost-benefit analysis is used increasingly in today's medical economic climate in the evaluation of screening programs. Cost-benefit analysis asks the following question: Is the cost of this test worth the outcome? The benefits of a particular test are evaluated by assessing safety, efficacy, and usefulness. The safety and efficacy of the test in detecting preclinical disease are evaluated by standard methods, but the usefulness of the test involves the benefit derived from the test versus the cost of the test to the individual and the health care system. To make this decision, both the cost and the benefit should ideally be measured in the same units, usually dollars.

Models can be developed that show the relationship between cost of the screening program and lives saved per patients screened (Fig. 23–1).[38] For a financial investment in a person, the average days of life saved for screening for cancer A is obviously greater than for screening for cancer B. In cancer A, with increasing

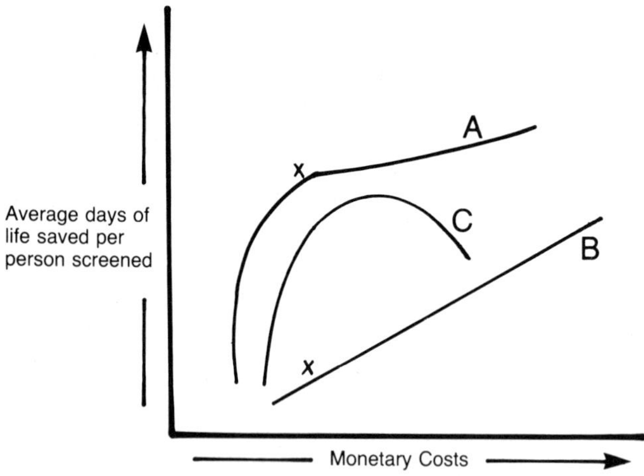

FIGURE 23–1. Screening for prostate cancer. (From Love RR: Principles of cancer screening. *In* Stoll BA [ed]: Screening and Monitoring of Cancer. Chichester, John Wiley & Sons, Ltd., 1985, p 15. Reprinted by permission of John Wiley & Sons, Ltd.)

costs a point (x) is reached at which increased frequency and subsequent increase in cost result in minimal benefit of life saved. For cancer A it would be most beneficial to identify point x and base costs on this point. For cancer B increasing cost continues to show increased lives saved. Another model relates to cancer C, in which increasing costs can have a negative effect and actually result in decreased saving of life. This may occur, for example, with use of cytologic examinations for bladder cancer or cervical cancer, in which laboratories would not be able to handle the case load and increasing error would result in wrong interpretation. Additionally, if the mortality of treatment is greater than the mortality of untreated disease, a curve similar to C evolves. The cost-benefit analysis of screening for prostate cancer is reviewed later in this chapter.

In summary, the characteristics of a successful screening program are many. The neoplasm being screened must have a preclinical phase of adequate length to allow time for detection and treatment, the neoplasm must represent a serious health risk, and early treatment must be effective. The screening test must be able to reliably differentiate a population into those with the neoplasm and those without by having a high sensitivity and specificity. A patient with a positive screening test must have a high likelihood of having the neoplasm, to avoid the potential morbidity and cost of unnecessary further testing. In other words, the specificity and prevalence of the neoplasm must ensure a high positive predictive value for the test. Ideally, the test should also be noninvasive, easy to perform, and inexpensive. The cost of the test and potential morbidity from the test and treatment should be worth the benefit achieved in quality of life and survival for those people screened. The only effective means to measure all of these factors of a screening program is performance of a randomized, controlled trial, as advocated by the International Union against Cancer.[51]

Prostate carcinoma has a long preclinical phase in which curative treatment is effective. It was the most common tumor found in men and the second leading cause of cancer death in 1991[3] and is therefore a significant health risk. We now examine the leading screening tests for prostatic carcinoma, specifically prostatic acid phosphatase (PAP), prostate-specific antigen (PSA), digital rectal examination (DRE), and transrectal ultrasonography (TRUS) and compare their value in detecting preclinical prostatic carcinoma.

ACID PHOSPHATASE

The acid phosphatases are a group of enzymes that hydolyze phosphate esters at an acidic pH, yielding inorganic phosphate. These enzymes occur normally in many body tissues, and the isoenzyme known as prostatic acid phosphatase (PAP) is produced in the glandular epithelium of the prostate. PAP is a sialoglycoprotein of molecular weight 100,000 with differing molecular forms based on variability of the sialic acid residues and carbohydrate content. These variations have led some to believe that multiple isoenzymes exist, although this view is not widely held.[25] After production in the acinar cells, PAP is secreted into the seminal fluid by the ductal system, allowing relatively little to enter the circulation. With release into the circulation, the enzyme is cleared with a first half-life of 0.5 to 2.5 hours and a second half-life of 11 days, most likely reflecting a slower rate of elimination because of protein binding of the enzyme.[66, 68] The small amount that is present in the serum can be detected by an enzyme assay as well as by a radioimmunoassay, although both tests have their deficiencies; for example, normal values or minor elevations may represent metastatic disease in the former assay, and the latter assay carries a high rate of false-positive results.

PAP was the first urologic serum tumor marker and has been used since 1938 in the evaluation and follow-up of patients with localized and metastatic prostate cancer.[24] Early work produced evidence that elevated PAP (enzyme assay) reflected occult or clinically apparent metastatic disease,[45, 60] and more recent work has confirmed that elevated PAP is associated with extraprostatic or metastatic disease.[2]

Foti and associates in 1977 suggested that the marker may be valuable in the detection of occult prostate cancer[19]; their group found elevated radioimmunoassays of PAP in 33 per cent of patients with Stage A disease and in 79 per cent of patients with Stage B disease. Of their controls with benign prostatic hyperplasia (BPH), only 6 per cent were found to have elevated assays. Watson and Tang reviewed their data and showed that although the sensitivity and specificity are 70 per cent and 94 per cent, respectively, the positive predictive value was only 0.41 per cent owing to the low prevalence of prostate cancer in an asymptomatic population.[73] In a large study, Vihko and associates measured the PAP in 771 asymptomatic men aged 54 to 76 years and found that PAP had a positive predictive value of 16.7 per cent for prostate carcinoma.[65]

A low prevalence of prostate cancer in a screening

population of older men has been confirmed by a number of investigators. Thompson and associates found an overall prevalence of prostate carcinoma of 0.55 per cent in screening 2005 men with DRE between the age of 40 and 70.[63] No patient with prostate cancer had an elevated PAP. Similiar results were found by Chodak and associates.[7]

In contrast to Foti's data, a recent review of the literature summarizes a number of studies that showed the low sensitivity of PAP in patients with localized prostate cancer.[25] A low specificity of PAP was demonstrated by Fleischmann and associates, who found elevated PAP in 17 of 295 men with histologically proven BPH.[18]

There is ample evidence that PAP used as a screening test in an asymptomatic population has low sensitivity, specificity, and predictive value and therefore cannot be recommended for detecting the preclinical phase of prostate cancer.

PROSTATE-SPECIFIC ANTIGEN

Since its discovery in 1979, PSA has received much attention for its use in the diagnosis and follow-up of men with prostate cancer. It was first isolated by injecting crude extracts of human prostate tissue into rabbits and recently was characterized as a serine protease (molecular weight 34,000) distinct both immunologically and biologically from PAP. PSA originates in the acinar and ductal cells of the prostate and is not found in other body tissues in the absence of metastatic prostate cancer.[44, 49] Yang laboratories and Hybritech have produced the two most widely used assays. The kit produced by Hybritech (Tandem-R) is a solid-phase immunoradiometric assay that uses two monoclonal antibodies specific for PSA. The kit from Yang Laboratories (Pros-Check) is a competitive radioimmunoassay in which displacement of radiolabeled antigen from a polyclonal antiserum is measured. A comparison of these two assays has shown a close linear relation, although values obtained by the Yang assay are nearly twice those measured by the Hybritech method.[27]

Studies have shown that PSA is proportional to both the volume of benign hyperplastic tissue and the volume of prostatic carcinoma. Stamey and associates showed that transurethral resection of the prostate (TURP) in patients with histologically benign disease reduced the serum PSA by 0.31 ng/ml/gram of hyperplastic tissue using the Yang assay.[59] In another study they compared the volume of prostatic carcinoma in 102 whole-mount radical prostatectomy specimens with the preoperative PSA and found an elevation of 3.5 ng/ml/gram of carcinoma, which is 10 times higher than the elevation for benign tissue.[57]

Early studies kindled interest in using serum PSA as a screening study. Seamonds and associates compared PSA in prostate cancer patients and age-matched controls and showed a 96 per cent sensitivity and a 96.8 per cent specificity.[55]

Subsequent studies have shown that PSA may not be as sensitive or specific as was initially thought. Ercole and Lange looked at the specificity of PSA and found that 21 per cent of 357 men with histologically proven BPH had an elevated level.[16] Guinan and Bhatti compared PSA in untreated prostate cancer patients and 69 patients with biopsy-proven BPH and found a sensitivity of 68 per cent and a specificity of 91 per cent.[23] A similar study revealed a sensitivity and specificity of 73 per cent and 83 per cent, respectively, and a positive predictive value of 58 per cent.[14] In these studies comparing patients with prostate cancer and BPH diagnosed by TURP assumes that even if all the resected tissue is examined, the TURP patients do not have cancer in the remainder of the gland. TURP samples only the transition zone, and absence of malignancy in the resected chips does not rule out the existence of carcinoma in the peripheral zone, which is the more common site for malignancy. These studies revealed sensitivities of 68 per cent to 73 per cent and specificities of 83 per cent to 91 per cent for PSA in patients with clinical prostate cancer or BPH but do not necessarily correlate with data for detecting prostate cancer in a screening population.

In a screening study of urologic clinic patients with abnormal DREs, Cooner and associates found that PSA had a sensitivity of 75 per cent and a specificity of 79.7 per cent for detecting prostate cancer.[11] In a more recent study, they measured the PSA in 835 patients with hypoechoic lesions on TRUS and found a positive predictive value of PSA to be 25.5 per cent to 61.8 per cent, depending on the DRE.[12] Lee and associates performed a similiar study and found a positive predictive value for PSA of 34 per cent in patients with a hypoechoic lesion on TRUS and a negative DRE.[36] These low positive predictive values were demonstrated in a population of patients presenting to a urologist's office. One would expect the positive predictive value of PSA to be even lower in a true screening population of older men.

Despite the encouraging sensitivity and specificity data of PSA, the poor predictive value of PSA even in a high-risk urologic clinic population makes it a poor screening test for prostate cancer. However, PSA has been clearly shown to be a more sensitive predictor of the volume of prostate carcinoma than PAP and is of value in monitoring the response to treatment of prostate carcinoma.[14, 16, 55, 57]

Other markers may in the future be compared with PSA and be of additional significance. Many markers have been examined and found to be nonspecific in that they are related to cancer in general or to tissue destruction as a result of metastatic disease. Substances such as alkaline phosphatase, polyamines, creatinine kinase B, lactic dehydrogenase, carcinoembryonic antigen, prostacyclin ribonuclease, urinary cholesterol, gamma-seminoprotein, and hydroxyproline have all been reported to be elevated in patients with prostatic carcinoma. These have not gained significant clinical recognition as useful adjuncts to our prostate tumor marker armamentarium.

DIGITAL RECTAL EXAMINATION

It is well recognized that the routine (e.g., yearly) use of the DRE is associated with the early detection of prostate carcinoma and that it represents the single most important step in the physical examination for detecting prostate cancer. With this in mind, it is interesting that DRE is not universally accepted as a screening modality for prostate cancer and that the value and frequency of the examination have yet to be clearly established.

One of the first studies to assess the DRE for screening of prostate cancer presented data on 5856 men who underwent 28,407 annual examinations between 1948 and 1964.[22] Seventy-five cases of prostate cancer were detected, 20 on the first examination (3.4 cases per 1000) and 55 cases on 22,551 subsequent examinations. The 5- and 10-year survivals of these patients were 77.3 per cent and 44 per cent, respectively, although only 64 per cent of patients had a full 10-year follow-up. In addition, no staging data were reported and patients were treated with a variety of modalities, including TURP, hormonal therapy, and total prostatectomy. Comparing contemporary survival data for unscreened prostate cancer patients revealed a 5- and 10-year survival of approximately 50 per cent and 33 per cent, which clearly shows that survival of the screened patients was improved. Despite the limitations of the study, it is the only published report with long-term survival data and it clearly demonstrates a survival advantage to screening by DRE.

More recent studies have compared the clinical stage distribution of prostate cancer diagnosed before the onset of screening with that found after screening by a routine annual DRE. Thompson and associates examined the stage distribution of newly diagnosed prostate cancer patients for the 5 years prior to screening compared with the subsequent 5 years of screening.[64] A statistically significant increase in clinical low-stage disease was detected during the period of screening. Although these data show that an increased number of patients with lower-stage prostate cancer is detected by a DRE screening program, we do not know if treatment of these patients will affect their survival unless a contemporary control group is used for comparison, as described earlier in the chapter.

Jenson and associates, in a screening study involving 4367 patients over 10 years, concluded that annual DRE was advantageous in asymptomatic men because the survival rate was markedly improved when prostate cancer was diagnosed in subsequent years compared with the initial year of screening.[29] The authors stated that malignancies identified after previously normal examinations are likely to be less advanced and more amenable to curative treatment. A recent review of 4843 patients undergoing screening examinations found a significant reduction in metastatic disease (43 per cent to 24 per cent) in patients who had undergone a previous screening examination within 18 months.[43] The results of these reports are affected by time in that annual examinations will detect preclinical disease at an earlier stage than in the patient detected on the first screening, but this does not prove that the subsequent patient has a survival advantage over unscreened patients. In order to prove that DRE is a beneficial screening test, one must show that treatment of these earlier-stage patients improves survival over that of a group of patients diagnosed when symptoms develop. In other words, these studies do not prove that screening affects the natural history of prostate cancer.

Some authors have shown that the ability of the DRE to detect localized, potentially curable cancer may be limited. Chodak and associates screened 2131 men with DRE and had a detection rate of 1.5 per cent with the initial examination.[6] However, surgical staging revealed that 50 per cent of the patients with clinical Stage B disease were upgraded to Stage C or D1. Other screening studies reveal that 42 to 58 per cent of tumors detected are found to be have spread beyond the confines of the prostate when they are surgically staged.[43, 63] Stamey and co-workers found extracapsular tumor in 18 per cent of patients with less than 3 cc of cancer volume, compared with 79 per cent of those with tumors greater than 3 cc.[58] Therefore, tumors of less than 3 cc volume are organ confined 82 per cent of the time, whereas tumors of greater than 3 cc volume have only a 21 per cent chance of being organ confined. These data suggest that the detection of small-volume tumors with a high likelihood of organ confinement is difficult to achieve using screening DRE.

Another potentially limiting factor in the use of screening by DRE alone is the overall detection rate of the malignancy. The percentage of cancers detected has been approximately 1 to 2 per cent in most reported screening series in the United States.[21] The European screening studies were markedly lower. Waaler and associates screened 480 men 45 to 67 years old and had a detection rate of 0.2 per cent.[67] Only 16 patients had an abnormal examination that warranted a biopsy. Similarly, Vihko and associates screened 771 men with DRE and PAP, and their detection rate was 1.2 per cent, but they performed only 66 prostate biopsies.[65] The rate of prostate biopsies was higher in the American studies, in which the detection rate was higher. The detection rate obviously varies depending on age, patient symptoms, rate of biopsy, and prevalence of the disease in each country.

In summary, no contemporary, large-scale, controlled trial of DRE screening for prostate cancer has been performed. Encouraging studies showing improved detection of lower-stage prostate cancer with annual examinations have not included survival data or have not been compared with studies of age-matched controls. Screening studies have shown a low prevalence of prostate cancer in an asymptomatic population, and approximately 50 per cent of those cancers detected, when they are staged pathologically, are not organ confined. Because survival data demonstrating improvement over control patients have not been proved, DRE used as a screening test for prostate cancer continues to be a subject of controversy. Most urologists believe it is of value and continue to recommend yearly examinations in men older than 40 years, but, as has been noted previously, controlled trials are needed to confirm the value of the examination.

These concepts take on greater impact in the light of recent reports of expectant management of patients with localized disease. Two studies documented the disease-specific survival of untreated patients with localized prostate cancer to be 93.8 per cent at 5 years,[30] and actuarial survival of 39 to 67 per cent at 15 years.[74] The favorable natural history of untreated localized prostate cancer reflected by these data calls into question the need for screening of localized disease.

TRANSRECTAL ULTRASONOGRAPHY

History

Dussik in Austria performed the first medical application of ultrasound when he used transducers in an attempt to locate brain tumors in the early 1940s.[15] He placed transducers on patients' craniums and recorded the through transmission of the sound beam. The first urologic application of ultrasound was reported in 1963 by Takahashi and Ouchi, who used A-mode scans to image the prostate.[62] Unfortunately, the presence of multiple tissue interfaces made these scans difficult to interpret and not clinically useful. One year later these investigators successfully obtained tomographic pictures of the prostate using a transrectal probe equipped with a radial scanning device, but these early tomograms were of poor quality and were thought to be of no clinical value.[61] Watanabe and his associates are credited with obtaining the first clinically useful transrectal ultrasonotomograms of the prostate in 1967.[69] The special concave transducer that they used was covered with a water-filled balloon, which provided good contact with the rectal wall and enhanced the imaging of the prostate, seminal vesicles, and bladder. A B-mode display was used in their studies, and reproducible prostate images were visualized on a black and white screen. In 1973 the first US report of TRUS of the prostate using similiar equipment was published by King and his associates, and subsequent studies showed that image quality was significantly improved when investigators from the same laboratory used the gray-scale technique.[4, 33] Since then further advances in instrumentation, including the refinement of gray-scale imaging, the development of high-frequency transducers, and the introduction of real-time imaging, have contributed to the enhanced resolution of transrectal sonographic images. Most investigators have concluded that the transrectal technique is preferable to the transabdominal, transperineal, or transurethral techniques for visualizing the prostate because of more consistent and reproducible imaging.[72]

Ultrasonographic Characteristics of Prostate Carcinoma

Unlike the usual homogeneous sonographic appearance of the normal prostate (Fig. 23–2), the ultrasonic

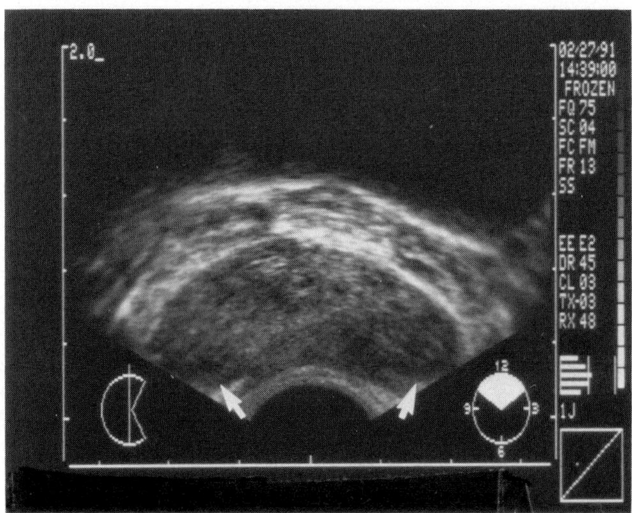

FIGURE 23–2. Scan demonstrating normal prostate with early benign hyperplasia. Lateral hypoechoic areas are due to refraction artifact *(arrows)* (7 mHz probe, transverse plane).

characteristics of carcinoma of the prostate are varied. Cancer originates and commonly is seen in the peripheral zone of the prostate, but it can be found in the transition zone as well.[39, 54] Some investigators have shown that prostatic malignancies appear as hypoechoic areas, whereas others have demonstrated that tumors can be hyperechoic, hypoechoic, isoechoic, or of mixed echogenicity.[26] Early investigators using B-mode and initial gray-scale imaging reported that prostatic carcinoma appeared as hyperechoic areas. With the development of 5- and 7-mHz transducers, it became evident that most peripheral zone tumors are hypoechoic.[37] Rifkin and associates evaluated 443 pathologically proven cases of benign and malignant prostate diseases with TRUS and found that in the large invasive tumors 69 per cent were hyperechoic, 27 per cent were of mixed echogenicity, and only 3 per cent were purely hypoechoic.[52] Other investigators have demonstrated that prostate cancers appear as hypoechoic areas in smaller, less invasive stages, and the higher stages may be isoechoic or of mixed echogenicity.[34]

These differing appearances can be explained by a number of factors. If the presence of collagen in the stroma of prostatic tissue determines echogenicity, prostate cancer may appear hypoechoic because the stroma is replaced by infiltrating glandular tumor elements (Fig. 23–3). Often associated with tumor growth and invasion is a desmoplastic reaction, and those changes certainly may contribute to the mixed pattern observed with advanced tumors.[53] Large prostate cancers can replace all of the normally isoechoic peripheral zone, thereby obliterating any ultrasonographic reference for normal tissues to contrast with the hypoechogenicity of the prostate cancer. Anterior tumors often cannot be distinguished reliably from the normal hypoechoic appearance of this region of the gland. Greater echogenicity seen in larger invasive tumors is likely secondary to the development of increased tissue interfaces that occur as the tumor grows and invades other areas of the prostate and surrounding tissues.

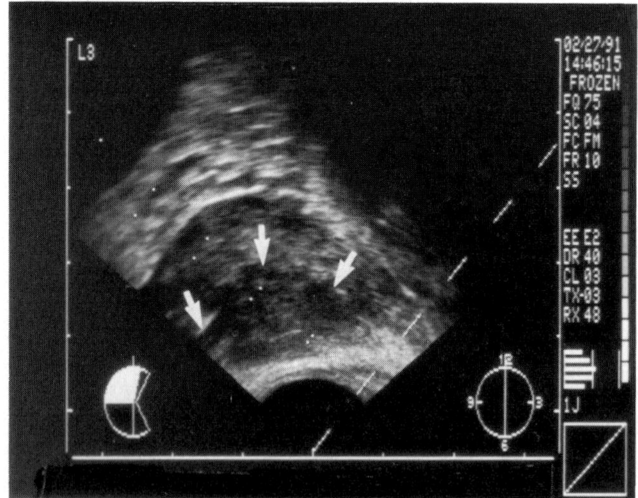

FIGURE 23–3. Scan demonstrating peripheral zone hypoechoic area *(arrows)*. Double-dotted line indicates path of biopsy needle (7 mHz probe, sagittal plane).

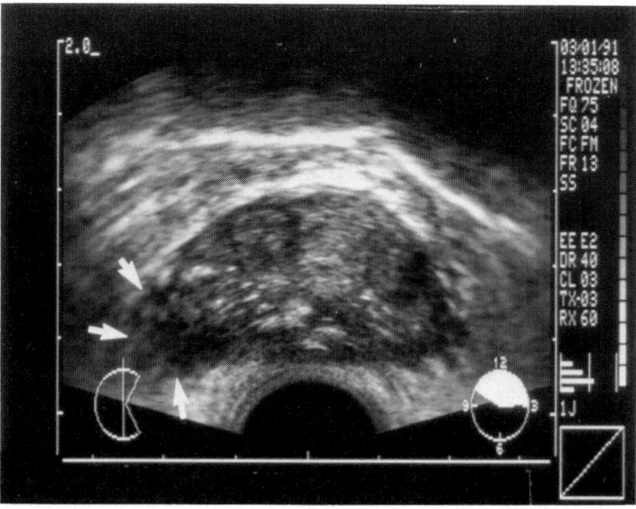

FIGURE 23–4. Scan demonstrating distortion of prostatic margin by peripheral zone tumor *(arrows)* (7 mHz probe, transverse plane).

In addition to the internal echo characteristics of the prostate, assessing capsular integrity and seminal vesicle symmetry is an important part of the ultrasonic evaluation of patients in whom carcinoma of the prostate is a possible diagnosis. The capsule of the prostate is usually well delineated circumferentially without distortion or disruption when prostate cancer has not spread beyond the confines of the capsule. In advanced cases of carcinoma of the prostate, the capsular integrity of the prostate is violated by invasive neoplastic cells, resulting in a loss of capsular symmetry and continuity that can be visualized sonographically (Fig. 23–4). The shape and echogenicity of the seminal vesicles change as they are invaded by local tumor spread. The distorted outline of the involved seminal vesicle is filled with dense echoes that are continuous with sonographic abnormalities of the prostate (Fig. 23–5). Occasionally, the image of the involved seminal vesicle is completely obliterated by tumor extension. Thus, any asymmetry in the sonographic appearance of the seminal vesicles is suspicious for advanced prostate carcinoma when seen in conjunction with disruption of the prostatic capsule.

Transrectal Ultrasonographic Screening for Prostate Carcinoma

TRUS is capable of detecting some prostate cancers that are not palpable. In addition, most palpable tumors are visible by ultrasonography. This knowledge has led to the evaluation of TRUS as a screening test for prostate carcinoma.

The only true large-scale screening study of asymptomatic, unselected men was performed by Watanabe and co-workers in 1984.[70] These studies were performed using a chair-mounted scanner and a 3.5-mHz probe on 1396 men. They found a detection rate of 0.6 per cent but did not report specificity data.

A group of studies have been performed comparing ultrasonographic results with pathologic findings obtained either by radical prostatectomy in relatively low-stage disease or by needle biopsy in a relatively mixed-stage population. In a recent study of low-stage disease pathologically confirmed by radical prostatectomy. Palken and associates showed that all but one carcinoma in the peripheral zone was hypoechoic, but they found it difficult to distinguish benign from malignant disease in the anterior or central zones.[47] They found TRUS to be a poor staging tool. It was inaccurate in estimating tumor volume and consistently understaged disease.

The sensitivity, specificity, and predictive value of a hypoechoic lesion seen by TRUS has been examined by a number of reports. Lee and co-workers evaluated 784 self-referred men using TRUS and DRE.[35] TRUS detected cancer in 2.6 per cent of the patients, compared

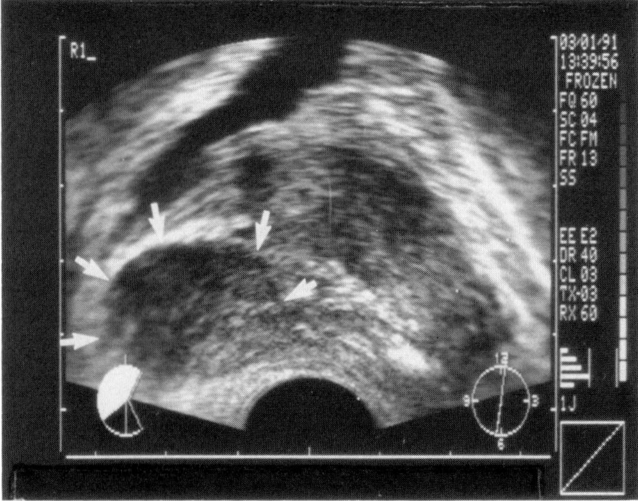

FIGURE 23–5. Scan demonstrating tumor involvement of right seminal vesicle *(arrows)* (7 mHz probe, sagittal plane).

with 1.3 per cent for DRE, suggesting that TRUS detects prostate cancer more often than DRE. However, twice as many biopsies were performed in the TRUS group, and the detection rate based on the number of biopsies was similar. Therefore, it is reasonable to conclude that the increased detection rate in the TRUS group was related to the number of biopsies performed rather than to the sensitivity of the study. The predictive values of both examinations were not significantly different in a number of earlier studies recently reviewed.[3]

Screening for prostate carcinoma with TRUS has been reported in a number of self-referral populations. These studies are not true screening populations, and therefore the prevalence is artificially elevated. Despite this advantage, the positive predictive values reported are a disappointing 30 to 35 per cent.[9, 35] Experience indicates that false-positive rates are high because TRUS cannot always reliably differentiate benign conditions (BPH, prostatic cysts, prostatic calculi, prostatic infarcts, and prostatitis) and normal tissue structures (blood vessels and muscle) from cancer.[72] There may be a 30 per cent overlap between benign and malignant lesions that have similiar acoustic appearances.[42]

The comparison of TRUS with both DRE and PSA for screening of prostate carcinoma has been studied in urologic referral populations. Cooner and associates biopsied 835 patients with hypoechoic lesions and found a positive predictive value as low as 9.3 per cent, if both PSA and DRE were normal, to 61.8 per cent if both tests were highly suspicious.[12] Similar results have been reported by Lee and associates.[36] Both studies confirm the belief that TRUS rarely detects cancer in patients with a normal DRE and a normal PSA.

The data show that TRUS detects prostate cancer that is not detected by DRE, but the rate of detection is related to the number of biopsies performed independent of the TRUS or DRE findings. When TRUS is used for screening a high-risk urologic clinic population, the positive predictive value has been shown to be disappointingly low. The other important consideration is the biologic potential of the nonpalpable tumors detected by TRUS. The old adage states that "more men die with prostate cancer than from prostate cancer," and it is not clear who will benefit from treatment and who should be left alone. It is also not clear whether tumors detected by TRUS are the ones destined to produce patient morbidity and mortality if left neglected or untreated. Studies are needed that compare screening for prostate cancer using TRUS in an asymptomatic population compared with age-matched controls and documenting long-term survival of both groups. Currently the data do not support the use of TRUS for screening of prostate cancer on a routine basis.

ECONOMICS OF SCREENING FOR PROSTATE CANCER

Cancer of the prostate, with an estimated 122,000 new cases detected in 1991, is the most common tumor found in men in the United States.[3] It caused an estimated 32,000 deaths in 1991, the second highest number of cancer deaths in American men. An increasing number of men are living into the age range at risk for prostate cancer, suggesting that an increase in incidence and mortality rates may be expected within the next decade. Often carcinoma of the prostate is diagnosed at an advanced stage: Nearly one third of patients have metastatic disease at the time of diagnosis.[71] A generally held belief in the success of curative treatments for organ-confined prostate cancer, combined with the large number of patients whose disease is diagnosed at a stage beyond which therapy is successful, has led to a concerted interest in screening for this disease.

Evidence from screening studies indicates that the low predictive values for the screening studies are in part due to the high false-positive rates of these screening tests. In the event that screening were implemented, a significant number of men would be diagnosed with prostate cancer who would subsequently be found not to have the disease. This fact calls into question the adverse affects of screening and diagnostic tests on these healthy men.

Admittedly, the adverse effects of the screening test are negligible, but all patients with an abnormal screening test would require a prostate biopsy. Although the average complication rate from a prostate biopsy may be only 2 per cent, in a screening program a large number of men would undergo this procedure. Chodak and associates estimate that if screening were performed, using the currently available screening tests, which have a positive predictive value of 13 to 35 per cent, for every two cases of cancer detected one complication would occur from a biopsy on a man without prostate cancer.[8] This morbidity would probably be acceptable if the value of the screening tests, i.e., reduction in mortality, could be conclusively proved.

A more serious concern is the morbidity and mortality that would result from the treatment of the significantly increased number of cases of organ-confined disease that would be detected by a screening program. On the basis of the DRE detection rate of 2 to 4 per cent, if all men over 50 in the United States were screened by DRE and TRUS, approximately 0.5 to 1.0 million cases of prostate cancer would be detected. If most of these cases were organ confined and most patients choose surgical treatment, with a mortality rate of approximately 1 per cent, then the screening program could result in 5,000 to 10,000 deaths.[5] Assuming that screening for prostate cancer is as effective as mammography screening (which has resulted in a 30 per cent reduction in mortality from breast cancer),[56] then almost as many lives would be lost from treatment as would be saved by screening, the net effect being that screening would have little impact on mortality. Furthermore, assuming an incontinence rate of only 2 per cent, 10,000 to 20,000 men could be made incontinent by surgery. This significant potential for morbidity and mortality is a strong reason to refrain from recommending routine screening unless clear proof of its efficacy is presented.

Another disadvantage of screening is the cost. Chodak

estimated that if a screening test required 15 minutes of a physician's time and cost $150, it would require 5000 physicians working 40 hours a week for more than 35 weeks to screen all men over 50. The annual cost would be more than $3 billion. Even if technicians performed the examinations, the cost would severely stress the health care system of this country. This would be impossible to justify in the absence of studies clearly supporting the value of screening.

Thompson and associates performed a detailed clinical decision analysis to estimate the potential cost of mass screening in the United States.[46] The parameters of the study included screening with DRE, TRUS, and biochemical markers all men aged 50 to 70 years who are not already at high risk for death from other causes. The estimated cost included screening, diagnostic biopsy in suspicious cases, staging of the cancer, and treatment of Stage B with radical prostatectomy, Stage C with external beam radiation therapy, and Stage D with bilateral orchiectomy. The cost of treating the complications of the above treatments was also included in the estimates.

The cost of screening by TRUS and treating an estimated total of 17,434,000 men in the first year was calculated to be $23.6 billion. Costs for DRE screening were calculated at $3.8 billion, and similiar costs were calculated for screening with PSA. Current total expenditure for these modalities in the same age group was estimated to be $25.5 million. Adoption of mass screening and anticipated treatment using TRUS would require an increase in the total United States health care budget from the current 0.06 per cent to more than 5 per cent. These costs may be underestimated because they are based on no patient having more than one complication. This obviously makes mass screening with these modalities prohibitively expensive.

With regard to complications, the use of mass screening was estimated to result in 266,271 cases of impotence; 61,618 cases of incontinence; more than 10,000 colostomies; and more than 20,000 treatment-related deaths during the first year. Current rates from these complications are 3354 cases of impotence, 908 cases of incontinence, 133 colostomies, and 220 treatment-related deaths according to Thompson's study. This 100-fold increase in treatment-related deaths is striking.

Prostate cancer has a variable natural history. A large population of patients with pathologically detectable prostate cancer exists who will never have clinical disease. Prostate cancer discovered as an incidental finding after cystoprostatectomy for bladder cancer ranges from 23 to 48 per cent.[32, 40, 50, 75] Autopsy studies have found that 30 per cent of men 50 to 59 years old and 67 per cent of men 80 to 89 years old who died of other causes had microscopic evidence of prostate cancer.[20] Using these data and the incidence of clinical prostate cancer, we find that only 0.3 per cent of patients with prostate cancer die of it. With the mortality rate this low, there is a serious disadvantage to developing a highly sensitive test to detect and treat all of these tumors.

It would be advantageous to develop a screening program that would detect clinically localized tumors with the ability to distinguish between small tumors that will never become clinically significant during a patient's lifetime and potentially lethal tumors that are also small.

In order to prove the clinical usefulness of any mass screening test for prostate cancer, a large, randomized, controlled clinical trial of the screening test is needed that would compare long-term survival in the screened and unscreened populations. Such a study, which has been recently approved and funded by the National Institutes of Health, will require 10 to 15 years to complete. Until that time, the value of screening for prostate cancer by any method remains unproved.

REFERENCES

1. Association for the Prevention and Relief of Heart Disease: First Report. New York, 1921.
2. Bahnson RR, Catalona WJ: Adverse implications of acid phosphatase levels in the upper range of normal. J Urol 137:427, 1987.
3. Boring CC, Squires TS, Tong T: Cancer Statistics, 1991. CA 41:19, 1991.
4. Boyce WH, McKinney WM, Resnick MI, Willard JW: Ultrasonography as an aid in the diagnosis and management of surgical disease of the pelvis. Ann Surg 184:477, 1976.
5. Chodak GW: Early detection and screening for prostate cancer. Urology 34 (Suppl 4):10, 1989.
6. Chodak GW, Keller P, Schoenberg HW: Assessment of screening for prostate cancer using the digital rectal examination. J Urol 141:1136, 1989.
7. Chodak GW, Schoenberg HW: Early detection of prostate cancer by routine screening. JAMA 252:3261, 1984.
8. Chodak GW, Schoenberg HW: Progress and problems in screening for carcinoma of the prostate. World J Surg 13:60, 1989.
9. Chodak GW, Wald V, Parmer E, et al: Comparison of digital rectal examination and transrectal ultrasonography for the diagnosis of prostate cancer. J Urol 135:951, 1986.
10. Cole P, Morrison AS: Basic issues in population screening for cancer. J Natl Cancer Inst 64:1263, 1980.
11. Cooner WH, Mosley BR, Rutherford CL, et al: Clinical application of transrectal ultrasonography and prostate specific antigen in the search for prostate cancer. J Urol 139:758, 1988.
12. Cooner WH, Mosley BR, Rutherford CL, et al: Prostate cancer detection in a clinical urologic practice by ultrasonography, digital rectal examination and prostate specific antigen. J Urol 143:1146, 1990.
13. Cramer DW: The role of cervical cytology in the declining morbidity and mortality of cervical cancer. Cancer 34:2018, 1974.
14. Drago JR, Nesbitt JA, Badalament RA, et al: Relative value of prostate-specific antigen and prostatic acid phosphatase in diagnosis and management of adenocarcinoma of the prostate: The Ohio State University experience. Urology 34:187, 1989.
15. Dussik KT: Uber die Moglichkeit hochfrequente mechanische Schwingungen als diagnostisches Hilfsmittel zu verwenden. Z Ges Neurol Psych 174:153, 1942.
16. Ercole CJ, Lange PH, Mathisen M, et al: Prostatic specific antigen and prostatic acid phosphatase in the monitoring and staging of patients with prostatic cancer. J Urol 138:1181, 1987.
17. Ferrer HP: Screening for health: Theory and Practice. London, Butterworth, 1968.
18. Fleischmann J, Catalona WJ, Fair WR, et al: Lack of value of radioimmunoassay for prostatic acid phosphatase as a screening test for prostate cancer in patients with obstructive prostatic hyperplasia. J Urol 129:312, 1983.
19. Foti AG, Cooper JF, Herschman H, Malavaez RR: Detection of prostate cancer by solid phase radioimmunoassay of serum prostatic acid phosphatase. N Engl J Med 297:1357, 1977.

20. Franks LM: Latent carcinoma of the prostate. J Pathol Bacteriol 68:603, 1954.
21. Gerber GS, Chodak GW: Digital rectal examination in the early detection of prostate cancer. Urol Clin North Am 17:739, 1990.
22. Gilbertson VA: Cancer of the prostate gland. Results of early diagnosis and therapy undertaken for cure of disease. JAMA 215:81, 1971.
23. Guinan P, Bhatti R, Ray P: An evaluation of prostate specific antigen in prostate cancer. J Urol 137:686, 1987.
24. Gutman AB, Gutman EB: An acid phosphatase occurring in the serum of patients with metastasizing carcinoma of the prostate gland. J Clin Invest 17:473, 1938.
25. Heller JE: Prostatic acid phosphatase: Its current clinical status. J Urol 137:1091, 1987.
26. Hernandez AD, Smith JA: Transrectal ultrasonography for the early detection and staging of prostate cancer. Urol Clin North Am 17:745, 1990.
27. Hortin GL, Bahnson RR, Daft M, et al: Difference in values obtained with 2 assays of prostatic specific antigen. J Urol 139:762, 1988.
28. Hutchison GB, Shapiro S: Lead time gained by diagnostic screening for breast cancer. J Natl Cancer Inst 41:665, 1968.
29. Jenson CB, Shahon DB, Wangensteen OH: Evaluation of annual examinations in the detection of cancer: Special reference to cancer of the gastrointestinal tract, prostate, breast, and female reproductive tract. JAMA 174:1783, 1960.
30. Johansson JE, Adame HO, Andersson SO, et al: Natural history of localised prostatic cancer. Lancet 1:799, 1989.
31. Jones WT, Resnick MI: Prostate ultrasound in screening, diagnosis, and staging of prostate cancer. Probl Urol 4:343, 1990.
32. Kabalin JN, McNeal JE, Price HM, et al: Unsuspected adenocarcinoma of the prostate in patients undergoing cystoprostatectomy for other causes: Incidence, histology, and morphometric observations. J Urol 141:1091, 1989.
33. King WW, Wilkiemeyer RM, Boyce WH, et al: Current status of prostate echography. JAMA 266:444, 1973.
34. Lee F, Gray JM, McLeary RD, et al: Prostatic evaluation by transrectal sonography: Criteria for diagnosis of early carcinoma. Radiology 158:91, 1986.
35. Lee F, Littrup PJ, Torp-Pedersen ST, et al: Prostate cancer: Comparison of transrectal US and digital rectal examinations for screening. Radiology 168:389, 1988.
36. Lee F, Torp-Pedersen S, Littrup PJ, et al: Hypoechoic lesions of the prostate: Clinical relevance of tumor size, digital rectal examination, and prostate specific antigen. Radiology 170:29, 1989.
37. Lee F, Torp-Pedersen ST, Siders DB, et al: Transrectal ultrasound in the diagnosis and staging of prostatic carcinoma. Radiology 170:609, 1989.
38. Love RR: Principles of cancer screening. *In* Stoll BA (ed): Screening and Monitoring of Cancer. New York, John Wiley and Sons, 1985, pp 3–18.
39. McNeal JE, Price HM, Redwine EA, et al: Stage A versus stage B adenocarcinoma of the prostate: Morphological comparison and biological significance. J Urol 139:61, 1988.
40. Montie JE, Wood DP, Pontes JE, et al: Adenocarcinoma of the prostate in cystoprostatectomy specimens removed for bladder cancer. Cancer 63:381, 1989.
41. Morrison AS: Screening in chronic disease. New York, Oxford University Press, 1985.
42. Morse RM, Resnick MI: Detection of clinically occult prostate cancer. Urol Clin North Am 17:567, 1990.
43. Mueller EJ, Crain TW, Thompson IM, Rodriguez FR: An evaluation of serial digital rectal examinations in screening for prostate cancer. J Urol 140:1445, 1988.
44. Nadji M, Tabei SZ, Castro A, et al: Prostatic specific antigen: An immunohistologic marker for prostate neoplasms. Cancer 48:1229, 1981.
45. Nesbit RM, Baum WB: Serum phosphatase determination in diagnosis of prostatic cancer: A review of 1,150 cases. JAMA 145:1321, 1951.
46. Optenberg SA, Thompson IM: Economics of screening for carcinoma of the prostate. Urol Clin North Am 17:719, 1990.
47. Palken M, Cobb OE, Warren BH, Hoak DC: Prostate cancer: Correlation of digital rectal examination, transrectal ultrasound and prostate specific antigen levels with tumor volumes in radical prostatectomy specimens. J Urol 143:1155, 1990.
48. Papanicolaou GN, Traut HF: Diagnosis of uterine cancer by the vaginal smear. New York, Commonwealth Fund, 1943.
49. Papsidero LD, Croghan GA, Wang MC, et al: Monoclonal antibody (F%) to human prostate antigen. Hybridoma 2:139, 1983.
50. Prichett TR, Moreno J, Warner NE, et al: Unsuspected prostatic adenocarcinoma in patients who have undergone radical cystoprostatectomy for transitional carcinoma of the bladder. J Urol 139:1214, 1988.
51. Prorok PC, Chamberlain J, Day NE, et al: UICC Workshop on the evaluation of screening programmes for cancer. Int J Cancer 34:1, 1984.
52. Rifkin MD, Friedland GW, Shortliffe L: Prostatic evaluation by transrectal endosonography: Detection of carcinoma. Radiology 158:85, 1986.
53. Rifkin MD, McGlynn ET, Choi HY: Echogenicity of prostate cancer correlated with histologic grade and stromal fibrosis. Radiology 170:549, 1989.
54. Salo JO, Rannikko S, Makinen J, Lehtonen T: Echogenic structure of prostate cancer imaged on radical prostatectomy specimens. Prostate 10:1, 1987.
55. Seamonds B, Yang N, Anderson K, et al: Evaluation of prostate-specific antigen and prostate acid phosphatase as prostate cancer markers. Urology 28:472, 1986.
56. Shapiro S, Venet W, Strax P, et al: Ten- to fourteen-year effect of screening on breast cancer mortality. J Natl Cancer Inst 69:349, 1982.
57. Stamey TA, Kabalain JN, McNeal JE, et al: Prostate specific antigen in the diagnosis and treatment of adenocarcinoma of the prostate. II. Radical prostatectomy treated patients. J Urol 141:1076–1083, 1989.
58. Stamey TA, McNeal JE, Freiha FS, et al: Morphometric and clinical studies on 68 consecutive radical prostatectomies. J Urol 139:1235, 1988.
59. Stamey TA, Yang N, Hay AR, et al: Prostate-specific antigen as a serum marker for adenocarcinoma of the prostate. N Engl J Med 317:909, 1987.
60. Sullivan TJ, Gutman EB, Gutman AB: Theory and application of the serum "acid" phosphatase determination in metastasizing prostatic carcinoma: Early effects of castration. J Urol 48:426, 1942.
61. Takahashi H, Ouchi T: The ultrasonic diagnosis in the field of urology. Proceedings of the 4th Meeting of the Japanese Society of Ultrasonic Medicine 2:35, 1964.
62. Takahashi H, Ouchi T: The ultrasound diagnosis in the field of biology. Jpn Med Ultrasonics 7:1, 1963.
63. Thompson IM, Ernst JJ, Gangai MP, Spence CR: Adenocarcinoma of the prostate: Results of routine urologic screening. J Urol 132:690, 1984.
64. Thompson IM, Rounder JB, Teague JL, et al: Impact of routine screening for adenocarcinoma of the prostate on stage distribution. J Urol 131:424, 1987.
65. Vihko P, Kontturi M, Lukkarinen O, et al: Screening for carcinoma of the prostate: Rectal examination, and enzymatic and radioimmunologic measurements of serum acid phosphatase compared. Cancer 56:173, 1985.
66. Vihko P, Schroeder FH, Lukkarinen O, et al: Secretion into and elimination from blood circulation of prostatic specific acid phosphatase, measured by radioimmunoassay. J Urol 128:202, 1982.
67. Waaler G, Ludvigsen TC, Runden TO, et al: Digital rectal examination to screen for prostate cancer. Eur Urol 15:34, 1988.
68. Wadstrom J, Wenk M, Huber P: Serum half life of prostatic acid phosphatase. Urol Res 13:131, 1985.
69. Watanabe H, Katoh H, Katoh J, et al: Diagnostic application of the ultrasonography for the prostate. Jpn J Urol 59:273, 1968.
70. Watanabe H, Ohe H, Inaba T, et al: A mobile mass screening unit for prostate disease. Prostate 5:559, 1984.
71. Waterhouse J, Muir C, Shanmugaratnam K, et al: Cancer inci-

dence in five continents. *In* Cancer Incidence. Lyon, France, International Agency For Research in Cancer, Publication 42, Vol 6, 1982.

72. Waterhouse RL, Resnick MI: The use of transrectal prostatic ultrasonography in the evaluation of patients with prostatic carcinoma. J Urol 141:233, 1989.

73. Watson RA, Tang DB: The predictive value of prostatic acid phosphatase as a screening test for prostatic cancer. N Engl J Med 303:497, 1980.

74. Whitmore WF, Warner JA, Thompson IM: Expectant management of localized prostatic cancer. Cancer 67:1091, 1991.

75. Winfield HN, Reddy PK, Lange PH: Coexisting adenocarcinoma of prostate in patients undergoing cystoprostatectomy for bladder cancer. Urology 30:100, 1987.

NERVE-SPARING RADICAL RETROPUBIC PROSTATECTOMY

HERBERT LEPOR

Radical retropubic prostatectomy was originally described and popularized by Millin[12] and subsequently modified by Campbell[2] and Walsh.[21] The retropubic approach to radical prostatectomy has several distinct advantages over the perineal approach. Urologists in general are more familiar with the retropubic anatomy. The retropubic approach provides the opportunity to perform a simultaneous staging pelvic lymphadenectomy. The anatomic relationships related to preservation of the autonomic innervation of the corpora cavernosa have been precisely delineated,[10] and the ability to preserve potency following nerve-sparing radical retropubic prostatectomy has been demonstrated.[3, 5] The retropubic approach provides the surgeon with the opportunity to obtain wider surgical margins. A theoretical advantage of retropubic prostatectomy is improved urinary continence, because the pelvic floor is not violated.[20] Advocates of the perineal approach emphasize that blood loss is less, operative time is shorter, and direct visualization of the membranous urethra and vesical neck facilitates the vesicourethral anastomosis. The anatomic approach to radical retropubic prostatectomy as detailed by Walsh has significantly reduced blood loss and operative time.[20] Proper positioning of the patient, meticulous hemostasis, and the use of a Foley catheter facilitate the urethrovesical anastomosis. The optimal surgical approach for radical prostatectomy is clearly dictated by the urologist's training, experiences, and personal preferences. The Walsh modifications have led to an even greater acceptance of the retropubic approach.

INDICATIONS FOR RADICAL PROSTATECTOMY

Radical prostatectomy has been advocated for the treatment of virtually every stage of prostate cancer. The indications for radical prostatectomy should reflect an understanding of the natural history of the disease, the projected survival of the patient, the stage of the disease at presentation, and the relative morbidity and efficacy of alternative therapeutic options. The natural history of prostate cancer remains poorly understood. A large series of untreated men with localized cancer of the prostate with long-term follow-up has not been reported in the literature. The relative morbidity and efficacy of the different therapies for carcinoma of the prostate are unknown because properly designed randomized clinical trials have not been performed. Comparative analysis of nonconcurrent studies are of limited value because staging criteria and statistical methods are not standardized. It is therefore difficult to reach definitive conclusions regarding the optimal treatment for any stage of carcinoma of the prostate.

Therapeutic intervention for carcinoma of the prostate is offered with the objective of achieving cure, local disease control, palliation of systemic metastases, and increased duration of survival. The cure of carcinoma of the prostate requires the complete excision or destruction of all malignant tumor cells. Hormonal therapy is a noncurative therapeutic modality owing to the development of hormone-resistant tumor cells.[8] An effective chemotherapeutic regimen has not been developed for the treatment of carcinoma of the prostate.[1] Owing to the limitations of hormonal therapy and chemotherapy, it is generally agreed that only carcinoma pathologically confined to the prostate is amenable to cure. Radical prostatectomy and radiation therapy represent the therapeutic options currently offered for the cure of organ-confined disease. The optimal curative treatment for carcinoma of the prostate represents one of the most controversial issues in urologic oncology.[13] Prostate cancer that is truly pathologically confined to the prostate is cured by radical prostatectomy. The persistence of biologically active prostate cancer indicates that radiation therapy does not consistently achieve cure when the carcinoma is organ confined.[7, 18, 19]

Radical prostatectomy may be offered with the objective of increasing survival for men with microscopic or macroscopic tumor extending beyond the prostate. No evidence exists to indicate that debulking the local tumor burden has a favorable impact on survival for men with carcinoma of the prostate. The impact of radical prostatectomy on survival rates for men with locally invasive disease will remain unknown until the natural history of carcinoma of the prostate is elucidated. A randomized clinical trial comparing survival rates following radical prostatectomy versus no treatment of Stage C, Stage D0, and Stage D1 disease would clarify the value of radical prostatectomy for disease that is not pathologically confined to the prostate.

Prostate cancer is a well-recognized cause of bladder outlet obstruction in aging men. It is unlikely that prostate cancer associated with infravesical obstruction is amenable to cure. The symptoms of prostatism may be relieved by radical prostatectomy, definitive radiation therapy, transurethral resection of the prostate (TURP), and orchiectomy. The relative efficacy of these therapeutic options for local disease control has never been examined critically. Orchiectomy and TURP are associated with relatively minimal morbidity. It is unlikely that the morbidity of radiation therapy and radical prostatectomy justify their use solely for local disease control.

PREOPERATIVE STAGING

The optimal candidate for radical prostatectomy harbors a tumor that is pathologically confined to the prostate gland.[23] The primary goal of preoperative staging is to exclude individuals who are unlikely to be rendered disease free by radical prostatectomy. It is generally agreed that the presence of seminal vesicle invasion, pelvic lymph node metastases, and bony metastases precludes a surgical cure. Gross seminal vesicle invasion is likely to be detected during a properly performed digital rectal examination. Although CT and transrectal ultrasonography (TRUS) are also able to detect gross seminal vesicle involvement, these imaging modalities are not sufficiently sensitive or specific to reliably detect microscopic capsular invasion and seminal vesicle invasion.[17] TRUS-directed seminal vesicle biopsy may ultimately prove to be a reliable method for detecting microscopic seminal vesicle invasion. At present, transrectal biopsy of the seminal vesicle should be performed only if a positive biopsy will preclude surgery.

CT is routinely used by many practicing urologists to stage the pelvic lymph nodes. Epstein et al[6] reported that approximately 10 per cent of subjects with clinically localized carcinoma of the prostate have positive pelvic lymph node involvement and that only a small proportion of these individuals have sufficient nodal disease to be detected by CT. CT is therefore not a useful modality for identifying lymph node metastasis in subjects with clinically localized carcinoma of the prostate.

The skeletal system is one of the primary sites of prostate cancer metastasis. The radionuclide bone scan has replaced plain film studies owing to increased sensitivity. Chybourski et al[4] recently reported that radionuclide bone scans were consistently negative in subjects with prostate-specific antigen (PSA) levels less than 15 ng/dl. I therefore do not routinely obtain a radionuclide bone scan on patients with PSA levels less than 15 ng/dl, provided that the tumor is not poorly differentiated.

The serum PSA and prostate acid phosphatase (PAP) levels should be obtained prior to biopsy. Several investigators have reported that serum PSA levels are of limited value for preoperative staging.[9, 14] Partin et al[14] reported that patients with PSA levels up to 70 ng/dl undergoing radical prostatectomy had no evidence of seminal vesicle invasion, nodal metastases, or capsular penetration in the surgical specimen. It is conceivable that subjects with significantly elevated PSA levels and apparent pathologically confined disease may experience disease progression. At the present time, PSA levels should not be routinely used to select patients for radical prostatectomy. Whitesel et al[24] reported that 79 per cent of subjects with clinically localized carcinoma of the prostate, elevated serum levels of PAP, and no evidence of lymph node metastasis following pelvic lymphadenectomy experienced disease progression within 2 years of diagnosis. Based upon this clinical experience, an elevated serum PAP level alone was thought to represent a contraindication to radical prostatectomy. Because these investigators did not perform radical prostatectomy in the subjects with elevated serum PAP levels, it is unclear whether the development of metastases occurred because the malignant prostate gland was not removed. Paulsen et al[15] has recently reported that disease progressed within 3 years in all subjects with an elevated serum PAP level who underwent radical prostatectomy. An elevated PAP indicates that a radical prostatectomy is ill advised.

In summary, the staging of clinically localized carcinoma of the prostate should include a PAP, PSA, and radionuclide bone scan if the PSA is greater than 15 ng/dl. Prostatic TRUS with biopsy of the seminal vesicle is optional. Routine CT should be discouraged.

PREOPERATIVE MEDICAL EVALUATION

Historically, radical prostatectomy has been offered to healthy individuals less than 70 years of age.[22] Deci-

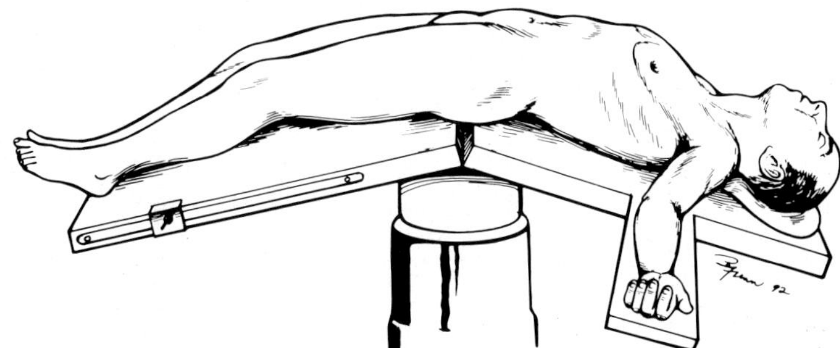

FIGURE 24–1. The patient is placed in the supine position, and the table is maximally flexed and placed in 20 degrees of Trendelenburg.

sions related to selecting surgical candidates should be based primarily on physiologic rather than chronologic age. It is my general rule to offer radical prostatectomy to individuals who have a high probability for 10-year survival. Middleton[11] has reported that healthy men in their late 70s have a relatively high probability of 10-year survival. Preoperative assessment by the urologist should include a complete history and physical examination. The history should be directed toward identifying significant cardiovascular and pulmonary disease and significant bleeding disorders. The physical examination should be directed toward identifying significant carotid bruits, chronic obstructive pulmonary disease, and inguinal hernias. The patient's primary care physician should be notified regarding the recommendation for radical prostatectomy. The decision to proceed with pulmonary function tests, cardiovascular stress test, and carotid Doppler ultrasonography should be made jointly by the urologist and primary care physician.

PREOPERATIVE PREPARATION

The patient is advised to provide 2 or 3 units of autologous or donor-directed blood prior to surgery. Patients are advised to discontinue aspirin, nonsteroidal anti-inflammatory drugs, and other drugs known to impair hemostasis. Iron supplements are administered to autologous blood donors. The patient is usually admitted to the hospital the day prior to surgery and chest radiography, electrocardiography, and routine blood and urine studies are done. Cleansing enemas are administered the evening prior to and the morning of surgery. A formal antibiotic and cleansing bowel preparation is not routinely administered. An intravenous line is placed the evening before surgery and 1 gm of cefazolin (Ancef) is administered at midnight and on call to the operating room.

SURGICAL PROCEDURE

Anesthesia

Radical prostatectomy may be performed under spinal or epidural anesthesia alone or in conjunction with a general anesthetic. The epidural approach is preferable because perioperative control of pain is facilitated by administering narcotics via the epidural catheter.

Positioning
(Fig. 24–1)

The patient is placed in the supine position. The midpoint between the umbilicus and pubic symphysis is positioned over the break in the table. The table is maximally flexed and placed in 20 degrees of Trendelenburg. The lower extremities are ultimately parallel with the floor of the operating room. The position facilitates exposure of the deep pelvis. The skin is prepped and draped in the usual sterile fashion. A number 22 Fr 30-ml balloon Foley catheter is inserted. The balloon is inflated with 45 ml of saline, and the catheter is draped into the operative field.

Incision
(Fig. 24–2)

A midline incision is made from the umbilicus to the pubic symphysis. The incision is sharply deepened through all layers of the abdominal wall. The superior and inferior aspects of the abdominal incision are completed following placement of the Balfour retractor. The transversalis fascia is incised, and the space of Retzius is bluntly developed. The external iliac veins are identified and the overlying peritoneum and peritoneal contents are mobilized in the cephalad direction. The vasa deferentia are identified and divided between surgical clips. The vas deferens lies immediately adjacent to the peritoneum, and therefore care should be taken not to create a peritoneotomy while isolating and dividing these structures. The spermatic cords are bluntly mobilized in order to create a pocket for the malleable blade of a Balfour retractor. The Balfour retractor is placed, and the superior and inferior aspects of the abdominal wall incision are completed. The abdominal incision is extended to the pubic symphysis, and the posterior sheath of the rectus fascia is sharply incised.

Staging Pelvic Lymphadenectomy
(Fig. 24–3*A*)

Exposure during the pelvic lymphadenectomy is achieved by the malleable Balfour blade superiorly, a deep sweetheart retractor reflecting the bladder medially, and a Gil Vernet vein retractor reflecting the

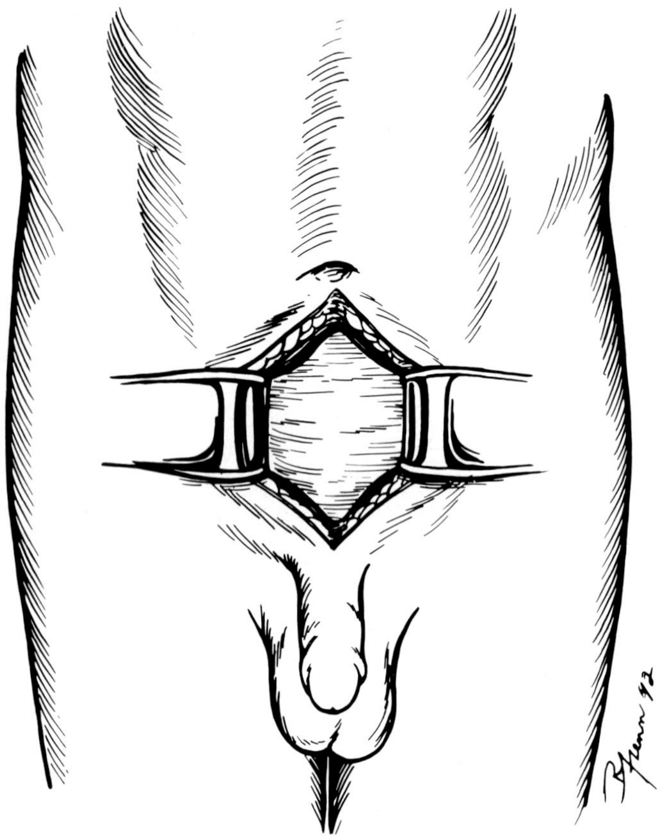

FIGURE 24–2. A midline incision is made from the umbilicus to the pubic symphysis, and the incision is sharply deepened through all layers of the abdominal wall.

external iliac vein laterally. The areolar tissue overlying the external iliac vein is sharply incised. The majority of the lymphadenectomy is performed using the metal suction tip. The obturator nodal package is bluntly mobilized from the pelvic sidewall. The obturator nerve is often visualized at this point and bluntly released from the nodal package (Fig. 24–3A). The surgeon should be cautious of an accessory obturator vein emptying into the distal aspect of the external iliac vein. The nodal package is divided above a large surgical clip at the level of the femoral canal. The nodal package is then bluntly mobilized and divided below a large surgical clip placed at the level of the bifurcation of the iliac vessels. The nodal package is submitted for frozen section analysis.

Division of the Puboprostatic Ligaments
(Fig. 24–3B and C)

An ampule of indigo carmine is administered prior to dividing the puboprostatic ligaments in order to provide sufficient time for filtration and eventual visualization of the ureteral orifices later in the procedure. The exposure for the division of the puboprostatic ligaments and the radical prostatectomy is achieved by trapping the Foley balloon in the malleable blade of the Balfour retractor. Moist, tightly rolled laparotomy sponges are placed on

either side of the malleable blade in order to secure the catheter balloon. The apical periprostatic areolar tissue is bluntly mobilized and excised. The midline superficial vein is carefully isolated and divided between 3-0 silk sutures.

The endopelvic fascia is sharply incised with Metzenbaum scissors as the fascia reflects over the obturator internus muscle (Fig. 24–3B). The endopelvic fascia is bluntly split to the level of the puboprostatic ligaments. The seminal vesicles should be palpated at this time in order to identify obvious clinical understaging. Occasionally, a venous tributary of the dorsal venous complex is identified lateral to the puboprostatic ligaments. The tributary, if present, is ligated between 3-0 silk suture ligatures. Troublesome bleeding may be encountered during division of the puboprostatic ligament if the adjacent tributaries of the dorsal venous complex are entered. The puboprostatic ligaments are sharply separated from these midline venous tributaries and divided under direct vision (Fig. 24–3C). Exposure of the puboprostatic ligament is facilitated by a sponge stick retracting the prostate in a cephalad direction.

Ligation of the Dorsal Venous Complex
(Fig. 24–3D)

Prior to division of the dorsal venous complex, the anesthesiologist should be alerted that significant bleeding may occur. The dorsal venous complex is enveloped by the lateral pelvic fascia.[16] Therefore, the lateral pelvic fascia must be perforated in order to isolate and divide the dorsal venous complex. The plane between the dorsal venous complex and the urethra is often easily discernible by palpation. The dorsal venous complex is grasped between the thumb and index finger so that only a thin tissue plane separates the dorsal venous complex and the anterior urethral wall. The plane between the dorsal venous complex and the urethra is perforated with a right-angle clamp. A generous plane between the dorsal venous complex and the urethra is developed with a right-angle clamp. A number 0 silk suture is placed around the dorsal venous complex and retracted in a cephalad direction. The jaws of the right-angle clamp are widely separated and a 0 chromic suture on a ⅝-inch tapered needle is placed into the midportion of the distalmost aspect of the dorsal venous complex (Fig. 24–3D). The 0 chromic suture is tied in order to prevent its cephalad migration. A free end of the chromic suture is grasped by the right-angle clamp. The entire dorsal venous complex is encircled by the 0 chromic suture following removal of the right-angle clamp. The distal chromic suture and the proximal silk sutures are tied. The dorsal venous complex is sharply incised between the two sutures (Fig. 24–3D). If troublesome bleeding occurs, the distal stump of the dorsal venous complex is oversewn with a 0 chromic suture. The backbleeding may be controlled with a figure-of-8 suture ligature.

Division of the Urethra
(Fig. 24–3*E* to *G*)

The neurovascular bundles are located immediately lateral to the membranous urethra. The plane between the urethra and the neurovascular bundle is developed sharply with Metzenbaum scissors (Fig. 24–3*E*). The plane between the posterior aspect of the urethra and the rectum is developed with a right-angle clamp, and the entire urethra is isolated with an umbilical tape. The anterior urethral wall is sharply incised, exposing the Foley catheter (Fig. 24–3*F*). The Foley catheter is elevated out of the urethral lumen, clamped, and transected. The catheter is subsequently used for retraction during mobilization of the prostate. The posterior urethral wall is sharply incised. The plane between the rectum and the prostate is developed in the midline using blunt finger dissection (Fig. 24–3*G*), which disrupts muscle fibers comprising the rectourethralis muscle and the rhabdosphincter mechanism (distal sphincter).

Ligation of the Neurovascular Innervation of the Prostate
(Fig. 24–3*H* and *I*)

The thin layer of the lateral pelvic fascia overlying the prostate is sharply incised. The plane between the prostate and the neurovascular bundle is easily defined. If nerve-sparing radical prostatectomy is indicated, the neurovascular bundle is divided immediately adjacent to the prostate (Fig. 24–3*H*). The objective of the nerve-sparing approach is to selectively ligate the neurovascular innervation to the prostate. The neurovascular innervation of the prostate is divided medial to surgical clips or 3-0 silk suture ligatures (Fig. 24–3*I*). The neurovascular pedicle to the prostate should not be divided en mass in order to avoid inadvertent entrapment of the neurovascular innervation to the corpora cavernosa. The neurovascular innervation to the prostate is most prominent at the base of the prostate. The plane between the seminal vesicle and neurovascular bundle is often difficult to identify. Therefore, I prefer to complete the division of the lateral pedicle following incision of Denonvilliers' fascia.

Mobilization of the Seminal Vesicle and Vas Deferens
(Fig. 24–3*J* to *L*)

The prostate is retracted cephalad and the anterior layer of Denonvilliers' fascia is incised in the midline at the level of ampulla of the vas deferens (Fig. 24–3*J*). Denonvilliers' fascia is bluntly mobilized off the seminal vesicle and vas deferens. The residual pedicle overlying the seminal vesicle is divided between suture ligatures or surgical clips (Fig. 24–3*K*). The plane between the seminal vesicle and bladder neck is bluntly developed (Fig. 24–3*L*). The mobilization of the seminal vesicles at this point simplifies subsequent division of the pos-

terior bladder neck. The vasa deferentia are bluntly developed to the level of the base of the seminal vesicle and divided above a large surgical clip. The prostate is elevated from the operative field, and the pedicles to the seminal vesicles are divided above large surgical clips.

Division of the Prostatovesical Junction
(Fig. 24–3*M*)

Traction on the Foley catheter facilitates identification of the anterior prostatovesical junction. The prostatovesical junction is divided using electrocautery. The anterior prostatovesical junction is divided and both ends of the Foley catheter are elevated from the operative field. A large right-angle clamp is placed within the previously developed plane between the seminal vesicles and the posterior bladder neck. The ureteral orifices are identified, and the posterior prostatovesical junction is divided with electrocautery above the clamp (Fig. 24–3*M*).

Bladder Neck Reconstruction
(Fig. 24–3*N*)

The bladder neck is reconstructed in a tennis racket fashion using interrupted 2-0 chromic sutures. The bladder neck is reconstructed to a caliber of approximately 22 Fr. The bladder mucosa is everted using interrupted 3-0 chromic sutures (Fig. 24–3*N*). The mucosa is anchored to adjacent detrusor muscle rather than perivesical fat. The creation of a stoma-like bladder neck is intended to reduce the incidence of postoperative bladder neck contracture.

Vesicourethral Anastomosis
(Fig. 24–3*O*)

A 20 Fr 5-ml Silastic Foley balloon catheter is inserted through the urethra. A silk suture is passed through the eye of the catheter to facilitate exposure of the urethral lumen. The anastomotic sutures of 2-0 chromic on a ⅝-inch tapered UR-5 needle are placed in a mucosa-serosa orientation at the 2, 4, 6, 8, and 10 o'clock positions of the transected urethra (Fig. 24–3*O*). The sutures incorporate the full thickness of the urethra. An effort must be made to exclude the adjacent neurovascular bundle. The two anterior sutures are elevated in order to facilitate placement of the posterior sutures. The five anastomotic sutures are positioned at the corresponding levels of the bladder neck. The Foley balloon is inflated with 15 ml of saline in order to ensure that the balloon is functioning properly. The Foley catheter is introduced into the bladder. The table is unflexed and placed in 20 degrees reverse Trendelenburg, and the Balfour retractor is removed. The assistant manually deflects the bladder toward the urethra in order to reduce tension while the anastomotic sutures are tied. The Foley bal-

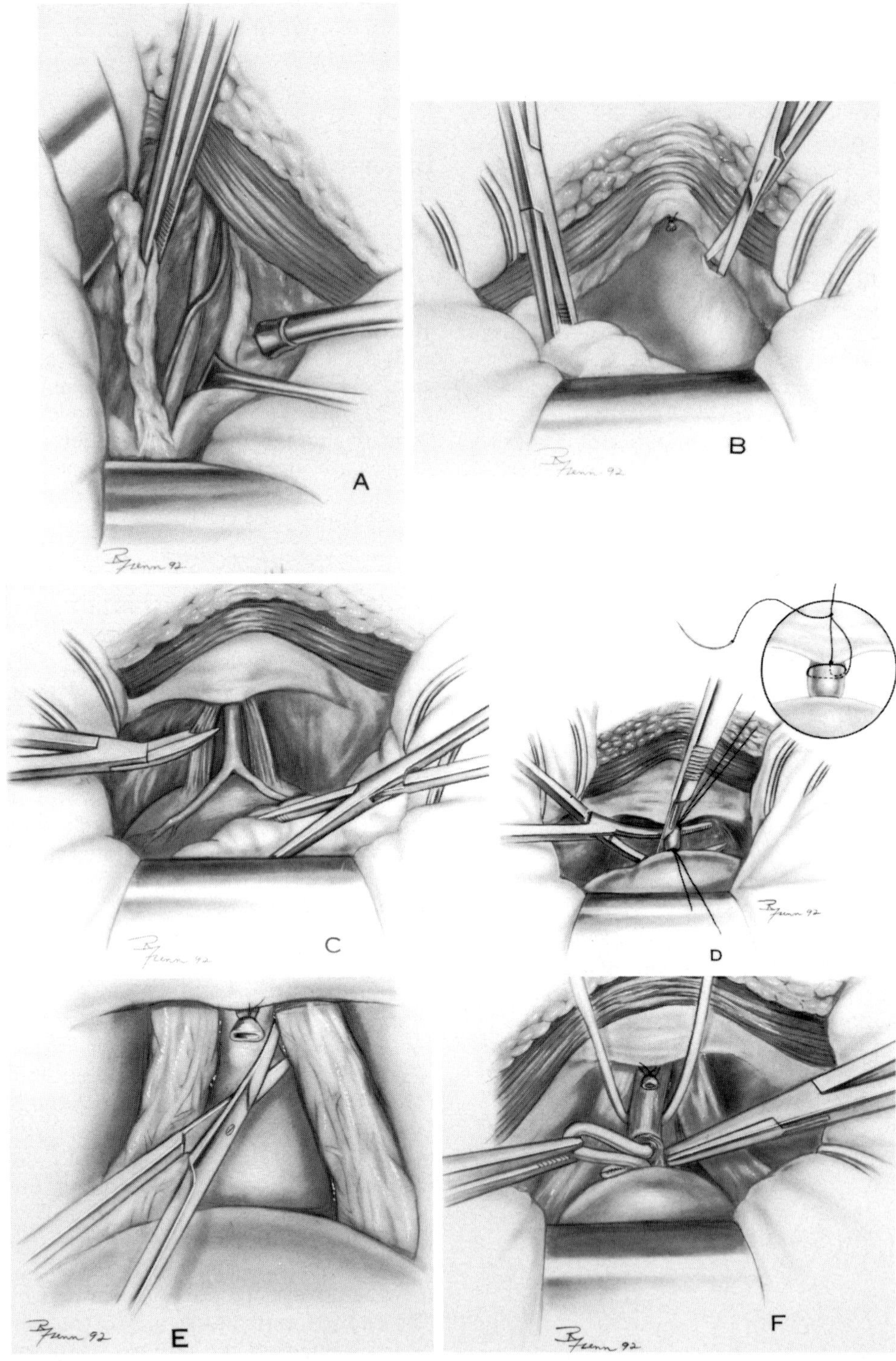

FIGURE 24–3. *A*, The areolar tissue overlying the external iliac vein is sharply incised, and the obturator lymph nodes are bluntly dissected. *B*, The endopelvic fascia is sharply incised as the fascia reflects over the obturator internus muscle. *C*, The puboprostatic ligaments are sharply separated from the midline venous tributaries and divided under direct vision. *D*, The plane between the dorsal venous complex and the urethra is perforated with a right-angle clamp. The most distal aspect of the dorsal venous complex is encircled by an 0 chromic suture placed as a suture ligature in order to prevent its displacement as the suture is tied. *E*, The plane between the urethra and the neurovascular bundle is developed sharply with Metzenbaum scissors. *F*, The Foley catheter is elevated out of the urethral lumen, clamped, and transected. The catheter is subsequently used for retraction during mobilization of the prostate.

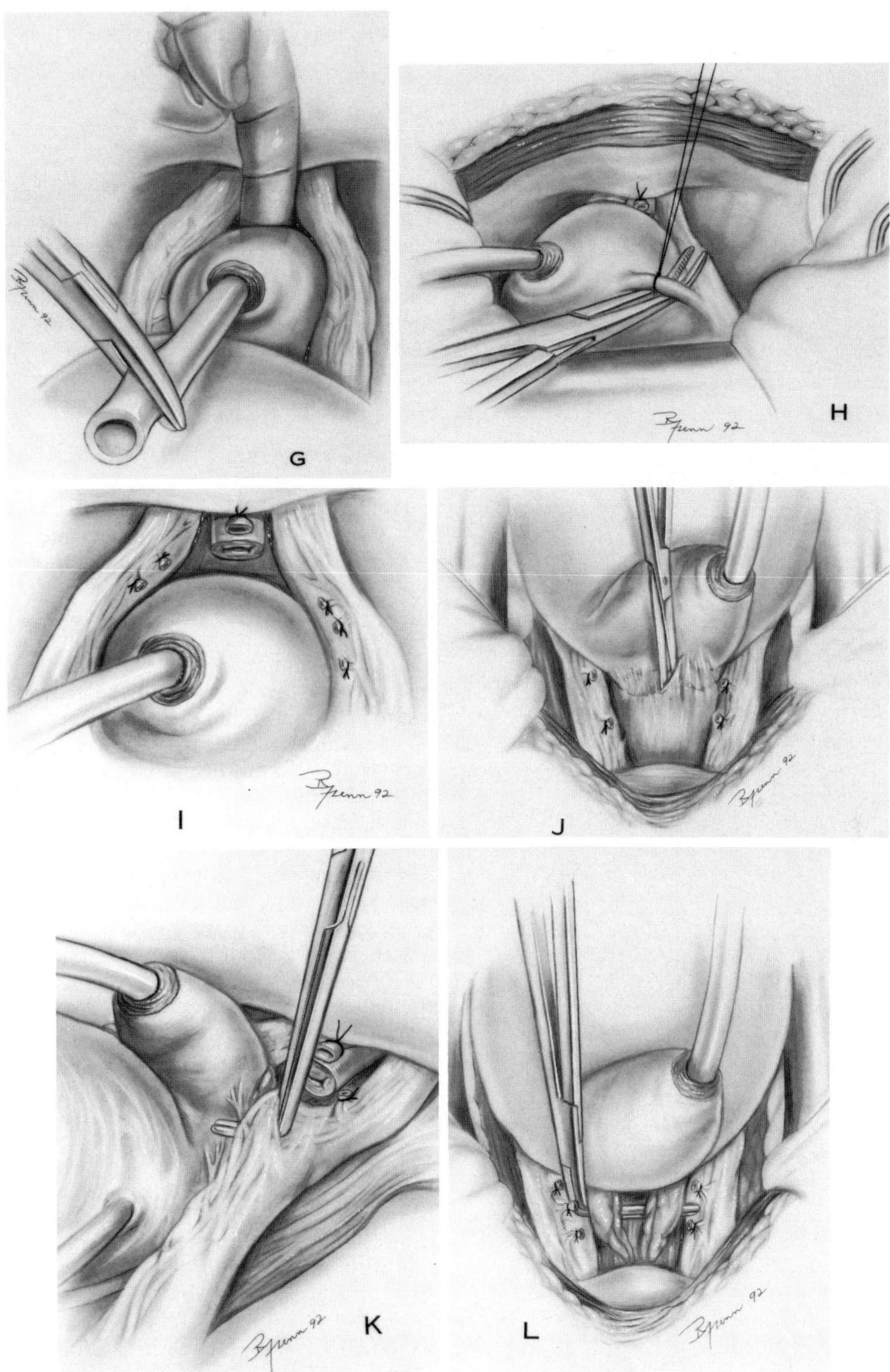

FIGURE 24–3 *Continued G*, The plane between the prostate and rectum is developed using blunt finger dissection. *H*, The neurovascular bundle at the apex of the prostate is divided immediately adjacent to the gland. *I*, The remainder of the neurovascular innervation to the prostate is divided between surgical clips and 2-0 silk suture ligatures. *J*, Denonvilliers' fascia is sharply incised at the level of the ampulla of the vasa. *K*, The residual pedicle overlying the seminal vesicle is divided between surgical clips following incision of the anterior layer of Denonvilliers' fascia. *L*, The seminal vesicles are bluntly separated from the posterior bladder neck.

Illustration continued on following page

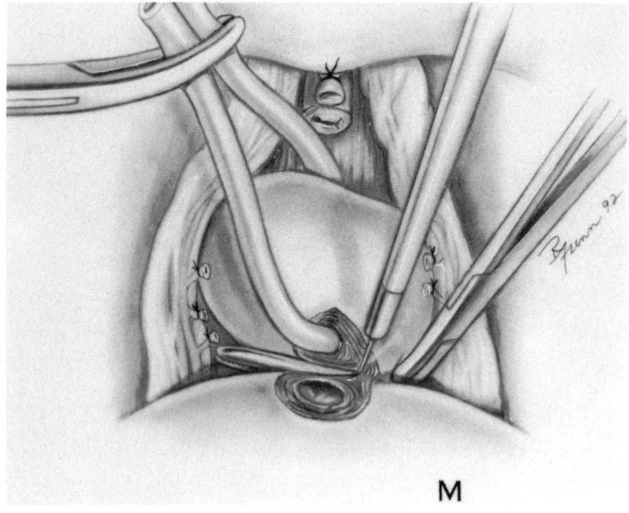

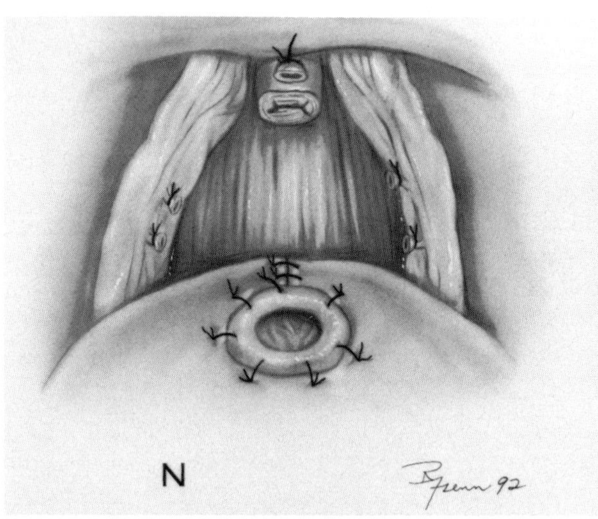

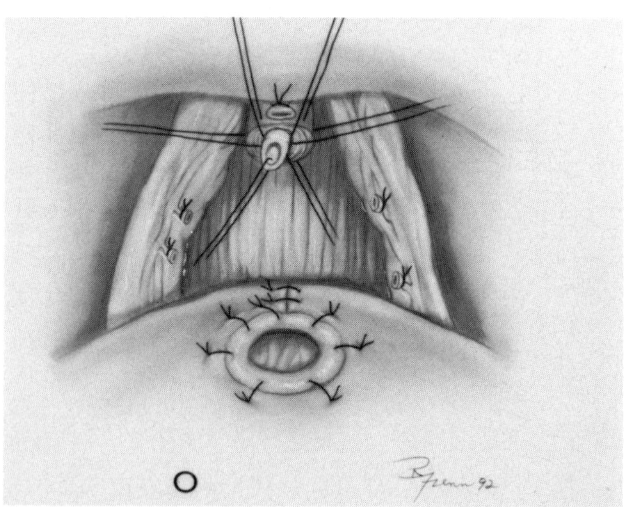

FIGURE 24–3 *Continued M,* The prostatovesical junction is divided using electrocautery. A large right-angle clamp is placed within the previously developed plane between the seminal vesicles and posterior bladder neck, and the posterior prostatovesical junction is divided. *N,* The bladder mucosa is everted using chromic sutures. *O,* The anastomotic sutures of 2-0 chromic are placed in a mucosa-serosa orientation at the 2, 4, 6, 8, and 10 o'clock positions of the transected urethra.

loon is inflated with 15 ml of saline and the bladder is distended with 150 ml of saline in order to ensure that a water-tight anastomosis has been accomplished. The pelvis is irrigated with an antibiotic irrigation solution.

Abdominal Wall Closure

Hemovac drains are positioned in the pelvis through separate stab incisions through all layers of the abdominal wall. The Hemovac drains are secured to the abdominal wall with a 2-0 silk suture. The midline rectus fascia is approximated with interrupted figure-of-8 0 chromic sutures. Alternatively, the rectus fascia may be approximated using a running 0 Vicryl suture. The skin is reapproximated with skin staples, and the Foley catheter is secured to the lower extremity.

PERIOPERATIVE MANAGEMENT

A hematocrit is obtained immediately upon arrival in the recovery room and the evening of surgery. In general, transfusions are administered only if the hematocrit is less than 25 per cent. The presence of significant coronary artery disease may alter the threshold for transfusion. Intravenous fluids are adjusted to maintain a minimum urine output of 30 ml. If the urine output is relatively low and the pelvic drainage high, the pelvic drainage fluid should be analyzed for glucose and creatinine in order to assess urine output more accurately. Parenteral antibiotics are administered for 48 to 72 hours and are discontinued when the patient initiates a liquid oral diet. They are eventually replaced by an oral antibiotic preparation such as Septra. The diet is advanced following the passage of flatus. The pelvic drains are removed when the combined 24-hour drainage is less than 50 ml. Typically, the pelvic drains are removed and oral intake is initiated on the third postoperative day. The skin staples are removed and the patient is discharged on the fifth or sixth postoperative day. Iron supplementation is offered if clinically indicated. The Foley catheter is removed on or about the 21st postoperative day. The patient is instructed to use disposable diapers until urinary control is achieved. Complete urinary control is typically achieved between 1 and 4 months postoperatively. The patient is instructed to spend several hours during the day attempting to increase the continence interval and to cognitively exert control of the external sphincter mechanism in association with timed voiding.

POSTOPERATIVE COMPLICATIONS

Walsh has reported the largest personal surgical experience addressing morbidity and outcome following radical retropubic prostatectomy.[20] The in-hospital mortality was zero. There were no rectal injuries or other bowel complications. One patient sustained a ureteral injury that was easily corrected at the time of surgery with no sequelae. Three of the first 100 patients developed pulmonary emboli, one of whom died 3 weeks postoperatively while at home. In the next 170 patients there were no recognized cases of thrombophlebitis or pulmonary emboli. No patient who was followed for a year or longer was totally incontinent, and no patient wore a urinary appliance or had undergone anti-incontinence surgery. Less than 5 per cent of patients wore a small pad in their trousers that required changing once or twice a day, and 70 percent of patients were potent.

SUMMARY

The indications for radical prostatectomy are highly controversial. The primary goal of radical prostatectomy is to cure carcinoma of the prostate. It is generally agreed that the majority of subjects with Stages A and B carcinoma of the prostate are cured by radical prostatectomy. The ability to cure clinically localized carcinoma must be balanced by the fact that a subset of these individuals, if left untreated, would not die of their malignancy. The proportion of patients who are currently overtreated is not known because the natural history of the disease is poorly understood. Unfortunately, there are no biochemical or imaging studies that predict the biologic activity of the tumor. On the other hand, a significant subset of patients with Stage B2 disease are understaged and have disease that is not amenable to cure. No biochemical or imaging studies can currently identify these clinically understaged patients preoperatively. The surgeon advocating radical prostatectomy must appreciate the limitations of the procedure, which are based primarily on factors unrelated to the technical aspects of the operation.

The ability to perform an anatomic nerve-sparing radical prostatectomy has greatly reduced the complications for patients unlikely to benefit from surgery. Owing to the pioneering work of Walsh, urologists offer radical prostatectomy with the expectation of favorably affecting the survival of the vast majority of candidates selected for the procedure. The majority of understaged candidates may also benefit from local disease control without significant compromise of their quality of life. The ability to perform radical prostatectomy with relatively low morbidity has encouraged some surgeons to extend the indication to include Stages C and D1. The therapeutic objective in these cases is local disease control. A prospective study critically evaluating radical prostatectomy versus conservative management (hormonal therapy/transurethral resection) must ultimately be performed before the indication is widely extended to Stages C and D1 patients.

Walsh's anatomic approach to radical prostatectomy represents the most significant advancement in the treatment of prostate cancer over the past several decades. Urologists may now approach surgical extirpation of the malignant prostate gland with a keen understanding of pelvic anatomy. The decision to preserve the neurovascular bundle should be made at the time of surgery. Critics who are uncomfortable with the nerve-sparing concept as it relates to surgical margins should perform the anatomic radical prostatectomy and simply excise the neurovascular bundles. The anatomic approach allows for greater surgical margins when clinically indicated.

The optimal therapy for clinically localized carcinoma of the prostate is highly controversial. The treatment options include radical prostatectomy, radiation therapy, and conservative management. Radical prostatectomy unequivocally represents the most effective therapy for disease that is truly confined to the prostate gland because the patient is guaranteed a cure. Historically, patients were discouraged from undergoing radical prostatectomy owing to the significant mortality and morbidity associated with the operative procedure. The ability to perform radical prostatectomy with low morbidity and limited impairment of quality of life should have a favorable impact on the application of this treatment alternative for prostate cancer.

REFERENCES

1. Benson MC: Management of primary Stage D prostatic cancer. *In* Murphy GP, Khoury S, Kuss R, et al (eds): Prostate Cancer, Part B: Imaging Techniques, Radiotherapy, Chemotherapy, and Management Issues. New York, Alan R. Liss, 1987, pp 411–428.
2. Campbell EW: Total prostatectomy with preliminary ligation of the vascular pedicle. J Urol 81:464, 1959.
3. Catalona WJ, Dresner SM: Nerve-sparing radical prostatectomy: Extraprostatic tumor extension and preservation of erectile function. J Urol 134:1149, 1985.
4. Chybourski FM, Larson K, Bergstralh EJ, Oesterling JE: Predicting radionuclide bone scan findings in patients with newly diagnosed untreated prostate cancer: Prostate specific antigen is superior to all other clinical parameters. J Urol 145:313, 1991.
5. Eggleston JC, Walsh PC: Radical prostatectomy with preservation of sexual function: Pathological findings in the first 100 cases. J Urol 134:1146–1148, 1985.
6. Epstein JI, Walsh PC, Eggleston JC: Frozen section detection of lymph node metastasis in prostatic carcinoma: Accuracy in grossly uninvolved pelvic lymphadenectomy specimens. J Urol 136:1234, 1986.
7. Freiha FS, Bagshaw MA: Carcinoma of the prostate: Results of post-irradiation biopsy. Prostate 5:19–25, 1984.
8. Isaacs JT: Antagonistic effect of androgen on prostatic cell death. Prostate 5:545, 1984.
9. Lange PH, Ercole CJ, Lightner DJ, et al: The value of serum prostate specific antigen determinations before and after radical prostatectomy. J Urol 141:873, 1989.
10. Lepor H, Crosby R, Gregerman M, et al: Precise localization of the autonomic nerves from the pelvic plexus to the corpora cavernosa: A detailed anatomical study of the adult male pelvis. J Urol 133:207, 1985.
11. Middleton AW Jr: Radical prostatectomy for carcinoma of the prostate in men more than 69 years of age. J Urol 138:1185, 1987.
12. Millin T: Retropubic urinary surgery. Baltimore, Williams & Wilkins, 1947.
13. National Institutes of Health Consensus Development Conference June 15–17, 1987. The management of clinically localized prostate cancer. J Urol 138:1369, 1987.
14. Partin AW, Carter HB, Chan DW, et al: Prostate specific antigen in the staging of localized prostate cancer: Influence of tumor differentiation, tumor volume, and benign hyperplasia. J Urol 143:747, 1990.
15. Paulson DF, Moul JW, Walther PJ: Radical prostatectomy for

clinical stage T_{1-2} N_0 M_0 prostatic adenocarcinoma: Long-term result. J Urol 144:1180, 1990.
16. Reiner WG, Walsh PC: A anatomical approach to the surgical management of the dorsal vein and Santorini's plexus during radical retropubic surgery. J Urol 121:198, 1979.
17. Salo JO, Kivisaari L, Rannikko S, Lehtonen T: Computerized tomography and transrectal ultrasound in the assessment of local extension of prostatic cancer before radical retropubic prostatectomy. J Urol 137:435–438, 1987.
18. Scardino PT, Wheeler TM: Prostatic biopsy after irradiation therapy for prostatic cancer. Urology 25 (Suppl):39–46, 1985.
19. Schellhammer PF, Ladaga LE, El-Mahdi A: Historical characteristics of prostatic biopsies after [125]iodine implantation. J Urol 123:700, 1980.
20. Walsh PC: Radical retropubic prostatectomy. *In* Walsh PC, Gittes RE, Perlmutter AD, Stamey IA (eds): Campbell's Urology, 5th ed. Philadelphia WB Saunders Co, 1986, pp 2754–2775.
21. Walsh PC, Donker PJ: Impotence following radical prostatectomy: Insight into etiology and prevention. J Urol 128:492, 1982.
22. Walsh PC, Jewett HJ: Radical surgery for prostatic cancer. Cancer 45:1906, 1980.
23. Walsh PC, Lepor H: The role of radical prostatectomy in the management of prostatic cancer. Cancer 60:526, 1987.
24. Whitesel JA, Donohue RE, Mani JH et al: Acid phosphatase: Its influence on the management of carcinoma of the prostate. J Urol 131:70, 1984.

Chapter 25

RADICAL PERINEAL PROSTATECTOMY

DAVID F. PAULSON

Radical perineal prostatectomy has long been a major curative procedure for the treatment of organ-confined adenocarcinoma of the prostate. The perineal approach fell from favor because of decreasing familiarity with the perineum as well as the perception that patients had more difficulty with impotence and cancer control with the perineal approach. Herein we describe our method for radical prostatectomy and various modifications that permit us to establish disease control with the same risks and benefits as the radical retropubic approach.

POSITIONING

The sacrum is placed at the edge of the table, the buttocks extending several inches over the edge of the table (Fig. 25–1). Padded shoulder braces placed against the acromial processes prevent stretch or pressure injury to the brachial plexus. The sacrum should be elevated on sand bags or folded towels. The legs are padded to prevent damage to the nerves and vessels. The arms may be taped to the legs rather than extended in order to reduce the risk of nerve injury to the brachial plexus. Correct positioning places the perineum parallel to the floor and provides optimal exposure.

EXPOSURE OF THE PROSTATE

The Lowsley prostatic tractor is passed retrograde into the bladder and the blades are opened (Fig. 25–2). If the Lowsley tractor cannot be passed into the bladder, a sound or a Foley catheter may be used. The skin incision is made anterior to the anal verge and curved posterolaterally on either side within the medial borders of the ischial tuberosities. The skin incision should be

extended posterolaterally to the posterior anal margin. The superficial perineal fascia is incised using the cautery, and the surgical space within the ischiorectal fossa is developed. The exposed superficial central muscles of the perineum may be divided with cautery (Fig. 25–3). The rectal sphincter is then visualized as a muscular

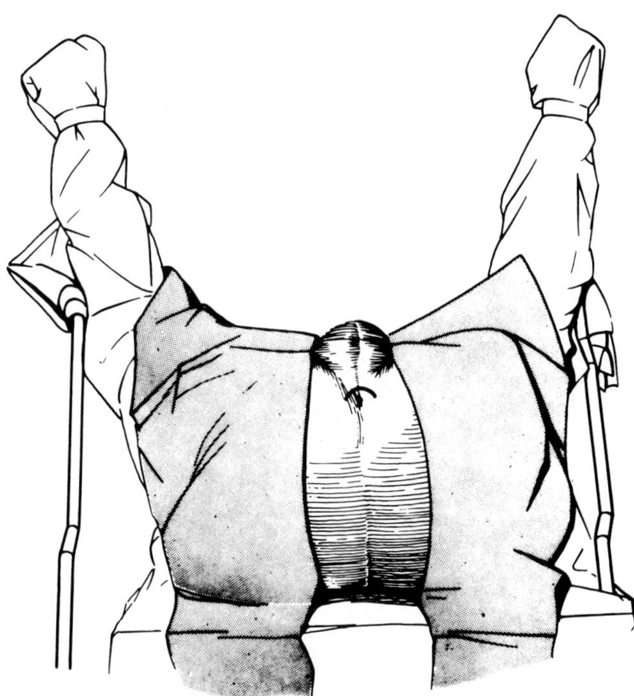

FIGURE 25–1. Exaggerated lithotomy position for radical perineal prostatectomy with line of incision indicated. (From Paulson DF: Technique of radical perineal prostatectomy. *In* Skinner DG, Lieskovsky G [eds]: Diagnosis and Management of Genitourinary Cancer. Philadelphia, WB Saunders Co, 1987, p 721.)

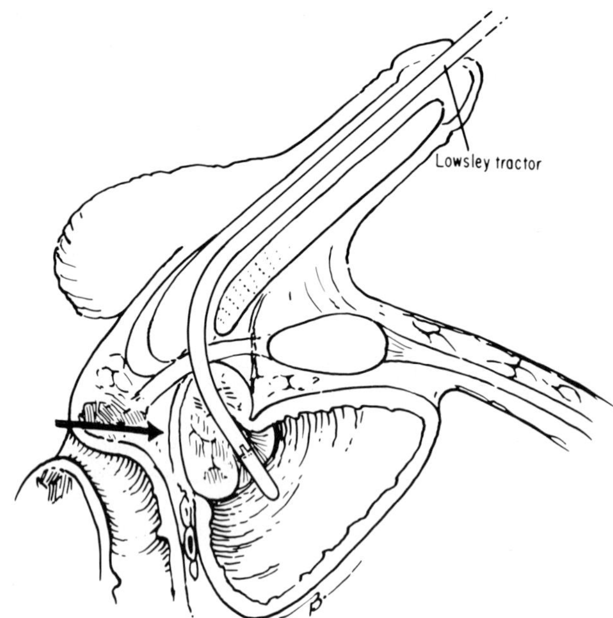

FIGURE 25–2. Positioning of Lowsley traction. The approach to the prostate is indicated by the heavy arrow. (From Paulson DF: Technique of radical perineal prostatectomy. *In* Skinner DG, Lieskovsky G [eds]: Diagnosis and Management of Genitourinary Cancer. Philadelphia, WB Saunders Co, 1987, p 721.)

FIGURE 25–3. The central tendon is the muscular sheet that extends anterior to the rectum and is superficial to the external anal sphincter. Incision of the central tendon along with division of the projection of the external sphincter to the perineal body permits the dissection to be carried out beneath the triangle formed by the superficial external anal sphincter. (From Paulson DF: Technique of radical perineal prostatectomy. *In* Skinner DG, Lieskovsky G [eds]: Diagnosis and Management of Genitourinary Cancer. Philadelphia, WB Saunders Co, 1987, p 721.)

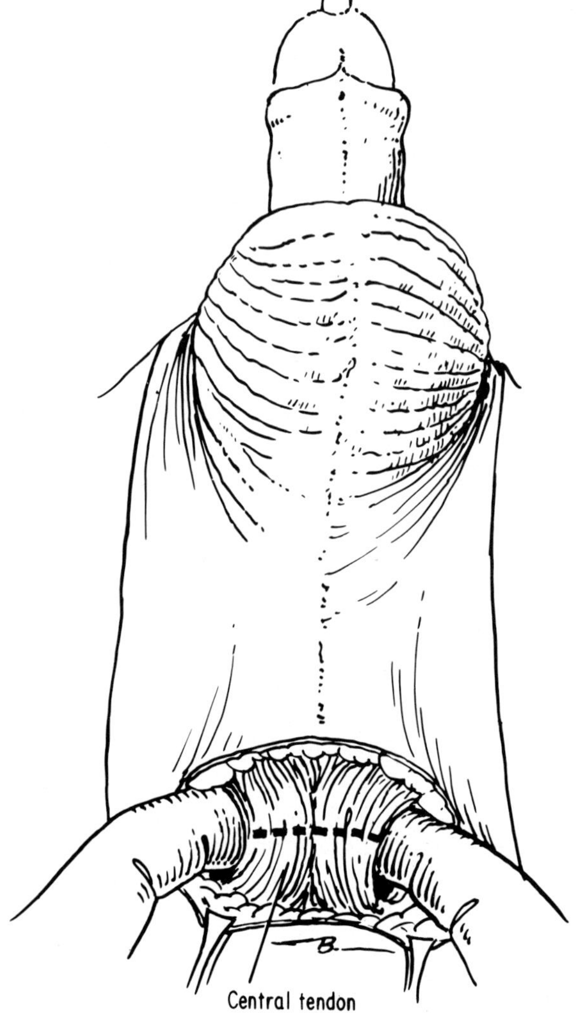

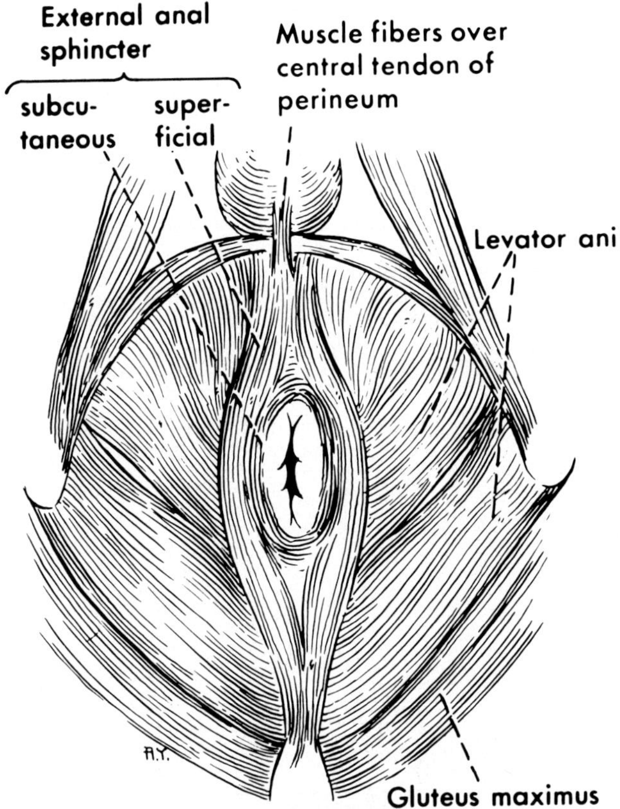

FIGURE 25–4. The fibers of the external anal sphincter can be visualized following division of the central tendon. A retractor can be placed in the triangle formed by the superficial external anal sphincter and those muscle fibers elevated to provide visualization of the rectal wall. (From Paulson DF: Technique of radical perineal prostatectomy. *In* Skinner DG, Lieskovsky G [eds]: Diagnosis and Management of Genitourinary Cancer. Philadelphia, WB Saunders Co, 1987, p 721.)

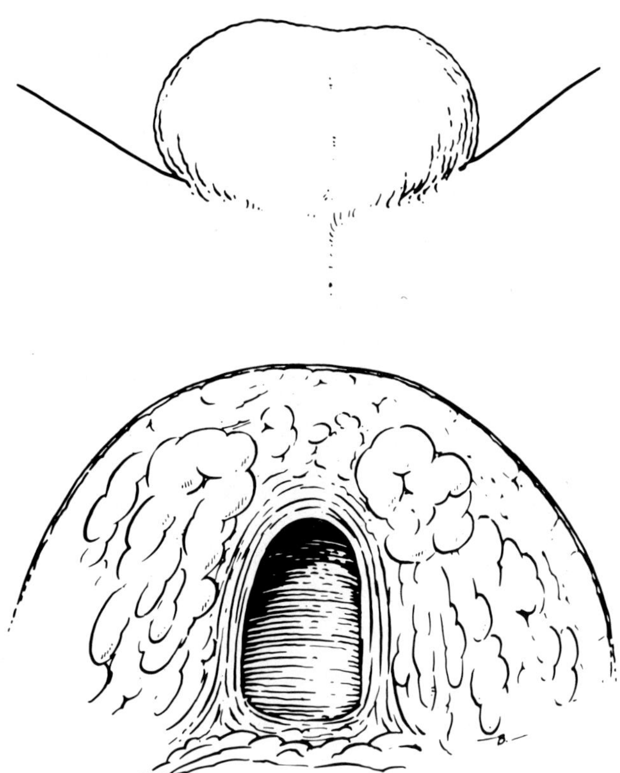

FIGURE 25–5. The anterior retractor has been removed for this diagrammatic representation of the subsphincteric approach. The anterior rectal fascia can be followed to the level of the rectourethralis. (From Paulson DF: Technique of radical perineal prostatectomy. *In* Skinner DG, Lieskovsky G [eds]: Diagnosis and Management of Genitourinary Cancer. Philadelphia, WB Saunders Co, 1987, p 721.)

arch overlying the rectum (Figs. 25–4 and 25–5). Dissection beneath this musculature reveals the white anterior rectal fascia, which should be used as a guide to the prostate. With blunt dissection the rectum can be mobilized on either side of the rectourethralis muscle. The rectum is tented upward by the rectourethralis (Fig. 25–6), and division of these muscle fibers permits posterior displacement of the rectum (Figs. 25–7 and 25–8).

THE CLASSIC PROSTATECTOMY

The rectum is displaced from the prostate by blunt dissection between Denonvilliers' fascia anteriorly and the rectal fascia posteriorly. Posterior retraction is maintained by a weighted posterior speculum. During division of the rectourethralis, the rectum may be identified by placing a finger in it. Blunt dissection then permits exposure of the lateral and anterior margins of the prostate (Fig. 25–9). The fascia overlying the prostate should be white and glistening. This fascia may be carried with the specimen, using the anterior rectal fascia to protect the rectum (Figs. 25–10 and 25–11).

The membranous urethra is exposed at the prostatic apex. A curved clamp is used to isolate the membranous

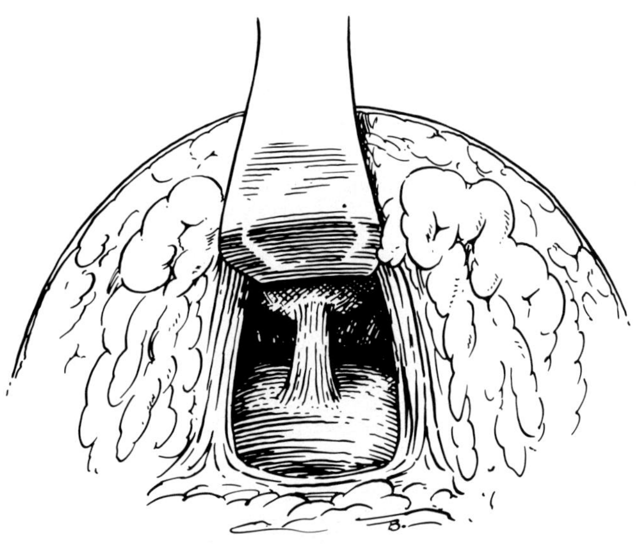

FIGURE 25–6. With the sphincter retracted superiorly (lateral retractor can be placed beneath the muscle to produce additional exposure), the rectourethralis muscle can be visualized. The extent of development of this muscle is variable. (From Paulson DF: Technique of radical perineal prostatectomy. *In* Skinner DG, Lieskovsky G [eds]: Diagnosis and Management of Genitourinary Cancer. Philadelphia, WB Saunders Co, 1987, p 721.)

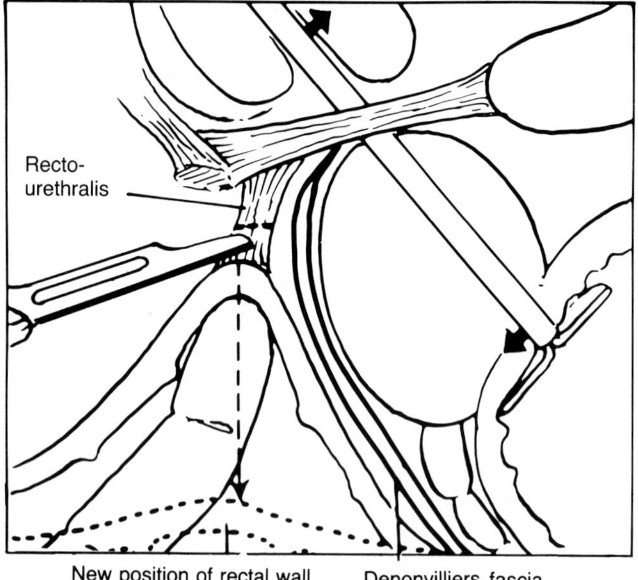

FIGURE 25–7. Lateral view of the rectourethralis muscle. The surgeon's finger has been placed in the rectum to assist in identification of the rectal wall. (From Paulson DF: Technique of radical perineal prostatectomy. *In* Skinner DG, Lieskovsky G [eds]: Diagnosis and Management of Genitourinary Cancer. Philadelphia, WB Saunders Co, 1987, p 721.)

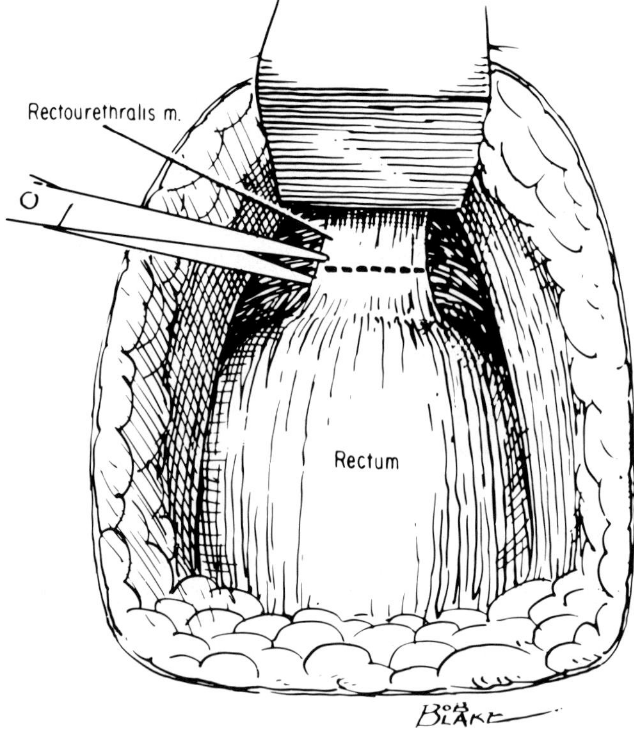

FIGURE 25–8. The line of incision of the rectourethralis muscle is identified. (From Paulson DF: Technique of radical perineal prostatectomy. *In* Skinner DG, Lieskovsky G [eds]: Diagnosis and Management of Genitourinary Cancer. Philadelphia, WB Saunders Co, 1987, p 721.)

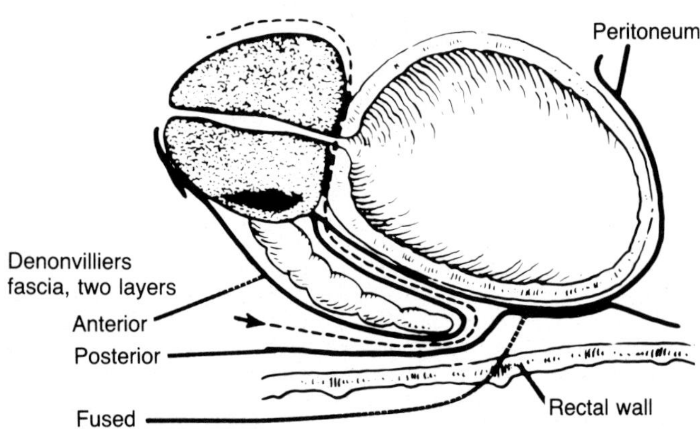

FIGURE 25–9. Limits of dissection for the radical prostatectomy. (From Paulson DF: Technique of radical perineal prostatectomy. *In* Skinner DG, Lieskovsky G [eds]: Diagnosis and Management of Genitourinary Cancer. Philadelphia, WB Saunders Co, 1987, p 721.)

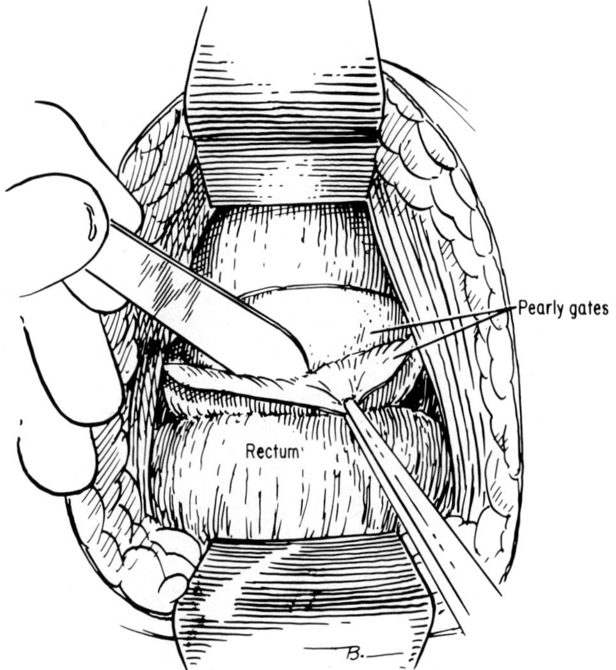

FIGURE 25–10. Incision of the overlying fascia (the pearly gates) to expose the true capsule of the prostate. (From Paulson DF: Technique of radical perineal prostatectomy. *In* Skinner DG, Lieskovsky G [eds]: Diagnosis and Management of Genitourinary Cancer. Philadelphia, WB Saunders Co, 1987, p 721.)

urethra distal to the prostatic apex, the Lowsley tractor is removed, and the urethra is divided (Fig. 25–12). A Young prostatic tractor is passed through the prostatic urethra into the bladder, and the blades are extended. A plane is developed beneath the venous plexus and between the bladder and the prostate anteriorly (Fig. 25–13) as the prostate is displaced from the bladder neck and the bladder neck fibers are identified (Fig. 25–14). Occasionally, the dissection can be carried laterally to the bladder neck such that the prostate is attached to the bladder only by the urethra at the level of the bladder neck. When this is not possible, the bladder is entered at 12 o'clock and the incision carried from 12 to 2 o'clock and from 12 to 10 o'clock, preserving

continuity of these bladder neck fibers. At this point, the Young tractor can be withdrawn and a Foley catheter of any appropriate size passed through the prostatic urethra and brought out superiorly through the line of incision between the prostate and bladder neck. Traction on this catheter permits the prostate to be displaced posteriorly (Fig. 25–15) and defines a line of cleavage between the bladder neck and prostate. This margin should be sharply divided until the prostate is attached only between 5 and 7 o'clock at the posterior bladder neck.

When visualization is difficult, digital examination allows the posterior bladder neck to be identified as a ridge by palpation. A transverse incision made at the

FIGURE 25–11. The solid arrow identifies the preferred plane of dissection above the anterior rectal fascia (the posterior fascia of Denonvilliers) and the fascia of the rectovesical septum (the anterior layer of Denonvilliers' fascia). The dashed arrow indicates a line of dissection beneath the rectal fascia that carries the hazard of rectal perforation. (From Paulson DF: Technique of radical perineal prostatectomy. *In* Skinner DG, Lieskovsky G [eds]: Diagnosis and Management of Genitourinary Cancer. Philadelphia, WB Saunders Co, 1987, p 721.)

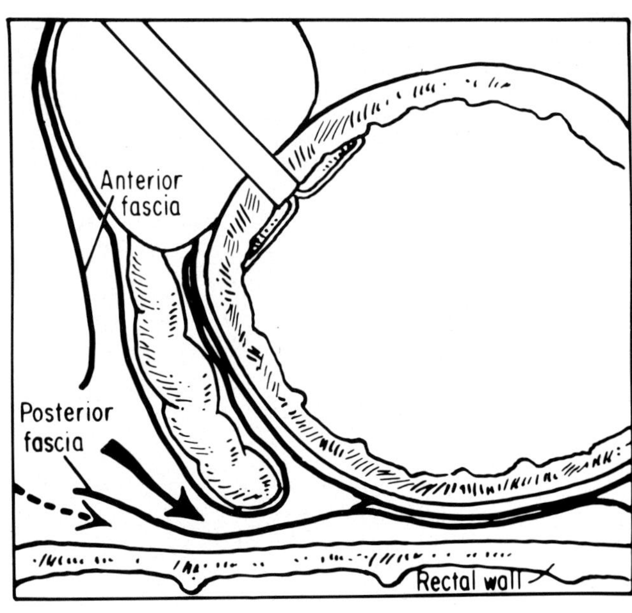

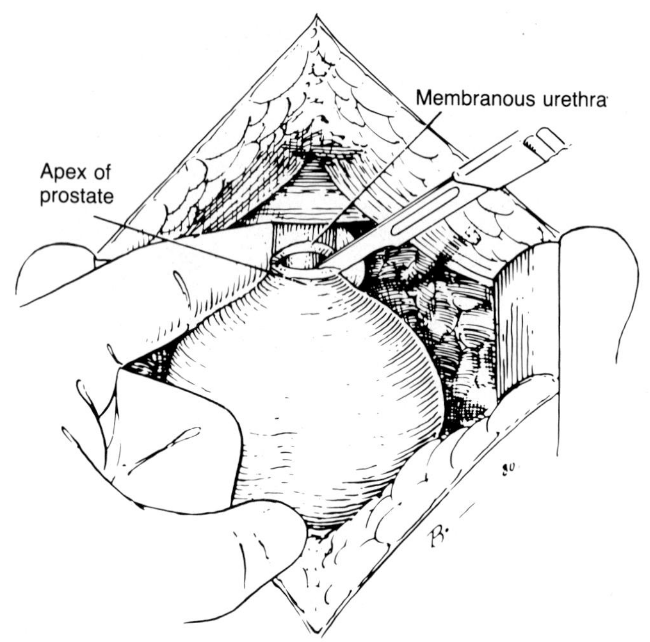

FIGURE 25–12. The apex of the prostate is identified and the membranous urethra sharply divided. (From Paulson DF: Technique of radical perineal prostatectomy. *In* Skinner DG, Lieskovsky G [eds]: Diagnosis and Management of Genitourinary Cancer. Philadelphia, WB Saunders Co, 1987, p 721.)

FIGURE 25–13. The solid arrow indicates the proper plane of dissection beneath the anterolateral fascia and the venous plexus. Dissection above this fascia (dashed arrow) carries the hazard of disruption of the venous sinus and troublesome bleeding. (From Paulson DF: Technique of radical perineal prostatectomy. *In* Skinner DG, Lieskovsky G [eds]: Diagnosis and Management of Genitourinary Cancer. Philadelphia, WB Saunders Co, 1987, p 721.)

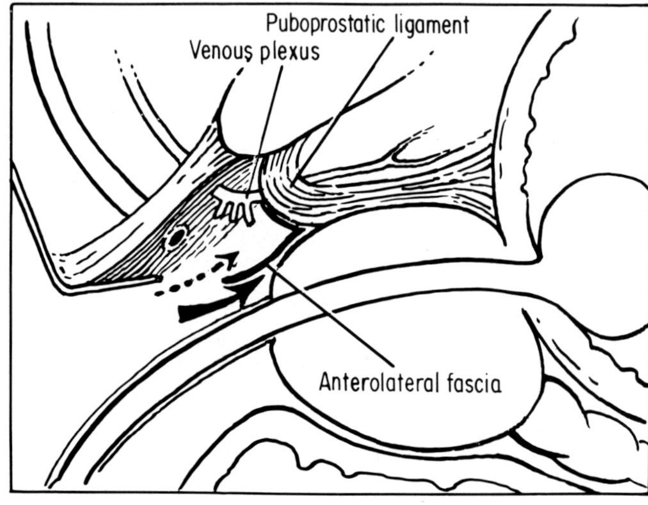

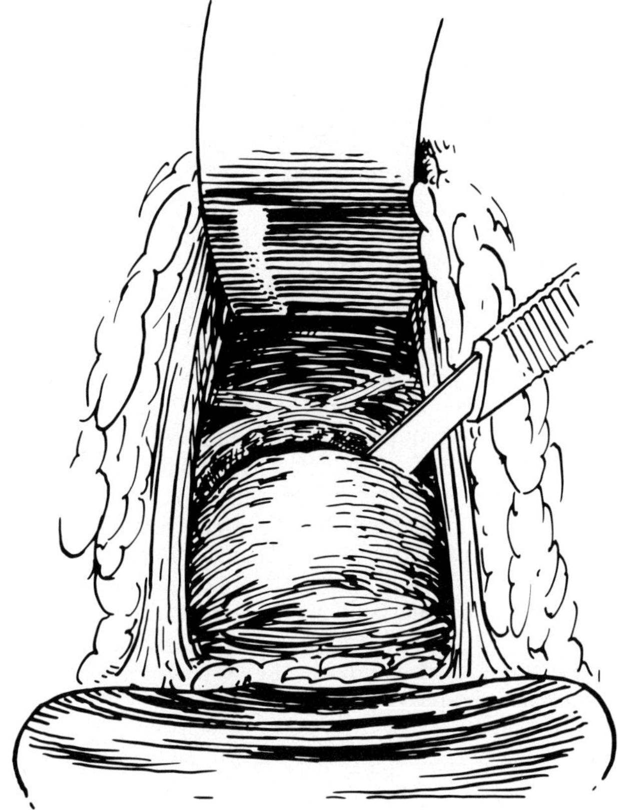

FIGURE 25–14. The prostate has been dissected off the bladder neck anteriorly, the bladder neck identified, and the prostate cut away from the bladder at this level. (From Paulson DF: Technique of radical perineal prostatectomy. *In* Skinner DG, Lieskovsky G [eds]: Diagnosis and Management of Genitourinary Cancer. Philadelphia, WB Saunders Co, 1987, p 721.)

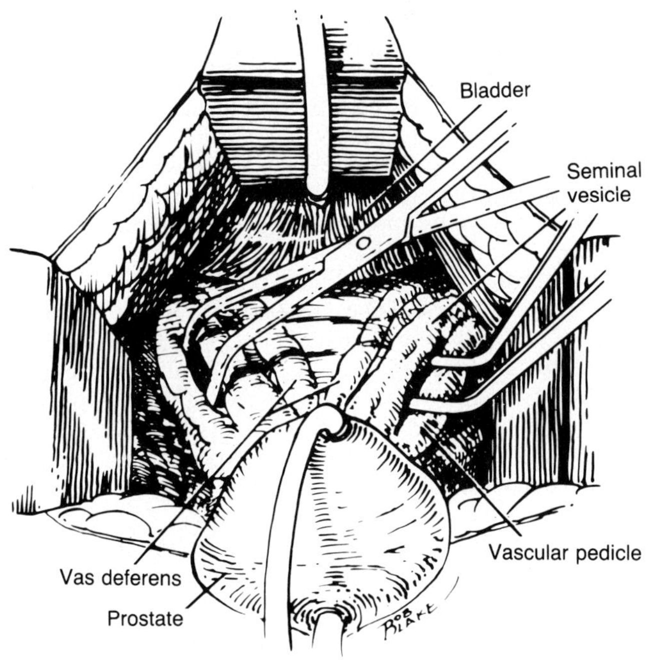

FIGURE 25–15. The posterior bladder neck has been cut away and the bladder allowed to retract separately. A plane is then developed between the bladder anteriorly and the prostate and seminal vesicles posteriorly. (From Paulson DF: Technique of radical perineal prostatectomy. *In* Skinner DG, Lieskovsky G [eds]: Diagnosis and Management of Genitourinary Cancer. Philadelphia, WB Saunders Co, 1987, p 721.)

level of the bladder neck and carried across the posterior aspect of the specimen separates the bladder neck fibers from the prostate. The posterior bladder neck then can be grasped with an Allis clamp and elevated. Dissection then proceeds between the bladder anteriorly and the seminal vesicles posteriorly. The remaining bladder fibers at 5 and 7 o'clock can be divided and the prostate cut away from the bladder neck. The prostate and the seminal vesicles remain secured posterolaterally by the vascular pedicles, but free from the bladder (Fig. 25–15). The vascular pedicles can be isolated at 5 and 7 o'clock and controlled with either surgical clips or absorbable sutures. Following division of the vascular pedicles bilaterally, the specimen is held only by the seminal vesicles and the vas deferens. The vasa deferentia are cross-clamped, divided, and either clipped or ligated. The seminal vesicles are removed with the specimen. The fibrofilamentous tissue overlying the seminal vesicles, which may contain small feeding vessels, can be divided with cautery. The glistening surface of the seminal vesicles assists in identification of the proper plane of dissection, and as these investing fibers are severed, the seminal vesicles are exposed (Fig. 25–16).

After hemostasis is secure, the vesicle neck should be reconstructed and continuity established between the

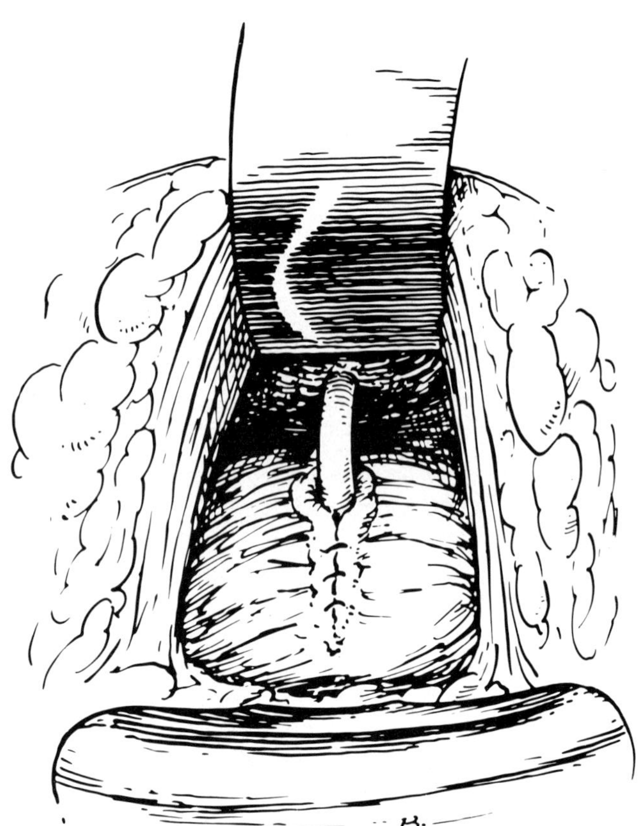

FIGURE 25–17. Closure of the bladder neck from 6 o'clock. (From Paulson DF: Technique of radical perineal prostatectomy. *In* Skinner DG, Lieskovsky G [eds]: Diagnosis and Management of Genitourinary Cancer. Philadelphia, WB Saunders Co, 1987, p 721.)

reconstructed bladder neck and the membranous urethra. This is done by a direct anastomosis between bladder neck and urethra, supported by a modification of the Vest traction sutures. This provides alignment between the reconstructed bladder neck and the membranous urethra and places minimum tension on the direct anastomosis. The bladder neck is closed from 6 to 12 o'clock with interrupted 0 chromic suture (Fig. 25–17). This permits the vesicourethral anastomosis to be done at maximal distance from the ureteral orifices. Inverting the racket handle rolls the posterior bladder neck and trigone into a tube and may occlude the ureteral orifices by incorporating them in the bladder closure.

The closure of the bladder neck should be snug, admitting an 18 Fr Foley catheter (Fig. 25–18). Mattress sutures of 0 chromic catgut are placed around the reconstructed bladder neck at 2, 5, 7, and 10 o'clock, outside-in, inside-out approximately 1.0 mm from the margin of the newly constructed bladder neck, tied loosely, and left long for subsequent placement beneath the perineal skin. Four sutures of 2-0 chromic catgut placed in the membranous urethra at 2, 4, 8, and 10 o'clock provide a mucosa-to-mucosa approximation of bladder neck to urethra. The 0 chromic catgut traction sutures, previously placed around the bladder neck, are drawn through on each side of the perineal body and tied subcutaneously to support the direct anastomosis

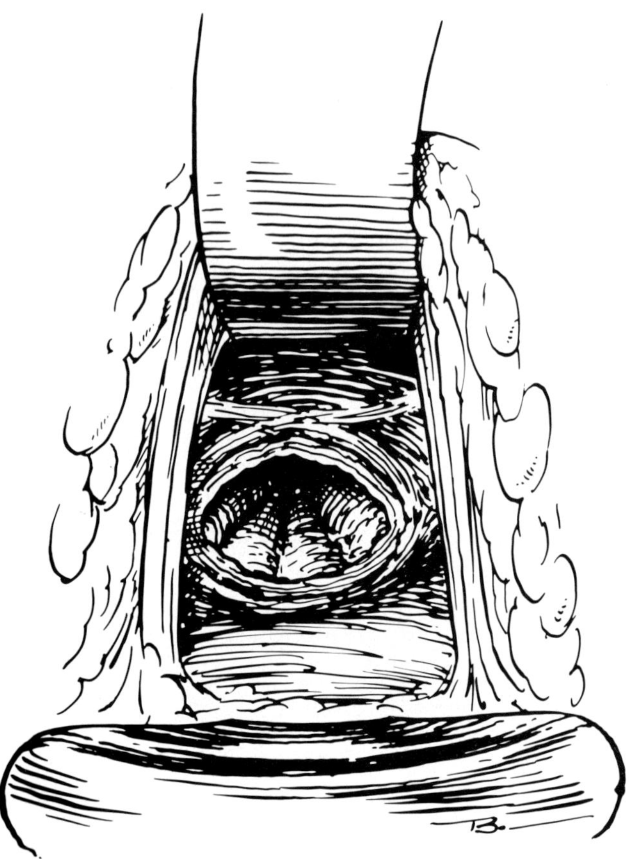

FIGURE 25–16. View of the bladder after removal of the specimen. The bladder neck fibers are preserved anteriorly but may be sacrificed posteriorly and laterally as necessary for removal of the tumor. (From Paulson DF: Technique of radical perineal prostatectomy. *In* Skinner DG, Lieskovsky G [eds]: Diagnosis and Management of Genitourinary Cancer. Philadelphia, WB Saunders Co, 1987, p 721.)

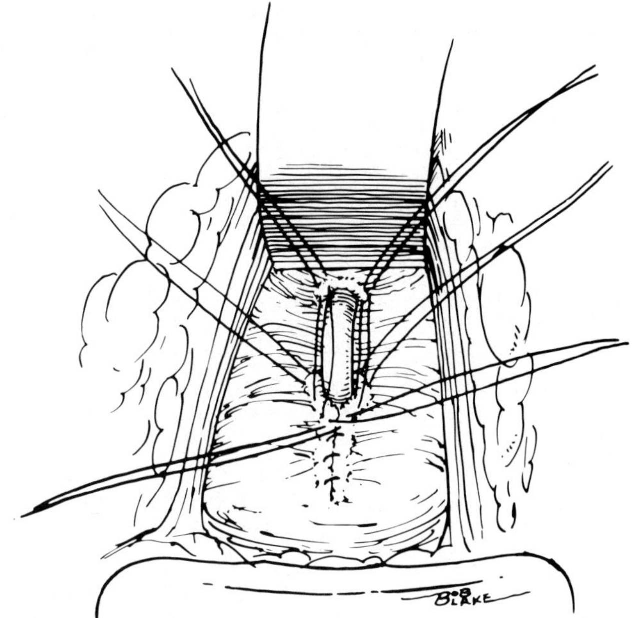

FIGURE 25–18. Placement of the Vest sutures at 2, 5, 7, and 10 o'clock of 0 chromic catgut, with placement of the sutures used for the direct anastomosis. (From Paulson DF: Technique of radical perineal prostatectomy. *In* Skinner DG, Lieskovsky G [eds]: Diagnosis and Management of Genitourinary Cancer. Philadelphia, WB Saunders Co, 1987, p 721.)

between the bladder neck and urethra. This anastomosis should be made without tension. The wound is drained with a Penrose drain, which may be brought out through either a stab wound or the lateral aspect of the incision. During closure, the levator ani musculature should be approximated in the midline with absorbable suture material. Reconstruction of this area supports the new bladder neck and reduces the likelihood of vesical and rectal incontinence.

WIDE-FIELD AND POTENCY-PRESERVING PERINEAL PROSTATECTOMY

For disease that is believed to have extended into or through the prostatic capsule, the surgeon may wish to extend the margins of the dissection in an attempt to establish specimen-confined disease. To accomplish this, the prostate is exposed as described previously. After the rectum has been dropped posteriorly, the surgeon develops a plane between the musculature pelvis, the levator ani sling laterally, and the fibrovascular fascia that surrounds the prostate medially (Fig. 25–19). This fascia is called the lateral pelvic fascia by Walsh, and it contains the neurovascular plexus associated with volitional or erectile function. Many large veins can be seen coursing through this fibrovascular tissue. Excessive bleeding may occur along the line of incision at the apex of the prostate and posteriorly as it sweeps off the rectum. However, this can be controlled with surgical clips. Even if the surgical clips become dislodged, the venous bleeding ceases once the prostate is removed and tension on the bladder neck fibers is released.

To accomplish a wide-field prostatectomy, a right-angle clamp is placed around the apex of the prostate

FIGURE 25–19. Dissection can be carried beneath or lateral to the tissue that has been described as the lateral pelvic fascia. When carried beneath the lateral pelvic fascia, the operation is established as originally described. When carried laterally, the neurovascular bundle is sacrificed; however, the margins of the procedure are increased by the width of the tissue encompassed in the surgical specimen.

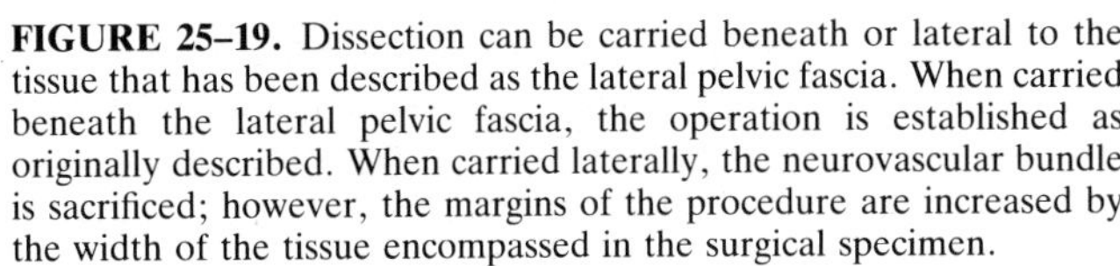

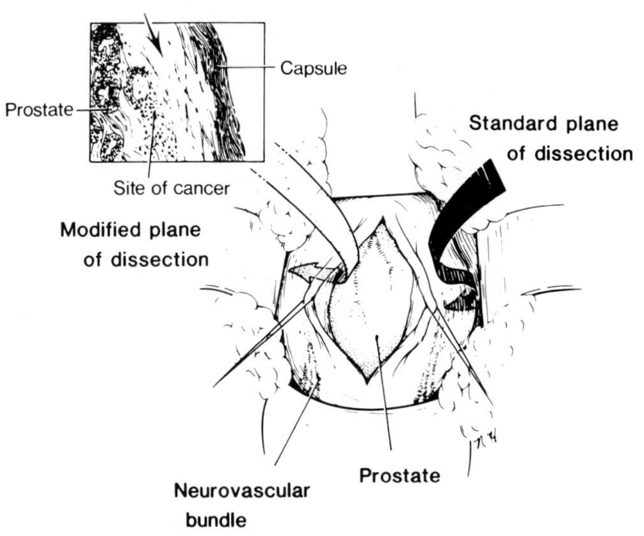

TABLE 25–1. RESULTS OF RADICAL PERINEAL PROSTATECTOMY

	GROUP 1 (233 pts.)		GROUP 2 (51 pts.)		P VALUES
	Median	Range	Median	Range	
Preoperative hematocrit (%)	43	(33–54)	42	(33–53)	0.845
Postoperative hematocrit (%)	36	(26–44)	34	(22–43)	0.012
Low hematocrit (%)	32	(24–41)	28.5	(23–41)	<0.001
Estimated blood loss (cc)	565	(150–1850)	2000	(600–10,000)	<0.001
Transfusions (No. units)	0	(0–4)	3	(0–27)	<0.001
Operative time (min)	203	(135–355)	225	(150–500)	0.001
Anesthesia time (min)	268	(185–435)	280	(190–555)	0.192
Hospital days	12	(6–27)	10	(7–20)	0.005
Catheter days	11	(8–42)	18	(10–86)	0.001
Weight of specimen (gm)	31.6	(7.2–106.8)	35	(12.4–95.5)	0.230

Adapted from Frazier HA, Robertson JE, Paulson DF: Radical prostatectomy: The pros and cons of the perineal vs. retropubic approach. J Urol 147:888–890, 1992, © by Williams & Wilkins, 1992; with permission.

TABLE 25–2. INCIDENCE OF INVOLVEMENT WITH PROSTATE CANCER

	GROUP 1 (122 pts)	GROUP 2 (51 pts)	P VALUES
Bladder involvement	21%	18%	0.591
Urethral involvement	25%	27%	0.696
Seminal vesicle involvement	23%	29%	0.373
Capsular penetration	43%	39%	0.682
Positive surgical margins	29%	31%	0.803

From Frazier HA, Robertson JE, Paulson DF: Radical prostatectomy: The pros and cons of the perineal vs. retropubic approach. J Urol 147:888–890, 1992, © by Williams & Wilkins, 1992; with permission.

TABLE 25–3. IN-HOSPITAL COMPLICATIONS OF RADICAL PERINEAL PROSTATECTOMY

	No. Pts.
Group 1 (4%)	
Epididymo-orchitis	1
Bacteremia	2
Abdominal incisional abscess	1
Perineal incisional abscess	1
Group 2 (4%)	
Aspiration pneumonia, myocardial infarction	1
Death secondary to cardiac arrest	1

From Frazier HA, Robertson JE, Paulson DF: Radical prostatectomy: The pros and cons of the perineal vs. retropubic approach. J Urol 147:888–890, 1992, © by Williams & Wilkins, 1992; with permission.

TABLE 25–4. LONG-TERM COMPLICATIONS OF RADICAL PERINEAL PROSTATECTOMY

	GROUP 1		GROUP 2	
	No.	(%)	No.	(%)
Stress incontinence	5	(4)	2	(4)
Anastomotic stricture	8	(7)	4	(8)
Bladder stones	0	(0)	1	(2)
Urethrorectal fistula	1	(1)	0	(0)
TOTALS	14	(12)	7	(14)

From Frazier HA, Robertson JE, Paulson DF: Radical prostatectomy: The pros and cons of the perineal vs. retropubic approach. J Urol 147:888–890, 1992, © Williams & Wilkins, 1992; with permission.

and the surrounding fibrovascular tissue, and this tissue and the membranous urethra are sharply incised as a single unit. As the prostate is mobilized anteriorly off the bladder, the reflection of the fibrovascular periprostatic tissue onto the bladder itself is sharply cut away. Taking the periprostatic fibrovascular tissue with the prostate itself increases the probability of a margin-negative specimen in patients with larger volume disease.

At the prostatic base, the two posterior layers of the periprostatic fascia must be incised to expose the seminal vesicles. The fibrovascular pedicles are taken as far from the prostatic base as possible. The surrounding neurovascular plexus, which contributes to volitional erection, is sacrificed both anteriorly at the prostatic apex and posteriorly at the right and left base.

In order to establish a potency-preserving prostatectomy, this periprostatic neurovascular plexus is incised in the midline and the prostate dissected from beneath this periprostatic fascia (Fig. 25–19). Conducting the dissection in this manner provides the potential for preservation of the neurovascular plexus. If a physician is concerned that there may be disease unilaterally, the periprostatic fascia may be unilaterally sacrificed. It is my custom to sacrifice the periprostatic fascia on the side of the palpable nodule of identified disease.

SUMMARY

We examined the relative impact of retropubic versus perineal prostatectomy. Between 1988 and 1989, 173 patients with organ-confined prostatic carcinoma (Stage A or B) were treated with radical prostatectomy. One hundred twenty-two patients underwent radical perineal prostatectomy (Group I) and 51 patients underwent radical retropubic prostatectomy (Group II). The estimated blood loss for Group I was 165 ml, and for Group II it was 2000 ml ($P < 0.001$) (Table 25–1).[1] Group I received a median of 0 units of blood during hospitalization, and Group II received a median of 3 units of blood ($P < 0.001$). The operative time was slightly shorter for Group I, but anesthesia time was similar for both patient populations. There was no difference in the incidence of positive surgical margins or in-hospital or long-term complication rates between the two groups (Tables 25–2 to 25–4).

Among the 122 patients in Group I, 74 were potent preoperatively. Of the 74, 22 were considered appropriate candidates for potency-preserving surgery and were so treated by preservation of either one or both neurovascular bundles. Of these 22 patients, 17, or 77 per cent, were potent postoperatively and able to have regular intercourse with vaginal penetration.

We conclude that radical perineal prostatectomy is an excellent operation for the treatment of adenocarcinoma clinically confined to the prostate. The perineal approach offers cancer control that seems to be equivalent to that of the retropubic approach and has a lesser transfusion requirement.

REFERENCE

1. Frazier HA, Robertson JE, Paulson DF: Radical prostatectomy: The pros and cons of the perineal vs. retropubic approach. J Urol 147:888–890, 1992.

Chapter 26

THE CHALLENGE OF RADIATION TREATMENT OF CARCINOMA OF THE PROSTATE

MALCOLM A. BAGSHAW

Except for skin cancer, carcinoma of the prostate is the most common malignancy in American men, having exceeded lung cancer in 1989.[2] Although not as lethal as lung or colon cancer,[3] prostatic carcinoma progresses relentlessly once it becomes symptomatic, and, by the time metastases have evolved, the median survival time is less than 2.5 years. Survival beyond 10 years after metastasis is rare[16] (Fig. 26–1). Although androgen deprivation may delay disease progression, substantial curability with hormone therapy has not been achieved. Conventional chemotherapy has had little impact on palliation, let alone cure; however, surgical extirpation can effect a cure in patients who have surgically resectable intracapsular disease.[28, 42, 51, 78, 91, 120] Radiation treatment of the primary tumor is associated also with long-term disease-free survival comparable to that achieved by total extirpation.[8, 10, 13, 14, 54, 95, 124] Long-term disease-free survival after irradiation can be correlated with the histopathologic grade, especially as determined by the Gleason score,[82] and the size and extent of the local neoplasm.[14, 19] More recently, prostate-specific antigen (PSA) levels[67] and perhaps changes in ploidy[36] have been shown to be important predictors of response to radiation of this neoplasm.

Milestones in the application of irradiation to the treatment of prostatic cancer are summarized in Table 26–1. A variety of radioactive isotopes have been applied either by intracavitary means or by direct implantation into prostatic tissue (brachytherapy). Early investigators used radium.[20, 38, 89, 90] Later, colloidal gold-198[44] and gold-198 seeds[26] were used. Permanently implanted encapsulated radioactive iodine-125[58] and palladium-103[22] (JC Blasko, personal communication) have been used, as have removable implants using iridium-192.[17, 22, 107] Prostatic cancer may also be treated by an external beam of high-energy x-rays,[15] by gamma rays from cobalt-60,[23, 37, 49] or by heavy particles, such as high-energy protons,[109] neon particles,[80] neutrons,[74] or negative pi mesons.[119]

Some of these ionizing radiations may be augmented by increasing the temperature of the target volume (hyperthermia),[17, 106] or possibly by the use of chemical

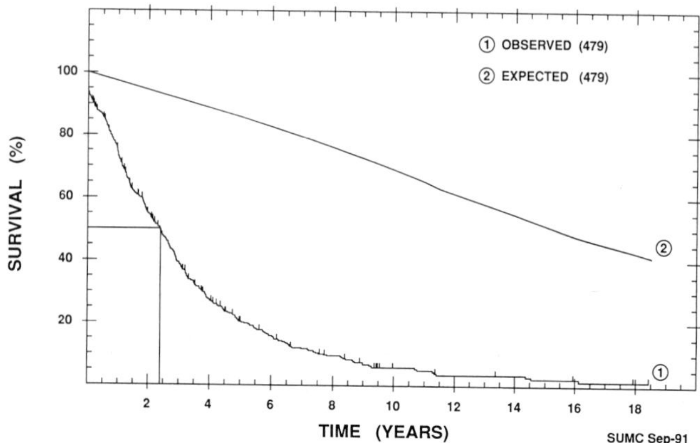

FIGURE 26–1. Survival after first evidence of metastasis of cancer of the prostate.

TABLE 26–1. MILESTONES IN THE APPLICATION OF RADIATION FOR THE TREATMENT OF PROSTATE CANCER

YEAR	AUTHORS	TREATMENT
1910	Paschkis and Tittinger[89] (Aust)	Cystoscopic radium source
1911	Pasteau[90] (Fr)	Catheter radium source
1915	Young and Fronz[123] (USA)	Various radium applications
1922	Barringer[20] (USA)	Radium needle implants
1934	Widmann[121] (USA)	Orthovoltage x-rays
1946	Hultberg[60] (Swed)	Radium teletherapy gamma rays
1952	Flocks et al[44] (USA)	Interstitial colloidal gold-198
1962	Bagshaw and Kaplan[15] (USA)	Linear accelerator x-rays
1964	Budhraja and Anderson[23] (UK)	Cobalt-60 teletherapy gamma rays
1972	Carlton et al[26] (USA)	Gold-198 seeds
1972	Hilaris et al[58] (USA)	Iodine-125 seeds
1979	Shipley et al[109] (USA)	Protons
1983	Syed et al[107] (USA)	Iridium-192
1985	Laramore et al[74] (USA)	Neutrons
1987	von Essen et al[119] (USA)	Negative pi-mesons

sensitizers, such as SR-2508, now under investigation as etanidazole.[32] High-energy x-rays and gamma rays, as well as implantable isotopes, such as radioactive gold seeds, iodine-125, colloidal gold solutions, and palladium, all produce sparsely ionizing radiations that interact in a similar way with neoplastic tissue and are assigned a relative biologic effectiveness (RBE) of 1.

Heavy-particle radiation consists of radiation beams generated by linear accelerators or cyclotrons, which produce beams of different characteristics depending upon the particle species. Protons and alpha particles, usually produced by cyclotrons, are charged nuclear fragments that can be collected by magnetic fields into beams, which may be sharply defined when penetrating tissue. This permits a more explicit control of dose distribution within the irradiated volume than can be achieved with photons from high-energy x-rays. These particles have an RBE of 1 or only slightly greater, similar to high-energy electrons, gamma rays, and x-rays. Neutrons are nuclear particles that are uncharged and cannot be focused or steered by electromagnetic fields. Therefore, the radiation dose distributions are less well controlled than those produced by protons and alpha particles. On the other hand, the neutron particle has a relatively higher RBE, thus causing more biologic damage in the target tissue per equivalent physical radiation unit. The RBE varies with a number of factors, such as relative energy and the amount of radiation delivered in a given dose (fraction size). However, for neutron beams that have been used to treat prostate cancer, the RBE is approximately 3.

Other charged nuclear particles include carbon and neon nuclei. Because of their positive charge, they can be steered by magnetic fields and are amenable to well-controlled dose distributions within the target tissue. They also share the property of a higher RBE, like the

neutrons.[80] Negative pi-mesons are lighter nuclear particles that hold a single negative charge and therefore may also be well focused within a treatment volume.[119] However, they cause a nuclear reaction within the absorbing tissue that releases a family of both high and low RBE particles and photons, which are less well confined to the target volume. The average RBE of pi-mesons is intermediate between those of high-energy photons and neutrons. In the ongoing trials at the Tri-University Meson Facility (TRIUMF) in Vancouver, British Columbia, the RBE of negative pi-mesons has been determined to be 1.5.[94]

All of these radiations have been used to treat prostate cancer, and evidence emerging from the cooperative neutron trials suggests that neutrons with the higher RBE are advantageous in increasing survival, disease-specific survival, and local control compared with high-energy x-rays of lower RBE.[73, 105] It is likely that any technique which can increase the biologic dose of radiation within the target volume without jeopardizing normal tissue will have increased effectiveness in sterilizing tumor cells. Heavy particle and neutron radiation therapies are considered experimental and are available only at a few research centers. Because of the widespread availability of the medical linear accelerator, high-energy x-irradiation is generally available and is the most common modality used today for radiation treatment of prostate cancer. Several implantable radioactive isotopes, such as gold-198, iodine-125, iridium-192, and palladium-103, also may be implanted into the prostate. However, effective exploitation of these agents depends upon skilled brachytherapists and a relatively sophisticated interstitial irradiation program.

This chapter is devoted mainly to the commonly employed application of external beam photon irradiation in the treatment of prostate cancer as exemplified by the extensive experience at Stanford University.[8, 13, 14, 16] In addition, preliminary experience with combined modality treatment using external beam x-rays, interstitial implants with iridium-192, and hyperthermia, is summarized.[17]

THE STANFORD EXPERIENCE IN THE RADIATION TREATMENT OF PROSTATIC CANCER

Although the Stanford series is described in detail, this experience is augmented with results of other studies of similar nature and scope where appropriate. The Stanford program began in 1956, at the time of the introduction of the first medical linear accelerator in the Western Hemisphere.[64] The original accelerator was operated at a nominal energy of 6 MV, and the patients were treated at a source/axis distance of 100 cm. The series should be considered contemporaneous rather than retrospective, and it continues to the present. Although the treatment program has evolved with time and techniques have improved, the radiation dose to the prostatic target volume has remained consistently at about 70 Gy (1 Gy = 100 rad).

Treatment Technique

The most widely used technique for external beam irradiation of prostate cancer employs four parallel opposed pelvic fields (pelvic box) designed to treat either the prostate only, the prostate and seminal vesicles, or the prostate, seminal vesicles, and first-echelon lymphatic drainage. Medium (6 MV) to high-energy (25 MV) linear accelerators are used. At the highest energies, some centers eliminate the lateral fields because the distribution of radiation dose from the anteroposterior (AP) and posteroanterior (PA) cross-fire tends to be homogeneous in the central region of the pelvis. Other centers maintain the lateral fields in order to protect the rectum. Still other centers[114] add oblique fields with special contouring of beam cross-sections to produce a more directly tailored "conformal" radiation pattern. The relative merits of contouring each field or extending the treatment program to include the next echelon of potential adenopathy, the para-aortic lymph nodes, are either experimental or controversial at present and beyond the scope of this presentation. A generally acceptable technique has evolved at Stanford, an abridged description of which follows. A more detailed technical exposition is presented elsewhere.[6, 7]

Patients are prepared for radiation therapy using a dedicated treatment simulator, the Ximatron (Varian Associates, Palo Alto, CA), and pelvic CT scans are performed in the treatment position, i.e., with the patient lying supine on a flat table top. The full pelvic radiation fields are opposed anterior and posterior, and right and left lateral. The radiation fields are shaped to confine the cross-section of the beam to the tumor target and to exclude vital structures, such as the anterior cortex of the pubic bone, the posterior wall of the rectum, the anus, and the anal sphincter (Fig. 26–2A and B). The anterior and posterior fields are fundamentally rectangular, with the corners trimmed to produce an octagonal shape similar to a stop sign. The lateral fields are contoured for each patient by the preparation of collimators molded from an alloy of low-melting-point Cerrobend.[103]

It is important to establish the position of the pelvic diaphragm because it determines the prostatic apex and the external sphincter. This is best demonstrated during simulation by the use of a static urethrogram.[52] After topical anesthesia is achieved with the instillation of urologic xylocaine, 50 per cent Hypaque (Winthrop Pharmaceuticals, Division of Sterling Drug, Inc., New York, NY) is instilled into the penile urethra and held in place by a Zipser clamp placed across the penis just proximal to the corona. This permits visualization of the proximal urethra, ensuring that approximately 1.5 cm of corpus urethra is included in the radiation field. Lange and Narayan[72] have emphasized that the region of the apex of the prostate, or the anastomotic site, is a frequent location for neoplastic cells, which persist after prostatectomy. Villers and associates[118] demonstrated that the perineural space serves as a conduit for neoplastic cells to penetrate the capsule at both the base and the apex of the prostate. A CT scan does not identify the prostatic apex well, but it is easily identified by the urethrogram or an MR scan. For irradiation of the prostate or the prostatic bed only, such as is the case for early postprostatectomy treatment or treatment in which there is no intention to treat all of the first-echelon lymph nodes, the inferior one half or one third of the APPA stopsign field is used. In the AP projection, this has the appearance of a keystone, with the base extending across the pelvis at the level of the acetabula (Fig. 26–3A and B). Since the mid-1970s, the lateral fields have been contoured by preparing Cerrobend collimators for each patient on an individual basis. This is a simple example of "conformal" radiation, which allows concentration of the radiation within the tumor volume and also permits a reduction in radiation to adjacent radiosensitive normal tissues.

Therefore, the radiation to the full pelvis is delivered to the four fields: anterior and posterior (stopsign technique) and left lateral and right lateral (customized collimators), taking care to treat each field every treatment day. The prostatic boost is delivered using the keystone technique for the anterior and posterior fields and the customized lateral fields, which limit irradiation to the prostate and seminal vesicles and spare the posterior wall of the rectum and the anterior cortex of the pubis. In practice, the first 26 Gy are delivered to the full four-field pelvic treatment, the next 20 Gy to the prostate and seminal vesicles only, and the final 24 Gy again to the full four-field pelvic region. This results in 70 Gy at 2 Gy per day, given over 7 weeks to the prostate and seminal vesicles, and 50 Gy at 2 Gy per day over 7 weeks to the regional adenopathy and permits a 2-week rest period at midcourse for the bowel and sigmoid colon. The key points of the technique include careful trimming of all radiation fields to minimize normal tissue exposure and confinement of the high-dose volume to the true target. It permits vital protection of the posterior wall of the rectum and anal sphincter. By applying treatment to all fields every day and inserting the prostatic boost during the middle one third of the therapy rather than at the end, the bowel is further protected by protracted fractionation of the radiation dose. It is unlikely that extending the overall time for the treatment of potentially involved lymph nodes from 50 Gy in 5 weeks to 50 Gy in 7 weeks in this technique would have a detrimental effect on the potential sterilization of lymph node metastases in the first-echelon drainage. Lai and associates[70] have recently shown that the overall treatment time for prostatic cancer does not impact on survival, survival with no evidence of disease, or local/regional control.

All patients accessioned into the study and their dispositions are accounted for in Table 26–2. Between October 1956 and December 1990, 1119 patients were treated with external beam irradiation alone. Figure 26–4 displays the distribution of age at treatment onset. The range was from 35 to 86 years, with a mean of 64.5 years and median of 65.0.

Staging

Staging by a TNM system was developed at Stanford in the early 1970s.[102] Unfortunately, many patients were

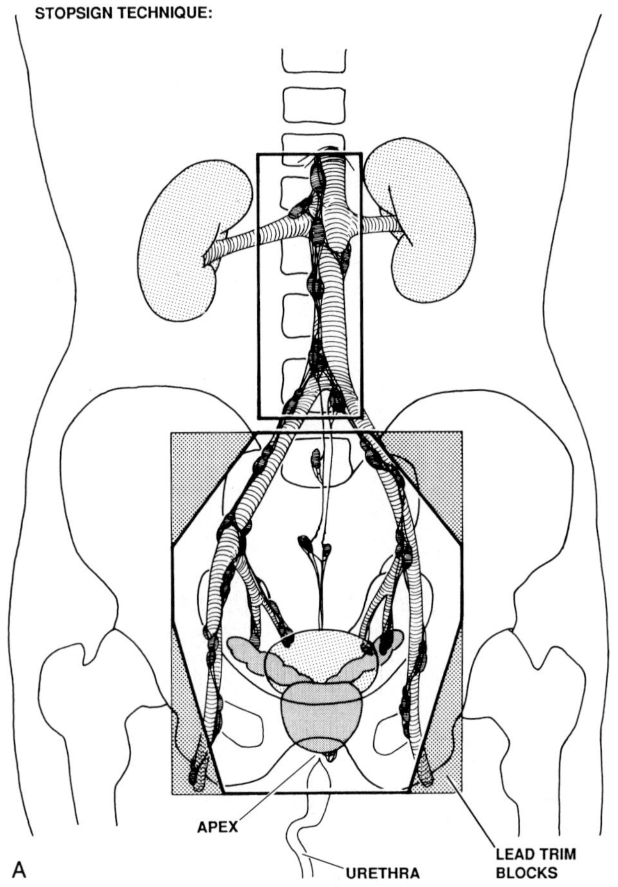

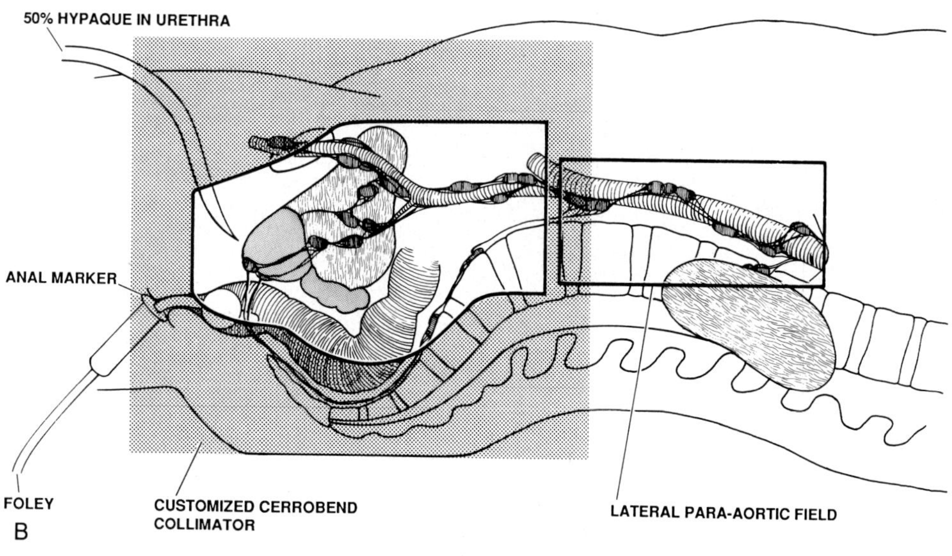

FIGURE 26–2. *A*, Diagrammatic representation of stopsign field. *B*, Diagrammatic representation of a lateral pelvic field, showing customized Cerrobend collimator. Note that the posterior wall of the rectum and the anterior cortex of the pubis are protected, and the first presacral lymph node station at S2 is within the radiation field.

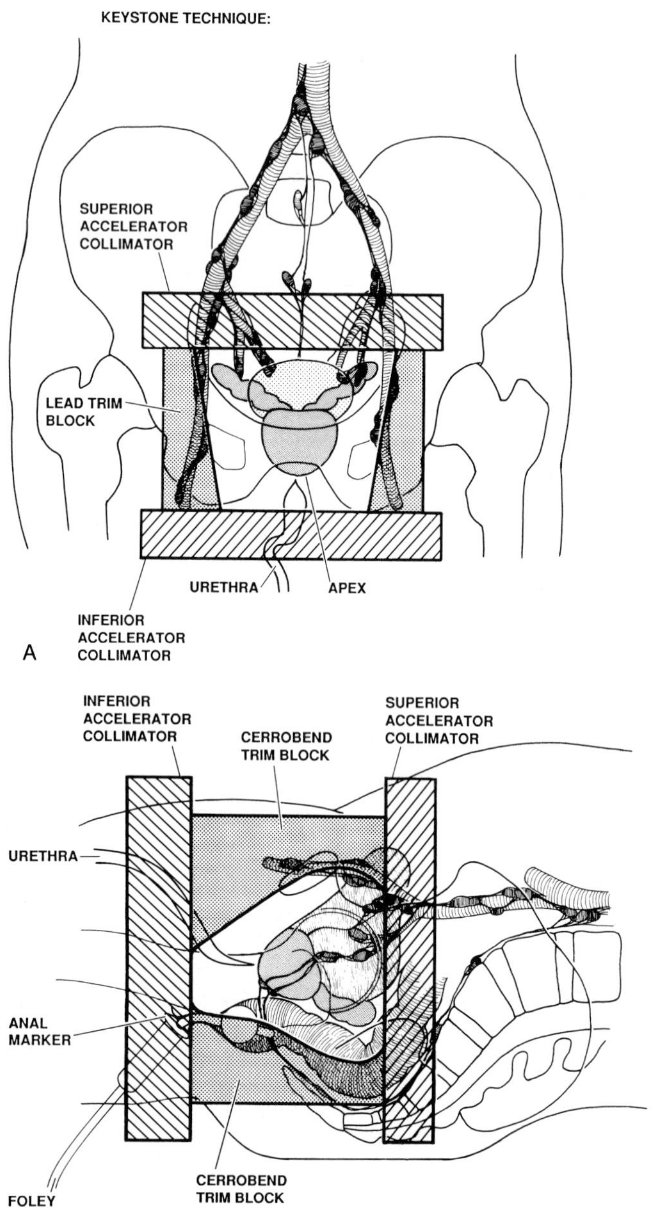

FIGURE 26–3. *A*, Diagrammatic representation of the keystone field. The superior and inferior margins of the radiation field are determined by the accelerator collimators. The left and right lateral margins are determined by lead trim blocks. The positions of the prostate and seminal vesicles are determined by a CT scan obtained in the treatment position. The diagram shows the urinary bladder to be empty; however, it is often possible to have the patient retain urine prior to the treatment so that the dome of the bladder may be protected by the superior collimator. *B*, Lateral field for the keystone technique, showing protection of the anterior pubis and posterior wall of the rectum. Note that the bladder is shown distended, and the dome of the bladder has moved behind the superior accelerator collimator.

TABLE 26–2. REFERRALS FOR TREATMENT OF PROSTATE CARCINOMA, OCTOBER 1956 TO DECEMBER 31, 1990

Total referrals		2549
Exclusions from analysis		
Consultation only	358	
Metastatic disease	716	
Subtotal		1074
Other		
Second primary tumor	91	
Prostatectomy	87	
Unusual primary tumor	6	
Questionable histology	4	
Previous irradiation	20	
Incomplete radiation therapy	24	
Implants	124	
Subtotal	356	
Total exclusions		1430
Treated by external beam radiation only		
Disease limited to prostate (Stages A and B)	= 673	
Extracapsular extension (Stage C)	= 446	
Total number of patients treated		1119

Some patients have had surgical staging of lymph nodes; however, unless otherwise indicated in the data sets, the status of the lymph nodes is considered unknown.

staged before either the Union Internationale Contre Le Cancer (UICC)[115] or the American Joint Committee TNM staging system[4] was available. The Stanford system in principle relates advancing stage to advancing tumor size and does not recognize histopathology. The histopathology is graded independently by the Gleason system.[82] Unfortunately, both the UICC and the American Joint Committee staging have undergone several alterations with time, and it has not been practical to retrospectively restage the hundreds of Stanford patients, all of whom have been staged consistently by the Stanford TNM system. Similarly, we have elected not to use the popular Urological ABC system, inasmuch as it has been defined differently at different institutions and at different times.

Currently, all patients are being staged by both the original Stanford system and by the current (1987) American Joint Committee procedure. We are hopeful that it will be possible to write a translation program to permit easy conversion and ultimately to phase out the parochial Stanford system. Meanwhile, it is necessary to relate the three systems to one another as best we can, and this relationship is presented in Table 26–3.

All patients were staged on the basis of a written description and diagram of the primary tumor as determined by digital rectal examination (DRE) at the time of the initial work-up. The staging data are reviewed and the final stage is assigned at the time of computer entry. No staging changes are permitted thereafter. The survival curves are generated from the last data entry on each patient. Approximately 75 per cent of the patients are followed at Stanford by the author. Post-treatment follow-up intervals are 1, 4, 8, and 12 months. Patients who manifest no clinical evidence of disease are followed at intervals of 6 months thereafter to 5 years, and then annually. Follow-up consists of a relevant history, an abbreviated physical examination with attention focused on the lymphatic and skeletal systems, and a DRE. Current laboratory tests include an initial complete blood count, serum prostate-specific antigen (PSA), and serum acid phosphatase determinations. Scintiscans of the skeleton are obtained prior to treatment and thereafter upon elevation of the PSA and/or for appropriate symptoms. Although 264 patients in the Stanford series have had post-therapeutic biopsies of the primary site, the determination of patient status for the series of curves described here is based upon clinical examination only, that is, DRE, and appropriate diagnostic radiographs or nuclear medicine studies. PSA is now used as a routine follow-up measure but was not available during most of the period of observation noted here. DRE is considered positive if, after an initial regression, there is progressive regrowth of tumor at the primary site or continuous growth without regression. The status of the prostate is diagrammed at each follow-up visit, and over time it is possible to chart recurrence. Patients not followed at Stanford are mailed a comprehensive questionnaire annually, and their status is updated accordingly. A similar questionnaire is also submitted to the patient's follow-up physician, and the patient's own report and the physician's report are then coordinated. Telephone follow-up is used if the questionnaires are not returned. Thus, the comprehensive computer file is continuously updated. Because of the frequent contacts with each patient, the data base is current and accurate.

Observations

The current survival for patients with incidental carcinoma of the prostate is presented in Figure 26–5.

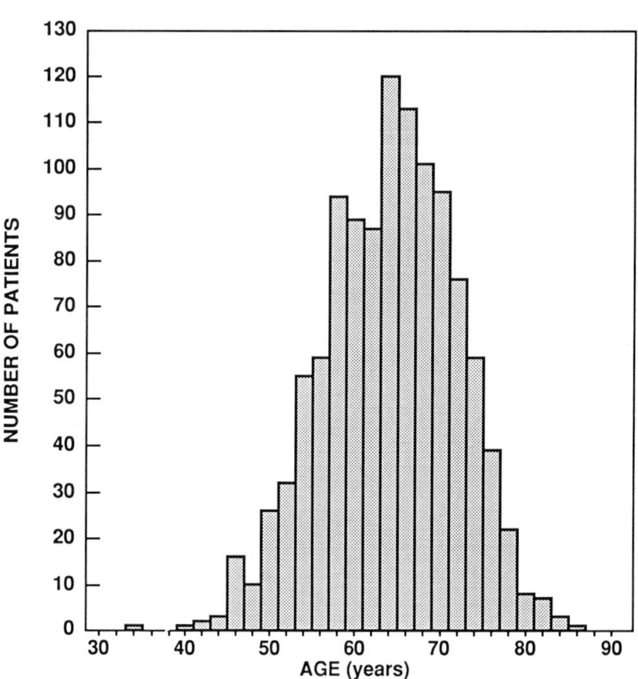

FIGURE 26–4. Distribution of patient age at the start of radiation treatment in the Stanford series of prostatic cancer. Mean age, 64.5; median age, 65.0; range, 35–86 years.

TABLE 26–3. COMPARISON OF STAGING SYSTEMS FOR PRIMARY TUMORS IN CARCINOMA OF THE PROSTATE

STANFORD STAGE	DESCRIPTION	AMERICAN JOINT COMMITTEE STAGE	DESCRIPTION	ABC
T0	Incidental carcinoma	T1	Incidental carcinoma	A1, A2
T1	Palpable tumor limited to prostate without distortion of prostatic capsule	T2	Tumor present clinically or grossly limited to gland	B
T1a	1.0-cm nodule	T2a	Tumor ≤1.5 cm in greatest dimension with normal tissue on at least three sides	B1
T1b	Nodule up to one half of lobe	T2b	Tumor >1.5 cm in greatest dimension or in more than one lobe	B1
T1c	Involvement of one entire lobe			B2
T1d	Involvement of both lobes			~B3
T2	Palpable tumor apparently limited to prostate with minimal distortion of the capsule		No comparable stage	
T2a	Palpable tumor occupying up to 50% of a lobe			
T2b	Palpable tumor occupying 50% of a lobe, multiple nodules limited to one lobe, or involvement of both lobes			
T3	Palpable tumor beyond capsule with or without seminal vesicle involvement	T3	Tumor invades into prostatic apex or into or beyond prostatic capsule, bladder neck, or seminal vesicle, but is not fixed	C1
T3a	Tumor involving <50% of a lobe			
T3b	Palpable tumor occupying >50% of a lobe, multiple nodules limited to one lobe, or involvement of both lobes			
T4	Palpable tumor extending beyond capsule with attachment to pelvic sidewall or rectal or bladder invasion	T4	Tumor is fixed or invades adjacent structures other than those listed in T3	C2

Incidental carcinoma is defined as carcinoma discovered incidentally in the specimen of patients who underwent transurethral resection of the prostate (TURP) for apparent benign hypertrophy (BPH). If less than 5 per cent of the chips contained carcinoma, they were scored as T0 focal (T0f) (A1); if 5 per cent or more of the chips were involved, they were scored as T0 diffuse (T0d) (A2). These are equivalent to the definitions of A1 and A2, as developed at Johns Hopkins University.[25] Microscopic disease is currently staged by the definition above and also by the American Joint Committee TNM system. Figure 26–5 demonstrates that survival is better for patients with T0f (A1) than for those with T0d (A2). The difference, however, is not statistically significant, and the expected survival of an age-matched cohort lies halfway between the observed survivals of patients with T0f (A1) and T0d (A2). Table 26–4 details the specific outcome for patients in each category at the time of last analysis.[66] Also, there was no significant difference between Stages T0f (A1) and T0d (A2) for disease-specific survival or for freedom from relapse. Similarly, for T0d (A2) patients, there was no difference in either survival or freedom from relapse, whether treatment was to the prostate only or to the prostate plus the pelvic lymph nodes. Patients older than 65 years tended to relapse more frequently than those less than 65 years, but the difference was not statistically significant. Gleason sums

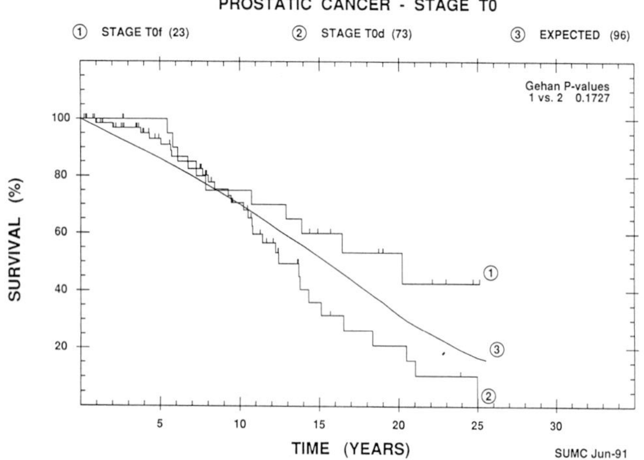

FIGURE 26–5. Survival of stage T0f (A1) and T0d (A2) patients following external beam irradiation of carcinoma of the prostate compared with the expected survival of an age-matched cohort. A downward step represents one death due to any cause. An upward tick represents a patient surviving at last follow-up, censored at the time indicated on the abscissa, and continuing in the follow-up program. The patient may or may not have residual or metastatic cancer.

TABLE 26–4. CURRENT STATUS OF ALL PATIENTS WITH STAGE T0f (A1) and T0d (A2)

	T0f		T0d		T0f		T0d	
	No.	(%)	No.	(%)	No.	(%)	No.	(%)
Alive without tumor					13	(59)	32	(49)
Alive with tumor					0	(0)	5	(8)
Intercurrent death					7	(32)	21	(32)
Without tumor	6	(27)	19	(29)				
After prior relapse	1	(5)	1	(2)				
With local tumor	0	(0)	1	(2)				
Dead with metastases					2	(9)	9	(14)
TOTAL					22		67	

were available for 55 patients. There was no difference in survival or in disease-specific survival between patients with Gleason scores of five or less and those with pattern scores greater than five. However, there was a highly significant decrease (Gehan $P=0.0000$) in the relapse rate favoring patients with Gleason scores of five or less (Fig. 26–6). This was undoubtedly due to the higher probability of early metastases to pelvic lymph nodes or distant sites in patients with the higher Gleason scores.

Figure 26–7 demonstrates the survival and disease-specific (cause-specific) survival of 383 patients who from the standpoint of stage (but not age, general condition, operability, or lymph node status) might have been considered to be candidates for radical prostatectomy. This includes all patients with incidental carcinoma (T0f, T0d, or A1 and A2), all patients with nodular disease confined to one lateral lobe (Stanford T1a, T1b, T1c), and all patients with nodular disease confined to one half of one lateral lobe (Stanford T2a) but with equivocal evidence of extracapsular extension on DRE. Figure 26–7 shows that the survival at 15 years was 47 per cent compared with 51 per cent for the expected survival of an age-matched cohort of California men.[85] The disease-specific survival was 73 per cent. Considering that the lymph node status was unknown for most of these patients and therefore was not considered in the staging process, the survival is remarkably close to that of the age-matched cohort.

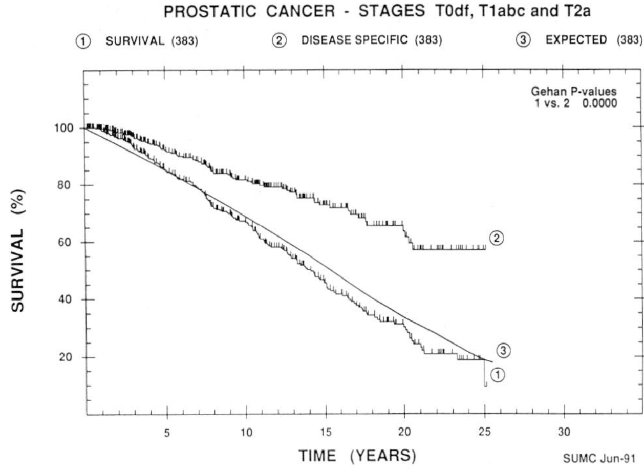

FIGURE 26–7. Survival and disease-specific survival for patients with stage T0f (A1) and T0d (A2) and nodular lesions, either apparently confined to one lobe (T1a, T1b, T1c) or confined to one lobe with distortion of the capsule (T2a), and unknown node status.

The survival status of all 1119 patients treated with external beam irradiation between 1956 and December 1990, and classified according to Stanford T stages, is presented in Figure 26–8. Patients who die of any cause are regarded as failing at the time of death; living patients are scored at the time of last follow-up and continue in the study. The significance of differences between actuarial curves was assessed by the generalized Wilcoxin test of Gehan.[48] The P values are presented with each data set.

Note that patients with Stanford T0 match the expected survival of an age-matched cohort and that, as might be expected, the survival systematically diminishes with advancing stage. The survival parameters for the several categories at 15 years are summarized in Table 26–5.

PROSTATIC CANCER - STAGE A

① **Gleason Score <= 5 (39)**

② **Gleason Score >= 6 (20)**

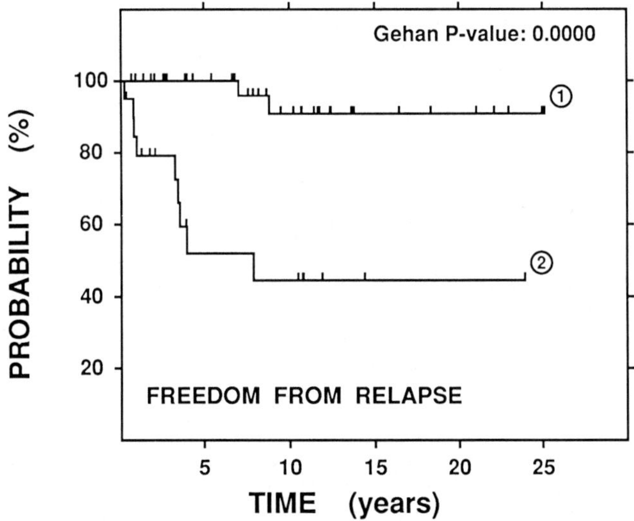

FIGURE 26–6. Freedom from relapse. A downward step indicates first evidence of recurrence, either at the primary site or at a metastatic site, as detected by either clinical observation or a positive biopsy. An upward tick represents a patient who was either observed to be disease free or died disease free at the time of last observation. Lymph node status is unknown.

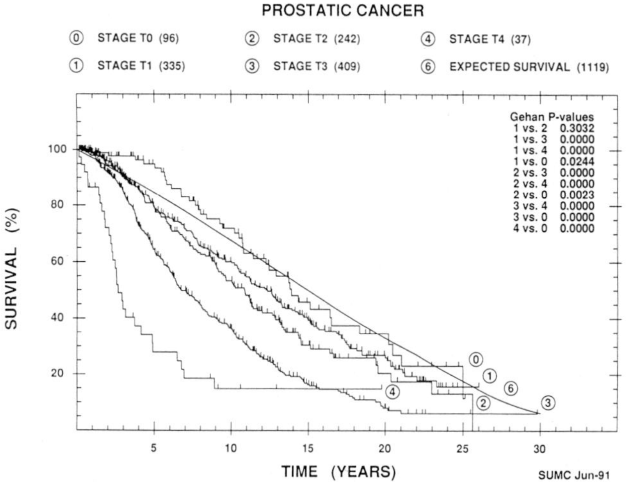

FIGURE 26–8. Survival curves as a function of clinical stage. A downward step represents death from any cause; an upward tick represents a patient surviving at last follow-up and censored at the time indicated on the abscissa. Patient may or may not have residual or metastatic cancer. Numbers in parentheses are the numbers of patients in each group. Nominal stage equivalents are as follows: T0 = A, T1 = B1 and B2, T2 = B3, T3 = C1, T4 = C2.

TABLE 26–5. PERCENTAGE OF PATIENTS SUCCEEDING* 15 YEARS AFTER TREATMENT FOR VARIOUS END-POINTS

END-POINTS	STAGE				
	T0	T1	T2	T3	T4
Survival	46	40	30	18	15
Disease-specific survival	84	66	46	30	26
Freedom from any relapse	75	46	28	18	16
Freedom from distant relapse	80	60	45	30	15
Clinical local control	93	65	49	47	72

*By Kaplan-Meier calculation. Refer to Table 26–3 for staging correlation.

The disease-specific (cause-specific) survival for all Stanford T stages is presented in Figure 26–9. Disease-specific survival for broader categories, that is, disease limited to the prostate or extracapsular extension, has been presented previously,[12] and more recently for patients staged according to the Stanford T categories.[13, 14] The curves presented here are updates for all patients entered through December 1990 and followed through June 1991.

Disease-specific survival is also termed cause-specific survival. In discussing the merits of using cause-specific survival to evaluate the outcome following various treatment modalities in prostate cancer, Lepor and associates[77] drew attention to the Stanford study[12] in which disease-specific survival for all patients with disease limited to the prostate was reported. One problem in using the Stanford data set for comparison with patients treated at Johns Hopkins is that the Stanford data included all patients with disease limited to the prostate, and this group of patients had more advanced tumor stages than the Johns Hopkins cohort of patients, which had been reported earlier by Walsh and Jewett.[120] The Hopkins cases were described as "B1" and defined as ". . . including palpable induration involving *less than* one lobe of the prostate." The Stanford patients also

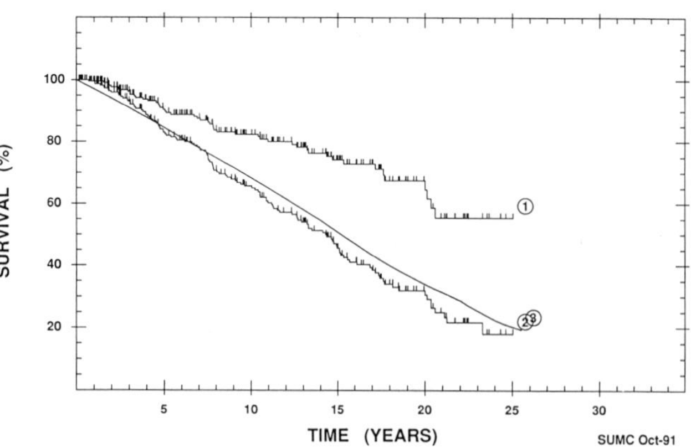

FIGURE 26–10. Disease- or cause-specific survival and all-cause survival for patients with nodular carcinoma of the prostate confined up to one entire lobe.

included all of the stage A patients, i.e., those with incidental carcinoma, both focal and diffuse, plus nodular lesions of 1 cm, nodular lesions occupying up to one half of one lobe, and nodular lesions involving an *entire lobe* of the prostate, or *both lobes* of the prostate.

Figure 26–10 demonstrates the current cause-specific survival for the 240 patients in the Stanford series with nodular disease in three categories: nodules 1 cm or less (Stanford T1a); nodules equal to one half of one lobe (Stanford T1b); and nodular disease involving an entire lobe (Stanford T1c). These patients are similar to those described by Lepor and associates[77] but still include some that are slightly more advanced, i.e., those with up to one lobe of involvement rather than those with involvement of "less than one lobe of the prostate." If one considers that 13 of the original 70 Hopkins patients were lost to follow-up, that diagnostic radiographs rather than nuclear scintiscans were used to evaluate the presence of bone metastases, and that there was no rigorous protocol, such as postmortem examination, for the determination of the cause of death, it seems unlikely that there is a significant difference in outcome between the two studies. Lepor and associates[77] made the point that the survival has plateaued beyond the 15th year in the Hopkins study, whereas they asserted that not to be the case in the Stanford study. However, that assertion was incorrect. There was one cause-specific death at the 18th or 19th year in each series,[12, 77] and although there have been a few more deaths attributed to prostate cancer in the current update of the Stanford series (Fig. 26–10), there are more than four times as many patients as in the older Hopkins data. Given the uncertainties of small numbers, extended periods of time, and differences in staging, we agree with Lepor's conclusion that these retrospective analyses have not resolved the controversy regarding the optimal management of localized prostatic cancer. Cause-specific survival may be a better end-point than survival for a comparison of treatment groups; however, more rigorous criteria for determining

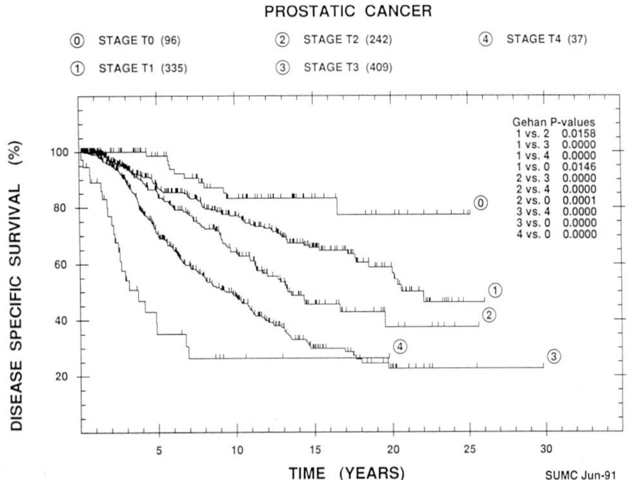

FIGURE 26–9. Disease- or cause-specific survival. A downward step indicates death from prostate cancer; an upward tick represents a patient who either died of intercurrent disease without evidence of prostatic cancer or was alive at the time of last follow-up; patient may or may not have had cancer at that time.

the cause of death, such as the requirement for a postmortem examination, than those found in most retrospective studies seems to be necessary. Today, PSA values may offer a better, or at least a supplementary, way to track the activity of prostatic cancer.

The clearest distinction between the staging grouping in the Stanford study is provided by tracking freedom from relapse (FFR), as presented in Figure 26–11, and freedom from distant relapse in Figure 26–12.

Clinical local control is presented in Figure 26–13. Inspection of Figure 26–13 shows a paradox, in that clinical local control appears better for the most advanced Stanford T4 lesions than for the Stanford T2 and Stanford T3 tumors. This is undoubtedly due to the small number of cases (37) and the aggressive nature of T4 disease, which terminates some patients secondary to the metastatic process before enough time has elapsed to manifest local recurrence.

In Figure 26–14, a semilogarithmic plot of FFR is presented. A dashed straight line has been drawn from the 100 per cent FFR point through the point representing FFR at 5 years for each clinical stage. These lines represent a constant risk of relapse equal to the average risk observed during the first 5 years of follow-up. It can be seen that the observed FFR curves bend upward relative to the straight lines, indicating that the risk of relapse decreases with time and that as the curves plateau, a cured subpopulation may exist in the groups for clinical stages T0 to T3. In Figure 26–15, the patients are grouped according to the sums of the Gleason pattern scores. A statistical comparison between the groups showed that the widest differences occurred when the Gleason sums were segregated as follows: 2, 3, 4, 5; 6; 7; 8, 9, 10. In an independent multifactorial analysis, the Gleason sum was the most powerful predictor of outcome, followed by clinical stage. Age was not significant.

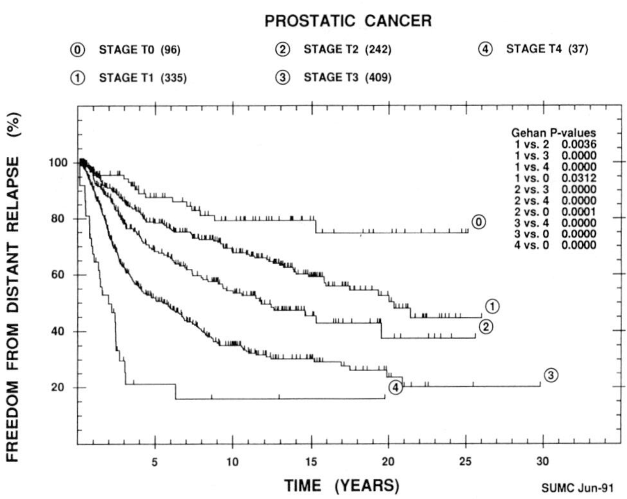

FIGURE 26–12. **Freedom from distant relapse.** A downward step indicates the first evidence of recurrence at a metastatic site as detected by clinical observation, including roentgenograms or scintigrams, or a positive biopsy. An upward tick represents a patient who was either observed to be disease free or died after being disease free at the time of last observation.

The Gleason pattern score is also important as a predictor of lymph node involvement. Pistenma and associates[102] correlated the incidence of lymph node involvement in a series of patients who had lymph nodes examined at the time of pelvic laparotomy. This distribution of lymph node involvement as a function of the Gleason pattern score was observed by several authors.[10] The observations reported can be reduced to a simple formula: The Gleason sum minus 4, times 15 = the percentage probability of pelvic lymph node involvement.[122] Unfortunately, lymph node involvement is associated with a marked decrease in survival (Fig. 26–

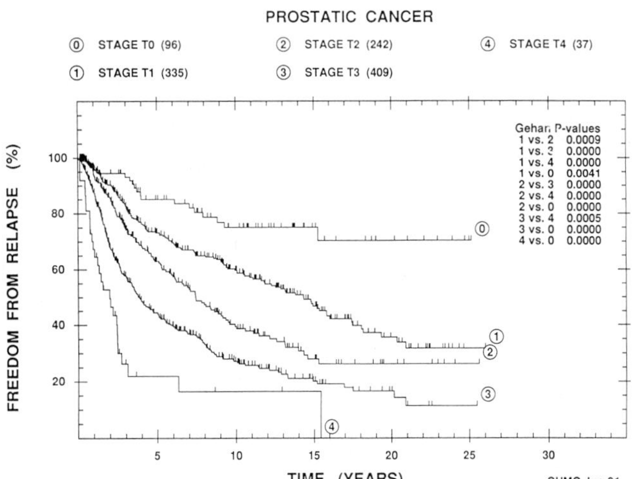

FIGURE 26–11. **Freedom from relapse.** A downward step indicates the first evidence of recurrence, either at the primary site or at a metastatic site as detected by clinical observation or a positive biopsy. An upward tick represents a patient who was either observed to be disease free or died after being disease free at the time of last observation.

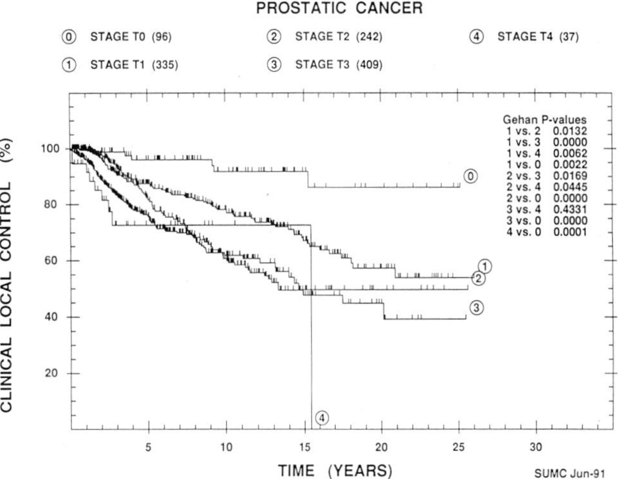

FIGURE 26–13. **Time course of local control.** A downward step indicates clinical evidence of local regrowth after initial regression of tumor or after an initial showing of no evidence of local neoplasm. An upward tick represents a patient who either demonstrated no clinical evidence of local tumor at last follow-up or died without clinical evidence of local neoplasm. Patient could have had evidence of metastatic tumor either while living or at death. Local control is paradoxically high for Stage T4 because many patients die of metastatic disease before lack of local control is manifest.

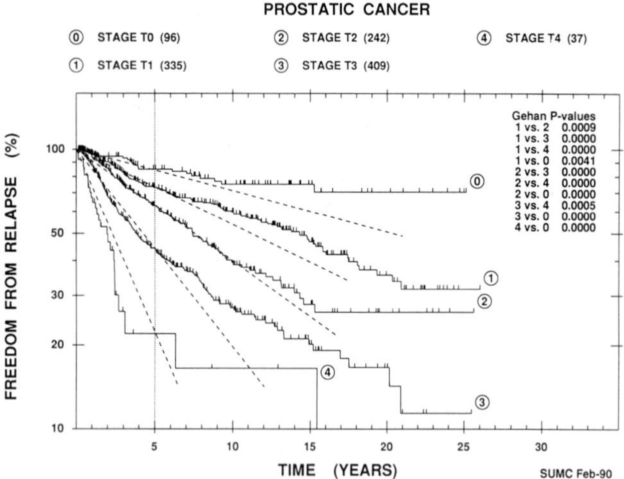

FIGURE 26–14. The logarithm of freedom from relapse as a function of primary tumor stage. The dashed lines represent a risk of relapse equal to the average risk observed during the first 5 years after radiation treatment. The upward-bending curves for each stage indicate that the risk of relapse decreases with time, and a cured subpopulation may exist in each stage except T4.

16), even in the face of radiation treatment to the first-echelon adenopathy.[11]

Similar overall survival patterns following irradiation in prostatic cancer have been observed at other centers. Several large series have been carefully followed over long periods, and these are generally in agreement with the Stanford data. These include the series from Mallinckrodt Institute of Radiology at Washington University School of Medicine[93] and the subsequent contribution, which details factors that influence the outcome of definitive radiation therapy for carcinoma of the prostate.[92] Prognostic factors in carcinoma of the prostate are analyzed for the Radiation Therapy Oncology Group (RTOG).[98] Another large single institution study has been reported from the M. D. Anderson Hospital and Tumor Institute.[124, 125] Allain and associates[1] reported

the combined experience of a consortium of French radiation therapy centers. The extensive data base generated by the Patterns of Care study (PCS) in the United States puts the general experience in the United States in perspective.[54, 56, 57, 76]

Hanks[54] has recently summarized data from the PCS (Fig. 26–17) and several RTOG trials. Notably, patients with relatively low tumor stage and negative lymph nodes demonstrate survival patterns indistinguishable from the expected survival of age-matched peer groups (Figs. 26–18 and 26–19). Figure 26–20 shows a remarkably similar outcome for patients with potentially resectable carcinoma of the prostate, even though the series were compiled at different institutions at different times and the patients were treated by different methods.[14] According to Hanks, surgery and radiation therapy appear to be equivalent in the treatment of low-volume T2a (stage B1) low-grade prostate cancer; and there is no evidence to suggest that surgical results at 10, 15, or 20 years after treatment of T2b (B2) prostate cancer approached those obtained with radiation in comparable patients. A summary of results from several institutions after irradiation for patients with stage C (T3 or T4) is given in Table 26–6.

Adjuvant Treatment

Because local control decreases with advancing stage and positive biopsies are common after radiation treatment, ways to increase the efficacy of prostatic irradiation have been investigated. One way might be to increase the RBE by using particle beams of a higher RBE.[74, 80, 94, 105, 119] Another way might be the use of radiation sensitizers, and these are now entering clinical trials.[32] Another way might be to increase the efficacy of the irradiation by supplementing it with concomitant or nearly concomitant hyperthermia. The prostate may

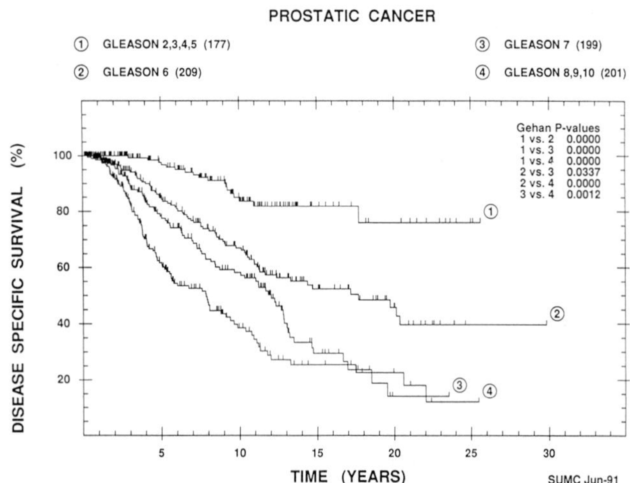

FIGURE 26–15. Disease- or cause-specific survival as a function of the sums of the Gleason pattern scores. Statistical analysis demonstrates that four distinct patterns of survival can be identified by grouping the Gleason sums as illustrated.

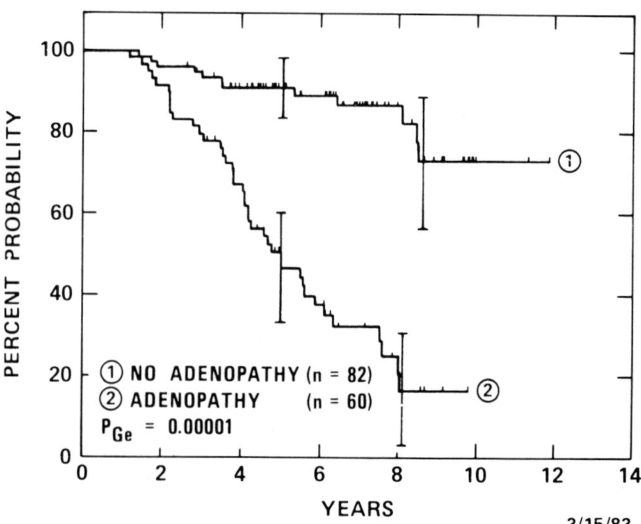

FIGURE 26–16. Influence of adenopathy on survival. The powerful difference in survival between patients with normal lymph nodes (curve 1) and those with adenopathy (curve 2) as established by surgical staging is demonstrated.

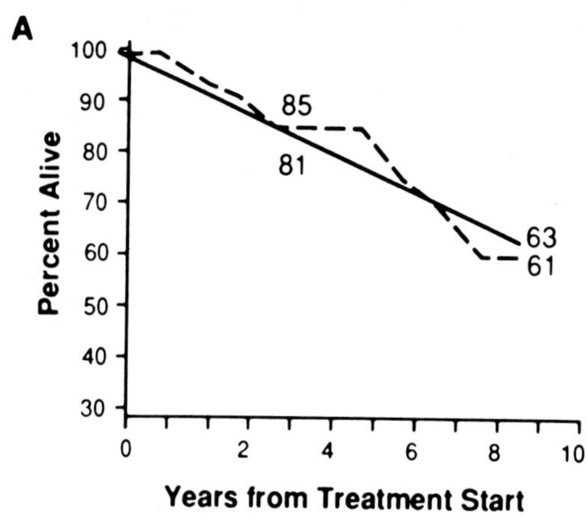

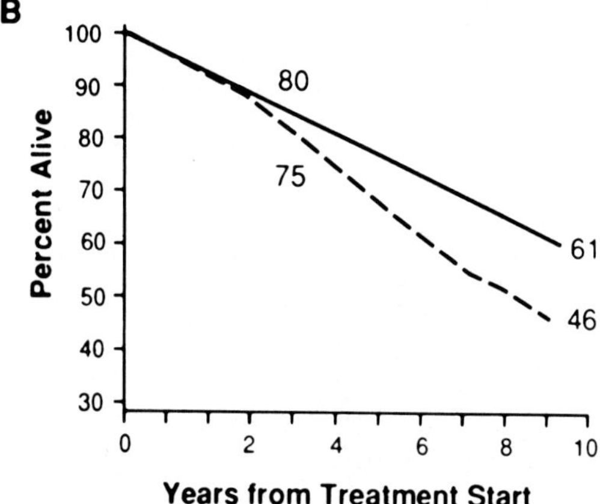

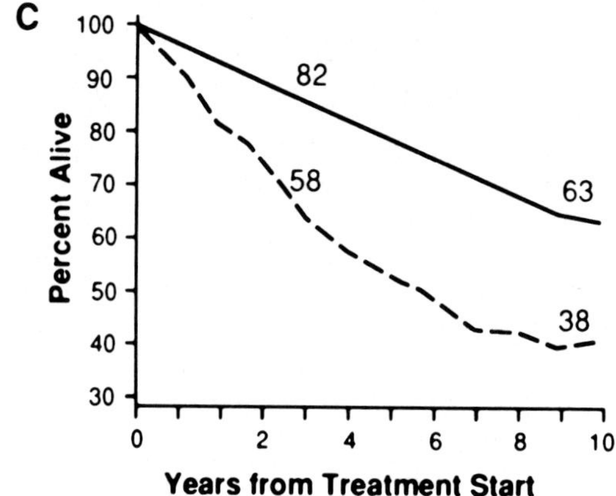

FIGURE 26–17. US national averages for survival (treated 1973, 1974). *A*, Stage A patients. *B*, Stage B patients. *C*, Stage C patients. Solid line = expected survival; dashed line = observed survival. (From Hanks GE: Radiotherapy or surgery for prostate cancer? Ten- and fifteen-year results of external beam therapy. Acta Oncol 30:231, 1991; with permission.)

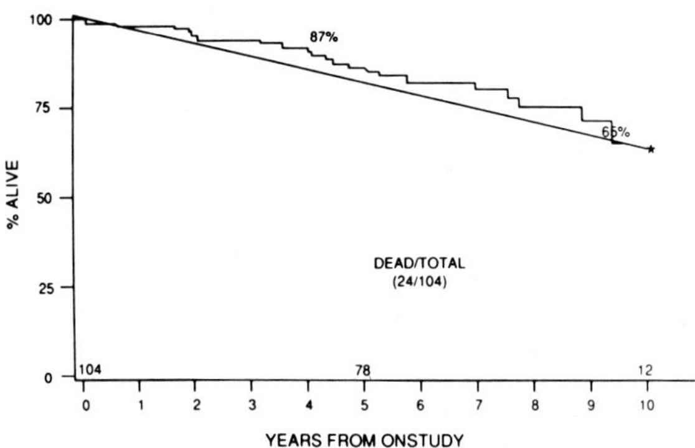

FIGURE 26–18. Survival of node-negative Stage A2, B patients after radiation therapy (RTOG 7706). Patients with laparotomy and normal SAP. * = Age-matched expected survival. (From Hanks GE: Radiotherapy or surgery for prostate cancer? Ten- and fifteen-year results of external beam therapy. Acta Oncol 30:231, 1991; with permission.)

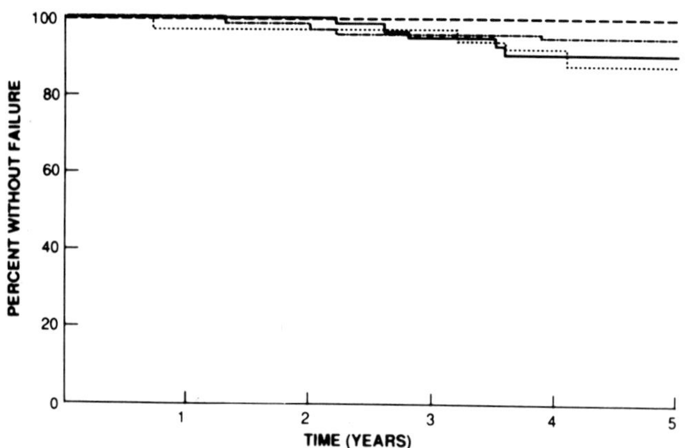

FIGURE 26–19. Any failure analysis for node-negative Stage A2, B patients. Solid line = Stanford (n = 51); dashed line = Mallinckrodt (n = 140); dashed-dotted line = RTOG (n = 104); dotted line = PCS (n = 37). (From Hanks GE: Radiotherapy or surgery for prostate cancer? Ten and fifteen-year results of external beam therapy. Acta Oncol 30:231, 1991; with permission.)

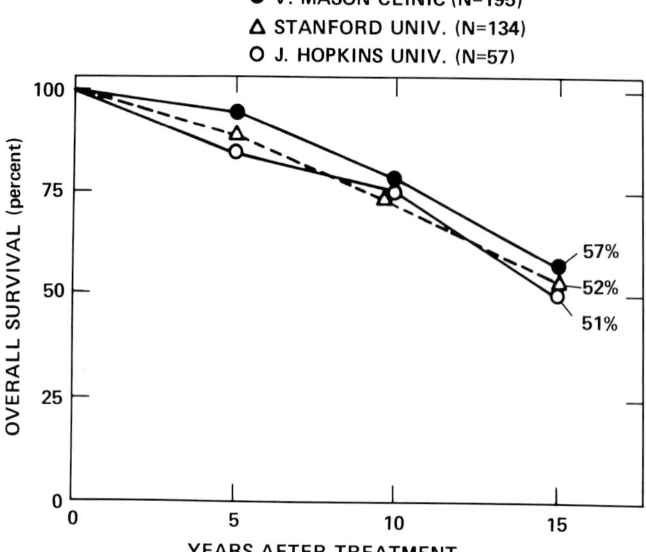

FIGURE 26–20. Comparison of long-term survival of patients in stage T2a (B1) treated by radiation therapy in the Stanford University series (134 patients; *open triangles*) and those treated by radical prostatectomy in the series at The Johns Hopkins Hospital (57 patients; *open circles*) and Virginia Mason Medical Center (195 patients; *solid circles*) according to a personal communication (WU Shipley).

be rendered homogeneously hyperthermic by the use of interstitial probes that deliver either radiofrequency or microwave radiation. An integrated system has been developed at Stanford which permits irradiation of the prostate with a removable iridium-192 interstitial implant and an appliance to elevate the temperature of the prostate to therapeutic temperatures, between 42.5 and 45.5°C. In this system, the trochars, which are inserted through the perineal skin and afterloaded with iridium-192 for the interstitial irradiation, can also be used as antennae for the application of radiofrequency power at 0.5 MHz. For this procedure, originally the prostate was exposed by a suprapubic incision. Now the trochars are inserted through a perineal template under ultrasound guidance. The template guarantees appropriate geometric spacing (Fig. 26–21). Upon recovery from anesthesia, the patient is transferred to the hyperthermia suite, where the trochars are energized at 0.5 MHz for 45 minutes, yielding a homogeneous temperature throughout the prostate of between 42.5 and 45.5°C. At the conclusion of the hyperthermia treatment, the trochars are loaded with a preplanned distri-

bution of iridium-192 which, during the next approximately 60 hours, homogeneously irradiates the prostate to a dose of 30 Gy (Fig. 26–22). In this technique, the patient has already received 50 Gy by external beam irradiation which has been delivered over a period of 5 weeks at the rate of 2 Gy per day. Following interstitial irradiation to the prescribed dose, the patient is returned to the hyperthermia suite where the iridium-192 sources are removed and the trochars are again connected to the 0.5 MHz radiofrequency source and energized. A second heating sequence is performed, again elevating the temperature of the prostate to 42.5 to 45.5°C for 45 minutes. Following this, the treatment is terminated and

TABLE 26–6. PROSTATE CANCER, STAGE C (T3 OR T4)

CENTER	NO.	5 YEARS		10 YEARS		15 YEARS	
		S	FFR	S	FFR	S	FFR
Stanford							
T3	348	64%	46%	35%	28%	18%	23%
T4	32	27%	17%	12%	17%	—	—
MD Anderson			DFS		DFS		DFS
Stage C	551	72%	59%	47%	45%	27%	40%
			NED		NED		
Washington University	328	65%	53%	35%	32%		
			NEDS		NEDS		
US national averages							
1973	296	58%	39%	38%	28%		
1978	237	65%	50%				

Abbreviations: S = survival; FFR = freedom from relapse; DFS = disease-free survival; NED = no evidence of disease; NEDS = no evidence of disease survival.
From Hanks GE: Radiotherapy or surgery for prostate cancer? Ten- and fifteen-year results of external beam therapy. Acta Oncol 30:231, 1991; with permission.

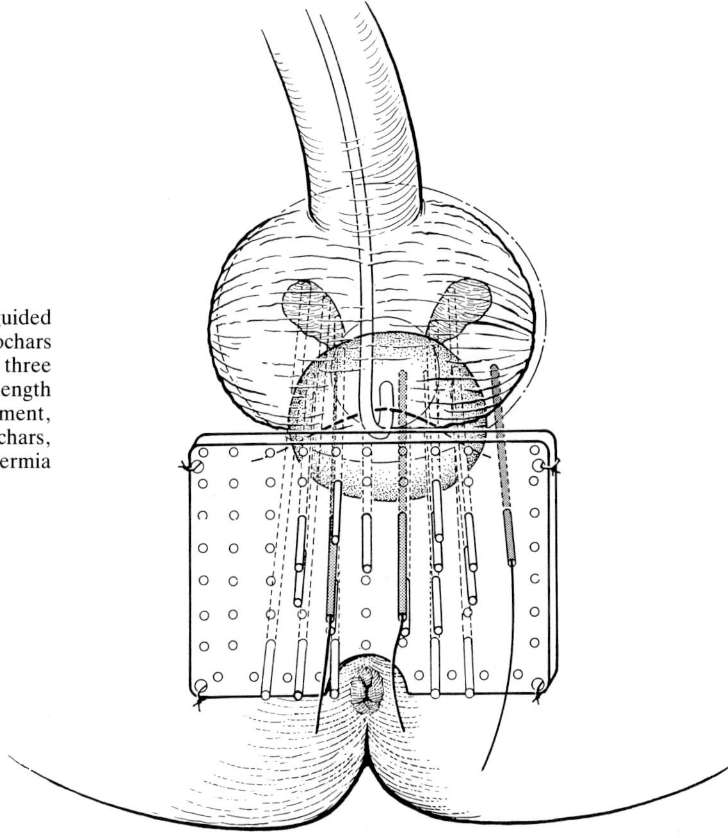

FIGURE 26–21. Diagrammatic representation of template-guided transperineal interstitial implant of the prostate. Note that trochars may extend through the prostate into the seminal vesicles. The three stippled trochars are used to measure the temperature along the length of the trochar. During the hyperthermia phase of the treatment, temperature detectors are placed in each of the metallic trochars, which also carry the radiofrequency current for the hyperthermia treatment.

the trochars are removed. Thus, the patient receives 5 weeks of external beam radiation, which delivers 50 Gy at the rate of 2 Gy per day, a 2- to 3-week rest period, followed by the interstitial implant which delivers an additional 30 Gy to the entire prostatic volume in a period of about 60 hours, plus two hyperthermia treatments. The procedure has been carried out in 16 patients; however, follow-up is too short to comment upon overall results. Basically, the technique accomplishes a higher dose to the prostate than can be delivered by

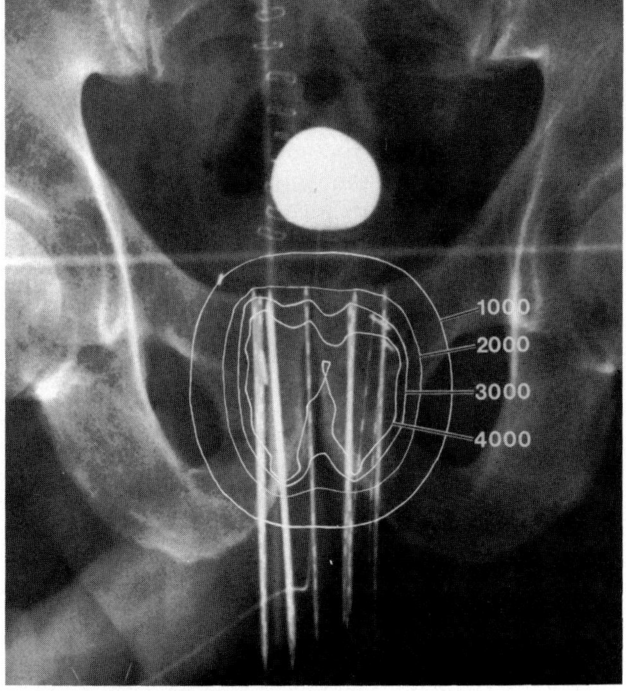

FIGURE 26–22. Localization film showing the transperineal trochars in place within the prostate. The isodose surfaces have been calculated, and the surface that surrounds the ^{192}Ir sources and encompasses the prostate received at least 3000 rad.

external beam irradiation alone, i.e., 50 Gy in 20 fractions in 5 weeks plus 30 Gy interstitial gamma radiation in about 60 hours versus 70 Gy in 35 fractions in 7 weeks. It also employs hyperthermia, adjuvant to the interstitial irradiation, which should add to the biologic effectiveness of the radiation treatments.

PROSTATE-SPECIFIC ANTIGEN AND RADIATION THERAPY

PSA has been shown to be a reliable marker of prostatic cancer activity under certain conditions. PSA is synthesized in prostatic tissue only, and therefore elevated serum PSA levels are found not only in patients with adenocarcinoma but also in those with prostatic hypertrophy or after DRE.[112] The level of serum PSA is also correlated with tumor burden.[59, 87, 111] However, PSA values cannot be used with certainty to distinguish between disease that is localized to the prostate and more extensive disease. Extreme elevations may indicate lymph node or bone metastases at presentation.[111] Two studies have suggested that normalization of the PSA after radiation therapy predicts tumor contol.[41, 71] In a group of 45 patients who received primary external beam radiation therapy for localized prostatic cancer (without hormonal therapy), the post-treatment trend of the PSA predicted the risk for the development of metastases.[67] Patients with a single rise in the PSA level greater than 120 per cent of the previous determination and out of the normal range were at intermediate risk. Two of six patients at intermediate risk developed distant metastases. Two consecutive rising PSA values at intervals of at least 3 months or greater, totaling more than 120 per cent of the nadir value and out of the normal range, placed the patient at high risk. Four of nine high-risk patients relapsed with distant metastases. In patients with a declining PSA, local or distant failure was not observed (0 of 28 patients). Consequently, bone scintiscans are not performed routinely but rather only on the escalation of the PSA or if indicated symptomatically.[67, 87] The kinetics of the decline of PSA after radiation therapy is much more gradual than after androgen deprivation treatment. PSA levels tended to decline over several months to years after radiation therapy, whereas after androgen ablation, the PSA declines rapidly.[67] This finding suggests that PSA synthesis is androgen dependent. Studies on human prostate carcinomas grown in nude mice confirm this observation: The rate of decline of PSA after castration is greater than the rate of tumor regression.[33] The ability of prostate carcinoma cells to constitutively express PSA may be a marker for hormonal resistance.[110]

RADIATION THERAPY FOLLOWING RADICAL PROSTATECTOMY

With the advent of the nerve-sparing radical prostatectomy, surgical treatment of prostatic cancer has become more common.[28, 42] Generally, nerve-sparing prostatectomy is advocated only when DRE or ultrasound examination indicates that the cancer is confined to the prostate.

However, in spite of serious efforts to resect tumors confined to the prostate, the incidence of pathologic upstaging after prostatectomy ranges widely and averages about 40 per cent (Table 26–7). The table also demonstrates that among the authors who reported long-term follow-up on upstaged patients, there was at least a 50 per cent decrease in survival compared with patients with tumors truly confined within the capsule. Moreover, for the three decades between 1953 and 1984, there was little improvement in the accuracy of preoperative staging. Post-prostatectomy radiation therapy has been shown to reduce the rate of local recurrence (Table 26–8). The impact of the improvement in local control with postoperative radiation on patient survival is difficult to ascertain, but perhaps not enough time has elapsed to establish its efficacy. Gibbons and associates[50] and Anscher and Prosnitz[5] have demonstrated a trend toward improved survival with post–radical prostatectomy radiation therapy. Furthermore, lack of local control is associated with the subsequent development of distant metastases.[47] However, if microscopic dissemination has occurred prior to treatment, improvement in local control would have no effect on the development of metastatic disease. If residual carcinoma is limited only to the surgical bed, post-prostatectomy radiation therapy has the potential to eliminate all remaining carcinoma. The efficacy of post-prostatectomy radiation therapy in patients with positive margins is currently being tested in a national intergroup protocol.

By using serial PSA determinations, the risk of developing a recurrence after post-prostatectomy irradiation can be determined. Patients treated with radiation therapy after prostatectomy, with a rising PSA, are at a high risk, and those with undetectable or falling levels of the tumor marker are at low risk.[65] In a group of 39 patients treated with radiation therapy after prostatectomy, 37 had detectable levels of PSA prior to irradiation. Follow-up ranged from 2 to 74 months, with a mean of 26.8 months. Eighteen patients demonstrated a rising PSA; nine of these patients have developed distant metastatic disease. In 17 patients, the PSA fell to and remained undetectable (with a minimum of 1 year follow-up). None of these patients has developed local recurrence or metastatic disease.[65]

PRE-EMPTIVE IRRADIATION

In the mid-1970s, it was observed that bone metastases from prostatic cancer occurred less commonly in bone that had been previously irradiated. In an analysis of 71 patients who had received para-aortic lymph node irradiation that coincidentally included the lumbar spine, and another group of 65 patients who received no lumbar irradiation but did receive pelvic irradiation only, the group that received incidental lumbar irradiation had a significantly lower rate and longer delay in the development of lumbar metastases[68] (Fig. 26–23). This observation has been corroborated recently.[62]

TABLE 26–7. PROSTATIC CANCER PREOPERATIVE UNDERSTAGING: CARCINOMA CONSIDERED CONFINED TO THE PROSTATE PRIOR TO RADICAL PROSTATECTOMY

YEAR	AUTHORS	CLINICAL STAGE	PATHOLOGIC CAPSULAR OR EXTRACAPSULAR DISEASE	No.	%	SEMINAL VESICLE INVASION (%)	IMPACT ON SURVIVAL AT	DECREASE From	To
1953	Colby[31]		25		71	36	5 years	52%	27%
1957	Turner and Belt[116]				45	—			—
1963	Vickery and Kerr[117]		—			47			—
1968	Culp[34] 1.5 cm	B1	Exceeded expectation		44	8			—
1972	Byar and Mostofi[24]				11	12	5 years	58%	33%
1974	Dahl et al[35]				22	—			—
1977	DeVere White et al[39]				29	—			—
1977	Boxer et al[21]				29	—	10 years	62%	29%
1980	Walsh and Jewett[120]	B1				16			
		B2				49	15 years	51%	5%
1982	Elder et al[43]	B2	Extracapsular		66	at least 13	15 years	50%	13%
1982	Catalona and Bigg[28]	A2	Extracapsular		11	—	5 pts. early		
		B1	Extracapsular		17	—	failure		
		B2	Extracapsular		39	—	Follow-up short		
			Overall		24	—	No data		—
1982	Middleton and Smith[83] node neg	B2			12	4			—
1983	Lange and Narayan[72]	A2 (6)	Extracapsular	(3)		3	Not stated		
		B1 (32)	Extracapsular	(25)	68	5	Used radiation therapy		
		B2 (25)	Extracapsular	(15)		9			
1984	Gibbons et al[51]	B			25	—			—

Adapted from Bagshaw MA, Cox RS, Ray GR: Status of radiation treatment of prostate cancer at Stanford University. NCI Monogr 7:47, 1988; with permission.

TABLE 26–8. RADIATION DOSE, LOCAL CONTROL, AND DISEASE-FREE SURVIVAL FOR PROSTATE PATIENTS TREATED WITH IRRADIATION FOLLOWING INCOMPLETE SURGICAL RESECTION

AUTHORS	NO. OF PTS.	DOSE/RAD	LOCAL CONTROL	DFS
Hanks and Dawson (1986)[55]	10	6000–7332	100% at 5 yrs	86% at 5 yrs
Pilepich and Walz (1983)[101]	27	6000–7000	96% mean follow-up 6 yrs	63% mean follow-up 6 yrs
Forman et al (1989)[45]	16	6500	100% at 5 yrs	91% at 5 yrs
Shevlin et al (1989)[108]	16	4500–7200	100% at 10 yrs	64% at 10 yrs
Ray et al (1984)[104]	13	7000	77% at 10 yrs	57% at 10 yrs
			Mean follow-up—5 yrs	
Carter et al (1989)[27]	31	4500–5500	97%	94%
			Mean follow-up—9.2 yrs	
Gibbons et al (1986)[50]	23	No XRT	70%	65%
	22	4900–7020	95%	77%
Jacobson et al (1987)[61]	24	No XRT	83% at 5 yrs	70% at 5 yrs
	26	5400–7000	100% at 5 yrs	69% at 5 yrs
Anscher and Prosnitz (1987)[5]	159	No XRT	32% at 15 yrs	28% at 15 yrs
	46	500–6500	96% at 15 yrs	40% at 15 yrs

DFS = Disease-free survival; XRT = radiation therapy.
Adapted from Kaplan ID, Bagshaw MA: Serum prostate-specific antigen after post-prostatectomy radiotherapy. Urology, 39:401, 1992.

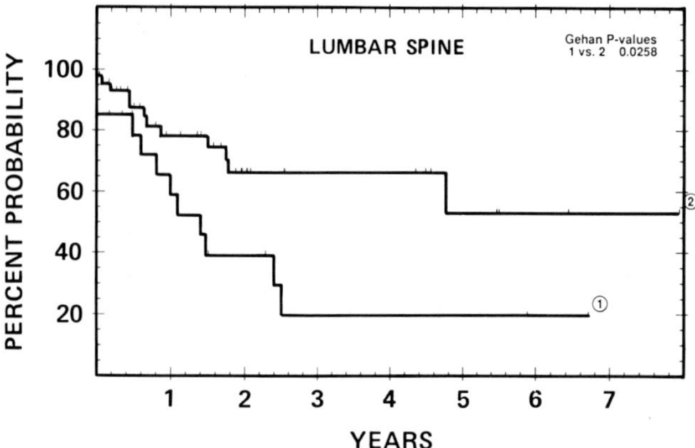

FIGURE 26–23. The actuarial freedom from metastases after the first evidence of recurrent disease, using the actuarial method of Kaplan and Meier (1958). Curve 1 represents patients receiving radiation to the pelvic and para-aortic regions. A statistically significant reduction in the incidence of metastatic involvement in the lumbar field was demonstrated among patients receiving extended field irradiation.

The mechanism by which prior irradiation reduces the subsequent development of metastases remains speculative. Radiation may either eradicate the "seed" (subclinical bone metastases) or alter the "soil" (the endothelial vascular matrix), or both, in order to prevent subsequent bone metastases.[88] On the basis of these observations, several patients with minimal metastatic disease have received pre-emptive total spinal irradiation. Progressive symptomatic lesions in the irradiated fields have been rare. The recent observation that patients with minimal metastases to bone have a significantly longer survival than those with more advanced metastases[69] supports the notion that early or pre-emptive irradiation of bone metastases executed before there has been structural damage or significant pain may be more efficacious in the palliation of metastatic disease to bone than the traditional concept of delaying treatment until metastatic disease is symptomatic.

RADIATION SEQUELAE ASSOCIATED WITH THE TREATMENT OF PROSTATIC CANCER

Complications associated with the radiation therapy of prostatic cancer have been reviewed in detail re-cently.[18] In that review, the Stanford experience is summarized along with that of other comprehensive studies (Table 26–9).[40, 53, 75, 96, 97, 99] The RTOG morbidity grading system is shown in Table 26–10. Only total dose to the prostate correlated with late urinary sequelae in the RTOG study. Patients receiving greater than 70 Gy to the prostate were significantly more likely to have grade 3 toxicity. By comparing the incidence of complications noted in the Stanford study presented here over three periods (1968–1971; 1972–1977; 1978–1985), Bagshaw noted that a gradual reduction in major sequelae took place with the passage of time.[18] This was undoubtedly due to improvements in technique, case selection, and supportive care. In contrast to the RTOG study, urinary incontinence in the Stanford series was significantly greater among patients who had TURP associated with irradiation (Table 26–11). An actuarial method for evaluating post-treatment erectile potency for the Stanford system has been reported and is updated in Figure 26–24.[9]

Data are presented which demonstrate no difference between the incidence of expected second malignancies and that actually observed in patients receiving radiation treatment for prostatic cancer (Table 26–12).

Morbidity associated with the radiation therapy of prostatic cancer may be reduced by the following:

1. Avoiding abdominal or pelvic exploration in association with radiation therapy, particularly if transperitoneal surgery is employed
2. Avoiding para–radiation therapy TURP
3. Avoiding an external beam radiation dose in excess of 70 Gy in 7 weeks
4. Tailoring the radiation fields to conform to the target volume to minimize the small bowel, rectal, and anal radiation doses
5. Delivering the radiation dose homogeneously to the target volume on each treatment day, especially avoiding single-field daily treatments
6. Careful attention to supportive care during irradiation, such as control of fluid intake, dietary management, and administration of appropriate medications, such as Anusol HC suppositories for rectal irritation or bleeding, imodium for diarrhea, phenoxybenzamine for urinary hesitancy, pyridium and ditropan for dysuria, and vigilance for secondary urinary infection and, if it occurs, appropriate antibiotic treatment.

TABLE 26–9. SUMMARY OF MODERATE AND SEVERE COMPLICATIONS IN FIVE MAJOR STUDIES

GROUP	PERIOD	TOTAL NO. CASES	NO. WITH COMPLICATIONS		
			Moderate	Severe	Death
Washington University	1967–1978	267	66	5	1
French	1975–1982	597	373/144*	17/16*	4
RTOG	1976–present	1020	110	27	2
PCS	1973–1975	662	17	14	2
Stanford University	1956–1985	914	106	22	3

*Complications/patients.
Modified from Bagshaw MA, Ray GR, Cox RA: Complications associated with radiotherapy of prostate cancer. *In* Smith RB, Ehrlich RM (eds): Complications of Urologic Surgery. Philadelphia, WB Saunders Co, 1990, pp 88–99.

TABLE 26–10. RTOG* MORBIDITY GRADING SYSTEM

Grade 1	Minor symptoms requiring no treatment
Grade 2	Symptoms responding to simple outpatient management, lifestyle (performance status) not affected
Grade 3	Distressing symptoms altering patient's lifestyle (performance status). Hospitalization for diagnosis or minor surgical intervention (such as urethral dilation) may be required.
Grade 4	Major surgical intervention (such as laparotomy, colostomy, cystectomy) or prolonged hospitalization required
Grade 5	Fatal complications

*Radiation Therapy Oncology Group.

Reprinted from Int J Radiat Oncol Biol Phys, Vol 13, MU Pilepich, JM Krall, WT Sause, et al., Correlation of radiotherapeutic parameters and treatment related morbidity in carcinoma of the prostate—analysis of RTOG study 75-06, p 351, Copyright 1987, with kind permission from Pergamon Press Ltd., Headington Hall, Oxford OX3 0BW, UK.

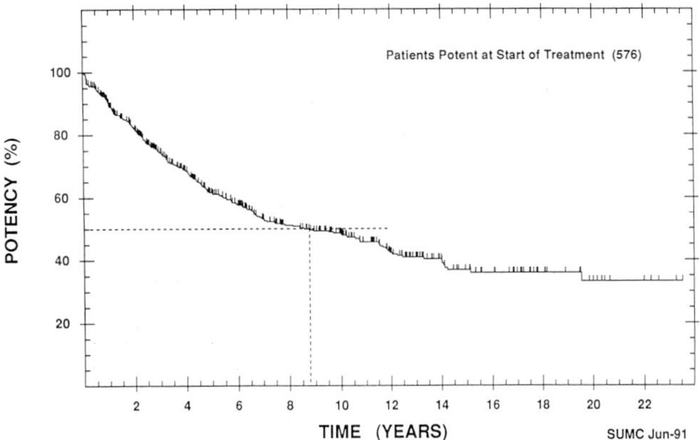

FIGURE 26–24. Kaplan-Meier calculation of the preservation of erectile potency after external beam irradiation. Note: Fifty per cent of the patients remained potent to 9 years, and 34 per cent remained potent to 23 years.

SUMMARY

Survival for patients following external beam irradiation of prostatic cancer is correlated with histopathologic differentiation as determined by the Gleason pattern score and clinical stage. As both the Gleason pattern score and the clinical stage escalate, survival deteriorates. For patients with Stanford T0 (Stage A) carcinoma of the prostate, survival did not deviate significantly from that of an age-matched peer group. For patients with Stanford Stages T1a, T1b, and T1c (B1 and B2), i.e., nodular disease that did not exceed involvement of one lateral lobe, survival was only 5 per cent less at 15 years than for that calculated for an age-matched group of California men. This was true even though the lymph node status and the true incidence of capsular penetration were not known. This survival pattern, following radiation doses that either were at or approached 70 Gy in 7 weeks, were found consistently in several large single-institution studies as well as several multi-institution studies in the United States and one in France. As these conservative selection criteria are shifted to include patients with more advanced stages, the likelihood of achieving 15-year survival diminishes; however, patients whose disease extends beyond the prostate and who seem too advanced for radical prostatectomy still may have a 20 to 30 per cent chance of 15-year survival following x-irradiation.

Postoperative irradiation is indicated for patients in whom careful examination of the specimen demonstrates transsection of tumor. This appears to be well tolerated and, at least in the Stanford experience described here, a post-prostatectomy rising PSA value may be expected to decrease to the normal range in many patients who receive treatment to the prostatic bed. Similarly, PSA values usually decline after irradiation of the primary tumor; however, serial determinations may show an upward reversal which, when present, usually indicates progressive disease, often at a metastatic site.

Irradiation of metastatic sites usually produces effective palliation of pain and, in bone, protects structural integrity. An analysis of bone coincidentally irradiated during the irradiation of para-aortic lymph nodes indicates that bone irradiation is most effective when the degree of involvement is minimal, giving rise to the concept of pre-emptive irradiation or the idea that it is more effective to achieve long-term palliation by irra-

TABLE 26–11. URINARY INCONTINENCE VERSUS PRE– AND/OR POST–RADIATION THERAPY TRANSURETHRAL RESECTION OF THE PROSTATE (TURP) (1956–1984)

	No. of Patients	No. With Persistent Incontinence (N = 39)
TURP	394	34* (8.6%)
No TURP	499	5* (1.0%)
TOTAL	893	39 (4.4%)

*$P = <0.01$.

From Bagshaw MA, Ray GR, Cox RA: Complications associated with radiotherapy of prostate cancer. *In* Smith RB, Ehrlich RM (eds): Complications of Urologic Surgery. Philadelphia, WB Saunders Co, 1990, pp 88–99.

TABLE 26–12. INCIDENCE OF SECOND CANCERS FOLLOWING PROSTATE CANCER*

TYPE OF CANCER	(1956–1985)		
	Observed	Expected	P Value
Lung	28	29.3	0.81
Colon	15	15.2	0.96
Bladder	11	10.2	0.80
Stomach	6	5.4	0.80
Rectum	4	7.4	0.21
Leukemia	4	3.8	0.92
Lymphoma	3	4.1	0.65
Pancreas	3	4.6	0.27
Kidney	1	2.9	0.26
Other	24	(24.0)	—
TOTAL	99 (10.8%)	106.9	0.48

*914 patients at risk for more than 7000 person-years.

Observed second cancers versus expected incidence as calculated by the method of Monson from SEER Program data for San Francisco Bay Area white males.

From Bagshaw MA, Ray GR, Cox RA: Complications associated with radiotherapy of prostate cancer. *In* Smith RB, Ehrlich RM (eds): Complications of Urologic Surgery. Philadelphia, WB Saunders Co, 1990, pp 88–99.

diating bone metastases soon after their detection, rather than awaiting the development of symptoms or structural deterioration. This concept may be especially appropriate in spinal irradiation in order to prevent vertebral deterioration and spinal cord compression.

A review of five extensive series, which detail serious complications attributed to the radiation treatment of prostatic cancer, indicates that these complications are uncommon and are becoming less so as radiation oncologists improve radiation therapy technique. Therapists more and more are striving to confine the radiation dose tightly to the target volume, using conformal techniques that protect normal tissues. It has been found that when a tumor dose of 70 Gy is exceeded, the incidence of complications becomes unacceptable. Various dose-escalation studies are in progress which are examining the trade-off of increasing the radiation dose to the target volume by reducing the dose to the adjacent normal tissues. The relatively high incidence of positive biopsies following irradiation indicates that it would be important to increase the biologic effectiveness of irradiation at the primary site. This is being examined by the use of conformal techniques to increase the radiation dose, the use of radiations of higher RBE such as neutrons and pi-mesons, the use of radiation-sensitizing agents, and the use of combinations of irradiation, such as external beam plus interstitial irradiation, with the addition of hyperthermia as a component of the interstitial treatment.

Radiation treatment of prostatic cancer is an alternative to surgery in relatively early disease, an adjuvant to surgery in patients who are incompletely resected, and a substitute for surgery in patients with disease advanced locally beyond criteria for local excision.

REFERENCES

1. Allain YM, Bolla M, Douchez J, et al: Cancer de la prostate: Resultats de la radiothérapie. Etude intercentres. Bull Cancer Paris 72:129, 1985.
2. American Cancer Society: Cancer statistics, 1989. CA, Vol 39, 1989.
3. American Cancer Society: Cancer statistics, 1991. CA 41:19, 1991.
4. American Joint Committee for Cancer Staging and End Results Reporting: Classification and staging of cancer by site. Chicago, Am Joint Comm 1983.
5. Anscher MS, Prosnitz LR: Postoperative radiotherapy for patients with carcinoma of the prostate undergoing radical prostatectomy with positive surgical margins, seminal vesicle involvement and/or penetration through the capsule. J Urol 138:1407, 1987.
6. Bagshaw MA: A technique for external beam irradiation of carcinoma of the prostate. *In* Levitt SH, Tapley N (eds): Technological Basis of Radiation Therapy: Practical Clinical Applications. Philadelphia, Lea & Febiger, 1984, pp 244–270.
7. Bagshaw MA: Carcinoma of the prostate. *In* Levitt S (ed): Technological Basis of Radiation Therapy: Practical Clinical Applications, 2nd ed. Philadelphia, Lea & Febiger, 1992, pp 300–322.
8. Bagshaw MA: Current conflicts in the management of prostatic cancer (1985 ASTRO Gold Medal Address). Int J Radiat Oncol Biol Phys 12:1721, 1986.
9. Bagshaw MA: Organ and function preservation after x-irradiation for prostatic cancer. *In* Smith PH, Pavone-Macaluso M (eds): EORTC Genitourinary Group Monograph 10, Urological Oncology: Reconstructive Surgery, Organ Conservation, and Restoration of Function. New York, Wiley-Liss, 1991, pp 257–268.
10. Bagshaw MA: Potential for radiotherapy alone in prostatic cancer. Cancer 55 (Suppl):2079, 1985.
11. Bagshaw MA: Radiotherapeutic treatment of prostatic carcinoma with pelvic node involvement. Urol Clin North Am 11:297, 1984.
12. Bagshaw MA: The role of radiation therapy in the management of prostatic carcinoma. Probl Urol 1:181, 1987.
13. Bagshaw MA, Cox RS, Ramback JE: Radiation therapy for localized prostate cancer. Urol Clin North Am 17:787, 1990.
14. Bagshaw MA, Cox RS, Ray GR: Status of radiation treatment of prostate cancer at Stanford University. NCI Monogr 7:47, 1988.
15. Bagshaw MA, Kaplan HS: Radical external radiation therapy of localized prostatic carcinoma. Proceedings of Tenth International Congress of Radiology, Montreal, Canada, September 1962.
16. Bagshaw MA, Kaplan HS, Sagerman RH: Linear accelerator supervoltage radiotherapy. VII. Carcinoma of the prostate. Radiology 85:121, 1965.
17. Bagshaw MA, Prionas SD, Goffinet DR, et al: External beam irradiation combined with the use of 192-iridium implants and radiofrequency-induced hyperthermia in the treatment of prostatic carcinoma. *In* Smith PH, Pavone-Macaluso M (eds): EORTC Genitourinary Group Monograph 10. Urological Oncology: Reconstructive Surgery, Organ Conservation and Function Restoration. New York, Wiley-Liss, 1991, pp 276–279.
18. Bagshaw MA, Ray GR, Cox RS: Complications associated with radiotherapy of prostate cancer. *In* Smith RB, Ehrlich RM (eds): Complications of Urologic Surgery. Philadelphia, WB Saunders Co, 1990, pp 88–99.
19. Bagshaw MA, Ray GR, Cox RS: Selecting initial therapy for prostate cancer. Radiation Therapy Perspective. Cancer 60:521, 1987.
20. Barringer BS: Carcinoma of prostate. Surg Gynecol Obstet 34:168, 1922.
21. Boxer RJ, Kaufman JJ, Goodwin WE: Radical prostatectomy for carcinoma of the prostate: 1951–1976. A review of 329 patients. J Urol 117:208, 1977.
22. Brosman SA: Iridium-192 implants in patients with large stage C prostate cancer. *In* Smith PH, Pavone-Macaluso M (eds): EORTC Genitourinary Group Monograph 10. Urological Oncology: Reconstructive Surgery, Organ Conservation, and Restoration of Function. New York, Wiley-Liss, 1991, pp 281–290.
23. Budhraja SN, Anderson JC: An assessment of the value of radiotherapy in the management of carcinoma of the prostate. Br J Urol 36:535, 1964.
24. Byar DP, Mostofi FK: Carcinoma of the prostate: Prognostic evaluation of certain pathologic features in 208 radical prostatectomies. Cancer 30:5, 1972.
25. Cantrell BB, DeKlerk DP, Eggleston JC, et al: Pathologic factors that influence prognosis in stage A prostatic cancer: The influence of extent versus grade. J Urol 125:516, 1981.
26. Carlton CE Jr, Dawoud F, Hudgins P, Scott R Jr: Irradiation treatment of carcinoma of the prostate: A preliminary report based on 8 years of experience. J Urol 108:924, 1972.
27. Carter GE, Lieskovsky G, Skinner DG, Petrovich Z: Results of local and/or systemic adjuvant therapy in the management of pathological stage C or D1 prostate cancer following radical prostatectomy. J Urol 142:1266, 1989.
28. Catalona WJ, Bigg SW: Nerve-sparing radical prostatectomy: Evaluation of results after 250 patients. J Urol 143:538, 1990.
29. Catalona WJ, Fleischmann J, Menon M: Pelvic lymph node status as predictor of extracapsular tumor extension in clinical stage B prostatic cancer. J Urol 129:327, 1983.
30. Chybowski FM, Keller JJL, Bergstralh EJ, Oesterling JE: Predicting radionuclide bone scan findings in patients with newly diagnosed, untreated prostate cancer: Prostate specific antigen is superior to all other clinical parameters. J Urol 145:313, 1991.

31. Colby FJ: Carcinoma of the prostate: Results of total prostatectomy. J Urol 69:797, 1953.

32. Coleman CN, Buswell L, Noll L, et al: The efficacy of pharmacokinetic monitoring and dose modification of etanidazole on the incidence of neurotoxicity: Results from a phase II trial of etanidazole and radiation therapy in locally advanced prostate cancer. Int J Radiat Oncol Biol Phys 22:565, 1992.

33. Csapo Z, Brand K, Walther R, Fokas K: Comparative experimental study of the serum prostate specific antigen and prostatic acid phosphatase in serially transplantable human prostatic carcinoma lines in nude mice. J Urol 140:1032, 1988.

34. Culp OS: Radical perineal prostatectomy: Its past, present and possible future. J Urol 98:618, 1968.

35. Dahl DS, Wilson CS, Middleton RG, Bourne HH: Pelvic lymphadenectomy for staging localized prostatic cancer. J Urol 112:245, 1974.

36. Deitch AD, deVere White RW: Flow cytometry as a predictive modality in prostate cancer. Hum Pathol 23:352, 1992.

37. Del Regato JA: Radiotherapy in the conservative treatment of operable and locally inoperative carcinoma of the prostate. Radiology 88:761, 1967.

38. Deming CL: Results in one hundred cases of cancer of the prostate and seminal vesicles treated with radium. Surg Gynecol Obstet 34:99, 1922.

39. deVere White R, Paulson DF, Glenn JF: The clinical spectrum of prostate cancer. J Urol 117:323, 1977.

40. Douchez J, Allain YM, Cellier P, et al: Cancer de la prostate: Intolerance et morbidité de la radiothérapie externe. Bull Cancer (Paris) 72:6:573, 1985.

41. Dundas GS, Porter AT, Venner PM: Prostate-specific antigen: Monitoring the response of carcinoma of the prostate to radiotherapy with a new tumor marker. Cancer 66:45, 1990.

42. Eggleston JC, Walsh PC: Radical prostatectomy with preservation of sexual function: Pathological findings in the first 100 cases. J Urol 134: 1146, 1985.

43. Elder JS, Jewett HJ, Walsh PC: Radical perineal prostatectomy for clinical stage B2 carcinoma of the prostate. J Urol 127:704, 1982.

44. Flocks RH, Kerr HD, Elkins HB, Culp D: Treatment of carcinoma of the prostate by interstitial radiation with radioactive gold (Au^{198}): A preliminary report. J Urol 68:510, 1952.

45. Forman JD, Wharam MD, Lee DJ, et al: Definitive radiotherapy following prostatectomy: Results and complications. Int J Radiat Oncol Biol Phys 12:185, 1989.

46. Fuks Z, Leibel SA, Wallner KE, et al: The effect of local control on metastatic dissemination. Clin Bull 2:94, 1972.

47. Fuks Z, Leibel SA, Wallner KE, et al: The effect of local control on metastatic dissemination in carcinoma of the prostate: Long-term results in patients treated with ^{125}I implantation. Int J Radiat Oncol Biol Phys 21:537, 1991.

48. Gehan EA: A generalized Wilcoxon test for comparing arbitrarily censored samples. Biometrika 52:202, 1965.

49. George FW, Carlton CE Jr, Dykhuizen RF, Dillon JR: Cobalt-60 telecurietherapy in the definitive treatment of carcinoma of prostate: A preliminary report. J Urol 93:100, 1965.

50. Gibbons RP, Cole BS, Richardson RG, et al: Adjuvant radiotherapy following radical prostatectomy: Results and complications. J Urol 135:65, 1986.

51. Gibbons RP, Correa RJ Jr, Brannen GE, Mason JT: Total prostatectomy for localized prostatic cancer. J Urol 131:73, 1984.

52. Haferman MD, Gibbons RP, Murphy GP: Quality control of radiation therapy in multi-institutional randomized clinical trials for localized prostate cancer. Urology 31:119, 1988.

53. Hanks GE: Optimizing the radiation treatment and outcome of prostate cancer (ASTRO 1984 Presidential Address). Int J Radiat Oncol Biol Phys 11:1235, 1985.

54. Hanks GE: Radiotherapy or surgery for prostate cancer? Ten and fifteen-year results of external beam therapy. Acta Oncol 30:231, 1991.

55. Hanks GE, Dawson AK: The role of external beam radiation therapy after prostatectomy for prostate cancer. Cancer 58:2406, 1986.

56. Hanks GE, Diamond JJ, Krall JM, et al: A ten year follow-up of 682 patients treated for prostate cancer with radiation therapy in the United States. Int J Radiat Oncol Biol Phys 13:499, 1987.

57. Hanks GE, Krall JM, Martz KL, et al: The outcome of treatment of 31 patients with T-1 (UICC) prostate cancer treated with external beam irradiation. Int J Radiat Oncol Biol Phys 14:243, 1988.

58. Hilaris BS, Whitmore WF, Grabstald H, O'Kelly PJ: Radical radiation therapy of cancer of the prostate: A new approach using interstitial and external sources. Clin Bull 2:94, 1972.

59. Hudson MA, Bahnson RR, Catalona WF: Clinical use of prostate specific antigen in patients with prostate cancer. J Urol 142:1011, 1989.

60. Hultberg S: Results of treatment with radiotherapy in carcinoma of the prostate. Acta Radiol 27:339, 1946.

61. Jacobson GM, Smith JA Jr, Stewart JR: Post-operative radiation therapy for pathologic stage C prostate cancer. Int J Radiat Oncol Biol Phys 13:1021, 1987.

62. Jacobsson H, Naslund I: Reduced incidence of bone metastases in irradiated areas after external radiation therapy of prostatic carcinoma. Int J Radiat Oncol Biol Phys 20:1297, 1991.

63. Kaplan EL, Meier P: Non-parametric estimations from incomplete observation. Am Stat Assoc J 53:457, 1958.

64. Kaplan HS, Bagshaw MA: The Stanford Medical Linear Accelerator. III. Application to clinical problems of radiation therapy. Stanford Med Bull 15:141, 1957.

65. Kaplan ID, Bagshaw MA: Serum prostate-specific antigen after post-prostatectomy radiotherapy. Urology 39:401, 1992.

66. Kaplan ID, Bagshaw MA, Cox CA, Cox RS: Radiotherapy for incidental adenocarcinoma of the prostate. *In* Altwein J, Faul P, Schneider W (eds): Incidental Carcinoma of the Prostate. Heidelberg, Springer-Verlag, 1991, pp 167–178.

67. Kaplan I, Prestidge BR, Cox RS, Bagshaw MA: Prostate specific antigen after irradiation for prostatic carcinoma. J Urol 144:1172, 1990.

68. Kaplan ID, Valdagni R, Cox RS, Bagshaw MA: Reduction of spinal metastases after preemptive irradiation in prostatic cancer. Int J Radiat Oncol Biol Phys 18:1019, 1990.

69. Knudson G, Grinis G, Lopez-Majano V, et al: Bone scan as a stratification variable in advanced prostate cancer. Cancer 68:316, 1991.

70. Lai PP, Pilepich MV, Krall JM, et al: The effect of overall treatment time on the outcome of definitive radiotherapy for localized prostate carcinoma: The radiation therapy oncology group 75-06 and 77-06 experience. Int J Radiat Oncol Biol Phys 21:925, 1991.

71. Landmann C, Hunig R: Prostate specific antigen as an indicator of response to radiotherapy in prostate cancer. Int J Radiat Oncol Biol Phys 17:1073, 1989.

72. Lange PH, Narayan P: Understaging and undergrading of prostate cancer. Urology 21:113, 1983.

73. Laramore GE, Krall JM, Thomas FJ, et al: Fast neutron radiotherapy for locally advanced prostate cancer: Final report of an RTOG randomized clinical trial. Radiother Oncol, in press.

74. Laramore GE, Krall JM, Thomas FJ, et al: Fast neutron radiotherapy for locally advanced prostate cancer: Results of an RTOG randomized study. Int J Radiat Oncol Biol Phys 11:1621, 1985.

75. Lawton CA, Won M, Pilepich MV, et al: Long-term treatment sequelae following external beam irradiation for adenocarcinoma of the prostate: Analysis of RTOG studies 7506 and 7706. Int J Radiat Oncol Biol Phys 21:935, 1991.

76. Leibel SA, Hanks GE, Kramer S: Patterns of care outcome studies: Results of the national practice in adenocarcinoma of the prostate. Int J Radiat Oncol Biol Phys 10:401, 1984.

77. Lepor H, Kimball AW, Walsh PC: Cause-specific actuarial survival analysis: A useful method for reporting survival data in men with clinically localized carcinoma of the prostate. J Urol 141:82, 1989.

78. Lepor H, Walsh PC: Long-term results of radical prostatectomy in clinically localized prostate cancer: Experience at the Johns Hopkins Hospital. NCI Monogr 8:117, 1988.

79. Lightner DJ, Lange PH, Reddy PK, Moore L: Prostate specific antigen and local recurrence after radical prostatectomy. J Urol 144:921, 1990.

80. Linstadt DE, Castro JR, Phillips TL: Neon ion radiotherapy:

Results of the phase I-II clinical trial. Int J Radiat Oncol Biol Phys 20:761, 1991.

81. Matzkin H, Lewyshon O, Ayalon D, Braf Z: Changes in prostate-specific markers under chronic gonadotrophin-releasing hormone analogue treatment of stage D prostatic cancer. Cancer 63:1287, 1989.

82. Mellinger GT, Gleason D, Bailar J: The histology and prognosis in carcinoma of the prostate. Front Radiat Ther Oncol 9:267, 1967.

83. Middleton RG, Smith JA Jr: Radical prostatectomy for stage B2 prostatic cancer. J Urol 127:702, 1982.

84. Middleton RG, Smith JA Jr, Melzer RB, Hamilton PE: Patient survival and local recurrence rate following radical prostatectomy for prostatic carcinoma. J Urol 136:422, 1986.

85. Monson RR: Analysis of relative survival and proportional mortality. Comput Biomed Res 7:325, 1974.

86. National Institutes of Health (NIH) (Biometry Branch, Division of Cancer Prevention and Control), Public Health Service, US Dept. of Health and Human Services. SEER Program: Cancer incidence and mortality in the United States 1973–1981. NIH Publication No. 85-1837, Rev. Nov. 1984.

87. Oesterling JE: Prostate specific antigen: A critical assessment of the most useful tumor marker for adenocarcinoma of the prostate. J Urol 145:907, 1991.

88. Paget S: Secondary growths in cancer of breast. Lancet, Mar. 23, 1889.

89. Paschkis R, Tittinger W: Radiumbehandlung eines prostatasarkoms. Wiener klinische Wochenschrift, Nr 48, 1910.

90. Pasteau O: Traitement du cancer de la prostate par le radium. Revue Malad Nutr 1911, p 363.

91. Paulson DF: Randomized series of treatment with surgery versus radiation for prostate adenocarcinoma. NCI Monogr 7:127, 1988.

92. Perez CA, Garcia D, Simpson JR, et al: Factors influencing outcome of definitive radiotherapy for localized carcinoma of the prostate. Radiother Oncol 16:1, 1989.

93. Perez CA, Pilepich MV, Garcia D, et al: Definite radiation therapy in carcinoma of the prostate localized to the pelvis: Experience at the Mallinckrodt Institute of Radiology. NCI Monogr 7:85, 1988.

94. Pickles T, Bowen B, Dixon P, et al: Pions—the potential for therapeutic gain in locally advanced prostate cancer. Dose escalation and toxicity studies. Int J Radiat Oncol Biol Phys 21:1005, 1991.

95. Pilepich MV, Bagshaw MA, Asbell SO, et al: Definite radiotherapy in resectable (stage A2 and B) carcinoma of the prostate—Results of a nationwide overview. Int J Radiat Oncol Biol Phys 13:659, 1987.

96. Pilepich MV, Krall J, George FW, et al: Treatment-related morbidity in phase III RTOG studies of extended-field irradiation for carcinoma of the prostate. Int J Radiat Oncol Biol Phys 10:1861, 1984.

97. Pilepich MV, Krall JM, Sause WT, et al: Correlation of radiotherapeutic parameters and treatment related morbidity in carcinoma of the prostate—analysis of RTOG study 75-06. Int J Radiat Oncol Biol Phys 13:351, 1987.

98. Pilepich MV, Krall JM, Sause WT, et al: Prognostic factors in carcinoma of the prostate—analysis of RTOG study 75-06. Int J Radiat Oncol Biol Phys 13:339, 1987.

99. Pilepich MV, Perez CA, Walz BJ, Zinuska FR: Complications of definitive radiotherapy for carcinoma of the prostate. Int J Radiat Oncol Biol Phys 7:1341, 1981.

100. Pilepich MV, Prasad SC, Perez CA: Computed tomography in definitive radiotherapy of prostatic carcinoma, Part 2: Definition of target volume. Int J Radiat Oncol Biol Phys 8:235, 1982.

101. Pilepich MV, Walz BJ: Postoperative irradiation in carcinoma of the prostate. Int J Radiat Oncol Biol Phys 9:105, 1983.

102. Pistenma DA, Bagshaw MA, Freiha FS: Extended-field radiation therapy for prostatic adenocarcinoma: Status report of a limited prospective trial. *In* Johnson DE, Samuels ML (eds): Cancer of the Genitourinary Tract. New York, Raven Press, 1979, pp 229–247.

103. Powers WE, Kinzie JJ, Demidecki AJ, et al: A new system of field shaping for external beam radiation therapy. Radiology 108:407, 1973.

104. Ray GR, Bagshaw MA, Freiha F: External beam radiation salvage for residual or recurrent local tumor following radical prostatectomy. J Urol 132:926, 1984.

105. Russell KJ, Laramore GE, Krall JM, et al: Eight years experience with neutron radiotherapy in the treatment of stages C and D prostate cancer: Updated results of the RTOG 7704 randomized clinical trial. Prostate II:183, 1987.

106. Syed AMN, Puthawala A, Rao J, et al: Temporary iridium-192 implant in the management of carcinoma of the prostate. Cancer 69:2515, 1992.

107. Syed AMN, Puthawala AA, Tansey LA, et al: Management of prostate carcinoma: Combination of pelvic lymphadenectomy, temporary Ir-192 implantation, and external irradiation. Radiology 149:829, 1983.

108. Shevlin BE, Mittal BB, Brand WN, Shetty RM: The role of adjuvant irradiation following primary prostatectomy, based on histopathologic extent of tumor. Int J Radiat Oncol Biol Phys 16:1425, 1989.

109. Shipley WU, Tepper JE, Prout GR, et al: Proton radiation as boost therapy for localized prostatic carcinoma. JAMA 241:1912, 1979.

110. Stamey TA, Kabalin JN, Ferrari M, Yang N: Prostate specific antigen in the diagnosis and treatment of adenocarcinoma of the prostate. IV. Anti-androgen treated patients. J Urol 141:1088, 1989.

111. Stamey TA, Kabalin JN, McNeal JE, et al: Prostate specific antigen in the diagnosis and treatment of adenocarcinoma of the prostate. II. Radical prostatectomy treated patients. J Urol 141:1076, 1989.

112. Stamey TA, Yang N, Hay AR, et al: Prostate-specific antigen as a serum marker for adenocarcinoma of the prostate. JAMA 317:909, 1987.

113. Tansey LA, Shanberg AM, Syed AMN, Puthawala A: Treatment of prostatic carcinoma by pelvic lymphadenectomy, temporary iridium-192 implant, and external irradiation. Urology 21:594, 1983.

114. Ten Haken RK, Perez-Tamayo C, Tesser RJ, et al: Boost treatment of the prostate using shaped, fixed fields. Int J Radiat Oncol Biol Phys 16:193, 1989.

115. TNM Classification of Malignant Tumors, 2nd ed. Geneva, Union Internationale Contre le Cancer, 1974.

116. Turner RD, Belt E: A study of 229 consecutive cases of total perineal prostatectomy for cancer of the prostate. J Urol 77:62, 1957.

117. Vickery AL Jr, Kerr WS Jr: Carcinoma of the prostate treated by radical prostatectomy. A clinicopathological survey of 187 cases followed for 5 years and 148 cases followed for 10 years. Cancer 16:1598, 1963.

118. Villers A, McNeal JE, Redwine EA, et al: The role of perineural space invasion in the local spread of prostatic adenocarcinoma. J Urol 142:763, 1989.

119. von Essen CF, Bagshaw MA, Bush SE, et al: Long-term results of pion therapy at Los Alamos. Int J Radiat Oncol Biol Phys 13:1389, 1987.

120. Walsh PC, Jewett HJ: Radical surgery for prostatic cancer. Cancer 45:1906, 1980.

121. Widmann BP: Cancer of the prostate. The results of radium and roentgen-ray treatment. Radiology 22:153, 1934.

122. Woo S, Kaplan I, Roach M, Bagshaw M: Formula to estimate risk of pelvic lymph node metastasis from the total Gleason score for prostate cancer [letter]. J Urol 140:387, 1988.

123. Young HH, Fronz WA: Some new methods in the treatment of carcinoma of the lower genitourinary tract with radium. J Urol 1:505, 1917.

124. Zagars GK, von Eschenbach AC, Johnson DE, Oswald MJ: The role of radiation therapy in stages A2 and B adenocarcinoma of the prostate. Int J Radiat Oncol Biol Phys 14:701, 1988.

125. Zagars GK, von Eschenbach AC, Johnson DE, Oswald MJ: Stage C adenocarcinoma of the prostate. Cancer 7:1489, 1987.

Chapter 27

HORMONAL THERAPY FOR PROSTATE CANCER

FRITZ H. SCHRÖDER

Endocrine treatment must be considered the best available palliation in this disease for those patients who respond favorably to the withdrawal of androgens from the prostate cancer cell. Nevertheless, many if not most issues in the field of endocrine treatment are unresolved. The endocrine dependence of the human prostate is dealt with in a separate chapter. The more basic aspects reviewed here are exclusively related to prostate cancer.

Early Developments

Great progress has been made in recent years concerning the understanding of clinical data and the organization of appropriate clinical studies. After the initial discovery by Huggins and his associates[42, 43] that disseminated prostate cancer favorably reacts to castration or to the administration of estrogenic hormones, a number of large clinical studies were conducted which determined clinical practice for a long period of time. All these studies followed the phase II pattern or used nonrandomized historical control groups for comparison. Nesbit and Baum[79] compared the results of endocrine treatment with those of a historical control group of the pre-endocrine era. They concluded from the differences encountered without an attempt to correct for prognostic factors that survival was prolonged by endocrine management. Ten years later, in 1960, Emmett et al[26] reviewed the very large Mayo Clinic experience of more than 714 patients who presented with nonmetastatic or metastatic disease and who were managed either by orchidectomy or transurethral resection of the prostate (TURP) combined with estrogens in 75 per cent of the cases. These authors found large differ-

ences in death rates from prostate cancer in favor of early orchidectomy. Furthermore, they concluded that orchidectomy was superior to estrogens in early management but that there was no difference in survival between treatments for patients who had already developed metastases. Five- and 10-year survival rates in this latter group amounted to 13.5 per cent and 3.2 per cent. Although the authors believed that survival is increased by endocrine treatment, the outcome in metastatic patients in spite of endocrine therapy "remains exceedingly poor."

The very favorable palliative effect in terms of inducing tumor regression in some patients and eliminating symptoms such as prostatic obstruction and pain was recognized early. It was probably because of these very favorable palliative results that the questions of prolongation of life and the best type of endocrine management were not dealt with until 30 years later. In 1967, the Veterans Administration Cooperative Urological Research Group (VACURG) reported on its first large randomized study, which was initiated in 1960 and which addressed in a four-arm protocol the question of whether diethylstilbestrol (DES), castration, or a combination of the two would produce better results in terms of survival in nonmetastatic and metastatic patients. Progression to metastatic disease in the nonmetastatic group was also evaluated. The most recent update of the results, which still remain very important for proper understanding of this field, is given by Byar and Corle.[16] The study group collected about 475 patients into each of the four groups, which included placebo. The most important result of this study (study 1) was that the 5-mg dose of DES led to an increased risk of death from cardiovascular causes. This excess toxicity appears within the first year and is manifested by a higher incidence of cardiovascular incidents and more pulmonary emboli. This effect was later confirmed in other studies.

Although this study was conducted according to methodology that would be unacceptable at this time, some important observations were made and carefully documented. In the placebo arm, 44 per cent of patients, most of them at the time of progression from the nonmetastatic to the metastatic state, were switched to endocrine treatment. This allowed a comparison of early versus delayed treatment. The data are shown in Figure 27–1. It was concluded that time to progression was significantly prolonged by early endocrine management. An advantage in survival, however, could not be detected. Contrary to early comparative studies, the combination of DES plus castration was not superior to either treatment alone.

In the third study of VACURG, placebo was compared with DES 0.2 mg, DES 1 mg, and DES 5 mg orally per day. In this study, the toxicity of 5 mg of DES was confirmed. It was shown that 1 mg of DES per day is significantly less toxic and that the rate of progression with 0.2 mg of DES is intermediate to placebo and 1 mg (Fig. 27–2). This important finding suggests a strictly dose-dependent relationship. DES 0.2 mg does not suppress plasma testosterone to castration levels. The group considered the fact that 1 mg of DES was as effective as 5 mg of DES in delaying progression while being associated with significantly fewer cardiovascular side effects to be the major result of their protocol.

With the reports of the VACURG studies, a great

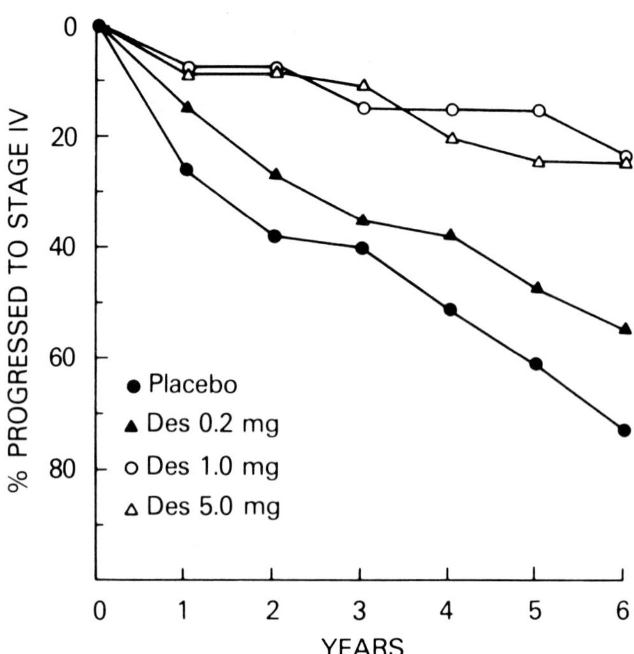

FIGURE 27–2. Actuarial curves for progression from Stage III to IV for patients in study 2. Note that the progression curve for DES 0.2 mg is intermediate to the placebo and the remaining endocrine treatment curves. (From Byar DP, Corle DK: Hormone therapy for prostate cancer: Results of Veterans Administration Cooperative Urological Research Group studies. NCI Monogr 7:165–170, 1988; with permission.)

interest was generated in the international urologic community to further develop and study details concerning endocrine management of prostate cancer. A large volume of prospective randomized studies was undertaken by the National Prostatic Cancer Project (NPCP), the European Organization for Research on Treatment of Cancer (EORTC), and other groups. Later, with the development of new treatment principles, the pharmaceutical industry started to conduct prospective studies of high quality. The results of such studies are the basis for the more detailed review of endocrine treatment given later in this chapter.

Cure and Prevention of Prostate Cancer by Endocrine Management

Cure of human prostate cancer can be achieved only by radical prostatectomy or by radiation therapy in the management of nonmetastatic, locally confined disease. The question of whether some patients can be cured by endocrine management has been subject to several reports. Johansson and Ljungren[49] reported on two cases of locally confined disease which were treated by means of polyestradiol phosphate injections. Both patients died of intercurrent disease after 9 and 12 years. Autopsy and careful histologic examination of the prostates were performed. In one patient no residual disease and in the other one only very small intraprostatic foci were found. The authors concluded that cure by endocrine treatment is possible.

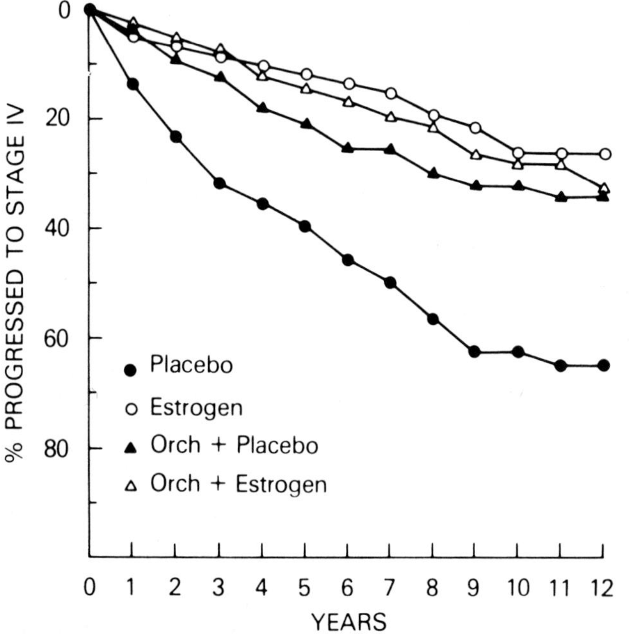

FIGURE 27–1. Actuarial survival curves for progression from Stage III to Stage IV for patients from VACURG study 1. Orch = Orchidectomy. (From Byar DP, Corle DK: Hormone therapy for prostate cancer: Results of the Veterans Administration Cooperative Urological Research Group studies. NCI Monogr 7:165–170, 1988; with permission.)

Reiner et al[88] reviewed five men with metastatic prostate cancer who were at risk under endocrine treatment for a period of at least 10 years. Four of the five eventually died of metastatic prostate carcinoma. The fifth died 15 years later with no clinical evidence of cancer. The authors concluded that they could not identify any parameters that would predict long-term survival and that cure of metastatic disease, if it ever occurs, is a rare event.

At this moment it is an open question whether very early endocrine ablation might cure prostate cancer. This possibility is suggested by anecdotal reports confirming at least the permissive role of androgens in the pathogenesis of this disease. Why should less androgenic stimulation for a long time period not be associated with a lower incidence of prostate cancer? Why should this mechanism not be useful in preventing the progression of this disease to advanced clinical stages?

It has been shown by Breslow et al[14] and Yatani et al[126] that the incidence of small, noninfiltrating, well-differentiated prostate cancer (focal disease) is equally high in parts of the world with a high and a low incidence of clinical prostate cancer. Although case control studies have not yet indicated the factors that promote prostate cancer in the high-incidence areas of the world, there is little doubt about the hypothesis that a "Western life style," besides other factors, promotes the pathogenesis of prostate cancer and its development to clinically relevant disease.[1] Migrants from low-incidence areas of the world (Japan) to Hawaii or to the United States slowly develop a higher incidence of clinically relevant prostatic carcinoma. Hämäläinen et al[36] have shown that a semivegetarian, low animal fat diet leads to a decrease of plasma androgen levels by about 10 per cent. Jong et al[52] found significantly lower testosterone (T), estradiol (E_2), and steroid hormone–binding globulin (T = SHBG) ratios in the plasma of the large age-matched male population of a Dutch-Japanese case control study of prostate cancer. Walsh and associates[121] recently suggested an association between higher plasma testosterone values and the later development of prostate cancer. On the other hand, several cases of adenocarcinoma in young body builders have been described which may be the result of long-term use of anabolic steroids, which may be metabolized to androgenic hormones.[90] Since methods have become available (5α-reductase inhibitors and pure, nonsteroidal antiandrogens) which are suitable for decreasing the androgenic stimulus to the target cell population in the human prostate and which, on the other hand, do not interfere with libido and potency, preventive applications may become possible in the future. Early results of the application of finasteride, a long-acting, orally active 5α-reductase inhibitor, have recently been reported by Gormley.[33]

PROSTATE CANCER AND HORMONES

The human prostate in its development and function depends on endocrine stimuli, mainly by androgens. It is unknown at this time what limits the effect of androgens and controls prostatic growth within the confines of its natural development. One consequence of malignant transformation of the normal human prostatic epithelial cell is that the unknown mechanisms determining homeostasis of prostatic growth do not seem to be active after cancerous transformation of prostatic epithelial cells. In addition to the traditional endocrine factors that are known to have an impact on growth and on functional parameters of prostate cancer cells (Fig. 27–3), autocrine and paracrine growth factors play an important role that is not yet fully understood.

Androgens

The normal development of the human prostate depends on the presence of testicular androgen production. The Leydig cells within the testes synthesize and secrete approximately 95 per cent of the circulating testosterone, 6 to 7 mg per day. Testosterone production in the Leydig cells is under the control of luteinizing hormone (LH) coming from the anterior pituitary, which again is under the control of luteinizing hormone–releasing hormone (LHRH) produced in the diencephalon. The remaining 5 per cent of the total circulating androgen levels of about 22 nmol/L are derived from adrenal secretion of precursor androgens dehydroepiandrosterone (DHEA) and androstenedione. Adrenal secretion and peripheral metabolism of adrenal androgens probably amount to 220 to 500 ng/day of testosterone. These data have recently been reviewed by Rommerts.[92] Only

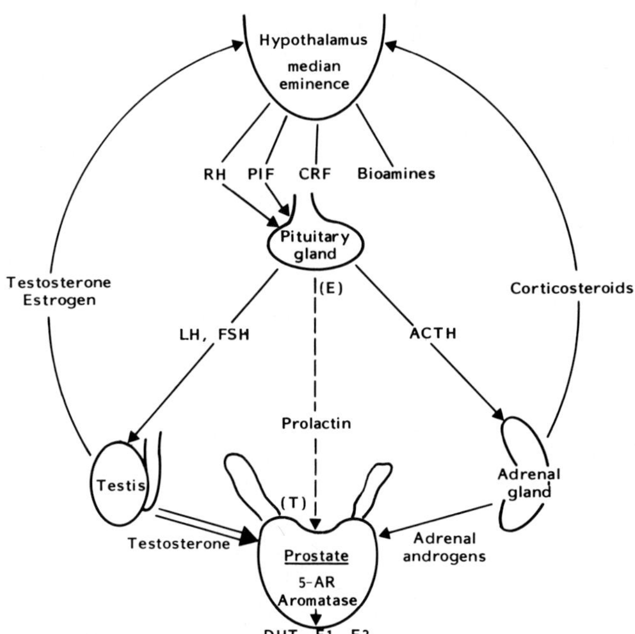

FIGURE 27–3. Endocrine factors regulating growth and function. RH = Releasing hormones; PIF = pituitary factor for prolactin; E = estrogen; LH = luteinizing hormone; FSH = follicle-stimulating hormone; ACTH = corticotropin; T = testosterone; DHT = 5 α-dihydrotestosterone; 5-AR = 5 α-reductase; CRF = corticotropin-releasing factor. (From Schröder FH: Cancer Surv 11:177–193, 1991.)

TABLE 27–1. CONCENTRATIONS OF TESTOSTERONE AND DIHYDROTESTOSTERONE (DHT) FOUND IN TISSUE OF NORMAL PROSTATE, BENIGN PROSTATIC HYPERPLASIA, AND PROSTATE CANCER*

AUTHORS	NORMAL PROSTATE		BENIGN PROSTATIC HYPERPLASIA		PROSTATE CANCER	
	Testosterone	DHT	Testosterone	DHT	Testosterone	DHT
Habib et al (1976)[35]	—	—	14	45	40	22
Ghanadian et al (1981)[31]	—	—	1.3	25	7	12
Geller et al (1978)[30]	—	7	—	18	—	10
Siiteri and Wilson (1970)[102]	4.0	4.5	4.0	20	—	—
Walsh et al (1983)[122]	4.0	18	6	18	—	—
Bolton et al (1986)[11]	—	—	0.9	18	—	—
Belis (1980)[6]	1.7	12	1.7	20	1.4	1.3

*Pmol/gram.

2 per cent of the total plasma testosterone level is biologically active. The remainder is bound to SHBG and albumin. Whereas corrected testosterone plasma levels decrease with aging, Vermeulen[116] and others have shown that SHBG levels increase with age. Only the free testosterone can be considered to be biologically active.

Within the prostate, but also in peripheral tissues such as liver and subcutaneous fat, testosterone is transformed to 5α-dihydrotestosterone (DHT) by 5α-reductase. DHT has a higher affinity for the androgen receptor system. It is generally accepted that DHT is the active intracellular androgen in prostatic cells, binding to the ligand-binding domain of the androgen receptor (AR). This process unmasks the DNA-binding domain of the receptor and triggers the release of a protein referred to as heat shock protein. This allows the binding of the DHT-AR complex to specific nuclear-type sequences of DNA in androgen-sensitive cells after dimerization, and the process of the gene transcription is effectively initiated, as described by Jones.[51] Adrenal androgens alone are not capable of maintaining prostate growth and function. This has been shown convincingly in a clinical investigation on hypopituitaric men by Oesterling et al.[81] Also, libido and potency in most instances are not maintained by adrenal androgens alone.

Although adrenal androgens are biologically weak compared with testosterone and DHT, enzyme systems are available within the prostate and in other tissues which can metabolize DHEA and androstenedione to testosterone and DHT. It was first reported by Geller[29, 30] that surprisingly large amounts of androgens can remain in prostatic tissue after castration. Probably the remaining androgen is of adrenal origin, as indicated by Bélanger et al.[5] Harper and associates[38] had shown as early as 1974 that steroids of adrenal origin are metabolized by human prostatic tissue and that DHT is one of the major resulting metabolites. Although there is no doubt that normal biologic functions within the prostate are not maintained by adrenal androgens in the absence of testicular androgen production, the possibility that cancerous tissue may show different androgen-sensitivity cannot be excluded. Labrie and Veilleux[68] showed that within the androgen-sensitive Shionogi mammary tumor line, cellular clones with a variable

androgen sensitivity can be identified. Experiments studying minimal amounts of androgen and adrenal androgens in the human prostatic tumor lines PC-82 and PC-EW in vivo in nude mice have not demonstrated clonal androgen "hypersensitivity" in these models. The available data, however, cannot be considered exclusive with respect to this possibility. An interesting observation that does not seem to fit this hypothesis at first glance was made by Harper et al[37] and confirmed by Hickey et al.[40] They found that patients who at the time of diagnosis of prostate cancer have a low plasma testosterone value (<8.3 nmol/L) have a significantly poorer prognosis than those with higher values. This phenomenon may be explained by the fact that such tumors have already been "treated" by partial androgen withdrawal, which may be constitutional or due to other causes. At the time of diagnosis in these cases, patients and urologists may be confronted more frequently and much earlier with progression due to hormone independence.

Unfortunately, the question of stimulation of prostate cancer tissue to proliferate by lower tissue concentrations of androgens remains controversial. Clinical data that correlate parameters for proliferation with testosterone and DHT levels in the prostatic tissue are unavailable. Androgen depletion and repletion experiments were carried out with the use of the PC-82 and PC-EW human prostate cancer lines in nude mice using various concentrations of androgens. DHT and testosterone were determined in the tumor tissue as well as in the plasma. In this model, DHT concentrations as they are found after castration in human prostate cancer tissue do lead to a growth arrest in these systems. Extremely low values, however, lead to a further volume reduction. Growth of the PC-82 tumor line requires more than 0.8 nmol/L of plasma testosterone corresponding to testosterone and DHT concentrations of 6 to 10 pmol/g and 3 to 4 pmol/g, respectively, as reported by Weerden.[125] These values are at or below concentrations achieved by castration in humans. However, the fact that mice lack SHBG must be considered.

Androgen concentrations in normal prostate, BPH, and prostate cancer tissue of untreated patients have been only scarcely studied. Some of the available data are summarized in Table 27–1. Some authors claim that prostate cancer tissue contains relatively more testosterone and less DHT. This is also confirmed by Krieg et al,[64] whose data are not shown in Table 27–1. Klein et al[60] find a lower activity of 5α-reductase in prostate cancer tissue but no difference in testosterone and DHT concentrations compared with benign prostatic hyperplasia (BPH).

Clinical evidence exists that large amounts of circulating androgens are capable of stimulating prostate cancer. The "flare" phenomenon, seen in the early phase of LHRH treatment coinciding with the associated rise in androgen production and the increase of prostatic acid phosphatase (PAP) noted by Klijn et al,[61] shows that tumor mass can increase with androgenic stimulation. Androgen depletion and repletion experiments using the Dunning R-3327-H carcinoma line show that with androgen repletion after castration, a significant increase in DNA synthesis and proliferation occurs. English and co-workers[27] have shown that in this situation a two- to four-fold increase in the proliferation rate occurs.

In summary, androgen-dependent human prostatic carcinoma is stimulated to grow by high androgen concentrations. Growth arrest and volume reduction occur after androgen production is reduced to castration level. This is associated with a functional suppression of prostate cancer cells reflected in a decrease of marker levels, prostatic acid phosphatase (PAP) or prostate-specific androgen (PSA). Adrenal androgens alone do not seem to support the growth of human prostate cancer cells in most patients. At this moment the possibility that the proliferation of some prostate carcinomas is maintained by adrenal androgens cannot be excluded. The mechanisms are unclear.

Estrogen

Circulating estrogen in the male originates largely from peripheral conversion of testosterone and of the adrenal androgen androstenedione to estradiol (E_2) and to estrone (E_1). Although plasma levels of testosterone in the aging male decrease, evidence shows that plasma E_2 concentrations rise in healthy men.[116] In the prostate very low concentrations of estrogen receptor and of natural estrogen are found mainly in the stroma, as shown by Krieg and co-workers.[64] The role of estrogens within the prostate is not entirely clear at this time. In the dog, prostate estrogens are synergistic with androgens in the induction of BPH. An extensive review of the older literature of actions of estrogens in the male is given by Mawhinney and Neubauer.[72] Besides regulating plasma testosterone levels by pituitary feedback, they strongly influence the availability of free testosterone in the plasma. Several authors, including Karr et al,[57] have shown that estrogen therapy and endogenous estrogens have a strong influence on the plasma levels of SHBG. Through this mechanism estrogen could decrease the bioavailability of androgens in addition to lowering total plasma androgens by increasing SHBG levels. This mechanism could explain some of the differences seen in prospective randomized trials comparing estrogens with castration. This information is dealt with later in this chapter.

In prostate cancer, estrogen treatment was one of the earliest available modalities. Clearly, estrogens exert their action by means of pituitary feedback and by suppression of LH production. Whether estrogens directly suppress growth of prostatic cancer cells is still a subject of debate. Several large clinical studies have shown that treatment with low-dose estrogens is equivalent to castration in the management of advanced prostate cancer. However, the question of whether very high doses of estrogens may exert additional effects has never been studied in a randomized prospective trial. Estrogens may also have a predictive effect in the pathogenesis of prostate cancer.

Vegetarian diet contains weak estrogenic hormones that may play a role in lowering the incidence of prostate cancer in non-Western countries, as suggested by Adlercreutz.[1] Definite proof of this hypothesis and the exact mechanism of action, however, are unavailable at this time.

Other Hormones and Prostate Cancer

Other pituitary hormones, namely prolactin and somatostatin, have been reported to be involved in the growth regulation of the normal prostate. These substances are discussed in the appropriate section on endocrine treatment.

The mechanism of action and the role of growth factors, mainly epidermal growth factor (EGF) and the transforming growth factors TGF-α and TGF-β, as well as fibroblast growth factors (FGF) and some others, in controlling prostate cancer growth, are subject to intensive investigation at this moment. Therapeutic implications for endocrine-dependent prostate cancer have not yet resulted from this field of research. There is also no doubt that stromal-epithelial interaction plays an important role. Cunha et al[21] have shown that urogenital mesenchyma regulates epithelial morphogenesis, differentiation, and growth of both normal and abnormal prostatic epithelium. Although this process is governed by androgens, growth factors are likely to play an important role. The mechanisms of mesenchymal control are undoubtedly multifactorial but remain unknown at this time.

Obviously, the ability to metastasize requires the ability to grow without stromal control. It has been shown recently by Gleave et al[32] that the human prostatic cancer cell line LNCaP requires prostatic stroma in order to grow in nude mice. Still, this very fascinating field of research has not yet yielded any therapeutic applications in the field of endocrine-dependent prostate cancer.

PRINCIPLES AND RESULTS OF ENDOCRINE TREATMENT

The goal of endocrine treatment is to achieve maximal palliation with treatment principles that are associated with minimal side effects and minimal costs.

Prognostic Factors and Response Criteria

Prognostic Factors. In judging the effects of endocrine treatment, it is crucial to realize that the natural course and the course of the treated disease are governed by very powerful prognostic factors. Some of these factors are directly tumor related, such as the extent of the primary tumor (T category), the estimated total tumor mass (M category), which can be judged by the extent of metastases on bone scans or by markers of tumor mass such as PSA, PAP, or alkaline phosphatase. Other prognostic factors are only indirectly tumor related but by no means less powerful. Voogt et al[120] have shown, in monovariate and multivariate analyses of combined EORTC trials of metastatic prostate cancer, that the WHO performance status is the most powerful prognostic factor in this disease. Consensus has emerged in recent years that it is impossible to correct for prognostic factors in historical comparison of treatment of prostate cancer patients. This review is therefore limited to information obtained from prospective randomized studies. The very strong influence of the performance status on survival in M1 patients with prostate cancer is shown in Figure 27–4.

Response to Endocrine Treatment. In the past, two major continuous attempts were made to define criteria for response and progression of prostate cancer under endocrine treatment which resulted in the availability of two slightly different sets of criteria, those of the NPCP summarized by Murphy and Slack[74] and those by the EORTC Genitourinary (GU) Group summarized by Schröder et al[97] and later by Newling.[80]

The big problem concerning the evaluation of response and progression in metastatic prostatic cancer lies in the fact that the most frequent metastatic sites—lymph nodes and bone—are usually not measurable but only evaluable. Serum markers, such as acid phosphatase, PAP, PSA, and alkaline phosphatases lack sufficient specificity to be recognized as valuable markers for progression. Too often, progression may occur in spite of improvement or normalization of the plasma levels of these substances.

Recently it has been shown by Cooper et al[18] that a rise of PSA under endocrine treatment may precede progression as evidenced by a bone scan for as long as 1 year. On the other hand, a recent study by Kadmon et al[55] showed that progression may occur without a rise of PSA in up to 25 per cent of cases. Considering the relative value of each individual available parameter for response and progression, the lack of measurable disease in following prostate cancer patients, and the great difference in time seen in occurrence of progression according to different parameters, the EORTC GU Group has now decided not to attempt any longer to use computations of the different parameters for response and progression. The individual parameters are now used **alone**. This results in the description of many different types of response and progression according to the individual parameters such as pain, quality of life, performance status, PSA, new bone lesions, soft tissue metastases, and so forth. The difficulty in clearly defining progression and the fact that PSA progression may occur a year earlier than other evidence of progression necessitates, on the one hand, the definition of end-points that should lead to change of treatment and, on the other hand, end-points that are more reliable in comparing clinical results such as death from prostate cancer and overall death rates. An example of the use of these various definitions of progression is given in the recent evaluation of EORTC study 30853, Zoladex and flutamide versus bilateral orchidectomy, by Keuppens et al.[59] As one would expect, marked variations in time to progression are seen with the use of the different parameters indicated above.

In studying response to endocrine treatment, pronounced differences are seen depending on the use of different types of response criteria. If subjective criteria are used and stable disease is considered an objective response, response rates may amount to 80 to 90 per cent. If the stricter EORTC GU Group criteria are applied and the no change category is not accounted for as a response to treatment, response rates will be only in the range of 30 to 40 per cent, as shown by Smith et al[104] and Pavone-Macaluso et al.[86] In the same studies, even with unsophisticated techniques, it became evident that the primary tumor is more likely to show a partial response than are metastatic deposits. Also, progression of the primary tumor occurs less frequently than does progression to metastases or metastatic disease. This is also evidenced by a recent longitudinal study by Sneller et al,[105] which reports on the monitoring of prostatic volume under endocrine treatment in 102 patients. More than a 20 per cent volume increase of the prostate occurred in 24 of these 102 patients, whereas during the same average period of follow-up (28.7 months), distant progression was seen in 61 of 102 patients (59.8 per cent).

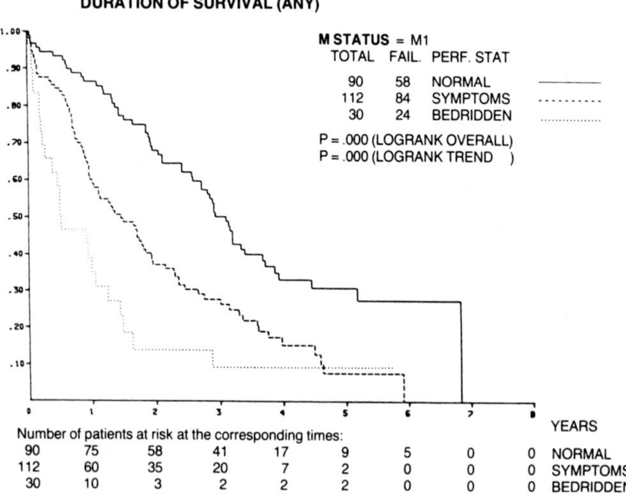

FIGURE 27–4. Survival and WHO performance status in 232 patients with M1 prostate cancer under endocrine treatment. Performance status was identified as being the most important prognostic factor in these studies. (Reprinted by permission from de Voogt HJ, Suciu S, Sylvester R, et al: Multivariate analysis of prognostic factors in patients with advanced prostatic cancer: Results from 2 European Organization for Research on Treatment of Cancer Trials. J Urol 141:883–888, 1989, © by American Urological Assoc., Inc.)

Pretreatment prediction of endocrine response has not been successfully achieved in prostate cancer. Small tumors seem to respond more frequently and for longer periods of time. Median times to progression in many recent studies of endocrine treatment of patients with bony metastases amount to 18 to 24 months, whereas the median time to progression after castration of patients with organ-confined disease metastases to regional lymph nodes was found to be in the range of 5 years by Bosch et al.[12] Although it has been shown by many authors early on that grade of differentiation is a poor predictor of endocrine response, the ploidy of the primary tumor was found to be an important determinator of response to endocrine treatment by Myers et al.[75] The monoclonal antibody Ki-67, which allows the staining of cells that have entered the proliferative phases of the cell cycle (G_1, S, M, and G_2), permits direct monitoring of the proliferative activity of primary tumors or metastatic deposits by the repeated study of aspiration biopsies. Preliminary findings suggest that endocrine response of the primary tumor can be predicted by this technique.[82] Unfortunately, determinations of the androgen receptor in prostatic tissue samples have not been found to be sufficiently predictive for routine clinical use. Brendler and co-workers[13] have used multiple variables to predict the response to endocrine treatment. Their parameters included the androgen receptor content in cytosol and nuclei and enzymes of steroid metabolism. The index separated responding and nonresponding groups of patients better than each parameter alone, but the index has not been used in clinical routines so far.

For all practical clinical purposes, monitoring of response and progression by means of subjective parameters such as pain and performance status, evaluation of the primary tumor either by rectal examination or by repeated ultrasonographic measurements, and repeated determinations of PSA, possibly together with acid phosphatase, are recommended. Clearly, bone scans are indicated only in patients with a PSA or other marker elevation or with subjective symptoms that point to a deterioration of the disease condition. Indications for the use of bone scans have been described by Smith et al.[103] The recommendation is to use the bone scan only at the time of diagnosis and when progression is suspected by other parameters. Bone radiography, because of its lower sensitivity, is usually limited to situations in which a bone scan is abnormal. It needs to be remembered, however, that roughly 10 per cent of all bony metastases may be lytic in nature and not visible on a bone scan. Other imaging techniques such as computer scans and MRI are limited to situations in which the evaluation of measurable disease is warranted (clinical trials) and in which complaints point toward symptomatic soft tissue metastases. In most situations these expensive techniques can be replaced by the cheaper ultrasonography.

Castration

Bilateral orchidectomy is probably still considered standard endocrine treatment of prostate cancer. The mutilating character of the operation can be diminished by using the technique of intracapsular orchidectomy described by Riba.[89] Several studies, including the one by Bergman et al,[7] have shown that intracapsular orchidectomy has the same effect on the levels of pituitary hormones and plasma testosterone as described earlier for bilateral orchidectomy. Castration has been used in a large number of prospective randomized studies as a control treatment. These studies are referred to below. Comparative studies with LHRH analogues have confirmed that the two treatment regimens are equivalent. A number of protocols, however, have revealed an advantage of estrogen treatment over castration. These studies are discussed below under estrogens.

Castration leads to an improvement of pain related to prostate cancers in 80 to 90 per cent of cases. This is usually associated with a clearly noticeable increase in the well-being of such symptomatic patients. Objective responses according to EORTC criteria are in the range of 25 to 40 per cent. Response of the primary tumor occurs more frequently and has a longer duration than response of metastatic disease. In spite of possible advantages of estrogen in preventing cancer progression and cancer death, as first described in the VACURG I study by Blackard et al,[9] estrogen is not commonly used at this time because of the pronounced side effects described by the same group.[16]

Castration is obviously a definitive treatment. The side effects are limited to the loss of libido and potency, which occur with all other treatment options that lower plasma testosterone to castration levels. Castration is inexpensive compared with many other available options. Nevertheless, patient preference seems to be limiting the use of castration with the advent of long-acting depot LHRH analogues.

Estrogen Treatment of Prostate Cancer

A large volume of literature on the management of prostate cancer patients by means of estrogenic hormones is available. This review is limited to prospective randomized comparative studies.

Application of Estrogens. The most common form of the application of estrogens is the use of diethylstilbestrol or related synthetic estrogens. Application once a day seems to be sufficient. In the past, dosages have varied between 5 mg and several hundred milligrams per day. After the side effects of 5 mg of DES per day were described by Mellinger et al,[73] DES was used at lower dosages, such as 1 or 3 mg/day. In Scandinavia and other parts of Europe, the use of polyestradiol phosphate alone or in combination with ethinyl estradiol is common. The drug is given monthly as an initial dose of 160 mg, followed by 80-mg intramuscular injections.[54] Another method of treatment is the intravenous application of diethylstilbestrol diphosphate. This drug was once given in very large dosages, ranging from 500 to 1000 mg over periods of 10 to 21 days. The issue of whether high-dose estrogen treatment may be superior to forms of management that aim at achieving castrate levels of plasma testosterone only has never been studied in a prospective randomized trial and must therefore be considered not to be settled. A recent review of this treatment modality is given by Susan et al.[110] Steg and Benoit[108] have suggested the percutaneous application of 17β-estradiol as an ointment and have shown that plasma testosterone can be reduced to castration levels. This treatment, however, has not found entry into clinical routine.

Because the main goal of estrogen treatment is the lowering of plasma testosterone to castrate levels, it is important to know with which dosages this goal can be achieved in a reliable fashion. A number of publications, including those by Kent et al[58] and Shearer et al,[101] have shown that only an incomplete suppression of plasma testosterone can be achieved with 1 mg of DES. The elevation of SHBG that results even from such low doses of DES may, however, compensate for the incomplete E_2 suppression and may also be related to the superior results obtained in some studies applying estrogen treatment to metastatic patient populations.

Toxicity. The lethal cardiovascular side effects of 5 mg of DES per day were first described within the VACURG studies by Mellinger et al[73] and later summarized by Byar and Corle.[16] The presence of such side effects was also confirmed for the lower dose of 3 mg of DES per day by the EORTC GU Group in protocol 30761, as reported by Pavone-Macaluso et al.[86] Although to a much lesser degree, cardiovascular side effects are also found with treatment of 1 mg of DES in the VACURG studies reported by Byar et al[16] and in EORTC GU Group protocol 30805 as reported by Robinson and Hetherington.[91] The cause of the increased rate of thromboembolism is not entirely clear. Water retention and electrolyte disturbances have been described, but reasons for toxicity remain controversial.

Results of Randomized Prospective Studies. The results of the studies of the VACURG have already been mentioned but must be considered historical for several reasons. The patient populations were poorly defined; for example, bone scans were not done and the metastatic status was assessed by means of serum acid phosphatase determinations. Roughly 40 per cent of patients from the placebo group were transferred upon evidence of progression to one of the three endocrine treatment groups in study I. For evaluation of disease-related and overall mortality, these patients were kept in the original randomly assigned group. It has therefore been concluded that the VACURG study I does not compare placebo with endocrine treatment, but rather delayed endocrine treatment with prompt endocrine treatment. Because there was no difference in overall survival between the original placebo and the endocrine treatment groups (DES 5 mg/day, castration, castration plus DES 5 mg/day), it was concluded that it would not matter whether endocrine treatment was begun immediately or after progression of or to metastatic disease had occurred. Because of the side effects of endocrine treatment, this option is still very widely used, although evidence is accumulating that early endocrine treatment may be preferable. The recent literature on this subject has been reviewed by Kozlowski et al.[63] The later dose-finding protocol of VACURG showed that the intermediate dose of 0.2 mg of DES is associated with a higher rate of progression to metastatic disease than 5 mg of DES (see Fig. 27–2).

The same study showed that actuarial estimates of death due to cardiovascular disease for patients with Stage III disease were as frequent in the 0.2 and 1.0 mg groups as in the placebo group but were significantly more frequent in the 5-mg DES group (Fig. 27–5).

A large number of studies are available which show that estrogen and other standard treatments produce equivalent results. These include protocols 30761 and 30762 of the EORTC GU Group as reported by Pavone-Macaluso et al[86] and Smith et al.[104] Protocol 30761 included 210 eligible patients with M0 and M1 disease randomized to receive cyproterone acetate, 250 mg/day, versus DES, 1 mg three times a day, versus medroxyprogesterone acetate with a priming dose of 500 mg intramuscularly for 8 days followed by an oral dose of 200 mg/day. There were, even after sophisticated corrections for prognostic factors, no differences in progression and survival rates between DES and cyproterone acetate. The medroxyprogesterone acetate group scored significantly worse by all evaluated parameters. At least this study has shown that there is such a thing as inadequate endocrine treatment. Unless stimulation by the drug is assumed, this result casts doubt on the finding of the VACURG studies that placebo may be equivalent to endocrine treatment. Also, the study

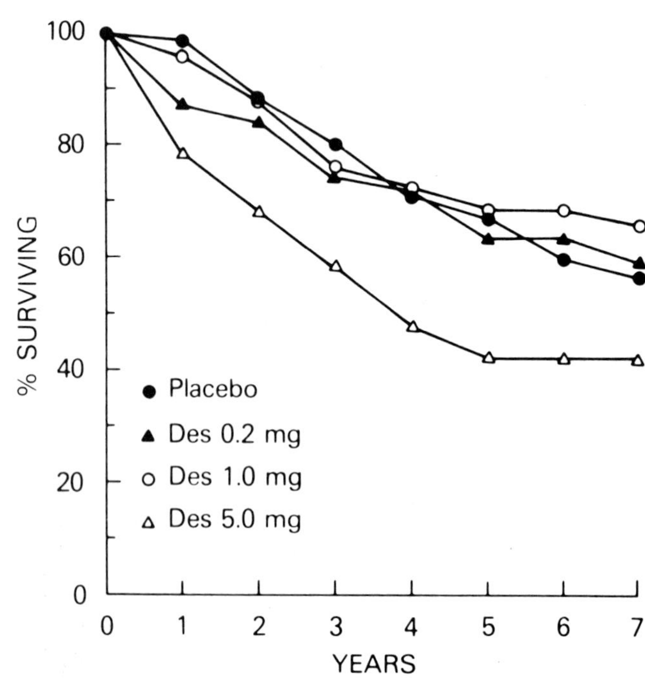

FIGURE 27–5. Actuarial survival curves for death due to cardiovascular disease only for patients in Stage III, VACURG study 2. Survival on DES 5 mg is poorer because of cardiovascular incidents. Note that the disadvantage of DES 0.2 mg in the progression curves (see Fig. 27–2) is not seen in comparing actuarial survival. (From Byar DP, Corle DK: Hormone therapy for prostate cancer: Results of the Veterans Administration Cooperative Urological Research Group studies. NCI Monogr 7:165–170, 1988; with permission.)

shows that adequate endocrine treatment prolongs life compared with less adequate endocrine management.

Protocol 30762 compared with a similar design 1 mg of DES three times a day and estramustine phosphate, 280 mg twice daily for 8 weeks and 140 mg twice daily thereafter. Again, no difference between the two treatment regimens was found. The cardiovascular side effects of both protocols were extensively analyzed and reported by Voogt.[119] Similar results with the use of estramustine phosphate (Estracyt) in the management of previously untreated metastatic prostate cancer were found in a comparative study using polyestradiol phosphate reported by Andersson.[3]

A number of studies conclude that treatment with DES, because of its side effects, is no longer warranted or at least requires careful consideration of the pretreatment cardiovascular status and special measures of observation. These include the reports by Henriksson and Edhag[39] and the report by Haapiainen et al[34] and the Finn Prostate Group. This study described a significant difference in time to progression in 200 prostate cancer patients in favour of orchiectomy over polyestradiol phosphate alone. This difference was explained by the fact that the recommended dose of polyestradiol phosphate is too low to maintain plasma testosterone at castration level. For this reason most authors subsequently add low-dose ethinyl estradiol to this depot, injectable estrogen. In another randomized comparison of polyestradiol phosphate plus ethinyl estradiol, 150 mg/day, with orchidectomy, Johansson et al[48] found a significantly better progression-free survival rate and similar survival rates but a significantly higher incidence of cardiovascular side effects in the estrogen-treated group. They concluded that estrogen treatment in this form cannot be recommended for the palliative treatment of prostate cancer.

Among the few protocols that show an advantage of estrogen treatment over orchidectomy is the study of 277 patients of the Finn Prostate Group reported by Haapiainen et al.[34] In this study polyestradiol phosphate plus low-dose ethinyl estradiol delayed progression significantly longer than castration did. There was no difference in overall survival.

In a number of other studies, estrogen treatment regimens are compared with newer treatment modalities. These studies are reviewed at the appropriate place. Estrogen treatment at this time probably has a limited clinical importance because of the cardiovascular side effects, which are extensively documented in the cited literature. Still, with appropriate follow-up and in appropriately selected patients, 1 mg of DES per day is probably still a viable treatment option. Also, a study comparing high-dose estrogens with castration or some other form of standard treatment should still be carried out. If estrogens have a direct toxic effect at the level of the prostate cancer cell, this may become evident only with high-dose estrogen treatment. There are several reports of uncontrolled studies in which subjective and objective response of prostate cancer progressing after castration or low-dose estrogen treatment was seen with high-dose DES phosphate.

Antiandrogens

Antiandrogens are substances which in vivo counteract exogenous hormones in the absence of relevant feedback mechanisms. Antiandrogens act by directly counteracting hormones at the target cell level. There are two classes of antiandrogens—pure antiandrogens and steroidal antiandrogens. The structural formulas of the four antiandrogens currently in clinical use are depicted in Figure 27–6. Cyproterone acetate, the oldest known antiandrogen, is steroidal and has some properties of a gestagen. It acts like an estrogen or an androgen at the level of the diencephalon by inhibiting LHRH secretion and thereby lowering plasma testosterone levels. Pure antiandrogens do not feed back at the diencephalic level. Because they counteract androgens at all target cells, including those of the pituitary feedback mechanism, these substances lead to a rise in LH and testosterone secretion. It is poorly understood why this rise is temporary, as recently described by Lund and Rasmussen.[71]

Some of the biologic effects are summarized in Table 27–2. If antiandrogens are used as monotherapy, they have different effects on the various biologic parameters listed. The fact that plasma testosterone remains high with the use of pure antiandrogens necessitates a higher dosage. The maintenance of libido and potency in most men who were potent prior to therapy is probably due to the high testosterone levels and incomplete blockage. It is poorly understood at this moment whether and by which mechanism pure antiandrogens may exert a long-term antiproliferative effect in men suffering from prostate cancer or BPH. It was shown by Stone et al[109] that over a 6-month period prostatic volume can be de-

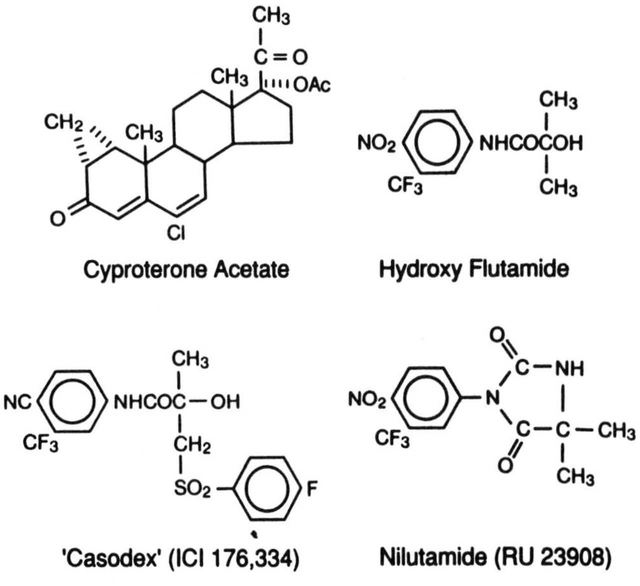

Furr (1988)

FIGURE 27–6. Structural formulas of cyproterone acetate, hydroxy-flutamide, Casodex, and Nilutamide. (From Furr BJA: The case for pure antiandrogens: Bailliere's Clin Oncol 2:581–590, 1988; with permission.)

TABLE 27–2. BIOLOGIC EFFECTS OF STEROIDAL AND "PURE" ANTIANDROGENS IN INTACT MALES

	PURE	STEROIDAL
Plasma testosterone	Rise	Decrease
Plasma dihydrotestosterone	Rise	Decrease
Luteinizing hormone	Rise	Decrease
Libido	Unchanged	Decreased
Potency	Unchanged	Decreased
Gynecomastia	Yes	No

creased by flutamide monotherapy in about the same way as by castration.

Antiandrogens can be used in monotherapy or in combination with treatment that eliminates testicular androgen production such as castration and antiandrogens. In this case, the rationale is that antiandrogens also counteract the adrenal androgens, which are the only remaining androgenic stimulus in this situation. Such regimens are called total androgen blockade or total androgen suppression and are dealt with in a separate section of this chapter.

All antiandrogens described here are orally active. Recent reviews of antiandrogens as monotherapy in prostate cancer are available by Pavone-Macaluso et al[85] and by Schröder.[96] In addition to their biologic activity, antiandrogens also differ in their pharmacology and side effects. Whereas cyproterone acetate is associated with a decrease of libido and potency, flutamide shows gynecomastia in about 40 per cent of cases as a sign of elevated plasma estrogens. Flutamide has a plasma half-life of 5 to 6 hours, whereas the plasma half-life of Anandron amounts to 45 hours and of Casodex to 5 to 7 days.

Only cyproterone acetate has been evaluated in prospective randomized studies reported by Pavone-Macaluso et al[86] in comparison with DES and medroxyprogesterone acetate and by Jacobi et al[46] also in comparison with an estrogen regimen. In the EORTC study reported by Pavone-Macaluso et al, cyproterone acetate was shown to be as effective as 3 mg of DES and at the same time to lack the cardiovascular side effects associated with estrogen treatment.[119] In a prospective randomized study comparing flutamide monotherapy with DES, unfortunately only a preliminary report by Neri and Kassem[78] is available. At the time of evaluation with incomplete recruitment, no significant difference between the two treatment regimens was found. Sogani et al[106] studied bone pain decrease, decrease in serum acid phosphatase, change in prostatic volume, improvement of hydronephrosis, improvement of soft tissue metastases, voiding symptoms, and improvement of the general condition separately in 72 patients with an average treatment duration of 12.5 months. Overall the response rate amounted to 68 per cent. It was concluded that at least for this period of time the treatment effects were satisfactory. Another phase II study of flutamide monotherapy on 40 patients revealed that 17 of 35 patients showed a partial response whereas 18 showed no change. Plasma testosterone and LH values were still elevated after 9 months but showed a decrease after 1

year.[23] Studies on Nilutamide and Casodex as monotherapy have not been reported.

Side effects of flutamide were evaluated within the randomized protocol NPCP 2400 on 109 patients in whom the substance was used as second-line endocrine management. Moderate or severe side effects were seen in terms of nausea (46 per cent), diarrhea (21 per cent), and gynecomastia (40 per cent).

Luteinizing Hormone–Releasing Hormone Agonists

Schally et al[93] discovered the decapeptide structure of the naturally occurring LHRH. Since that time several thousand LHRH analogues have been synthesized. It was found that the substitution at position 6 of the decapeptide of D-leucine in place of glycine greatly enhances the potency of such analogues. Although naturally occurring LHRH leads to an increase of plasma testosterone, the synthetic hyperactive LHRH analogues, after inducing a short initial rise of LH and testosterone production of about 1 week duration, lead to a lowering of LH and testosterone levels which is compatible as far as the testosterone goes with the castrate situation. This paradoxic effect of strong LHRH analogues was apparently first described by Labrie et al.[65] LHRH antagonists are still under development. Several compounds are available for experimentation but have not reached the stage of routine clinical use. A complete review of the early development of LHRH agonists and antagonists is given by Schally et al.[94]

Phase I–II Studies in Prostate Cancer. The endocrine and clinical effects in prostate cancer patients were initially studied in a series of phase I–II studies which used short-acting preparations for daily subcutaneous injection. Redding and Schally[87] showed the effectiveness of a D-Trp[6] analogue of LHRH in suppressing growth of the endocrine-dependent H-line of the R3327 Dunning rat adenocarcinoma and of other similar tumor models. The endocrine effects in the rat were described. No castrate control group was used in this study, however.

The first clinical studies appeared during 1981 and 1982. Again, one of the first comprehensive studies describing the endocrine effects of LHRH analogues and also the clinical effects on metastatic disease came from Schally's group.[113] All these early studies, which included the first reports on all LHRH analogues now in clinical use, showed clearly and in agreement that there is an early rise of plasma testosterone to two to three times normal values, with a maximum occurring on days 3 to 5. It was clearly shown by Klijn et al[61] that PAP follows this rise, indicating a stimulation of tumor mass during the initial phase of LHRH analogue treatment. This rise follows a similar elevation of LH. Adrenal androgens were studied under LHRH treatment, but changes observed by Schröder et al[98] do seem to follow the progression of the disease rather than being related to the effect of the LHRH analogue buserelin used in this study. The effects on primary tumor and metastatic deposits seen in these early phase II studies were considered similar to those seen after castration and are described in reports by Jacobi et al[47] and Trachtenberg.[114] Tayek et al[111] analyzed the nutritional and metabolic effects of an LHRH analogue in men with prostate cancer. They confirmed earlier observations concerning LH, testosterone, and DHT in plasma. They also found, however, a significant decrease of cortisol and a significant increase in triiodothyronine (T_3) and free T_3. They reported significant reductions in hepatic glycose production rates and significant increases of body weight, cholesterol, and overall fat mass. Body water content was not significantly increased after the 12-month period. The significant weight gain was therefore related to an actual increase in fatty body mass.

The first preparations available for clinical use of LHRH agonists were applied by daily subcutaneous injection or as nasal spray (buserelin). The need to develop suitable depot preparations was immediately recognized. The first such preparation was a tablet that had to be implanted subcutaneously through a small incision.[124] This concept did not prove to be clinically viable. One-month depots were soon developed by incorporating LHRH analogues into lactide-glycolide copolymers as either injectable rods or injectable microcapsules. Early reports on the feasibility of the use of such preparations have been made by Debruyne et al[22] and Sharifi et al,[100] among others. Recently, 3-month and 2-month depot preparations using the rod principle have been described.

The "Flare" Phenomenon. It was recognized early on with the use of LHRH agonists that patients with a heavy tumor load or metastatic disease in critical locations were likely to suffer an increase of symptoms during the initial phase of the rise of plasma testosterone. This syndrome was called the "flare syndrome."[123] Three early deaths from prostate cancer were reported by Schröder et al,[98] which might have been due to such early exacerbation under stimulation of prostate cancer by excessive testosterone. Thompson et al[112] recently reviewed nine different series and found an early death rate which might have been caused by disease flare in 14 of 765 patients (1.8 per cent). Several authors recognized that the use of a steroidal antiandrogen a few days prior to the initiation of LHRH analogue treatment[10] or simultaneously with such treatment[61] can prevent disease flare. Similar effects may be expected from pure antiandrogens. The initial rise of plasma testosterone, however, is not suppressed by these substances. Flare can be documented by an increase of symptoms as originally described but also by a rise of tumor markers and quantitative alterations visible on bone scans (scintigraphic flare).[50] If prostate cancer is treated with LHRH agonists alone in an attempt to replace castration, it is advisable to use an antiandrogen during the first months of treatment and to preferably start the antiandrogen 1 week prior to the initiation of the LHRH analogue.

Randomized Comparative Phase III Studies of LHRH Agonists. Early phase III studies of LHRH agonists had the goal of establishing the new treatment in comparison with standard forms of treatment such as castration or

3 mg of DES. Total androgen blockade studies are reviewed in the following section.

Comparison with DES was reported in two large studies, by the Leuprolide Study Group[69] and by Citrin et al.[17] Suppression of plasma testosterone values was found to be identical in the treatment groups. Castration levels were, however, reached more rapidly in the DES group. These studies are of crucial importance because leuprolide has been used without antiandrogen protection during the initial phase of treatment. Unfortunately, in the Leuprolide Study Group's report, in which 12 patients progressed, as opposed to only two in the DES group, it is not entirely clear whether the early-progression patients, who are likely to have suffered from flare, are excluded from the statistical analysis of progression by the original treatment group. The evaluation of survival is complicated by a cross-over treatment policy. The study by Citrin et al[17] is an open prospective comparative nonrandomized study and does not have the statistical power necessary to justify conclusive treatment comparisons.

The largest study reporting a comparison of the LHRH analogue buserelin by daily injection or monthly depot application versus castration is the one by the British Prostate Study Group reported by Kaisary et al.[56] In this study 358 patients with previously untreated metastatic prostate carcinoma were included and randomized between the two treatment arms. A similar study was conducted by the Zoladex Prostate Study Group and reported by Soloway et al.[107] In both studies no differences in plasma testosterone after castration or LHRH analogue application were found. No differences in response rates, time to response, median duration of response, median time to progression, and survival were found. This study is mature enough to be considered conclusive. Median times to progression and median survival have been posted. The study by Soloway et al[107] is statistically less powerful but comes to similar conclusions. Interestingly, Huben et al[41] found a difference in progression-free survival in a large prospective randomized study when DES or orchidectomy was compared with buserelin nasal spray. Sneller et al[105] found in a comparative study that with buserelin nasal spray prostatic volume reduction was significantly less pronounced than in a similar group of castrated patients.

Earlier protocols comparing the D-Trp[6] LHRH preparation in the form of microcapsules were reported by Parmar.[83, 84] Again, in these studies no differences in results between the treatment groups are described. LHRH analogue treatment, usually in the form of one of the available monthly depot preparations, is applied to clinical situations in which castration is indicated but not accepted by the patient for whatever reason. If antiandrogen protection is used during the initial treatment phase (1 month), the results will be identical to those with castration. Plasma testosterone levels can be checked as a parameter for compliance and correct injection technique. Escape or resistance against depot LHRH analogues has not been reported but must be considered. A progressing patient with an elevated plasma testosterone value may respond to second-line endocrine treatment.

TABLE 27–3. PROSPECTIVE RANDOMIZED STUDIES OF TOTAL ANDROGEN BLOCKADE VERSUS AN LHRH ANALOGUE IN PRIMARY TREATMENT OF M0-M1 PROSTATE CANCER

AUTHORS	DESIGN	NO. OF PATIENTS	TIME TO PROGRESSION	CORRECTED SURVIVAL	TOTAL SURVIVAL	COMMENTS
Crawford et al (1989)[20]	Leuprolide + FLU vs leuprolide + placebo	603	+3.0 mo ($P = 0.039$)	— —	+7.1 mo ($P = 0.035$)	Mature, subgroup analysis
Fourcade et al (1991)[28]	Zoladex + FLU vs Zoladex + placebo	245	NS	NS	NS	Mature study
Tyrrell et al (1991)[115]	Zoladex depot vs Zoladex + FLU	589	NS	NS	NS	44/393 pts. in FLU arm withdrawn (side effects)
de Voogt plus EORTC (1990)[118] Protocol 30843	Orchiectomy vs buserelin vs buserelin + CPA	349	NS	NS	NS	Nasal spray buserelin + CPA for 2 wks; preliminary data
Di Silverio et al (1990)[24]	Zoladex vs Zoladex + FLU	328	NS	NS	NS	Study immature in 1990
Crawford (1990)[19]	Leuprolide + FLU vs leuprolide + placebo	392	NS	NS	NS	Immature in 1990
		2506				

Abbreviations: FLU = flutamide; CPA = cyproterone acetate; NS = not significant.

Total Androgen Blockade

Total androgen blockade (TAB) and total androgen suppression (TAS) indicate treatment regimens that aim at the exclusion of testicular androgens simultaneously with adrenal androgens. Adrenalectomy or measures that exclude adrenal androgens as second-line endocrine treatment in patients progressing after castration or other first-line forms of management were frequently used in the past with moderate success. The data on second-line use of adrenal androgen suppression have been summarized by Schröder.[95] Objective and subjective response rates of 34 and 74 per cent, respectively, with a duration of 2.5 months and 4.0 months, were reported in 116 patients after bilateral adrenalectomy. The term *total androgen blockade* was propagated in the medical literature and in the lay press by Labrie et al[67] after an initial publication on the subject. In this report on a phase II study, the fate of 29 patients under TAB achieved by means of an LHRH agonist combined with a pure antiandrogen was described. The results do not contribute to the problem of whether TAB is a better treatment.

The first randomized study using TAB was conducted by the EORTC GU Group and initiated in 1980. In protocol 30805, castration was compared with 1 mg of DES and with castration plus cyproterone acetate. The preliminary results, as reported by Robinson and Hetherington,[91] and also the final results of this large and well-conducted study, which are in the process of being submitted, do not show a difference in time to progression and in survival between the three treatment arms. This is especially remarkable because 1 mg of DES is considered to be a marginally effective treatment that does not suppress plasma testosterone to castration values in all patients. Strong public pressure resulted from early reports on TAB to use this expensive treatment without a sufficient body of reliable information concerning its merits above standard treatment such as castration. The arguments for and against TAS are summarized in reviews by Labrie and co-workers[66] and

by Schröder and van Steenbrugge.[99] Although clear evidence exists that adrenal androgens in the absence of testicular androgen production are not capable of maintaining the morphology and function of the prostate in men and do not provide sufficient androgenic stimulation to preserve libido and potency, the possibility could never be excluded that adrenal androgens may stimulate growth of prostate cancer cells in at least some patients. Also, adrenal androgens have never been studied as a pretreatment parameter in large series of patients to properly exclude the possibility that some men have higher levels of adrenal androgens than others. Fortunately, in recent years a large body of information resulting from well-conducted randomized prospective phase III studies has become available. These studies compare standard treatment by means of either castration or LHRH agonists with TAB. Still, as the following review shows, the situation is not entirely clear, and it cannot be concluded that TAB represents better endocrine treatment than castration or LHRH alone.

Randomized Comparative Studies of TAB. In order to evaluate TAB, only the results of prospective randomized studies can be used. Quite obviously, the very large differences predicted by Labrie et al[67] and in later publications from the same group are not seen as adequate comparative studies. TAB can be achieved in various ways. Any treatment principle that reduces to castration levels or counteracts completely at the target cells testicular androgens together with adrenal androgens is suitable. The two approaches most frequently applied are an LHRH analogue alone and in combination with a pure or steroidal antiandrogen. On the other hand, in roughly an equal number of prospective randomized studies, castration is used as a control.

Results of TAB Using LHRH Analogues as Control. The data on prospective randomized trials that use an LHRH analogue with or without placebo as a control are summarized in Table 27–3. The large intergroup study 0036 reported by Crawford et al[20] has shown a statistically significant difference in favor of the LHRH analogue leuprolide applied in daily injections in combination with flutamide as opposed to leuprolide alone.

The differences in median times to progression and survival amount to 3.0 months and 7.1 months, respectively. These differences are statistically significant. In this study subgroups of patients with more favorable as opposed to less favorable prognostic factors (performance status, pain, acid phosphatase levels, "extent of metastases") were identified and compared. The subgroup with more favorable prognostic factors (41 patients in each arm) were found to benefit more from the combination treatment. Leuprolide was used without antiandrogen protection during the first weeks of treatment. The possibility that early disease exacerbation (flare) plays a role in determining time to progression and survival in the control group has never been entirely excluded. The intergroup is now studying castration versus castration plus flutamide.

Unfortunately, the favorable results seen in intergroup study 0036 have not been reproduced by any of the other protocols. At least two of the studies, the ones reported by Fourcade et al[28] and Tyrrell et al,[115] can be considered mature and have been finally analyzed. No trends are visible in these protocols. It is remarkable that with a total of 2506 patients, only one study shows significant differences. It will be important to await maturity and meta-analysis of the remaining studies.

Studies of TAB Using Castration as the Control. The studies using castration as a control are summarized in Table 27–4. These studies exclude the possibility that the results in the control arm may be adversely influenced by flare due to the initial rise of plasma testosterone related to the use of an LHRH analogue. A total of 2372 patients are summarized in this table. There is one study, EORTC protocol 30853, which shows a significant difference in time to progression and in the most recent analysis also in corrected survival. Overall survival shows a clear trend which at this time is not significant ($P = 0.06$). The difference in median survival between the two treatment arms amounts to about 11 months. None of the remaining studies shows a significant difference in overall survival. It is remarkable that the DAPROCA study,[45] which used identical selection criteria to protocol 30853, shows an excellent match of prognostic factors but does not reproduce the differences seen in EORTC protocol 30853. The study of the International Anandron Group (1990) shows a difference in time to progression and corrected survival in favor of the combination treatment. The seven studies using Nilutamide in addition to castration with castration as a control were run according to identical protocols. These studies have been subject to a meta-analysis, which has recently been reported by Bertagna.[8] From this meta-analysis it was concluded that there was a significantly higher incidence of early partial or complete tumor regression in favor of the combination treatment, as measured by objective and subjective (pain) parameters. In comparison with the castration-only group, there was a significantly reduced risk of progression ($P = 0.05$). There was also a trend toward an improved

TABLE 27–4. PROSPECTIVE RANDOMIZED STUDIES OF TOTAL ANDROGEN BLOCKADE VERSUS CASTRATION IN THE PRIMARY TREATMENT OF M0-M1 PROSTATE CANCER

AUTHORS	DESIGN	NO. OF PATIENTS	TIME TO PROGRESSION	CORRECTED SURVIVAL	TOTAL SURVIVAL	COMMENTS
Robinson et al (1986, 1992)[91] EORTC 30805	Castration vs castration + CPA vs 1 mg DES	241	NS	NS	NS	Final analysis (oral communication) shows identical results; mature
de Voogt + EORTC (1990)[118] Protocol 30843	Castration vs buserelin vs buserelin + CPA	349	NS	NS	NS	Nasal spray buserelin + CPA for 2 wks, in buserelin arm; immature
Keuppens et al (1990)[59] EORTC 30853	Zoladex + FLU vs castration	327	$P = 0.032$ $P = 0.01$*	NS $P = 0.04$*	NS $P = 0.06$*	*Oral communication Denis et al: American Association of Genitourinary Surgeons
Iversen et al (DAPROCA) (1990)[45]	Zoladex + FLU vs castration	264	NS	NS	NS	Mature study, same as EORTC 30853
Béland et al (1991)[4]	Castration + NIL vs castration + placebo	208	NS	NS	NS	
Navratil (1991)[77]	Same as Béland et al (1991)	122	NS	NS	NS	
Brisset (1990)[15]	Same as Béland et al (1991)	191	NS	NS	NS	
Namer et al (1990)[76]	Same as Béland et al (1991)	151	NS	NS	NS	
Knönagel et al (1990)[62]	Same as Béland et al (1991)	51	NS	NS	NS	
International Anadron Group (1990)	Same as Béland et al (1991)	457				
Du Plessis (1990)[25]	Same as Béland et al (1991)	11				
		2372				

Abbreviations: CPA = cyproterone acetate; DES = diethylstilbestrol; FLU = flutamide; NIL = Nilutamide; NS = not significant.

corrected and overall survival, which, however, was not statistically significant. The meta-analysis claims a benefit for the use of Nilutamide in combination with orchidectomy, which in the author's thinking justifies the routine use of this combination treatment.

Again, most of the studies cited do not show significant differences concerning time to progression, corrected survival, and overall survival. Some of the studies are immature, and final analyses are still pending. None of the studies using the steroidal antiandrogen cyproterone acetate show any advantage of TAB over standard treatment. The reasons for this are unclear. Although cyproterone acetate has been reported to be an antiandrogen with about 50 per cent of the potency of flutamide, this disadvantage should be compensated by the fact that it lowers plasma testosterone and has been shown to produce excessively high levels in prostatic tissue.[53] A possible explanation could be that most of the studies are older, and the only recent protocol[118] is still too immature for final analysis.

In protocol 30853,[59] a subgroup analysis according to more and less favorable prognostic factors has been carried out. This analysis confirms the findings of Crawford et al[20] that most benefit is present in the relatively small subgroups of patients with favorable prognostic factors. In fact, in the EORTC study the statistically significant advantage in survival disappears for the remaining group after elimination of the patients with favorable prognostic factors. This more favorable group amounts to only 20 per cent of all patients recruited into the study. This proportion is very similar to that of intergroup protocol 0036. The identification of subgroups that benefit from TAB should have high research priority and may lead to a more rational approach to the use of this aggressive and very expensive mode of treatment. At this moment, it is therefore not clear whether TAB should be used routinely and in all patients with prostate cancer.

FUTURE—UNRESOLVED QUESTIONS

It remains an open question whether endocrine management may prolong survival. It appears that subgroups of patients with more favorable prognostic factors may have more benefit from aggressive endocrine treatment by TAB than from other types of withdrawal of testicular androgens. Findings in this respect, however, are contradictory in several similar prospective studies. Why should that be the case? If early metastatic disease, such as in patients identified to have microscopically positive lymph nodes at the time of attempted radical prostatectomy, is treated by endocrine means, time to progression can be prolonged in a highly significant way. However, at this moment it is not known whether such prolongation will be associated with prolonged survival.

Why do virtually all human prostate cancers progress to the hormone-independent stage if the patient outlives his disease? The genetic changes that give rise to hormone independence are likely to become clinically relevant by clonal overgrowth of hormone-independent

cell populations. In what stage of development do such changes occur? Is there a very early stage in the natural development of this disease during which all tumor cells are hormone dependent, and escape to hormone independence would not occur if early treatment occurred? Is it really true, as the studies of the VACURG[117] suggest, that it does not matter whether endocrine treatment is begun in a metastatic but asymptomatic as opposed to a symptomatic state of the disease? If this is so, can we assume from such data that early treatment, if applied to earlier stages, is not superior to delay of endocrine management? Is there a place for preventive endocrine management? Can progression to hormone independence in some way be influenced by endocrine suppression of growth and function in a very early stage of the development of prostate cancer? Is there a type of minimal endocrine suppression that would achieve such a goal without causing the most relevant side effects: loss of libido and potency? These are some of the questions relevant to the management of human prostate cancer that will have to be answered in the future. This list could be continued by including the issues of growth factors, endocrine control of cell death, and the identification and eventual manipulation of genetic changes, which may be shown in the future to be relevant to the progression of prostate cancer from endocrine dependence to endocrine independence.

REFERENCES

1. Adlercreutz H: Western diet and western diseases: Some hormonal and biochemical mechanisms and associations. Scand J Clin Lab Invest (Suppl)201:3–23, 1990.
2. Anandron International Study Group: Reported by Bertagna C: Rencontres d'Urologie, Montreal, May 31, 1990.
3. Andersson L: Estrogens and estramustine phosphate. *In* Denis L (ed): The Medical Management of Prostate Cancer. Heidelberg, Springer-Verlag, 1988, pp 37–42.
4. Béland G, Elhilali M, Fradet Y, et al: Total androgen ablation: Canadian experience. Urol Clin North Amer 18:75–82, 1991.
5. Bélanger B, Bélanger A, Labrie F, et al: Comparison of residual C-19 steroids in plasma and prostatic tissue of human, rat and guinea pig after castration: Unique importance of extratesticular androgens in men. J Steroid Biochem 32:695–698, 1989.
6. Belis JA: Methodologic basis for the radioimmunoassay of endogenous steroids in human prostatic tissue. Invest Urol 17:332–336, 1980.
7. Bergman B, Damber JE, Tomic R: Effects of total and subcapsular orchidectomy on serum concentrations of testosterone and pituitary hormones in patients with carcinoma of the prostate. Urol Int 37:139–144, 1982.
8. Bertagna C: Oral communication. Rencontres d'Urologie, Montreal, May 31, 1990.
9. Blackard CE, Byar DP, Jordan WP: Orchiectomy for advanced prostatic carcinoma. Urology 1:553–560, 1973.
10. Boccon-Gibod L, Laudat MH, Dugue MA, Steg A: Cyproterone acetate lead-in prevents initial rise of serum testosterone induced by luteinizing hormone–releasing hormone analogues in the treatment of metastatic carcinoma of the prostate. Eur Urol 12:400–402, 1986.
11. Bolton NJ, Lukkarinen O, Vikho R: Concentrations of androgens in human benign prostatic hypertrophic tissues incubated for up to three days. Prostate 9:159–167, 1986.
12. Bosch RJLH, Kurth KH, Schröder FH: Surgical treatment of locally advanced (T3) prostatic carcinoma—early results. J Urol 138:816–822, 1987.
13. Brendler CB, Isaacs JT, Follansbee AL, Walsh PC: The use of

multiple variables to predict response to endocrine therapy in carcinoma of the prostate: A preliminary report. J Urol 131:694–700, 1984.

14. Breslow N, Chan CW, Dhom G, et al: Latent carcinoma of prostate at autopsy in seven areas. Int J Cancer 20:680–688, 1977.

15. Brisset JM: Reported by Bertagna C: Rencontres d'Urologie, Montreal, May 31, 1990.

16. Byar DP, Corle DK: Hormone therapy for prostate cancer: Results of the Veterans Administration Cooperative Urological Research Group studies. NCI Monogr 7:165–170, 1988.

17. Citrin DL, Resnick MI, Guinan P, et al: A comparison of Zoladex and DES in the treatment of advanced prostate cancer: Results of a randomized, multicenter trial. Prostate 18:139–146, 1991.

18. Cooper EH, Armitage TG, Robinson MRG, Prostatic specific antigen and the prediction of prognosis in metastatic prostatic cancer. Cancer 66(Suppl):19–22, 1990.

19. Crawford ED: Combination studies with leuprolide. Eur Urol 18(Suppl 3):30–33, 1990.

20. Crawford ED, Eisenberger MA, McLeod DG, et al: A controlled trial of leuprolide with and without flutamide in prostatic carcinoma. N Engl J Med 321:419–424, 1989.

21. Cunha GR, Hayashi N, Wong YC: Regulation of differentiation and growth of normal adult and neoplastic epithelia by inductive mesenchyme. *In* Isaacs JT (ed): Cancer Surveys, 11: Prostate Cancer: Cell and Molecular Mechanisms in Diagnosis and Treatment. Imperial Cancer Research Fund. New York, Cold Spring Harbor Laboratory Press, 1991, p. 73–90.

22. Debruyne FMJ, Denis L, Lunglmayer G, et al: Long-term therapy with a depot luteinizing hormone–releasing hormone analogue (Zoladex) in patients with advanced prostatic carcinoma. J Urol 140:775–777, 1988.

23. Delaere KPJ, van Thillo EL: Flutamide monotherapy as primary treatment in advanced prostatic carcinoma. Semin Oncol 18(Suppl 6):13–18, 1991.

24. Di Silverio F, Serio M, D'Eramo G, Sciarra F: Zoladex versus Zoladex plus cyproterone acetate in the treatment of advanced prostatic cancer: A multicenter Italian study. Eur Urol 18 (Suppl 3):54–61, 1990.

25. Du Plessis: Reported by Bertagna C: Rencontres d'Urologie, Montreal, May 31, 1990.

26. Emmett JL, Greene LF, Papantoniou A: Endocrine therapy in carcinoma of the prostate gland: 10 year survival studies. J Urol 83:471–483, 1960.

27. English HG, Kloszewski ED, Valentine EG, Santen RJ: Proliferative response of the Dunning R3327-H experimental model of prostatic adenocarcinoma to conditions of androgen depletion and repletion. Cancer Res 46:839–844, 1986.

28. Fourcade RO, Cariou G, Coloby P, et al: Total androgen blockade in the treatment of advanced prostatic carcinoma: Final report of a double blind placebo controlled study using Zoladex and flutamide [abstract]. J Urol 145:426A, 1991.

29. Geller J, Albert JD, Nachtsheim DA, Loza D: Comparison of prostatic cancer tissue dihydrotestosterone levels at the time of relapse following orchiectomy or estrogen therapy. J Urol 132:693–696, 1984.

30. Geller J, Albert JD, Loza D, et al: DHT concentrations in human prostate cancer tissue. J Clin Endocrinol Metabol 46:440–444, 1978.

31. Ghanadian R, Masters JRW, Smith CB: Altered androgen metabolism in carcinoma of the prostate. Eur Urol 7:169–170, 1981.

32. Gleave ME, Hseih JT, von Eschenbach AC, Chung LWK: Prostate and bone fibroblasts induce human prostate carcinoma growth in vivo: Implications for bidirectional stromal-epithelial interaction in prostate carcinoma growth and metastases [abstract]. J Urol 145:213A, 1991.

33. Gormley G: Role of 5-α-reductase inhibitors in the treatment of advanced prostatic carcinoma. Urol Clin North Am 18:93–98, 1991.

34. Haapiainen R, Rannikko S, Ruutu M, et al: Orchiectomy versus oestrogen in the treatment of advanced prostatic cancer. Br J Urol 67:184–187, 1991.

35. Habib FK, Lee IR, Stitch SR, Smith PH: Androgen levels in the plasma and prostatic tissues of patients with benign hypertrophy and carcinoma of the prostate. J Endocrinol 7:99–107, 1976.

36. Hämäläinen E, Adlercreutz H, Puska P, et al: Diet and serum sex hormones in healthy men. J Steroid Biochem 20:459–464, 1984.

37. Harper ME, Pierrepoint CG, Griffiths K: Carcinoma of the prostate: Relationship of pre-treatment hormone levels to survival. Eur J Cancer Clin Oncol 20:477, 1984.

38. Harper ME, Pike A, Peeling WB, Griffiths K: Steroids of adrenal origin metabolized by human prostatic tissue both in vivo and in vitro. J Endocrinol 60:117–125, 1974.

39. Henriksson P, Edhag O: Orchidectomy versus oestrogen for prostatic cancer: Cardiovascular effects. Br Med J 293:413–415, 1986.

40. Hickey D, Todd B, Soloway MS: Pre-treatment testosterone levels: Significance in androgen deprivation therapy. J Urol 136:1038–1040, 1986.

41. Huben RP, Murphy GP, and the investigators of the National Prostatic Cancer Project: A comparison of diethylstilbestrol or orchiectomy with buserelin and with methotrexate plus diethylstilbestrol or orchiectomy in newly diagnosed patients with clinical stage D2 cancer of the prostate. Cancer 62:1881–1887, 1988.

42. Huggins C, Hodges CV: Studies on prostate cancer. I. The effect of estrogen and of androgen injection on serum phosphatases in metastatic carcinoma of the prostate. Cancer Res 1:293–297, 1941.

43. Huggins C, Stevens RE, Hodges CV: Studies in prostatic cancer. II. The effects of castration on advanced carcinoma of the prostate gland. Arch Surg 43:209, 1941.

44. Iversen P, Christen MG, Friis E, et al: A phase III trial of Zoladex and flutamide versus orchiectomy in the treatment of patients with advanced carcinoma of the prostate. Cancer 66:52–60, 1990.

45. Iversen P, Suciu S, Sylvester R, et al: Zoladex and flutamide versus orchiectomy in the treatment of advanced prostatic cancer. A combined analysis of two European studies— EORTC 30853 and DAPROCA 86. Cancer 66:61–67, 1990.

46. Jacobi GH, Altwein JE, Kurth KH, et al: Treatment of advanced prostatic cancer with parenteral cyproterone acetate: A phase III randomised trial. Br J Urol 52:208–215, 1980.

47. Jacobi GH, Wenderoth UK: Gonadotropin-releasing hormone analogues for prostate cancer: Untoward side effects of high-dose regimens acquire a therapeutic dimension. Eur Urol 8:129–134, 1982.

48. Johansson JE, Andersson SO, Holmberg L, Bergström R: Primary orchiectomy versus estrogen therapy in advanced prostatic cancer—a randomized study: Results after 7 to 10 years of follow-up. J Urol 145:519–523, 1991.

49. Johansson S, Ljunggren E: Prostatic carcinoma cured with hormonal treatment. Scand J Urol Nephrol 15:331–332, 1981.

50. Johns WD, Garnick MB, Kaplan WD: Leuprolide therapy for prostate cancer. An association with scintigraphic "flare" on bone scan. Clin Nucl Med 15:485–487, 1990.

51. Jones N: Transcriptional regulation by dimerization: Two sides to an incestuous relationship. Cell 61:9–11, 1990.

52. Jong FH de, Oishi K, Hayes RB, et al: Peripheral hormone levels in controls and patients with prostatic cancer or benign prostatic hyperplasia: Results from the Dutch-Japanese case-control study. Cancer Res 51:3445–3450, 1991.

53. Jong FH de, Reuvers PJ, Bolt-de Vries J, et al: Androgens and androgen-receptors in prostate tissue from patients with benign prostatic hyperplasia: Effects of cyproterone acetate. J Steroid Biochem Mol Biol 42:49–55, 1992.

54. Jönsson G: Treatment of prostatic carcinoma with polyestradiol phosphate combined with ethinylestradiol. Scand J Urol Nephrol 5:97–102, 1971.

55. Kadmon D, Thompson TC, Lynch GR, Scardino PT: Elevated plasma chromogranin-A concentrations in prostatic carcinoma. J Urol 146:358–361, 1991.

56. Kaisary AV, Tyrrell CJ, Peeling WB, Griffiths K: Comparison of LHRH analogue (Zoladex) with orchiectomy in patients with metastatic prostatic carcinoma. Br J Urol 67:502–508, 1991.

57. Karr JP, Wajsman Z, Kirdani RY, et al: Effects of diethylstilbestrol and estramustine phosphate on serum sex hormone binding globulin and testosterone levels in prostate cancer patients. J Urol 124:232–236, 1980.

58. Kent JR, Bischoff AJ, Arduino LJ, et al: Estrogen dosage and suppression of testosterone levels in patients with prostatic carcinoma. J Urol 109:858–860, 1973.

59. Keuppens F, Denis L, Smith PH, et al: Zoladex R and flutamide versus bilateral orchiectomy: A randomized phase III EORTC 30853 study. Cancer 66:39–51, 1990.

60. Klein H, Bressel M, Kastendieck H, Voigt KD: Androgens, adrenal androgen precursors, and their metabolism in untreated primary tumors and lymph node metastases of human prostatic cancer. Am J Clin Oncol (CCT) 11(Suppl 2):30–36, 1988.

61. Klijn JGM, de Voogt HJ, Schröder FH, de Jong FH: Combined treatment with busereline and cyproterone acetate in metastatic prostatic carcinoma [letter]. Lancet 2:493, 1985.

62. Knönagel et al: Reported by Bertagna C: Rencontres d'Urologie. Montreal, May 31, 1990.

63. Kozlowski JM, Ellis WJ, Grayhack JT: Advanced prostatic carcinoma. Early versus late endocrine therapy. Urol Clin North Am 18:15–24, 1991.

64. Krieg M, Bartsch W, Janssen W, Voigt KD: A comparative study of binding, metabolism and endogenous levels of androgens in normal, hyperplastic and carcinomatous human prostate. *In* Coffey DS, Isaacs J (eds): Prostate Cancer. UICC Technical Report Series 48, Geneva 1979. J Steroid Biochem 10:93–111, 1979.

65. Labrie F, Auclair C, Cusan L, et al: Inhibitory effects of GnRH and its agonists on testicular gonadotropin receptors and spermatogenesis in the rat. Int J Androl Suppl 2:303, 1978.

66. Labrie F, Bélanger A, Veilleux R, et al: Rationale for maximal androgen withdrawal in the therapy of prostate cancer. Bailliere's Clin Oncol 2:597–619, 1988.

67. Labrie F, Dupont A, Bélanger A, et al: New approaches in the treatment of prostate cancer: Complete instead of partial withdrawal of androgens. Prostate 4:579–594, 1983.

68. Labrie F, Veilleux R: A wide range of sensitivities to androgens develops in cloned Shionogi mouse mammary tumor cells. Prostate 8:293–300, 1986.

69. Leuprolide Study Group: Leuprolide versus diethylstilbestrol for metastatic prostate cancer. N Engl J Med 311:1281–1286, 1984.

70. Lipsett B: Interaction of drugs, hormones and nutrition in the causes of cancer. Cancer 43:1967–1981, 1979.

71. Lund F, Rasmussen F: Flutamide versus stilbestrol in the management of advanced prostatic cancer. Br J Urol 61:140–142, 1988.

72. Mawhinney MG, Neubauer BL: Actions of estrogen in the male. Invest Urol 16:409–420, 1979.

73. Mellinger GT, as member of the Veterans Administration Cooperative Urological Research Group: Treatment and survival of patients with cancer of the prostate. Surg Gynecol Obstet 124:1011–1017, 1967.

74. Murphy GP, Slack NH: Response criteria to the prostate of the USA National Prostatic Cancer Project. Prostate 1:375–382, 1980.

75. Myers RP, Larson-Keller JJ, Bergstralh EJ, et al: Hormonal treatment at time of radical retropubic prostatectomy for stage D1 prostate cancer: Results of long-term follow-up. J Urol 147:910–915, 1992.

76. Namer M, et al: Reported by Bertagna C: Rencontres d'Urologie. Montreal, May 31, 1990.

77. Navratil H: Reported by Bertagna C: Rencontres d'Urologie. Montreal, May 31, 1991.

78. Neri RO, Kassem NY: Biological and clinical properties of antiandrogens. Progr Cancer Res Ther 31:507–518, 1984.

79. Nesbit RM, Baum WC: Endocrine control of prostatic carcinoma. JAMA 143:1317–1320, 1950.

80. Newling DWW: Criteria of response to treatment in advanced prostatic cancer. Bailliere's Clin Oncol 2:505–519, 1988.

81. Oesterling JE, Epstein JI, Walsh PC: The viability of adrenal androgens to stimulate the adult human prostate: An autopsy, evaluation of men with gonadotropic hypogonadism and panhypopituitarism. J Urol 136: 1030–1034, 1986.

82. Oomens EHGM, van Steenbrugge GJ, van der Kwast TH, Schröder FH: Application of the monoclonal antibody Ki-67 on prostate biopsies to assess the proliferative cell fraction of human prostatic carcinoma. J Urol 145:81–85, 1991.

83. Parmar H, Edwards L, Phillips RH, et al: Orchiectomy versus long-acting D-Trp-6-LHRH in advanced prostatic cancer. Br J Urol 59:248–254, 1987.

84. Parmar H, Lightman SL, Allen L, et al: Randomised controlled study of orchidectomy versus long-acting D-TRP-6-LHRH microcapsules in advanced prostatic carcinoma. Lancet 2:1201–1205, 1985.

85. Pavone-Macaluso M, Pavone M, Serretta V, Dapricello G: Antiandrogens alone or in combination for treatment of prostate cancer: The European experience. Urology 34 (Suppl 4): 27–36, 1989.

86. Pavone-Macaluso M, de Voogt HJ, Viggiano G, et al: Comparison of diethylstilbestrol, cyproterone acetate and medroxyprogesterone acetate in the treatment of advanced prostatic cancer: Final analysis of a randomized phase III trial of the European Organization for Research on Treatment of Cancer Urological Group. J Urol 136:624–631, 1986.

87. Redding TW, Schally AV: Inhibition of prostate tumor growth in two rat models by chronic administration of D-Trp[6] analogue of luteinizing hormone–releasing hormone. Proc Natl Acad Sci USA 78:6509–6512, 1981.

88. Reiner WG, Scott WW, Eggleston JC, Walsh PC: Long-term survival after hormonal therapy for stage D prostatic cancer. J Urol 122:183–184, 1979.

89. Riba LW: Subcapsular castration for carcinoma of prostate. J Urol 48:384–387, 1942.

90. Roberts JT, Essenhigh DM: Adenocarcinoma of prostate in 40-year-old body-builder. Lancet 2:742, 1986.

91. Robinson MRG, Hetherington J: The EORTC studies: Is there an optimal endocrine management for M1 prostatic cancer? World J Urol 4:171–175, 1986.

92. Rommerts FFG: Testosterone: An overview of biosynthesis, transport, metabolism and action. *In* Nieschlag E, Behre HM (eds): Testosterone. Action Deficiency Substitution. Berlin, Springer-Verlag, 1990, pp 1–22.

93. Schally AV, Arimura A, Baba Y, et al: Isolation and properties of the FSH and LH-releasing hormone. Biochem Biophys Res Commun 43:393–399, 1971.

94. Schally AV, Arimura A, Coy DH: Recent approaches to fertility control based on derivatives of LH-RH. *In* Munson PL, Diczfalusy E, Glover J, Olson RE (eds): Vitamins and Hormones, Advances in Research and Applications. New York, Academic Press, 1980, pp 257–323.

95. Schröder FH: Total androgen suppression in the management of prostatic cancer. A critical review. *In* Schröder FH, Richards B (eds): Progress in Clinical and Biological Research, Volume 185A. EORTC GU Group Monograph 2, Part A. Therapeutic Principles in Metastatic Prostatic Cancer. New York, Alan R. Liss, 1985, pp 307–317.

96. Schröder FH (ed): Treatment of Prostatic Cancer, Facts and Controversies. Progress in Clinical and Biological Research 359, EORTC Genitourinary Group Monograph 8. New York, Wiley-Liss, 1990.

97. Schröder FH, European Organization on Research on Treatment of Cancer Urological Group: Treatment response criteria for prostatic cancer. Prostate 5:181–191, 1984.

98. Schröder FH, Lock MTWT, Chadha DR, et al: Metastatic cancer of the prostate managed with buserelin versus buserelin plus cyproterone acetate. J Urol 137:912–918, 1987.

99. Schröder FH, van Steenbrugge GJ: Rationale against total androgen withdrawal. Bailliere's Clin Oncol 2:621–633, 1988.

100. Sharifi R, Soloway M, Leuprolide Study Group: Clinical study of leuprolide depot formulation in the treatment of advanced prostate cancer. J Urol 143:68–71, 1990.

101. Shearer RJ, Hendry WF, Sommerville IF, et al: Plasma testosterone an accurate monitor of hormone treatment in prostatic cancer. Br J Urol 45:668–677, 1973.

102. Siiteri PK, Wilson JD: The formation and content of dihydrotestosterone in the hypertrophic prostate of man. J Clin Invest 49:1737–1745, 1970.

103. Smith PH, Bono A, Calais da Silva F, et al: Some limitations of

the radioisotope bone scan in patients with metastatic prostatic cancer. A subanalysis of EORTC trial 30853. Cancer 66:3–10, 1990.

104. Smith PH, Suciu S, Robinson MRG, et al: A comparison of the effect of diethylstilbestrol with low dose estramustine phosphate in the treatment of advanced prostatic cancer: Final analysis of a phase III trial of the European Organization for Research on Treatment of Cancer. J Urol 136:619–623, 1986.

105. Sneller ZW, Hop WCJ, Carpentier PJ, Schröder FH: Prognosis and prostatic volume changes during endocrine management of prostate cancer: A longitudinal study. J Urol 147:962–966, 1992.

106. Sogani PC, Minoo R, Vagaiwala R, Whitmore WS: Experience with flutamide in patients with advanced prostatic cancer without prior endocrine therapy. Cancer 54:744–750, 1984.

107. Soloway MS, Chodak G, Vogelzang NJ, et al: Zoladex versus orchiectomy in treatment of advanced prostate cancer; a randomized trial. Zoladex Prostate Study Group. Urology 37:46–51, 1991.

108. Steg A, Benoit G: Percutaneous 17-β-estradiol in treatment of cancer of prostate. Urology 14:373–375, 1979.

109. Stone NN, Krongrad A, Chodak GW, et al: A double-blind randomized controlled study of the effect of flutamide on benign prostatic hypertrophy: Clinical efficacy [abstract]. Urol Res 17(5):338, 1989.

110. Susan LP, Roth RB, Adkins WC: Regression of prostatic cancer metastasis by high doses of diethylstilbestrol diphosphate. Urology 7:598–601, 1976.

111. Tayek JA, Byerley LO, Steiner B, et al: Nutritional and metabolic effects of gonadotropin-releasing hormone agonist treatment for prostate cancer. Metabolism 39:1314–1319, 1990.

112. Thompson IM, Zeidman EJ, Rodriguez FR: Sudden death due to disease flare with luteinizing hormone–releasing agonist therapy for carcinoma of the prostate. J Urol 144:1479–1480, 1990.

113. Tolis G, Ackman D, Stellos A, et al: Tumor growth inhibition in patients with prostatic carcinoma treated with luteinizing hormone–releasing hormone agonists. Proc Natl Acad Sci USA 79:1658–1662, 1982.

114. Trachtenberg J: The treatment of metastatic prostatic cancer with a potent luteinizing hormone releasing hormone analogue. J Urol 129:1149–1152, 1983.

115. Tyrrell CJ, Altwein JE, Klippel F, et al: A multicenter randomized trial comparing the luteinizing hormone–releasing hormone analogue goserelin acetate alone and with flutamide in

116. Vermeulen A: Androgens and male senescence. *In* Nieschlag E, Behre HM (eds): Testosterone. Action Deficiency Substitution. Berlin, Springer-Verlag, 1990, pp 261–276, 1990.

117. Veterans Administration Cooperative Urological Research Group (VACURG): Treatment and survival of patients with cancer of the prostate. Surg Gynecol Obstet 124:1011–1017, 1967.

118. Voogt HJ de, Klijn JGM, Studer U, et al: Orchidectomy versus buserelin in combination with cyproterone acetate, for 2 weeks or continuously, in the treatment of metastatic prostatic cancer. Preliminary results of EORTC trial 30843. J Steroid Biochem Mol Biol 37:965–971, 1990.

119. Voogt HJ de, Smith PH, Pavone-Macaluso M, et al: Cardiovascular side effects of diethylstilbestrol, cyproterone acetate, medroxyprogesterone acetate and estramustine phosphate used for the treatment of advanced prostatic cancer: Results from European Organization for Research on Treatment of Cancer trials 30761 and 30762. J Urol 135:303–307, 1986.

120. Voogt HJ de, Suciu S, Sylvester R, et al: Multivariate analysis of prognostic factors in patients with advanced prostatic cancer: Results from 2 European Organization for Research on Treatment of Cancer trials. J Urol 141:883–888, 1989.

121. Walsh PC, Carter HB, Metter EJ, et al: Longitudinal evaluation of serum androgen levels in men with and without prostate cancer [abstract]. Proceedings American Association of Genitourinary Surgeons Meeting, Hot Springs, Virginia, 1992, p 37.

122. Walsh PC, Hutchins GM, Ewing LL: Tissue content of dihydrotestosterone in human prostatic hyperplasia is not supranormal. J Clin Invest 72:1772–1777, 1983.

123. Waxman J, Man A, Hendry WF, et al: Short reports. Importance of early tumor exacerbation in patients treated with long acting analogues of gonadotrophin releasing hormone for advanced prostatic cancer. Br Med J 291:1387–1388, 1985.

124. Waxman JH, Sandow J, Man A, et al: The first clinical use of depot buserelin for advanced prostatic carcinoma. Cancer Chemother Pharmacol 18:174–175, 1986.

125. Weerden WM, van Steenbrugge GJ, van Kreuningen A, et al: Assessment of the critical level of androgen for growth response of transplantable human prostatic carcinoma (PC-82) in nude mice. J Urol 145:631–634, 1991.

126. Yatani R, Chigusa I, Akazaki K, et al: Geographic pathology of latent prostatic carcinoma. Int J Cancer 29:611–616, 1982.

Chapter 28

MANAGEMENT OF ANDROGEN-INDEPENDENT PROSTATE CARCINOMA

CHRISTOPHER J. LOGOTHETIS

Androgen-independent growth of prostatic carcinoma is a clinically virulent disease that has a short survival. The median survival of patients with metastatic and hormone-independent prostate cancer is less than 2 years in the majority of patients.[2] Unfortunately, therapeutic strategies have resulted in a limited benefit. Clinical trials have not resulted in a high enough response rate to consider any of the published therapies as standard. Therefore, patients with metastatic adenocarcinoma of the prostate exhibiting androgen-independent growth are candidates for investigational therapy. The difficulty in measuring response to therapy, the absence of routinely used prognostic criteria, and the absence of uniform criteria for patient entry into clinical trials have made interpretation of available clinical data difficult. Because of these limitations, patients with prostatic carcinoma have not benefited from the extensive phase II evaluations of novel agents.

At The University of Texas M. D. Anderson Cancer Center (UTMDACC), we have adopted a uniform approach to the study of patients' androgen-independent prostate cancer. The purpose of the prospective studies is not only to test the value of the therapy being used but also to test the validity of the parameters of response we have adopted. The use of a uniform method of studying such patients will assess the validity of response criteria, prognostic parameters, and the criteria for protocol entry. Guidelines for protocol entry at UTMDACC are designed to strictly identify patients who truly have androgen-independent growth of their prostatic cancer. By definition, patients must have a serum testosterone level within castrate range and objective evidence of tumor growth as documented by new sites of metastasis. Suggestive evidence exists both clinically and preclinically that tumors exhibiting androgen-independent growth continue to be sensitive to the mitogenic effects of androgens. We therefore require continued suppression of the serum testosterone levels as a part of the treatment of such patients. The criterion of objective evidence of progression manifested by new sites of metastases or deterioration in the symptom status excludes that small subset of patients who have an indolent clinical course and avoids the initiation of potentially morbid investigational therapy (Table 28–1).

The need for continued suppression of the serum testosterone level in patients who are androgen independent has been reported in the literature.[5] This need for continued suppression is based on the evidence that androgen-independent growth of prostatic carcinoma does not preclude the ability of the adenocarcinoma of the prostate to be stimulated by testosterone.

Volume of disease is a very important factor in predicting response to therapy. This prediction occurs for both androgen-independent and androgen-dependent prostatic carcinoma.[3, 10] In order to ensure an equal distribution of tumor volume and adequately describe the study populations, we have divided the patients into four categories determined by extensive organ involve-

TABLE 28–1. UTMDACC CRITERIA FOR PROTOCOL ENTRY INTO INVESTIGATIONAL TRIALS FOR ANDROGEN-INDEPENDENT PROSTATIC CARCINOMA

1. Objective evidence of progressive disease in 6-month period prior to protocol entry
2. Castrate level of serum testosterone
3. Expected survival of greater than 6 months for either objectively evaluable disease or elevated serum prostate-specific androgen

TABLE 28–2. STAGING OF DISSEMINATED PROSTATE CANCER

STAGE	SITE OF METASTASIS
Osseous I* (O_I)	Axial skeleton
Osseous II (O_{II})	Axial skeleton plus diaphyseal and distal extremity involvement
Visceral I* (V_I)	Parenchymal lung metastasis
Visceral II (V_{II})	Visceral other than lung (usually liver, brain, and mediastinum)

*Patients with bone marrow failure due to tumor infiltration or renal failure (creatinine > 2 mg/dl) are placed in corresponding Stage II. Nodal metastases other than mediastinal do not influence stage.

ment and volume of disease in osseous sites (Table 28–2). The value of this staging system has been reported and confirmed by others.[3, 10]

The treatment approaches for such patients can basically be divided into three broad groups: (1) secondary hormonal therapy, (2) novel therapies (growth factor inhibition), and (3) cytotoxic chemotherapy. Each of these is discussed separately.

HORMONAL THERAPY FOR ANDROGEN-INDEPENDENT PROSTATE CANCER

Salvage hormonal therapy by further inhibition of the androgen stimulation among patients who have progressive prostate cancer is ineffective. Transient palliative responses have been seen, but they possess little clinical utility.[2] The use of agents inhibiting the peripheral effects (flutamide) have not achieved responses in patients with progressive disease.

Adrenalectomy and hypophysectomy have each been used with little success. Overall, the beneficial response rate has been relatively low, of short duration, and only for that subset of patients who have minimally progressive disease.

Glucocorticoids have recently been reported to have antitumoral activity in patients with hormone-refractory prostatic carcinoma. This report suggests that this response has been associated with elevated levels of serum dehydroepiandrosterone (DHEA) and dehydroepiandrosterone sulfate (DHEAS). The suppression of these by exogenous steroids is the presumed mechanism of such responses.[14]

Pituitary ablation, bromocriptine, and adrenalectomy have all been used, and all result in significant responses in small numbers of patients. Overall, in progressive trials these response rates are of relatively low frequency and short duration. Response rates associated with this approach to therapy have unfortunately been of short duration and have minimal benefit. Future directions for the use of further hormonal blockade in patients with prostatic carcinoma may require specific inhibition of other pathways of hormonal stimulation (somatostatin).[8] Intriguing preclinical data exist for the use of somatostatin in prostatic carcinoma. A clinical trial performed at our institution has failed to demonstrate significant antitumoral activity in such patients. In pa-

tients selected by the criteria employed at the UTM-DACC for inclusion in the trial, no evidence of antitumoral activity was noted with somatostatin. It is possible that the use of this analogue specifically was responsible for this lack of benefit or that this approach to the treatment of patients is ineffective. Further studies with the use of other analogues are required.

At present, standard hormonal approaches to the therapy of prostatic carcinoma with further inhibition of the androgen-mediated pathway are likely to be fruitless, and the addition of other growth hormone blockades (somatostatin and bromocriptine) are interesting therapies that need to be investigated further. In summary, secondary hormonal therapy has been used as a palliative therapeutic approach but rarely achieves responses that are either reproducible or of durable clinical benefit for the majority of the patients.

CYTOTOXIC CHEMOTHERAPY

The use of cytotoxic chemotherapy in the treatment of prostatic carcinoma has not produced an increased rate of survival. It should be emphasized that responses have been achieved in prostatic carcinoma at a frequency ranging from 20 to 40 per cent. The quality of the response and the frequencies related impartially to the intensity of therapy, the selection of antitumoral agents, and the response criteria used. Yagoda has reported that response rates with similar agents but using different criteria were markedly different and could account for the differences in response rate treated. It is generally accepted that "stabilization" is no longer a valid criterion for the treatment of this disease.[17]

Responses among patients with bidimensionally measurable disease occur regularly. Its relatively high response rate in soft tissue disease, compared with that in bone disease, could be accounted for by the greater sensitivity to measurement of the more prevalent osseous metastases. Another explanation for this difference may be that soft tissue disease is a unique clinical phenotype that possesses an increased sensitivity to cytotoxic therapy.

The single agents considered to be most active in the treatment of this disease are listed in Table 28–3. Although these agents have traditionally achieved responses, combination chemotherapy regimens have

TABLE 28–3. CHEMOTHERAPY TRIALS IN BIDIMENSIONALLY MEASURABLE PROSTATE CANCER

AGENT	NO. OF PATIENTS	PARTIAL RESPONSE (%)
Cisplatin	22	12
Amsacrine	18	0
Doxorubicin (Adriamycin)	39	5
Mitomycin-C	22	25
Mitoguazone (MGBG)	25	24
Etoposide (VP-16-213)	20	5
Gallium nitrate	20	10
Doxorubicin (weekly)	32	12
5-Fluorouracil	73	10

**TABLE 28–4. CHEMOTHERAPY DOSAGES,
1980 TO 1986**

NO. OF PATIENTS	CHEMOTHERAPY	
	Agent	**Dosage**
78	Doxorubicin	50 mg/m^2 C1* $\times$ 1
	Mitomycin-C	5 mg/m^2 $\times$ 2
	5-Fluorouracil	750 mg/m^2 $\times$ 2
22	Vinblastine	1.5 mg/m^2 C1 $\times$ 5
27	Doxorubicin	50 mg/m^2 C1 $\times$ 1
	Vinblastine	1.5 mg/m^2 C1 $\times$ 5
32	Adriamycin	50 mg/m^2 C1 $\times$ 1
	Vinblastine	1.5 mg/m^2 C1 $\times$ 5
	Mitomycin-C	10 mg/m^2 $\times$ 1

*C1 = Course one.

failed to increase this response rate substantially. This can be accounted for by the relatively low response rate of each individual drug and the lack of significant synergistic antitumoral activity.

Chemotherapy at the UTMDACC has been based on the use of intensive combination therapy. The drugs considered to be most active are vinblastine, doxorubicin, and mitomycin-C. Although a large number of patients were treated, we were unable to show any definite evidence for long-term tumor-free survival in such patients (Tables 28–4 and 28–5). The clinical responses and their durability were directly related to the volume of disease, as measured by the clinical stages of our study patients. Striking responses in patients with visceral metastases have occurred frequently. In addition, patients with painful osseous metastases experienced significant relief of symptoms. This contrast between the clinical relief of symptoms and objective evidence of response is characteristic of many therapies in hormone-refractory prostate cancer.

To summarize the results of chemotherapy in prostate cancer, one can conclude that frequent objective antitumor activity is encountered but the response rate is not of sufficient clinical benefit to justify its routine use. The two most effective single agents in published available data are mitomycin-C and doxorubicin.[4, 9, 11] Although cytotoxic therapy is of limited value in patients with androgen-independent classic adenocarcinoma, cytotoxic therapy is of definite value in patients with small-cell subtypes of prostate cancer.

The future role of cytotoxic therapy in the treatment of prostate cancer will need to be investigated in novel settings and early in the therapy. Isaacs has suggested that early cytotoxic therapy may result in an increased response rate.[6] In our own experience in a single-arm pilot trial, we saw long-term tumor-free survival in a fraction of patients, but this cannot be interpreted as definite evidence of benefit because of the study design of that trial. An ongoing prospective randomized trial is trying to confirm these data in large populations. The use of androgen priming to increase the response rate with chemotherapy has been published by a number of investigators. Unfortunately, this results in an occasionally severe and rapidly progressive disease whose course cannot be ameliorated by cytotoxic therapy. Although

androgen priming may increase sensitivity to chemotherapy in vitro, the lack of benefit clinically is probably attributable to the relative ineffectiveness of the cytotoxic agents currently available for the treatment of hormone-refractory prostatic carcinoma.

Despite the relative ineffectiveness of cytotoxic chemotherapy in achieving a survival advantage for patients with metastatic hormone-refractory prostatic carcinoma, it is frequently a valuable palliative regimen for relieving painful symptoms attributed to this disease and can achieve responses in a significant portion of patients. Although cytotoxic therapy cannot be routinely recommended for patients with prostatic carcinoma, its incorporation into therapeutic schemas combining different therapeutic modalities should be considered.

Although classic adenocarcinoma of the prostate with diffuse bony metastases is relatively resistant to cytotoxic therapy, other histologic subtypes are more responsive to chemotherapy. The true frequency of small cell carcinoma of the prostate is unknown, but this subtype of prostatic carcinoma has been characterized by a unique sensitivity to cytotoxic therapy, a visceral spread, and a unique pattern of marker distribution.[1] It is characterized by early visceral metastases, relatively low prostate-specific antigen and prostatic acid phosphatase with a relatively high frequency of elevated serum carcinoembryonic antigen. The cytotoxic regimens employed at our institution are similar to those used for small cell carcinomas of other sites and have resulted in a high response rate. Patients treated at the UTMDACC receive initial chemotherapy of the histologic tissue to confirm the presence of small cell carcinoma.[1] This is being reported with increasing frequency at our institution because of awareness of the pathology of this lesion.

The future role of cytotoxic therapy in prostatic carcinoma will obviously be in those histologic subtypes that possess a unique sensitivity to these agents and perhaps in the treatment of early disease. Cytotoxic therapy should not be neglected as a potential agent in combination with other therapeutic strategies for the treatment of this disease.

KETOCONAZOLE

Ketoconazole was initially reported by Trachtenburg and Pont to possess antitumoral activity clinically in prostatic carcinoma.[15] It was theorized that the blocking of adrenal androgens was partially responsible for these responses. Studies have shown that direct cytotoxic effects of ketoconazole exist in vitro. The response rates

**TABLE 28–5. RESPONSE RATE OF HORMONE-
REFRACTORY PROSTATIC CARCINOMA**

REGIMEN	PARTIAL RESPONSE	GREATER THAN 50% DECLINE IN PSA (%)
Ketoconazole + doxorubicin	7/11 (64%)	13/23 (57%)
Estramustine + vinblastine	3/11 (24%)	11/23 (48%)

TABLE 28–6. COMPARISON OF RESPONSE RATE BY STAGE AND PROTOCOL

STAGE	TOTAL PATIENTS	CHEMOTHERAPY				P Value
		Doxorubicin + Vinblastine	DMF*	Vinblastine	VAM†	
O_I	70	3/11 (27.3%)	15/34 (44.1%)	4/11 (36.4%)	5/14 (35.71%)	0.77707 (NS)‡
O_{II}	48	0/6 (0%)	6/25 (24%)	1/6 (16.7%)	5/11 (45.45%)	0.19596 (NS)
V_I	19	3/4 (75%)	8/10 (80%)	3/5 (60%)	—	0.70751 (NS)
V_{II}	23	6/22 (33.3%)	3/9 (33.3%)	0/1 (0%)	3/7 (42.86%)	0.86186 (NS)
Total	160	8/27 (29%)	32/78 (41%)	8/23 (35%)	13/32 (41%)	(NS)
P value		0.88810	0.02199	0.42022	0.87766	

*DMF = Doxorubicin, mitomycin-C, and 5-fluorouracil.
†VAM = Vinblastine, Adriamycin (doxorubicin), and mitomycin-C.
‡NS = Not significant.

have varied but have all been reported to be higher than 30 per cent.[7, 16] The antitumoral activity of ketoconazole is established in patients with castrate levels of serum testosterone and does not influence serum DHEA level. It is therefore likely that this is one of the significant agents for the treatment of this disease. Ketoconazole for hormone-refractory prostatic carcinoma is being studied in combination with doxorubicin at the UTM-DACC, and very promising early data exist for this treatment[2] (Table 28–6). Ketoconazole very clearly should be developed as a cytotoxic agent and incorporated into regimens for prostatic carcinoma. Classifying ketoconazole as hormonal therapy is probably inaccurate, and its future role or its analogues may be expanded.

Inhibiting the progression of prostatic carcinoma can be achieved by interrupting the communication between growth factors and their ligands on the prostate epithelium. Suramin was the first agent investigated as a putative inhibitor of growth factor–mediated progression.[13] Responses with this agent are definite and occur in truly hormone-refractory patients. Unfortunately, suramin is a toxic agent and has limited antitumor activity. The future role of this agent is unlikely to be significant unless responses occur to a much higher degree in patients with earlier disease. The development of analogues may be a therapeutic strategy of significant future value.

REFERENCES

1. Amato RJ, Logothetis CJ, Hallinan R, et al: Chemotherapy for small cell carcinoma of prostatic origin. J Urol 147:935–937, 1992.
2. Crawford ED, Eisenberger MA, McLeod DG, et al: A controlled trial of leuprolide with and without flutamide in prostatic carcinoma. N Engl J Med 321:419–424, 1989.
3. Eisenberger M, Crawford ED, Blumenstein B, et al: Significance of pre-treatment stratification by extent of disease (ED) in stage D₂ prostate cancer (PC) patients treated with leuprolide + flutamide (LF) or leuprolide + placebo (LP). Proc Am Soc Clin Oncol 8:132, 1989.
4. Eisenberger MA, Abrams JS: Chemotherapy for prostatic carcinoma. Semin Urol 6:303–310, 1988.
5. Gittes RF: Carcinoma of the prostate. N Engl J Med 324:236–245, 1991.
6. Isaacs JT: Relationship between tumor size and curability of prostatic cancer by combined chemo-hormonal therapy in rats. Cancer Res 49:6290–6294, 1989.
7. Johnson D, Babaian R, von Eschenbach A, et al: Ketoconazole therapy for hormonally refractive metastatic prostate cancer. Urology 31:132, 1988.
8. Liebow C, Lee MT, Schally A: Antitumor effects of somatostatin mediated by the stimulation of tyrosine phosphatase. Metabolism 39(Suppl 2):163–166, 1990.
9. Logothetis CJ, Dexeus F, Chong CDK, et al: Cytotoxic chemotherapy for hormone-refractory metastatic prostate cancer. *In* Johnson DE, Logothetis CJ, von Eschenbach AC (eds): Systemic Therapy for Genitourinary Cancers. Chicago, Year Book Medical Publishers, 1989, pp 234–238.
10. Logothetis CJ, Samuels ML, von Eschenbach A, et al: Doxorubicin, mitomycin-C, and 5-fluorouracil (DMF) in the treatment of metastatic hormonal refractory adenocarcinoma of the prostate, with a note on the staging of metastatic prostate cancer. J Clin Oncol 1:368–379, 1983.
11. Scher HI, Smart-Curley T, Dershaw DD, et al: Cytotoxic chemotherapy for advanced cancer of the prostate: Memorial Sloan-Kettering Cancer Center Experience. *In* Johnson DE, Logothetis CJ, von Eschenbach AC (eds): Systemic Therapy for Genitourinary Cancers. Chicago, Year Book Medical Publishers, 1989, pp 228–233.
12. Sella A, Kilbourn R, Amato R, et al: A phase II study of ketoconazole (KC) combined with weekly doxorubicin (DOX) in patients (PTS) with hormone refractory prostate cancer (PC) results in a high response rate. Proc Am Soc Clin Oncol 11:219, 1992.
13. Stein CA, LaRocca RV, Thomas R, et al: Suramin: An anticancer drug with a unique mechanism of action. J Clin Oncol 7:499–508, 1989.
14. Tannock I, Gospodarowicz M, Meakin W, et al: Treatment of metastatic prostatic cancer with low-dose prednisone: Evaluation of pain and quality of life as pragmatic indices of response. J Clin Oncol 7:590–597, 1989.
15. Trachtenberg J, Pont A: Ketoconazole therapy for advanced prostate cancer. Lancet 2:433–435, 1984.
16. Trump DL, Havlin KH, Messing EM, et al: High-dose ketoconazole in advanced hormone-refractory prostate cancer: Endocrinologic and clinical effects. J Clin Oncol 7:1093–1098, 1989.
17. Yagoda A: Cytotoxic agents on prostate cancer: An enigma. Semin Urol 1:311–321, 1983.

Chapter 29

TREATMENT OF LOCALIZED CARCINOMA OF THE PROSTATE (CLINICAL STAGES A AND B)

DAVID F. PAULSON

Considerable controversy exists over the relative impact of surgery and radiation for the treatment of prostatic carcinoma clinically confined to the organ of origin. Much of this controversy arises because of the variable biologic course of prostatic malignancy and the difficulty in predicting the biologic outcome of apparent organ-confined disease. The variation in the biologic course of the disease has even prompted concern that observation could be appropriate in certain circumstances. Many institutional trials using a single modality were developed to examine the impact of that single therapy, and these results were then compared with those of other nonrandomized groups alternatively treated. Many of these efforts were flawed because of variation in the patient population, presumably derived from a biased segregation of populations of high and low biologic risk. In the last decade, a series of observations from both randomized and nonrandomized trials has been published. These observations have brought about the current enthusiasm for the use of radical surgery in the management of T1 and T2 prostatic malignancy.

OBSERVATION 1: CURRENT TECHNOLOGY SHOULD PERMIT DETERMINATION OF DISEASE EXTENT IN THE HOST AT RISK

In the early 1970s a large multi-institutional study involving investigators at 13 major medical centers and their associated Veterans Administration Hospitals set out to determine the accuracy of staging studies to assess the anatomic distribution of malignant disease in the host at risk and, upon identification of the anatomic extent of disease, to compare the relative efficacy of surgery, radiation, and observation in altering the outcome of the disease progress.[10, 11] Patient accession in this study began in February 1975, and the last patient was entered in September 1978. In this study, 509 men with newly diagnosed, biopsy-proven prostatic adenocarcinoma were assigned a preliminary clinical stage based upon digital rectal examination (DRE), colorimetric serum acid phosphatase level, a plain chest radiograph, and a metastatic bone survey. Staging studies, each designed to determine the anatomic distribution of disease with progressive focus on the prostate itself, were sequenced to progress from studies that showed widely disseminated disease to those that demonstrated regional or local extension. All men who had an elevated serum acid phosphatase by colorimetric assay were believed to have systemic disease and were excluded from the randomization schema.

All men who demonstrated no evidence of osteoblastic disease on their skeletal bone films were subjected to a technetium-99 bone scan. Approximately 25 per cent of all patients with no bone disease identified on routine skeletal radiographs had bone disease determined by isotopic bone scanning. The frequency of detectable bone metastases increased as the volume of local disease increased (Fig. 29–1). After exclusion of disease in the axial and appendicular skeleton by isotopic

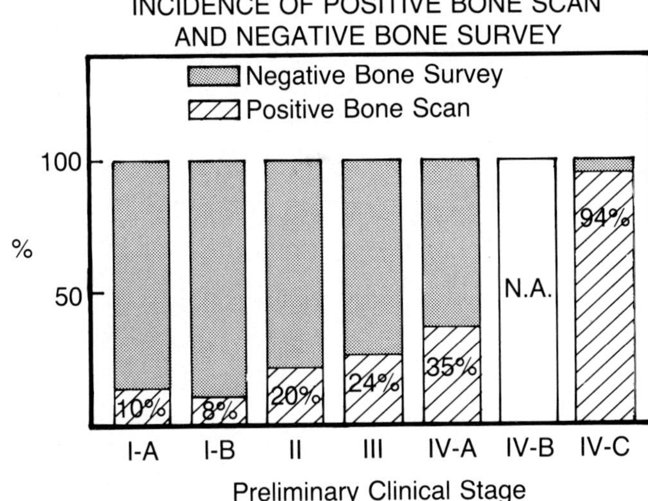

FIGURE 29–1. Patients with bone disease detected by radioisotopic scanning who were considered disease free by skeletal survey.

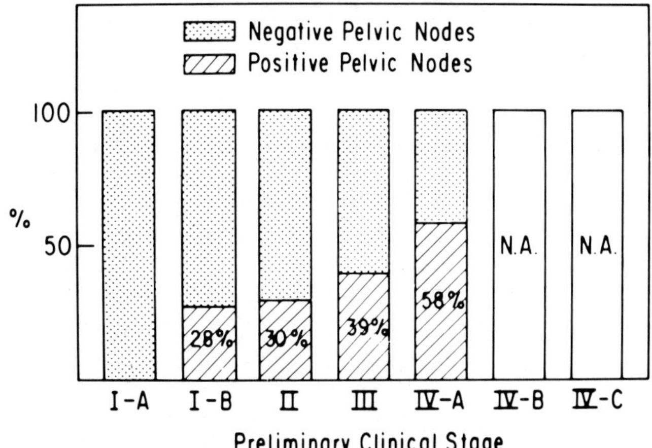

FIGURE 29–3. Incidence of pelvic node extension as a function of preliminary clinical stage in patients with no bone disease as determined by isotopic bone scan.

bone scanning, attention was turned to the nodes of the prostatic lymphatics. All patients underwent either lymphangiography, or later CT, and were then subjected to a pelvic lymphadenectomy. The margins of the node dissection were limited to the triangle bordered by the external iliac vasculature, the pelvic floor, and the hypogastric vasculature; all node-bearing tissue in this area was removed, including the node-bearing tissue surrounding the obturator nerves and vessels (Fig. 29–2). As anticipated, the incidence of node-positive disease was found to increase as the volume of local disease increased (Fig. 29–3). Further study was incorporated into this staging schema. In an attempt to determine whether histopathologic characteristics of the tumor tissue biopsied to establish the diagnosis of cancer could be used to predict the presence or absence of nodal extension, an analysis of the incidence of positive nodes as a function of Gleason sum was carried out. The analysis demonstrated that both high- and low-grade disease (as determined by the Gleason sum) functioned

as relatively accurate predictors of the presence of node-positive disease, equivalent to that of the imaging modalities of lymphangiography and CT. Eighty-seven per cent of patients with a Gleason sum of less than 5 had node-negative disease, whereas 100 per cent of those with a Gleason sum of 9 or 10 had node-positive disease (Table 29–1). With minor variations, this general trend has been substantiated by subsequent investigators. However, as disease has been detected at smaller and smaller volumes by careful early DRE or by transrectal ultrasonography (TRUS), currently we do identify patients with a Gleason 9 or 10 in their prostatic primary who do not have detectable nodal extension.

Thus, these series of staging studies did present a mechanism by which a clinician could assess the extent of disease in the host at risk with relative accuracy and determine the potential for disease control using treatments designed to control malignancy confined to the prostate itself.

OBSERVATION 2: THE RELATIVE BENEFIT OF RADIATION THERAPY AND SURGERY IN THE MANAGEMENT OF CLINICALLY CONFINED DISEASE

In the trial described above, patients whose disease was clinically confined to the prostate as determined by DRE and who had no evidence of bone- or node-positive

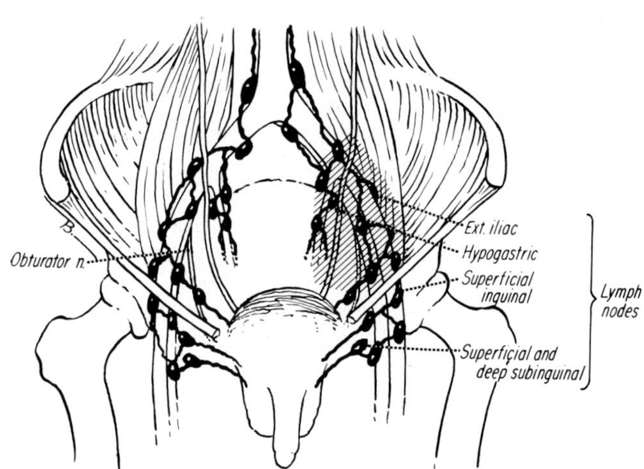

FIGURE 29–2. Shaded area indicates area of limited pelvic lymph node dissection for staging of prostate carcinoma.

TABLE 29–1. NODE BIOPSY

GLEASON SUM	POSITIVE	NEGATIVE	N/GROUP
2–5	13.9%	86.1%	36
6	32.4%	67.6%	34
7	49.9%	50.1%	21
			($P < 0.0005$)
8	75.0%	25.0%	12
9–10	100.0%	0%	7
No diagnosis	33.0%	66.1%	12

disease were assumed to have organ-confined disease and were randomized to radical prostatectomy or external beam radiation therapy. These patients with clinical Stage A2 or Stage B (T1-2NOMO) disease were randomized in balanced groups of four by institution to either radical prostatectomy or megavoltage radiation therapy.[8] Any patient with an occult focal carcinoma was excluded from this randomization scheme, as were any patients who had clinical Stage C (T3NOMO) disease. Prostatectomy could be accomplished by either a perineal or a retropubic route; however, the anatomic limits of the dissection had to include the apex of the prostate and the seminal vesicles (Fig. 29–4). Patients assigned to radiation therapy were treated with megavoltage equipment, i.e., the highest available energy (cobalt-60, linear accelerator, and/or betatron x-ray beam), with a minimum surface-to-axis distance of 80 cm. The field was to include the prostate, periprostatic region, and pelvic lymph nodes as determined by lymphograms and localization films. The upper margin of the radiation field was at the level of the iliac crest, the lateral margin at least 1 cm beyond the external iliac nodal chains, and the lower margin 1 cm below the inferior margin of the prostate. All fields were treated with a total tumor dose of 4500 to 5000 rad in 40 days total elapsed time. The dose was specific from the appropriate isodose curve as a minimum dose in the volume of the prostate. An additional treatment boost of 2000 rad was delivered to a reduced volume, which had to include the prostate.

Patients were followed at 2-month intervals for the first year and 3-month intervals thereafter. Serum biochemical profiles with acid phosphatase determinations by colorimetric or enzymatic assay, Karnofsky's performance ratings, and physical examination were performed at each follow-up; chest radiographs and isotopic bone scans were obtained at 6-month intervals. The effectiveness of the treatment in controlling the cancer was determined using first evidence of treatment failure as the end-point. The investigators chose to use the first evidence of recurrent disease rather than survival to avoid confounding the impact of first therapy by the subsequent application of a second therapy that could

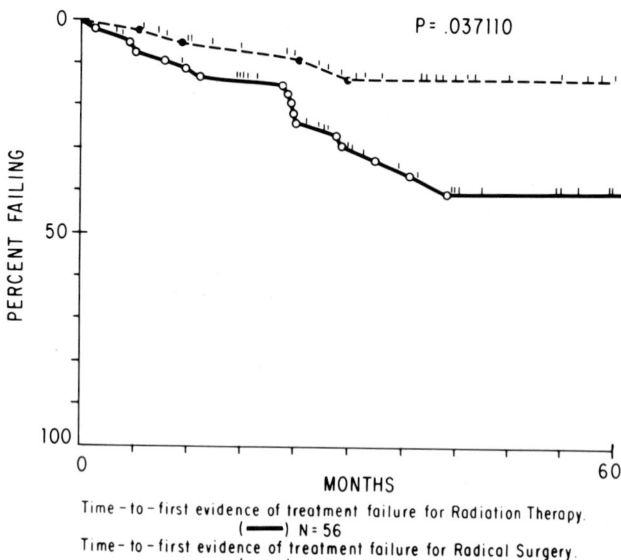

FIGURE 29–5. Time to treatment failure for patients randomized to radiation therapy or radical surgery whose disease is confined to the prostate. (From Paulson DF, Lin GH, Hinshaw W, et al: Radical surgery vs. radiotherapy for Stage A2 and Stage B (T1-2MONO) adenocarcinoma of the prostate. J Urol 128:502, 1982, © by Williams & Wilkins, 1982; with permission.)

alter the survival experience. Subsequent studies used to evaluate the impact of treatment in prostatic carcinoma have used this same end-point but have chosen to call it by the less cumbersome title of disease-free survival. Survival data were not accrued in this study because funding was withdrawn by the National Cancer Institute prior to completion of the study and patient follow-up and data analysis could not be completed as originally projected. Treatment failure (or disease progression) was identified by acid phosphatase elevation on two consecutive follow-ups or by the appearance of bony or other parenchymal disease with or without concomitant acid phosphatase elevation. New appearance or increased radioisotopic uptake on bone scan was identified as progression. Identification of cancer within the prostate on follow-up biopsy of those patients who received radiation did not signify failure within this study. Curves representing nonparametric estimates of first evidence of treatment failure were generated according to the Kaplan-Meier method.[6] Censored values representing patients without evidence of treatment failure at the time of last follow-up are presented on all graphs by a single vertical tick. Treatment efficacy in pairs of subgroups was assessed for differences by the Cox-Mantel test.[3] Fifty-six patients received external beam radiation therapy and 41 underwent radical prostatectomy. Analysis of the time-to-failure curves of the two treatment groups demonstrated that radical surgery provided a distinct advantage over radiation therapy in controlling disease (increasing the progression-free interval), and this was significant at the 0.037 level (Fig. 29–5). This study was enthusiastically embraced by the urologic community but critiqued by the radiation therapy community. Detractors argued that patients with more aggressive disease had been assigned to radiation

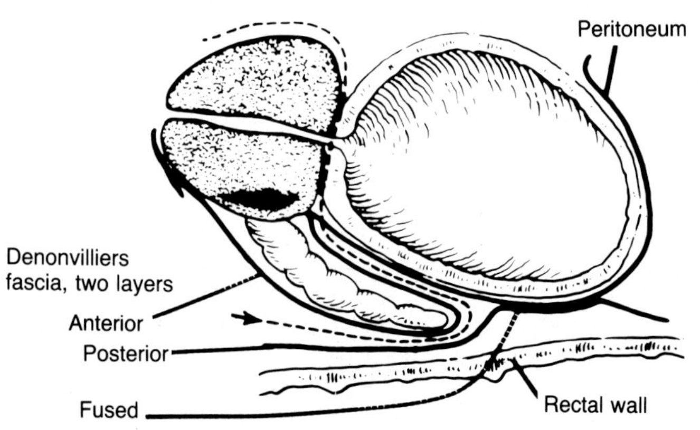

FIGURE 29–4. Limits of dissection for a radical prostatectomy. (From JB DeKernion and DF Paulson: Genitourinary Cancer Management. Philadelphia, Lea & Febiger, 1987. Used with permission.)

therapy and their length of follow-up was too short. It should be noted that the study design required that all patients be examined prior to randomization by both radiation therapists and urologists and that both had to agree that the disease was organ-confined. Analysis of the relative Gleason grade between the two groups demonstrated that the average Gleason sum of the radiation therapy arm was 5.1, and the average Gleason sum of the radical surgery arm was 5.5. If Gleason sum functions as an indicator of biologic aggressiveness, the two groups seem equivalent. An additional 20 months of follow-up continued to demonstrate a disease control advantage of radical surgery over radiation therapy.[6]

OBSERVATION 3: DEMONSTRATION THAT ERECTILE POTENCY COULD BE PRESERVED BY MODIFICATION OF THE SURGICAL PROCEDURE

The third major observation made in the 1980s which further strengthened the position for radical prostatectomy in the management of prostatic adenocarcinoma was the observation by Donkers and Walsh that, by modifying the technical conduct of radical prostatectomy, one could preserve the neurovascular structures that surround the prostate and contribute to corporal innervation and erectile potency. Drawing on information gathered from a series of cadaveric dissections, Walsh cleverly and adroitly applied and modified the technique of radical retropubic prostatectomy, demonstrating a method for early control of the dorsal venous complex, thus reducing blood loss in what had previously been a procedure with less than optimal hemostatic control while modifying the local dissection in such a way as to preserve the neurovascular periprostatic plexus which contributed to corporal innervation (Fig. 29–6). Walsh was able to translate this operative procedure into preservation of erectile potency in a large number of men who previously would most likely have been rendered impotent. Walsh clearly demonstrated that modification of the radical prostatectomy procedure could preserve erectile potency and that preservation of

erectile potency appeared to be a function of volume of tumor size, extent of local tumor, and age of the patient.

These three observations did much to increase the enthusiasm for radical prostatectomy. The first observation had demonstrated that it was possible to determine the extent of disease with reasonable accuracy. The second observation demonstrated that radical prostatectomy provided an enhanced disease-control advantage over that provided by external beam radiation therapy. Last, the observation of Walsh and co-workers removed the argument that radical prostatectomy always resulted in loss of erectile potential, whereas the radiation approach had the prospect of preserving erectile function following definitive radiation therapy.

HOW SHOULD ONE MANAGE THE PATIENT WITH NEWLY DIAGNOSED, APPARENTLY CLINICALLY CONFINED PROSTATIC CARCINOMA?

When presented with the patient whose clinical history is suspicious for prostatic carcinoma or whose physical examination is suspicious for the presence of prostatic carcinoma, the physician should immediately take steps to confirm or deny the presence of disease.

WHAT CLINICAL SITUATIONS SHOULD INCREASE THE INDEX OF SUSPICION OF PROSTATIC MALIGNANCY?

A patient who has a family history of prostatic carcinoma should immediately be placed in a high-suspicion group. This is specifically true for patients whose fathers or brothers have been diagnosed with the malignancy. Young men (under 55 to 60 years of age) who present with the sudden onset of obstructive outflow should be considered as high-risk candidates for evaluation. Patients who present with irritative prostatic outflow symptoms and who have acquired the working diagnosis of prostatitis but whose prostate feels normal on DRE should be similarly classified. Finally, men who experi-

FIGURE 29–6. Schematic diagram of the correct site for ligation of the lateral pedicle.

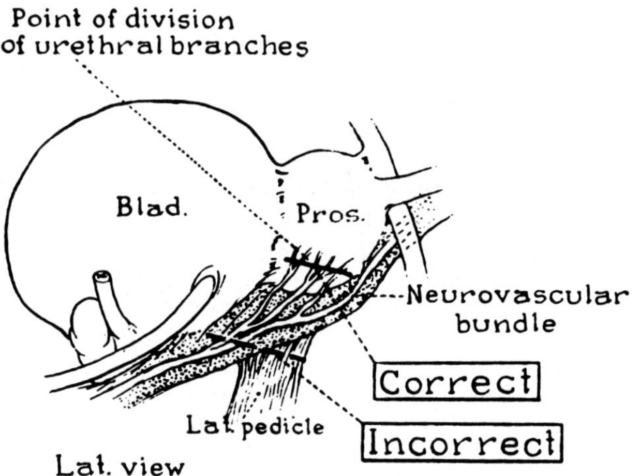

ence a change of volume or force in their ejaculatory pattern should be considered high-risk candidates.

WHAT PHYSICAL SIGNS PROMPT EVALUATION?

Any patient who has any area of increased consistency or firmness of the gland should be considered for evaluation.

SHOULD ANY LABORATORY FINDINGS PROMPT EVALUATION?

Prostate-specific antigen (PSA), a glycoprotein produced by prostatic epithelial cells which can be detected in the circulation, has been considered by many to be a reasonable marker for screening. Unfortunately, as a single entity, PSA elevations are not sufficient to confirm the presence of malignancy. However, the use of PSA for the selection of patients for TRUS and biopsy may be appropriate. Although many argue that the data accrued by Cooner and co-workers are biased in that the detection rate of prostatic carcinoma is unnaturally high, their data do provide information of interest.[2] They divided their patient population into those who had a normal or abnormal DRE and those who had a PSA of less than 4 ng/ml, between 4 and 10 ng/ml, and greater than 10 ng/ml. Both PSA elevation alone and DRE alone were significant predictors of the presence of prostatic carcinoma (Tables 29–2 and 29–3). However, when PSA was used in combination with DRE, the ability to predict the presence of prostatic carcinoma was markedly increased (Table 29–4). It is the duty of the responsible physician to determine the detection rate of clinical importance. The data strongly suggest that it is not appropriate to biopsy patients who have a normal DRE and a PSA less than 4 ng/ml. However, patients whose PSA is above 4 but less than 10.0 ng/ml have a cancer detection rate of 5.5 per cent. This means that 1 of every 20 patients with this finding has prostatic carcinoma. Does this detection rate of 1 of 20 make it reasonable to pursue biopsy in this category? My opinion is that it does. Patients who fall into this category should undergo TRUS and biopsy. Thus, PSA should be used to derive need for TRUS and biopsy rather than as a single screening tool.

TABLE 29–2. CANCER DETECTION RATE RELATED TO DIGITAL RECTAL EXAMINATION IN 2634 PATIENTS

DIGITAL RECTAL EXAMINATION	NO. CANCERS/NO. PATIENTS
+	288/884 (32.6%)
−	95/1750 (5.4%)

From Cooner WH: Prostate specific antigen, digital rectal examination and transrectal ultrasonic examination of the prostate in prostate cancer detection. Monogr Urol 12:1–13, 1991; with permission.

TABLE 29–3. CANCER DETECTION RATE RELATED TO LEVEL OF SERUM PROSTATE-SPECIFIC ANTIGEN

PROSTATE-SPECIFIC ANTIGEN* (ng/ml)	NO. CANCERS/NO. PATIENTS
≤ 4	77/1711 (4.5%)
> 4	306/923 (33.2%)
4.1–10	93/535 (17.4%)
> 10	213/400 (53.3%)

*Hybritech.
From Cooner WH: Prostate specific antigen, digital rectal examination and transrectal ultrasonic examination of the prostate in prostate cancer detection. Monogr Urol 12:1–13, 1991; with permission.

CAN PROSTATE-SPECIFIC ANTIGEN PREDICT THE EXTENT OF DISEASE?

PSA elevations do not provide accurate information with respect to extent of disease. Our own data indicate that patients who had preoperative PSA determinations prior to radical surgery demonstrated too broad a range of levels to be useful in detecting local extent of disease. Patients with organ-confined disease had preoperative PSAs that ranged from 0.3 to 44.6 ng/ml, with a mean of 9.4 ng/ml, whereas patients who had specimen-confined disease had PSAs that ranged from 3.1 to 122, with a mean of 20.7, and patients who had margin-positive disease had PSAs that ranged from 0.3 to 213, with a mean of 34.7. Thus, PSA alone should not be used to select treatment.

CONTROVERSY OF THE ENHANCED BENEFIT OF TRANSRECTAL ULTRASONOGRAPHY OVER DIGITAL RECTAL EXAMINATION

In the early data from the national screening trial to evaluate the efficacy of DRE versus TRUS to detect prostatic carcinoma, 2427 patients were subjected to both studies. Two thousand thirty-two of these patients were found to have no evidence of disease by either examination. Three hundred ninety-five patients were found to have findings suspicious of prostatic carcinoma

TABLE 29–4. CANCER DETECTION RATE RELATED TO BOTH LEVELS OF SERUM PROSTATE-SPECIFIC ANTIGEN AND DIGITAL RECTAL EXAMINATION IN 2634 PATIENTS

PROSTATE-SPECIFIC ANTIGEN* (ng/ml)	DIGITAL RECTAL EXAMINATION (NO. CANCERS/NO. PATIENTS)	
	Positive	**Negative**
≤ 4	46/446 (10.3%)	31/1265 (2.5%)
> 4	242/438 (55.3%)	64/485 (13.2%)
4.1–10	74/194 (38.1%)	19/343 (5.5%)
> 10	168/256 (65.6%)	45/144 (31.3%)

*Hybritech.
From Cooner WH: Prostate specific antigen, digital rectal examination and transrectal ultrasonic examination of the prostate in prostate cancer detection. Monogr Urol 12:1–13, 1991; with permission.

by either DRE or TRUS. A breakdown of the relative efficacy of these two demonstrated that of the 395 patients 65 had suspicion of disease only on DRE, 242 had disease identified only by TRUS, and 88 had disease identified by both modalities. Thus, DRE detected a total of 153 of 395 suspicious patients, with TRUS identifying an additional 242 suspicious for malignancy.

Three hundred twenty-nine patients were subjected to biopsy directed by TRUS. Fifty-one of 329 patients were identified with malignancy. Of the 51 patients with a positive biopsy, 33 had a suspicious DRE. Thus, 18 of 51 patients would not have been detected if DRE had been the only method for evaluating the presence of disease in these patients at risk.

WHAT IS THE ANTICIPATED OUTCOME IN PATIENTS WITH CLINICALLY LOCALIZED PROSTATIC CANCER?

At the time of last review, 470 patients, personally operated by the senior author, with histologically proven prostatic adenocarcinoma were staged by serum acid phosphatase determinations, by isotopic bone scan, and by staging pelvic lymphadenectomy. All patients without evidence of bony extension and without histologic evidence of nodal extension were then subjected to radical perineal prostatectomy. Eighteen of these 470 patients had microscopic nodal disease and are excluded from the analysis of the T1-2NOMO population. Eleven additional patients had no evidence of bony and nodal disease but did have an elevated serum acid phosphatase by colorimetric or enzymatic assay. These 11 patients are also excluded from the analysis of the T1-2NOMO disease. All histopathologic specimens were reviewed and categorized by pathology as to the extent of local disease and segregated into organ-confined, specimen-confined, or margin-positive groups. Capsular invasion without penetration was classified as organ-confined. Two patients could not be categorized because of distribution of the surgical specimen for research purposes prior to histopathologic examination. For this review, patients were followed at 3-month intervals during the

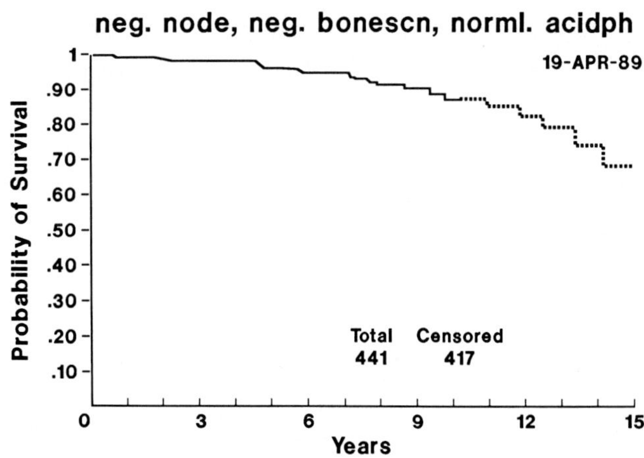

FIGURE 29–8. Probability of survival for the total population undergoing radical prostatectomy.

first year and 6-month intervals thereafter, progress being monitored by DRE and determination of serum acid phosphatase and PSA. Bone scans were obtained only after acid phosphatase elevations had been detected or when patients appeared with symptoms compatible with bony disease. Failure time was calculated from the first date of acid phosphatase elevation, from the first date of bony or parenchymal extension by imaging, or from the date local recurrence was detected by DRE and confirmed by biopsy. Curves representing nonparametric estimates of time to first evidence of treatment failure (disease-free survival) were generated using the Kaplan-Meier method. Censored values representing patients without evidence of disease failure at the time of latest follow-up were represented by single vertical ticks on the graph. Treatment efficacy in pairs of subgroups were tested for difference by the Cox-Mantel test. All curves are marked at 10 years to reflect that valid confidence limits could not be obtained after the 10-year interval.

Among the 442 T1-2NOMO patients, 28 per cent had failed at 10 years, but only 12 per cent had died (Figs.

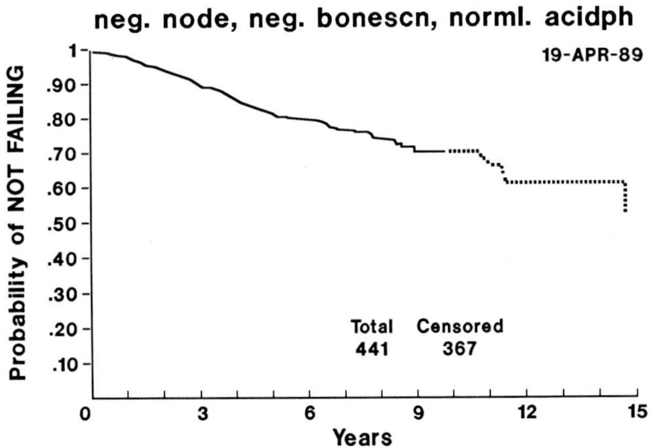

FIGURE 29–7. Probability of not failing for the total population undergoing radical prostatectomy.

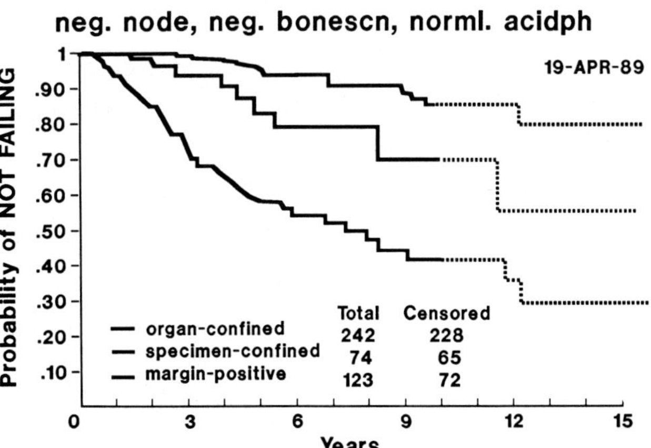

FIGURE 29–9. Probability of not failing as a function of organ-confined disease, specimen-confined disease, and margin-positive disease (organ- versus specimen-confined, $P<0.002$; organ-confined versus margin-positive, $P<0.0001$; specimen-confined versus margin-positive, $P<0.001$).

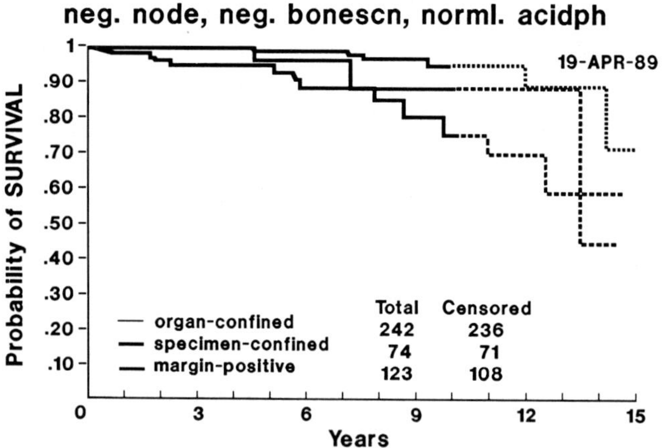

FIGURE 29–10. Probability of surviving as a function of organ-confined disease, specimen-confined disease, and margin-positive disease (organ-confined versus margin-positive, $P<0.001$).

29–7 and 29–8).[9] When the population was segregated according to local extent of disease and analyzed as a function of being either organ confined or specimen or margin positive, statistically significant differences were identified in both time to failure and survival time (Figs. 29–9 and 29–10). Two hundred forty-two had organ-confined disease with a failure rate of 12 per cent at 10 years. Thirty per cent of 74 patients with specimen-confined disease had failed at 10 years, whereas 60 per cent of 123 patients with margin-positive disease failed at 10 years. However, when one examines survival experience, at 10 years only 8 per cent of the organ-confined patients, 12 per cent of the specimen-confined patients, and 30 per cent of the margin-positive patients had died. As demonstrated previously, Gleason grading continued to predict the potential for failure. Only 23 per cent of patients whose Gleason sum was 7 or less had failed by 10 years, as opposed to 80 per cent of the patients who had a Gleason sum of greater than 7 (Fig. 29–11). The Gleason sum could not be assessed in 14 of the 442 patients.

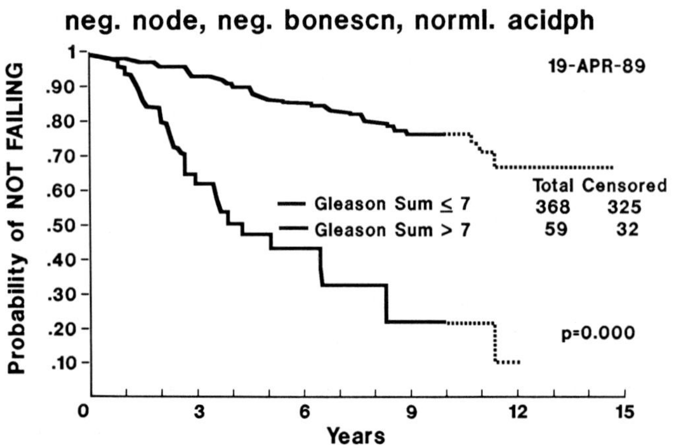

FIGURE 29–11. Probability of not failing as a function of Gleason sum.

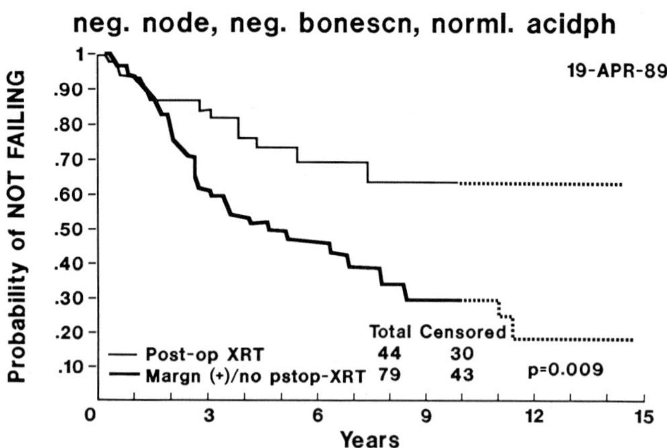

FIGURE 29–12. Probability of not failing among margin-positive patients who received postoperative radiation therapy or not.

THE HAZARDS OF MARGIN-POSITIVE DISEASE

Although Walsh and others have stated that preservation of the neurovascular bundle does not provide an enhanced risk for the potential of margin-positive residual disease, there is concern among many students of the disease that such modification of the operative procedure has the potential to increase the incidence of margin-positive disease. How does one handle margin-positive disease when it is identified? Is any treatment of specific benefit? Among the patients identified above, 44 margin-positive patients received adjunctive postoperative radiation, whereas 79 margin-positive patients did not. The Gleason sum averaged 6.9 for both groups. Eleven of the 44 patients who received adjunctive radiation failed distantly only, and 37 of 79 nonradiated patients failed either locally or distantly and/or locally (Fig. 29–12). Nine of the 79 nonirradiated patients failed with only local recurrence. Excluding these 9 patients from analysis, no statistically significant difference in time to failure can be identified between the radiated and nonradiated patients (Fig. 29–13). Thus, we con-

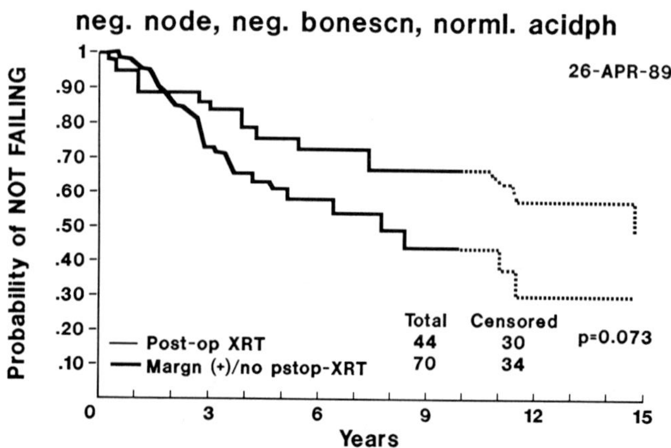

FIGURE 29–13. Probability of survival among margin-positive patients who received postoperative radiation therapy or not.

TABLE 29–5. 114 MARGIN-POSITIVE PATIENTS

SITE	RADIATED FAILED	NOT RADIATED FAILED	TOTAL FAILED
Capsule only	3/14	14/38	17/52
Seminal vesicle only	2/4	1/6	3/10
Capsule and seminal vesicle	10/26	22/35	32/61

From Paulson DF, Moul JW, Walther PJ: Radical prostatectomy for clinical T1-2NOMO prostatic adenocarcinoma: Long term results. J Urol 144:1180, 1990, © by Williams & Wilkins, 1990; with permission.

clude that no survival advantage can be achieved by postoperative adjunctive radiation.

No relationship of failure by site of margin-positive disease and by adjunctive radiation received could be identified, suggesting that no specific site of residual disease is a high predictor for failure (Table 29–5).[9]

DOES EARLY ADJUNCTIVE ANDROGEN DEPRIVATION PROVIDE ANY SIGNIFICANT ADVANTAGE?

Early in their operative experience at the Duke University Medical Center, patients with margin-positive disease were subjected to either immediate androgen deprivation or delayed androgen deprivation provided when failure was identified. An analysis of the time to failure among the margin-positive patients who received immediate androgen deprivation compared with those who did not demonstrated that early androgen deprivation delayed the appearance of subsequent disease recurrence. However, when survival was examined, no difference in survival could be identified between the two groups.

Thus, it appears that neither adjunctive radiation nor immediate androgen deprivation provides any survival

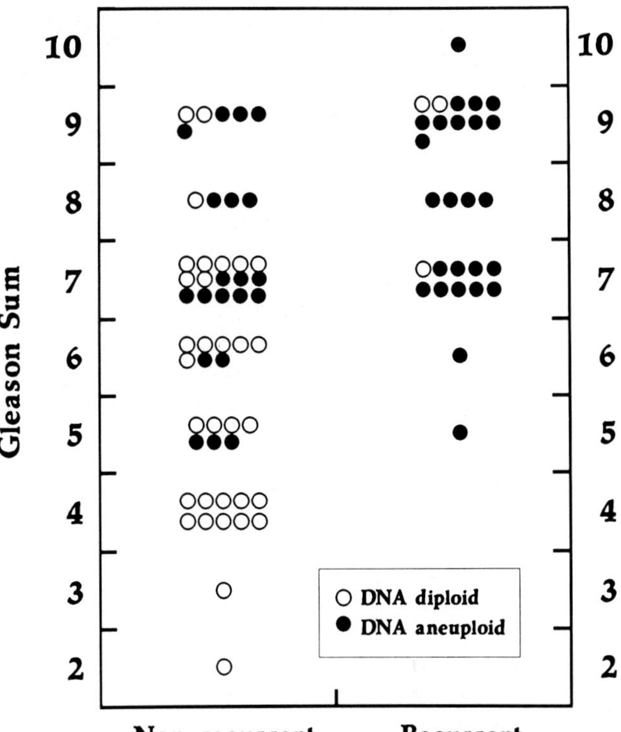

FIGURE 29–15. Graphic representation of Gleason sum in patient population as function of disease recurrence. Note association of aneuploidy and higher Gleason sums with recurrence. (From Lee SE, Currin SM, Paulson DF, Walther PJ: Flow cytometric determination of ploidy in prostatic adenocarcinoma: A comparison of seminal vesicle involvement and histopathological grading as a predictor of clinical recurrence. J Urol 140:769–774, 1988, © by Williams & Wilkins, 1988; with permission.)

advantage when one considers these two treatment modalities in patients who have margin-positive residual disease. Last, we must ask why there is no apparent survival advantage among margin-positive patients treated with radiation therapy. It appears that radiation reduces local recurrence rates without actually providing total cell kill. When one uses PSA as an indicator of local disease, one finds that PSA levels are driven down, often becoming undetectable in the early period following local radiation for margin-positive recurrence. However, with time, most of these patients almost uniformly demonstrate rising PSA levels, indicating that disease has recurred, presumably at a local level (Fig. 29–14).

IS THERE A WAY TO PREDICT OUTCOME IN PATIENTS WHO HAVE RADICAL PROSTATIC SURGERY?

Previous studies have demonstrated that Gleason histopathologic grading provides a reasonable predictor of outcome after radical prostatectomy in node-negative, bone-negative patients. Patients with Gleason sums of 7 or less consistently fare better than patients with Gleason sums of 8, 9, or 10. The Gleason sum is criticized for being subjective and difficult to reproduce.[1, 12, 14]

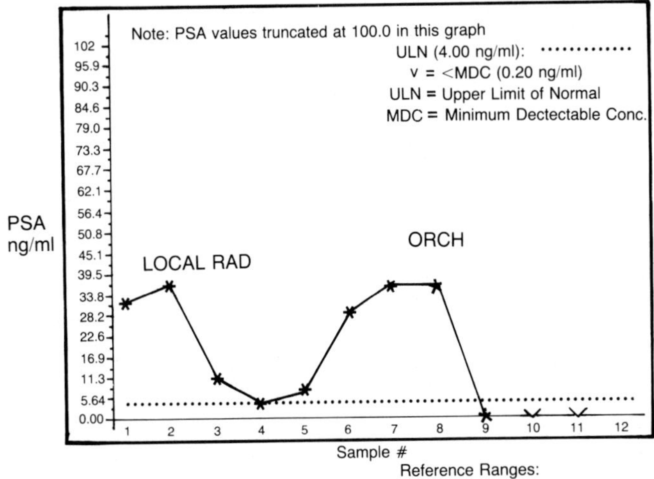

FIGURE 29–14. Curve depicting PSA response after radiation therapy in a patient with margin-positive recurrent disease following radical prostatectomy.

More importantly, the predictive value of the Gleason score among patients with intermediate-grade tumors is reduced. Walther and co-workers, in an attempt to determine a more accurate method of predicting biologic risk of prostatic carcinoma, undertook the analysis of 88 deparaffinized radical prostatectomy specimens in order to determine the relative predictive value for disease recurrence on the basis of tumor ploidy, Gleason sum, and seminal vesicle involvement (stage).[7] Ninety-four patients who underwent radical prostatectomy as primary treatment were selected. Sixty-five patients demonstrated seminal vesicle invasion by light microscopy. An additional 29 patients without seminal vesicle involvement were selected on the basis of the Gleason sum cluster alone in order to adequately represent the diverse spectrum of histopathologic grade in prostatic cancer. Nine tumors were of Gleason sum 2 to 4, 14 were of Gleason sum 5 to 7, and 6 were of Gleason sum 8 to 10. All patients were T1-2N0M0 patients at the time they were subjected to radical prostatectomy. First evidence of failure was determined by the appearance of biopsy-proven local recurrence, by positive scan, or by the appearance of an elevation in serum prostatic acid phosphatase. No patient received any adjunctive therapy until distant disease was identified. The methods for ploidy analysis were as previously described.[4, 5, 7, 13] Examination for the occurrence of treatment failure when stratified by Gleason sum and ploidy demonstrated that the predominance of aneuploidy occurred in the recurrent disease group (Fig. 29–15). Recurrent disease was noted with a marked increase in frequency among patients with seminal vesicle involvement and in patients with aneuploidy (Table 29–6). Although the incidence of recurrence in the total population as a function of Gleason sum also was statistically significant, this signif-

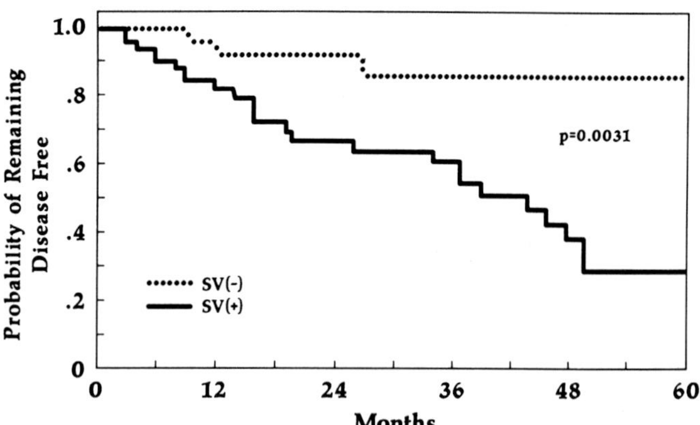

FIGURE 29–16. Kaplan-Meier plot demonstrates significant difference in probability of remaining free of disease between seminal vesicle–positive [SV($+$)] and seminal vesicle–negative [SV($-$)] disease. (Reprinted with permission from Lee SE, Currin SM, Paulson DF, Walther PJ: Flow cytometric determination of ploidy in prostatic adenocarcinoma: A comparison of seminal vesicle involvement and histopathological grading as a predictor of clinical recurrence. J Urol 140:769–774, 1988, © by Williams & Wilkins, 1988; with permission.)

icance occurred at a lower confidence level. When the entire population was stratified into positive and negative seminal vesicle cohorts, ploidy appeared as a significant predictor of recurrence in patients with seminal vesicle involvement.

A Kaplan-Meier analysis was used to determine the probability of remaining disease free as a function of seminal vesicle status and ploidy. The probability of remaining free of disease at 60 months when seminal vesicle invasion occurred was only 28 per cent, as opposed to 87 per cent in the absence of seminal vesicle involvement (Fig. 29–16). When ploidy alone was examined, only 9 per cent of aneuploid patients remained disease free at 60 months, as opposed to 85 per cent of those with diploid tumors (Fig. 29–17).

TABLE 29–6. RECURRENCE AS FUNCTION OF PLOIDY, GLEASON SUM, AND SEMINAL VESICLE STATUS

	RECURRENCE		
	Yes	No	P Value
Seminal vesicle positive			
DNA diploid	3	14	
DNA aneuploid	22	13	<0.005
Gleason ≤ 7	11	20	
Gleason > 7	14	7	<0.05
Seminal vesicle negative			
DNA diploid	0	18	
DNA aneuploid	3	7	<0.025
Gleason ≤ 7	1	22	
Gleason > 7	2	3	<0.025
Total population			
DNA diploid	3	32	
DNA aneuploid	25	20	<0.001
Gleason ≤ 7	12	42	
Gleason > 7	16	10	<0.05
Seminal vesicle negative	3	25	
Seminal vesicle positive	25	27	<0.005

From Lee SE, Currin SM, Paulson DF, Walther PJ: Flow cytometric determination of ploidy in prostatic adenocarcinoma: A comparison of seminal vesicle involvement and histopathological grading as a predictor of clinical recurrence. J Urol 140:769–774, 1988, © by Williams & Wilkins, 1988; with permission.

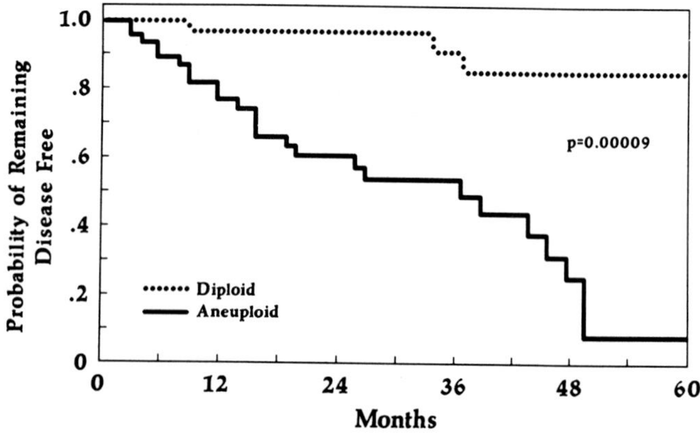

FIGURE 29–17. Kaplan-Meier plot demonstrates marked difference in probability of remaining free of disease between patients with diploid versus aneuploid tumors. (Reprinted with permission from Lee SE, Currin SM, Paulson DF, Walther PJ: Flow cytometric determination of ploidy in prostatic adenocarcinoma: A comparison of seminal vesicle involvement and histopathological grading as a predictor of clinical recurrence. J Urol 140:769–774, 1988, © by Williams & Wilkins, 1988; with permission.)

Patients were segregated into four groups based on ploidy and seminal vesicle status. No failures were seen in the best prognostic group, the 18 diploid patients with negative seminal vesicles. Examination of the prostatic parameters analyzed within this study reveal that ploidy and seminal vesicle status have similar prognostic significance with very high negative predictive values. Thus, ploidy as assessed by flow cytometric analysis of deparaffinized prostatic carcinoma, Gleason sum, and seminal vesicle status are important predictors of disease progression. However, ploidy as the objective measurement of malignant potential and seminal vesicle status as the objective measurement of pathologic stage seem equally important when one examines the negative predictive value.

Unfortunately, we are not yet at a stage where we can exclude patients with diploid tumors from radical surgical intervention. We do know from previous studies that approximately 50 per cent of patients with metastatic disease have diploid tumors. Thus, other factors must be involved if we are to use biologic markers as indicators in the selection of therapy.

REFERENCES

1. Barzell W, Bean MA, Hilaris BS, Whitmore WF: Prostatic adenocarcinoma: Relationship of grade and local extent to the pattern of metastases. J Urol 118:278, 1977.
2. Cooner WH: Prostate specific antigen, digital rectal examination and transrectal ultrasonic examination of the prostate in prostate cancer detection. Monogr Urol 12:1–13, 1991.
3. Cox DR: Regression models and life tables. JR Stat Soc 34:187–220, 1972.
4. Fossa SD, Thorud E, Shoaib MC, Pettersen EO: DNA flow cytometry of cells obtained from old paraffin-embedded specimens. A comparison with results of scanning absorption cytometry (a methodological study). Path Res Pract 181:200, 1986.
5. Hedley DW, Friedlander ML, Taylor IW, et al: Method for analysis of cellular DNA content of paraffin-embedded pathological material using flow cytometry. J Histochem Cytochem 31:1333, 1983.
6. Kaplan EL, Meier P: Nonparametric estimation from incomplete observations. J Am Stat Assoc 53:457–481, 1958.
7. Lee SE, Currin SM, Paulson DF, Walther PJ: Flow cytometric determination of ploidy in prostatic adenocarcinoma: A comparison of seminal vesicle involvement and histopathological grading as a predictor of clinical recurrence. J Urol 140:769–774, 1988.
8. Paulson DF, Lin GH, Hinshaw W, et al: Radical surgery vs. radiotherapy for stage A2 and stage B (T1-2MONO) adenocarcinoma of the prostate. J Urol 128:502–504, 1982.
9. Paulson DF, Moul JW, Walther PJ: Radical prostatectomy for clinical T1-2NOMO prostatic adenocarcinoma: Long term results. J Urol 144:1180, 1990.
10. Paulson DF, Uro-Oncology Research Group: The impact of current staging procedures in assessing disease extent of prostatic adenocarcinoma. J Urol 121:300–305, 1979.
11. Paulson DF, Uro-Oncology Research Group: Predictors of lymphatic spread in prostatic adenocarcinoma. J Urol 123:697–699, 1980.
12. Sagalowsky AL, Milam H, Reveley LR, Silva FG: Prediction of lymphatic metastases by Gleason histologic grading in prostatic cancer. J Urol 128:951, 1982.
13. Schutte B, Reynders MMJ, Bosman FT, Blijham GH: Flow cytometric determination of DNA ploidy level in nuclei isolated from paraffin-embedded tissue. Cytometry 6:26, 1985.
14. Wilson JWL, Morales A, Bruce AW: The prognostic significance of histological grading and pathological staging in carcinoma of the prostate. J Urol 130:481, 1983.

Chapter 30

MANAGEMENT OF LOCAL RECURRENCE OF PROSTATE CANCER

VAHAN S. KASSABIAN and PETER T. SCARDINO

Even though the majority of patients dying of prostate cancer succumb to generalized disease, local recurrence of prostate cancer after definitive therapy can cause substantial morbidity and occasional mortality. Studies of the natural history of prostate cancer and of the outcome of treatment trials indicate that failure to control the local tumor eventually leads to distant metastases and death from prostate cancer.[22]

Historically, local recurrence was manifested by increasing lower tract obstructive symptoms, hematuria, ureteral obstruction with or without septicemia, or chronic renal failure. Today with the advent of PSA measurement, ultrasonography, and transrectal needle biopsy, local recurrence after either radiation therapy or radical prostatectomy is detected more frequently and is often found in an otherwise asymptomatic patient.

Natural History of Untreated Prostate Cancer

The natural history of prostate cancer has been summarized elsewhere.[56] All studies that have followed patients for long periods show that progression is inexorable, with local recurrence often preceding distant metastases.[24]

In a group of patients from the United Kingdom with known prostate cancer of varying stages, treatment was deferred after diagnosis until symptomatic progression occurred. Eighteen per cent of the patients died of other causes without needing treatment, and 17 per cent died of prostate cancer without ever being treated. Within 5 years of diagnosis, 49 per cent of patients required further treatment, and in this group local progression occurred twice as often as distant progression. It be-

comes apparent that with a deferred treatment policy, a high proportion of patients eventually require treatment. However, deaths from other causes are common in elderly men.[24]

Failure to control the tumor locally leads eventually to distant metastases and death from prostate cancer if patients live long enough. Fuks et al[22] studied the long-term results in patients with localized prostate cancer treated with ^{125}I seed implantation. They observed that the relative risk of metastatic spread subsequent to local failure was four times the relative risk in patients without evidence of local relapse. In patients with local failure, distant metastases occurred chronologically at a later date than in patients who developed distant metastases without local relapse. Treatment failure in patients without local relapse seems, therefore, to result from pre-existing micrometastases, whereas treatment failure (and distant metastases) in patients with local recurrence arises later, when distant metastases result from local relapse of the tumor. Early and complete eradication of the primary tumor is important, therefore, in order to achieve long-term cure. Kaplan et al[33] also demonstrated the importance of local control in prostate cancer. In patients treated with external beam radiation therapy, the risk of dying of prostate cancer was significantly less in patients with local control than in patients with local recurrence (Fig. 30–1 and 30–2).

LOCAL RECURRENCE AFTER RADIATION THERAPY

Definition

Clinical local recurrence means progressive local growth of the primary tumor after radiation therapy and

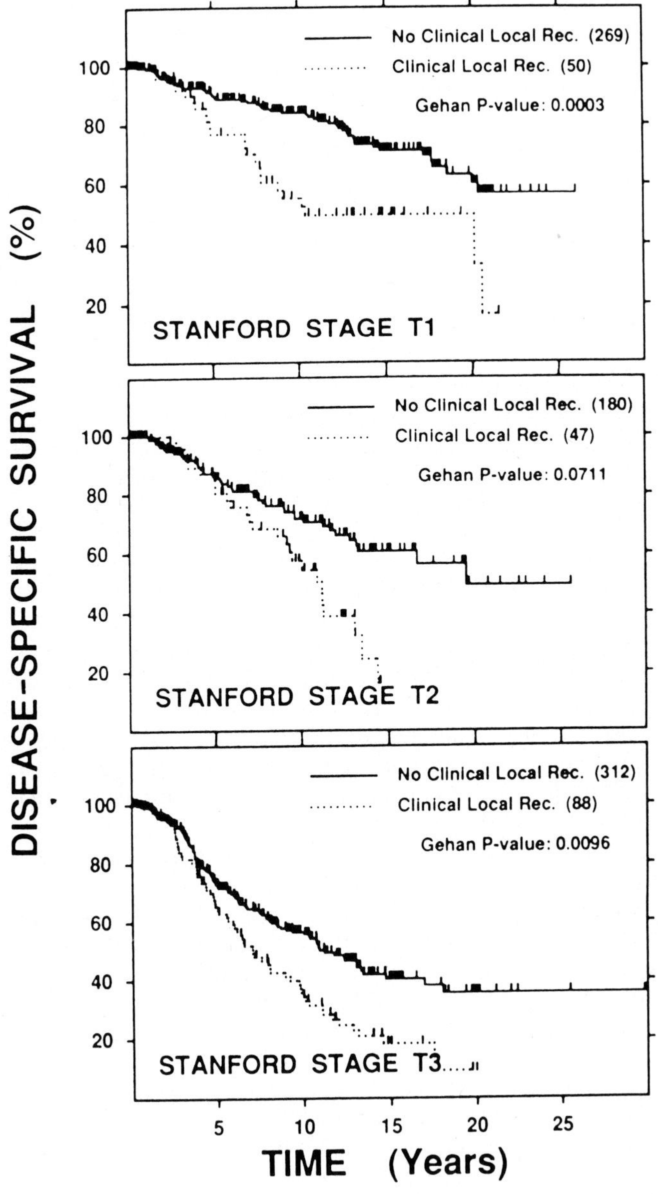

FIGURE 30–1. Disease-specific survival for patients with Stanford stages T1, T2, and T3 disease with or without clinical local recurrence. (From Kaplan ID, Prestidge BR, Bagshaw MA, Cox RS: The importance of local control in the treatment of prostatic cancer. J Urol 147:917–921, 1992, © by American Urological Assoc. Inc.; with permission.)

tation alone and no evidence of recurrence, 32 per cent had at least one positive biopsy. Also, a positive biopsy correlated strongly with eventual recurrence. Lee et al[41] found an 81 per cent positive biopsy rate in patients treated with ^{125}I seed implantation. In their series, only hypoechoic areas were biopsied regardless of other findings, and 88 per cent of the patients had such lesions on transrectal ultrasonography (TRUS). Although the significance of a positive biopsy result may be debated, it is clear that a positive biopsy in the presence of new local symptoms, rising prostate-specific antigen (PSA) level, or an enlarging lesion on TRUS or digital rectal examination (DRE) signifies local recurrence. However, a positive biopsy in the absence of any associated

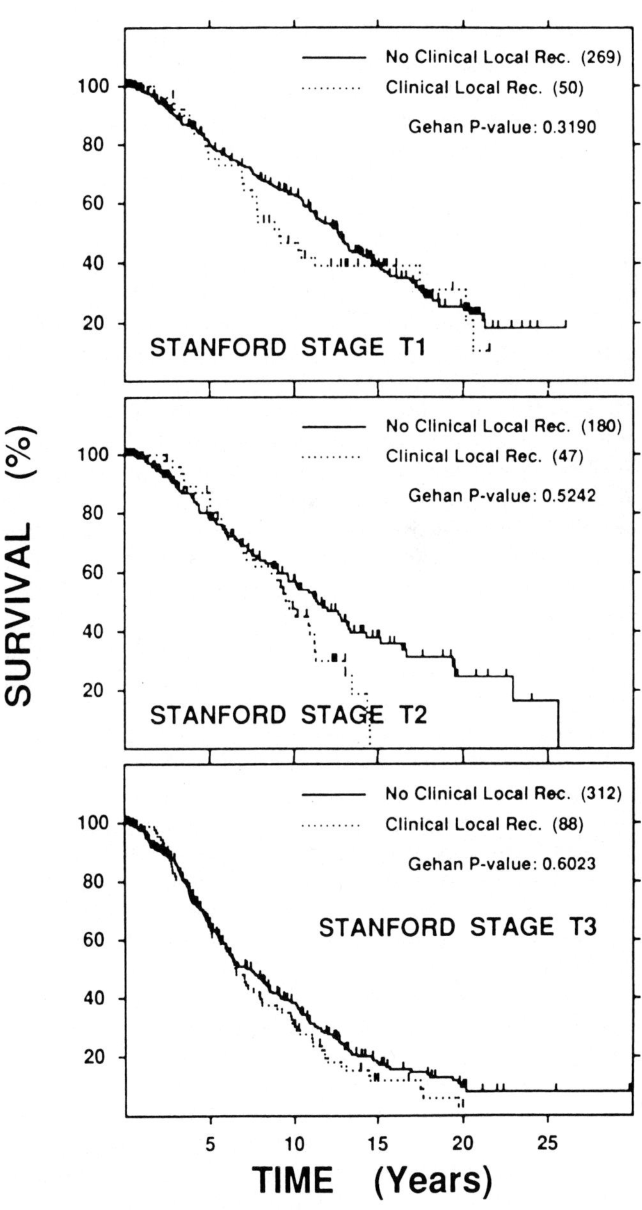

FIGURE 30–2. Survival for patients with Stanford stages T1, T2, and T3 disease with or without clinical local recurrence. (From Kaplan ID, Prestidge BR, Bagshaw MA, Cox RS: The importance of local control in the treatment of prostatic cancer. J Urol 147:917–921, 1992, © by American Urological Assoc. Inc.; with permission.)

is best defined as a morbid clinical phenomenon manifested by signs or symptoms (for example, obstruction of the bladder outlet or ureter) and proved by biopsy. Using such strict clinical criteria, Holzman et al[27] found a 53 per cent local recurrence rate in clinical Stage C (T3) patients treated with gold seeds and external beam radiation therapy. Clinical local recurrence is less common after radiation therapy in patients with clinical Stage A and B (T1-2) tumors.[7, 33] In an effort to predict clinical local recurrence, needle biopsy of the prostate has been performed 1 to 2 years after radiation therapy in patients with no clinical evidence of local treatment failure.[58] Of 140 patients treated with gold seed implan-

findings may not be sufficient for institution of further therapy. Although controversy still exists regarding the significance of such biopsy results, there is no dispute about the disturbingly high incidence of positive biopsy results. Kabalin et al[31] performed multiple systematic biopsies in patients with a rising PSA following radiation therapy and found a 93 per cent positive biopsy rate at least 18 months after treatment. The source of the unusually high rate is unclear and is contrary to previous reports from the same institutions[63–65]; however, most of the patients in the recent series had an elevated or rising PSA level.

Incidence

Several factors affect the local recurrence rate of prostate cancer reported in the literature. These factors include the stage and grade of the tumor, the age and health of the patient, the duration of follow-up, and the effects of other treatments, especially hormonal therapy.

Stage and grade of the primary tumor have been repeatedly shown to affect the local recurrence rate,[59] whether after radical prostatectomy or following definitive radiation therapy. Local recurrence is more likely in patients with high-stage or high-grade cancers.

Prostate cancer is a disease of the elderly, and many patients have concomitant disease. In a Swedish study of untreated prostate cancer in men with a mean age of 72 years, a substantial proportion of patients diagnosed with clinically localized prostate cancer died with their cancer, rather than of it, before local progression occurred.[30] In younger patients, however, the outcome is different. We reported that 17 per cent of patients died of causes other than prostate cancer among 360 patients with a mean age of 66 who were treated with radioactive gold seeds and external beam irradiation for clinical stages A2, B, and C1 disease and followed for a mean of 7.3 years.[42] During this same period, 21 per cent died of prostate cancer.

Prostate cancer is a slow-growing tumor with a doubling time of about 2 years[63–65] and a long natural history. Treatment with radiation therapy or hormonal therapy may delay the appearance of local recurrence even further. Consequently, the local failure rate reported in a given series depends largely on the length of follow-up. Local failure occurs as long as 15 to 20 years after therapy, so that the length of follow-up affects the reported rate of local recurrence.

The concomitant use of hormonal therapy has a profound effect on the apparent rate of local recurrence. Many urologists have seen dramatic reduction in the size of the primary tumor after hormonal therapy alone. On DRE the nodule usually becomes nonpalpable within several months, and the degree and rate of shrinkage have been precisely measured by ultrasonography.[8] Studies have shown that after hormonal therapy, a biopsy converts to negative in 36 to 47 per cent of patients.[10, 13]

Despite these effects on local recurrence, the incidence of local failure after definitive therapy has been extensively reviewed by Schellhammer and co-workers.[59] Clinical local failure occurred in 4.6 and 19 per cent of patients with clinical Stage A and B tumors, respectively, after radiation therapy and in 28 per cent with Stage C prostate cancer over 5 to 10 years in the absence of hormonal therapy. At our institution, 53 per cent of the clinical Stage C patients treated with gold seeds and external beam radiation therapy developed a clinical local recurrence at a mean of 8.1 years[27] (Table 30–1).

DIAGNOSIS OF LOCAL RECURRENCE

Although the diagnosis of local recurrence in the presence of an enlarging palpable mass or in those with urinary symptoms may be straightforward, the diagnosis of local recurrence by DRE is difficult in an irradiated field. By the time clinical symptoms and signs appear, it is often too late for curative therapy.[58] Consequently, physicians have sought earlier and more objective indicators of local control in the absence of overt local progression manifested clinically. Needle biopsies of the prostate after radiation therapy have generated intense controversy. Histologic examination of irradiated prostate biopsies is difficult. Residual carcinoma may be confused with radiation-induced atypia. Cox and co-workers[11, 12] have stated that histologic examination of lethally irradiated cancer cells cannot distinguish viable from nonviable cells. However, Bostwick et al,[6] after studying the issue, have clearly defined specific criteria for post-irradiation biopsy specimens to distinguish irradiation-induced atypia from carcinoma. They refute the theory of "nonviable cancer" and support the concept that it should not be applied to post-irradiation biopsy of the prostate and point out that no such entity exists in other cancers. Furthermore, Musselman et al[47a] examined the in vitro characteristics of cancer cells harvested from prostate biopsies 2 years after radiation therapy and demonstrated monolayer growth, confirming their viability. Another important factor in the

TABLE 30–1. LOCAL RECURRENCE FOLLOWING PRIMARY TREATMENT WITH RADIATION THERAPY

	CLINICAL STAGE	ACTUARIAL LOCAL RECURRENCE (%)	FOLLOW-UP (Years)
Kaplan, 1992	B (Stanford T1a)	17.0	15
	(T1b–T1d)	22.0	15
	(T2)	35.0	15
Holzman, 1991*	C	53.0	8
Schellhammer, 1990*	A	4.6	5–10
	B	19.0	5–10
	C	28.0	5–10
Shipley, 1988	B	8.0	8
	C	28.0	8
Hanks, 1988	B	23.0	7
	C	36.0	7

*Excluding use of hormone therapy.

interpretation of a post-irradiation biopsy is the timing of the biopsy following irradiation. Figure 30–3 shows the correlation of biopsy at least 12 months after radiation therapy and clinical local recurrence as defined by a morbid event. There was a strong correlation between a positive biopsy and eventual clinical local recurrence.

Studies that compare the rate of distant metastases and survival between patients with positive and negative post-irradiation biopsies suggest several conclusions. For these comparisons to be valid, however, patients in both groups must be similar. Staging must be accurate and must include pelvic lymph node dissection; biopsy must be done when a reasonable time has elapsed since radiation therapy; hormonal therapy must not begin until there is evidence of progression, and follow-up must be adequate. Most of these studies do not satisfy these important criteria. Freiha and Bagshaw[20] studied patients after external beam irradiation for localized prostate cancer and found that 72 per cent of patients with a positive biopsy subsequently developed metastases, compared with 24 per cent of patients with a negative biopsy. Also, of patients with a positive biopsy, 53 per cent were alive, compared with 89 per cent of patients with a negative biopsy. The length of follow-up was similar in both groups at 4.5 years but included patients treated with DES at the time of distant recurrence. Other studies using external beam irradiation have found similar results.

At our institution, in studies of patients treated with gold seed and external beam irradiation, the correlation between biopsy results and eventual recurrence was highly significant, especially when the cancer was advanced in stage.[58] Of patients with a positive biopsy, 60 per cent developed local recurrence defined as a morbid clinical phenomenon, such as bladder outlet obstruction or hydronephrosis, compared with 19 per cent with a

negative biopsy. The mean follow-up was 8.6 years. At 10 years the actuarial values increased to 72 and 30 per cent, respectively. Patients who were treated with hormonal therapy at the time of failure were excluded from the analysis.

Schellhammer et al[60] reported patients treated with either ¹²⁵I implantation or external beam radiation therapy. Biopsies were performed at least 18 months later, and follow-up was a minimum of 3 years. Although no patient was hormonally manipulated before progression of disease, patients who received external beam irradiation were not surgically staged. Despite the probable understaging in some patients, those with a positive biopsy had a significantly greater incidence of local recurrence, distant metastases, and death than those with a negative biopsy.

Transrectal Ultrasonography

After radiation therapy there is a steady decrease in prostatic size over 3 to 6 months.[51] Fujino and Scardino[21] evaluated ultrasonography after gold seed and external beam radiation therapy and noted a resumption of a more normal symmetric prostate, thickening and reformation of the prostatic capsule, and a decrease in the volume of extracapsular extension including normalization of the seminal vesicles. Maximum reduction of about 25 per cent occurred 9 months after therapy. Similar findings were reported by Carpentier et al[8] in 24 patients, with a reduction of about 20 per cent at 9 months.

In 1985 Lee et al[40] showed that prostate cancer is typically hypoechoic on TRUS. They later showed an 81 per cent positive biopsy rate of hypoechoic lesions following ¹²⁵I seed implantation.[41] From our institution, Egawa et al[16, 18] reported that, after radiation therapy, prostate cancer retained its hypoechoic appearance and could still be identified sonographically in 66 per cent. Foci of cancer affected by radiation retained their hypoechogenicity in 25 per cent of cases, compared with 72 per cent of foci of cancer not affected by radiation. The same authors[17] later showed that TRUS-guided needle biopsy performed in these persistently hypoechoic areas revealed residual cancer in 59 per cent.

Kabalin et al[31] examined 27 men by transrectal ultrasound-guided needle biopsies at least 18 months after radiation therapy. Overall, 93 per cent had positive biopsies, and five of five with induration noted on DRE were positive. The extraordinarily high incidence of positive biopsies in this series is difficult to explain. This was not a consecutive series of patients treated with radiation therapy, but patients who had returned for follow-up in the urology clinic. All except four of these men had an elevated serum PSA level at the time of the biopsy, now known to be a poor prognostic factor (see below), and multifocal ("systematic") biopsy samples were taken. In this series, the correlation between findings on ultrasonography and pathology was poor. Hypoechoic areas were positive for carcinoma in 67 per cent, and isoechoic areas were positive in 65 per cent.

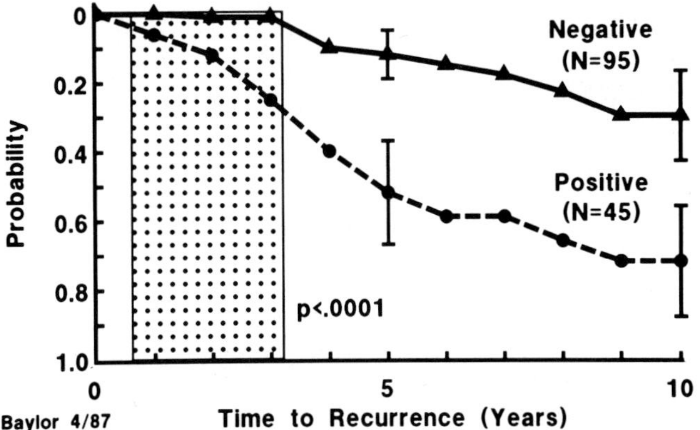

FIGURE 30–3. Actuarial analysis showing that probability of clinical local recurrence was significantly greater if the result of routine needle biopsy performed 6 to 36 months [shaded areas] after completion of therapy was positive for cancer. (From Scardino PT, Wheeler TM: Local control of prostate cancer with radiotherapy: Frequency and prognostic significance of positive results of post-irradiation prostate biopsy. NCI Monogr 7:95, 1988.)

However, because prostate cancer is multifocal and not all foci are hypoechoic,[16, 18] it would not be surprising to find multiple biopsies positive for cancer in a series in which 93 per cent of the patients had a persistent cancer.[63–65]

Prostate-Specific Antigen

The use of PSA as an important clinical tumor marker for prostate cancer cannot be overemphasized, and it is most useful in the follow-up of patients treated with radical prostatectomy. However, the role of PSA in patients treated with radiation therapy is not yet fully defined.[34]

PSA levels do decline rapidly after radiation therapy and usually reach a nadir by 3 to 6 months. Zagars et al[70] observed a significant decline in PSA values by 3 months in 98 per cent. Mean and median PSA values fell to levels less than 4 ng/ml (Hybritech). In most patients, PSA continued to decline for up to 12 months and stabilized by 21 months, but it was detectable in all patients. If PSA levels do not decrease to normal by 6 to 12 months the prognosis is poor, but a decrease to normal values does not guarantee success.

Pretreatment PSA levels are perhaps the best prognostic factor for prostate cancer patients treated with primary irradiation therapy. Russell et al[54] found that pretreatment PSA levels increased with increasing tumor stage, but not with increasing Gleason sum. The probability of remaining a complete responder decreased with increasing stage, but not with increasing Gleason score. Of the patients with a pretreatment PSA level of less than four times the upper limit of normal, 83 per cent remained complete responders, compared with 30 per cent of those with a higher pretreatment PSA level.

If PSA levels do rise after radiation therapy in a consistent manner, clinical recurrence is inevitable and the increase in PSA levels precedes clinical recurrence by months or years. Stamey et al[63–65] demonstrated that an increasing PSA level after radiation therapy correlated with disease progression and with a positive biopsy of the prostate. A cohort of patients included those treated with external beam radiation therapy and iodine seed implantation but excluded patients with prior hormonal therapy. Results demonstrated that 82 per cent had decreasing PSA levels in the first 12 months, but only 8 per cent continued to decrease after 1 year. Of those patients evaluated for more than 1 year, 51 per cent had increasing PSA levels and 41 per cent had stable values. Nine of 41 patients (22 per cent) with increasing PSA levels 12 months after therapy underwent biopsy. Interestingly, eight of these nine patients had flat, symmetric prostates and unsuspicious DREs, but all nine had positive biopsies. Dundas et al[15] also demonstrated the usefulness of PSA monitoring after radiation therapy in that none of the patients who failed with local or distant recurrence experienced a return to normal PSA values, whereas normal values had returned in the remaining 73 per cent of patients.

Results of biopsies of irradiated prostates are more frequently positive in patients with elevated PSA levels than in patients with PSA levels in the normal range. Dugan et al[14] found 71 per cent of biopsies positive if the PSA was greater than 2.5 ng/ml, compared with 21 per cent if the PSA was less than 2.5 ng/ml. A positive biopsy in a patient with a rising PSA and no evidence of distant metastases currently is the best documentation of local recurrence at an early stage when other curative treatments are still possible.

However, a positive biopsy in a patient with a normal or falling PSA level and no clinical evidence of local recurrence is problematic. It is possible that irradiation suppresses PSA production in some cancers without controlling cancer growth.[61]

Meek et al[45] calculated the half-life of PSA after radiation therapy to be 43 ± 11 days. In this series the half-life of PSA after radiation therapy was an independent prognostic factor compared with stage, grade, or pretreatment PSA level. It was proposed that if the PSA is greater than one half of the pretreatment PSA level at the end of therapy, it should be considered abnormal.

In our institution, patients treated with radiation therapy for localized prostate cancer are followed with DRE and marker results (PSA, prostatic acid phosphatase [PAP]) every 3 months for the first year, every 3 to 6 months thereafter, and finally once a year after 5 years. Imaging studies are performed if PSA increases consistently or if clinical symptoms warrant suspicion of bony metastases. If distant metastases are documented, hormonal therapy is commenced. If there is no evidence of metastases, then the local tumor is evaluated by rectal examination, ultrasonography, and ultrasound-guided needle biopsy of the prostate. If the biopsy is positive in the presence of a rising or elevated serum PSA level, local recurrence is diagnosed and treatment instituted. Most such patients are candidates for palliative therapy alone, and hormonal therapy or transurethral resection of the prostate (TURP) to relieve obstructive symptoms is appropriate. Few patients with radiorecurrent prostate cancers are candidates for definitive treatment.

SALVAGE RADICAL PROSTATECTOMY

Indications

When local recurrence is diagnosed by a rising PSA level and positive biopsy results, the patient may be a candidate for salvage prostatectomy. For a successful outcome of this difficult operation, the initial tumor must have been clinically confined to the prostate and the pelvic lymph nodes must have been negative if a lymphadenectomy was performed at the time of the initial treatment. Candidates should be in excellent general health with a life expectancy of at least 10 years and should not have received recent or long-term hormonal therapy that might mask the present stage of the disease. Staging studies should include PSA, PAP, chest radiography, bone scan, and CT scans of the pelvis. Candidates for this operation should be well motivated and willing to accept the possibility of incontinence and the certainty of impotence in an attempt at surgical cure (Table 30–2).

We evaluate these patients thoroughly, using both cystoscopy and bimanual examination with the patient under general anesthesia, to assess the degree of local pathology, including mobility of the prostate, and to look for evidence of radiation cystitis. Transurethral biopsies are performed on any suspicious tissue at the bladder neck because results might preclude performance of prostatectomy. Patients also undergo proctoscopy for assessment of the degree of radiation proctitis. The patient may need to be warned of the possibility of a temporary or permanent colostomy if damage to the rectum occurs during surgery. TRUS of the prostate is performed to aid in evaluation of the extent of the tumor. The upper urinary tracts should be evaluated by either excretory urography or renal ultrasonography, as well as by determination of serum creatinine concentration. Lower urinary tract function should be assessed with cystometrograms, flow rates, and determination of postvoid residual urine.

Surgical Technique

Because of the risk of rectal injury, all patients should receive mechanical and antibiotic bowel preparation preoperatively. Because the posterior prostatic fascia and the anterior rectal wall are densely adherent after radiation therapy, we often initiate the operation through a perineal incision to separate the rectum from the prostate and decrease the incidence of rectal injury and to ensure removal of the maximum amount of periprostatic tissue (everything is removed except the rectal wall). To ensure that the perineum is resting in a position parallel to the operating room floor, the buttocks are placed on a pad that extends them over the edge of the operating table. The thighs must be flexed to rest on the patient's abdomen, parallel to the ground. A drape is sewn over the anterior anal verge to isolate the rectum from the field and to allow the surgeon to place a finger inside the rectum to aid in its dissection. A Lowsley prostatic retractor is passed through the urethra and the wings are opened. This permits adequate mobilization of the prostate during dissection. The incision is created in curvilinear fashion as classically described by Belt et al[4] by incising approximately 2 cm anterior to the anal verge and extending the incision laterally within the ischial tuberosities. The ischial rectal space is then defined and the central tendon of the perineum taken down with cautery. Dissection continues

directly on top of the anterior rectal wall, with care taken to dissect beneath the external sphincter muscle. Dissection along this plane with adequate lateral retraction allows identification of the apex of the prostate. With the Lowsley retractor used to mobilize the prostate, the anterior wall of the rectum is dissected free from the posterior prostatic fascia by sharp and blunt dissection until the seminal vesicles are identified. At this point, we have found it helpful to transect the urethra just distal to the apex of the prostate while it is under direct vision so that a smooth, concise division can be made. The Lowsley retractor is then removed, the bladder drained, and the incision closed in a standard fashion.

The patient is then placed in the supine position with the table anteflexed slightly over the pubis. A longitudinal midline incision from the pubis to the umbilicus is preferred, usually through the scar of the previous operation. Most patients have previously undergone a lymphadenectomy and tissue planes are severely obliterated. The bladder often is adherent to the undersurface of the abdominal wall, pelvic side walls, iliac vessels, and obturator nerve. If pelvic surgery has not been performed previously, the tissue planes are surprisingly normal, and mobilization of the bladder and prostate can be performed without difficulty. The combination of previous surgery and radiation therapy, however, often results in marked fibrosis, so that mobilization of the bladder and identification of the lateral border of the prostate and the endopelvic fascia are extremely difficult. When necessary, we do not hesitate to open the peritoneum above the bladder to improve the exposure and to aid in the dissection of the bladder away from the pelvic side walls and iliac vessels. If an adequate pelvic lymphadenectomy has not been performed previously and the nodal tissue is not densely adherent to the iliac vessels, a limited lymphadenectomy can be performed, with the limits of the dissection being the bifurcation of the common iliac artery superiorly and the circumflex iliac vein inferiorly. Nodal tissue medial to the external iliac artery is removed and the obturator nodal tissue is dissected free, with care taken to preserve the obturator nerve. All lymphatic vessels are clipped proximally and distally.

Once the bladder is mobilized, dissection around the prostate is begun. The tissue planes anterior and lateral to the prostate often are obliterated. Dissection is facilitated by using electrocautery, with care taken to dissect widely along the undersurface of the pubic periosteum anteriorly and into the levator muscles laterally, to minimize the risk of incising into tumor. Once the anterior dissection is completed, the prostate is almost always completely mobilized, as the difficult posterior and apical dissection have already been performed through the perineal incision. The anterior bladder neck is then divided, with the remainder of the procedure performed much like a standard radical or retropubic prostatectomy. No attempt is made to spare the cavernosal nerves, which are encased in the periprostatic fibrous reaction and are difficult to identify after radiation therapy. Occasionally, we perform the prostatic

TABLE 30–2. SALVAGE RADICAL PROSTATECTOMY: PATIENT SELECTION

Biopsy-proven tumor 1 year or longer after definitive radiation treatment
Negative metastatic evaluation
No recent hormonal therapy
Excellent health with extended life expectancy
Well motivated

TABLE 30–3. SALVAGE RADICAL PROSTATECTOMY: INDICATIONS FOR BIOPSY

	N	PER CENT
Nodule	22	73
Abnormal ultrasonography or elevated PSA	4	13
Incidentally discovered after TURP	3	10
Routine post-irradiation biopsy	1	3
TOTAL	30	100

dissection in an antegrade manner, as described by Campbell.[6a]

Once the prostate is removed, the bladder neck mucosa is dissected from the muscularis of the bladder anterolaterally and closed back onto itself using a Lembert stitch to create a mucosal eversion. The bladder neck is closed in two layers to a 24 Fr catheter and a vesicourethral anastomosis is performed, usually with five interrupted absorbable sutures over a 20 Fr silicone Foley catheter. We routinely cut a small side hole into the catheter proximal to the balloon to further aid in drainage of urine near the vesicourethral anastomosis. Jackson-Pratt drains are left in the obturator fossa and removed when the drainage is less than 30 ml a day.

Results

Recently we reviewed the first 30 patients treated at our institution with salvage radical prostatectomy. The indications for biopsy are presented in Table 30–3 and the type of prior radiation therapy previously received is presented in Table 30–4. These were heavily pretreated patients. Twenty-two patients had a palpable nodule on DRE at the time of recurrence; seven had an abnormal ultrasonogram, elevated PSA, or lower tract obstructive symptoms, and one had no clinical or biochemical evidence of recurrence.

The operation was generally more difficult and time consuming and carried a higher complication rate than standard radical retropubic prostatectomy. The mean operative time was 4.5 hours (range 2.8 to 7); the mean estimated blood loss was 1010 ml (range 350 to 2200); the mean number of blood transfusions was 1.56 (range 0 to 8); and the mean postoperative hospital stay was 9.8 days (range 6 to 16).

The complication rate was significant. Rectal injury occurred in 20 per cent of patients, and a stricture at the level of the anastomosis occurred in 23 per cent of

patients, including two who required a repeat optical urethrotomy. Unusual complications, including ureteral transection and ureterovesical junction stricture, occurred in one patient each (Table 30–5).

The pathology specimens were analyzed carefully using the whole-mount technique. Forty per cent of the patients had tumor confined either to the gland or to the immediate periprostatic tissue. Twenty-seven per cent had microscopic seminal vesical invasion without positive surgical margins, and 27 per cent had positive surgical margins, of which all but one had seminal vesicle invasion. Two patients had positive lymph nodes.

With a mean follow-up of 32 months, two patients are dead, one of prostate cancer. Of the remaining 27 patients, 16 have no evidence of recurrence, but there are no PSA data for two of them. The remaining 11 have elevated PSA and/or positive bone scans.

In conclusion, salvage radical prostatectomy is a potential option and feasible in a small subset of patients failing definitive radiation therapy. Surgical experience is required for performance of the difficult operation with little morbidity. Most major complications in our patients occurred early in our series, but still occur more frequently than in simple radical prostatectomies. Although 50 per cent of the patients in our series have no evidence of disease, the follow-up is short, and we expect recurrences at a later date. Some patients will be cured by this procedure, however, and we will attempt to better define and predict outcome by longer follow-up.

Exenterative Surgery

Patients with locally advanced and symptomatic prostate cancers without distant metastases are difficult to manage and suffer significant morbidity. Fortunately, such patients are not encountered frequently.

Anterior exenteration (cystoprostatectomy) or total exenteration may serve as a suitable alternative despite a high surgical morbidity. However, residual cancer rates and local control usually are not improved and survival is short. Zincke[71] presented a salvage surgery series of 62 patients who had failed radiation therapy only locally. Thirty patients had an anterior exenteration and seven had total exenteration. Progression and cancer death were related to aneuploid status and in particular to hormonal treatment. Salvage radical prostatec-

TABLE 30–4. SALVAGE RADICAL PROSTATECTOMY: PRIOR THERAPY

	N	PER CENT
PLND, [198]Au seeds, XRT	18	60
PLND, ^{125}I seeds	3	10
PLND, XRT	2	7
XRT alone	7	23
Total	30	100

PLND = pelvic lymph node dissection.
XRT = radiation therapy.

TABLE 30–5. SALVAGE RADICAL PROSTATECTOMY: COMPLICATIONS

TYPE	NO. PATIENTS
Rectal injury	6 (20)
Closed without complications	4
Rectal injury leading to further surgery (colostomy, vesicorectal fistula repair)	2
Anastomotic stricture*	7 (23)
Ureteral transection	1 (3)
Ureterovesical junction stricture	1 (3)

*Two patients developed two strictures.

tomy seemed to benefit some patients, but salvage exenterative surgeries seemed to have little or no effect on distant recurrence or death. The median time to progression after salvage radical prostatectomy was 7.5 years, compared with 1.3 years in exenterative procedures.

In a smaller series by Ahlering et al[1] the authors concluded that salvage surgery is feasible but that exenterative procedures, although perhaps better than hormonal therapy alone, are not very helpful. We do not recommend exenterative surgery because patients do poorly and survival does not seem to be altered.

Palliative Treatment

If patients are not suitable candidates for salvage operations for local failure after radiation, either because of the presence of distant metastases or because of medical contraindications, simple measures may alleviate local problems.

Severe lower tract obstructive symptoms including urinary retention can be managed by indwelling catheters or preferably by intermittent catheterization. Channel TURP procedures improve flow rates but are associated with complications, including hemorrhage, incontinence secondary to damage or invasion by tumor of the external sphincter,[27] and the possibility of metastatic dissemination. The issue of metastatic spread by TURP in patients with prostate cancer is controversial. Sandler and Hanks[55] suggest the spread via mechanical dissemination of tumor, but in our institution, metastatic spread was correlated with tumor grade and stage, TURP being simply more frequent in tumors of higher stage and grade. TURP was done in patients with obstructive symptoms, and these patients have a worse prognosis.[44]

Hormone therapy also controls local symptoms by decreasing tumor burden and shrinking prostate volume, but improvement in symptoms may be slow and unpredictable. Catalona et al[9] treated 35 patients in urinary retention for advanced prostate cancer. Twenty-six per cent of the patients voided within 1 week after hormonal therapy (this group included four patients in retention due to presumed edema following needle biopsy), but 46 per cent were able to void only after 21 to 60 days of catheter drainage. TURP was still necessary in 29 per cent of the patients.

LOCAL RECURRENCE AFTER RADICAL PROSTATECTOMY

Definition

Classically, local recurrence after radical prostatectomy was defined as a palpable mass detected on DRE and proven by biopsy. Symptoms of local recurrence are uncommon but include late development of obstructive voiding symptoms such as a decreased size and force of stream, the development of continence in an otherwise incontinent patient, hematuria, and local pain. Local failure is less common than distant metastases, but the two occur concomitantly in some patients.

Incidence

A review of the reported incidence of local failure is shown in Table 30–6. For tumors pathologically confined to the prostate without concomitant hormonal therapy, local failure at 15 years occurred in 16 per cent of patients in Jewett's series[29] and 17 per cent in Schellhammer's series.[59] For tumors extending beyond the prostate pathologically, again without hormonal therapy, local recurrence rates were higher. In Schellhammer's series of 13 patients with pathologic Stage C tumors, 30 per cent had local recurrence at 15 years. The relative effects of extracapsular extension, positive surgical margins, or seminal vesicle invasion on local recurrence have not been well quantified. However, Morton et al[46] reviewed the results of cancer control a median of 4 years after radical prostatectomy. The actuarial 5-year rate of clinical local recurrence for pathologically organ-confined tumors was 2 per cent (with or without distant metastases). Specimen-confined tumors (extracapsular extension or seminal vesicle invasion with negative surgical margins) demonstrated a 9 per cent rate of local recurrence. Tumors with positive surgical margins had a 31 per cent recurrence rate. The relative effects of differing pathologic features on recurrence in general (local and/or distant) or on survival have been extensively studied. Paulson et al[50] documented a failure (any recurrence) rate for positive surgical margins equivalent to that of patients with positive lymph nodes (60 per cent at 10 years), compared with a failure rate of 30 per cent for specimen-confined disease and 12 per cent for organ-confined disease.

Certain other important criteria influence the rate of

TABLE 30–6. LOCAL RECURRENCE FOLLOWING TREATMENT WITH RADICAL PROSTATECTOMY

	PATHOLOGIC STAGE	ACTUARIAL LOCAL RECURRENCE (%)	FOLLOW-UP (Years)
Schellhammer, 1990	B	17	15
	C	30	15
Blute, 1989	B	22*	15
Jewett, 1976	B	16	15

*Projected.

local recurrence or tumor progression after radical prostatectomy. The grade of the primary tumor affects prognosis, especially at the extremes of Gleason grade.[50, 59] Other forms of treatment, especially hormone therapy, which has been used in several series, cloud the true progression and local recurrence rate. The time of follow-up is also important. The frequency of late clinical recurrence (more than 6 years after treatment) emphasizes the need for long-term follow-up.[9]

Diagnosis

In the past, detection of local recurrence was based on a needle biopsy of a newly palpable mass evident on DRE in a patient with or without local symptoms. Today with the advent of PSA measurement and ultrasound-guided biopsy of the anastomosis, local recurrence can be detected earlier and appears to occur more frequently than once thought. Routine DRE after radical prostatectomy was important in searching for nodules in the prostatic fossa to detect local recurrence early and, along with the change in voiding symptoms, was virtually the only way local recurrence was detected. Today we know that a rising PSA or a PSA that never declines to undetectable range after radical prostatectomy signifies residual disease.[48, 63–65]

Although most patients with an elevated PSA after radical prostatectomy have unremarkable DREs, some of these patients do indeed have tumor identified by biopsy in the area of the anastomosis. Interestingly, Lightner et al[43] evaluated 63 patients with increased PSA levels 6 to 240 months after radical prostatectomy. All patients were evaluated by DRE, bone scan, and CT scan of the abdomen and pelvis and were thought to be otherwise free of disease. Of the 63 patients, six had evidence of either metastatic bone disease or lymphadenopathy or both, and five of the six had positive ultrasound-guided biopsies of the anastomosis. Of the remaining 57 patients with a negative metastatic work-up, 42 per cent had a positive biopsy of the anastomotic area. In a second group of 30 patients with an undetectable PSA after radical prostatectomy, none of the patients had a positive biopsy. The author has wisely cautioned that the unexpectedly high prevalence of local recurrence found by using PSA levels and ultrasound-guided biopsies awaits further study. In the same series the DRE was not a good predictor of the presence of local tumor or of the biopsy results.

At our institution we have developed a standard algorithm for following patients after radical retropubic prostatectomy. If the PSA remains at 0.4 ng/ml or less and the patient is asymptomatic with a negative DRE, the patient is considered free of disease and biopsies of the anastomotic area are not performed. If the PSA is greater than 0.4 ng/ml and consistently rises on three or more occasions, biopsies are performed if the metastatic evaluation (bone scan, CT scan, PAP) is negative. Radiation therapy to the prostatic bed is offered only if biopsies are positive and metastatic work-up is negative, suggesting microscopic local recurrence. If biopsies are

negative, the patient may be followed with examinations repeated every 6 to 12 months, or empiric hormonal therapy may be offered.

THERAPY FOR LOCAL RECURRENCE

Indications

The definitive indication for salvage radiation therapy after radical prostatectomy includes "clinical" local recurrence (palpable mass) or "microscopic" local recurrence (positive biopsy only) in patients with no evidence of distant metastases.

Results

Ray et al[52] compared two groups of patients receiving radiation therapy because of either incomplete tumor excision or palpable local recurrence following radical prostatectomy. Hanks and Dawson[25] also compared patients receiving radiation therapy before and after local recurrence. In both series, the first group had the greater number of patients with seminal vesicle invasion, bladder neck involvement, or positive surgical margins, whereas the latter had more documented palpable local recurrence without distant metastases. PSA data were not available. Both studies were nonrandomized and contained small samples but found that radiation therapy following radical prostatectomy was safe and well tolerated and might be more effective before development of palpable local recurrence than after such recurrence had become clinically manifest.

Anscher et al[2] showed a better local control rate in patients treated with radiation therapy for extraprostatic disease than in patients who had no treatment. Although in their series the rates of disease-free survival were not improved with adjuvant treatment, early deaths from cancer were reduced and there was a meaningful increase in survival.

Interestingly, Lange et al[37] treated patients who had an elevated PSA 9 to 95 months after radical prostatectomy but who otherwise had no evidence of disease by the usual criteria. Most (66 per cent) of these patients surprisingly had positive random biopsies of the anastomosis. In 82 per cent, PSA decreased by 50 per cent after radiation therapy, and in 43 per cent the PSA became undetectable. This suggests that local disease may be the only site of disease in such patients and supports the notion that distant metastases result from failure of local control. However, the long-term results of such treatment are unknown.

ADJUVANT RADIATION THERAPY

Pathologic Risk Factors for Recurrence

Patients with extracapsular extension, positive surgical margins, and seminal vesical invasion are at increased risk for local recurrence after radical prostatectomy. Yet, there is no consensus on the use of adjuvant therapy to prevent eventual clinical local recurrence in these patients. There is, however, general agreement that patients with a pathologically confined tumor and an undetectable PSA need no other therapy after radical prostatectomy.

A positive surgical margin can occur in two ways: Either the surgeon has cut into the tumor within the prostate or the tumor extends through the capsule into the periprostatic tissues beyond the plane of surgical dissection. In both cases, it is likely that tumor has been left behind. We consider a surgical margin positive if there are malignant cells at the inked border of the specimen. Of course, this policy presumes that tumor exists beyond the inked margin, but this is not always the case.[68] A positive surgical margin, however defined, is associated with an increased risk of local recurrence and of progression (Fig. 30–4), especially if identified by an increased postoperative PSA level.[46, 49]

The prognostic significance of the extent of capsular invasion or penetration has not been clearly demonstrated. Complete capsular penetration in the absence of positive surgical margin has not been shown to place the patient at significantly greater risk of local recurrence.[49]

Seminal vesicle invasion, on the other hand, is clearly associated with a poor prognosis. Mukamel et al[47] showed that patients with seminal vesicle invasion had a less favorable prognosis than those without, and most of their patients (57 per cent) with seminal vesicle invasion did not have lymph node involvement. Both local recurrence and distant metastases are more common in patients with seminal vesicle invasion.[9] Villers et al[67] found a strong correlation between seminal vesicle invasion and cancer volume, with only 6 per cent of the tumors of less than 4 cc showing invasion. The root of invasion in most of the cases in their series involved direct tumor spread into the mid-base region near the ejaculatory ducts. Wheeler et al[69] studied seminal vesicle invasion in detail and found three different mechanisms. Although 70 per cent of patients had direct extension via the ejaculatory ducts or through the prostatic capsule, 30 per cent had isolated metastases to the seminal vesicle but no direct continuation from the intraprostatic tumor. These patients had a very favorable prognosis.

Thus, seminal vesicle invasion signifies a greater risk of both distant metastases and local recurrence. It is not clear whether adjuvant radiation therapy in patients with seminal vesicle invasion but negative surgical margins reduces the subsequent rate of local recurrence and of death from prostate cancer. Reports to date give little reason for optimism,[23] but a properly controlled study has not been done. A finding of positive lymph nodes during radical prostatectomy generally means an increased risk of metastases rather than clinical local recurrence, despite the higher rate of positive surgical margins or seminal vesicle invasion in patients with positive lymph nodes. Historically, such patients are better treated with early or delayed hormonal therapy than with an attempt to control the tumor locally.

Recently, we reported that seminal fluid seen at the apex of the prostate during radical prostatectomy may contain malignant cells, as demonstrated by cytology in 14 per cent of cases. This mechanism of seeding may account for certain cases of local recurrence.[36]

Results

There is no clear evidence that adjuvant radiation therapy improves survival in any group of patients. Gibbons et al[23] also demonstrated a lower rate of clinical local recurrence when postoperative adjuvant radiation therapy was used than when no adjuvant treatment was used in patients with extension of tumor outside the prostate. However, there was no decrease in the rate of distant metastases or of death from prostate cancer. Paulson et al,[49] using failure or death as endpoints, did not identify any benefit of adjuvant radiation therapy following perineal prostatectomy.

Elevated PSA levels after radical prostatectomy, regardless of pathologic stage, indicate residual disease even if conventional studies such as bone scan, radiography, CT scan, MRI, or even ultrasound-guided biop-

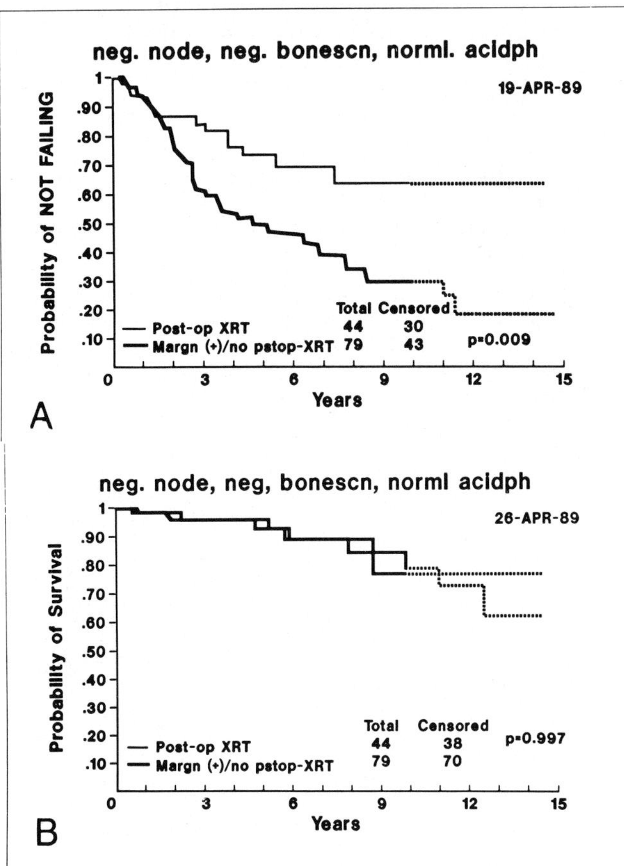

FIGURE 30–4. Probability of not failing (*A*) and probability of survival (*B*) among margin-positive patients who did and did not receive postoperative radiation therapy. (From Paulson DF, Moul JW, Walther PJ: Radical prostatectomy for clinical stage T1-2 N0M0 prostatic adenocarcinoma: Long-term results. J Urol 144:1180, 1990, © by American Urological Assoc. Inc.; with permission.)

sies are negative. Oesterling et al[48] demonstrated that PSA is a sensitive marker for detection of residual disease after radical prostatectomy and subsequent recurrence on long-term follow-up. In his group of patients with tumors confined to the prostate or extracapsular extension, only 91 per cent had undetectable PSA compared with only 19 per cent of patients with seminal vesicle invasion or positive lymph nodes. Also, all of the patients with a documented clinical recurrence had an elevated PSA. In an early study, Hudson and Catalona[28] demonstrated the potential benefit of using PSA to monitor the response of adjuvant radiation following radical prostatectomy.

The effect of adjuvant radiation therapy in patients with an elevated PSA after radical prostatectomy was studied by Lange et al.[37] A significant number of their patients had a decrease of the PSA to undetectable levels, but no long-term follow-up is available. Interestingly, 18 of 32 patients had microscopic lymph node involvement, and all but one had a decrease in the serum PSA. Of note, however, is that nine of these pathologic Stage D1 patients had undetectable PSAs prior to radiation therapy. The follow-up was short, and some patients eventually had recurrence. Some patients with microscopic lymph node involvement following radical prostatectomy may benefit from adjuvant radiation therapy, but no long-term data are available to argue for this mode of therapy.

More recently, Stein et al,[66] by using PSA levels as an indication of failure, showed that adjuvant radiation therapy has a beneficial effect after radical prostatectomy in patients with local tumor extension

Local recurrences may also be treated with hormonal therapy, especially if there is a high suspicion of distant metastases or the patient is not a good candidate for radiation therapy. Such a regimen is considered palliative rather than curative but avoids the complications associated with radiation therapy. Anscher et al[3] compared results of salvage radiation therapy with those of hormonal therapy in patients with palpable biopsy-proven local recurrences. Local control was better in the radiation therapy–treated group (88 per cent) than in the hormonally treated group (4 per cent). However, no difference in survival was noted, and complications occurred more frequently after radiation therapy.

The timing of adjuvant radiation therapy after radical prostatectomy is important. It is best to wait at least 6 weeks (Catalona[9a]) to ensure better "healing" of the vesicourethral anastomosis and to reduce the complication rate. It probably is also better to await return of continence, which usually occurs 3 to 4 months postoperatively.[36] The complications of salvage radiation therapy have been fully described by Lange et al[38, 39] and include both acute and chronic complications affecting the gastrointestinal tract, mostly anorectal disease, irritative urinary symptoms due to radiation cystitis, urethral stricture, lymphedema, impotence, and rarely cutaneous erythema. The complications of adjuvant therapy are well documented, but no controlled study has been performed demonstrating a survival advantage of radiation therapy.

An ongoing protocol by SWOG 8794 randomizes patients who have either extracapsular extension, seminal vesicle invasion, or positive surgical margins after radical prostatectomy either to receive 6400 cGy of external beam radiation therapy in 32 fractions or to be observed. It is hoped that this will clarify the indications for adjuvant radiation therapy.

SUMMARY

Adjuvant radiation therapy for extraprostatic disease has not been shown to influence survival more than radical prostatectomy alone. However, because seminal vesicle invasion and positive surgical margins are known to affect local recurrence and because local failure eventually leads to distant metastasis and death, adjuvant radiation therapy should be offered to such high-risk patients, especially if the PSA is elevated. It is better to wait at least 6 weeks and, if possible, until the return of continence to minimize the effect of radiation on the sphincter mechanism.

Also, recent studies using PSA and ultrasound-guided biopsies demonstrate a higher local recurrence rate than once expected, and early discovery of these recurrences when tumor burden is still low may prevent or at least delay distant metastases or death. The surgeon must be aware of the potential complications of such therapy and explain the controversy to each patient.

REFERENCES

1. Ahlering TE, Laskowski G, Skinner D: Salvage surgery plus androgen deprivation for radioresistant prostatic adenocarcinoma. J Urol 147:900, 1992.
2. Anscher MS, Prosnitz LR: Postoperative radiotherapy for patients with carcinoma of the prostate undergoing radical prostatectomy with positive surgical margins, seminal vesicle involvement and/or penetration through the capsule. J Urol 138:1407, 1987.
3. Anscher MS, Prosnitz LR: Radiotherapy vs. hormonal therapy for the management of locally recurrent prostate cancer following radical prostatectomy. Int J Radiat Oncol Biol Phys 17:953, 1989.
4. Belt E, Ebert CF, Surber AC: A new anastomotic approach in perineal prostatectomy. J Urol 41:482, 1939.
5. Blute ML, Nativ O, Zincke H, et al: Pattern of failure after radical retropubic prostatectomy for clinically and pathologically localized adenocarcinoma of the prostate: Influence of tumor deoxyribonucleic acid ploidy. J Urol 142:1262, 1989.
6. Bostwick DG, Egbert BM, Fijardo LF: Radiation injury of the normal and neoplastic prostate. Am J Surg Pathol 6:541, 1982.
6a. Campbell EW: Total prostatectomy with preliminary ligation of the vascular pedicle. J Urol 81:464, 1959.
7. Carlton CE Jr, Scardino PT: Long-term results after combined radioactive gold seed implantation and external beam radiotherapy for localized prostate cancer. *In* Coffey DF, Resnick MI, Dorr SA, Karr JP (eds): A Multidisciplinary Analysis of Controversies in the Management of Prostate Cancer. New York, Plenum Publishing Corp, 1988.
8. Carpentier PJ, Schroeder SH, Blaum JH: Transrectal ultrasonography in the follow-up of prostatic carcinoma patients. J Urol 128:742, 1982.
9. Catalona WJ, Miller ER, Kavoussi LR: Intermediate-term survival result in clinically understage prostate cancer patients following radical prostatectomy. J Urol 140:540, 1988.
9a. Catalona WJ, Scott WW: Carcinoma of the prostate. *In* Walsh PC, Gittes, RF, Perlmutter AD, Stamey TA (eds): Campbell's Urology, 5th ed. Philadelphia, WB Saunders, 1986, p 1499.
10. Cosgrove MD, George GW III, Terry R: The effects of treatment

on a local lesion of carcinoma of the prostate. J Urol 109:861, 1973.

11. Cox JD, Kline RW: Do prostatic biopsies 12 months or more after external irradiation for adenocarcinomas, stage III predict long-term survival? Int J Radiat Oncol Biol Phys 9:299, 1983.

12. Cox JD, Stoffel TJ: The significance of needle biopsy after irradiation for stage C adenocarcinoma of the prostate. Cancer 40:156, 1977.

13. Dhom G, Degro S: Therapy of prostatic cancer and histopathologic follow-up. Prostate 3:531, 1982.

14. Dugan TC, Shipley WU, Young RH, et al: Biopsy after external beam radiation therapy for adenocarcinoma of the prostate: Correlation with original histological grade and current prostate specific antigen levels. J Urol 146:1313, 1991.

15. Dundas GS, Porter AT, Venner PM: Prostate specific antigen: Monitoring the response of carcinoma of the prostate to radiotherapy with a new tumor marker. Cancer 66:45, 1990.

16. Egawa S, Carter S St C, Wheeler TM, Scardino PT: Sonographic monitoring of prostate cancer after definitive radiotherapy. Urology, May 1991.

17. Egawa S, Wheeler TM, Greene DR, Scardino PT: Detection of residual prostate cancer after radiotherapy by sonographically guided needle biopsy. Urology 39:358, 1992.

18. Egawa S, Wheeler TM, Scardino PT: The sonographic appearance of irradiated prostate cancer. Br J Urol 68:172, 1991.

19. Fleischmann JD, Catalona WI: Endocrine therapy for bladder outlet obstruction from carcinoma of the prostate. J Urol 134:498, 1985.

20. Freiha FS, Bagshaw MA: Carcinoma of the prostate: Result of postirradiation biopsy. Prostate 5:19, 1984.

21. Fujino A, Scardino PT: Transrectal ultrasonography for prostatic cancer: Its value and staging in monitoring the response to radiotherapy and chemotherapy. J Urol 133:806, 1985.

22. Fuks KS, Leibel SA, Wallner KE, et al: The effect of local control on metastatic dissemination in carcinoma of the prostate: Long-term results in patients treated with I^{125} implantation. Int J Radiat Oncol Biol Phys 21:537, 1991.

23. Gibbons RP, Cole S, Richardson G, et al: Adjuvant radiotherapy following radical prostatectomy: Results and complications. J Urol 135:65, 1986.

24. Handley R, Karr TW, Travis D, et al: Deferred treatment for prostate cancer. Br J Urol 62:249, 1988.

25. Hanks GE, Dawson AK: The role of external beam radiation therapy after prostatectomy for cancer. Cancer 58:2406, 1986.

26. Hanks GE: External beam radiation therapy for clinically localized prostate cancer: Patterns of care studies in the United States. NCI Monogr 7:75, 1988.

27. Holzman M, Carlton CE Jr, Scardino PT: The frequency and morbidity of local tumor recurrence after definitive radiotherapy for stage C prostate cancer. J Urol 146:1578, 1991.

28. Hudson MA, Catalona WJ: Effect of adjuvant radiation therapy on prostate specific antigen following radical prostatectomy. J Urol 143:1174, 1990.

29. Jewett HJ: Radical perineal prostatectomy for prostatic cancer. *In* Marberger H (ed): Prostatic Disease. New York, Alan R. Liss, 1976, pp 205–218.

30. Johansson JE, Adami HO, Andersson SO, et al: High 10-year survival rate in patients with early, untreated prostatic cancer. JAMA 267:2191, 1992.

31. Kabalin JN, Hodge KK, McNeal JE, et al: Identification of residual cancer in the prostate following radiation therapy: Role of transrectal ultrasound, guided biopsy and prostate specific antigen. J Urol 142:326, 1989.

32. Kaplan ID, Bagshaw MA: Serum prostate-specific antigen after post-prostatectomy radiotherapy. Urology 34:401, 1992.

33. Kaplan ID, Prestidge BR, Bagshaw MA, Cox RS: The importance of local control in the treatment of prostatic cancer. J Urol 147:917, 1992.

34. Kaplan ID, Prestidge BR, Cox RS, Bagshaw MA: Prostate specific antigen after irradiation for prostatic carcinoma. J Urol 144:1172, 1990.

35. Kassabian VS, Bottles K, Weaver R, et al: Possible mechanisms for seeding of tumor during radical prostatectomy. J Urol (in press).

36. Kassabian VS, Collini MP, Seale-Hawkins C, et al: Anatomical radical prostatectomy: Comparison of morbidity in the earliest and most recent 100 patients [abstract]. J Urol 147:4, 1992.

37. Lange PH, Lightner DJ, Medini E, et al: The effect of radiation therapy after radical prostatectomy in patients with elevated prostate specific antigen levels. J Urol 144:927, 1990.

38. Lange PH, Moon TD, Narayan P, Medini E: Radiation therapy as adjuvant treatment after radical prostatectomy: Patient tolerance and preliminary results. J Urol 136:45, 1986.

39. Lange PH, Reddy PK, Medini E, et al: Radiation therapy as adjuvant treatment after radical prostatectomy. NCI Monogr 7:141, 1988.

40. Lee F, Gray JM, McLeary RD, et al: Transrectal ultrasound in the diagnosis of prostate cancer: Location, echogenicity, histopathology and staging. Prostate 7:117, 1985.

41. Lee F, Torp-Pedersen S, Meiselman L, et al: Transrectal ultrasound that is diagnosing and staging of local disease after I^{125} seed implantation for prostate cancer. Int J Radiat Oncol Biol Phys 15:1453, 1988.

42. Lerner SP, Seale-Hawkins C, Carlton CE Jr, Scardino PT: The risk of dying of prostate cancer in patients with clinically localized disease. J Urol 146:1040, 1991.

43. Lightner DJ, Lange PH, Reddy PK, Moore L: Prostate specific antigen and local recurrence after radical prostatectomy. J Urol 144:921, 1990.

44. Meacham RB, Scardino PT, Hoffman GS, et al: The risk of distant metastases after transurethral resection of the prostate versus needle biopsy in patients with localized prostate cancer. J Urol 142:320, 1989.

45. Meek AG, Park PL, Oberman E, Wielopolski L: A prospective study of prostate specific antigen levels in patients receiving radiotherapy for localized carcinoma of the prostate. Am J Radiat Oncol Biol Phys 15:733, 1990.

46. Morton RA, Steiner MS, Walsh PC: Cancer control following anatomical radical prostatectomy: An interim report. J Urol 145:1197, 1991.

47. Mukamel E, deKernion JB, Hannah J, et al: The incidence and significance of seminal vesicle invasion in patients with adenocarcinoma of the prostate. Cancer 59:1535, 1987.

47a. Musselman PW, Tubbs R, Connely RW, et al: Biological significance of prostatic carcinoma after definitive radiation therapy. J Urol 137:114A, 1987.

48. Oesterling JE, Chan DW, Epstein JI, et al: Prostate specific antigen in the preoperative and postoperative evaluation of localized prostatic cancer treated with radical prostatectomy. J Urol 139:766, 1988.

49. Paulson DF, Moul JW, Robertson JE, Walther PJ: Postoperative radiotherapy of the prostate for patients undergoing radical prostatectomy with positive margins, seminal vesicle involvement and/or penetration through the capsule. J Urol 143:1178, 1990.

50. Paulson DF, Moul JW, Walther PJ: Radical prostatectomy for clinical stage T1-2 N_0M_0 prostatic adenocarcinoma: Long-term results. J Urol 144:1180, 1990.

51. Pontes JE, Ohe H, Watanabe H, Murphy GP: Transrectal ultrasonography of the prostate. Cancer 53:1369, 1984.

52. Ray GR, Bagshaw MA, Freiha F: External beam radiation salvage for residual or recurrent local tumor following radical prostatectomy. J Urol 132:926, 1984.

53. Robey EL, Schellhammer PS: Local failure after definitive therapy for prostatic cancer. J Urol 137:613, 1987.

54. Russell KJ, Dunatov C, Hafermann MD, et al: Prostate specific antigen in the management of patients with localized adenocarcinoma of the prostate treated with primary irradiation therapy. J Urol 146:1046, 1991.

55. Sandler HM, Hanks GE: Analysis of the possibility that transurethral resection promotes metastasis in prostate cancer. Cancer 62:2622, 1988.

56. Scardino PT: Early detection of prostate cancer. Urol Clin North Am 16:635, 1989.

57. Scardino PT, Frankel JM, Wheeler TM, et al: The prognostic significance of post-irradiation biopsy results in patients with prostatic cancer. J Urol 135:510, 1986.

58. Scardino PT, Wheeler TM: Local control of prostate cancer with radiotherapy: Frequency and prognostic significance of positive results of post-irradiation prostate biopsy. NCI Monogr 7:95, 1988.

59. Schellhammer PF, El-Mahdi AM: Local failure and related complications after definitive treatment of carcinoma of the prostate by irradiation or surgery. Urol Clin North Am 17:835, 1990.
60. Schellhammer PH, El-Mahdi AM, Higgins EM, et al: Prostate biopsy after definitive treatment by interstitial iodine-125 implant or external beam radiation therapy. J Urol 137:897, 1987.
61. Schellhammer PF, Schlossberg SM, El-Mahdi AM, et al: Prostate specific antigen levels after definitive irradiation for carcinoma of the prostate. J Urol 145:1008, 1991.
62. Shipley WU, Prout GR, Coachman NM: Radiation therapy for localized prostate carcinoma: Experience at the Massachusetts General Hospital (1973–1981). NCI Monogr 7:67, 1988.
63. Stamey TA, Kabalin JN: Prostate specific antigen in the diagnosis and treatment of adenocarcinoma of the prostate. I. Untreated patients. J Urol 141:1070, 1989.
64. Stamey TA, Kabalin JN, Ferrari M: Prostate specific antigen in the diagnosis and treatment of adenocarcinoma of the prostate. III. Radiation treated patients. J Urol 141:1084, 1989.
65. Stamey TA, Kabalin JN, McNeal JE, et al: Prostate specific antigen in the diagnosis and treatment of adenocarcinoma of the prostate. II. Radical prostatectomy treated patients. J Urol 141:1076, 1989.
66. Stein A, deKernion JB, Dorey F, Smith RB: Adjuvant radiotherapy in patients post-radical prostatectomy with tumor extending through capsule or positive seminal vesicles. Urology 39:59, 1992.
67. Villers AA, McNeal JE, Redwine EA, et al: Pathogenesis and biological significance of seminal vesicle invasion in prostatic adenocarcinoma. J Urol 143:1183, 1990.
68. Walsh PC, Epstein JI, Lowe FC: Potency following radical prostatectomy with wide unilateral excision of the neurovascular bundle. J Urol 138:823, 1987.
69. Wheeler TM: Anatomic considerations in carcinoma of the prostate. Urol Clin North Am 16:623, 1989.
70. Zagars GK, Sherman NE, Babaian RJ: Prostate specific antigen and external beam radiation therapy in prostate cancer. Cancer 67:412, 1991.
71. Zincke H: Radical prostatectomy and exenterative procedures for local failure after radiotherapy with curative intent: Comparison of outcomes. J Urol 147:894, 1992.

Chapter 31

TREATMENT OF LOCALLY ADVANCED PROSTATE CANCER

RICHARD G. MIDDLETON

Prostate cancer that is confined within the prostatic capsule is potentially curable by radical prostatectomy. Clinical Stage C cancer is traditionally defined as tumor that palpably extends locally beyond the margins of the capsule—usually laterally into the pedicle of the prostate toward the pelvic sidewall or cephalad into the seminal vesicles and bladder neck. Lateral and upward local tumor extension is common. Less common is tumor extension distally into the membranous urethra and urogenital diaphragm. Tumor that reaches the pelvic lymph nodes is Stage D1, and Stage D2 prostate cancer indicates bone metastasis.

Clinical staging, in this case the important differentiation between localized tumor (Stage B) and cancer that has penetrated the prostatic capsule to extend beyond the prostate (Stage C), has traditionally been based on careful digital rectal examination (DRE). In equivocal or borderline cases, staging by DRE is notoriously unreliable. Overstaging and particularly understaging have been all too common. Prostatic acid phosphatase (PAP) determination has rarely been helpful in separating clinical Stage B from locally extensive Stage C prostatic carcinoma. Also, CT scanning and MRI have generally been unhelpful. The most useful adjuncts to DRE have been transrectal ultrasound scanning (TRUS) and prostate-specific antigen (PSA) determination. As experience is accumulating with TRUS, it seems increasingly possible to detect extracapsular extension, including seminal vesicle tumor invasion, ultrasonographically and to prove the presence of extracapsular tumor by guided needle biopsies. PSA has become an increasingly valuable adjunct in tumor staging. Elevation of the PSA level has been reported in 65 to 100 per cent of patients

with clinical Stage C prostatic cancer. Stamey and associates have reported that in a group of patients with PSA levels over 50 ng/ml, 90 per cent had seminal vesicle tumor involvement and two thirds had positive pelvic lymph nodes.[16] In another study, the mean value for PSA in patients with clinical Stage C cancer was 67 ng/ml.[3] The mean level for patients with Stage D2 prostatic cancer was 292 ng/ml.

Once prostate cancer has penetrated the capsule to extend locally, tumor involvement of the pelvic lymph nodes increases dramatically. The incidence of positive pelvic lymph nodes in clinical Stage C lesions ranged widely from 15 to 85 per cent in seven reported series. (IM Thompson, unpublished report, 1991) Commonly, the incidence of nodal metastasis has been 40 to 50 per cent.[14] In high-grade Stage C cancers, more than 90 per cent have been reported to have involvement of the pelvic lymph nodes. Although certain factors—tumor size, grade, and PSA level—allow prediction of the likelihood of pelvic nodal metastasis, pelvic lymphadenectomy has been necessary to determine accurately the state of the pelvic nodes in an individual patient. Occasionally, lymphadenectomy can be omitted when a CT scan identifies an enlarged node that can be assessed by percutaneous node biopsy or aspiration.

Current trends suggest that laparoscopic pelvic lymphadenectomy will be an increasingly useful staging maneuver in the future. For now, assessment of the value of therapy of Stage C prostate cancers is difficult because many of the data reported in the medical literature are based on inadequately staged case material, i.e., usually the absence of histologic examination of pelvic lymph nodes. At least half of reported cases of Stage C prostate cancer are actually cases of Stage D1 cancer unless the patients have undergone staging pelvic lymphadenectomy.

Unlike Stage A and B prostate cancer, which can be indolent or slow to progress at times, Stage C or locally extended prostatic carcinoma is usually progressive, and most tumors that extend beyond the prostate capsule are of intermediate or high grade. When these tumors are treated by hormonal measures and transurethral resection of the prostate (if necessary), 5-year survival is in the 45 to 69 per cent range, and 70 per cent of those who survive 5 years progress to bony metastases.[4, 6, 18] Ten-year survival is in the range of 17 to 20 per cent.

RADICAL PROSTATECTOMY

Shroeder and Belt in 1975 reported a large experience with radical perineal prostatectomy for Stage C cancers that seemed "locally removable."[12] Of 213 Stage C patients, 70 (33 per cent) had seminal vesicle tumor invasion histologically. In all Stage C patients subjected to surgery, about 55 per cent survived 5 years; 10-year survival was approximately 37 per cent. These patients were operated on before staging pelvic lymphadenectomy had become commonplace, but we know from many reports in the urologic literature that half or more of these reported cases were likely Stage D, and some were even more advanced.

Tomlinson et al reported an experience with radical perineal prostatectomy for clinical Stage C lesions.[17] No claim was made for extending survival, but radical prostatectomy was advocated for decreasing the manifestations of local tumor recurrence and improving quality of life. Other reports have disputed the value of radical prostatectomy in controlling local disease. Flocks has reported radical prostatectomy supplemented with Au-198 with apparently some delay in tumor progression.[5] Recurrence, tumor progression, and mortality are clearly higher with Stage C than Stage B tumors, making the value of surgical excision in Stage C cancers highly questionable. More extended pelvic resection has been considered and employed. Radical cystoprostatectomy including wide excision of the membranous and bulbous urethra plus the urogenital diaphragm has been carried out.[15] Total pelvic exenteration for local extension into the rectal wall has also been tried. Extended pelvic surgery such as anterior and total pelvic exenteration is in disfavor generally; results have not been significantly better than in comparable cases treated with hormone measures only.

HORMONAL DOWNSTAGING PLUS RADICAL PROSTATECTOMY

Significant shrinkage or reduction in size and induration of a local prostate cancer is rather common after hormonal therapy is begun. A locally extended tumor, clinical Stage C, often seems by DRE to be a smaller and more localized lesion, or the prostate may even feel soft and benign after 3 or 4 months of DES, luteinizing hormone–releasing hormone analogue treatment, or bilateral orchiectomy. Does this hormonal effect make the lesion more likely to be curable? Can the surgeon totally encompass the prostate cancer which once seemed unresectable? Scott and Boyd reported delayed radical prostatectomy after hormonal treatment with 61, 51, and 29 per cent 5-, 10-, and 15-year progression-free survivals.[13] Actual survival with and without progressive disease was 74, 61, and 29 per cent at 5, 10, and 15 years. Patients subjected to the combined treatment were selected from those who responded best to the hormone treatment. Also, because lymph nodes were not examined histologically, the selection process was compromised.

Interest in attempted hormone downstaging has been renewed with enthusiasm in some circles. Certainly radical prostatectomy that includes pelvic lymphadenectomy and whole-mount examination of the radical prostatic specimen will ultimately give us a better idea of the value of this type of combined treatment. A carefully conducted study with adequate numbers of cases and randomization of patients to combined therapy versus early hormone therapy alone should clarify the usefulness of this treatment concept. A staging pelvic lymphadenectomy by open surgical or laparoscopic technique will be necessary at the onset to identify patients who clearly have Stage C disease. Those with positive pelvic lymph nodes are unsuitable for consideration of tumor downstaging. Insufficient evidence is available currently to recommend hormonal downstaging followed by radical prostatectomy as a useful therapeutic modality, but neither are adequate data available to dismiss the concept.

RADICAL PROSTATECTOMY AND ADJUVANT HORMONAL TREATMENT

Zincke et al from the Mayo Clinic have advocated radical prostatectomy with early adjuvant hormone treatment for clinical Stage C disease.[19] Results at 5 years are encouraging, but that is no surprise from knowledge of outcomes of untreated prostatic cancer patients and the anticipated temporary benefits from hormonal treatment. Further data and long-term outcomes of these patients will clarify the benefits of radical prostatectomy plus adjuvant hormonal therapy.

PATHOLOGIC STAGE C CANCER

On occasion during the performance of radical prostatectomy, the surgeon recognizes that he is cutting across tumor as he divides the prostatic capsule from the prostatic pedicles—usually near the bladder neck. Firm, fibrous-like tissue surrounding the seminal vesicles, making dissection of these structures more difficult than usual, may also represent locally extensive prostate cancer. If histologic examination confirms periprostatic tumor extension, incomplete tumor excision is to be expected. Much more subtle microscopic tumor extension beyond the prostate is more common (in carefully selected patients), making careful histologic examination of the radical prostatectomy specimen of great importance. Whole-mount techniques with step sections of the surgical specimen have led to the realization that microscopic tumor at the periphery is more common than was previously appreciated. Level III capsular penetration is defined as thorough penetration through the capsule into the periprostatic tissue. Level II is tumor invasion close to the outer capsular surface, and level I is a lesser degree of tumor invasion of the capsule.

Histologic tumor extension into the seminal vesicles also varies and is difficult to quantify. Small clusters of adenocarcinoma sometimes can be seen in the wall of the seminal vesicles. Much more ominous is tumor in the soft tissue surrounding the seminal vesicle, a true proximal positive margin in the author's opinion.

Positive margins, capsular involvement and penetration, and seminal vesicle invasion are all terms commonly used to identify histologic tumor at the periphery of the resected prostate. Some difference exists in the interpretation of margins and the level of capsular involvement, but it is imperative for the urologist to review the data carefully with the pathologist. Capsular involvement and seminal vesicle invasion do not mean that local recurrence is inevitable, but knowing the extent and level of local extension can allow the urologist to make an estimate of the likelihood of local tumor recurrence. At the University of Utah we recently reviewed our 10-year follow-up results after radical prostatectomy, including pelvic lymphadenectomy (RG Middleton, unpublished data, 1991). Of those with localized tumors, clinical and pathologic Stages A and B, 55 per cent survived 10 years without tumor recurrence, whereas only 30 per cent with extracapsular extension (pathologic Stage C) survived free of recurrence for 10 years. These data indicate that the outcome is clearly worse for pathologic Stage C tumors, yet some of these patients seem to benefit from the surgery and ultimately may be cured of prostate cancer.

PSA determination in recent years has proved to be a marvelous tool to assess residual disease and early local recurrence in the patient following radical prostatectomy.[8] With a locally extensive tumor at radical prostatectomy and a rising PSA in the early months after surgery, the presence of residual tumor is certain. What treatment is to be advised? A number of authors have advocated postoperative radiation treatment to the prostatectomy site in patients with positive margins, complete capsular penetration, and microscopic seminal vesicle tumor invasion.[7, 9–11] An elevated and rising PSA in the months after radical prostatectomy gives objective evidence of residual tumor. Local tumor recurrence is clearly suppressed by the radiation therapy, and the rising PSA is reversed in more than half of the patients so treated. It is not known whether radiation treatment actually produces long-range benefits such as a measurable delay in tumor progression and a prolonged patient survival. Early or delayed hormonal therapy also suppresses local recurrence and reverses the rising PSA.

The ultimate value of radiation treatment in this setting requires time and a large randomized clinical study. Potential benefits of post-prostatectomy radiation therapy must be measured against the potential complications of radiation in this situation—an increased incidence of incontinence, bladder neck and urethral stricture, radiation cystitis, and proctitis.

EXTERNAL RADIATION THERAPY

It has been extremely difficult to evaluate the efficacy of external radiation in Stage C prostate cancer. There are no good randomized controlled studies dealing with this issue. Further, most patients who have been treated have had presumed Stage C cancer in the absence of staging pelvic lymphadenectomy; statistically, at least half of these patients have positive pelvic nodes. With high-grade Stage C cancers, the overwhelming majority have pelvic nodal metastases. Additional factors obscuring the problem of determining treatment effectiveness are the fact that many patients are treated concurrently with hormonal measures, and many patients, once treated, have positive prostatic biopsies when evaluated thereafter. The frequency of biopsy in postradiation patients varies greatly from one reported series to another.

In a report of his large series from Stanford, Bagshaw reports survivals after radiation therapy for T3 (smaller Stage C lesions) and T4 (large Stage C lesions that extend to the pelvic sidewall or have rectal or bladder invasion).[2] For the smaller C tumors, survival at 5, 10, and 15 years was 65, 40, and 20 per cent, respectively. For the large C lesions, survival at 5 and 10 years was 35 and 20 per cent, respectively. Babaian et al from MD Anderson Hospital reported a 77 per cent 10-year disease-free survival in well-differentiated C lesions treated by external beam radiation therapy.[1] A 10-year disease-free survival of 50 per cent was achieved in moderately well-differentiated tumors, and only a 20 per cent disease-free survival was accomplished in high-grade tumors.

Thompson conducted a review of 22 reported series, including 3031 patients who had external beam radiation for Stage C disease (IM Thompson, unpublished report, 1991). Only 3 per cent of these patients had staging pelvic lymphadenectomy. Overall survival was 63, 39, and 24 per cent at 5, 10, and 15 years. From Bagshaw's report, 74 per cent of treated patients have positive prostate biopsies at 2 years. Complications from radiation therapy included 2.4 per cent with rectal injury, 3.9 per cent with urethral stricture, 8 per cent with chronic proctitis, 2.9 per cent with incontinence, and 5 per cent with chronic genital edema. External beam radiation therapy overall produced results somewhat better than those reported with various types of interstitial radiation.

Does pelvic radiation provide a better outcome than observation and delayed hormone therapy? The answer is not known, and the question is unlikely to be resolved without a large randomized study. Is radiation therapy justified even without providing a survival advantage if it controls local tumor progression and reduces recurrent hemorrhage, pain, the need for subsequent prostate resection, and the rate of ureteral obstruction? The urologic literature is mixed on this question.

STAGE D1 PROSTATE CANCER

Stage D1 prostate cancer is defined as cancer with metastasis to the pelvic lymph nodes but no extension to bones or other distant sites. Accurate identification of nodal metastasis is usually made at pelvic lymphadenectomy; various imaging techniques—lymphangiography, ultrasonography, CT scanning, and MRI—are unreliable. An elevated acid phosphatase level is common but not consistently so with Stage D1 prostate tumors. Positive pelvic nodes are commonly found when the PSA exceeds 20 ng/ml, and positive nodes have been reported in two thirds of patients with a PSA that exceeds 50 ng/ml. The incidence of positive pelvic lymph nodes also is associated with the clinical stage and tumor grade, as seen in Table 31–1, a review of 452 pelvic lymphadenectomies performed at the University of Utah.

The discovery of positive pelvic nodes is ominous, and disease progression and length of survival seem to depend mostly upon tumor grade, probably DNA ploidy and tumor growth rate. Whether or not radical prostatectomy is performed does not seem to be a major factor in the patient's outcome. Only 50 to 60 per cent of patients are likely to survive 5 years. Those who survive 5 years usually have disease progression, and few reach the 10-year milestone. Because radical prostatectomy has little influence on the patient's outcome, I advise that radical prostatectomy not be carried out when nodal metastasis is confirmed.

Pelvic radiation therapy is commonly used in patients with Stage D1 cancer, but evidence from several studies suggests that tumor progression and survival rates are similar in those who do and do not receive radiation treatment. Considering the morbidity, expense, and ineffectiveness of radiation therapy in controlling Stage D1 prostate tumor, there seems to be no advantage for the patient to receive this therapy.

Enthusiasm for radical prostatectomy with early adjuvant hormonal therapy, namely, bilateral orchiectomy, has come from the Mayo Clinic in recent years. Zincke recently reported the Mayo Clinic experience with 380 patients treated since 1967.[20] He has found progression-free survival rates of 80 and 77 per cent at 5 and 10 years for these patients, and they have done significantly better than patients receiving radical prostatectomy with delayed hormonal therapy at the time of recurrence. Further information, particularly more data on long-term progression-free rates and survival, is necessary to evaluate the advantages of this method for treating Stage D1 prostate cancer.

SUMMARY

No clear-cut guidelines are available for directing the treatment of the patient with locally extensive prostatic cancer. Treatment of clinical Stage C tumors has generally been carried out with inadequate tumor staging, i.e., the absence of pelvic lymphadenectomy. Radical prostatectomy, both initially and after "tumor downstaging," radiation therapy, and early and delayed hormonal therapy have been advocated. Combinations of surgery, radiation, and hormonal manipulation have been recommended, but large and carefully conducted randomized treatment trials are still necessary if we are to determine the optimal management of this lesion. Treatment options are available, but no scientifically sound treatment guidelines or recommendations.

For pathologic Stage C lesions with a rising PSA level, postoperative radiation or the institution of hormone therapy at some point is likely to be helpful in suppressing the PSA value and controlling local recurrence for an uncertain period. Each method of treatment is an option and is reasonable; neither at this point can be preferred over the other.

For Stage D1 prostate cancer, it is still unclear whether treatment methods and combination treatments hold any advantage over early or delayed institution of hormonal measures. Tumor grade, DNA ploidy, and tumor growth potential (an unmeasurable factor) seem to affect the patient's outcome more than the specific therapeutic method employed. However, the early good results reported from the Mayo Clinic with radical

TABLE 31–1. INCIDENCE OF PELVIC NODE METASTASIS BY HISTOLOGIC GRADE AND CLINICAL STAGE

	GRADE						
	Well Differentiated		Moderately Differentiated		Poorly Differentiated		TOTALS
	No./Total (%)		No./Total (%)		No./Total (%)		No./Total (%)
Stage							
A1	0/28		0/12		0/1		0/41	
A2	0/7		5/19	(26)	3/7	(43)	8/33	(24)
B1	2/53	(4)	13/94	(14)	3/9	(33)	18/156	(12)
B2	5/27	(18)	29/106	(27)	9/21	(43)	43/154	(28)
C	5/10	(50)	18/44	(41)	13/14	(93)	36/68	(53)
Totals	12/125	(10)	65/275	(24)	28/52	(54)	105/452	(23)

prostatectomy and early orchiectomy require further evaluation of this approach to treatment.

REFERENCES

1. Babaian RJ, Zagars GK, Ayala AG: Radiation therapy of stage C prostate cancer: Significance of Gleason grade to survival. Semin Urol 8:225, 1990.
2. Bagshaw MA, Cox RS, Ramback JE: Radiation therapy for localized prostate cancer. Urol Clin North Am 17:787, 1990.
3. Barak M, Meca Y, Luri A, et al: Evaluation of prostatic specific antigen as a marker for adenocarcinoma of the prostate. J Lab Clin Med 113:598, 1989.
4. deVere White R, Paulson DF, Glenn JF: The clinical spectrum of prostate cancer. J Urol 117:323, 1977.
5. Flocks RH: The treatment of stage C prostatic cancer with special reference to combined surgical and radiation therapy. J Urol 109:461, 1973.
6. Ganem EJ: Carcinoma of the prostate gland: 5-year survival following antiandrogenic treatment. J Urol 74:804, 1955.
7. Hudson MA, Catalona WJ: Effect of adjuvant radiation therapy on prostate specific antigen following radical prostatectomy. J Urol 143:1175, 1990.
8. Lange PH, Ercole CJ, Lightner DJ, et al: The value of serum prostate specific antigen determinations before and after radical prostatectomy. J Urol 141:873, 1989.
9. Link P, Freiha FS, Stamey TA: Adjuvant radiation therapy in patients with detectable prostate and specific antigen following radical prostatectomy. J Urol 145:532, 1991.
10. Morgan WR, Zincke H, Rainwater LM, et al: Prostate specific antigen values after radical retropubic prostatectomy for adenocarcinoma of the prostate: Impact of adjuvant treatment (hormonal and radiation). J Urol 145:319, 1991.
11. Paulson DF, Moul JW, Robertson JE, Walther PJ: Post-operative radiotherapy of the prostate for patients undergoing radical prostatectomy with positive margins, seminal vesicle involvement and/or penetration through the capsule. J Urol 143:1178, 1990.
12. Schroeder FH, Belt E: Carcinoma of the prostate: A study of 213 patients with Stage C tumors treated by total perineal prostatectomy. J Urol 114:257, 1975.
13. Scott WW, Boyd HL: Combined hormone control and radical prostatectomy in the treatment of selected cases of advanced carcinoma of the prostate. J Urol 101:86, 1969.
14. Smith JA Jr, Seaman JP, Gleidman JB, Middleton RG: Pelvic lymph node metastasis from prostatic cancer: Influence of tumor grade and stage in 452 consecutive patients. J Urol 130:290, 1983.
15. Spaulding JT, Whitmore WW Jr: Extended total excision of prostatic adenocarcinoma. J Urol 120:188, 1978.
16. Stamey TA, Kabalin JN, McNeal JE, et al: Prostate specific antigen in the diagnosis and treatment of adenocarcinoma of the prostate. II Radical prostatectomy treated patients. J Urol 141:1076, 1989.
17. Tomlinson RL, Currie DP, Boyce WH: Radical prostatectomy: Palliation for stage C carcinoma of the prostate. J Urol 117:85, 1977.
18. The Veterans Administration Co-operative Urological Research Group: Treatment and survival of patients with cancer of the prostate. Surg Gynecol Obstet 124:1011, 1967.
19. Zincke H, Utz DC, Taylor WF, et al: Bilateral pelvic lymphadenectomy for clinical stage C prostatic cancer: Role of adjuvant treatment of residual cancer and in disease progression. J Urol 135:1199, 1986.
20. Zincke H: Combined surgery and immediate adjuvant, hormonal treatment for stage D_1 adenocarcinoma of the prostate: Mayo Clinic experience. Semin Urol 8:175, 1990.

Section IV

PROSTATITIS

Chapter 32

HISTOPATHOLOGY AND CYTOLOGY OF PROSTATITIS

BETSY D. BENNETT, PATTI H. RICHARDSON, and WILLIAM A. GARDNER, JR.

PROSTATITIS—INTRODUCTION

Inflammation of the prostate is one of the most common conditions in urologic practice, accounting for over 1 million office visits in 1991. Although many of these patients are treated with antibiotics, the cause of their prostatitis probably will not be identified with certainty. Many develop multiple recurrences of their symptoms and carry the clinical diagnosis of "chronic prostatitis" throughout the rest of their lives.

The true prevalence of histologic prostatitis in the absence of other prostatic disease is difficult to determine for two reasons: (1) Most histologic studies of prostatitis have used specimens obtained at surgery or at autopsy of hospitalized patients over age 40. In the surgical series, all patients had known prostatic disease (hyperplasia or carcinoma), which could be expected to alter the prostatic architecture and contribute to the development of inflammation. In the autopsy series, in addition to the effects of age and hyperplasia, the patients were frequently victims of chronic debilitating illness that may have influenced findings in the prostate. (2) The definitions of prostatitis used by various investigators were not uniform. In some studies, the presence of lymphocytes in prostatic stroma was considered to represent a form of prostatitis, whereas in others more stringent criteria were used. In addition, in many series it is quite difficult to determine the frequency of acute versus chronic versus mixed inflammatory infiltrates because the number of cases that contain a mixed pattern is rarely noted. With these caveats in mind, the prevalence of prostatitis has been reported to be between 35 and 98 per cent.[4, 42, 59, 65, 71, 72, 93]

In a more recent study,[6] prostates were obtained at forensic autopsies in males aged 16 to 42 in an effort to determine the prevalence of disease in a presumably healthy, asymptomatic population. A diagnosis of prostatitis in these cases required association of the inflammatory infiltrate with glandular epithelium. Stromal lymphocytes alone were not included. One hundred fifty cases were evaluated, and prostatitis was found in 110 (73 per cent). A mixed pattern of acute and chronic inflammation was the most common, occurring in 46 cases. Cases of focal and multifocal chronic prostatitis were next in frequency, with 33 and 28 cases, respectively. The proportion of positive cases was highest in the 26 to 30 and 36 to 42 age groups (82 and 86 per cent) and lowest in the 21 to 25 age group (64 per cent). Causes of these cases were not addressed in this study.

The cause of prostatitis is an area replete with conflicting and confusing data. In the majority of cases a causative agent is never determined. In cases of proven bacterial prostatitis, the organisms involved are those causing urinary tract infections in general, with *Escherichia coli* being responsible for 80 per cent of cases.[51, 58] The frequency of this organism is explained by the presence of receptors on human transitional epithelial cells which interact with P-fimbriae of *E. coli*.[20] Additional organisms identified as common causative agents of acute and chronic prostatitis are other gram-negative rods and enterococci.[51, 58]

Mycobacterial infection of the prostate produces granulomatous prostatitis and is seen in association with disseminated disease.[10, 51, 57, 106] The incidence of mycobacterial prostatitis in the United States has decreased with improved diagnosis and therapy of pulmonary tuberculosis. The incidence of tuberculosis, however, is increasing in immunosuppressed patients, and the prevalence of granulomatous prostatitis due to typical and atypical mycobacteria is expected to follow this trend. The histologic appearance of granulomatous prostatitis due to tuberculosis or atypical organisms is histologically identical to the prostatitis that develops in patients who have received intravesical bacille Calmette-Guérin (BCG) as therapy for transitional cell carcinoma of the urinary bladder.[50, 66, 73]

The majority of cases of prostatitis have a nonbacterial origin. Presumably, these represent a mixture of infectious and noninfectious causes.

Mycotic infection of the genitourinary system is uncommon and almost always represents systemic hematogenous dissemination. The most commonly involved genitourinary organs are the kidneys, prostate, epididymis, and testes in descending order of frequency. Fungal disease of the prostate is often overlooked until it is discovered incidentally by cultures or by histologic examination of surgical specimens.[78] Over the last several decades there has been an increase in genitourinary tract fungal infections attributable to the widespread use of antibiotic, immunosuppressive, and antineoplastic drugs, to the prolonged life span in patients with underlying serious diseases, and more recently to acquired immunodeficiency syndrome (AIDS).

Viral and parasitic agents have been implicated in a few cases of prostatitis, but an established diagnosis is uncommon.[45, 51, 58] *Ureaplasma* species, for example, have been implicated as agents responsible for significant numbers of cases of chronic prostatitis.[13, 60] This hypothesis has been questioned by other investigators based on serologic and epidemiologic studies and results of antibiotic therapy.[56, 58, 77] *Trichomonas vaginalis* has also been implicated as a causative agent of chronic prostatitis based on clinical association and the long-held belief that the prostate serves as a reservoir for trichomonads in males. The role of *T. vaginalis* in the development of prostatitis remains controversial, however.[31, 41] The organism has been demonstrated in cases of chronic prostatitis by immunochemical methods, but definitive organisms are seen only rarely.[31]

Evidence that *Chlamydia trachomatis* causes some cases of nonbacterial prostatitis is much stronger, although the relative importance of this agent remains to be clarified. Numerous studies have proposed this association on the basis of serologic evidence and results of antibiotic therapy.[58] Culture-proven chlamydial infection of the prostate is less frequently identified, although conflicting data are present in the literature.[12, 21, 41] Typical intracytoplasmic inclusion bodies and positive immunofluorescent stains for chlamydia have been identified in some cases.[12, 82] More recently, Shurbaji and colleagues have demonstrated chlamydial antigens in tissue sections of urinary bladder and prostate with chronic inflammatory disease.[96, 97] Abdelatif et al used in situ hybridization to demonstrate chlamydial antigen in 7 of 23 cases of chronic abacterial prostatitis.[1] Although these studies lend strong support to the role of chlamydia in prostatitis, the numerical significance of this organism remains unclear.[2, 95] The majority of cases

of nonbacterial prostatitis continue to resist specific etiologic definition. It is assumed, therefore, that these represent true noninfectious cases.

Multiple causes of noninfectious prostatitis have been postulated and are supported by a variety of experimental and clinical data. Studies by Naslund and Coffey and by Robinette have demonstrated the effects of age, genetic background, and hormonal imbalance in the development of nonbacterial prostatitis in rats.[67, 68, 87] These investigators have shown that changes in sex hormone levels during the neonatal period can affect development of prostatitis in adulthood.[67]

A role for chronic stress in the induction of nonbacterial prostatitis is also supported by experimental and clinical studies. Gatenbeck et al and Aronsson et al have shown that exposure of rats to standardized stress results in histologic changes similar to those of chronic nonbacterial prostatitis in humans.[3, 32] These results are in accord with observations of Miller and others, who have identified patients with chronic prostatitis whose most satisfactory therapy was based on management of stress. They proposed the term *stress prostatitis* for this condition. Further, they suggested that the causative relationship is based on autonomic innervation of the prostate, which is similar to that of other organs on which the effects of stress are well documented.[34, 64]

Clinically, other physiologic and pathophysiologic events have been postulated to be associated with the development of prostatitis. A role for urinary reflux, demonstrated to occur during micturition in some patients, has been proposed for both bacterial and abacterial prostatitis. In the latter case, reflux may contribute to the formation of prostatic calculi. Chemical irritation from urine may also initiate and maintain an inflammatory process in the prostate.[40] Allergic and autoimmune phenomena have also been postulated to be causative factors in prostatitis. Allergic prostatitis is found predominantly in patients with a history of asthma and is characterized by an eosinophilic infiltrate, granulomatous inflammation, and, in some cases, necrotizing vasculitis. Symptoms of prostatitis in these patients generally coincide with exacerbations of asthma.[25, 106] A similar histologic pattern, however, has been described following transurethral resection and probably represents a local reaction to prostatic antigens exposed as a result of the surgical procedure.[25, 26, 43, 62, 83] Other "physiologic" events shown or postulated to result in chronic prostatitis include (1) erosion of prostatic epithelium by corpora amylacea with ensuing chronic and/or granulomatous reaction in adjacent stroma[29] (Fig. 32–1); (2) reflux of sperm into the prostate with production of spermiophages and chronic inflammation[69] (Fig. 32–2); and (3) persistence of unstimulated or hypoplastic foci with presumably abnormal amounts or composition of prostatic secretions[30] (Fig. 32–3).

HISTOPATHOLOGY

Acute Prostatitis. Although considerable variation exists with regard to the histologic classification of chronic inflammation, most pathologists agree on the

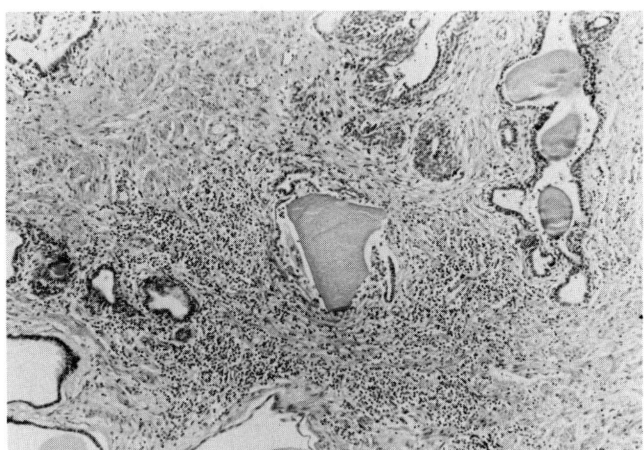

FIGURE 32–1. An irregular corpus amylaceum has eroded through the prostatic epithelium into the stroma. Note the giant cell in the lumen with chronic inflammation in the remaining epithelium as well as in the surrounding stroma (hematoxylin and eosin, original magnification × 100).

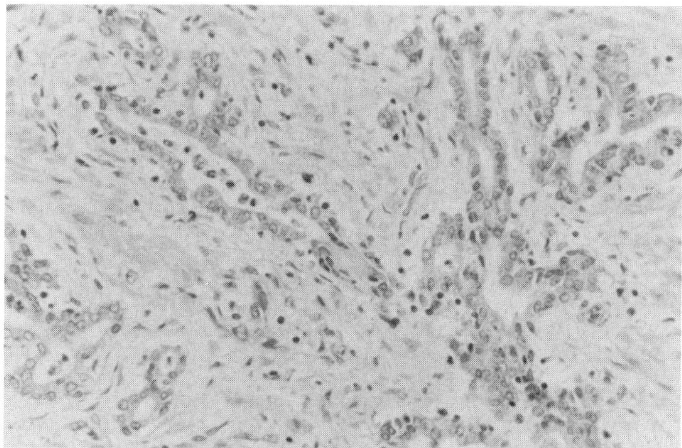

FIGURE 32–3. A focus of undeveloped (hypoplastic) glandular tissue in the prostate of an adult male. Mild acute and chronic inflammation is present within and around the gland (hematoxylin and eosin, original magnification × 100).

basic definition of acute prostatitis. Opinions differ only with regard to frequency and relationship to bacterial infection and to chronic prostatitis.

Acute prostatitis is characterized by the presence of polymorphonuclear leukocytes within glandular or ductular lumina, their epithelium, and/or adjacent stroma[4, 6, 42, 59, 72, 93] (Fig. 32–4). The degree of stromal involvement varies, usually increasing in association with the density of the intraluminal infiltrate.[4, 42] Pure acute inflammation, unaccompanied by any chronic inflammatory component, is unusual, occurring in 11 of 84 and 2 of 110 cases of prostatitis in reported series.[6, 42] In other series, the exact number of cases of pure acute inflammation is difficult to determine but again appears to be uncommon.[4, 72] In the majority of cases, luminal infiltration by polymorphonuclear cells is accompanied by periglandular accumulations of lymphocytes, monocytes, and occasional plasma cells mixed with varying degrees of acute inflammation.[4, 6, 42, 93] Some studies have suggested that acute and chronic prostatitis are more frequent in peripheral areas of the prostate and spill over into the central, periurethral zone.[52] Other studies have failed to support this difference.[4, 6, 42, 59, 93]

In most cases of acute prostatitis, little, if any, tissue necrosis is present, although focal areas of epithelial loss are frequent. Occasionally severe acute inflammation results in microabscess or abscess formation. Even in severe cases, however, acute prostatitis tends to be focal or multifocal rather than diffuse.[6, 42]

Although acute prostatitis as defined above is commonly assumed to be of bacterial origin, such an assumption has not been supported by culture. Indeed, studies have shown that the presence and/or severity of acute inflammation does not correlate with bacteriuria at or near the time of biopsy, recurrent urinary tract infections, cystitis, the presence of an indwelling catheter, or even clinical symptoms.[14, 42, 72]

Chronic Nonspecific Prostatitis. As noted above, the definition of chronic prostatitis is more variable than that of acute prostatitis. Although some studies do not provide a morphologic definition of chronic prostatitis,[65, 76] the majority of reports require a mono-

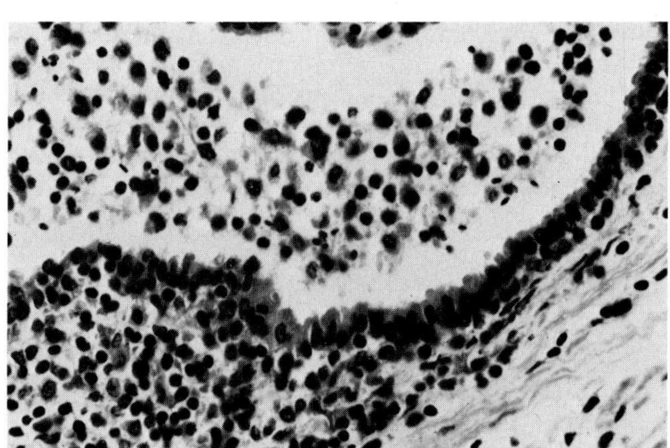

FIGURE 32–2. Numerous spermatozoa and macrophages are present in the lumen of this prostatic gland. Chronic inflammation with prominent plasma cells is located in adjacent stroma (hematoxylin and eosin, original magnification × 400).

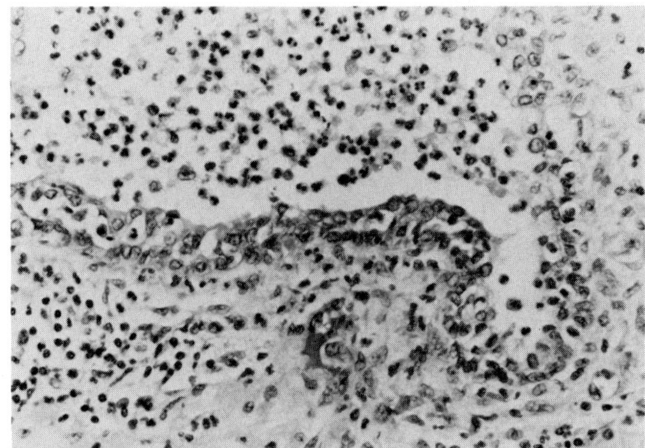

FIGURE 32–4. In this case of acute prostatitis the inflammatory infiltrate has partially destroyed the glandular epithelium. Polymorphonuclear leukocytes are noted within the remaining epithelium as well as within the glandular lumen and surrounding stroma (hematoxylin and eosin, original magnification × 400).

nuclear cell infiltrate (lymphocytes, monocytes, plasma cells) in the stromal connective tissue around a gland or duct[4, 6, 42, 71, 72, 93] (Fig. 32–5). In some cases a diffuse infiltrate composed of sheets of mononuclear cells is present, effacing normal stroma and enveloping glands. In other cases only focal inflammation is present. Whether or not chronic urethritis is included in these studies is not stated in most reports. In one series,[6] 14 of 33 cases of pure focal chronic inflammation were confined to the periurethral prostate. Most commonly the infiltrate is multifocal and shows an irregular distribution.[4, 6, 42, 93] Although all observers note the presence of collections of lymphocytes scattered randomly throughout the stroma (Fig. 32–6), only one study defines these as a pattern of prostatitis.[42] Whether or not these lymphocytic nodules are included in some other studies is not clear.[65, 76] Most studies specifically exclude them from consideration.[4, 6, 9, 72, 93] Approximately one half of reported series state that chronic inflammatory cells were present in glandular epithelium and lumina in some cases,[4, 6, 9] whereas the remainder state that they were not.[42, 72, 93] In some prostates, especially those obtained at autopsy, sloughed epithelial cells may be present in glandular lumina and must be distinguished from luminal histiocytes (Fig. 32–7A and B). In contrast to acute prostatitis, in which the majority of cases are associated with chronic inflammation, most cases of chronic prostatitis are not accompanied by acute inflammation.[4, 6, 9, 65, 71, 72] A follicular variant of chronic prostatitis has been described and may be present in association with other forms of chronic prostatitis (Fig. 32–8). The significance of this pattern has not been demonstrated. Although some studies have suggested an association between follicular inflammation and chlamydial infection in the cervix,[17, 36, 79, 107, 108] this relationship has not been supported in the prostate.

There is little or no correlation between the histologic presence of chronic prostatitis and clinical symptoms. No association has been demonstrated between chronic prostatitis and cystitis, indwelling catheters, recurrent

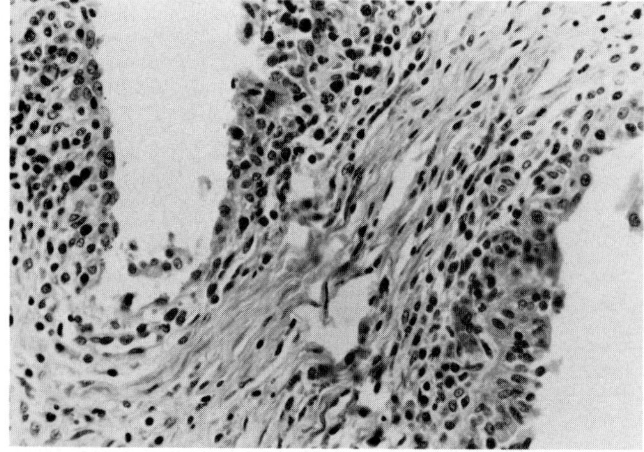

FIGURE 32–5. Chronic prostatitis with a lymphohistiocytic infiltrate in the epithelium and adjacent stroma. A few histiocytes are present in the lumen of the gland on the left (hematoxylin and eosin, original magnification × 400).

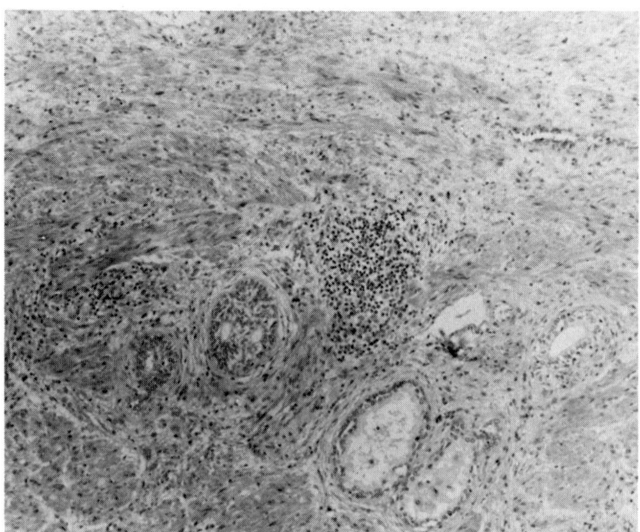

FIGURE 32–6. A collection of lymphocytes is noted within the prostatic stroma. Such accumulations of lymphocytes are *not* considered to represent chronic prostatitis (hematoxylin and eosin, original magnification × 100).

urinary tract infection, or positive culture at the time of biopsy.[14, 71, 72, 93] Some studies have shown an increased frequency with age and the occurrence of hyperplasia. In these cases, inflammation is especially prominent at the junction of hyperplastic nodules and adjacent atrophic glands.[9, 59] Chronic prostatitis has been identified in all age groups, including patients under the age of 20, and in its pure form has been shown to be most prevalent in patients less than 30 years old.[6] Organisms have not been demonstrated by tissue Gram stains, even in cases in which cultures were positive.[4, 71]

Histologic findings associated with chronic prostatitis include architectural distortion of glands,[24] attenuation and focal disruption of epithelium,[4] loss of epithelial secretory activity,[42] and hyperchromasia and polymorphism of epithelial cell nuclei accompanied by increased cytoplasmic basophilia[103] (Fig. 32–9). These "dysplastic" changes may be misinterpreted as carcinoma of the prostate if the association with chronic prostatitis is not recognized. Increased proliferative activity of the epithelium of glands involved by chronic prostatitis has been demonstrated by radiolabeling techniques.[103] Squamous metaplasia is also a frequent occurrence in areas of chronic prostatitis. Various mechanisms have been postulated to account for these changes.[99] The relationship, if any, between chronic prostatitis and the development of prostatic carcinoma remains to be explored.

Mycotic Prostatitis. *Blastomyces dermatitidis* is the most common of the deep mycoses to involve the prostate.[78, 94] Genitourinary involvement occurs in 20 to 30 per cent of cases of systemic blastomycosis,[23] but only a small percentage of these patients present with symptoms related to the genitourinary tract. The enlarged, boggy, and tender prostate may yield fungal organisms with massage.

The inflammation associated with blastomyces prostatitis may be suppurative, granulomatous, or mixed. Yeast forms can be found in and around ducts and

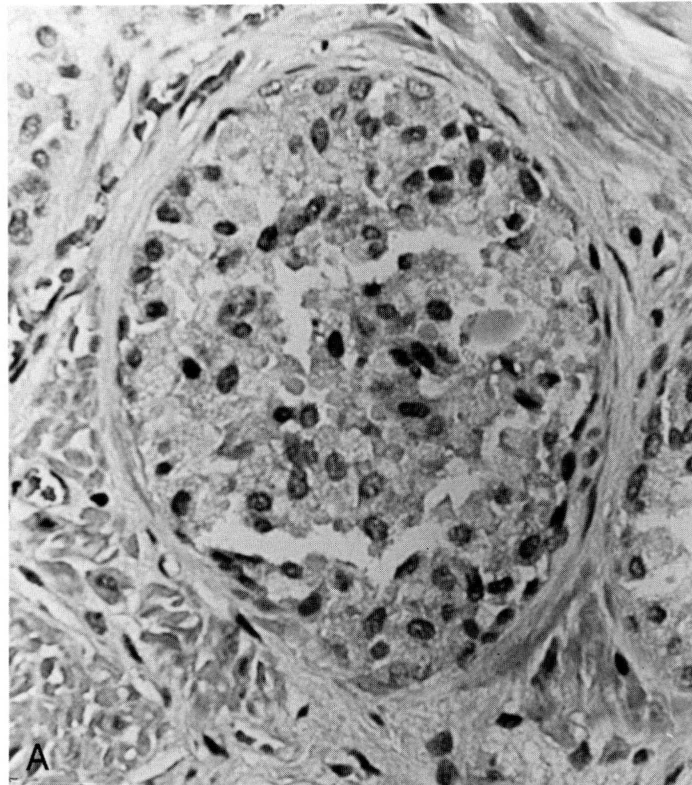

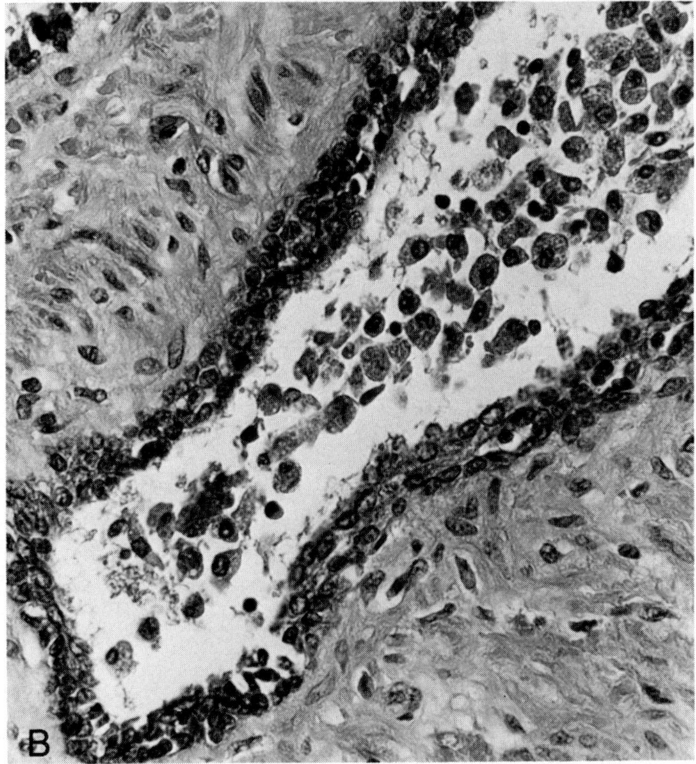

FIGURE 32–7. The superficial histologic similarity between sloughed, autolytic epithelial cells in the prostatic lumen and histiocytes may result in overdiagnosis of chronic prostatitis. *A,* Sloughed prostatic epithelial cells fill the lumen. This finding represents autolytic change and is most often seen in prostates obtained at autopsy. *B,* Histiocytes in the lumen of this gland involved by chronic prostatitis can be identified by their sharp cell borders, clear nuclear image, and round cell outlines. In questionable cases, immunoperoxidase identification of lysozyme within histiocytes may provide the correct interpretation (hematoxylin and eosin, original magnification × 400).

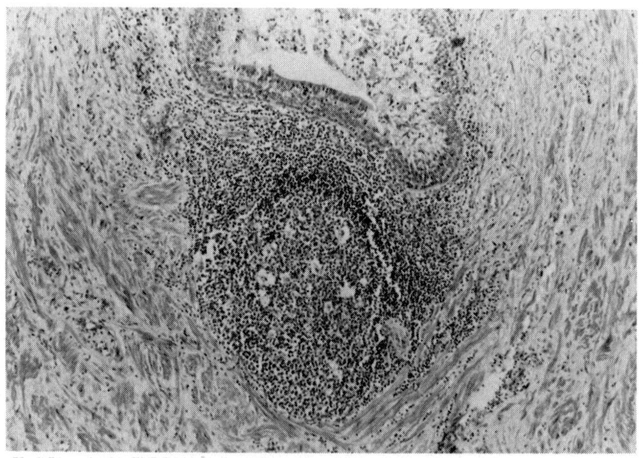

FIGURE 32–8. Chronic prostatitis involves the lumen, epithelium, and stroma adjacent to this prostatic gland. Note the stromal lymphoid follicle with germinal center (hematoxylin and eosin, original magnification × 100).

glands in association with varying degrees of inflammation, including abscess formation. In severe cases, the glandular lumina may appear packed with easily recognizable organisms (Fig. 32–10). Older lesions consist of granulomata with necrosis. In these cases *B. dermatitidis* can be seen within giant cells, in histiocytes, or free in the tissue.

The histologic diagnosis of blastomycosis is made by demonstrating the spherical, thick-walled, broad-based, budding yeasts 8 to 15 μ in diameter. The yeasts are sharply defined and have a refractile double-contoured wall. With hematoxylin and eosin, the cytoplasm stains basophilic and is usually separated from the unstained cell wall by a clear space. This appearance is sufficiently distinctive that special stains are not usually required, although Gomori methenamine silver (GMS), Gridley fungus, and periodic acid–Schiff (PAS) can be used to stain the organisms.

Coccidioides immitis is associated with extrapulmonary dissemination in less than 1 per cent of affected patients.[16, 47, 85] Immunosuppression, dark skin, age less than 5 or greater than 50, and pregnancy are risk factors for dissemination.[16, 22, 85]

The incidence of prostatic involvement is difficult to assess owing to the paucity of reported cases. Forbus and Bestebreurtje[27] reported an autopsy series of 50 cases with 6 per cent involvement of the prostate. Rohn, in a review of 214 cases, reported 1.8 per cent involvement of the prostate.[88] Petersen et al described 12 cases of coccidioiduria, four of which had coccidioidal prostatitis.[80] Patients with the antemortem diagnosis of coccidioidomycosis usually demonstrate symptoms of bladder outlet obstruction, a tender prostate, or hematuria.[47]

Tissue reaction to this organism may be suppurative and/or granulomatous. Generally, any given field contains a mixed reaction. The stage of the fungus in part dictates the inflammatory reaction. A localized purulent reaction occurs when numerous endospores are released, as in rapidly disseminating disease. As the endospores mature into spherules, the purulent reaction is replaced by a granulomatous response. Spherules can be seen in histiocytes and giant cells within granulomata. When these spherules rupture, polymorphonuclear leukocytes infiltrate into the granulomata. The histologic diagnosis is made by demonstrating the typical 20 to 200 μ in diameter, thick-walled spherules. The hematoxylin

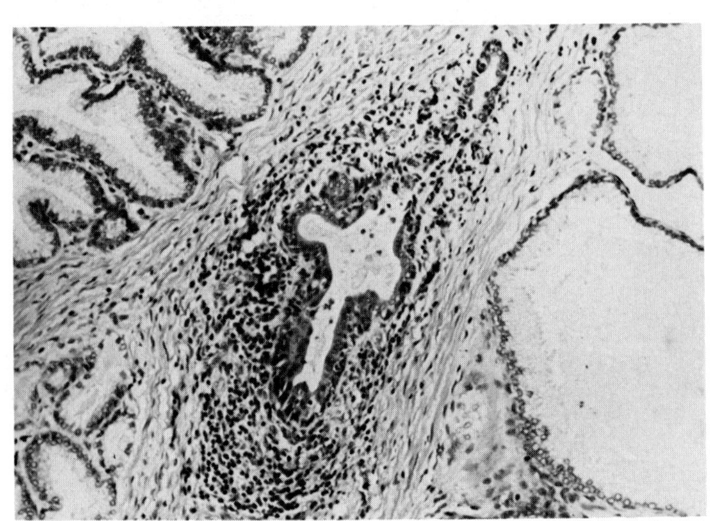

FIGURE 32–9. Epithelial changes noted in this gland involved by chronic prostatitis include enlargement and irregularity of the nuclei and increased basophilia of the cytoplasm compared with normal glands at left and right (hematoxylin and eosin, original magnification × 100).

and eosin procedure stains both the endospores and cell wall of the spherule, as does the GMS stain. PAS stains the endospores but not the cell wall of the spherule.

Cryptococcal prostatitis is usually part of disseminated disease with central nervous system and renal involvement.[78, 90] Rare cases have been reported in which the prostate was the only organ involved.[37, 63, 74] Involvement of the prostate may be clinically silent.[48, 90]

The tissue response to *Cryptococcus neoformans* is varied. At one end of the spectrum is mild chronic inflammation, and at the other end is a marked granulomatous response with variable suppuration. In some cases the organisms can be present in sufficient numbers to impart a mucoid appearance to the tissue.

The histologic diagnosis of cryptococcal prostatitis is made by finding the relatively pleomorphic yeasts, which are 2 to 20 μ in diameter. The mucopolysaccharide capsule stains red with Mayer's mucicarmine. Because of its variable size and shape and the fact that unencapsulated forms may be prominent, *C. neoformans* should be considered in the differential diagnosis of any fungal prostatitis. If the histologic diagnosis is in doubt, fluorescent antibody stains are generally useful.

Isolated cases of prostatitis due to *Histoplasma capsulatum*, *Candida* species, *Aspergillus flavus,* and *Paracoccidioides brasiliensis* have also been reported.[5, 35, 39, 54, 61, 74, 78, 88, 89]

Viral Prostatitis. Although viruses are postulated as causative agents for nonbacterial prostatitis, little evidence exists that viral infection of the prostate is clinically important.[8, 46, 58] Documented cases of herpetic or cytomegalic prostatitis have been reported, but such cases are exceedingly rare.[8, 15] The chronic inflammatory response associated with viral prostatitis may be similar to that seen with other viral infections. In AIDS patients, however, viral prostatitis is increasing in frequency and, as is true for other organisms, there may be a virtual absence of any inflammatory response (Fig. 32–11).

Parasitic/Protozoal Prostatitis. Documented cases of prostatitis caused by parasites or protozoa other than

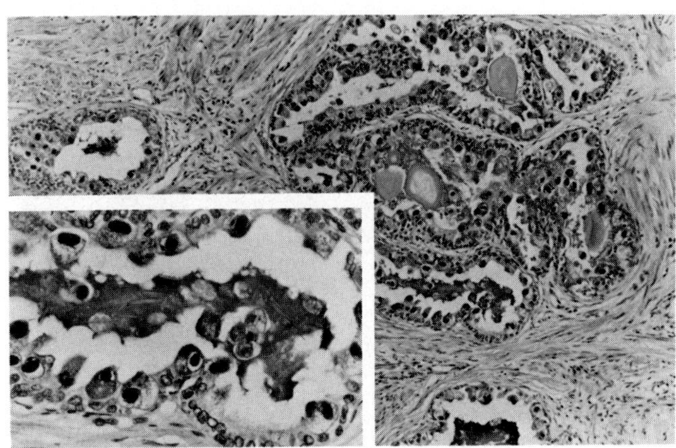

FIGURE 32–11. Inclusions characteristic of cytomegalovirus infection are seen in various stages of development in glands within the prostate of this patient with AIDS. Note the absence of significant inflammation within or around the glands (hematoxylin and eosin, original magnification × 100; inset, original magnification × 400). (Courtesy of Russell Harley, M.D., Charleston, SC.)

Schistosoma hematobium are rare. The latter is endemic in Africa and the Middle East. Genitourinary schistosomiasis is common, especially in the seminal vesicles and bladder, with prostatic involvement being relatively rare. During the active stage of the disease, the inflammatory response may be diffuse granulomatous inflammation with an eosinophilic and neutrophilic component or may take the form of discrete granulomata that form around a central egg. In the inactive stage, calcified eggs are found in dense connective tissue with little if any remaining inflammation.[45]

Prostatitis due to the protozoan *Trichomonas vaginalis* has long been postulated, but the evidence is largely indirect. Using immunoperoxidase techniques, rare organisms have been identified in intraepithelial vacuoles associated with chronic prostatitis.[31] Whether or not this organism plays a significant role in chronic prostatitis remains controversial.[46, 58]

One case of amebic prostatitis has been reported, but evidence was circumstantial and no tissue was available for study.[33]

Chlamydial Prostatitis. An increasing body of evidence points to chlamydia as a definite causative agent for some cases of chronic nonbacterial prostatitis. The proportion of these cases attributable to chlamydia, however, remains to be determined. Several studies have detected chlamydia by tissue culture and/or immunofluorescent techniques. Typical chlamydial inclusions have also been seen in expressed prostatic secretions from men with symptoms of chronic prostatitis.[11, 12, 70, 82] Although some investigators have been unsuccessful in immunofluorescent demonstration of organisms in prostate tissue,[21] recent immunohistochemical or in situ hybridization studies have identified chlamydial antigens in tissue sections showing typical histologic changes of chronic prostatitis (Fig. 32–12*A* and *B*). These changes consisted of an intense mixed mononuclear cell infiltrate around prostatic ducts and acini, partial distortion of the glands by the inflammatory process, and neutrophils and histiocytes in the lumina.[1, 2, 95, 97] In other sites, chlamydiae have been demonstrated

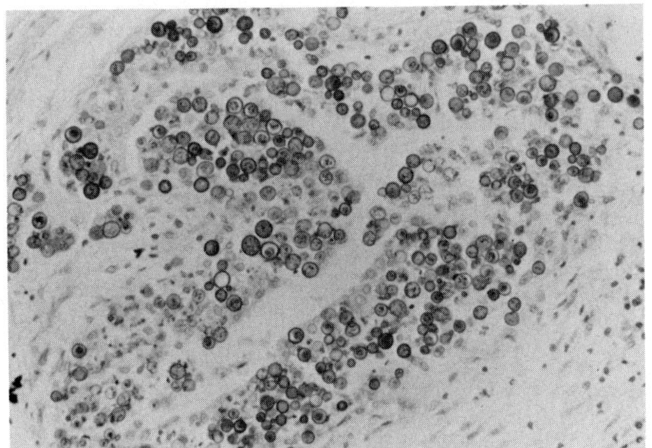

FIGURE 32–10. Yeast forms of *Blastomyces dermatitidis* can be easily identified in this prostatic gland. Residual epithelium is largely hidden by the combination of organisms and inflammatory reaction (periodic acid–Schiff, original magnification × 400).

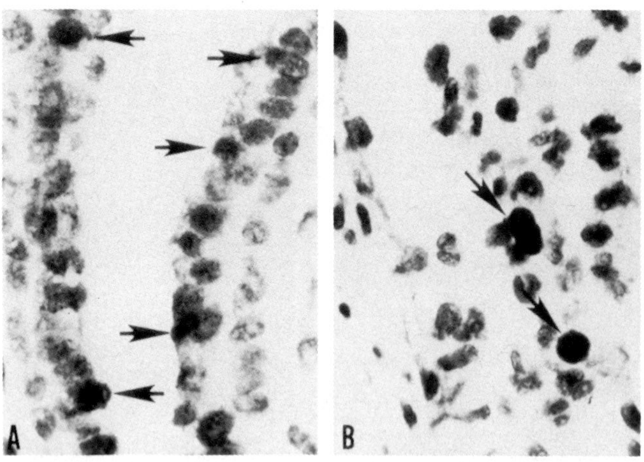

FIGURE 32–12. Colorimetric in situ hybridization for *Chlamydia trachomatis* in formalin-fixed, paraffin-embedded prostate tissue. Dark signal *(arrows)* demonstrates *(A)* numerous chlamydia bodies within epithelial cells of prostatic duct (nuclear fast red counterstain, original magnification × 100), and *(B)* intracellular *(top arrow)* and extracellular *(bottom arrow)* chlamydia bodies within the lumen of a dilated acinus (nuclear fast red counterstain, original magnification × 100). (From Abdelatif OMA, Chandler FW, McGuire BS: *Chlamydia trachomatis* in chronic abacterial prostatitis: Demonstration by color in situ hybridization. Hum Pathol 22:43, 1991; with permission.)

to be associated with severe chronic, often follicular inflammation, as well as with significant epithelial atypia.[17, 36, 79, 107] Similar changes in the prostate have not yet been demonstrated.

Granulomatous Prostatitis. Granulomatous inflammatory reactions in the prostate may produce an irregular, firm, often fixed gland on physical examination—findings indistinguishable from those of prostatic carcinoma. Since granulomatous prostatitis was first described,[105] numerous attempts at classification of its various forms have been made. A recently proposed classification scheme is based on a combination of etiologic and histologic criteria.[106] Granulomatous prostatitis is thereby described as infectious, idiopathic, post-surgical, or allergic.

Infectious granulomatous prostatitis is primarily due to *Mycobacterium tuberculosis* and is associated with disseminated disease. The histologic appearance is similar to that of tuberculosis in other locations—i.e., granulomata composed of epithelioid cells, histiocytes, and giant cells surrounded by lymphocytes and fibroblasts. Central caseous necrosis is often identified. Patients present with obstructive symptoms and an enlarged, firm prostate. Acid pyuria is frequently present and provides a clue to the specific diagnosis. A history of tuberculosis may be elicited, but genitourinary symptoms may occur many years after the initial diagnosis of tuberculosis.[10, 24, 45, 51, 57, 75, 100, 104, 106]

A histologically identical process may be seen in the prostates of patients who have received intravesicular BCG for therapy of transitional cell carcinoma of the urinary bladder. Organisms instilled into the bladder spread locally, producing prostatic lesions in virtually all patients who have been followed by biopsy. As with tuberculosis, a spectrum of lesions occurs ranging from vaguely nodular collections of histiocytes to ca-

seating granulomata (Fig. 32–13). Organisms are readily demonstrated by acid-fast stains and can be cultured from the genitourinary tract up to 1 year after therapy.[29, 50, 66, 73]

Malakoplakia is an unusual type of granulomatous prostatitis, occurring in association with gram-negative infections of the genitourinary tract, usually due to *E. coli*. It is characterized by large numbers of distinctive macrophages (von Hansemann cells) with occasional lymphocytes and plasma cells. Michaelis-Gutman bodies (laminated, round inclusions that stain positively for calcium and iron) occur in the cytoplasm of some of the macrophages[38, 55, 102] (Fig. 32–14).

Other specific infectious causes of granulomatous prostatitis include brucella and a variety of fungi as discussed above. The most frequent type of granulomatous prostatitis is the nonspecific, idiopathic form that accounts for 50 to 75 per cent of reported series. The clinical presentation is similar to that of other forms. Histologically, the prostate shows a chronic inflammatory infiltrate composed primarily of histiocytes and epithelioid cells with lymphocytes, plasma cells, and occasional giant cells. The inflammation may form discrete granulomata or may occur as sheets of cells "infiltrating" the prostatic stroma. In the latter setting, the histologic findings mimic those of adenocarcinoma, and immunocytochemical stains for lysozyme may be helpful in differentiating the histiocytes from malignant epithelial cells[84] (Fig. 32–15). The granulomata are noncaseating, and no organisms are demonstrated by special stains. Liquefactive necrosis may be present in areas of intense inflammation.[25, 28, 29, 92, 106]

Granulomatous prostatitis also occurs in patients who have undergone prostate surgery. In this setting, the granulomata may resemble classic rheumatoid nodules. The lesions are well circumscribed with a central area of fibrinoid necrosis which is frequently stellate or linear. This area is surrounded by palisading epithelioid histiocytes accompanied by lymphocytes, occasional giant cells, and varying numbers of eosinophils (Fig. 32–16). These distinctive lesions may be accompanied by the more usual forms of noncaseating granulomata. Occasional cases show necrotizing vasculitis. Some cases with large numbers of eosinophils and associated vasculitis may be histologically indistinguishable from cases of "allergic prostatitis." Knowledge of the patient's history of recent prostatic surgery is required to make the appropriate diagnosis.[24–26, 43, 45, 62, 83]

Eosinophilic granulomatous lesions may occur in two forms, either of which may be associated with a history of allergy. The first is similar to that of idiopathic granulomatous prostatitis except for the presence of large numbers of eosinophils. No vasculitis is present, and these patients have a uniformly good prognosis. The second form of eosinophilic granulomatous prostatitis is histologically similar to the post-surgical lesions described above. These cases show granulomata with central fibrinoid necrosis, intense eosinophilic infiltrate, and often necrotizing vasculitis. Systemic vasculitis may be present. In addition to asthma, this condition has been reported in association with drug allergies and in patients with systemic vasculitides such as Wegener's

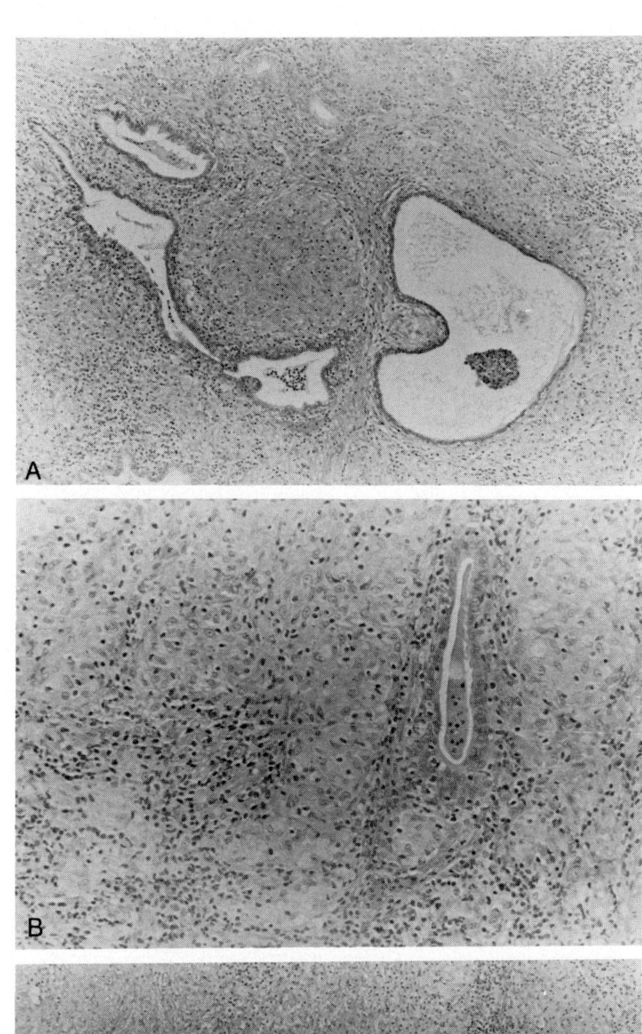

FIGURE 32–13. Spectrum of granulomatous lesions seen after intravesical therapy with BCG. These are histologically indistinguishable from those seen in cases of tuberculosis of the prostate. *A,* A small granuloma with a central giant cell and no necrosis. A chronic lymphohistiocytic infiltrate involves both glands and stroma. The granuloma produces minimal distortion of the prostatic architecture and no significant destruction (hematoxylin and eosin, × 100). *B,* Diffuse granulomatous inflammation in which prostatic architecture is distorted and only one gland is identifiable within this field (hematoxylin and eosin, × 400). *C,* A large granuloma with central caseous necrosis associated with typical epithelioid cell and lymphocytic infiltrate. One small prostate gland is identifiable in the lower right (hematoxylin and eosin, original magnification × 400).

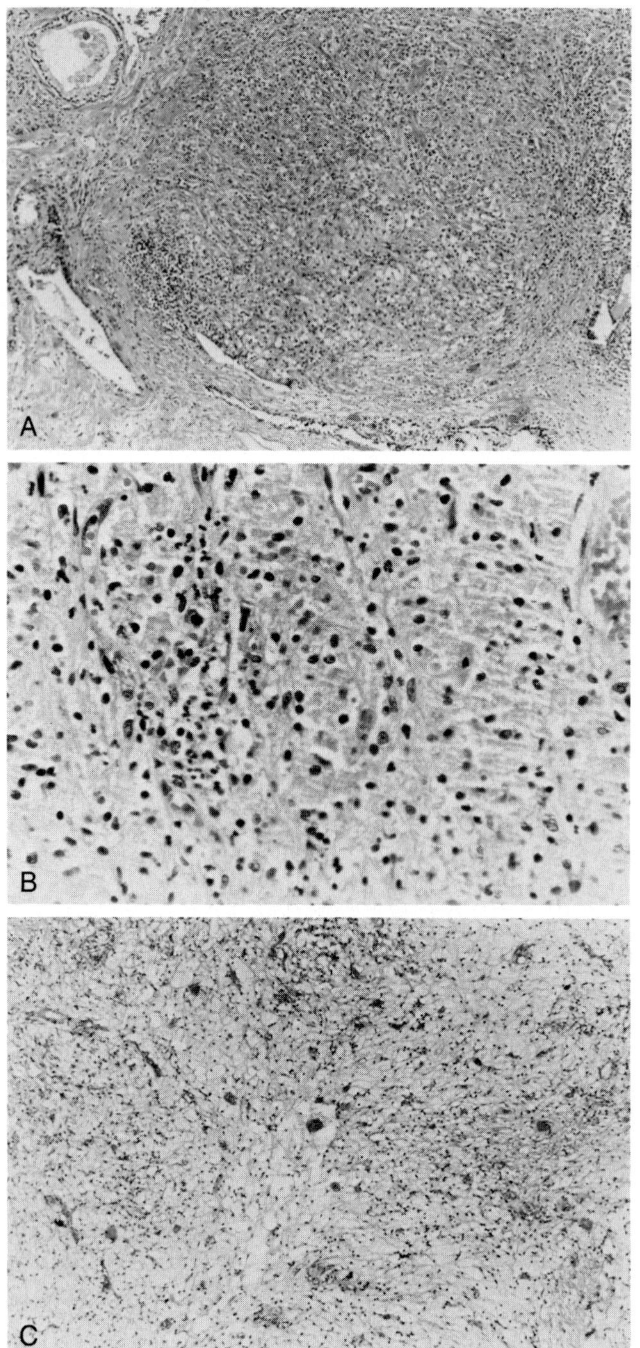

FIGURE 32–14. Malakoplakia of the prostate is characterized by the presence of foamy or granular macrophages with associated Michaelis-Gutman bodies. *A,* A nodular area of histiocytes and lymphocytes produces mild distortion of prostatic architecture (hematoxylin and eosin, × 100). *B,* Large numbers of macrophages with a granular eosinophilic cytoplasm (von Hansemann cells) contain numerous Michaelis-Gutman bodies (hematoxylin and eosin, × 400). *C,* In another field the macrophages have a clear, foamy cytoplasm. Michaelis-Gutman bodies are not identifiable at this magnification (hematoxylin and eosin, original magnification × 100).

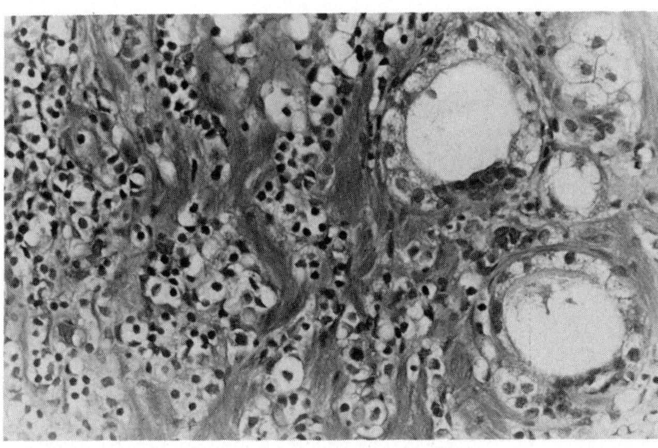

FIGURE 32–15. Histiocytes with clear cytoplasm are seen infiltrating the prostatic stroma. At low power, the resulting pattern resembles the malignant epithelial cells of adenocarcinoma. In difficult cases, immunohistochemical demonstration of lysozyme allows recognition of the histiocytes (hematoxylin and eosin, original magnification × 100).

granulomatosis, polyarteritis nodosa, and Churg-Strauss syndrome. The prognosis is variable and is less favorable in those cases associated with systemic vasculitis.[19, 25, 86, 92, 106, 109]

CYTOLOGY OF PROSTATITIS

Examination of expressed prostatic secretions has been used extensively in evaluating patients with sus-

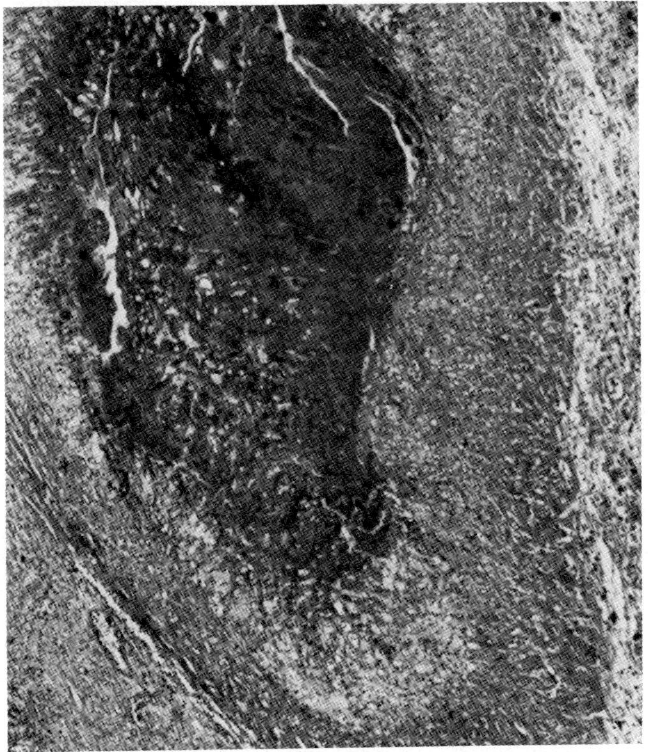

FIGURE 32–16. Post-transurethral resection granuloma with central fibrinoid necrosis and palisading epithelioid histiocytes surrounded by mild chronic inflammation (hematoxylin and eosin, original magnification × 85). (From Epstein JI, Hutchins GM: Granulomatous prostatitis: Distinction among allergic, nonspecific, and post-transurethral resection lesions. Hum Pathol 15:821, 1984; with permission.)

pected prostatitis. More recently, the appearance of specimens obtained by fine-needle aspiration (FNA) from patients with prostatitis has been described. FNA is contraindicated in cases of symptomatic acute prostatitis because of the associated risk of sepsis, especially in patients with underlying rheumatologic diseases.[44, 53] Findings of acute and/or chronic prostatitis may, however, be seen in patients who undergo FNA of the prostate because of physical findings suggestive of prostatic carcinoma. Prostatitis may be incidental in these patients or may be found to be responsible for gross abnormalities detected in the gland on physical examination.

Both prostatic secretions and fine-needle aspirates may be obtained by office procedures. These procedures provide specimens for cytologic diagnosis in a reliable, inexpensive, and, in experienced hands, relatively painless and atraumatic manner.

Prostatic Secretions. Normal prostatic fluid obtained by massage is sterile, thin, and milky. On microscopic examination, there are fat globules (lecithin granules), less than 10 to 15 white blood cells per high-power field, occasional epithelial cells, and corpora amylacea. Rare red blood cells may be present. Sperm may also be seen, but neither their presence nor their absence is of clinical significance.[7, 91, 98] Microscopic examination of expressed prostatic secretions is often helpful in the diagnosis of prostatitis. In order to be meaningful, however, the findings should be compared with smears of urethral and midstream urine specimens obtained just prior to prostatic massage.

In acute bacterial prostatitis, expressed prostatic fluid is thick and purulent, containing excessive numbers of white blood cells and oval fat bodies. Chronic prostatitis is characterized by greater than 15 white blood cells per high-power field and numerous oval fat bodies. Microscopic examination cannot reliably distinguish chronic bacterial from nonbacterial prostatitis[18, 81] (Fig. 32–17).

Fine-Needle Aspiration. Normal epithelial cells in prostatic aspirates occur in sheets of varying size in a clear background. The individual cells have sharp borders producing a honeycomb pattern. Small spindle-

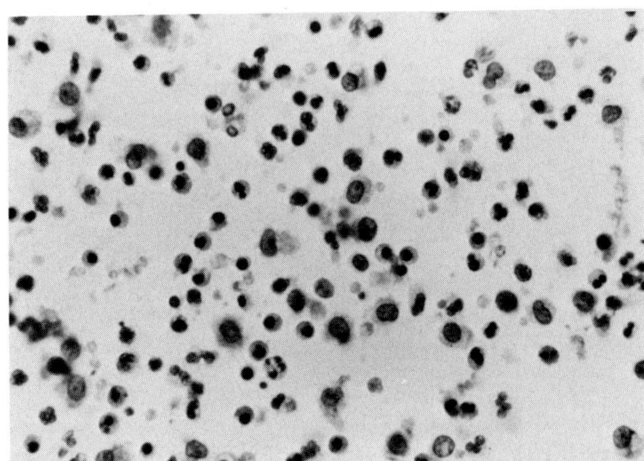

FIGURE 32–17. Smear of expressed prostatic secretions of a patient with acute prostatitis. Large numbers of polymorphonuclear leukocytes are accompanied by amorphous debris and several oval fat bodies (Papanicolaou stain, original magnification × 400).

shaped nuclei representing myoepithelial cells may occasionally be seen within the sheets. Isolated epithelial cells, secretions, and stromal cells are rare.

The nuclei of prostatic epithelial cells are round to oval and centrally located and have smooth nuclear membranes. The nuclear chromatin is finely granular and evenly distributed throughout the nucleus. In normal prostatic epithelial cells, nucleoli are inconspicuous. Epithelial cytoplasm is clear to finely granular with the Papanicolaou stain and may contain small eosinophilic granules with the May-Gruenwald-Giemsa stain.[41, 49]

Aspiration biopsy in the presence of prostatitis produces a very cellular smear with large numbers of inflammatory cells and epithelial cells in sheets and clusters. Inflammatory cells may infiltrate the prostatic epithelium. A few isolated inflammatory cells outside of the sheets of prostatic epithelium are not sufficient for a diagnosis of prostatitis.

Varying degrees of epithelial atypia occur in prostatitis. Mild atypia may involve only minor changes in nuclear arrangement. More striking epithelial atypia, characterized by nuclear crowding and overlapping cell borders, may be seen. Individual nuclei may be hyperchromatic, vary somewhat in size and shape, and may contain prominent nucleoli.

In the presence of marked atypia, the distinction between carcinoma and prostatitis may be difficult. Caution should be exercised when making the diagnosis of carcinoma in the presence of inflammation. In such cases, a second biopsy after treatment with antibiotics is warranted.[41, 44, 49, 53]

In acute prostatitis, abundant polymorphonuclear leukocytes dominate the picture. These cells infiltrate sheets of epithelial cells and are scattered throughout the smear individually or in clumps. Histiocytes and lymphocytes may occasionally be seen. Debris is present in the background. The epithelial cells show degenerative changes, such as cytoplasmic vacuolization and nuclear pyknosis. Reactive changes, including nuclear

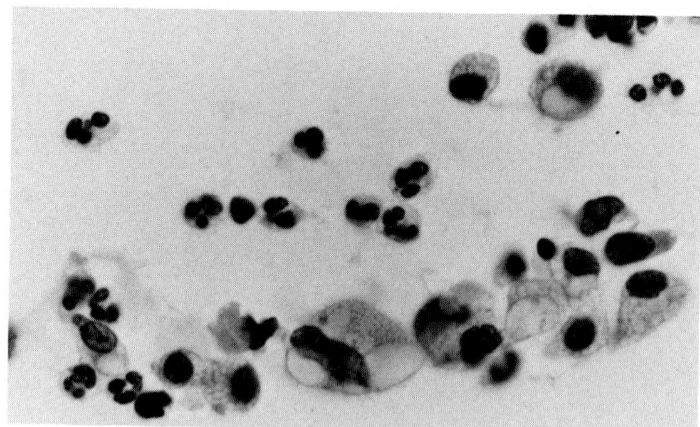

FIGURE 32–19. Smear of a fine-needle aspirate showing the predominant inflammatory cells in chronic prostatitis. Typical foamy histiocytes and scattered polymorphonuclear leukocytes are visible (Papanicolaou stain, original magnification × 1000). (Courtesy of G. Fred Worsham, M.D., Charleston, SC.)

crowding and overlap, can occur. Nucleoli may be present, but nuclear membranes are smooth (Fig. 32–18).

The predominant inflammatory cell in chronic prostatitis is the foamy histiocyte, which frequently contains phagocytized material (Fig. 32–19). Lymphocytes, plasma cells, occasional eosinophils and polymorphonuclear leukocytes, and rare giant cells can be found. The epithelial cells may manifest changes suggestive of malignancy. Sheets and clusters with decreased cohesion and nuclear crowding may be seen as well as microacini composed of clusters of 3 to 10 cells shaped into rings or crescents with eccentric variable size nuclei.[41, 44, 49, 53]

As with other forms of prostatitis, aspirate smears from patients with granulomatous prostatitis are quite cellular. Epithelial groups are generally abundant. The inflammatory cells are similar to those seen in chronic prostatitis with the addition of epithelioid cells and increased numbers of multinucleate giant cells. Giant cells are not specific for granulomatous prostatitis; rather, epithelioid cells are required for the definitive diagnosis[44, 53, 101, 106] (Fig. 32–20).

There are several pitfalls in the cytologic as well as the clinical differentiation between granulomatous prostatitis and carcinoma. Both giant cells and epithelioid histiocytes can have prominent nucleoli. Giant cells can form pseudoglandular structures that may be mistaken for malignant acini (Fig. 32–21), and epithelioid cells can be mistaken for individual malignant cells.

Epithelial atypia may be quite pronounced with nuclear hyperchromasia, crowding, and anisonucleosis. Many of the epithelial cells contain nucleoli, some of which are quite prominent. Despite these changes, the inflammatory background should prevent overdiagnosis of carcinoma.[41, 44, 49, 53]

The cause of granulomatous prostatitis can often be established with special stains for bacteria, fungi, or acid-fast bacilli, and with clinical correlation with a history of previous prostatectomy, BCG immunotherapy, systemic granulomatous disease, or an allergic disorder.[53] It has been reported that tuberculous pros-

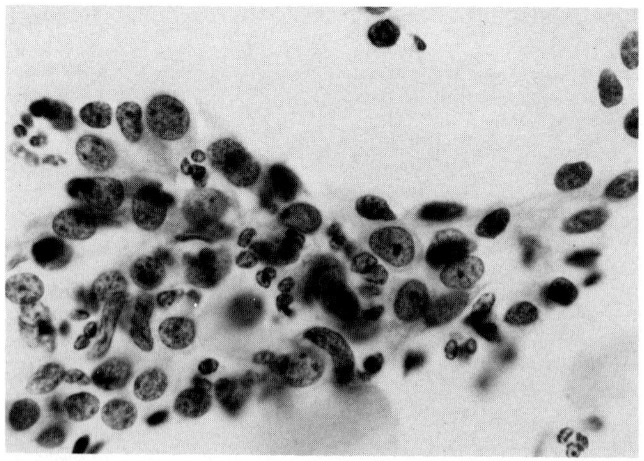

FIGURE 32–18. Smear of a fine-needle aspirate of the prostate in acute prostatitis showing polymorphonuclear leukocytes infiltrating a sheet of epithelial cells. There is nuclear crowding and overlap. Nucleoli are present in some cells, but nuclear membranes are smooth (Papanicolaou stain, original magnification × 1000).

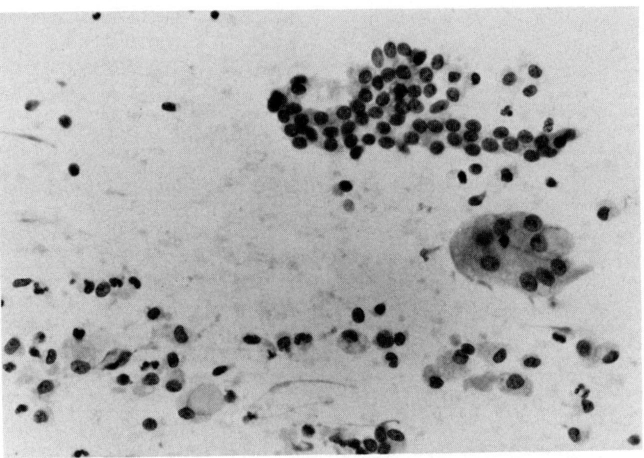

FIGURE 32–20. Smear of a fine-needle aspirate in granulomatous prostatitis. A sheet of relatively normal prostatic epithelial cells in the upper right is accompanied by a giant cell and numerous epithelioid histiocytes (Papanicolaou stain, original magnification × 400). (Courtesy of G. Fred Worsham, M.D., Charleston, SC.)

tatitis can be reliably differentiated from other forms of granulomatous prostatitis by the presence of severe epithelial atypia and large collections of histiocytes and epithelioid cells in a dirty background of amorphous material representing caseous debris.[49]

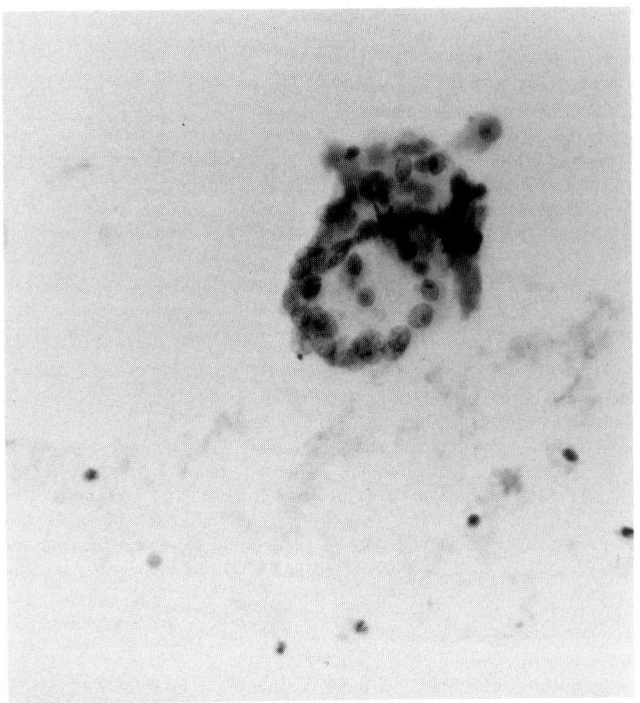

FIGURE 32–21. A giant cell with peripheral localization of nuclei in a smear of a fine-needle aspirate of granulomatous prostatitis. "Pseudoglandular" structures formed in this way may be mistaken for malignant acini if other indicators of inflammation are not noted (Papanicolaou stain, original magnification × 1000). (Courtesy of G. Fred Worsham, Charleston, SC.)

PROSTATITIS—UNANSWERED QUESTIONS

Although a large amount of data is available on prostatitis, numerous important aspects of the disorder(s) remain to be clarified. As noted, the cause is never determined for many cases of both acute and chronic prostatitis. The role of a variety of microbiologic agents (e.g., chlamydiae, trichomonads) in these cases and the causes of truly noninfectious cases of prostatitis are areas that require further study.

Of equal or possibly greater importance are the consequences of prostatitis. One area for investigation is the recently proposed hypothesis that prostatitis may play a role in sexual transmission of human immunodeficiency virus (HIV) and/or evolution of clinical AIDS in the seropositive male.[29] A second area requiring additional study is the morphologic outcome of prostatitis. The familiar histologic sequelae of inflammation are evident in many prostates examined post-surgically or at autopsy. The most common change is glandular atrophy with stromal fibrosis, usually accompanied by mild residual inflammation. Epithelial changes are also frequent and range from squamous metaplasia to the dysplastic changes described above. Largely unexamined is the question of the relationship, if any, between prostatitis and prostatic carcinoma. In other epithelia, the association between chronic inflammation and the development of epithelial neoplasms has been well demonstrated. Such a connection has not been documented in the prostate but remains an area of speculation.

REFERENCES

1. Abdelatif OMA, Chandler FW, McGuire BS: *Chlamydia trachomatis* in chronic abacterial prostatitis: Demonstration by color in situ hybridization. Hum Pathol 22:41, 1991.
2. Abdelatif OMA, Chandler FW, McGuire BS: *Chlamydia trachomatis* in chronic abacterial prostatitis [letter]. Hum Pathol 22:625, 1991.
3. Aronsson A, Dahlgren A, Gatenbeck L, Stromberg L: Predictive sites of inflammatory manifestation in the prostatic gland: An experimental study on nonbacterial prostatitis in the rat. Prostate 13:17, 1988.
4. Attah E: Nonspecific inflammatory lesions of the prostate. Int Surg 60:158, 1975.
5. Bartkowski DP, Lanesky JR: Emphysematous prostatitis and cystitis secondary to *Candida albicans*. J Urol 139:1063, 1988.
6. Bennett BD, Culberson DE, Petty CS, Gardner WA: Histopathology of prostatitis. J Urol 143:265A, 1990.
7. Berger RE, Krieger JN, Kessler D, et al: Case-control study of men with suspected chronic idiopathic prostatitis. J Urol 141:328, 1989.
8. Boldogh I, Baskar JF, Mar EC, Huang ES: Human cytomegalovirus and *herpes simplex* type 2 virus in normal and adenocarcinomatous prostate glands. J Natl Cancer Inst 70:819, 1983.
9. Bostrom K: Chronic inflammation of human male accessory sex glands and its effect on the morphology of the spermatozoa. Scand J Urol Nephrol 5:133, 1971.
10. Brooker WJ, Aufderheidi AC: Genitourinary tract infections due to atypical mycobacteria. J Urol 124:242, 1980.
11. Bruce AW, Chadwick P, Willett WS, O'Shaughnessy M: The

role of chlamydiae in genitourinary disease. J Urol 126:625, 1981.

12. Bruce AW, Reid G: Prostatitis associated with *Chlamydia trachomatis* in 6 patients. J Urol 142:1006, 1989.

13. Brunner H, Weidner W, Schiefer H: Quantitative studies on the role of *Ureaplasma urealyticum* in non-gonococcal urethritis and chronic prostatitis. Yale J Biol Med 56:545, 1983.

14. Cameron K: Pathology of the prostate. Br J Hosp Med 11:348, 1974.

15. Clason AE, McGeorge A, Garland C, Abel BJ: Urinary retention and granulomatous prostatitis following sacral herpes zoster infection. A report of 2 cases with a review of the literature. Br J Urol 54:166, 1982.

16. Conner WT, Drach GW, Bucher WC: Genitourinary aspects of disseminated coccidioidomycosis. J Urol 113:82, 1975.

17. Crum C, Mitao M, Winkler B, et al: Localizing chlamydial infection in cervical biopsies with the immunoperoxidase technique. Int J Gynecol Pathol 3:191, 1984.

18. Daniels GS, Grayhack JT: Physiology of prostatic secretions. *In* Chisholm GD, Fair WR (eds): Scientific Foundations of Urology. Chicago, Year Book Medical Publishers, 1990, pp 351–357.

19. Delaney WE, Burros HM, Bhisitkul I: Eosinophilic granulomatous prostatitis simulating carcinoma. J Urol 87:169, 1962.

20. Dilworth JP, Neal DE Jr, Fussell EN, Roberts JA: Experimental prostatitis in nonhuman primates: I. Bacterial adherence in the urethra. Prostate 17:227, 1990.

21. Doble A, Thomas BJ, Walker MM, et al: The role of *Chlamydia trachomatis* in chronic abacterial prostatitis: A study using ultrasound-guided biopsy. J Urol 141:332, 1989.

22. Drutz DJ, Catanzaro A: Coccidioidomycosis. Part II. Am J Respir Dis 117:727, 1978.

23. Eickenberg HU, Amin M, Lich R: Blastomycosis of the genitourinary tract. J Urol 113:650, 1975.

24. Epstein JI: Prostate Biopsy Interpretation. New York, Raven Press, 1989.

25. Epstein JI, Hutchins GM: Granulomatous prostatitis: Distinction among allergic, nonspecific, and post-transurethral resection lesions. Hum Pathol 15:818, 1984.

26. Eyre RC, Aaronson AG, Weinstein BJ: Palisading granulomas of the prostate associated with prior prostatic surgery. J Urol 136:121, 1986.

27. Forbus WD, Bestebreurtje AM: Coccidioidomycosis: Study of 95 cases of disseminated type with special reference to pathogenesis of disease. Mil Surg 99:633, 1946.

28. Fox H: Nodular histiocytic prostatitis. J Urol 96:372, 1966.

29. Gardner WA, Bennett BD: The prostate—Overview: recent insights and speculations. *In* Weinstein RS, and Gardner WA (eds): Pathology and Pathobiology of Urinary Bladder and Prostate. Baltimore, Williams & Wilkins, 1992, pp 129–148.

30. Gardner WA, Culberson DE: Atrophy and proliferation in the young adult prostate. J Urol 137:53, 1987.

31. Gardner WA, Culberson DE, Bennett BD: *Trichomonas vaginalis* in the prostate gland. Arch Pathol Lab Med 110:432, 1986.

32. Gatenbeck L, Aronsson A, Dahlgren S, et al: Stress stimuli-induced histopathological changes in the prostate: An experimental study in the rat. Prostate 11:69, 1987.

33. Goff DA, Davidson RA: Amebic prostatitis. South Med J 77:1053–1054, 1984.

34. Goldstein AMB, Padma-Nathan H: Stress prostatitis [letter]. Urology 33:449, 1989.

35. Goodwin RA, Shapiro JL, Thurman GTT, et al: Disseminated histoplasmosis: Clinical and pathologic correlations. Medicine 59:1, 1990.

36. Hare MJ, Toone E, Robinson-Taylor D, et al: Follicular cervicitis—colposcopic appearances and association with *Chlamydia trachomatis*. Br J Obstet Gynecol 88:174, 1981.

37. Hinchey WW, Someren A: Cryptococcal prostatitis. Am J Clin Pathol 75:257, 1981.

38. Hoffmann E, Garrido M: Malakoplakia of the prostate: Report of a case. J Urol 92:311, 1964.

39. Khawand N, Jones G, Edson M: Aspergillosis of the prostate. Urology 34:100, 1989.

40. Kirby RS, Lowe D, Bultitude MI, Shuttleworth KED: Intra-

prostatic urinary reflux: An aetiological factor in abacterial prostatitis. J Urol 54:729, 1982.

41. Kline TS: Guides to Clinical Aspiration Biopsy: Prostate. New York, Igaku-Shoin, 1985.

42. Kohnen PW, Drach GW: Patterns of inflammation in prostatic hyperplasia: A histologic and bacteriologic study. J Urol 121:755, 1979.

43. Kopolovic J, Rivkind A, Sherman Y: Granulomatous prostatitis with vasculitis. Arch Pathol Lab Med 108:732, 1984.

44. Koss LG, Woyke S, Schreiber K, et al: Thin-needle aspiration biopsy of the prostate. Urol Clin North Am 11:237, 1984.

45. Kovi J: Surgical Pathology of Prostate and Seminal Vesicles. Boca Raton, FL, CRC Press, 1989.

46. Krieger JN: Prostatitis syndromes: Pathophysiology, differential diagnosis, and treatment. Sex Transm Dis 11:100, 1984.

47. Kuntze JR, Hermann MH, Evans SG: Genitourinary coccidioidomycosis. J Urol 140:370, 1988.

48. Larsen RA, Bozzette S, McCuthan A, et al: Persistent cryptococcal neoformans infection of the prostate after successful treatment of meningitis. Ann Intern Med 111:125, 1989.

49. Leistenschneider W, Nagel R: Atlas of Prostatic Cytology. New York, Springer-Verlag, 1984.

50. Linn R, Klimberg IW, Wajsman Z: Persistent acid-fast bacilli following intravesical Bacillus Calmette-Guerin. J Urol 141:1197, 1989.

51. Lopez-Plaza I, Bostwick DG: Prostatitis. *In* Bostwick DG (ed): Pathology of the Prostate. New York, Churchill Livingstone, 1990, pp 15–30.

52. MacNeal JE: Regional morphology and pathology of the prostate. Am J Clin Pathol 49:347, 1968.

53. Maksem JA, Park CH, Johenning PW, et al: Aspiration biopsy of the prostate gland. Urol Clin North Am 15:555, 1988.

54. Marans HY, Mandell W, Kislak JW, et al: Prostatic abscess due to *Histoplasma capsulatum* in the acquired immunodeficiency syndrome. J Urol 145:1275, 1991.

55. McClure J: Malakoplakia of the prostate: A report of two cases and a review of the literature. J Clin Pathol 32:629, 1979.

56. McCormack WC: Epidemiology of *Mycoplasma hominis*. Sex Transm Dis 10:261, 1983.

57. Meares EM, Jr: Prostatitis and related diseases. Urology 26(8):1, 1980.

58. Meares EM, Jr: Prostatitis—acute and chronic. *In* Paulson DF (ed): Prostatic Disorders. Philadelphia, Lea & Febiger, 1989, pp 71–106.

59. Mehlhorn VJ: Die prostatitis aus morphologischer sicht—eine sektionsanalyse. Z Urol Nephrol 80:253, 1987.

60. Meseguer MA, Martinez-Ferre M, de Rafael L, et al: Differential counts of *Ureaplasma urealyticum* in male urologic patients. J Infect Dis 149:657, 1984.

61. Michigan S: Genitourinary fungal infections. J Urol 116:390, 1976.

62. Mies C, Balogh K, Stadecker M: Palisading prostate granulomas following surgery. J Surg Pathol 8:217–221, 1984.

63. Milchgrub S, Visconti E, Avellini J: Granulomatous prostatitis induced by capsule deficient cryptococcal infection. J Urol 143:160, 1965.

64. Miller HC: Stress prostatitis. Urology 32:507, 1988.

65. Mostofi FK, Sesterhenn I: Plenary Lecture. Lymphocytic infiltrate in relationship to urologic tumors. NCI Monogr 49:133, 1976.

66. Mukamel E, Konichezky M, Engelstein D, et al: Clinical and pathological findings in prostates following intravesical Bacillus Calmette-Guerin instillations. J Urol 144:1399, 1990.

67. Naslund MJ, Coffey DS: The differential effects of neonatal androgen, estrogen and progesterone on adult rat prostate growth. J Urol 136:1136, 1986.

68. Naslund MJ, Strandberg JD, Coffey DS: The role of androgens and estrogens in the pathogenesis of experimental nonbacterial prostatitis. J Urol 140:1049, 1988.

69. Nelson G, Culberson DE, Gardner WA: Intraprostatic spermatozoa. Hum Pathol 19:541, 1988.

70. Nelsson S, Johannisson G, Lycke E: Isolation of *Chlamydia trachomatis* from the urethra and from prostatic fluid in men with signs and symptoms of acute urethritis. Acta Dermatol Venereol 61:456, 1981.

71. Nielsen ML, Asnaes S, Hattel T: Inflammatory changes in the non-infected prostate gland. A clinical microbiological and histological investigation. J Urol 110:423, 1973.

72. Nielsen ML, Christensen P: Inflammatory changes of the hyperplastic prostate. Scand J Urol Nephrol 6:6, 1972.

73. Oates RD, Stilmant MM, Freedlund MC, Siroky MB: Granulomatous prostatitis following Bacillus Calmette-Guerin immunotherapy of bladder cancer. J Urol 140:751–754, 1988.

74. O'Connor FJ, Fousha JHS, Cox CE: Prostatic cryptococcosis. J Urol 94:160, 1965.

75. O'Dea MJ, Moore SB, Greene LG: Tuberculous prostatitis. Urology 11:483, 1978.

76. Odunjo EO, Elebute EA: Chronic prostatitis in benign prostatic hyperplasia. Br J Urol 43:333, 1971.

77. Oriel JD: Role of genital mycoplasmas in nongonococcal urethritis and prostatitis. Sex Transm Dis 10:263, 1983.

78. Orr WA, Mulholland SG, Walzak MP: Genitourinary tract involvement with systemic mycosis. J Urol 107:1047, 1972.

79. Paavonen J, Vesterinen E, Meyer B, Saksela E: Colposcopic and histologic findings in cervical chlamydial infection. Obstet Gynecol 59:712, 1982.

80. Petersen EA, Friedman BA, Crowder ED, Rifkind D: Coccidioidouria: Clinical significance. Ann Intern Med 85:34, 1976.

81. Pfau A, Caine M: Prostatitis. *In* Spring-Mills E, Hafez ESE (eds): Human Reproductive Medicine. Male Accessory Sex Glands. Amsterdam, Elsevier/North Holland Biomedical Press, 1980, pp 357–372.

82. Phillips WR, Biggs A: The incidence of cytoplasmic and nuclear inclusions in non-specific genital infections in men. J Urol 104:470, 1970.

83. Pieterse AS, Aarons I, Jose JS: Focal prostatic granulomas rheumatoid-like probably iatrogenic in origin. Pathology 16:174, 1984.

84. Presti B, Weidner N: Granulomatous prostatitis and poorly differentiated carcinoma. Their distinction with the use of immunohistochemical methods. Am J Clin Pathol 95:330, 1991.

85. Price MJ, Lewis EL, Carmalt JE: Coccidioidomycosis of the prostate gland. Urology 29:653, 1982.

86. Redman JF, Downs RA: Simple eosinophilic granulomatous prostatitis. J Urol 132:358, 1984.

87. Robinette CL: Sex-hormone-induced inflammation and fibromuscular proliferation in the rat lateral prostate. Prostate 12:271, 1988.

88. Rohn JG: Urogenital aspects of coccidioidomycosis of the prostate gland. Urology 65:660, 1951.

89. Rubin H, Furolow ML, Yates JL, Brasher CA: Seminar on mycotic infections. Am J Med 27:278, 1959.

90. Salyer WR, Salyer DC: Involvement of the kidney and prostate in cryptococcosis. J Urol 109:695, 1973.

91. Schaeffer AJ, Wendel EF, Dunn JK, Grayhack JT: Prevalence and significance of prostatic inflammation. J Urol 125:215, 1981.

92. Schmidt JD: Non-specific granulomatous prostatitis: Classification, review, and report of cases. J Urol 94:607, 1965.

93. Schmidt JD, Patterson MC: Needle biopsy study of chronic prostatitis. J Urol 90:519, 1966.

94. Schwarz J: Mycotic prostatitis. Urology 19:1, 1982.

95. Shurbaji MD: *Chlamydia trachomatis* in chronic abacterial prostatitis. Hum Pathol 22:625, 1991.

96. Shurbaji MS, Dumler JS, Gage WR, et al: Immunochemical detection of chlamydia antigens in association with cystitis. Am J Clin Pathol 93:363, 1990.

97. Shurbaji MS, Gupta PK, Myers J: Immunohistochemical demonstration of chlamydial antigens in association with prostatitis. Mod Pathol 1:348, 1988.

98. Simmons PD, Thin RN: A method for recognizing non-bacterial prostatitis: Preliminary observations. Br J Vener Dis 59:306–310, 1983.

99. Smith CJ, Gardner WA: Inflammation-proliferation: Possible relationships in the prostate. *In* Coffey D, Bruchovsky N, Gardner W, et al (eds): Current Concepts and Approaches to the Study of Prostate Cancer. New York, Alan R. Liss, 1987, pp 317–325.

100. Sporer A, Auerbach O: Tuberculosis of prostate. Urology 4:362–365, 1978.

101. Stanley MW, Horwitz CA, Sharer W, et al: Granulomatous prostatitis. A spectrum including nonspecific, infectious, and spindle cell lesions. Diagn Cytopathol 7:508, 1991.

102. Sterrett GF, Heenan PJ, Wyche P, Papadimitriou JM: Malakoplakia of the prostate: A morphological and biochemical study. Pathology 7:139, 1975.

103. Stiens R, Helpap B, Bruhl P: The proliferation of prostatic epithelium in chronic prostatitis. Urol Res 3:21, 1975.

104. Stoller JK: Late recurrence of *Mycobacterium bovis* genitourinary tuberculosis: Case report and review of literature. J Urol 134:565, 1985.

105. Tanner FH, McDonald JR: Granulomatous prostatitis. A histologic study of a group of granulomatous lesions collected from prostate glands. Arch Pathol 36:358, 1943.

106. Tuero JG, Campa JA, Lacort LP, et al: Granulomatous prostatitis. Urol Int 43:97, 1988.

107. Winkler B, Crum CP: *Chlamydia trachomatis* infection of the female genital tract. Pathol Ann 22:193, 1987.

108. Winkler B, Gallo L, Reumann W, et al: Chlamydial endometritis. A histological and immunohistochemical analysis. Am J Surg Pathol 8:771, 1984.

109. Yonker RA, Katz P: Necrotizing granulomatous vasculitis with eosinophilic infiltrates limited to the prostate. Am J Med 77:362, 1984.

Chapter 33

CLINICAL MANIFESTATIONS AND DIAGNOSIS OF PROSTATITIS

ANTHONY J. SCHAEFFER

Prostatitis is one of the most commonly encountered inflammatory diseases in urologic practice. The clinical manifestations range from asymptomatic to acute toxic presentations. The diagnosis centers on microscopic and microbiologic evaluation of expressed prostatic fluid. It is agreed that microscopic examination of expressed prostatic fluid is the essential initial observation to identify prostatic inflammation and that microbiologic localization of bacteria to the prostatic fluid must be performed to differentiate bacterial from nonbacterial prostatitis.

DEFINITION

To define prostatitis, one must first determine the degree of inflammatory change that can be found in normal prostate fluid. Traditionally, an abnormal number of leukocytes in prostatic fluid has been defined arbitrarily as greater than 10, 15, or 20 white blood cells per high-power microscopic field.[3, 4, 6, 7, 13, 18] Although Anderson and Weller[1] found a mean count of approximately 10 white blood cells per high-power field in prostatic fluid from normal controls, other studies suggest that the prostatic expressate from normal controls has considerably less inflammation.[1, 2, 17] We addressed this question by assessing the degree of inflammation in consecutive prostatic fluid specimens from patients without urinary tract disease and from those with symptoms or findings of infectious or noninfectious urologic abnormalities.[20] Prostatic fluid samples were collected at the initial presentation from 325 consecutive men. The patients' ages ranged from 19 to 82 years, with a mean of 47 years. The first 10 ml of voided urine representative of the urethral washout was obtained, and then a second voided specimen was collected late in the urinary flow. Prostatic fluid was obtained by digital massage 10 to 30 minutes after voiding and was collected on a glass slide. The residual fluid was collected on a glass slide, placed under a coverslip, and examined with the high-power ($\times 43$) microscopic lens for cells and particles in three to five fields. The average number of white blood cells per high-power field was recorded.

Prostatic inflammation can also be assessed by identifying changes in biochemical indicators of epithelial cellular damage. Lactate dehydrogenase (LDH) is an enzyme that reversibly catalyzes the reduction of pyruvate to lactate in the presence of nicotinamide adenine dinucleotide plus. Electrophoretic separation and semi-quantitation of LDH have identified isoenzyme fractions 1 through 5. One of the characteristics of LDH is a shift to predominantly LDH-5 in the presence of malignancy or inflammation.[5, 10] Previous studies have shown that ratios of LDH-5/LDH-1 in prostatic fluid are greater than 2 in 80 per cent of patients with identifiable prostatic malignancy, in greater than 10 per cent of patients with benign prostatic hyperplasia (BPH), and in many patients with prostatitis.[11, 12] The LDH isoenzyme concentrations were determined by acrylamide disk electrophoresis,[6] and the ratio of LDH-5/LDH-1 was calculated.

White Blood Cells per High-Power Field and LDH Isoenzyme Ratio in Fluids from Normal Patients

Of the 325 patients studied, 119 (37 per cent) had no history, symptoms, or physical findings (excluding prostatic fluid evaluation) of urinary tract inflammation, normal prostate glands by digital rectal examination (DRE), and two or more white blood cells per high-power field in the first 10 ml of voided urine and no or insignificant growth on urine culture. Of these 119 patients, 31 judged to have no urologic disease had prostatic fluid containing 0.7 ± 0.41 white blood cells per high-power field and 88 with a variety of noninflammatory urologic diseases had 3.8 ± 0.83 white blood cells per high-power field in the prostatic fluid. There were two or more white blood cells per high-power field observed in 97 per cent of the patients with no urologic disease and in 75 per cent with noninflammatory urologic diseases and normal prostate glands by DRE. Only 13 of the 119 patients in these two groups had prostatic fluid with 10 or more white blood cells per high-power field. The LDH-5/LDH-1 ratio was elevated (greater than 2) in 3 of 17 specimens (18 per cent) from patients with no urologic disease and 10 of 39 specimens (26 per cent) from patients with noninflammatory urologic disease. A significant, linear association of prostatic fluid leukocyte count and LDH-5/LDH-1 ratio was observed. Thus, high leukocyte counts were associated with elevated LDH-5/LDH-1 ratios.

The impact of other factors on prostatic fluid and LDH ratio was evaluated. A significant but weak (nonlinear) association of patient age and prostatic fluid LDH-5/LDH-1 ratio was identified, but no correlation was noted between the age of the patient and the prostatic fluid leukocyte count. The influence of other factors on prostatic fluid was assessed by determining the degree of leukocytosis associated with individual diagnosis.

In 18 infertile men (mean fertility index 16, range 0 to 75), the leukocyte count was 8.3 ± 2.43 per high-power field, significantly higher than the value of 0.7 ± 0.41 white blood cells per high-power field observed for patients with no urologic disease. Seven infertile men had greater than 10 white blood cells per high-power field in the prostatic fluid. The LDH-5/LDH-1 ratio of the infertile group was not significantly elevated. Fertile patients with varicoceles had no significant elevation of the prostatic fluid leukocyte count or LDH isoenzyme ratio.

The effect of noninflammatory prostatic disease on the prostatic fluid leukocyte count and LDH isoenzyme ratio was also investigated. The prostatic fluid contained less than 10 white blood cells per high-power field in 46 (88 per cent) of the patients with BPH. The LDH-5/LDH-1 ratio of 30 of these 46 patients was 3.4 ± 0.85. Taken together, these studies support the concept that clinically significant inflammation is present when the prostatic fluid contains 10 or more white blood cells per high-power field.

The misconception that prostatic fluid from normal men frequently contains 10 or more white blood cells per high-power field has been based on studies of less well defined populations.[4, 18] The possibility that in these earlier studies inclusion of patients with BPH or urethritis could have an increased prostatic fluid leukocyte count is underscored by our observation that 10 or more white blood cells per high-power field occurred in 6 (12 per cent) of 52 patients with BPH. In addition, Bourne

and Frishette[3] showed that 15 (57 per cent) of 26 patients with BPH had prostatic fluid containing 15 or more white blood cells per high-power field in the absence of bacterial infection, and Kohnen and Drach[14] found inflammation in 98 per cent of surgically resected prostates. Patients with even minimal urethral inflammation also can have significantly elevated prostatic fluid leukocyte counts. Thus, in our series,[20] 22 (64 per cent) of the 34 patients with two or more white blood cells per high-power field in the first 10 ml of voided urine had prostatic fluid containing 10 or more white blood cells per high-power field.

The clinical significance of prostatic inflammation in asymptomatic patients has been questioned.[3, 18] Our data indicate that an increased prostatic fluid leukocyte count probably is indicative of an underlying disease and/or prostatic cellular damage. Normal controls rarely had inflammatory cells in the prostatic secretions, whereas identifiable groups of patients had significantly increased leukocyte counts in the prostatic expressate. For example, infertile patients in our study had an unexpectedly high mean prostatic fluid leukocyte count compared with patients with no urologic disease. These data support the observation of Eliasson and Johannisson[8] that 20 (52 per cent) of 38 infertile men with palpably normal prostates had prostatic fluid with 10 or more white blood cells per high-power field. The absence of bacterial infection and biochemical evidence of cellular damage in our studies suggest an immune rather than an inflammatory response. The prostatic expressate of patients with urethritis or BPH also had significantly increased leukocyte counts. Furthermore, significant linear correlation was demonstrated between prostatic fluid leukocyte counts and LDH-5/LDH-1 ratios in patients with palpably normal prostate glands and no bacterial infection; this suggests that elevated leukocyte counts can be associated with epithelial cellular damage.

CLASSIFICATION

The distinguishing characteristics of patients with bacterial and nonbacterial prostatitis are summarized in Table 33-1. Patients with bacterial and nonbacterial prostatitis have evidence of inflammation in their expressed prostatic secretions and therefore they cannot be distinguished by inflammatory cells. In addition to white blood cells, prostatic secretions from patients with prostatitis usually contain large macrophages laden with cholesterol particles. The size of these macrophages varies from that of a white blood cell to several times the diameter of a white blood cell. They appear dark brown under the low-power microscopic field and are sometimes called "oval brown bodies." Patients with bacterial prostatitis, both acute and chronic, are distinguished from those with nonbacterial prostatitis based on microbiologic rather than inflammatory parameters of the prostatic secretion. Patients with bacterial prostatitis have documented urinary tract infections and prostatic secretions containing bacteria. On the other hand, patients with nonbacterial prostatitis have 10 or

TABLE 33–1. CLASSIFICATION OF PROSTATITIS

	PROSTATODYNIA*	EVIDENCE OF INFLAMMATION (EPS)†	CULTURE POSITIVE (EPS)	CULTURE POSITIVE (BLADDER)	COMMON ETIOLOGIC BACTERIA	RECTAL EXAMINATION (PROSTATE)
Acute bacterial prostatitis	+	+	+	+ ‡	Entero-bacteriaceae	Abnormal
Chronic bacterial prostatitis	±	+	+	+ §	Entero-bacteriaceae	Normal
"Nonbacterial" prostatitis	±	+	0	0	?	Normal
Pelviperineal pain	±	0	0	0	0	Normal

*Pain in the prostate.
†EPS = Expressed prostatic secretion.
‡Acute bacterial prostatitis is nearly always accompanied by bladder infection.
§Characterized by recurrent bacteriuria, at varying intervals up to several months, after stopping antimicrobial therapy.
From Stamey TA: Pathogenesis and Treatment of Urinary Tract Infections. Baltimore, The Williams & Wilkins Co., 1980.

more white blood cells per high-power field but no history of urinary tract infections or bacterial growth in cultures of prostatic secretions. The cause of nonbacterial prostatitis is unknown, but some infectious agents that can infect the urethra, such as *Chlamydia,* may also infect the prostatic ducts or gland and cause both urethritis and/or "nonbacterial" prostatitis.

Patients with "pain in the prostate" have traditionally been said to have prostatodynia. This classification assumes that the patient's symptoms, which include urinary urgency, dysuria, poor urinary flow, and prostatic discomfort, are due to an unrecognized inflammation in the prostate. The assumption that these symptoms are always of prostatic origin may be erroneous, however. Many patients probably are unable to differentiate pelvic or perineal symptoms owing to musculoskeletal or psychiatric abnormality from true prostatic pathology. Therefore, the term *pelviperineal pain* is suggested as a more accurate description of this symptom complex that may be but is not invariably of prostatic origin.

Segmental Bacterial Localization Cultures

In order to differentiate microbiologically bacterial from nonbacterial prostatitis, sequential, quantitative bacteriologic cultures of the urethra, bladder urine, and prostatic secretion must be obtained[16] (Fig. 33–1). The voided urine is partitioned into urethral (VB1—voided bladder 1, that is, the first voided 5 to 10 ml), bladder (VB2—voided bladder 2, or midstream), and postprostatic massage (VB3—voided bladder 3, first voided 10 ml after massage). Culture of the expressed prostatic secretion (EPS) is helpful when the VB1 and VB3 aliquots are equivalent in bacterial number. Bladder urine must show no growth at the time of sampling. If the patient has an infection, all specimens show bacterial growth and therefore localization is not possible. In such a case the patient should be treated with an antimicrobial drug such as nitrofurantoin or oral penicillin G that will eradicate the bladder infection and clear the urethra of prostatic organisms but not alter the prostatic microbial flora. Under these circumstances localization cultures can be obtained with the patient on antimicrobial therapy.

In order to obtain localization cultures, the patient must have a full bladder to ensure an adequate urinary stream. If the patient is circumcised, no preparation of the meatus is required. If the patient is uncircumcised, the foreskin must be in the retracted position throughout the collection. The glans is washed with an antiseptic and cleaned with water in order to prevent false-negative cultures owing to antiseptic contamination of the specimens. The first VB1 and VB2 specimens are collected, and then the patient is instructed to stop voiding. Prostatic fluid is obtained by digital massage and collected on a glass slide. This allows confirmation of prostatic inflammation. Additional drops of fluid are then collected for culture, and immediately after prostatic massage the patient voids again and the VB3 is collected in a manner similar to that for VB1.

Routine urinalysis and a prostatic fluid examination are performed. Cultures are performed on a blood agar plate (for growth of most gram-negative and gram-positive bacteria) and either eosin–methylene blue or MacConkey agar culture plates (for growth of gram-negative organisms). If the volume of EPS is too small, a bacteriologic loop or pipette can be used to deliver 0.01 ml. Interpretation of culture results depends upon quantitative comparison of the number of bacteria in each specimen. When the bacterial counts in the urethral

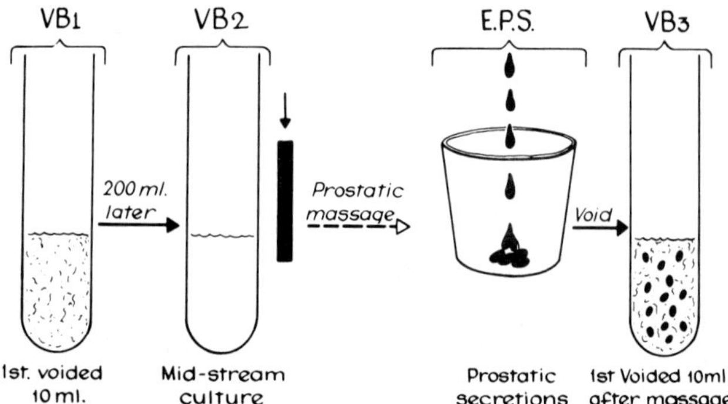

FIGURE 33–1. Segmental culture technique for localizing urinary infections in the male to the urethra or the prostate. (Reprinted with permission from Meares EM, Stamey TA: Bacteriologic localization of patterns in bacterial prostatitis and urethritis. Invest Urol 5:492, 1968, © by Williams & Wilkins Company, 1968.)

specimen are greater than those in the EPS or the VB3 specimens, bacterial urethritis is present. For accurate diagnosis of bacterial prostatitis, the bacterial count in the EPS and VB3 should exceed those in the VB1 by at least one logarithm. When the difference is small, the culture should be repeated to be sure that the data are reproducible. Demonstration of bacteria in the VB3 and/or EPS when the VB1 and VB2 specimens show no growth is most diagnostic of bacterial prostatitis.

Quantitative cultures of the ejaculate have been performed if prostatic fluid secretions cannot be obtained. However, this technique is inappropriate for diagnosing prostatitis because the cultures contain an admixture of fluids from various glands and sites. Furthermore, proper interpretation cannot be obtained because quantitative cultures of the urethra and bladder specimens are usually not available.

CLINICAL MANIFESTATIONS OF BACTERIAL PROSTATITIS

Etiology and Pathogenesis

Bacterial prostatitis is caused by the same organisms that cause urinary tract infections. *Escherichia coli* and other members of the Enterobacteriaceae family predominate; *Pseudomonas* species and *Enterococcus faecalis* are less common. Infections involving two or more strains or classes of microorganisms are not rare. Grampositive organisms such as coagulase-negative streptococci and diptheroids that are normally found in the urethra are probably very uncommon causes of bacterial prostatitis. The pathogenesis of bacterial prostatitis is unclear. The ascending urethral route of infection probably accounts for the majority of infections, but direct extension from the rectum to the prostate or by lymphogenous or hematogenous routes is also possible. Colonization by urinary tract pathogens on the vaginal introitus of women with urinary tract infections is common, and sexual intercourse may lead to seeding of the male urethra and subsequent development of chronic bacterial prostatitis.

Once the bacteria enter the urethra, they may reflux into the prostatic ducts. Evidence for this is supported by the observation that prostatic calculi contain constituents commonly found in urine but foreign to prostatic secretions. These calculi may become colonized with bacteria and thereby remain protected from the action of antimicrobial drugs and act as a bacterial focus for recurrent prostatitis.

A natural defense mechanism of the prostate against uropathogenic bacteria was first observed by Youmans and his associates in 1938.[23] They observed a bactericidal effect of canine prostatic fluid. Later Stamey et al[21] and Fair et al[9] identified an antibacterial factor in normal prostatic fluid of adults and found it to be a zinc salt. They observed that men with chronic bacterial prostatitis average about 50 μg of zinc per milliliter of prostatic fluid, compared with levels in healthy controls of 450 μg/ml. Furthermore, serum levels of zinc were normal in patients with bacterial prostatitis, and depressed prostatic levels could not be elevated by oral exogenous zinc.

Acute bacterial prostatitis usually has a dramatic presentation that is diagnosed easily by clinical symptoms and physical examination and is associated with acute urinary tract infection. The patient presents with malaise, fever, low back or perineal pain, and myalgia for several days prior to onset of symptoms of urinary frequency, dysuria, urgency, and varying degrees of bladder outlet obstruction. Palpation of the prostate, which must be done carefully, reveals a hard, tender, irregular gland that is warm to touch. Prostatic fluid should not be obtained by massage because of the risk of bacteremia. Because cystitis is associated with acute bacterial prostatitis, the responsible bacterial pathogen can be isolated from bladder urine.

Chronic bacterial prostatitis is a subtle disease characterized by relatively asymptomatic periods between episodes of recurrent acute urinary tract infections. It is impossible to diagnose by physical examination. Although some patients are asymptomatic, most present with symptoms associated with bacteriuria such as dysuria, frequency and urgency, low back or perineal discomfort, or painful ejaculation with or without hematospermia. The prostate feels normal on palpation, and excretory urography and cystoscopy are usually unremarkable.

NONBACTERIAL PROSTATITIS

Nonbacterial prostatitis is approximately eight times more common than bacterial prostatitis.[19] Patients with nonbacterial prostatitis are characterized by irritative or obstructive voiding symptoms or back or pelvic pain radiating to the perineum or scrotum. However, approximately one third of patients with nonbacterial prostatitis are asymptomatic and identified only by examination of expressed prostatic fluid. Leukocyte counts in the prostatic secretions do not differentiate bacterial from nonbacterial prostatitis. However, patients with nonbacterial prostatitis never have bacteriuria.

Etiology and Pathogenesis

Efforts to identify the cause of nonbacterial prostatitis have been futile. Organisms such as fungi, anaerobic bacteria, trichomonads, and various viral agents including cytomegalovirus, *Herpesvirus hominis,* rubella virus, and varicella-zoster virus have been ruled out.[15] *Ureaplasma urealyticum* has been suggested as a potential pathogen in nonbacterial prostatitis,[22] but data have not been reproduced. The fact that *Chlamydia trachomatis* is responsible for the majority of nongonococcal urethritis has led to speculation that it may be a pathogen in nonbacterial prostatitis. Furthermore, approximately one third of patients with nonbacterial prostatitis have associated urethritis. However, clear-cut evidence supporting this postulate is not forthcoming.

The clinical significance of evidence of prostatic inflammation, particularly in asymptomatic patients, has been questioned. The natural history of the disease is also not clear. Some studies indicate that nonbacterial prostatitis may persist for long periods of time or alternatively may be of relatively short duration. However, recognition that identifiable groups of patients, particularly those with other conditions such as infertility, may have significantly elevated leukocyte counts could indicate that nonbacterial prostatitis is a predictor of significant underlying disease.

PROSTATODYNIA (PELVIPERINEAL PAIN)

As indicated, the origin of this condition is unknown and the term *prostatodynia* may frequently be misleading. Musculoskeletal abnormalities have been implicated and are probably responsible for many of the symptoms. Conversely, urethral dysfunction may lead to painful urination and reflux of urine into the prostatic ducts. Some patients have emotional disturbances.

SUMMARY

The manifestations of prostatitis vary, and therefore the diagnosis must be precise. Initial evaluation of expressed prostatic fluid is mandatory to identify patients with significant prostatic inflammation. In addition, urine cultures and bacterial localization studies must be performed to differentiate bacterial from nonbacterial prostatitis. Acute bacterial prostatitis is dramatic in presentation. A history of recurrent urinary tract infections and segmental localization cultures of the urethra, bladder urine, and expressed prostatic secretions identify patients with chronic bacterial prostatitis. Nonbacterial prostatitis is the most common type of prostatitis. Because its cause is unknown, the treatment is empiric. Pelviperineal pain may be of prostatic origin, but other nonprostatic causes should be sought.

REFERENCES

1. Anderson RU, Weller C: Prostatic secretion leukocyte studies in non-bacterial prostatitis (prostatosis). J Urol 121:292, 1979.
2. Blacklock NJ: Some observations on prostatitis. *In* Williams DC, Briggs MH, Stanford M (eds): Advances in the Study of the Prostate. London, William Heinemann Medical Books, 1969, pp 37–55.
3. Bourne CW, Frishette WA: Prostatic fluid analysis and prostatitis. J Urol 97:140, 1967.
4. Bowers JE, Thomas GB: The clinical significance of abnormal prostatic secretion. J Urol 79:976, 1958.
5. Carvajal HF, Passey RB, Berger M, et al: Urinary lactic dehydrogenase isoenzyme 5 in the differential diagnosis of kidney and bladder infections. Kidney Int 8:176, 1975.
6. Dietz AA, Lubrano T, Rubinstein HM: LDH isoenzymes. *In* Cooper GR (ed): Standard Methods of Clinical Chemistry, Vol 7. New York, Academic Press, 1972, pp 49–61.
7. Drach GW, Fair WR, Meares EM, Stamey TA: Classification of benign diseases associated with prostatic pain: Prostatitis or prostatodynia? [letter] J Urol 120:266, 1978.
8. Eliasson R, Johannisson E: Cytological studies of prostatic fluids from men with and without abnormal palpatory findings of the prostate. Int J Androl 1:582, 1978.
9. Fair WR, Couch J, Wehner N: Prostatic antibacterial factor. Identity and significance. Urology 7:169, 1976.
10. Goldman RD, Kaplan NO, Hall TC: Lactic dehydrogenase in human neoplastic tissue. Cancer Res 24:389, 1964.
11. Grayhack JT, Wendel EF, Lee C, et al: Lactate dehydrogenase isoenzymes in human prostatic fluid: An aid in recognition of malignancy? J Urol 118:204, 1977.
12. Hein RC, Grayhack JT, Goldberg E: Prostatic fluid lactic dehydrogenase isoenzyme patterns of prostatic cancer and hyperplasia. J Urol 113:511, 1975.
13. Jameson RM: Sexual activity and the variations of the white cell content of the prostatic secretion. Invest Urol 5:297, 1967.
14. Kohnen PW, Drach GW: Patterns of inflammation in prostatic hyperplasia: A histologic and bacteriologic study. J Urol 121:755, 1979.
15. Meares EM: Prostatitis syndromes: New perspectives about old woes. J Urol 123:141, 1980.
16. Meares EM, Stamey TA: Bacteriologic localization patterns in bacterial prostatitis and urethritis. Invest Urol 5:492, 1968.
17. Oates JK: Diagnosis of chronic prostatitis. Br J Vener Dis 34:250, 1958.
18. O'Shaughnessy EJ, Parrino PS, White JD: Chronic prostatitis—fact or fiction? JAMA 160:540, 1956.
19. Schaeffer AJ: Prostatitis and prostatodynia. AUA Update Series, Vol II, Lesson 30, 1983, pp 2–7.
20. Schaeffer AJ, Wendel EF, Dunn JK, Grayhack JT: Prevalence and significance of prostatic inflammation. J Urol 125:215, 1981.
21. Stamey TA, Fair WR, Timothy MM, Chung HD: Antibacterial nature of prostatic fluid. Nature 218:444, 1968.
22. Weidner W, Brunner H, Krause W: Quantitative culture of *Ureaplasma urealyticum* in patients with chronic prostatitis or prostatosis. Read at annual meeting of American Urological Association, New York, New York, May 13–17, 1979.
23. Youmans GP, Liebling J, Lyman RY: The bactericidal action of prostatic fluid in dogs. J Infect Dis 63:117, 1938.

Chapter 34

NONBACTERIAL PROSTATITIS AND PROSTATODYNIA

EDWIN M. MEARES, JR.

Prostatic inflammations and infections are rare in boys but are exceedingly common in adult men. It has been reported that prostatitis is responsible for about 25 per cent of annual office visits by men in the United States.[16] Unfortunately, despite this common incidence of prostatitis, many clinicians remain confused about the cause, pathogenesis, pathophysiology, and clinical significance of inflammations and infections of the prostate. Investigations have recently shown that prostatitis occurs in several distinct forms, or syndromes. Recognized specific types of prostatitis include the following:

Common forms
    Acute bacterial prostatitis
    Chronic bacterial prostatitis
    Nonbacterial prostatitis
    Prostatodynia
Uncommon forms
    Gonococcal prostatitis
    Tuberculous prostatitis
    Parasitic prostatitis
    Mycotic prostatitis
    Nonspecific granulomatous prostatitis
        Noneosinophilic variety
        Eosinophilic variety
Suspected but unproved forms
    Prostatitis due to ureaplasmas or mycoplasmas
    Prostatitis due to *Chlamydia trachomatis*
    Prostatitis due to viruses

Many clinical features of the common varieties of prostatitis are similar, but each type has certain unique characteristics. Bacterial prostatitis is associated with urinary tract infection (UTI), positive cultures localizing a bacterial pathogen to the prostatic secretions, and excessive numbers of inflammatory cells (white blood cells and lipid-laden macrophages) in the prostatic secretions. Acute bacterial prostatitis (ABP) is an abrupt, febrile illness with marked irritative and obstructive urinary voiding dysfunction plus various constitutional signs and symptoms. Chronic bacterial prostatitis (CBP) is a less pronounced illness associated with relapsing recurrent UTI caused by persistence of the bacterial pathogen in the prostatic secretory system despite courses of antimicrobial therapy. In contrast, men with nonbacterial prostatitis (NBP) have various symptoms of prostatitis and excessive numbers of inflammatory cells in the prostatic secretions but negative histories of documented UTI and negative cultures. Patients with prostatodynia have certain symptoms of prostatitis, but have no associated UTI, negative prostatic fluid cultures, and typically no excessive numbers of inflammatory cells in their prostatic secretions.

In 1983, Brunner et al[7] reported the results of an evaluation of about 600 men attending a special prostatitis clinic in Germany: About 5 per cent had bacterial prostatitis, 64 per cent had NBP, and 31 per cent had prostatodynia. In 1991, Weidner et al[35] updated this series to include 1461 patients, and found that at least 90 per cent had nonbacterial forms of prostatitis. Some similarities and differences in clinical features of these common prostatitis syndromes are shown in Table 34–1.

ETIOLOGY AND PATHOGENESIS

Whereas ABP and CBP are caused by specific pathogenic bacterial organisms, usually coliforms, and are

TABLE 34–1. CLINICAL FEATURES OF COMMON PROSTATITIS SYNDROMES

SYNDROME	HISTORY OF CONFIRMED UTI	PROSTATE ABNORMAL ON RECTAL EXAM	EXCESSIVE WBCs IN EPS	POSITIVE CULTURE OF EPS	COMMON CAUSATIVE AGENTS	RESPONSE TO ANTIMICROBIAL TREATMENT	IMPAIRED URINARY FLOW RATE
Acute bacterial prostatitis	Yes	Yes	Yes	Yes	Coliform bacteria	Yes	Yes
Chronic bacterial prostatitis	Yes	±	Yes	Yes	Coliform bacteria	Yes	±
Nonbacterial prostatitis	No	±	Yes	No	None ? *Chlamydia* ? *Ureaplasma*	Usually no	Often
Prostatodynia	No	No	No	No	None	No	Yes

Abbreviations: UTI = urinary tract infection, WBCs = white blood cells, EPS = expressed prostatic secretions.
Modified from Meares EM Jr: Prostatitis and related disorders. *In* Walsh PC, Retik AB, Stamey TA, Vaughan ED Jr (eds): Campbell's Urology, 6th ed. Philadelphia, WB Saunders Co, 1992.

associated with relapsing recurrent UTIs caused by the prostatic pathogen, NBP and prostatodynia are characterized by negative cultures and no history of documented UTIs. It therefore appears that nonbacterial forms of prostatitis are caused by unidentified pathogenic organisms or represent noninfectious inflammations of the prostate.

Men with NBP sometimes have higher counts of gram-positive bacteria (other than *Enterococcus faecalis* and *Staphylococcus aureus,* which are known to cause bacterial prostatitis) in their prostatic fluid cultures than in their urethral cultures. These organisms include non–group D streptococci, *S. epidermidis,* micrococci, *S. saprophyticus,* and diphtheroids. Most investigators, however, believe that these bacteria are not causative agents in prostatitis for several reasons: The localization culture results usually are not reproducible; these gram-positive organisms produce no immune response in the prostatic fluid; and, in contrast to gram-negative prostatic pathogens, these gram-positive bacteria do not lead to relapsing recurrent UTI in untreated patients.[18]

Studies of the cause of noninfectious forms of prostatitis have usually excluded as causative agents various fungi, obligate anaerobic bacteria, trichomonads, and viruses.[18] Likewise, most studies indicate that mycoplasmas and ureaplasmas are not causative agents in cases of NBP.[18] In 1983, however, Brunner et al[7] reported a 10-fold or greater increase in quantitative counts of *Ureaplasma urealyticum* in prostatic cultures compared with urethral cultures in 82 (13.7 per cent) of 597 patients who appeared to have NBP. Most of these patients were said to respond favorably to therapy with tetracycline drugs. In 1991, Weidner et al[35] reported finding bacteriologic culture localization evidence of a "ureaplasma-associated" prostatitis in 131 (9 per cent) of 1461 prostatitis patients. In a few cases, *Mycoplasma hominis* also appeared to be a causative agent in prostatitis. Unfortunately, these culture results were not confirmed by the demonstration of an antigen-specific immune response in the prostatic secretions of these patients; therefore, ureaplasmas and mycoplasmas remain unconfirmed pathogens in prostatitis.

C. trachomatis is the most controversial putative agent in prostatitis. Both Mardh et al[17] and Berger and associates[5] studied 50 or more men with NBP and found little or no evidence that *C. trachomatis* is a causative

agent. Subsequently, Poletti et al[25] performed transrectal aspiration biopsies of the prostate in 30 men with NBP and reported isolating *C. trachomatis* in tissue cultures from 10 men (33 per cent). In an accompanying editorial, however, Schachtar[27] expressed concerns about the authors' methods of identifying *Chlamydia* and about the observation that all 30 men had positive urethral cultures for *Chlamydia,* which indicates possible contamination of the specimens. More recently, Doble et al[8] reported a study of 50 men with NBP, only one of whom had *Chlamydia* detected in the urethra by an immunofluorescence technique. Each patient underwent prostatic needle biopsy under transrectal ultrasonic control. *Chlamydia* was detected in none of these patients despite the use of McCoy tissue culture and immunofluorescence techniques. The most significant evidence that *Chlamydia* is not an important causative agent in prostatitis was reported by Shortliffe et al,[29] who found no significant antigen-specific antibody elevations against *Chlamydia* in the prostatic secretions of their patients with NBP. It therefore appears that *Chlamydia* is an insignificant agent in prostatitis.

Intraprostatic Urinary Reflux

The intraprostatic reflux of urine occurs commonly and may play an important role in the pathogenesis of all types of prostatitis, including NBP and prostatodynia. Sutor and Wooley[33] and Rameriz et al[26] studied prostatic calculi by crystallographic analysis and discovered that many contained constituents found only in urine, not in prostatic secretions. Intraprostatic urinary reflux therefore is implicated in the formation of these stones. In 1982, Kirby and associates[14] reported direct proof of intraprostatic urinary reflux. A carbon-particle solution was instilled into the bladders of 10 men just prior to transurethral prostatectomy and of 5 men who were diagnosed as having NBP. The surgical specimens showed carbon particles within the prostatic acini and ductal system in 7 (70 per cent) of the 10 men who underwent surgery. In addition, each of the five men with NBP had numerous macrophages studded with intracellular carbon particles in their prostatic expressates 3 days after bladder instillation of the carbon-particle solution. It therefore is postulated that intraprostatic urinary reflux, causing a "chemical" prostatitis, may play an important role in the pathogenesis of both NBP and prostatodynia.[20]

Autoimmune Theory

Speculation but little proof exists that NBP may be an autoimmune form of prostatic inflammation. In 1985, Anderson and Ma[1] reported a study measuring a humoral antiprostate antibody titer in normal controls compared with patients with NBP. Only 1 (7 per cent) of 14 normal controls had a humoral titer of greater than 1:32, whereas 24 (71 per cent) of 34 patients with NBP had a titer greater than 1:32. This difference was statistically significant (P = <0.01).

Recent studies by Fowler et al[10] and Neal and associates[24] have demonstrated, respectively, Tamm-Horsfall protein deposits in the lamina propria of the bladder in patients with interstitial cystitis and elevated serum antibodies against Tamm-Horsfall protein in patients with interstitial cystitis compared with controls. This suggests that when Tamm-Horsfall protein penetrates the normal surface layer of the urinary bladder, it is immunogenic and possibly produces an autoimmune reaction, namely, interstitial cystitis. Because Tamm-Horsfall protein is a normal constituent of urine, and because men with NBP have intraprostatic urinary reflux (containing Tamm-Horsfall protein), is NBP an autoimmune disease? This intriguing question obviously deserves careful study.

METHODS OF DIAGNOSIS

Fundamental to the diagnosis of noninfectious forms of prostatitis is exclusion of the diagnosis of bacterial prostatitis. The clinical manifestations of ABP are sufficiently florid that the clinician usually has no difficulty in establishing the diagnosis. Unfortunately, the signs and symptoms of CBP and NBP are too variable and inexact to allow differentiation on the basis of the history and physical examination alone. A history of relapsing recurrent UTI suggests the diagnosis of CBP but does not confirm it. Likewise, radiologic studies, prostatic imaging studies, and cystourethroscopy do not confirm a diagnosis or assist in differentiating one chronic prostatitis syndrome from another. Even the histologic examination of prostatic biopsy specimens cannot distinguish CBP from NBP.[15]

Analysis of Prostatic Fluid and Semen

Microscopic examination of the expressed prostatic secretions is important in the diagnosis and classification of prostatitis. For proper interpretation, however, the condition of the urethra must be evaluated simultaneously. For example, the urethral surface sheds inflammatory cells freely in cases of urethritis, urethral strictures, or urethral diverticula. These inflammatory cells can contaminate the prostatic secretions obtained by prostatic massage and give the false impression that the prostate is inflamed. Furthermore, the leukocyte count in prostatic fluid often rises significantly in healthy men for several hours after normal ejaculation.[13]

To localize the site of inflammation to the urethra or prostate, one must always compare the microscopic appearance of the prostatic expressate with smears of the spun sediment of the first voided 10 ml of urine (urethral sample) and the midstream urine (bladder sample) that are obtained immediately prior to prostatic massage. Despite some controversy, most clinicians agree that more than 15 white blood cells per high-power field represents an abnormal number of leukocytes in prostatic secretions.[19] Provided that the urethral and midstream samples show insignificant pyuria, the finding of more than 15 white blood cells per high-power field in the prostatic expressate is diagnostic of prostatic inflammation.

The finding of both excessive numbers of leukocytes and macrophages containing fat droplets (oval fat bodies) is the most convincing sign of prostatic inflammation. These fat-laden macrophages are not seen in urethritis alone, are seldom noticed in the prostatic secretions of healthy men, but are prominent in the prostatic secretions of patients with bacterial prostatitis and NBP.[19] It must be emphasized that "inflamed" prostatic fluid merely indicates prostatic inflammation and is not diagnostic of bacterial prostatitis.

Isolated microscopy and culture of the semen are potentially even more misleading than isolated analysis and culture of the prostatic expressate. Not only is urethral contamination a concern, but the ejaculate is a mixture of prostatic secretions and fluids that arise from several other glands and sites. Furthermore, immature sperm forms are difficult to distinguish from leukocytes by microscopy. When semen is used to diagnose prostatitis, the clinician must simultaneously examine urethral and bladder samples to rule out inflammation or infection at these sites.

Bacteriologic Cultures for Localization of Infection

The diagnosis of bacterial prostatitis is confirmed when quantitative bacteriologic cultures clearly localize pathogenic bacteria to the prostate.[22] This methodology is discussed in detail by Schaeffer in Chapter 33.

Immune Response in Prostatitis

Both acute and chronic bacterial prostatitis caused by various coliform bacteria and *Pseudomonas* species produce a profound antigen-specific antibody response (immunoglobulins A and G) in the prostatic secretions of infected patients.[30, 31] In contrast, Shortliffe et al[29] have found insignificant antigen-specific antibody elevations against ureaplasmas and chlamydiae in the prostatic fluid of their patients with NBP. A causative role for these organisms in prostatitis therefore seems doubtful.

NONBACTERIAL PROSTATITIS

Clinical Features

Nonbacterial prostatitis, also called abacterial prostatitis or prostatosis, is the most common prostatitis syndrome. Although patients with NBP have no identifiable infectious cause, they typically have excessive numbers of leukocytes (greater than 15 white blood cells per high-power field) and macrophages containing fat in their prostatic secretions.[1, 19] The symptoms of NBP vary but include urinary urgency and frequency, nocturia, dysuria, and pain or discomfort perceived in the pelvic, suprapubic, and genital areas. Painful ejaculation is sometimes a prominent feature. Physical examination is nonspecific. Tender or boggy prostates are unreliable indicators of prostatitis. Typically, the signs and symptoms of NBP wax and wane. Many patients with NBP and prostatodynia notice a worsening of symptoms related to the ingestion of alcoholic beverages. Because most patients with these noninfectious prostatitis syndromes experience intraprostatic and ejaculatory duct urinary reflux, and because alcohol is excreted in the urine, it is not surprising that alcohol ingestion may intensify the symptoms.

Treatment

When cultures exclude the usual bacterial pathogens and the clinician suspects prostatitis caused by ureaplasmas, mycoplasmas, or chlamydiae, it is reasonable to prescribe a trial of tetracycline, erythromycin, or the new fluoroquinolone ofloxacin, which has good activity against these organisms. Recommended therapy consists of minocycline, 100 mg orally twice daily for 14 days; doxycycline, 100 mg orally twice daily for 14 days; erythromycin, 500 mg orally four times daily; or ofloxacin, 400 mg orally twice daily for 14 days. Unless the clinical response is definitely favorable, however, additional treatment using antimicrobial agents is unwarranted.

Once other forms of prostatitis are excluded, the diagnosis of NBP is established. A frank discussion with the patient about his condition is always important. It is helpful to reassure the patient by comparing NBP with other noninfectious inflammatory conditions, such as arthritis or bursitis. These infirmities cause chronic or intermittent symptoms of variable intensity, but they are not infectious or contagious diseases, and they do not lead to cancer or other serious consequences.

In 1990, Barbalias[3] reported performing video-urodynamic studies on men with NBP and prostatodynia and finding the same abnormalities in both groups of patients. My own experience has been the same: Regardless of the presence or absence of "inflamed" prostatic expressates, patients with NBP usually have the same abnormalities on video-urodynamic studies as those found in patients with prostatodynia. It therefore is reasonable to use alpha-blocking agents as the mainstay of therapy in patients with NBP (see the section on prostatodynia).

The main management plan is to control symptoms and relieve anxieties and worry. Normal sexual activity should be encouraged, and dietary restrictions are advised only if spicy foods or alcoholic beverages appear to cause or make symptoms worse. Painful symptomatic episodes often are relieved by hot sitz baths. Pain and discomfort may respond to short courses of nonsteroidal anti-inflammatory agents, such as ibuprofen, 600 mg orally four times daily. Irritative voiding dysfunction may respond to the use of an anticholinergic agent, such as oxybutynin chloride, 5 mg orally three times daily. The efficacy of oral zinc preparations and megavitamins is unproven.

PROSTATODYNIA

Clinical Features

By definition, the patient with prostatodynia has symptoms of prostatitis, but no history of documented UTI, no infectious pathogen identifiable by culture, and normal prostatic secretions at microscopy. As many as 25 per cent of patients with prostatodynia, however, at times show excessive leukocyte counts in their prostatic expressates.[20] Furthermore, the same video-urodynamic abnormalities are found in patients with NBP ("inflamed" prostatic expressates) and patients with prostatodynia (normal prostatic expressates).[4, 20] Thus NBP and prostatodynia are prostatitis syndromes with more similarities in cause and effect than was appreciated in 1978 by Drach and associates.[9]

The patient with prostatodynia typically is young to middle-aged. Although most patients complain of variable signs and symptoms of obstructive and irritative voiding dysfunction, the prominent complaints relate to pain and discomfort in a pelvic pain distribution.[20] Symptoms of abnormal urinary flow include hesitancy, interrupted flow (often voiding in pulses), diminution in stream force and size, and postvoid dribbling. Irritative voiding dysfunction symptoms include urinary urgency, frequency, and nocturia. Pain and discomfort may be perceived in the perineum, groin, testicles, low back, and suprapubic areas, but especially in the penis and urethra.

Some patients with prostatodynia have "tight" anal sphincters, tender prostates, or tender paraprostatic muscles and tendons on rectal examination; otherwise, general physical and neurologic examinations are normal. At cystoscopy, mild to moderate bladder neck obstruction and variable bladder trabeculation are often appreciated.

Video-Urodynamic Studies

Clinical and video-urodynamic findings in patients with prostatodynia and NBP evaluated in my department indicate that most have a "spastic" dysfunction of the bladder neck and prostatic urethra, that is, the internal urinary sphincter.[4, 20, 21] These studies demonstrate depressed urinary flow rates associated with incomplete relaxation of the bladder neck and abnormal narrowing of the urethra just proximal to the external urinary sphincter (EUS). Urethral pressure profiles typically show a high maximum urethral closure pressure in the area of the EUS, despite electrical silence of the EUS on electromyography (Table 34–2). Because these patients are otherwise normal neurologically, an acquired functional disorder is suggested.

Barbalias[3] has described the same video-urodynamic findings in patients with prostatodynia and NBP whom he has studied in Greece. He emphasizes that the basic pathophysiology is "urethral hypertonia" and suggests using the term "painful male urethral syndrome" instead of prostatodynia. It is his theory that untreated patients may eventually develop chronic NBP.

Our preference is to call this condition a bladder neck/urethral spasm (BN/US) syndrome, which is a form of bladder–internal sphincter dyssynergia.[20] The postulated basis of signs and symptoms in these patients is as follows: Some event triggers smooth muscle spasm of the bladder neck and prostatic urethra, which causes elevated pressures in the prostatic urethra, leading to intraprostatic and ejaculatory duct urinary reflux, which results in a chemical prostatitis, seminal vesiculitis, and even epididymitis. In this regard, Hellstrom et al[12] reported three patients with NBP/PD whose intraprostatic and ejaculatory duct urinary reflux was so severe that it was demonstrated easily by voiding cystourethrography.

Other Types of Prostatodynia

Some patients with prostatodynia suffer mainly from tension myalgia of the pelvic floor muscles.[28, 32, 34] Symptoms in these patients are thought to arise from habitual contraction and spasms of the pelvic floor skeletal muscles. Pelvic pain is associated with sitting, running, or other physical activities that lead to fatigue of the perineal muscles. On rectal examination, the anal sphincter and paraprostatic muscles and tendons, but not the prostate gland, are tender.

Emotional stress and psychosocial or psychosexual difficulties often characterize patients with prostatodynia. Indeed, many clinicians believe that "stress" and psychological factors play a primary role in the development of prostatodynia.[6, 23] The difficulty is in distinguishing whether stress is a cause or an effect of prostatodynia.

Whatever initiates prostatodynia, the symptoms seem to be a result of nonrelaxation (or spasm) of the internal urinary sphincter and the pelvic floor striated muscles, alone or in combination, leading to elevated prostatic urethral pressures and intraprostatic (and possible ejaculatory duct) urinary reflux.

Treatment

The smooth muscle of the bladder neck and prostate is rich in alpha-adrenergic receptors,[11] and alpha-blocking agents are effective in treating most patients with prostatodynia, especially those who have the BN/US syndrome.[6, 20] To avoid adverse side effects, one must prescribe these agents in low doses and then gradually increase the dosage until the desired therapeutic effects are achieved. Because it is available in low-dose capsules and is better tolerated than phenoxybenzamine, prazosin currently is the preferred alpha-blocking agent for the treatment of prostatodynia (and most cases of NBP). My preference is to begin prazosin, 1 mg orally once daily at bedtime for 7 days, followed by 1 mg twice daily for 7 days, followed by 2 mg twice daily. Patients vary considerably in their tolerance and response to this drug; therefore, the dosage must be individualized carefully. The dosage should be gradually increased to achieve efficacy without causing significant adverse side effects. Provided that they are able to tolerate the medication in proper dosage, most patients respond favorably to prazosin therapy. Because most patients relapse soon after stopping the prazosin, it generally is necessary for responders to continue the medication indefinitely. It is not unusual for responders to require a slightly higher dosage with time to maintain good relief of symptoms.

Patients with tension myalgia of the pelvic floor muscles respond best to treatment using diazepam, 5 mg orally three times daily, alone or in combination with prazosin. The liberal use of hot sitz baths and the selected use of other therapies, as discussed in the treatment of NBP, is sometimes beneficial. Those who respond poorly to medical management or who have significant emotional problems should be referred to a psychiatrist or psychologist.

TABLE 34–2. PROSTATODYNIA: VIDEO-URODYNAMIC FINDINGS

Normal
  Neurologic examination
  Pudendal nerve function
  Urethral reflexes
  Synergistic voiding
  Bladder capacity
  Bladder contractions
Abnormal
  VCUG: bladder neck obstructed or incompletely funnelled
  VCUG: prostatic urethra narrowed in area of EUS despite EMG silence of the EUS
  Urethral pressure profile: increased maximal urethral closure pressure (at rest)
  Urinary flow rate: decreased peak and average flow

Abbreviations: EUS = external urethral sphincter, EMG = electromyography, VCUG = voiding cystourethrography.

REFERENCES

1. Anderson RU, Ma SH: Immunological studies in abacterial prostatitis. *In* Brunner H, Krause W, Rothauge CF, Weidner W (eds): Chronic Prostatitis. Stuttgart, FK Schattauer Verlag, 1985, pp 113–120.

2. Anderson RU, Weller C: Prostatic secretion leukocyte studies in non-bacterial prostatitis (prostatosis). J Urol 121:292, 1979.
3. Barbalias GA: Prostatodynia or painful male urethral syndrome? Urology 36:146, 1990.
4. Barbalias GA, Meares EM Jr, Sant GR: Prostatodynia: Clinical and urodynamic characteristics. J Urol 130:514, 1983.
5. Berger RE, Krieger JN, Kessler D, et al: Case control study of men with suspected chronic idiopathic prostatitis. J Urol 141:328, 1989.
6. Blacklock NJ: Urodynamic and psychometric observations and their implications in the management of prostatodynia. *In* Weidner W, Brunner H, Krause W, Rothauge CF (eds): Therapy of Prostatitis. Munich, W. Zuckschwerdt Verlag, 1986, pp 201–206.
7. Brunner H, Weidner W, Schiefer HG: Studies of the role of *Ureaplasma urealyticum* and *Mycoplasma hominis* in prostatitis. J Infect Dis 147:807, 1983.
8. Doble A, Thomas BJ, Walker MM, et al: The role of *Chlamydia trachomatis* in chronic abacterial prostatitis: A study using ultrasound guided biopsy. J Urol 141:332, 1989.
9. Drach GW, Fair WR, Meares EM Jr, Stamey TA: Classification of benign disease associated with prostatic pain: Prostatitis or prostatodynia? J Urol 120:266, 1978.
10. Fowler JE Jr, Lynes WL, Lau JLT, et al: Interstitial cystitis is associated with intraurothelial Tamm-Horsfall protein. J Urol 140:1385, 1988.
11. Gosling JA, Dixon JS, Lendon RG: The autonomic innervation of the male and female bladder neck and proximal urethra. J Urol 118:302, 1977.
12. Hellstrom WJG, Schmidt RA, Lue TF, et al: Neuromuscular dysfunction in nonbacterial prostatitis. Urology 30:183, 1987.
13. Jameson RM: Sexual activity and the variations of white cell content of the prostatic secretion. Invest Urol 5:297, 1967.
14. Kirby RS, Lowe D, Bultitude MI, et al: Intraprostatic urinary reflux: An aetological factor in abacterial prostatitis. Br J Urol 54:729, 1982.
15. Kohnen PW, Drach GW: Patterns of inflammation in prostatic hyperplasia: A histologic and bacteriologic study. J Urol 121:755, 1979.
16. Lipsky BA: Urinary tract infections in men. Ann Intern Med 110:138, 1989.
17. Mardh P-A, Ripa KT, Colleen S, et al: Role of *Chlamydia trachomatis* in non-acute prostatitis. Br J Vener Dis 54:330, 1978.
18. Meares EM Jr: Prostatitis. Med Clin North Am 75:405, 1991.
19. Meares EM Jr: Prostatitis syndromes: New perspectives about old woes. J Urol 123:141, 1980.
20. Meares EM Jr: Prostatodynia: Clinical findings and rationale for treatment. *In* Weidner W, Brunner H, Krause W, Rothauge CF (eds): Therapy of Prostatitis. Munich, W. Zuckschwerdt Verlag, 1986, pp 207–212.
21. Meares EM Jr, Barbalias GA: Prostatitis: Bacterial, nonbacterial, and prostatodynia. Semin Urol 1:146, 1983.
22. Meares EM, Stamey TA: Bacteriologic localization patterns in bacterial prostatitis and urethritis. Invest Urol 5:492, 1968.
23. Miller HC: Stress prostatitis. Urology 32:507, 1988.
24. Neal DE Jr, Dilworth JP, Kaack MB: Tamm-Horsfall autoantibodies in interstitial cystitis. J Urol 145:37, 1991.
25. Poletti F, Medici MC, Alinovi A, et al: Isolation of *Chlamydia trachomatis* from the prostatic cells in patients affected by nonacute prostatitis. J Urol 134:691, 1985.
26. Rameriz CT, Ruiz JA, Gomez AZ, et al: A crystallographic study of prostatic calculi. J Urol 124:840, 1980.
27. Schachter J: Is *Chlamydia trachomatis* a cause of prostatitis? [editorial] J Urol 134:711, 1985.
28. Segura JW, Opitz JL, Greene LF: Prostatosis, prostatitis or pelvic floor tension myalgia? J Urol 122:168, 1979.
29. Shortliffe LMD, Elliott KM, Sellers RG, et al: Measurement of chlamydial and ureaplasma antibodies in serum and prostatic fluid of men with nonbacterial prostatitis [abstract]. J Urol 133(4), part 2:276A, 1985.
30. Shortliffe LMD, Wehner N: The characterization of bacterial and nonbacterial prostatitis by prostatic immunoglobulins. Medicine 65:399, 1986.
31. Shortliffe LMD, Wehner N, Stamey TA: The detection of a local prostatic immunologic response to bacterial prostatitis. J Urol 125:509, 1981.
32. Sinaki M, Merritt JL, Stillwell GK: Tension myalgia of the pelvic floor. Mayo Clin Proc 52:717, 1977.
33. Sutor DJ, Wooley SE: The crystalline composition of prostatic calculi. Br J Urol 46:533, 1974.
34. Thompson JM: Tension myalgia as a diagnosis at the Mayo Clinic and its relationship to fibrositis, fibromyalgia, and myofascial pain syndrome. Mayo Clin Proc 65:1237, 1990.
35. Weidner W, Schiefer HG, Krause H, et al: Chronic prostatitis: A thorough search for etiologically involved microorganisms in 1,461 patients. Infection 19 (Suppl 3):S119, 1991.

INDEX